THROMBOSIS
in
CARDIOVASCULAR DISORDERS

THROMBOSIS
in
CARDIOVASCULAR
DISORDERS

Edited by

VALENTIN FUSTER, M.D., Ph.D.

Mallinckrodt Professor of Medicine, Harvard Medical School
Chief, Cardiac Unit
Massachusetts General Hospital
Boston, Massachusetts

MARC VERSTRAETE, M.D., Ph.D.

Professor of Medicine, University of Leuven
Center for Thrombosis and Vascular Research
Leuven, Belgium

W.B. SAUNDERS COMPANY

A Division of Harcourt Brace & Company

Philadelphia / London / Toronto / Montreal / Sydney / Tokyo

W.B. SAUNDERS COMPANY
A Division of
Harcourt Brace & Company

The Curtis Center
Independence Square West
Philadelphia, Pennsylvania 19106

Library of Congress Cataloging-in-Publication Data

Thrombosis in cardiovascular disorders / edited by Valentin Fuster,
Marc Verstraete.
    p.   cm.
  ISBN 0-7216-4012-5
    1. Thrombosis—Chemotherapy.   2. Anticoagulants (Medicine).
3. Cardiovascular system—Diseases—Complications and sequelae.
I. Fuster, Valentin.   II. Verstraete, M. (Marc).
    [DNLM: 1. Anticoagulants—therapeutic use.   2. Heparin—
therapeutic use.   3. Thrombosis—drug therapy.   WG 300 T5301]
RC684.C6T44   1992   616.1′35—dc20
DNLM/DLC   91-33823

Thrombosis in Cardiovascular Disorders   ISBN   0-7216-4012-5

Last digit is the print number: 9   8   7   6   5   4   3   2

Dedicated to the present and former members of the Center for Thrombosis and Vascular Research, University of Leuven, Belgium.

MARC VERSTRAETE

Dedicated to the medical staff, fellows, research fellows and alumni of The Division of Cardiology at the Mount Sinai Medical Center, New York.

VALENTIN FUSTER

Contributors

JUAN JOSE BADIMON, Ph.D.
Harvard School of Medicine; Assistant Physiologist, Cardiac Unit, Massachusetts General Hospital, Boston, Massachusetts
Pathogenesis of Thrombosis

LINA BADIMON, Ph.D.
Harvard School of Medicine; Associate Physiologist, Cardiac Unit, Massachusetts General Hospital, Boston, Massachusetts
Pathogenesis of Thrombosis

HENRI BOUNAMEAUX, M.D.
Privat Dozent, University of Geneva; Chief, Angiology Unit, University Hospital of Geneva, Geneva, Switzerland
Peripheral Arterial Occlusion: Thromboembolism and Antithrombotic Therapy

JOHN A. CAIRNS, M.D., F.R.C.P.C.
Professor of Medicine, McMaster University; Chairman of Medicine, McMaster University, Ontario, Canada
Unstable Angina—Antithrombotics and Thrombolytics

ROBERT M. CALIFF, M.D.
Associate Professor of Medicine, Duke University School of Medicine; Director, Cardiac Care Unit, Duke Medical Center, Durham, North Carolina
Percutaneous Transluminal Coronary Angioplasty: Prevention of Occlusion and Restenosis

JAMES H. CHESEBRO, M.D.
Professor of Medicine, Mayo Medical School; Consultant in Cardiovascular Disease and Internal Medicine, Mayo Clinic and Foundation, Rochester, Minnesota
Chronic Coronary Disease; Coronary Artery Bypass Surgery: Antithrombotic Therapy; Valvular Heart Disease and Prosthetic Heart Valves

MARC COHEN, M.D.
Associate Professor of Medicine, Division of Cardiology, Department of Medicine, Hahnemann University, Philadelphia, Pennsylvania
Unstable Angina—Antithrombotics and Thrombolytics

DÉSIRÉ COLLEN, M.D., Ph.D.
Professor of Medicine, University of Leuven; Director, Center of Thrombosis and Vascular Research, University of Leuven, Leuven, Belgium
Thrombolytic Agents

MICHAEL J. DAVIES, M.D.
Professor of Cardiovascular Pathology, St. Georges Hospital Medical School, University of London, London, United Kingdom
Interrelationship between Atherosclerosis and Thrombosis

STEVEN M. FRUCHTMAN, M.D.
Assistant Professor of Medicine, Mount Sinai School of Medicine; Director, Bone Marrow
Transplantation Service, Mount Sinai Hospital, New York, New York
Disseminated Intravascular Coagulation

VALENTIN FUSTER, M.D., Ph.D.
Mallinckrodt Professor of Medicine, Harvard Medical School, Chief, Cardiac Unit, Massachusetts
General Hospital, Boston, Massachusetts
*Antiplatelet and Anticoagulant Therapy in Evolving and Myocardial Infarction and Primary Prevention;
Clinical Pharmacology of Platelet Inhibitors; Decision Making Based on Pathogenesis and Risk;
Pathogenesis of Thrombosis; Valvular Heart Disease and Prosthetic Heart Valves*

JEFFREY S. GINSBERG, M.D.
Assistant Professor, Department of Medicine, McMaster University Medical Centre; Director,
Thromboembolism Unit, Chedoke-McMaster Hospitals, Ontario, Canada
Anticoagulants During Pregnancy

SAMUEL Z. GOLDHABER, M.D.
Associate Professor of Medicine, Harvard Medical School; Associate Physician, Cardiovascular
Division, Brigham and Women's Hospital, Boston, Massachusetts
Treatment of Venous Thrombosis and Pulmonary Embolism

STEVEN GOLDMAN, M.D.
Professor of Internal Medicine, University of Arizona; Chief of Cardiology, Tucson VA Medical
Center, Tucson, Arizona
Coronary Artery Bypass Surgery: Antithrombotic Therapy

JONATHAN L. HALPERIN, M.D.
Associate Professor of Medicine, Mount Sinai School of Medicine of the City University of New
York; Associate Attending Physician for Cardiology, Director of Clinical Services, Division of
Cardiology, Mount Sinai Medical Center, New York, New York
Thrombosis in the Cardiac Chambers: Ventricular Dysfunction and Atrial Fibrillation

LAURENCE A. HARKER, M.D.
Blomeyer Professor of Medicine; Director, Division of Hematology and Oncology, Emory
University School of Medicine, Atlanta, Georgia
Thrombosis and Fibrinolysis

ROBERT G. HART, M.D.
Associate Professor of Medicine, University of Texas Health Science Center at San Antonio;
Staff Neurologist, Medical Center Hospital, San Antonio, San Antonio, Texas
Stroke and Transient Ischemic Attack: Thromboembolism and Antithrombotic Therapy

PATRICIA HEBERT, Ph.D.
Instructor in Medicine, Department of Medicine, Brigham and Women's Hospital, Harvard
Medical School, Boston, Massachusetts
Antiplatelet and Anticoagulant Therapy in Evolving and Myocardial Infarction and Primary Prevention

CHARLES H. HENNEKENS, M.D., DrPH
Professor of Medicine and Preventive Medicine, Acting Chair, Department of Preventive
Medicine, Harvard Medical School; Physician, Brigham and Women's Hospital, Boston,
Massachusetts
Antiplatelet and Anticoagulant Therapy in Evolving and Myocardial Infarction and Primary Prevention

JACK HIRSH, M.D.

Professor of Medicine, McMaster University; Director, Hamilton Civic Hospitals Research Centre, Henderson General Hospital, Ontario, Canada

Anticoagulants During Pregnancy; Hemorrhagic Complications of Long-Term Antithrombotic Treatment; Optimal Therapeutic Ranges for Oral Anticoagulation; Optimal Therapeutic Ranges for Unfractionated Heparin and Low Molecular Weight Heparins

RUSSELL D. HULL, M.B.B.S., M.Sc.

Professor of Medicine, University of Calgary; Head, Division of General Internal Medicine, Foothills Hospital, Alberta, Canada

Prevention of Venous Thrombosis and Pulmonary Embolism

JAN J. C. JONKER, M.D.

Thrombosis Foundation and Laboratory, Department of Medicine, Ysselland Hospital, Rotterdam, The Netherlands

Chronic Coronary Disease

VIJAY V. KAKKAR, M.D., F.R.C.S., F.R.C.S.E.

Professor of Surgical Science, University of London; Director, Thrombosis Research Institute, London, England

Prevention of Venous Thrombosis and Pulmonary Embolism

J. WARD KENNEDY, M.D.

Professor of Medicine, School of Medicine, University of Washington; Director, Division of Cardiology, University of Washington, Seattle, Washington

Myocardial Infarction—Thrombolytic Therapy in the Prehospital Setting

MARK N. LEVINE, M.D., M.Sc., F.R.C.P.(C.)

Associate Professor, Medicine and Clinical Epidemiology and Biostatistics, McMaster University; Head, Medical Oncology, Ontario Cancer Foundation, Hamilton Regional Centre, Ontario, Canada

Hemorrhagic Complications of Long-Term Antithrombotic Treatment

KENNETH G. MANN, Ph.D.

Professor and Chairman, Department of Biochemistry, University of Vermont College of Medicine, Burlington, Vermont

Thrombosis and Fibrinolysis

THOMAS W. MEADE, D.M., F.R.C.P.

Director, MRC Epidemiology and Medical Care Unit, Northwick Park Hospital, Harrow, United Kingdom

Characteristics Associated with the Risk of Arterial Thrombosis and the Prethrombotic State

G. J. MILLER, M.D., F.R.C.P.

Senior Clinical Scientific Staff, U.K. Medical Research Council, Epidemiology and Medical Care Unit, Northwick Park Hospital, Harrow, England

Characteristics Associated with the Risk of Arterial Thrombosis and the Prethrombotic State

PALLE PETERSEN, M.D., Ph.D.

Associate Professor of Neurology, University Hospital, Copenhagen, Denmark

Thrombosis in the Cardiac Chambers: Ventricular Dysfunction and Atrial Fibrillation

LEON POLLER, D.Sc., M.D., F.R.C.Path.

Honorary Professor, University of Manchester; Director, UK Reference Laboratory for Anticoagulant Reagents and Control, Withington Hospital, Manchester, United Kingdom

Optimal Therapeutic Ranges for Oral Anticoagulation

JACOB H. RAND, M.D.
Associate Professor of Medicine, Mount Sinai School of Medicine; Director, Coagulation Laboratory, Mount Sinai Hospital, New York, New York
Disseminated Intravascular Coagulation

GARY E. RASKOB, M.Sc.
Instructor, Department of Medicine, College of Medicine; Instructor, Department of Biostatistics and Epidemiology, College of Public Health, University of Oklahoma, Oklahoma City, Oklahoma
Prevention of Venous Thrombosis and Pulmonary Embolism

ROBERT D. ROSENBERG, M.D., Ph.D.
Professor of Biology, Massachusetts Institute of Technology, Cambridge, Massachusetts; Professor of Medicine, Harvard Medical School and Beth Israel Hospital, Boston, Massachusetts
Characteristics Associated with the Risk of Arterial Thrombosis and the Prethrombotic State

ALLAN M. ROSS, M.D.
Professor of Medicine; Director, Division of Cardiology, George Washington University, Washington, DC
Myocardial Infarction: Adjunctive Antithrombotic Therapy to Thrombolysis

PHILIP A. ROUTLEDGE, M.D., F.R.C.P.
Professor of Clinical Pharmacology, University of Wales College of Medicine, Cardiff, United Kingdom; Consultant Physician, Llandough Hospital, South Glamorgan, United Kingdom
Computer-Assisted Anticoagulation

DAVID G. SHERMAN, M.D.
Professor of Medicine, Division of Neurology, University of Texas Health Science Center; Chief of Neurology, Audie L. Murphy Veterans Administration Hospital, San Antonio, Texas
Stroke and Transient Ischemic Attack: Thromboembolism and Antithrombotic Therapy

HAMSARAJ G. M. SHETTY, B.Sc., M.B.B.S., M.R.C.P.
Lecturer in Clinical Pharmacology and Therapeutics, University of Wales College of Medicine, Cardiff, United Kingdom; Honorary Senior Registrar in Medicine, Llandough Hospital, South Glamorgan, United Kingdom
Computer-Assisted Anticoagulation

PÅL SMITH, M.D.
Head of Coronary Care Unit, Department of Cardiology, Ullevål Hospital, Oslo, Norway
Antithrombotic Therapy in the Chronic Phase of Myocardial Infarction

BURTON E. SOBEL, M.D.
Director, Cardiovascular Division, Washington University School of Medicine; Cardiologist-in-Chief, Barnes Hospital, St. Louis, Missouri
Thrombolysis in the Treatment of Acute Myocardial Infarction

HERVÉ SORS, M.D., M.Sc.
Professor of Medicine, University Paris V, Paris, France; Department of Pulmonary Medicine and Intensive Care, Laennec Hospital, Paris, France
Treatment of Venous Thrombosis and Pulmonary Embolism

BERNARDO STEIN, M.D.
Assistant Professor of Medicine, Baylor College of Medicine; Director, Cardiac Catheterization Laboratories and Interventional Cardiology, Veterans Affairs Medical Center, Houston, Texas
Clinical Pharmacology of Platelet Inhibitors; Decision Making Based on Pathogenesis and Risk

RAYMOND VERHAEGHE, M.D.

Professor of Medicine, University of Leuven, Leuven, Belgium; Consultant in Vascular Diseases, University Hospital, Gyasthuisberg, Belgium

Peripheral Arterial Occlusion: Thromboembolism and Antithrombotic Therapy

MARC VERSTRAETE, M.D., Ph.D., F.R.C.P.(Edin), F.A.C.P.(Hon)

Professor of Medicine, University of Leuven; Center for Thrombosis and Vascular Research, University of Leuven, Leuven, Belgium

Drug Interference with Heparin and Oral Anticoagulants; Heparins and Oral Anticoagulants; Thrombolytic Agents; Novelties in Antithrombotic and Thrombolytic Therapy: A Latest Update

W. DOUGLAS WEAVER, M.D.

Associate Professor of Medicine, School of Medicine, University of Washington; Acting Director, Division of Cardiology, University of Washington School of Medicine, Seattle, Washington

Myocardial Infarction—Thrombolytic Therapy in the Prehospital Setting

STANFORD WESSLER, M.D.

Professor of Medicine, New York University School of Medicine; Attending Physician, University Hospital, New York, New York

Drug Interference with Heparin and Oral Anticoagulants; Heparins and Oral Anticoagulants

JAMES T. WILLERSON, M.D.

Professor and Chairman, Department of Internal Medicine, University of Texas Medical School at Houston; Director of Cardiology Research, Texas Heart Institute, Houston, Texas

Percutaneous Transluminal Coronary Angioplasty: Prevention of Occlusion and Restenosis

NEVILLE WOOLF, M.B., Ch.B., M.Med.(Path), Ph.D., F.R.C.Path.

Bland-Sutton Professor of Histopathology, University College and Middlesex School of Medicine; Honorary Consultant Pathologist, The Middlesex Hospital, London, United Kingdom

Interrelationship between Atherosclerosis and Thrombosis

Foreword

Progress in science and medicine is often greatest at the interface between what were once separate disciplines. Such "hybrid" fields include some of the most exciting scientific realms: physical chemistry, bioengineering, immunogenetics, astrophysics, neurobiology, and electrophysiology, to name just a few. In clinical medicine, an important area of growth, as well as the subject of *Thrombosis in Cardiovascular Disorders*, involves two separate specialties: hematology and cardiology. Although the role of thrombosis, which leads to both chronic cardiovascular disease and acute, life-threatening complications, has been recognized for more than a century, critical developments in the last dozen years have helped illuminate the pathophysiological changes in both thrombosis and thrombolysis as well as our ability to modify these processes.

Together, these advances are revolutionizing cardiovascular therapeutics. Among the relatively recent landmark events in this field are the following:

1. The observation—in the *living patient*—that coronary thrombosis is the proximate cause of all (or virtually all) instances of acute transmural myocardial infarction and that it frequently plays a critical role in the development of unstable angina as well.

2. The unequivocal demonstration that thrombolytic therapy, when delivered in a timely and appropriate manner, substantially improves the immediate survival of patients with acute myocardial infarction and that this improvement is sustained.

3. Advances in molecular biology that allow the production, by recombinant methods, of substances that exert profound effects on various aspects of the coagulation process in sufficient quantities for clinical trials and widespread use. These substances include thrombolytic agents such as tissue-type plasminogen activator and saruplase, and antithrombotics such as hirudin and activated protein C.

4. The successful completion of clinical trials demonstrating that aspirin—an inexpensive, readily available drug–is effective in both the *primary* prevention of acute myocardial infarction, in the *secondary* prevention of unstable angina pectoris and myocardial infarction, and in improving survival in patients with acute myocardial infarction.

To apply these and many other important developments to the clinical arena, physicians must have more than a nodding acquaintance with thrombosis and thrombolysis and the many conditions and drugs that can affect these processes. However, except for investigators and subspecialists who deal with disorders of coagulation and bleeding, most physicians (including cardiologists) are uncomfortable with this complex field and have had difficulty understanding it. Therefore, *Thrombosis in Cardiovascular Disorders* comes along at a most opportune time. It is among the first books yet written on this important subject, and I believe it is the most ambitious and best. It is designed to aid physicians in all specialties as they apply recent information about the coagulation system to the care of patients with cardiovascular disease. The editors are highly respected world leaders in this field whose backgrounds, formidable personal contributions, and deep knowledge of the subject complement each other remarkably. Dr. V. Fuster, an eminent American cardiologist with a thorough understanding of thrombosis, and Dr. M. Verstraete, a distinguished European hematologist with an intense interest

Preface

There can be no doubt, unfortunately, about the importance of thrombosis in medicine today. For decades, the nonspecialist has been bewildered by the profusion and complexity of ideas on the mechanism of clotting, and perhaps mentally deafened by the controversy which surrounds even factual observations. He may have lost sight of the simplest of all observations—the fact that normal blood does not clot in normal blood vessels. For every patient who dies because of the failure of his blood to clot, many thousands of people die because of the failure of their blood to remain fluid in vital parts of the circulation.

The thrombotic diseases are unusual in that they are included in the practice of most doctors, whether they are general physicians, cardiologists, neurologists, surgeons or, of course, hematologists. Traditionally, scientists and specialists have communicated regularly with other workers in their particular discipline while remaining curiously isolated from those in other fields. To achieve an interdisciplinary approach, two editors, an American cardiologist and a European hematologist, recruited outstanding scientists/clinicians from diverse fields and from different geographical areas. In doing so, the editors' hope was not to reach a consensus on all issues, but rather to present a volume of complementary and balanced views which, by allowing for differences of opinion, actually gives the reader a clearer understanding of thrombosis in medicine today.

At a time when the pace of advances in the biomedical field and in communication is staggering, traditional means of publishing seem incapable of keeping up. Books are often substantially out of date even before they appear in print. The chapters contained within this volume represent the hard work of authors who not only accepted a three-month deadline, but actually met that deadline in fine style. Thus, in less than six months after we received the first manuscript, the project was complete, demonstrating that at least one of the objections to a multiauthored book can be circumvented. Another objection is that books are disreputable for their lack of peer review. The two editors have independently and vigorously refereed each chapter, most of which were resubmitted in a revised form. There remains a refreshing variation in emphasis and opinion among chapters, although some slight overlaps were unavoidable. Remembering that history does not repeat itself but that historians do, we asked the authors to free themselves from the fetters of lengthy historical material. One should take the fire from the altar of the past, not the ashes.

Toward the end of the book the reader might agree that the greater the island of knowledge, the greater the shoreline of the unknown. However, authors and editors hope that the reader will also be left with a belief in the interconnectedness of facts and a better understanding of the subject at hand.

The editors wish to thank the authors, the real producers of this book, who have endured our pressing demands, adhered to a tight schedule, and enthusiastically collaborated in a cost-ineffective undertaking. Their best reward would be that this book is avidly read, warmly received, and that it provides good competition for its rivals.

MARC VERSTRAETE
VALENTIN FUSTER

Contents

1

THROMBOSIS AND FIBRINOLYSIS

LAURENCE A. HARKER and KENNETH G. MANN

Thrombotic and thromboembolic occlusions of diseased arteries cause life-threatening heart attacks, strokes, and peripheral ischemia. Venous thrombosis and thromboembolism also lead to serious disability and death. Thus, the diagnosis, therapy, and prevention of thrombotic events are important public health priorities.

Normally, blood constituents do not interact with intact vascular endothelium. However, the exposure of flowing blood to disrupted vasculature or to cardiovascular devices initiates complex mechanisms that give rise to the rapid deposition of platelets, insoluble fibrin, leukocytes, and entrapped erythrocytes in variable flow-dependent patterns, to produce localized mechanical masses. Arterial flow conditions give rise to platelet-rich ("white") thrombi, and static venous flow yields fibrin- and red cell-rich ("red") thrombi. Developing thrombi may occlude vascular blood flow locally, or detach and embolize to occlude downstream. Endogenous fibrinolysis gradually removes already formed thrombus, and physiologic mechanisms limit the threat of propagating thrombus.[1-3]

The site, size, and composition of thrombi and thromboemboli are determined by: (a) mechanical hemodynamic blood flow effects; (b) amount and thrombogenicity of exposed endovascular surface components; (c) concentrations and reactivity of responding plasma and cellular blood constituents; and (d) effectiveness of the physiologic protective mechanisms, particularly fibrinolysis.[1-5] In this overview, the complex integrated reactions constituting these thrombotic processes and their regulation will be discussed.

HEMODYNAMIC EFFECTS

Blood normally flows with a characteristic streaming flow pattern in which flow of concentric cylindrical layers of blood is minimal at the vessel wall and successively more rapid toward the central stream. Because the cellular components are mutually repelled by their common negative electrical charges, the innermost stream of red cells tends to displace the smaller platelets toward the vascular wall.[4,6] Since velocities are minimal close to the vessel wall, formed elements have little tendency for inward radial migration. Thus, platelet masses once formed may have extended residence times and greater likelihood of attaching to the wall. Moreover, when flow is disturbed, such as in the vortex patterns produced distal to sites of stenosis, activated species of platelets and coagulation factors, or factors that induce vascular damage, may be concentrated and retained at the vessel wall.[4-6]

On the other hand, platelet-rich thrombus forming at sites of arterial narrowing tends to embolize because of the increased shear forces. Moreover, the increased flow velocity removes and dilutes activated species more quickly, thereby limiting the extent of platelet deposition. Thus, it is difficult for an occlusive thrombus to form until blood flow is disturbed and retarded. However, when flow is ultimately arrested by an occlusive platelet-rich thrombus, blood distal and proximal to the occlusion is stagnant, giving rise to propagated fibrin- and red cell-rich thrombus.

In veins, flow is characteristically slow, and at times, interrupted. Venous thrombi generally begin at sites of maximum stasis, often as platelet aggregates in the pockets of vein

1

valves or in the intramuscular venous sinuses of the legs.[7] When stasis is combined with focal vessel injury, venous thrombi form more readily because of the consequent local activation of platelets and coagulation proteins.[5] Additionally, impaired protective mechanisms predispose to venous thrombotic events, as illustrated by hereditary deficiencies of antithrombins, proteins C and S, and fibrinolytic factors. Similarly, if stasis is associated with circulating prothrombotic species, as is the case with some malignancies or with remote tissue damage, the likelihood of venous thrombosis increases considerably. By combining stasis with both local vessel injury and systemically activated platelets and coagulation factors, the development of venous thrombosis is typical, as illustrated by the high probability of venous thrombosis complicating hip surgery or knee replacement.

PLATELET DEPOSITION

Platelets attaching to nonendothelialized surfaces undergo adherence by activation and spreading and subsequent recruitment to form rapidly enlarging platelet thrombi.[3,4,8–10] These processes involve: (a) platelet attachment to collagen or exposed surface adhesive proteins; (b) platelet activation and intracellular signaling, the expression of platelet membrane integrins as receptors for adhesive proteins, and the initiation of the contractile processes leading to shape change and granular secretion; (c) platelet aggregation by interplatelet fibrinogen bridging; and (d) platelet self-amplifying recruitment mediated by thrombin, thromboxane A_2 (TxA_2), and adenosine diphosphate (ADP), three potent, independent but interactive agonists (Fig. 1–1).

Platelet Adhesion

The process of adhesion involves the diffusive transport of platelets to the reactive surface and the interaction of platelet surface glycoprotein (GP) receptors with subendothelial structural elements of the injured vascular wall or biomaterial surface.[4,8] Collagen is the most important platelet-reactive subendothelial extracellular matrix constituent, although adhesive matrix proteins (fibronectin, von Willebrand factor, laminin, vitronectin, and thrombospondin) may also facilitate

adhesion.[8] The membrane glycoprotein receptors and their respective coupling extracellular ligand(s) that are capable of mediating platelet adhesion include: (a) glycoprotein Ib-IX–von Willebrand factor; (b) glycoprotein Ia-IIa–collagen; (c) glycoprotein Ic-IIa–fibronectin; (d) glycoprotein Ic-IIa–laminin; (e) vitronectin receptor–vitronectin/von Willebrand factor/fibronectin/thrombospondin; (f) glycoprotein IIb-IIIa–fibronectin/thrombospondin/vitronectin; and (g) glycoprotein IV–thrombospondin/collagen (Table 1–1).

Localized adhesion of unactivated platelets occurs despite the presence of constitutively expressed receptors on platelets.[8] The local reaction is assured because: (a) the subendothelial adhesive matrix proteins are only exposed to platelets after denuding vascular injury (that is, collagen, laminin, thrombospondin, and vitronectin); or (b) the adhesive proteins become conformationally altered during their binding to subendothelial constituents or biomaterial surface enabling the modified adhesive molecules to react with unactivated platelets, particularly under high shear conditions; that is, von Willebrand factor and fibronectin.

The glycoprotein Ib-IX heterodimeric complex is the most prominent sialoglycoprotein of platelet membranes (25,000 copies per platelet) and contributes to their negative charge.[8,11] Glycoprotein Ib-IX mediates platelet adhesion by serving as the receptor for von Willebrand factor immobilized on exposed vascular subendothelium (Table 1–1). Two discontinuous sequences in the native disulfide-linked glycoprotein Ib-alpha molecule constitute the binding domains for von Willebrand factor,[12] residues 251 to 279, and sequences in the tryptic fragment 449 to 728. The cytoplasmic domain of glycoprotein Ib-IX links the platelet membrane to actin-binding proteins that crosslink with the polymerizing actin filaments of the submembranous skeleton upon activation.[13] Protease cleavage of platelet glycoprotein Ib-IX complex releases glycocalicin,[14] the large extracellular domain of glycoprotein Ib, leaving the membrane-bound fragment linked to glycoprotein IX. Patients who lack glycoprotein Ib-IX (Bernard-Soulier syndrome) have a bleeding disorder[1,2] caused by the dysfunctional platelets (large globular platelets that do not bind von Willebrand factor and fail to form effective hemostatic plugs). Similarly, patients with reduced or dysfunctional von Willebrand factor (von Willebrand's disease)

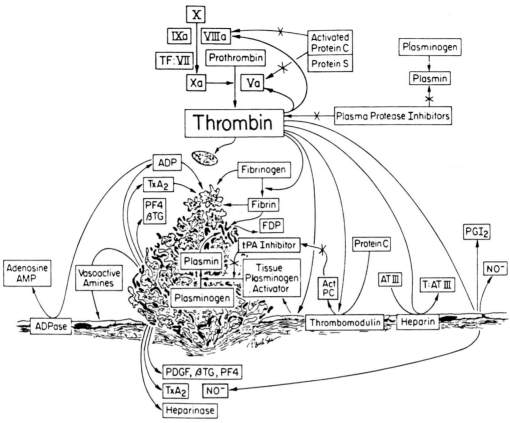

FIGURE 1–1. Schematic representation of the interactive mechanisms giving rise to thrombus formation, its regulation, and dissolution. (Reproduced from Harker LA. Pathogenesis of thrombosis. In: Williams WJ, ed. Hematology. 4th ed. New York: McGraw-Hill, 1990:1559–81, with permission.)

manifest impaired hemostatic plug-forming capability.[1,2]

Upon platelet exposure to subendothelial connective tissue structures, four minor platelet integrins, glycoprotein Ia-IIa, glycoprotein Ic-IIa, laminin receptors, and vitronectin receptors, may also participate in adhesion with collagen, fibronectin, laminin, and vitronectin/thrombospondin, respectively (Table 1–1). Glycoprotein IV serves as the principal platelet receptor for thrombospondin and may be an alternative receptor for collagen.[8] It is a highly glycosylated major platelet surface glycoprotein that is also ex-

TABLE 1–1. Platelet Membrane Glycoproteins and Their Function

GLYCOPROTEIN	RECEPTOR	PLATELET FUNCTION
Ib-IX	von Willebrand factor and thrombin	Adhesion
Ia-IIa ($\alpha^2\beta_1$)	Collagen	Adhesion
Ic-IIa ($\alpha^5\beta_1$)	Fibronectin	Adhesion
Ic-IIa ($\alpha^6\beta_1$)	Laminin receptor	Adhesion
Vitronectin receptor ($\alpha^v\beta_3$)	Vitronectin, von Willebrand factor, fibrinogen, and thrombospondin	Adhesion
IV (GP IIIb)	Thrombospondin and collagen	Adhesion
IIb-IIIa ($\alpha^{IIb}\beta_3$)	Fibrinogen, von Willebrand factor, fibronectin, thrombospondin, and vitronectin	Aggregation
GMP-140	?	Platelet-leukocyte interaction

pressed by monocytes (assigned the cluster designation CD 36) and endothelial cells.

The integrin membrane glycoproteins comprise a family of molecules consisting of two subunits, alpha and beta.[9] At present 11 alpha subunits and 6 beta subunits are known, and others are likely to be identified. The ligand-binding site of integrins appears to be formed by sequences from both subunits and their cytoplasmic domains that connect with the cytoskeleton, thereby integrating the extracellular matrix reactions with the intracellular cytoskeletal responses. The glycoprotein Ib-IX complex, a member of the leucine-rich glycoprotein family, has similarities with the integrins.[8] Glycoprotein IV is unrelated to any known gene family. Glycoprotein IIb-IIIa is restricted to megakaryocytes and their platelet products, while the vitronectin receptor is also expressed by macrophages and a broad range of nonhematopoietic cells.

Platelet Activation by Thrombin

Thrombin is the most potent and physiologically important activator of platelets and is pivotal in the process of platelet recruitment into thrombus forming after vascular injury.[15,16] The thrombin receptor on platelets is a 425-amino-acid seven-transmembrane molecule with a large aminoterminal extracellular extension that undergoes thrombin-mediated activation cleavage at arginine 41 in the LDPR/S amino acid sequence.[15] Cleavage of the receptor's aminoterminus creates a new receptor aminoterminus that activates the receptor as a tethered ligand to effect signal transduction (Fig. 1–2). A synthetic peptide sequence beginning SFLL ... , reproducing the new

aminoterminus created by thrombin proteolysis of the receptor tail, activates platelet thrombin receptors directly. The LDPR/S cleavage sequence in the thrombin receptor closely resembles the thrombin cleavage site LDPR/I in the zymogen protein C (see later). Carboxyl to the thrombin cleavage site is the highly acidic sequence EPFWEDEEKNES, similar to hirudin's binding sequence for thrombin's anion exosite, implying that this exosite may participate in thrombin's binding to the receptor. This thrombin receptor is also present on endothelium and smooth muscle cells, and is similar to the seven-membrane beta$_2$-adrenergic receptor for epinephrine on platelets.[15] Because the proteolytic activation of the thrombin receptor is not reversible, the threshold/dose-response characteristics of platelet activation by thrombin implies that each activated thrombin receptor generates some short-lived second messenger before the receptor is inactivated.

Mechanisms of Platelet Recruitment

Platelet attachment to collagen and other extracellular matrix proteins or stimulation by agonists arising from other activated platelets, and thrombin, initiates platelet signaling with subsequent expression of functional membrane receptors and contractile responses constituting platelet spreading and platelet–platelet interactions.[8,9] The platelet membrane integrin glycoprotein IIb-IIIa becomes conformationally reconfigured to create functional membrane receptors for fibrinogen.[17] Calcium-dependent interplatelet linkages may then form between the activa-

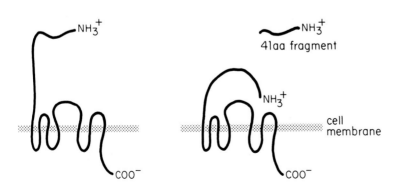

FIGURE 1–2. Platelet thrombin receptor. The aminoterminal extracellular portion of the unactivated thrombin receptor is cleaved by thrombin, exposing a new aminoterminus and releasing an activation receptor fragment. The newly generated aminoterminus, the sequence $S_{42}F_{43}$ ..., then functions as a receptor agonist after binding to another region of the thrombin receptor; that is, a peptide receptor containing its own ligand.

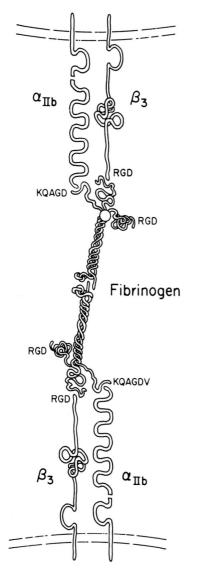

α_{IIb} β_3

RGD

KQAGD

RGD

Fibrinogen

RGD

KQAGDV

RGD

β_3 α_{IIb}

FIGURE 1–3. Glycoprotein IIb-IIIa structure and interactions binding platelets via divalent fibrinogen.

tion-expressed platelet receptors and bivalent fibrinogen (Fig. 1–3). The glycoprotein IIb-IIIa receptor is promiscuous in that it also binds with von Willebrand factor, fibronectin, vitronectin, and thrombospondin. Because of the relative plasma concentrations of these adhesive proteins, fibrinogen generally functions as the ligand. When fibrinogen is deficient or defective, von Willebrand factor may substitute for fibrinogen as the bridging ligand. However, receptor binding with fibronectin, thrombospondin, and vitronectin normally also appears to contribute toward the usual process of platelet recruitment.

Platelets generally contain about 50,000 copies of glycoprotein IIb-IIIa (1 to 2 per cent of the total platelet protein) distributed randomly on the surface of resting platelets.[8] The glycoprotein IIb subunit (molecular weight = 140,000 daltons) consists of a large chain (molecular weight = 125,000 daltons) linked by a disulfide bond to a light chain (molecular weight = 22,000 daltons). Only the light chain has a transmembrane domain. The large chain contains four repeating segments of about 65 amino acids, each containing a 12-residue sequence characteristic of the calcium-binding domains of calmodulin.[18] The glycoprotein IIIa subunit is a single polypeptide chain (molecular weight = 105,000 daltons) that contains a 29-residue transmembrane domain and a 41-residue cytoplasmic tail. The extracellular portion of glycoprotein IIIa contains 31 cysteine residues clustered in four tandemly repeated segments of about 40 amino acids each. The glycoprotein IIb-IIIa complex is present as a calcium-dependent heterodimer, noncovalently associated on the platelet surface. The heterodimer consists of a globular head and two rod-like tails extending from the globular domain.[8]

The Arg-Gly-Asp (RGD) sequence is the integrin recognition sequence present in the adhesive proteins fibrinogen, von Willebrand factor, fibronectin, thrombospondin, laminin, vitronectin, and collagen.[8,9,17,19] The capability of glycoprotein IIb-IIIa to bind to many different adhesive proteins is due to the common presence of the Arg-Gly-Asp sequence. Fibrinogen contains Arg-Gly-Asp sequences[20] in each alpha chain, one near the N-terminus (residues 95 to 97) and a second near the C-terminus (residues 572 to 574). An additional site on fibrinogen that binds to glycoprotein IIb-IIIa is the carboxyterminal dodecapeptide of each gamma chain.[21] This sequence is not found in other adhesive proteins and does not contain the Arg-Gly-Asp sequence. Peptides containing either Arg-Gly-Asp or dodecapeptide sequences inhibit platelet aggregation. The fibrinogen binding domains in the glycoprotein IIb-IIIa complex include residues 109 to 171 and residues 211 to 222 in glycoprotein IIIa. In contrast, the gamma chain dodecapeptide crosslinks with glycoprotein IIb within the sequence bounded by residues 294 to 314 (Fig. 1–4). In patients, a heterogeneous array of genetic defects affecting either glycoprotein IIb or glycoprotein IIIa or both

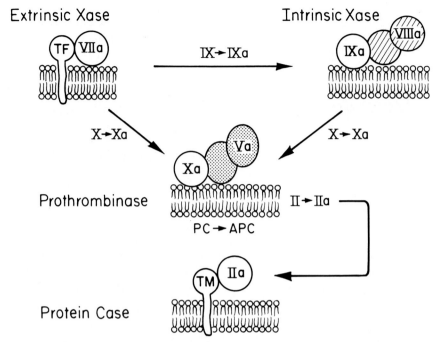

FIGURE 1–4. Schematic representation of the vitamin K-dependent complexes of coagulation. Each serine protease is shown in association with the appropriate cofactor protein on the membrane surface.

subunits may cause the Glanzmann disease phenotype, which is manifest as a disorder of platelet hemostatic plug formation with abnormal bleeding.

The conformational alterations in both glycoprotein IIb and glycoprotein IIIa are dependent on ligand occupancy and lead to clustering of the ligand-occupied receptors. The conformational change in glycoprotein IIb-IIIa is evidenced by the appearance of ligand-induced binding sites (LIBS), as detected by monoclonal antibodies.[22] The expression of glycoprotein IIb-IIIa fibrinogen-binding determinants are under intracellular control, being inhibited by increases in cytoplasmic cyclic adenosine monophosphate (cAMP).

The conformational changes in glycoprotein IIb-IIIa initiate intracellular signaling, as shown by (a) tyrosine-specific phosphorylation of threonine residues in glycoprotein IIIa, and (b) linkage between glycoprotein IIb-IIIa and the cytoskeleton.[8] The signal transduction induces metabolic activation within the cell, involving G protein-dependent phospholipase C activation, generation of inositol 1,4,5-triphosphate (IP_3) and diacylglycerol, protein kinase C activation, and

intracellular release of cytosolic Ca^{2+} from the dense tubular system.[8,9,23]

Importantly, through these activation processes there is an enhancement of the ongoing production of two potent platelet agonists, thromboxane A_2 (also a potent inducer of vasoconstriction) generated via arachidonic acid conversion to diacylglycerol and cyclic endoperoxides, and adenosine diphosphate secreted through dense granule release. Through the release of thromboxane A_2 and adenosine diphosphate, together with platelet-dependent production of thrombin, platelet recruitment becomes self-amplifying.[3,8,23] Thrombin, adenosine diphosphate, and thromboxane A_2 bind to specific receptors, initiate signaling, reduce cyclic adenosine monophosphate activity, induce shape change, and activate platelet contractile elements to form irregular extending pseudopodia and to secrete granular contents thereby perpetuating platelet recruitment (adenosine diphosphate, adenosine triphosphate, serotonin, and Ca^{2+} from dense granules, and adhesive proteins and coagulation factors from alpha-granules). Although epinephrine and possibly serotonin are weaker platelet agonists at physiologic concentrations, they may promote platelet aggregation in combination with other stimulatory agents. Collagen and thrombin are clearly the most potent and relevant inducers of platelet activation.

ACTIVATION OF COAGULATION FACTORS

Thrombin is rapidly generated in response to vascular injury (Fig. 1–1), and plays a central role in platelet recruitment and in the formation of the associated insoluble fibrin network.[24] The thrombotic response is localized, amplified, and modulated. Localized reactions of the blood coagulation cascade are achieved by the reversible binding of circulating coagulation proteins to damaged vascular cells, elements of the exposed subendothelium (especially collagen), platelets, and monocytes/macrophages. These binding events lead to the assembly of enzyme complexes that rapidly deliver products locally, whereby small initiating stimuli become greatly amplified to yield high levels of terminal products. The formation of membrane-bound enzyme complexes, the membrane binding properties of the substrates, and the resistance of the bound complexes to potent inhibitory systems are important features of these localized amplification processes.

Surface-dependent reactions convert the vitamin K-dependent zymogens to the respective serine protease. Each complex comprises a vitamin K-dependent serine protease and an accessory or cofactor protein in association with a membrane surface (Fig. 1–4). The presence of calcium is essential for the assembly and activity of these enzyme complexes. While each enzyme complex exhibits discreet substrate and proteolytic specificity, the complexes share several common features: (a) the complex constituents are functionally and structurally homologous; (b) the complexes assemble in similar patterns; (c) the assembled complexes greatly amplify the localized catalytic rates by regulating the conversion of the membrane-bound proenzyme to active proteases, the proteolytic activation of cofactors to their active forms, activated factors V and VIII, the expression of the integral membrane protein cofactors tissue factor and thrombomodulin, and the expression and function of the cellular membrane reactivity for these complex enzymes.

Both thrombin and activated factor X (fXa) amplify their own formation rates by catalyzing the activation of factor VII to activated factor VII and the activation of factors V and VIII to activated factors V and VIII, respectively. In addition, thrombin activates the expression of cellular binding sites for assembly of the vitamin K-dependent complexes.[24]

Vitamin K-Dependent Zymogens

Vitamin K-dependent zymogens are formed by the liver and are characterized by (a) the aminoterminal "Gla-domain" containing 9 to 12 glutamic acid residues that undergo post-translational gamma carboxylation and mediate calcium-dependent binding to phospholipid membranes, and (b) the carboxyterminal serine protease domain similar in general structure to chymotrypsin. Prothrombin also includes two "kringle" structural domains that facilitate its binding to activated factors X and V constituents in the prothrombinase complex.[25] The other vitamin K-dependent zymogens factors VII, IX, X, and protein C substitute two "epidermal growth factor-like" domains to mediate their unique binding properties in complex assembly.[26] Prothrombin, factor VII, and factor IX are synthesized and circulate as single-chain proteins, while factor X and protein C circulate in plasma as two-chain proteins because of proteolytic cleavages during synthesis and secretion. During proteolytic activation, factor X, factor IX, and protein C release specific activation peptides.[24] Current findings indicate that factor VII is also activated by limited proteolytic cleavage (at Arg-152 when complexed with the cofactor cell-bound tissue factor), similar to other vitamin K-dependent enzyme precursors in blood.[24,27]

Calcium-dependent binding of the vitamin K-dependent factors to acidic phospholipid membranes involves conformational transition of the aminoterminal residues 1 to 35.[24,28] This conformational reconfiguration depends on the post-translational gamma carboxylation of the glutamate sites. Interruption of this carboxylation process by either dietary deficiency of vitamin K or by the administration of vitamin K antagonists such as warfarin produces molecules that are unable to interact with membranes, and eliminates their participation in the formation of enzyme complexes.[24] The kinetic properties of the vitamin K-dependent proteins are presented in Table 1–2.

TABLE 1–2. Properties of Human Clotting Factors

Clotting Factor	Molecular Weight (Number of Chains)	Normal Plasma Concentration (Micromoles/Liter)	Active Form
Intrinsic System			
Factor XII	80,000 (1)	0.4	Serine protease
Prekallikrein	80,000 (1)	0.6	Serine protease
High molecular weight kininogen	105,000 (1)	0.7	Cofactor
Factor XI	160,000 (2)	0.25	Serine protease
Factor IX	68,000 (1)	0.09	Serine protease
Factor VIII	265,000 (1)	0.004	Cofactor
von Willebrand Factor	1–15,000,000*	†	Cofactor
Extrinsic System			
Factor VII	47,000 (1)	0.01	Serine protease
Tissue factor	46,000 (1)	0	Cofactor (cell bound)
Common Pathway			
Factor X	56,000 (2)	0.17	Serine protease
Factor V	330,000 (1)	0.02	Cofactor
Prothrombin	72,000 (1)	1.4	Serine protease
Fibrinogen	340,000 (6)	7.5	Clot structure
Factor XIII	320,000 (4)	0.05	Transglutaminase
Anticoagulant Pathway			
Protein C	56,000 (2)	0.08	Serine protease
Protein S	67,000 (1)	0.14	Serine protease
Thrombomodulin	35,000 (1)	0	Cofactor (cell bound)

* Subunit molecular weight of factor VIII/von Willebrand Factor is approximately 220,000 with a series of multimers found in circulation.

† Cannot be calculated because of wide variations in molecular weight.

Cofactor Proteins

Of the four proteins providing coagulant complex cofactor activity, factors V and VIII circulate as inactive plasma proteins, while tissue factor and thrombomodulin are integral membrane proteins anchored via transmembrane domain in adherent cells. Tissue factor is an integral membrane protein and does not require activation. It consists of a cysteine-containing cytoplasmic domain, transmembrane domain, and extracellular macromolecular ligand-binding domain.[29,30] Tissue factor is abundant on extravascular cells and may also be expressed on blood monocytes and possibly endothelial cells when stimulated by chemicals, cytokines, and endotoxin, although tissue factor expression by endothelial cells has not been documented directly in vivo.[31] Tissue factor is an important trigger for initiating coagulation in ruptured arterial atheromatous lesions because of its abundant presence in these intimal plaques and exposure to blood following disruption of the vascular intima.[31]

Factors V and VIII are homologous proteins sharing a common structural configuration of triplicated "A" domains and duplicated "C" domains with structurally divergent "B" domains connecting the A_2 and A_3 domains.[24] Factor V circulates in plasma as a single-chain protein at a concentration of 20 nanomoles/liter, while factor VIII circulates in a multiplicity of fragmented species in a tightly associated complex with von Willebrand factor at a concentration of 1 nanomole/liter (Table 1–2). During activation by thrombin or activated factor X, the "B" domains are excised, leading to the association of A_1A_2 with $A_3C_1C_2$ domains. In the case of activated factor V the active species is a heterodimer composed of aminoterminal-derived heavy chain (A_1A_2) and carboxyterminal-derived light chain ($A_3C_1C_2$) that interact tightly and noncovalently in the presence of divalent cations.[24] In contrast, thrombin acts on factor VIII which results in the removal of a peptide at the NH_2-terminal of the A_3 domain and the release from von Willebrand factor. Factor VIII activation occurs by a cleavage between the A_1 and A_2 domains, resulting in the unstable heterotrimeric activated factor VIII molecule.[32] Activated factors V and VIII both bind tightly to membranes containing acidic phospholipids via the light chains of the molecules. The binding site appears to reside in the A_3 domain which is in the light chains of the molecules. While the heavy chain of activated factor V is responsible for binding prothrombin, activated factor X binding depends on both the heavy and light chain of the activated factor V molecule.[24] Activated factors V and VIII may both be inactivated by plasmin, forming polydisperse smaller peptides, and by activated protein C by cleaving activated factor V at two sites and activated factor VIII at a single site to produce inactive proteins.[24]

The formation of the prothrombinase complex on membrane surfaces initially involves the independent binding of activated factors V and X to the membrane. This is followed by surface-facilitated complexing of the proteins[33] and leads to a tight complex with a dissociation constant of about 1 nanomole/liter. This membrane reaction constant is three orders of magnitude greater than that observed for the solution phase reaction between activated factors V and X. This enhancement may be due to a conformational change in the two proteins or reduction in the permissible orientations of the reacting molecules. The intrinsic factor IX and factors X activation complexes also appear to assemble and function in a facilitated and coordinated fashion. The addition of cofactors and the assembly of the appropriate membrane-bound enzyme complex leads to profound enhancement of reaction rates. For example, the activation of prothrombin by activated factor X is enhanced 300,000-fold by the addition of saturating concentrations of activated factor V and acidic phospholipid membranes.[34]

Membrane-bound prothrombinase complex initially cleaves Arg-323, producing the intermediate meizothrombin, followed by cleavage of Arg-274 to yield alpha-thrombin.[35] Meizothrombin remains membrane-bound through the retained Gla-domain linkage and activates protein C, but lacks procoagulant properties including the capacity to activate platelets and cleave fibrinogen.[24]

For the sequentially-linked reactions comprising the coagulation cascade, it has been hypothesized that the shuttling of product between reaction centers appears to take place on the same membrane surface with channeling of products between assembled complexes without dissociating from the membrane surface.[24] This type of mechanism increases the efficiency of the interactions by several orders of magnitude. Moreover, single-membrane channeling protects critical intermediate products from the inactivating effects of potent plasma inhibitors (for example, antithrombin III, heparin cofactor II, alpha$_2$-macroglobulin, alpha$_1$-antitrypsin), the inactivating effects of activated protein C (see later), and the rapid and inactivating dissociation of unstable cofactor activated factor VIII as well as from dilution by blood flow over the generating thrombus.[24]

Fibrin Formation

The final phase of thrombus formation in vivo involves the generation of a stable fibrin network that provides the structural support for the blood cellular elements comprising the thrombus and the scaffolding for subsequent cellular remodeling (Fig. 1–5). In this process, thrombin cleaves fibrinopeptides A and B from soluble circulating fibrinogen, producing fibrin monomers that multimerize to form soluble fibrillar strands of fibrin. This process is followed by an orderly fibrillar assembly, branching, lateral association, and covalent crosslinking to form the mature fibrin network (Fig. 1–6). Thrombin-activated factor XIII (fXIIIa) stabilizes fibrin by forming covalent bonds through transamidation between adjacent fibrin strands.[36]

Fibrinogen is a tridomainal disulfide-bridged molecule comprising two symmetric half-molecules, each consisting of one set of three different polypeptide chains termed Aα, Bβ, and gamma (Fig. 1–5). The two half-molecules are joined in the central aminoterminal domain in an antiparallel manner by three interchain disulfide bridges, two of which are between gamma chains at positions 8 and 9 and the other at Aα 28. Release of fibrinopeptide A (FPA) and fibrinopeptide B (FPB) exposes binding sites in the aminoterminal regions of the fibrin monomer that function cooperatively in the self-assembly process. Fibrinopeptide A release exposes a polymerization site in the central region of the molecule (E domain) that subsequently aligns with a complementary site in the outer region (D domain) of another molecule to form staggered overlapping two-stranded fibrils (Fig. 1–6). The slower fibrinopeptide B release also exposes an independent polymerization site that is used in a similar complementary alignment of the fibrin polymer.

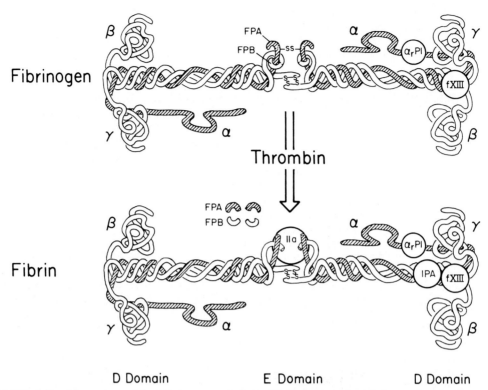

D Domain   E Domain   D Domain

FIGURE 1–5. Schematic model of fibrinogen and fibrin. Fibrinogen consists of three pairs of polypeptide chains, Aα, Bβ, and gamma, joined by disulfide bonds to form a symmetric dimeric structure (A). The NH₂-terminal regions of all six chains form the central domain (E Domain) of the molecule containing fibrino-peptide A and fibrinopeptide B sequences that are cleaved by thrombin during enzymatic conversion to fibrin. Enzymatic conversion of fibrinogen to fibrin (B) by thrombin cleavage results in release of fibrinopeptide A and fibrinopeptide B. A binding site for thrombin is present in the central domain of alpha, beta-fibrin, and depends largely on the presence of the beta-15 to 42 sequence. Binding sites for activated factor II, tissue-type plasminogen activation, factor XIII, and alpha₂-antiplasmin, respectively, are indicated on the fibrinogen or fibrin molecule.

Polymerization of the A-chains involves the peptide sequences Aα 17 to 20 and a second sequence in the aminoterminal region of the Bβ chain near the thrombin cleavage site at position 14. Thus, fibrin polymer assembly begins with the formation of double-stranded fibrils through noncovalent intermolecular interactions between outer D and central E domains in a staggered overlapping manner (Fig. 1–6). Subsequently, lateral association of fibrils occurs, increasing fiber thickness.[36] The branching structures consist of laterally associated double-stranded fibrils that form a four-stranded fiber (Fig. 1–6).

Structural stability and integrity of the fibrin network is achieved through covalent crosslinking. Fibrin molecules undergo interchain linkages in the presence of activated factor XIII and calcium ions by forming covalent epsilon-(gamma-glu)lys isopeptide bonds.[37] Intermolecular gamma chain cross-linking within fibrils forms gamma dimers, which occur as reciprocal bridges between lysine at position 406 of one gamma chain and glutamine at position 398 of another gamma chain. Slower crosslinking among alpha-chains and between gamma and alpha-chains also creates covalent polymers. In addition, gamma trimers and tetramers have been identified.[38]

Thrombin binds with fibrin through its exosite and the central molecular domain of fibrin.[39,40] The fibrin-bound thrombin retains its catalytic coagulant and platelet-activating capabilities.[40] Moreover, the fibrin-bound thrombin is protected from inactivation by heparin-antithrombin III complexes.[41] Thus, in arterial thrombi, thrombin bound to fibrin continues to mediate platelet-dependent thrombus formation despite heparin or thrombolytic therapies.

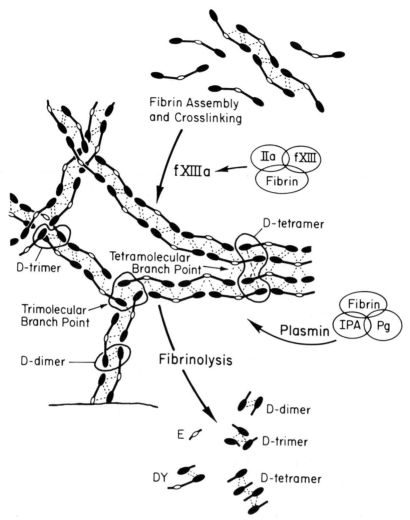

FIGURE 1–6. Schematic model of fibrin assembly, crosslinking, and fibrinolysis. Fibrin molecules are represented by trimolecular structures having a central E domain and two outer D domains. After enzynmatic conversion of fibrinogen to fibrin, fibrin monomeric units assemble in a staggered overlapping manner by noncovalent interactions between the E and D domains to form two-stranded fibrils. Polymerization of alpha-fibrin forms similar fibrils. The fibrils undergo noncovalent lateral associations to form thicker fibers, and trimolecular and tetramolecular branch points to form a three-dimensional matrix. In the presence of activated factor XIII, assembled fibrin undergoes covalent crosslinking by formation of epsilon gamma glutamyl-lysl isopeptide bonds, mainly between gamma chains and alpha chains. When crosslinked fibrin undergoes fibrinolysis, the peptides joining the D and E domains are cleaved, leading to generation of fragment E(E), fragment E and D-containing fragments (DY), and fragment D-containing products containing crosslinked multimeric D domains that reflect the type of gamma-chain crosslinking that has occurred (D-dimer, D-trimer, D-tetramer).

Endogenous Inhibitors of Thrombus Formation

The potentially devastating effects of uncontrolled extension of thrombus throughout the vascular system is prevented by the multiple processes designed to limit thrombus formation to the site of vascular injury.[3] Although activating species that diffuse out of forming thrombus into flowing blood are rapidly diluted and subsequently removed during passage through the liver, multiple additional active mechanisms are in place to ensure protection. In general, these protective mechanisms are endothelial-dependent and thrombin-mediated (Fig. 1–1). Since the ratio of endothelial surface area to blood volume is very high in the microcirculation compared with the large vessels, the efficacy of the endothelial-related mechanisms will be greatest in the microcirculation.

Endothelial cells exhibit both active and passive antithrombotic properties.[3] The negative charge of endothelial cells together with the essentially nonreactive luminal glycosaminoglycan and glycoprotein endothelial coat largely insulates the vessel wall from elements of circulating blood.[42] Additionally, intact endothelial cells adjacent to the site of injury reduce the reactivity of ambient platelets by membrane-bound adenosine diphosphatase-mediated degradation of proaggregatory adenosine diphosphate derived from thrombus-associated activated platelets and the rapid removal of proaggregatory vasoactive amines. The most important mechanisms for limiting thrombus extension are related to the inactivation of thrombin activity, the reduction in thrombin generation, and the thrombin-stimulated production of antithrombotic and vasodilating factors by intact endothelium.

Thrombin entering the circulation is directly inactivated by plasma protease inhibitors.[42] Heparin and antithrombin III, a 58,000-dalton plasma protein present at a concentration of 3 micromoles/liter, inhibits thrombin and activated factors XI, X, and IX (but not activated factor VII). Whereas antithrombin III alone inactivates these serine proteases slowly, the process is markedly accelerated (at least three orders of magnitude) when it is bound to heparin. Inactivation by antithrombin III is similarly greatly facilitated by the heparin-like glycosaminoglycan heparin sulfate abundantly present on the luminal surface of endothelial cells,[42] and possibly by thrombomodulin-mediated enhancement. On average, there are approximately 200,000 equivalent binding sites on each cell, and these cells regulate this protective mechanism by modulating the synthesis of heparin sulfate.[42] Antithrombin III may be regarded as a constitutive regulation of blood clotting. The genetic reduction in the level of plasma antithrombin III predisposes affected individuals to venous thrombotic and thromboembolic events. Alpha$_1$-antitrypsin and alpha$_2$-macroglobulin provide additional backup inhibitory capability. Activated factor VII is inactivated by the formation of a complex involving the lipid-associated coagulation inhibitor (LACI), tissue factor, activated factor X phospholipids, and calcium ions.[43] While the LACI-TF-fVIIa-fXa complex has the capacity of tightly binding and inhibiting activated factors X and VII, it is not clear whether the formation of this complex serves to inactivate these proteases or to maintain dissociable and protected pools in whole blood.

Thrombin in association with intact endothelium induces the production and release from vascular endothelial cells of two highly potent local antiaggregatory vasodilators, prostacyclin[10] and nitric oxide (endothelial-derived relaxing factor).[44] These molecules are thought to provide significant antithrombotic protection for microcirculatory beds adjacent to sites of thrombus formation.

Thrombin arising locally from forming thrombus induces the production and release of tissue-type plasminogen activator (t-PA) from adjacent intact endothelium.[3,45] Tissue-type plasminogen activator binds with the fibrin present in thrombus and forms a trimeric complex with bound or circulating plasminogen, which results in the production of plasmin and increased fibrinolysis, particularly in the microcirculation (see later).

Thrombin, when complexed with protein C and thrombomodulin, activates the natural antithrombotic zymogen protein C by cleaving the heavy chain to produce an aminoterminal dodecapeptide.[46] Thrombomodulin is a constitutive vascular endothelial membrane protein (100,000 copies per endothelial cell) comprising six epidermal growth factor-like domains that resemble the low-density lipoprotein receptor.[46] The epidermal growth factor repeats 2 through 6 of thrombomodulin facilitate the activation of protein C by thrombin, and repeats 5 and 6 provide the site for thrombin binding. Protein C is a 56,000-dalton vitamin K-dependent plasma zymogen that circulates at a concentration of about 0.1 micromoles/liter. Both protein C and activated protein C possess gamma-carboxyglutamic and beta-hydroxyaspartic acid residues, thereby retaining the formed calcium-dependent complexes bound to endothelial cell surfaces.[24,46] Activated protein C inhibits thrombin formation by inactivating surface-bound activated factor V and activated factor VIII through proteolytic cleavages. The importance of protein C activation in protecting against unwanted thrombus formation is evident from the life-threatening thrombotic consequences in newborns with homozygous deficiency and the predisposition to thrombosis in some kindreds with heterozygous individuals. Protein S is the cofactor for the activation of protein C on both platelets and endothelium.[46] Protein S enhances the efficacy of protein C inactivation of membrane-bound activated factor V and activated factor VIII. Protein S circulates in the blood as the active free protein and in noncovalent association with a large, multisubunit protein of the complement system, C4bBP, in an inactive state. Heterozygous hereditary deficiency states are predisposed to thrombotic events. In summary, the protein C/thrombomodulin/protein S pathway provides an important thrombin-dependent protective mechanism initiating negative feedback regulation for decreasing thrombin's own production. In addition, since the generation of activated protein C is directly linked to the extent of thrombin production, the pathway is reactive rather than constitutive.

Blood Leukocytes

Blood leukocytes may be involved in thrombus formation and its regulation.[1-3] For example, monocytes/macrophages express tissue factor or a direct prothrombin activator when stimulated by endotoxin, the cytokines interleukin-1 and tissue necrosis factor, or platelet-derived growth factor, thereby giving rise to thrombin production. Additionally, platelets may be activated directly by granulocyte-released cathepsin G, thromboxanes, prostaglandins, or acetylglyceryl ether phosphorylcholine. Furthermore, both cathepsin G and elastase may degrade endothelial barrier function. On the other hand, granulocyte-secreted serine proteases degrade extracellular matrix proteins and mediate nonplasminogen-dependent fibrinolysis. Conversely, activated platelets may recruit granulocytes into actively forming thrombus by expressing GMP-140, a receptor for platelet-neutrophil binding, and by releasing platelet basic protein, which undergoes proteolytic cleavage to form neutrophil activating peptide-2.[47]

FIBRINOLYSIS

Fibrinolysis plays an important role in the dissolution of thrombi and in maintaining the vascular system patent, as illustrated by the clinical occurrence of thrombosis in patients with constitutive or acquired hypofi-

brinolysis.[45] The fibrinolytic system removes thrombi by proteolytically degrading fibrin into soluble fragments (Fig. 1–6). In this process, the serine protease plasmin is formed from the zymogen plasminogen by the action of either tissue-type plasminogen activator (t-PA) or urokinase-type plasminogen activator (u-PA). Plasmin cleaves fibrin to produce progressively smaller degradation products, typically containing two D domains (D-dimer), each from different monomers of fibrin that are covalently linked through activated factor XIII-mediated transamidation during the stabilization of fibrin, and therefore resistant to lysis by plasmin. Physiologic inhibition of fibrinolysis may occur at the level of the tissue-type plasminogen activator and urokinase-type plasminogen activator by specific plasminogen activator inhibitors (PAI-1 and PAI-2), or at the level of plasmin, by alpha$_2$-antiplasmin. Some of the properties of this system are outlined in Table 1–3.

Plasminogen, a 92,000-dalton molecule, exhibits four functional domains: (a) the carboxyterminal serine protease domain, (b) the aminoterminal finger domain (homologous to the finger domains in fibronectin), (c) epidermal growth factor domain (homologous to growth factors), and (d) the domain containing the five triple-looped sulfide-bonded kringle structures. Native plasminogen has an aminoterminal glutamic acid. Limited proteolysis at Arg-67 may convert it to the more reactive Lys-plasminogen. Plasminogen binds specifically to fibrin through the lysine binding sites contained in the first three kringles, particularly with the first kringle structure. Its activation involves the cleavage of Arg-560, creating the two-chain proteolytically active plasmin. Intrinsic activation involves contact factor complex formation (factor XII, prekallikrein, high molecular weight kininogen). This pathway may be involved in single-chain urokinase-type plasminogen activator (saruplase) activation, but its physiologic importance is uncertain.

Tissue-type plasminogen activator is a 70,000-dalton molecule comprising a carboxyterminal serine protease domain, an aminoterminal finger domain, epidermal growth factor domain, and two kringle domains.[48] It is synthesized mainly by endothelium, and circulates at a concentration of about 1 nanomole/liter. Plasmin quickly converts tissue-type plasminogen activator to a two-chained molecule. Binding of tissue-type plasminogen activator to fibrin is essential for effective

TABLE 1–3. **Properties of the Main Components of the Fibrinolytic System***

Component	Catalytic Triad	Reactive Site	Molecular Weight ($\times 10^3$)	Plasma Concentration (micrograms/milliliter)
Plasminogen	—	—	92	200
Plasmin	His 602, Asp 645, Ser 740	—	85	—
t-PA	His 322, Asp 371, Ser 478	—	68	0.005
scu-PA	His 204, Asp 255, Ser 356	—	54	0.008
α_2-antiplasmin	—	Arg 364-Met 365	70	70
PAI-1	—	Arg 346-Met 347	52	0.05
PAI-2	—	Arg 358-Thr 359	60,47	<0.005

* The numbering of amino acid residues is usually based on these initially determined incorrect values.

t-PA = tissue-type plasminogen activator; scu-PA = single-chain urokinase-type plasminogen activator (saruplase), pro-urokinase; PAI-1 = plasminogen activator inhibitor-1; PAI-2 = plasminogen activator inhibitor-2.

plasmin generation. The binding is mediated via the finger and second kringle domains. Fibrin provides a surface on which tissue-type plasminogen activator and plasminogen absorb in a sequential and ordered way, yielding a cyclic ternary complex. Since the plasmin formed on fibrin retains its lysine binding sites, plasmin generally remains bound and therefore resists inactivating complex formation with alpha₂-antiplasmin. However, when plasmin ultimately degrades fibrin, lysis may be enhanced because of increased binding by both tissue-type plasminogen activator and plasminogen.

Saruplase is a 54,000-dalton protein exhibiting an aminoterminal epidermal growth factor domain and a single kringle domain with a carboxyterminal catalytic domain.[49] Saruplase (as opposed to two-chain urokinase-type plasminogen activator) has significant fibrin specificity, that is due to neutralization by fibrin of components in plasma that impair plasminogen activation. Alternatively, saruplase has been claimed to be inactive toward circulating plasminogen, but active toward conformationally altered plasminogen bound to partially digested fibrin. It circulates at about 1 nanomole/liter and is synthesized by many cells of different origin.

Platelets promote fibrinolysis. Plasminogen binds with platelets, facilitating the conversion of plasminogen to plasmin by plasminogen activators; this binding is enhanced by thrombin activation. Saruplase also binds with platelet receptors, and plasmin induces platelet aggregation and release.

Alpha₂-antiplasmin, a 70,000-dalton protein present in plasma at concentration of about 1 micromole/liter, belongs to the serpin family of inhibitors and is a potent and rapid inhibitor of unbound plasmin.[45] Plasminogen activator inhibitors-1 and -2 are also serpin-type inhibitors.

In general, plasmin generation occurs locally and is confined to the vicinity of the thrombotic mass without significant plasmin escape into the systemic circulation. The mechanisms to ensure that plasmin does not act systemically include: (a) the local release of plasminogen activators from intact adjacent endothelial cells by the action of thrombin; (b) the activation of plasminogen activators within thrombi due to affinity for fibrin in the case of tissue-type plasminogen activator and by some less well understood mechanism for saruplase; and (c) the inactivation of free plasmin in the circulation by antiplasmin, and the inhibition of tissue-type plasminogen activate and saruplase by plasminogen activator inhibitor-1 and plasminogen activator inhibitor-2.[50,51]

In conclusion, vascular damage initiates a localized, amplified, and regulated assembly of localized insoluble thrombus that physiologically prevents excessive blood loss caused by invasive injuries without impairing blood's fluidity. In disease states, the formation of occlusive thrombi or thromboemboli in veins or diseased arteries threatens the viability of dependent tissues. Initial localization is achieved by the focal deposition of platelets. Amplification is dependent on the assembly of highly efficient interactive enzyme-cofactor complexes on the membrane surfaces of deposited cells, and is modulated by the expression of membrane-binding activity, cofactor activation, and zymogen activation. Regulation is mediated by (a) inactivation and removal as inhibitor-enzyme complexes, (b) destruction of membrane cofactor activities by activated protein C, (c) thrombin-induced release of antithrombotic products (prostacyclin, nitric oxide, and tissue-type plasminogen activator), and (d) enhanced fibrinolysis. Resolution proceeds by fibrinolysis and healing. In recent years, our understanding of thrombosis, its pathogensis, detection, evaluation, prevention, and management has greatly expanded. This volume highlights many of these advances. (See also Chapter 10.)

REFERENCES

1. Colman RW, Hirsh J, Marder VJ, Salzman EW, eds. Hemostasis and thrombosis: basic principles and clinical practice. 2nd ed. Philadelphia: JB Lippincott, 1987.
2. Bloom AL, Thomas DP, eds. Haemostasis and thrombosis. 2nd ed. Edinburgh: Churchill Livingstone, 1987.
3. Harker LA. Pathogenesis of thrombosis. In: Williams WJ, ed. Hematology. 4th ed. New York: McGraw-Hill, 1990: 1559–69.
4. Turitto VT, Baumgartner HR. Platelet-surface interactions. In: Colman RW, Hirsh J, Marder VJ, Salzman EW, eds. Hemostasis and thrombosis: basic principles and clinical practice. 2nd ed. Philadelphia: JB Lippincott, 1987: 555–71.
5. Virchow R. Phlogose und Thrombose im efäss-system. In: Virchow R, ed. Gesammelte abhandlungen zur wissenschaflichen medicin. Frankfurt: Von Meidinger Sohn, 1856: 458–636.
6. Turitto VT. Blood viscosity, mass transport, and thrombogenesis. In: Spaet TH, ed. Progress in hemostasis and thrombosis. New York: Grune & Stratton, 1982: 139.
7. Sevitt S. The structure and growth of valve-pocket thrombi in femoral veins. J Clin Pathol 1974; 27: 517–28.
8. Kieffer N, Phillips DR. Platelet membrane glycoproteins: functions in cellular interactions. Ann Rev Cell Biol 1990; 6: 329–57.
9. Ruoslahti E. Integrins. J Clin Invest 1991; 87: 1–5.
10. Moncada S, Palmer RMJ, Higgs EA. Prostacyclin and endothelium-derived relaxing factor: biological interactions and significance. In: Verstraete M, Vermylen J, Lijnen R, Arnout J, eds. Thrombosis and haemostasis. Leuven: Leuven University Press, 1987: 505–23.
11. Fressinaud E, Baruch D, Rothschild C, Baumgartner HR, Meyer D. Platelet von Willebrand factor: evidence for its involvement in platelet adhesion to collagen. Blood 1987; 70: 1214–7.
12. Vincente V, Houghten RA, Ruggeri ZM. Identification of a site in the α chain of platelet glycoprotein Ib that participates in von Willebrand factor binding. J Biol Chem 1990; 265: 274–80.
13. Fox JEB, Reynolds CC, Johnson MM. Identification of glycoprotein Ibβ as one of the major proteins phosphorylated during exposure of intact platelets to agents that activate cyclic AMP-dependent protein kinase. J Biol Chem 1987; 262: 12627–31.
14. Clemetson KJ, Capitanio A, Lüscher EF. High resolution two-dimensional gel electrophoresis of the proteins and glycoproteins of human blood platelets and platelet membranes. Biochim Biophys Acta 1979; 553: 11.
15. Thien-Khai HV, Hung DT, Wheaton VI, Coughlin SR. Molecular cloning of a functional thrombin receptor reveals a novel proteolytic mechanism of receptor activation. Cell 1991; 64: 1057–68.
16. Hanson SR, Harker LA. Interruption of acute platelet-dependent thrombosis by the synthetic antithrombin D-phenylalanyl-L-prolyl-L-arginyl chloromethylketone. Proc Natl Acad Sci USA 1988; 85: 3184–8.
17. Ginsberg MH, Loftus JC, Plow EF. Cytoadhesins, integrins, and platelets. Thromb Haemost 1988; 59: 1–6.
18. Poncz M, Eisman R, Heidenreich R, et al. Structure of the platelet membrane glycoprotein IIb: homology to the α subunits of the vitronectin and fibronectin membrane receptors. J Biol Chem 1987; 262: 8476–82.
19. Ruoslahti E, Pierschbacher MD. New perspectives in cell adhesion: RGD and integrins. Science 1987; 238: 491–7.
20. Doolittle RF, Watt KWK, Cottrell BA, Strong DD, Riley M. The amino acid sequence of the α-chain of human fibrinogen. Nature 1979; 280: 464–7.
21. Kloczewiak M, Timmons S, Lukas TJ, Hawiger J. Platelet receptor recognition site on human fibrinogen. Synthesis and structure-function relationship of peptides corresponding to the carboxyterminal segment of the γ chain. Biochemistry 1984; 23: 1767–74.
22. Frelinger AL, Lam SC-T, Plow EF, Smith MA, Loftus JC, Ginsberg MH. Occupancy of an adhesive glycoprotein receptor modulates expression of an antigenic site involved in cell adhesion. J Biol Chem 1988; 263: 12397–402.
23. Brass LF. The biochemistry of platelet activation. In: Hoffman R, Benz EJ Jr, Shattil SJ, Furie B, Cohen HJ, eds. Hematology: basic principles and practice. New York: Churchill Livingstone, 1991: 1176–97.
24. Mann KG, Nesheim ME, Church WR, Haley P, Krishnaswamy S. Surface-dependent reactions of the vitamin K-dependent enzyme complexes. Blood 1990; 76: 1–16.
25. Magnusson S, Sottrup JL, Petersen TE, Dudek WG, Claeys H. Homologous "Kringle" structures common to plasminogen and prothrombin. Substrate specificity of enzymes activating prothrombin and plasminogen. In: Ribbons DW, Brew K, eds. Proteolysis and physiological regulation. New York: Academic Press, 1976: 203.
26. Doolittle RF, Feng DF, Johnson MS. Computer-based characterization of epidermal growth factor domains. Nature 1984; 307: 558.
27. Williams EB, Kirshnaswamy S, Mann KG. Zymogen/enzyme discrimination using peptide chloromethyl ketones. J Biol Chem 1989; 264: 7536.
28. Soriano-Garcia M, Park CH, Tulinsky A, Ravichandran KG, Skrzypczak-Jankun E. Structure of Ca^{2+} prothrombin fragment 1 including the conformation of the Gla domain. Biochemistry 1989; 28: 6805.
29. Spicer EK, Horton R, Bloem L, et al. Isolation of cDNA clones coding for human tissue factor: primary structure of the protein and cDNA. Proc Natl Acad Sci USA 1987; 84: 5148.
30. Morrissey JH, Fakhrai H, Edgington TS. Molecular cloning of the cDNA for tissue factor. Cell 1987; 50: 129.
31. Wilcox JN, Smith KM, Schwartz SM, Gordon D. Localization of tissue factor in the normal vessel wall and in the atherosclerotic plaque. Proc Natl Acad Sci USA 1989;86:2839.
32. Lollar P, Parker CG. Subunit structure of thrombin-activated porcine factor VIII. Biochemistry 1989; 28: 666.
33. Krishnaswamy S. Prothrombinase complex assembly: contributions of protein-protein and protein-membrane interactions towards complex formation. J Biol Chem 1990; in press.
34. Nesheim ME, Taswell JB, Mann KG. The contribution of bovine Factor V and Factor Va to the activity of prothrombinase. J Biol Chem 1979; 254: 10952.
35. Krishnaswamy S, Mann KG, Nesheim ME. The prothrombinase-catalyzed activation of prothrombin proceeds through the intermediate meizothrombin in an ordered, sequential reaction. J Biol Chem 1986; 261: 8977.
36. Mosesson MW. Fibrin polymerization and its regulatory role in hemostasis. J Lab Clin Med 1990; 116: 8–17.
37. Olexa SA, Budzynski AZ. Evidence for four different polymerization sites involved in human fibrin formation. Proc Natl Acad Sci USA 1980; 77: 1374–8.
38. Mosesson MW, Siebenlist KR, Amrani DL, DiOrio JP. Identification of covalently linked trimeric and tetrameric D domains in crosslinked fibrin. Proc Natl Acad Sci USA 1989; 86: 1113–7.
39. Fenton JW II, Olson TA, Zabinski MP, Wilner GD. Anion-binding exosite of human α-thrombin and fibrin (ogen) recognition. Biochemistry 1988; 27: 7106–12.
40. Kaminski M, McDonagh J. Inhibited thrombins: interactions with fibrinogen and fibrin. Biochem J 1987; 242: 881–7.
41. Hogg PJ, Jackson CM. Fibrin monomer protects thrombin from inactivation by heparin-antithrombin III: implications

for heparin efficacy. Proc Natl Acad Sci USA 1989; 86: 3619–23.

42. Rosenberg RD. The heparin-antithrombin system: a natural anticoagulant mechanism. In: Colman RW, Hirsh J, Marder VJ, Salzman EW, eds. Hemostasis and thrombosis: basic principles and clinical practice. Philadelphia: JB Lippincott, 1987: 1373–92.

43. Broze GJ Jr, Warren LA, Novotny WF, Higuchi DA, Girard JJ, Miletich JP. The lipoprotein-associated coagulation inhibitor that inhibits the factor VII-tissue factor complex also inhibits factor Xa: insight into its possible mechanism of action. Blood 1988; 71: 335.

44. Palmer RMJ, Ferrige AG, Moncada S. Nitric oxide release accounts for the biological activity of endothelium-derived relaxing factor. Nature 1987; 327: 524.

45. Collen D, Lijnen HR. Molecular and cellular basis of fibrinolysis. In: Hoffman R, Benz EJ Jr, Shattil SJ, Furie B, Cohen HJ, eds. Hematology: basic principles and practice. New York: Churchill Livingstone, 1991: 1232–42.

46. Esmon CT. The roles of protein C and thrombomodulin in the regulation of blood coagulation. J Biol Chem 1989; 264: 4743.

47. Larsen E, Cell A, Gilbert GE, et al. PADGM protein: a receptor that mediates the interaction of activated platelets with neutrophils and monocytes. Cell 1989; 59: 306–12.

48. Pennica D, Holmes WE, Kohr WJ, et al. Cloning and expression of human tissue-type plasminogen activator cDNA in E. coli. Nature 1983; 301: 214.

49. Holmes WE, Pennica D, Blaber M, et al. Cloning and expression of the gene for pro-urokinase in Escherichia coli. Biotechnology 1985; 3: 923.

50. Schleef RR, Loskutoff DJ. Fibrinolytic system of vascular endothelial cells. Role of plasminogen activator inhibitors. Haemostasis 1988; 18: 328.

51. Francis CW, Marder VJ. Physiologic regulation and pathologic disorders of fibrinolysis. In: Colman RW, Hirsh J, Marder VJ, Salzman EW, eds. Hemostasis and thrombosis: basic principles and clinical practice. Philadelphia: JB Lippincott, 1987: 358–79.

2

PATHOGENESIS OF THROMBOSIS

LINA BADIMON, JUAN JOSE BADIMON, and VALENTIN FUSTER

Although coronary thrombotic occlusion causing acute myocardial infarction was suspected at the turn of the century,[1] only over the last few years have clinical and pathologic observations and experimental investigation led to a better understanding of how a thrombus forms and its incidence in the acute ischemic coronary events. The groups of de Wood,[2,3] Falk,[4-6] and Davies[7-10] have clearly shown that thrombus formation, usually secondary to atherosclerotic plaque disruption, plays a fundamental role in the development of the acute coronary syndromes. In addition, recent evidence indicates that mural thrombosis, also at the site of plaque rupture, is an important mechanism in the progression of atherosclerosis even when symptoms are absent. This chapter will be divided into three sections: Evolving Concepts in Thrombosis; Arterial Thrombosis; and, very briefly, Venous Thrombosis. In the first section we will analyze the evolving concepts on the mechanisms of thrombosis, particularly arterial, including: (a) a brief description of the pathophysiology of thrombus formation; (b) mural thrombus formation and organization on atherosclerotic plaque; and (c) occlusive thrombosis and thrombogenic risk factors. The second section will analyze the clinical manifestations of atherosclerotic vascular disease including (a) coronary thrombosis, (b) cerebrovascular thrombosis, (c) peripheral arterial disease, and (d) thrombosis in the cardiac chambers.

EVOLVING CONCEPTS IN THROMBOSIS

Pathophysiology of Thrombus Formation

We will briefly discuss the role of platelets and coagulation in thrombosis (see also Chapter 1). After plaque rupture, exposed collagen, in addition to other mediators, induces platelet aggregation. Most platelet agonists seem to act through the hydrolysis of platelet membrane phosphatidylinositol by phospholipase C, which results in the mobilization of free calcium from the platelet-dense tubular system. Calcium, in turn, is an important mediator of platelet activation.[11,12]

PLATELET ACTIVATION

Exposed collagen from the vessel wall and thrombin generated by the activation of the coagulation cascade as well as circulating epinephrine are powerful platelet activators. Another pathway of platelet aggregation is mediated by adenosine diphosphate, which may be released from hemolyzed red cells in the area of vessel injury. Each agonist stimulates the discharge of calcium from the platelet-dense tubular system and promotes the contraction of the platelet, with the subsequent release of its granule contents. Platelet-released adenosine diphosphate and serotonin stimulate adjacent platelets, further enhancing the process of platelet activation. Arachidonate, which is released from the platelet membrane by the stimulatory activity of collagen, thrombin, adenosine diphosphate, and serotonin, is another platelet agonist. Arachidonate is converted to thromboxane A_2 by the sequential action of cyclooxygenase and thromboxane synthetase. Thromboxane A_2 not only promotes further platelet aggregation, but also is a potent vasoconstrictor (Fig. 2–1).

Any or all of these pathways induce the subsequent exposure of platelet receptors, namely, the glycoprotein IIb-IIIa.[13,14] Adhesive macromolecules including fibrinogen, von Willebrand factor (vWF), and fibronectin bind to glycoprotein IIb-IIIa and form bridges between neighboring platelets, thereby playing an essential role in the process of platelet aggregation.

The receptor-mediated mechanisms relating to the platelet interaction in the thrombotic process around stenoses have not been directly studied as yet; however, two glycoproteins (GP) on the surface of the platelet have been identified as being important in platelet–vessel wall interaction. Platelet glycoprotein Ib is necessary for normal platelet adhesion to subendothelium at high shear rates,[15,16] presumably through its interaction with von Willebrand factor.[17,18] Von Willebrand factor has been shown to bind to platelet glycoprotein IIb-IIIa,[19,20] and a role for this platelet glycoprotein in both adhesion and in the platelet–platelet interactions leading to thrombus formation has been suggested by perfusion studies conducted at high shear rates.[15,21–26] The present consensus is that, at high shear rate conditions, platelet glycoproteins Ib and IIb-IIIa both appear to be involved in the events of platelet adhesion, whereas glycoprotein IIb-IIIa may be involved predominantly in platelet–platelet interactions, although a role of glycoprotein Ib in the latter interactions has not been investigated as yet. These mechanisms have not been evaluated with respect to events in the vicinity of a geometrically created stenosis, but are currently under investigation by our group, utilizing antibodies antiglycoprotein IIb-IIIa (Fig. 2–2).

The specific plasma proteins which are involved in platelet–platelet interactions under various shear conditions remain to be determined. The absence of platelet aggregation (observed using low shear and nonflow systems) in thrombasthenia has been ascribed to inability of platelets to bind fibrinogen, since platelets are known to require fibrino-

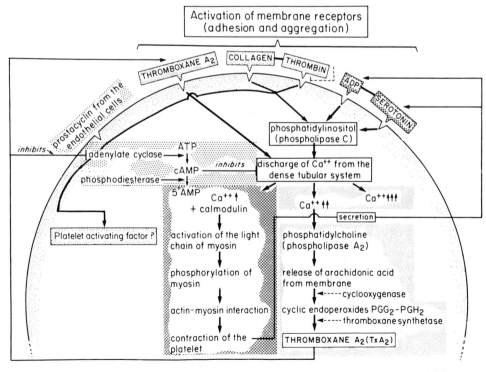

FIGURE 2–1. Diagram of platelet activation pathways. (Modified from Stein B, et al. Inhibitor agents in cardiovascular disease: an update. J Am Coll Cardiol 1989; 14:813–36.)

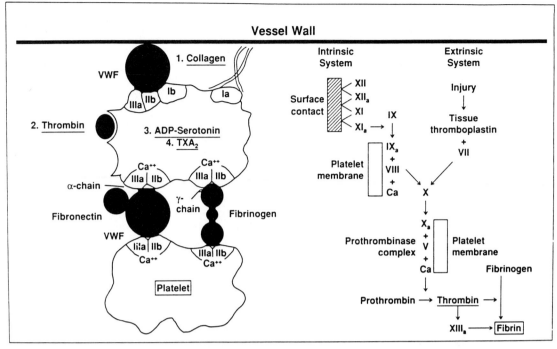

FIGURE 2–2. Left, scheme of the biochemical interactions between platelet membrane receptors, vessel wall, and adhesive macromolecules during the processes of platelet adhesion and aggregation. Right, scheme of the biochemical activation of the coagulation system. (From Fuster V, et al. Circulation 1988; 77: 1213, with permission.)

gen for aggregation in plasma or buffer; however, this requirement is not absolute.[27,28] Recent perfusion studies have indicated that platelet attachment or aggregate buildup (thrombus formation) on subendothelium is normal in afibrinogenemia under a wide variety of shear conditions.[16,29,30] Antibodies to fibrinogen, even when added to afibrinogenemic blood in order to remove any small trace of residual fibrinogen, did not inhibit the platelet interaction with the vessel wall,[31] although they did reduce aggregation with adenosine diphosphate and collagen when tested in an aggregometer. Blocking the glycoprotein IIb-IIIa receptor site on platelets with either an antibody (LJ–CP8) which blocks the general binding of adhesive proteins, or with various peptides which simulate the sequence Arg-Gly-Asp (RGD) present in a variety of adhesive proteins inhibits both platelet adhesion and thrombus formation in flowing blood at high shear rates. These findings reinforce the importance of the glycoprotein IIb-IIIa site in platelet–vessel wall interaction and suggest that fibrinogen is not always a necessary component for such interactions. Moreover,

the results are also consistent with previous perfusion studies which demonstrated the importance of von Willebrand factor in both platelet–platelet and platelet–vessel wall interactions.[15,16,22–24,32] Additional direct support for the ability of adhesive proteins other than fibrinogen to participate in platelet–platelet interactions has been obtained from studies conducted with a monoclonal antibody (LJ–P5) to glycoprotein IIb-IIIa which blocks the binding of von Willebrand factor and other adhesive proteins, but not of fibrinogen, to platelets.[33] In presence of this antibody levels of both platelet–vessel wall and platelet–platelet interaction on subendothelium were reduced, suggesting that von Willebrand factor or one of the other proteins blocked by the antibody could participate in thrombotic events occurring in flowing blood. A peptide-specific monoclonal antibody that inhibits von Willebrand factor binding to glycoprotein IIb-IIIa [152B6] without affecting the binding of other RGD-dependent glycoproteins has been shown to significantly inhibit platelet deposition to human atherosclerotic vessel wall,[34] suggesting a key role for von Willebrand factor in platelet–vessel wall interaction. Pigs that have normal fibrinogen levels but are congenitally deficient in von Willebrand factor showed a significantly reduced ability to deposit platelets in subendothelium[22] and collagen type I bundles,[23] using a variety of in vivo and in vitro perfusion conditions at high and low local shear rates.[26] The importance of such mechanisms in atherosclerotic disease is currently being evaluated by our group in pigs with von Willebrand's disease and with antibodies to von Willebrand factor.

ACTIVATION OF THE COAGULATION SYSTEM

During plaque rupture, in addition to platelet deposition in the injured area, the clotting mechanism is activated by the exposure of the deendothelialized vascular surface and the release of tissue factor. The activation of the coagulation cascade leads to the generation of thrombin which, as mentioned before, is a powerful platelet activator that also catalyzes the formation and polymerization of fibrin. Fibrin is essential in the stabilization of the platelet thrombus and allows it to resist removal by high intravascular pressure and shear rate. These basic concepts have clinical relevance in the context of the acute coronary syndromes where plaque rupture exposes collagen, which activates platelets and the coagulation system and results in the formation of a fixed and occlusive platelet–fibrin thrombus (Fig. 2–2).

The efficacy of fibrinolytic agents pointedly demonstrates the importance of fibrin-related material in the thrombosis associated with myocardial infarction.[35] However, few studies have considered the influence of flow on procoagulant activity either in laminar or nonparallel streamline conditions. The observation that fibrin formation is diminished at increasing shear rates[18] is currently unexplained. While dilution of procoagulant moieties has generally been proposed as the mechanism by which flow minimizes coagulative events at surfaces, such a mechanism has never been verified experimentally and, in fact, there are theoretical grounds to suspect the validity of such an hypothesis.[36] It is quite plausible to suspect that flow may have direct effects on certain enzyme or polymerization kinetics involved in thrombosis, in addition to the well-defined effect that flow has in enhancing transport of reactants and products to and from the vessel wall.[37] Such effects of flow on immobilized

enzymes have been occasionally observed, but never studied with respect to coagulative processes.[38,39] It is interesting to note that venous thrombosis, which is predominantly constituted by fibrin clots, occurs in areas of stasis and low shear rate conditions typical of the venous system. Therefore, the low local shear rate conditions and flow recirculations developing in the poststenotic areas may explain fibrin accumulation. Recently, it has been shown that vascular subendothelium which is completely devoid of endothelial cells is able to clot whole plasma and more specifically activate factor X in the presence of factor VII.[40] This activity results in the deposition of fibrin on the subendothelium at low shear conditions which can be blocked by monoclonal antibody to tissue factor.[40] Thus, tissue factor appears to be a major procoagulant factor in the vascular space immediately underlying the endothelial lining of arteries, a site which might be readily accessible upon local injury or upon rupture of an atherosclerotic plaque. Recently, we have shown that under the same blood conditions, local fibrin formation on the damaged vessel wall will be dependent on the severity of the damage. The exposure of deep layers of the vessel wall to blood will stimulate local fibrin formation even in the presence of a considerable amount of heparin dosages (1 to 2 international units heparin/mililiter plasma).[41]

Mural Thrombus and its Contribution to the Progression of Atherosclerosis

Following plaque rupture or vascular damage, it has been postulated that platelets, releasing platelet-derived growth factor (PDGF) and other mitogenic factors, play a role in the myofibrotic response of atherosclerosis.[42] This hypothesis was substantiated by observations in pigs with homozygous von Willebrand's disease that showed reduced tendency to develop thrombosis[22–26,43,44] (Fig. 2–3) and resistance to atherosclerosis.[45–47] In order to confirm that these findings were due to abnormal platelet–vessel wall interaction and platelet aggregation, and not due to a congenital anomaly of the arterial wall, an exchange aortic transplantation study was performed.[46] When aortic segments from von Willebrand pigs were transplanted into normal pigs, a myofibrotic response devel-

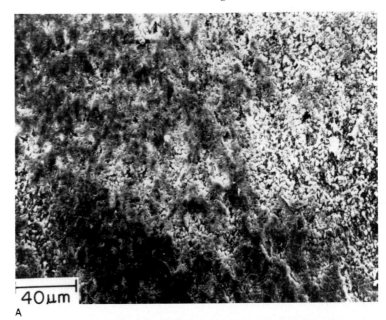

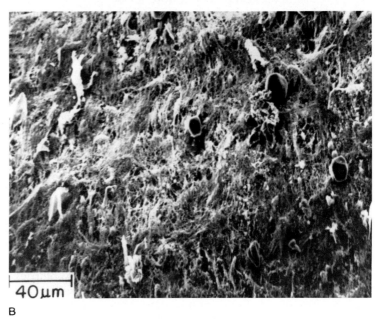

FIGURE 2–3. Scanning electron microscopy of platelet attachment to deendothelialized vessel wall perfused for ten minutes at a local wall shear rate of 1690 second. (*A*) Normal pig blood and (*B*) von Willebrand's disease pig blood. Note the lighter platelet density on the vessel wall when perfused by von Willebrand blood.

oped at the same rate as transplanted controls; however, when aortic segments from normal pigs were transplanted into von Willebrand animals, the fibrotic response was virtually absent. Similar evidence of the importance of platelets in the myofibrotic vascular response following damage and mural thrombosis derives from two earlier studies in which thrombocytopenic rabbits subjected to balloon arterial abrasion exhibited significantly less intimal thickening than control animals with normal platelet counts.[48,49]

More recently, using the pig and the rat carotid balloon injury-thrombosis models, three phases in the process of myofibrosis have been distinguished.[50,51] Phase 1 is characterized by the deposition of platelet thrombi, which occurs within minutes and reaches a stable state within 24 hours. At approximately 24 hours, smooth muscle cell proliferation in the media, as detected by increased deoxyribonucleic acid (DNA) synthesis, begins. Phase 2 is characterized by the onset of smooth muscle cell migration from the media to the intima and is initiated at approximately day 4; smooth muscle cells continue to migrate and then to proliferate up until day 14, at which point the cell population number has reached its maximum. During phase 3 (day 14 to 3 months) intimal thickening progresses, but this progression is due entirely to accumulation of extracellular matrix, which contributes to the fibrotic organization and configuration of the thrombi.

Because the initiation of medial smooth muscle proliferation occurs within hours of platelet deposition at the site of injury, it has been suspected that the primary role of the platelet is the induction of such medial smooth muscle cell replication. However, carotid artery intimal lesion formation following balloon injury was investigated in rats made thrombocytopenic.[52] At two days after injury, messenger ribonucleic acid (mRNA) for ornithine decarboxylase, a marker for early replication events, was found to be elevated to a degree similar to that seen in arteries from control animals; such early medial smooth muscle cell replication has been subsequently considered to result from the direct mechanical trauma, releasing intracellular non–platelet-dependent platelet-derived growth factor or inducing a pathway of autocrine and self-stimulating non–platelet-dependent platelet-derived growth factor.[53] But importantly, contrary to the control animals, in animals kept thrombocytopenic throughout the seven-day observation period, no intimal hyperplasia was observed, leading the investigators to conclude that platelets are important in the formation of vascular lesions in that they stimulate cell migration into the intima. That is, platelets may induce smooth muscle migration by secreting platelet-derived growth factor, which is known to have chemotactic as well as mitogenic activities.[54] Thus, rather than chemotactic and mitogen factors produced in the media, it is reasonable to think that platelet-derived growth factor released at the luminal surface by platelets would better establish the concentration gradient necessary to direct movement of smooth muscle cells from the media to the intima. As in the early medial smooth muscle cell proliferation, smooth muscle cells (after their migration to the intima) may be involved in a non–platelet-dependent autocrine pathway of intimal proliferation. It has been demonstrated that there is a tenfold increase in the production of platelet-derived growth factor-like proteins by smooth muscle cells isolated from arterial intima two weeks following balloon injury, compared to cells derived from non-injured media.[55] In addition, using the sensitive technique of in situ hybridization, Wilcox et al.[56] demonstrated the presence of platelet-derived growth factor messenger ribonucleic acid in mesenchymal-appearing cells localized within thrombus material undergoing fibrotic organization at the surface of human carotid plaques removed by endarterectomy. Furthermore, this capacity to produce endogenous, potentially self-stimulating growth factors, has been recently demonstrated in smooth muscle cells isolated from atheroma.[57]

The above-mentioned non–platelet-dependent early medial and late intimal smooth muscle cell proliferative response and other stages of the myofibrotic reaction can also in part be related to the original thrombus; specifically, to the enzyme thrombin. Thus, experimental evidence suggests that alpha-thrombin, which has a central bioregulatory function in hemostasis and is generated at high concentrations during blood clotting, is able to bind specifically to the subendothelial extracellular matrix where it remains functionally active, localized, and protected from inactivation by its major circulating inhibitor: antithrombin III.[58] Incorporated in the extracellular matrix or into clots,[59] thrombin may be released gradually in active form during spontaneous fibrinolysis, or during the stages of thrombus organization. Surface-bound fibrin in particular may act as a reservoir for enzymatically active thrombin.[59,60] A reservoir of slowly released thrombin, with its known ability to bind to platelet membrane receptors and produce platelet activation, may help explain how, following significant vascular damage, platelets come to be involved in the relatively delayed process of smooth muscle cell migration; and, as adjunctive to the above-mentioned autocrine or self-stimulating process, such thrombin–platelet interaction may also play a role in the subsequent intimal smooth muscle proliferation. In addition, recent studies have shown thrombin to be a potent activator of multiple growth-related signals in smooth muscle cells, including the expression of the c-fos oncogene which may be related to the significant increase in protein synthesis and hypertrophy.[61] Such hypertrophy of the smooth muscle cells may be important in the early stages of medial smooth muscle cell activation, but most importantly, may be one of the triggers for the synthesis and secretion of the late intimal extracellular matrix of thrombus organization. In fact, such formation of fibrous tissue in the arteries contributes significantly to the composition of the growing atherosclerotic plaques.[42,62-64] The elements that make up this fibrous tissue are collagen, proteoglycans, elastin, and glycoproteins.

Disruption of small atherosclerotic plaques, with subsequent mural thrombosis and fibrotic organization of the thrombus, seems to contribute to the progression of atherosclerosis. Although at the present time it is unknown how prevalent this process is, it has potential clinical significance because of its possible inhibition by platelet inhibitor or anticoagulant therapy. In this regard, we have recently completed a five-year trial of platelet inhibitor therapy in the angiographic progression of coronary disease. The preliminary results of this trial are promising.[65] (See also Chapter 3.)

Occlusive Thrombus and Thrombogenic Risk Factors

Numerous pathologic and angiographic[2,3,7,66-70] and several angioscopic[71-74] reports have documented the presence of intraluminal thrombi both in unstable angina and in acute myocardial infarction. In contrast with the very high incidence of thrombi in acute myocardial infarction, the incidence in unstable angina varied significantly among different studies, related in part to the interval between the onset of symptoms and the angiographic study.[75-79] Accordingly, when cardiac catheterization was delayed for weeks, the incidence of thrombi was low; on the other hand, angiography early after the onset of symptoms revealed the presence of thrombi in approximately two thirds of cases. Presumably, the thrombus is occlusive at the time of anginal pain and later may become subocclusive and slowly lysed or digested. Local and systemic "thrombogenic risk factors" at the time of coronary plaque disruption may favor the degree and time length of thrombus deposition and so the different pathological and clinical syndromes (Table 2-1). Some of the local and systemic factors that contribute to the degree of thrombogenicity following plaque rupture are described below.

TABLE 2-1. Thrombogenesis—Evolving Local and Systemic Risk Factors

Local factors
  Degree of damage (collagen, tissue factor)
  Degree of stenosis (change in geometry)
  Surface residual thrombus (thrombin)
Systemic factors
  Epinephrine levels (stress, circadian, smoking)
  Cholesterol levels
  Lipoprotein (a) and plasminogen activator inhibitor levels (impaired fibrinolysis)
  Fibrinogen and factor VII levels

Low risk: mural thrombus, progressive disease.
Medium risk: labile occlusive thrombus, unstable angina, non-Q wave infarction.
High risk: fixed occlusive thrombus, Q wave infarction.

SEVERITY OF VESSEL WALL DAMAGE

To investigate the dynamics of platelet deposition and thrombus formation following vascular damage and to study the influence of various biochemical and physical factors, Badimon et al. have developed and characterized a sensitive and specific computer-assisted nuclear scintigraphic method with an extracorporeal perfusion system to study the process of platelet deposition on various degrees of vascular stenosis and injury in both in vitro and in vivo perfusion conditions[80-83] (Fig. 2-4). Exposure of deendothelialized vessel wall (thus mimicking mild type II vascular injury or damage) to blood at high shear rate (mimicking a stenosed coronary artery) induced platelets' deposition to the exposed vessel[80] (Fig. 2-5). The deposition of platelet reached a maximum within five to ten minutes of exposure, and thrombus formation occurred. However, thrombus that was formed could be dislodged from the substrate by the flowing blood, suggesting that the thrombus was labile. Exposure of fibrillar collagen (thus mimicking a deep type III injury or damage) to blood produced platelet deposition of more than two orders of magnitude greater than on subendothelium[81] (Fig. 2-6). Even at high shear rate, platelet thrombus formed was not dislodged but remained adherent to the surface. Similar experimental quantitative information on the importance of the degree of vascular damage on the degree and stability of thrombus formation has now been documented by varying degrees of stenosis.[82,83] Importantly, besides the fibrillar collagen,[81] exposed thromboplastin or tissue factor[84,85] also contribute to the high thrombogenicity when deep or severe injury occurs.

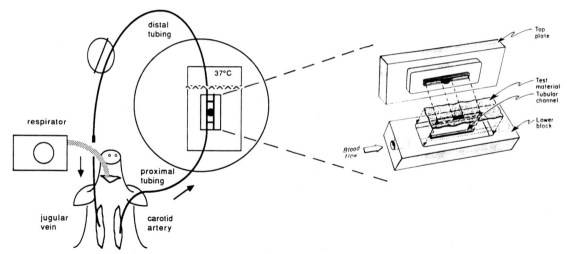

FIGURE 2–4. Diagram of the experimental system used for the dynamic monitoring of platelet–vessel wall interaction under rheologically controlled flow conditions. The substrate, severely damaged vessel wall, is placed in the chamber and exposed to flowing blood (*right*). Deposited platelets are continuously detected by the gamma camera and stored in an imaging computer during the 50-minute perfusion (*left*).

In the clinical context, aside from the previously-mentioned angiographic data showing transient thrombosis,[76–79,86] Hirsh et al.[87] showed a temporal relation between chest pain in unstable angina and increases in transcardiac concentration of thromboxane A_2, lending support to the hypothesis that thromboxane A_2 release was associated with transient or labile platelet aggregation in patients with unstable angina. These early observations were confirmed by other investigators[88,89] who demonstrated an increase in thromboxane metabolites in patients with unstable ischemic coronary syndromes. Furthermore, another product of platelet secretion—serotonin—was increased in some patients with frequent angina and complex coronary artery lesion morphology.[90] Al-though these observations do not prove a causal relation, they suggest that transient platelet activation and secretion occur in unstable coronary syndromes. Overall, it is likely that when injury to the vessel wall is mild, the thrombogenic stimulus is relatively limited, and the resulting thrombotic occlusion is transient, as occurs in unstable angina. On the other hand, deep vessel injury secondary to plaque rupture or ulceration results in exposure of collagen, tissue factor, and other elements of the vessel media, leading to relatively persistent thrombotic occlusion and myocardial infarction.[9]

INFLUENCE OF STENOSIS

Using the same above-mentioned computer-assisted extracorporeal perfusion sys-

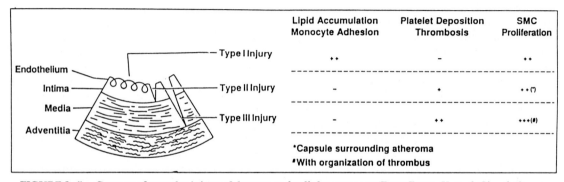

	Lipid Accumulation Monocyte Adhesion	Platelet Deposition Thrombosis	SMC Proliferation
Type I Injury	+ +	–	+ +
Type II Injury	–	+	+ + (*)
Type III Injury	–	+ +	+ + + (#)

*Capsule surrounding atheroma
#With organization of thrombus

FIGURE 2–5. Concept of vascular injury of damage and cellular response (From Fuster V, et al. Circulation 1988; 77: 1213, with permission.)

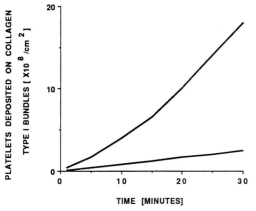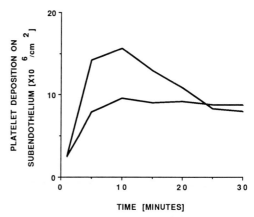

FIGURE 2–6. Platelet deposition on different biological vessel wall components at controlled rheological conditions. *Left,* Platelet deposition on collagen type I fibers at shear rate 1690 second (*upper line*) and 212 second (*lower line*). *Right,* Platelet deposition on deendothelialized vessel wall at shear rate 1690 second (*upper line*) and 212 second (*lower line*). Note that deendothelialized vessel wall is a mild thrombogenic stimulus showing labile platelet deposition at the highest shear rate, the maximum platelet deposition reached at about ten minutes is transient and followed by a plateau of single layer of platelets. However, exposure of collagen fibers, as in deep wall injury, induces fixed platelet deposition and there is a continuous increase in platelet deposition (Note the different ordinate scales used in both panels). (From Badimon L, et al. Z Kardiol 1990; 3: 133, with permission.)

tem in which the rheology of the blood flow can be controlled and varying degrees of stenosis can be produced on severely damaged vessel wall, Badimon et al.[82,83] found that platelet deposition increased significantly with a higher stenosis, indicating a shear-induced cell activation (Fig. 2–7). In addition, analysis of the axial distribution of platelet deposition indicated that the apex, and not the flow recirculation zone distal to the apex, was the segment of greatest platelet accumulation. These data suggest that the severity of the acute platelet response to plaque disruption depends in part on the sudden changes in degree of stenosis following the rupture.

THROMBOGENICITY OF RESIDUAL THROMBUS

Spontaneous lysis of thrombus does occur, not only in unstable angina,[91] but also in acute myocardial infarction.[92,93] In these patients, as well as in those undergoing thrombolysis for acute infarction, the presence of a residual mural thrombus predisposes to recurrent thrombotic vessel occlusion.[94–97] Two main contributing factors for the development of rethrombosis have been identified.

First, a residual mural thrombus may encroach into the vessel lumen resulting in increased shear rate, which facilitates the activation and deposition of platelets on the lesion. As mentioned previously, using an experimental animal model of ex vivo perfusion, it has been shown that platelet deposition is higher with increasing degrees of vessel stenosis[82,83] (Fig. 2–8).

Second, the presence of a fragmented thrombus appears to be one of the most powerful thrombogenic surfaces. This was also evaluated in the ex vivo perfusion model, where platelet deposition was assessed by continuous scintigraphic imaging of indium-111-labeled platelets.[82,83] A gradual increase in platelet deposition in the area of maximal stenosis was observed, followed by an abrupt drop, probably owing to spontaneous thrombus embolization or platelet disaggregation. This was immediately followed by a rapid increase in platelet deposition, suggesting that the remaining thrombus was markedly thrombogenic. In fact, platelet deposition is increased two to four times on residual thrombus compared with deeply injured arterial wall;[82] and thrombus continues to grow during heparin therapy, but is inhibited by other specific antithrombin.[98,99] Supporting the observations of a highly thrombogenic surface and the role played by thrombin, Fitzgerald and Fitzgerald[100] reported that the reocclusion of a recanalized artery in a canine model of coronary thrombolysis was mainly related to the high local thrombin activity on the surface of the fragmented thrombus.

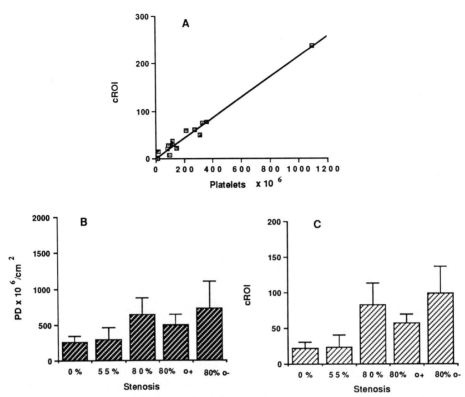

FIGURE 2–7. Effect of increasing degree of stenosis on platelet deposition. (A) Correlation of data obtained by continuous imaging (cROI, counts in the region of interest) versus gamma-well counting (platelet counting); (B) total platelet deposition/square centimeter versus degree of stenosis; and (C) platelet deposition by continuous imaging versus stenosis. Data of 80 per cent stenosis includes data of total occlusion (80 per cent +) and nonocclusive (80 per cent −) perfusions.

Indeed, experimentally, when thrombus breaks, the thrombin bound to fibrin becomes exposed.[101] Thus, following lysis of thrombus, thrombin may become exposed to the circulating blood, leading to platelet and clotting activation, and further thrombosis. In the above-mentioned experimental conditions, the antithrombin activity of heparin is limited for three main reasons.[99–102] First, a residual thrombus contains active thrombin bound to fibrin, which is thus poorly accessible to the large heparin-antithrombin III complexes; second, a platelet-rich arterial thrombus releases large amounts of platelet factor 4, which inhibits heparin; third, fibrin II monomer, formed by the action of thrombin on fibrinogen, also inhibits heparin. Conversely, molecules of hirudin and other specific antithrombins are at least ten times smaller than the heparin-antithrombin III complex, have no natural inhibitors, and therefore, have greater accessibility to thrombin bound to fibrin. Finally, aside from the clot itself being the source for active throm-

bin, recent studies have suggested that platelet or thrombin activity is enhanced by the thrombolytic agents themselves. These observations were based on the presence of increased plasma and urinary metabolites of thromboxane A_2,[103] an increase in fibrinopeptide A[104] which results from the action of thrombin on fibrinogen, and most importantly, an increase in thrombin-antithrombin III complexes. However, these phenomena result from the activation of platelets and thrombin on the surface of the clot undergoing lysis, rather than from a direct effect of the lytic agents on platelets and the coagulation system.

These experimental results clarify the clinical observations in patients with acute myocardial infarction undergoing thrombolysis, which have shown that residual stenosis is in part related to residual nonlysed thrombus.[96,105–107] Such residual stenosis[108–110] or intracoronary thrombi[110,111] were associated with an increased risk of thrombotic reocclusion.

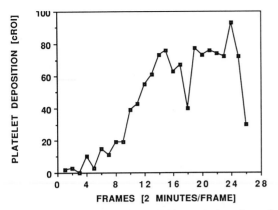

FIGURE 2–8. Continuous scintigraphic imaging of the events occurring during perfusion of severely damaged vessel wall with 80 per cent stenosis. Platelet deposition was measured as corrected count acquired in the region of interest versus perfusion time (50 minutes). Note that at approximately 30 minutes of perfusion there is an abrupt decrease in counts followed by a rapid increase. This suggests that partial rupture of an evolving thrombus is followed by massive rethrombosis on the affected area. (From Badimon L, et al. Circulation 1988; 78: 1431, with permission.)

Systemic Thrombogenic Risk Factors

As discussed above, it is now well recognized that focal thrombosis can lead to a local hypercoagulable or thrombogenic state of the circulation that may favor progression or recurrence of the thrombi. In addition, there is increasing experimental and clinical evidence that a primary hypercoagulable or thrombogenic state of the circulation exists which can favor focal thrombosis. Thus, experimentally, platelet aggregation and the generation of thrombin may be activated by circulating catecholamines;[80,112,113] this interrelationship could be of importance in humans because it may be a link between conditions of emotional stress or circadian variation (early morning hours)[114] with catecholamine effects[115–117] and the development of myocardial infarction. Of importance is the increasing evidence of enhanced platelet reactivity in cigarette smokers,[118–120] which may or may not be related to catecholamine stimulus;[121,122] indeed, in agreement with the thrombogenic role of cigarette smoking, after discontinuation of smoking it has been observed that there is a sharp decrease in acute vascular events most often associated with thrombosis.[123–125]

Of no less importance is the increasing clinical and experimental evidence of hyper-coagulability (fibrinogen, factor VII, poor fibrinolysis) in patients with progressive coronary disease[126] and of enhanced platelet reactivity at the site of vascular damage in experimental hypercholesterolemia,[127] which supports previous clinical observation;[128,129] in addition, enhanced platelet reactivity has also been documented in young patients with strong family history of coronary disease, related or not to hyperlipidemia.[119] Within this context of metabolic abnormalities in young patients with coronary disease, high plasma levels of homocysteine after methionine loading and of lipoprotein(a) are also beginning to be identified as powerful "thrombogenic risk factors." Homocystinuria or homocystinemia in its heterozygous trait is now being identified as an important risk factor for atherosclerotic disease in young individuals with a strong family history of coronary disease.[130–132] This metabolic condition can be considered as an atherogenic rather than thrombogenic risk factor because homocystinemia induces endothelial damage with a subsequent proliferative response in experimental studies.[133] Lipoprotein (a), which is very similar to low-density lipoproteins (LDL) in its configuration,[134] has been shown to be an important risk factor for ischemic heart disease, presumably for thrombotic occlusion (Wilcken DEL, personal communication), and particularly in familial hypercholesterolemia.[135–137] Apoprotein (a) is a glycoprotein that is present in lipoprotein (a) and has close structural homology with plasminogen,[138] both genes being clearly linked on the long arm of chromosome 6.[139] There is suggestive evidence that the close homology of lipoprotein (a) with plasminogen results in competitive inhibition of the fibrinolytic properties of plasminogen,[140–145] thus predisposing to thrombotic complications.

The above discussion on metabolic abnormalities (specifically, the role of lipoprotein (a) in coronary disease) supports the concept of deficient fibrinolysis as a thrombogenic risk factor in coronary disease patients. Since available methods to study fibrinolysis are not sensitive or specific, it has not been proven yet that definite fibrinolysis is an important thrombogenic risk factor in coronary disease patients. One of the closest parameters of fibrinolysis now being measured is plasminogen activator inhibitor-1 (PAI-1) levels; although some studies suggest high levels of plasminogen activator inhibitor-1 as a risk factor for ischemic heart disease[146,147] and myocardial infarction,[148,149] other studies may be less convincing.[126,150] Finally, aside from the possibility that true defective fibrinolysis with high plasminogen activator inhibitor-1 levels is a thrombogenic risk factor, other hemostatic parameters, specifically fibrinogen and factor VII levels, have also been implicated. (See Chapter 4).

ARTERIAL THROMBOSIS: THE CLINICAL MANIFESTATIONS OF ATHEROSCLEROTIC VASCULAR DISEASE

Atherosclerotic disease in the coronary artery system may manifest in the form of stable or unstable angina, acute myocardial infarction, or sudden cardiac death. Atherosclerotic disease in the cerebral arterial system (including the intracranial and extracranial arteries) can manifest in the form of transient ischemic attack (TIA) and cerebral ischemic infarction. In contrast to that of acute coronary syndromes, the pathophysiologic process leading to acute cerebral ischemia is less well defined, but appears to involve multiple etiologic mechanisms. Atherosclerotic disease of the abdominal or leg arteries can result in acute and chronic ischemia of the extremities and usually involves thrombosis or embolism or both originating from atherosclerotic plaques. This section will discuss thrombosis in the acute coronary syndromes, thrombosis in cerebrovascular disease, thrombosis in peripheral arterial disease, and, thrombosis in the cardiac chambers.

Thrombosis in the Acute Coronary Syndromes

Fissuring or rupture of an atherosclerotic plaque in the coronary arteries plays a fundamental role in the development of the acute coronary syndromes, as has been clearly shown in patients who died suddenly or shortly after an episode of unstable angina or myocardial infarction. Disrupted atherosclerotic plaques are commonly associated with the formation of mural or occlusive thrombi, usually anchored to fissures in the ruptured or ulcerated plaque. Angiographic studies have documented the presence of intraluminal thrombi both in unstable angina and acute myocardial infarction. The incidence of thrombi in unstable angina varied

TABLE 2–2. Proposed Hypothesis of Pathogenesis of the Acute and Subacute Coronary Syndromes

SYNDROME	PLAQUE DAMAGE	THROMBUS Fixed	THROMBUS Labile
Unstable angina	+	+ *	+ + +
Non-Q wave myocardial infarction	+ +	+ + *	+ +
Q wave myocardial infarction	+ + +	+ + + †	+

* Vasoconstriction (may contribute to coronary occlusion).
† Collaterals (may decrease extension of infarction).
+ = mild; + + = moderate; + + + = severe.

significantly among different studies, in part related to the interval between anginal symptoms and arteriographic study. The shorter this interval, the higher the likelihood of finding occlusive thrombi.

Severity of vessel wall damage is probably the most important of all the previously mentioned "thrombogenic risk factors" in the acute coronary syndromes. It is likely that when injury to the vessel wall is mild, the thrombogenic stimulus is relatively limited and the resulting thrombotic occlusion transient, as occurs in unstable angina. On the other hand, deep vessel injury secondary to plaque rupture and ulceration results in exposure of collagen, lipids, and other elements of the vessel media, leading to relatively persistent thrombotic occlusion and myocardial infarction (Table 2–2).

Although a substantial proportion of episodes of unstable angina and acute myocardial infarction are caused by plaque fissuring or rupture with superimposed thrombosis, other mechanisms that alter the balance between myocardial oxygen supply and demand need to be considered.[151] Hemodynamic, electrocardiographic, and angiographic monitoring suggested that coronary vasospasm plays an important role in the pathogenesis of ischemic heart diseases. Vasospasm appears to be an important contributor to intermittent coronary occlusion in patients with acute myocardial infarction treated with intracoronary streptokinase, which responds, in some cases, to administration of nitrates.

In patients with stable coronary disease, angina commonly results from increases in myocardial oxygen demand beyond the ability of stenosed coronary arteries to increase its delivery. In contrast, unstable angina, non-

Q wave myocardial infarction, and Q wave myocardial infarction represent a continuum of the disease process, and are usually characterized by an abrupt reduction in coronary flow. In unstable angina, disruption of an atherosclerotic plaque may lead to acute changes in plaque morphology and reduction in coronary flow. Transient episodes of thrombotic vessel occlusion at the site of plaque injury may occur, leading to angina at rest. This thrombus is usually labile, resulting in only temporary vessel occlusion. In addition to plaque disruption, other mechanisms contribute to reduced coronary flow. Platelets attach to the damaged endothelium or to exposed media and release vasoactive substances including thromboxane A_2 and serotonin, leading to aggregation of neighboring platelets and vasoconstriction. Alterations in perfusion and myocardial oxygen supply probably account for two thirds of episodes of unstable angina; the rest may be caused by transient increases in myocardial oxygen demand.

In non-Q wave infarction, the angiographic morphology of the responsible lesion is similar to that seen in unstable angina, suggesting that plaque disruption is common to both syndromes. About one fourth of patients with non-Q wave infarction have a completely occluded infarct-related vessel at early angiography, with the distal territory usually supplied by collaterals. The presence of ST segment elevation in the electrocardiogram, early peak in plasma creatine kinase, and high angiographic patency rate of the involved vessel, suggest that complete coronary occlusion followed by early reperfusion (within the first two hours) or resolution of vasospasm, are pathogenetically important in non-Q wave infarction.

In Q wave infarction, plaque rupture is commonly associated with deep arterial injury or ulceration, resulting in the formation of a fixed and persistent thrombus, leading to abrupt cessation of myocardial perfusion and necrosis. The coronary lesion responsible for the infarction is frequently only mild to moderately stenotic, which suggests that plaque rupture with superimposed thrombosis is the primary determinant of acute occlusion rather than of the severity of the underlying lesion.[105,152,153] While severe preexisting lesions often lead to complete vessel occlusion, myocardial infarction does not commonly supervene, perhaps owing to adequate collateral flow. In perhaps one fourth of patients, coronary thrombosis results from superficial intimal injury or blood stasis in areas of high-grade stenosis.

In sudden cardiac death, two mechanisms predominate.[10] First, fatal ventricular arrhythmias are common in patients after extensive myocardial infarction or other forms of cardiomyopathy, in whom a substrate for the generation and maintenance of ventricular tachycardia or fibrillation exists. Second, sudden death related to ischemia probably involves a rapidly progressive coronary lesion in which plaque rupture and resultant thrombosis lead to myocardial hypoperfusion and fatal ventricular arrhythmias. Absence of collateral flow to the myocardium distal to the occlusion or platelet microthrombi may contribute to the development of sudden ischemic death.

Thrombosis in Cerebrovascular Disease

Clinical manifestations of atherosclerotic disease in the cerebral circulation (intracranial and extracranial) results in a spectrum of acute cerebral ischemic syndromes ranging from transient ischemic attacks to full-blown cerebral infarction. Similar to the pathogenesis of acute coronary syndromes, thrombosis over a disrupted plaque plays a key pathogenic role in the majority of patients suffering from these vascular events. However, in contrast to acute coronary syndromes, other pathogenic mechanisms such as intracranial hemorrhage, subarachnoid hemorrhage, and cardiogenic embolism also play a role in a substantial proportion of these patients. The relative importance of these pathogenic mechanisms remains undefined because of the lack of well-designed prospective pathologic studies. In this section, we will discuss the pathogenic roles of thrombosis and disrupted plaques in two major syndromes: (a) transient ischemic attacks (TIAs), and (b) acute cerebral infarction. Cardiogenic embolism and its role in transient ischemic attacks and acute stroke will also be discussed. Pathogenic mechanisms such as intracerebral hemorrhage and subarachnoid hemorrhage, although important, are beyond the scope of this chapter. (See also Chapter 22.)

TRANSIENT ISCHEMIC ATTACKS

Transient ischemic attacks are brief episodes of focal loss of brain function, thought to be due to ischemia, that can usually be localized to that portion of brain supplied by one vascular system, and to which no other cause can be found. Though arbitrary, by convention, episodes lasting less than 24 hours are classified as transient ischemic attacks although the longer the episode, the greater the likelihood of finding a cerebral infarct by computer tomography. Transient ischemic attacks commonly last 2 to 15 minutes and are rapid in onset. Each transient ischemic attack leaves no persistent deficit, and there are often multiple attacks. Most patients have transient ischemic attacks that include motor symptoms. It is common for amaurosis fugax (monocular blindness) to occur without other symptoms during the episode. In general, transient ischemic attacks evolve from two causes: focal low blood flow and embolism. The mechanism of focal low flow in transient ischemic attacks is not well defined. Probably, a critical stenotic or occluded artery reduces flow to a focal area of normal brain. Certainly, poor collateral circulation to the ischemic area plays a prominent role, but factors such as viscosity, vessel wall compliance, and other unknown factors are needed to explain why the reduction is transient.

Pathologic studies of carotid endarterectomy specimens of atherosclerotic plaques in patients with transient ischemic attacks demonstrated that the carotid residual lumen was less than 1 millimeter in 98 per cent of patients studied. Imparato et al.[154] also demonstrated severe carotid artery stenosis in over 75 per cent of patients with repetitive transient ischemic attacks. More recently, O'Holleran et al.[155] reported a long-term follow-up of asymptomatic, untreated individuals who had ultrasonic carotid studies. Over a five-year period the cumulative stroke and transient ischemic attack rate was 65 per cent in patients with greater than 75 per cent stenosis, and only 12.5 per cent in those with less than 75 per cent stenosis. Also using ultrasonographic data, Sterpetti et al.[156] found that hemispheric symptoms were almost four times as frequent in patients with greater than 50 per cent stenosis, while only one sixth of all asymptomatic patients had more than 50 per cent stenosis. In addition, as the degree of stenosis increased beyond 70 per cent, the incidence of new symptoms also showed a sharp increase. Similarly, Weinberger et al.[157] reported that development of ischemic symptoms in patients whose plaques

progressed was more frequent (25 per cent) than in those whose plaques regressed or had not changed (8 per cent). In addition, plaques that became obstructive and disrupted flow were associated with a higher frequency of symptoms (40 per cent) than those that did not (13 per cent). In most pathological series, the occurrence of transient ischemic attacks correlates best with the severity of carotid luminal stenosis (lumen of 1 millimeter or less or greater than 75 per cent narrowing).

The presence of fibrin or fibrin–platelet mural thrombus was found overlying an atherosclerotic plaque in 77 per cent of cases with hemispheric transient ischemic attacks. In contrast, evidence of ulceration on the plaques, which were widely regarded as sources of emboli, was found in only 24 per cent of the cases with transient neurological deficit as compared to an identical 27 per cent of the asymptomatic cases. That the incidence of ulceration was about the same in transient ischemic attack and asymptomatic groups appeared to preclude an important role for ulceration as the etiology of repetitive transient ischemic attacks. Intraplaque hemorrhage was present in about 39 per cent of cases of transient ischemic attacks. This hemorrhage, however, was usually small, and in less than 3 per cent of cases were the hemorrhages of large enough size to constitute one quarter of the volume of the plaque. Future investigation into the pathogenesis of carotid intraplaque hemorrhage might indicate that this is the result of small plaque fissuring and dissection, as recently demonstrated in acute coronary syndromes.

Overall, the evidence from these pathologic studies indicate that probably in a substantial proportion of these patients, transient ischemic attacks result from progressive luminal narrowing leading to precarious hemodynamic insufficiency. One can also infer that mural thrombi at the subocclusive stage can either contribute to the obstruction or give rise to emboli. Large plaque ulceration or intraplaque hemorrhage did not correlate well with clinical ischemic events, but probably play a role in plaque growth.

It has been assumed that fragments of mural thrombi of extracranial atheromatous plaque break and cause transient ischemic attacks. However, the proportion of patients with transient ischemic attacks of embolic origin is not clearly defined. As discussed previously, pathologic studies in patients with transient ischemic attack indicated that about

30 per cent of endarterectomy specimens obtained demonstrated no overlying thrombi. Furthermore, probably in a substantial proportion of patients with transient ischemic attacks, cardiogenic emboli (emboli from cardiac chambers) appears to be the pathogenic mechanism. Clinical data indicated that at least 25 per cent of all cerebral ischemic events and more than a third of cerebral ischemic events in the elderly are associated with atrial fibrillation.[158] In addition, about one in three patients with atrial fibrillation will experience a cerebral ischemic event during lifetime. A recent arteriographic study[159] of 12 consecutive patients with atrial fibrillation and acute cerebral ischemia suggested a cardioembolic etiology in as many as 75 per cent of the patients. In addition, two autopsy studies[160,161] reported that 50 to 70 per cent of patients with atrial fibrillation were associated with cerebral ischemic events. These confounding data have complicated our understanding of the pathogenic mechanisms involved in transient ischemic events. Further prospective clinical studies are needed in order to assess the relative importance of various pathogenic processes in different risk groups and to formulate therapeutic strategies.

ACUTE CEREBRAL INFARCTION

The clinical hallmark of an acute cerebrovascular accident (CVA), or stroke, is the abrupt development of a focal neurologic deficit explainable by ischemia or bleeding in a particular territory. Intracerebral or subarachnoid hemorrhage accounts for 15 per cent of strokes and is suspected by the history and physical examination and confirmed by computed tomographic scan or lumbar puncture or both. The vast majority of strokes (up to 85 per cent) are ischemic, arising from atherosclerotic large and small cerebral arterial disease. Clinical studies[162] suggested that about 15 per cent (range 6 to 23 per cent) of all ischemic strokes were cardioembolic in origin. A large multicenter stroke databank project[163] recently reported a 19 per cent prevalence of cardioembolic stroke, based on carefully defined clinical criteria. The prevalence of presumed cardioembolic stroke varied between 13 and 34 per cent at the four centers participating in this study, suggesting either patient population differences or intercenter variability in application of diagnostic criteria. In addition to the lack of validated, reliable clinical diagnostic criteria for differentiating cardioembolic and nonembolic ischemic stroke, a significant proportion of the patients have risks for both mechanisms of stroke. Thus, according to recent reports,[159,164,165] about 30 per cent of patients with acute ischemic stroke will have a potential cardiac source of embolism, but about one third of these patients will also have concomitant cerebrovascular atherosclerosis that could also be responsible for brain ischemia.

Thrombosis in Peripheral Arterial Disease

The incidence of intermittent claudication tends to vary with age, sex, and perhaps, geographical influences. For men aged 50 to 59, claudication rates range from 0.8 per cent to 3.1 per cent in the general population.[166] The reported incidence appears to be higher in 50 to 60-year-old Scandinavian men, with rates as high as 5.8 per cent.[167] In the Framingham study, the overall incidence of intermittent claudication was 0.8 per cent in men and 0.4 per cent in women aged 50 to 74.[168] Other studies confirm a 3- to 13-fold higher incidence of intermittent claudication in men,[167] and a fourfold greater incidence in diabetics.[169] Because peripheral arterial disease is frequently asymptomatic for long periods, the frequency of intermittent claudication is likely to underestimate the incidence of significant peripheral arterial disease. One study using noninvasive testing of peripheral arterial flow and pressure found an 11.7 per cent prevalence of large vessel peripheral arterial disease with only about 2 per cent of patients reporting claudication.[166]

Not surprisingly, peripheral artery and coronary artery disease often occur together. In the Framingham study, the presence of intermittent claudication increased the risk of new occurence of coronary symptoms by 2.3- and 5.4-fold in men and women, respectively.[168] The actual incidence of underlying symptomatic or latent coronary disease is very high in patients with symptomatic peripheral arterial disease. In an angiographic study of 381 patients with lower extremity ischemia, 90 per cent of patients had coronary disease, which was advanced in 57 per cent.[170] Because it is a marker for extensive coronary atherosclerosis, intermittent claudication is associated with a poor long-term prognosis. Age-adjusted mortality, mostly cardiovascular, is twofold higher for men and women with intermittent claudication in the Framingham and other studies.[168,171] When sensitive noninvasive tests are used to detect latent peripheral arterial disease (PAD), those with evidence of significant impairment have a four- to fivefold increase in mortality,[172] comparable to that seen with evidence of myocardial ischemia on exercise testing. In a study by Lassila et al.[173] of 312 patients with peripheral arterial disease followed for ten years, 69 per cent of patients had died during follow-up, nearly 70 per cent of cardiovascular causes. Survival was significantly worse in patients with advanced ischemia in the limb. Of patients undergoing aortic aneurysm repair or lower extremity revascularization, 50 to 70 per cent of operative deaths are due to myocardial infarction. Conversely, of patients with known coronary artery disease, the incidence of peripheral arterial disease is much lower: intermittent claudication occurred at about 25 per cent the incidence of coronary artery disease in the Framingham study,[168] and peripheral arterial disease was diagnosed noninvasively in only 12 and 17 per cent of male and female survivors of myocardial infarction, respectively.

The risk factor most closely associated with the development of peripheral arterial disease is cigarette smoking.[174] In autopsy studies, cigarette smoking is consistently linked with aortic atherosclerosis. Cigarette smokers demonstrate more extensive intimal involvement and a much higher incidence of fibrous, calcified, and ulcerated plaques in the aorta.[175] In the iliofemoral circulation, cigarette smoking was associated with severe diffuse fibrocalcific atherosclerosis, and significant stenotic lesions were essentially absent in nonsmokers. Diabetes mellitus is also commonly associated with iliofemoral disease, but also shows a strong correlation with distal arterial disease in the leg.[169] This site of involvement appears to be related more to the duration and severity of diabetes and presence of microvascular disease than to the other well-recognized risk factors for atherosclerosis. Of patients presenting with symptomatic peripheral arterial disease for therapeutic intervention, 90 to 100 per cent are current smokers.[175]

The most characteristic symptom of peripheral arterial disease is intermittent claudication, which occurs when the oxygen demand of exercising skeletal muscle exceeds the flow reserve of the diseased limb arteries.

This usually occurs first in the gastrocnemius muscle, because of its high oxygen requirement during ambulation. Characteristically, intermittent claudication occurs reproducibly with exercise at a given workload and is relieved by rest. Thus, intermittent claudication represents the skeletal muscle counterpart to stable angina pectoris. Peripheral arterial disease tends to be slowly progressive and may remain asymptomatic for long periods, particularly when collateral circulation is well developed.

An abrupt onset of ischemic rest pain or sudden worsening of intermittent claudication may be due to thromboembolism, or thrombosis in situ complicating an atherosclerotic lesion. Embolism in a previously healthy artery is more likely when symptoms occur suddenly in a patient without prior claudication, and with risk factors for thromboembolism (such as atrial fibrillation, left ventricular failure, prosthetic heart valves, or aortic aneurysm). When this occurs, advanced ischemia is common, owing to inadequate time for development of collateral circulation. A syndrome of microembolization may also occur, commonly with atherothrombotic materials released from a proximal arterial lesion (such as an aortic aneurysm). The clinical presentation associated with microembolization is that of digital pain, cyanosis, or gangrene, with preserved pulses and skin temperature in the extremity. This may also occur as a complication of arterial catheterization. Sudden worsening of intermittent claudication, or progression of intermittent claudication to rest pain or gangrene, is often seen with thrombotic or embolic occlusion of a preexisting stenotic lesion. When in situ thrombosis complicates an existing lesion, the presumed mechanism in many cases is plaque rupture or fissuring as previously described, but is also probably due to stasis of blood flow with a severely stenotic lesion in some cases. The clinical outcome in such cases is most dependent on the adequacy of the collateral circulation.

In comparison to the limited overall cardiovascular prognosis of patients with peripheral arterial disease, the risk of progression of local symptomatology is not as great. Nevertheless, most studies reveal a rate of progression to advanced ischemia requiring amputation in 1 to 3 per cent of patients per year,[171,176] with higher rates among diabetics. Higher rates of progression are also seen in selected nondiabetic populations, particularly those with symptoms severe enough to come to the attention of the vascular surgeon. In a series from the Cleveland Clinic, patients with a total of 1,850 ischemic limbs were followed for an average of four years.[177] Up to 30 per cent of patients with femoropopliteal disease experienced sudden worsening of intermittent claudication or new onset of rest pain or gangrene. In most studies, progression correlated inversely with segmental limb blood pressure:[171] the major risk factors for progression are continued tobacco use and diabetes. Cessation of tobacco use may result in improvement in symptoms in 85 per cent of individuals, presumably because of withdrawal of the vasoactive effects of nicotine. In fact, a number of studies showed no further progression to rest pain or amputation in patients who stop smoking, compared to an 11 to 16 per cent risk of these outcomes in five to seven-year follow-up in patients who continue to smoke.[178] Continued smoking after arterial reconstruction is highly correlated with progressive ischemia and risk of subsequent amputation.[179] In one study, heavy smokers had a tenfold higher rate of amputation after attempted revascularization compared to moderate or light smokers. (See also Chapter 23.)

Thrombosis in the Cardiac Chambers

In this section, we will distinguish: (a) Thrombosis of left ventricular and left atrial chambers, and (b) prosthetic heart valves and thromboembolism.

THROMBOSIS OF LEFT VENTRICULAR AND LEFT ATRIAL CHAMBERS

Intracavitary mural thrombi develop frequently in patients with acute myocardial infarction, chronic left ventricular infarction, chronic left ventricular aneurysm, dilated cardiomyopathy, and atrial fibrillation. The clinical significance of thrombosis in the cardiac chambers derives from its potential for systemic embolism, which also depends on dynamic forces of the circulation (as described before).

In the first few days after acute myocardial infarction, leukocyte infiltration separates endothelial cells from their basal lamina.[180] The resulting exposure of subendothelial tissue to blood serves as the nidus for thrombus development. Specific endocardial abnor-malities have also been identified histologically in surgical and postmortem specimens from patients with left ventricular aneurysms[181] and at necropsy in patients with idiopathic dilated cardiomyopathy.[182]

Both experimental and clinical[183-185] studies have emphasized the importance of wall-motion abnormalities in the development of left ventricular thrombi, and it seems clear that stasis of blood in regions of akinesis or dyskinesis is the essential factor. Similarly, stasis is important in the development of atrial thrombi[186] when effective mechanical atrial activity is impaired, as occurs in atrial fibrillation, atrial enlargement, mitral stenosis, and cardiac failure. Stasis is paramount to conditions of low shear rate in which activation of coagulation factors rather than of platelet leads to fibrin formation and constitutes the predominant pathogenic mechanism in the development of intracavitary thrombi.

One study of patients with acute myocardial infarction found a significantly greater incidence of thromboembolism in cases of increased serum fibrinogen levels,[187] suggesting a hypercoagulable tendency in this condition. Although a hypercoagulable state is controversial, it is conceivable that a systemic procoagulant tendency arises during the acute stage of myocardial infarction and predisposes to thromboembolic events. More relevant is experimental evidence that the surface of a fresh thrombus is itself highly thrombogenic, producing at least a local, if not a systemic, hypercoagulable state.[188]

The problems of thromboembolism originating from the cardiac chambers prompt consideration of the balance between the effects of regional injury, stasis, and procoagulant factors, which favor thrombus formation; and dynamic forces of the circulation, which are responsible for the migration of thrombotic material into the systemic circulation. Even though stasis favors thrombus formation within the sac of a left ventricular aneurysm, isolation from dynamic circulatory forces protects against embolic migration.[188,189] In diffusely dilated cardiomyopathy, on the other hand, mural thrombus is not isolated from the circulation, and the embolic risk is higher.

PROSTHETIC HEART VALVES AND THROMBOEMBOLISM

Mechanical Prosthesis. The pathologic events leading to thromboembolism develop already during surgery. The damaged peri-valvular tissue and prosthetic materials acti-vate platelets as soon as blood starts flowing across the valve, and immediate platelet dep-osition results.[190,191] A Dacron sewing ring is common to all prosthetic valves, both me-chanical and bioprosthetic. Platelet deposi-tion on this ring can be demonstrated by use of indium-III-labeled platelets within the first 24 hours after operation when either a mechanical or a bioprosthetic valve is placed.[190,191] More importantly, prosthetic materials can activate the intrinsic clotting system,[192] with subsequent fibrin formation. In addition, the abnormal hemodynamic characteristics of mechanical prosthetic de-vices promote mainly fibrin generation and, less importantly, platelet activation. Finally, the process of fibrin thrombus formation can be facilitated in areas with stasis and de-creased blood flow, such as in the left atrium during atrial fibrillation and in the left ven-tricle during low cardiac output state second-ary to left ventricular dysfunction.

Biologic Prosthesis. Bioprosthetic valves are considerably less thrombogenic,[193] mainly because of the biologic properties of materials used in their construction and also because of characteristic axial flow profile and leaflet pliability.[194]

VENOUS THROMBOSIS

While arterial thrombi are predominantly formed by platelets, venous thrombi are in-travascular deposits composed predomi-nantly of fibrin and red cells, with a variable platelet and leukocyte component.[195,196] These thrombi usually form in regions of slow or disturbed flow and begin as small deposits that frequently arise in large venous sinuses in the calf, in valve cusp pockets either in the deep veins of the calf or thigh,[197,198] or in venous segments that have been exposed to direct trauma.[199] The major predisposing factors to venous thrombosis are activation of blood coagulation and venous stasis,[200] while vascular wall damage is less important than in arterial thrombosis. Nevertheless, wall damage may predispose to venous thrombosis in special circumstances. Venous thrombosis and its pathogenesis and clinical complica-tions are presented in chapters 24 and 25.

REFERENCES

1. Herrick JB. Clinical features of sudden obstruction of the coronary arteries. JAMA 1912; 59: 2015–20.
2. DeWood MA, Spores J, Notske R, et al. Prevalence of total coronary occlusion during the early hours of transmural myocardial infarction. N Engl J Med 1980; 303: 897–902.
3. DeWood MA, Stifter WF, Simpson CA, et al. Coronary arteriographic findings soon after non-Q wave myocardial infarction. N Engl J Med 1986; 315: 417–23.
4. Falk E. Plaque rupture with severe pre-existing stenosis precipitating coronary thrombosis. Characteristics of cor-onary atherosclerotic plaques underlying fatal occlusive thrombi. Br Heart J 1983; 50: 127–34.
5. Falk E. Morphologic features of unstable atherothrombotic plaques underlying acute coronary syndromes. Am J Car-diol 1989; 63: 1114E–20E.
6. Falk E. Unstable angina with fatal outcome, dynamic cor-onary thrombosis leading to infarction and/or sudden death: autopsy evidence of recurrent mural thrombosis with pe-ripheral embolization culminating in total vascular occlu-sion. Circulation 1985; 71: 699–708.
7. Richardson PD, Davies MJ, Born GVR. Influence of plaque configuration and stress distribution on fissuring of coro-nary atherosclerotic plaques. Lancet 1989; 2: 941–4.
8. Davies MJ, Bland MJ, Hartgartner WR, et al. Factors in-fluencing the presence or absence of acute coronary thrombi in sudden ischemic death. Eur Heart J 1989; 10: 203–8.
9. Davies MJ. A macro and micro view of coronary vascular insult in ischemic heart disease. Circulation 1990; 82(suppl II): 38–46.
10. Davies MJ, Thomas AC. Plaque fissuring—The cause of acute myocardial infarction, sudden ischemic death and crescendo angina. Br Heart J 1985; 53: 363–373.
11. Colman RW, Walsh PN. Mechanisms of platelet aggrega-tion. In: Colman RW, Hirsh J, Marder VJ, Salzman EW, eds. Haemostasis and thrombosis. Philadelphia: JB Lippin-cott Co., 1987:594–605.
12. Huang EM, Detwiler TC. Stimulus-response coupling mechanisms. In: Philips DR, Shuman MC, eds. Biochem-istry of platelets. New York: Academic Press, Inc., 1986:1–68.
13. Hawiger J. Formation and regulation of platelet and fibrin hemostatic plug. Hum Pathol 1987; 18: 111–22.
14. Kunicki TJ. Organization of glycoproteins within the plate-let plasma membrane. In: George JN, Nurden AT, Philips DR, eds. Platelet membrane glycoproteins. New York: Plenum Press, 1985:87–101.
15. Sakariassen KS, Nievelstein PF, Coller BS, Sixma JJ. The role of platelet membrane glycoproteins Ib and IIb/IIIa in platelet adherence to human artery subendothelium. Br J Haematol 1986; 63: 681–91.
16. Weiss HJ, Turitto VT, Baumgartner HR. Effect of shear rate on platelet interaction with subendothelium in citrated and native blood. I. Shear rate-dependent decrease of adhe-sion in von Willebrand's disease and the Bernard-Soulier syndrome. J Lab Clin Med 1978; 92: 750–4.
17. Sixma JJ. In: Bloom AL, Thomas DP, eds. Hemostasis and thrombosis. New York: Churchill Livingstone, 1987:283–302.
18. Turitto VT, Baumgartner HR: In: Colman R, Hirsh J, Mar-der V, Salzman E, eds. Hemostasis and thrombosis, basic principles and clinical practice. 2nd ed. New York: JB Lip-pincott Co., 1987:555–71.
19. Ruggeri ZM, Bader R, de Marco L. Glanzmann thrombas-thenia; deficient binding of von Willebrand Factor to throm-bin-stimulated platelets. Proc Natl Acad Sci USA 1982; 79: 6038–41.
20. Ruggeri ZM, de Marco L, Gatto L, et al. Platelets have more than one binding site for von Willebrand Factor. J Clin In-vest 1983; 72: 1–12.
21. Sakariassen K, Bolhuis PA, Sixma J. Human blood platelet adhesion to artery subendothelium is mediated by Factor VIII-von Willebrand factor bound to the subendothelium. Nature 1979; 636–638.
22. Badimon L, Badimon JJ, Turitto VT, Fuster V. Platelet

deposition in von Willebrand Factor deficient vessel wall. J Lab Clin Med 1987; 110: 634–47.

23. Badimon L, Badimon JJ, Turitto VT, Vallabhajosula S, Fuster V. Platelet thrombus formation on collagen type I. Influence of blood rheology, von Willebrand Factor and blood coagulation. Circulation 1988; 78: 1431–42.

24. Badimon L, Badimon JJ, Chesebro JH, Fuster V. Inhibition of thrombus formation: blockage of adhesive glycoprotein mechanisms versus blockage of the cyclooxygenase pathway. J Am Coll Cardiol 1988; 11: 30A.

25. Badimon L, Badimon JJ, Turitto VT, Fuster V. Platelet interaction to vessel wall and collagen. Study in homozygous von Willebrand's disease associated with abnormal collagen aggregation in swine. Thromb Haemost 1989; 61: 57–64.

26. Badimon L, Badimon JJ, Turitto VT, Fuster V. Role of von Willebrand factor in mediating platelet-vessel wall interaction at low shear rate; the importance of perfusion conditions. Blood 1989; 73: 961–7.

27. Cattaneo M, Kinlough-Rathbone R, Lecchi A, Bevilacqua C, Packham MA, Mustard JF. Fibrinogen-independent aggregation and deaggregation of human platelets: studies in two afibrinogenemic patients. Blood 1987; 70: 221–16.

28. Soria J, Soria C, Borg JY, et al. Platelet aggregation occurs in congenital afibrinogenaemia despite the absence of fibrinogen or its fragments in plasma and platelets, as demonstrated by immunoenzymology. Br J Haematol 1985; 60: 503–10.

29. Turitto VT, Weiss JH, Baumgartner HR. Platelet interaction with rabbit subendothelium in von Willebrand's disease: altered thrombus formation distinct from defective platelet adhesion. J Clin Invest 1984; 74: 1730–41.

30. Weiss HJ, Turitto VT, Vicic WJ, Baumgartner HR. Fibrin formation, fibrinopeptide A release, and platelet thrombus dimensions on subendothelium exposed to flowing native blood: greater in Factor XII and XI than in Factor VIII and IX deficiency. Blood 1984; 63: 1004–14.

31. Weiss HJ, Hawiger J, Ruggeri ZM, Turitto VT, Thiagarajan I, Hoffman T. Fibrinogen-independent interaction of platelets with subendothelium mediated by glycoprotein IIb-IIIa complex at high shear rate. J Clin Invest 1989; 83: 288–97.

32. Badimon L, Badimon JJ, Cohen M, Chesebro J, Fuster V. Thrombosis in stenotic and laminar flow conditions: effect of an antiplatelet GPIIb/IIIa monoclonal antibody fragment [7E3F(ab′)₂] (abstr). Circulation 1989; 80(suppl): II–422.

33. Lombardo VT, Hodson E, Roberts JR, Kunicki TJ, Zimmerman TS, Ruggeri ZM. Independent modulation of von Willebrand factor and fibrinogen binding to the platelet membrane glycoprotein IIb/IIIa complex as demonstrated by monoclonal antibody. J Clin Invest 1985; 76: 1950–8.

34. Badimon L, Badimon J, Ruggeri Z, Fuster V. A peptide-specific monoclonal antibody that inhibits von Willebrand factor binding to GPIIb/IIa [152B6] inhibits platelet deposition to human atherosclerotic vessel wall (abstr). Circulation 1990; 82(4): III–370.

35. Rentrop KP, Feit F, Blanke H, et al. Effects of intracoronary streptokinase and intracoronary nitroglycerin infusion on coronary angiographic patterns and mortality in patients with acute myocardial infarction. N Engl J Med 1984; 311: 1457–63.

36. Basmadjian D, Sefton MV. A model of thrombin inactivation in heparinized and non-heparinized tubes with consequences for thrombus formation. J Biomed Mater Res 1986; 20: 633–51.

37. Goldsmith HL, Turitto VT. Rheological aspects of thrombosis and haemostasis: basic principles and applications. Thromb Haemost 1986; 55: 415–36.

38. Charm SE, Wong BL. Enzyme inactivation with shearing. Biotechnol Bioeng 1970; 12: 1103–9.

39. Charm SE, Lai CJ. Comparison of ultrafiltration systems for concentration of biologicals. Biotechnol Bioeng 1971; 12: 185–202.

40. Weiss HJ, Turitto VT, Baumgartner HR, Nemerson Y, Hoffmann T. Evidence for the presence of tissue-factor activity on subendothelium. Blood 1989; 73: 968–75.

41. Badimon L, Badimon JJ, Lassila R, Heras M, Chesebro JH, Fuster V. Thrombin regulation of platelet interaction with damaged vessel wall and isolated collagen type I at arterial flow conditions in a porcine model. Effects of hirudins, heparin and calcium chelation. Blood 1991. In press.

42. Ross R. The pathogenesis of atherosclerosis: an update. N Engl J Med 1986; 314: 488–500.

43. Nichols TC, Bellinger DA, Tate DA, et al. von Willebrand factor and occlusive arterial thrombosis. Arteriosclerosis 1990; 10: 449–61.

44. Fuster V, Griggs TR. Porcine von Willebrand disease: implications for the pathophysiology of atherosclerosis and thrombosis. Prog Hemost Thromb 1986; 56: 159–83.

45. Fuster V, Bowie JW, Lewis JC, Fass DN, Owen CA, Brown AL. Resistance to atherosclerosis in pigs with von Willebrand's disease. Spontaneous and high cholesterol diet-induced arteriosclerosis. J Clin Invest 1978; 61: 722–30.

46. Fuster V, Fass DN, Kaye MP, Josa M, Zinmeister AR, Bowie EJW. Arteriosclerosis in normal and von Willebrand pigs. Long-term prospective study and aortic transplantation. Circ Res 1982; 51: 587–93.

47. Badimon L, Steele P, Badimon JJ, Bowie EJW, Fuster V. Aortic atherosclerosis in pigs with heterozygous von Willebrand disease. Comparison with homozygous von Willebrand and normal pigs. Arteriosclerosis 1985; 5: 366–70.

48. Cohen P, McComb HC. Platelets and atherogenesis. II. Amelioration of cholesterol atherogenesis in rabbits with reduced platelet counts as a result of P(32) administration. J Atheroscler Res 1968; 8: 389–93.

49. Friedman RJ, Stemerman MB, Wenz B, et al. The effect of thrombocytopenia on experimental arteriosclerotic lesion formation in rabbit. J Clin Invest 1977; 60: 1191–201.

50. Steele PM, Chesebro JH, Stanson AW, et al. Balloon angioplasty: natural history of the pathophysiologic response to injury in a pig model. Circ Res 1985; 57: 105–12.

51. Clowes AW, Clowes MM, Fingerle J, Reidy MA. Regulation of smooth muscle cell growth in injured artery. J Cardiovasc Pharmacol 1989; 14(suppl 6): S12–15.

52. Fingerle J, Johnson R, Clowes A, Majesky M, Reidy MA. Role of platelets in smooth muscle cell proliferation and migration after vascular injury in rat carotid artery. Proc Natl Acad Sci USA 1989; 86: 8412–6.

53. Fingerle J, Tina Au YP, Clowes AW, Reidy MA. Intimal lesion formation in rat carotid arteries after endothelial denudation in absence of medial injury. Arteriosclerosis 1990; 10(6): 1082–7.

54. Ross R, Raines EW, Bowen-Pope DF. The platelet derived growth factor. Cell 1986; 46: 155–69.

55. Walker LN, Bowen-Pope DF, Ross R, Reidy MA. Production of platelet-derived growth factor-like molecule by cultured arterial smooth muscle cells accompanied proliferation after arterial injury. Proc Natl Acad Sci USA 1986; 83: 7311–5.

56. Wilcox JN, Smith KM, Williams CT, Schwartz JM, Gordon D. Platelet-derived growth factor mRNA detection in human atherosclerotis plaques by in-situ hybridization. J Clin Invest 1988; 82: 1134–43.

57. Libby P, Warner SJC, Salomon RN, Birinyi LK. Production of platelet-derived growth factor-like mitogen by smooth muscle cells from human atheroma. N Engl J Med 1988; 318: 1493–8.

58. Bar-Shavit R, Amiram E, Vlodavsky I. Binding of thrombin to subendothelial extracellular matrix. Protection and expression of functional properties. J Clin Invest 1989; 84: 1096–104.

59. Weitz JI, Hudoba M, Massel D, Maraganore J, Hirsh J. Clot-bound thrombin is protected from inhibition by heparin-antithrombin III but is susceptible to inactivation by antithrombin III-independent inhibitors. J Clin Invest 1990; 86: 385–91.

60. Wilner GD, Danitz MP, Mudd MS, Hsieh KH, Fenton JW. Selective immobilization of alpha-thrombin by surface-bound fibrin. J Lab Clin Med 1981; 97: 403–11.

61. Berk BC, Taubman MB, Griendling KK, Cragoe E, Fenton J. Thrombin-stimulated events in cultured vascular smooth muscle cells. J Biol Chem 1990; 265: 17334–40.

62. Schwartz SM, Reidy MA. Common mechanism of proliferation of smooth muscle in atherosclerosis and hypertension. Hum Pathol 1987; 18: 240–7.

63. Wight LN. Cell biology of arterial proteoglycans. Arteriosclerosis 1989; 9: 1–20.

64. Yea-Herttuala S, Sumuvuori H, Karkola K, Mottonen M, Nikkari P. Glycosaminoglycans in normal and atherosclerotic human coronary arteries. Lab Invest 1986; 54: 402–8.

65. Webster MWI, Chesebro JH, Smith HC, et al. Myocardial infarction and coronary artery occlusion: a prospective 5-years angiographic study (abstract). J Am Coll Cardiol 1990; 15(suppl): 281A.

66. Rentrop P, Blanke H, Karsch KR, Kaiser H, Kostering H, Leitz K. Selective intracoronary thrombolysis in acute myocardial infarction and unstable angina pectoris. Circulation 1981; 63: 307–17.

67. Benson RL. The present status of coronary arterial disease. Arch Pathol 1926; 2: 876–916.

68. Constantinides P. Plaque fissures in human coronary thrombosis. J Atheroscler Res 1966; 6I: 1–17.

69. Friedman M, van den Bovenkamp GJ. The pathogenesis of coronary thrombosis. Am J Pathol 1966; 48: 19–31.

70. Rehr R, Disciascio G, Vetrovec G, Crowley M. Angiographic morphology of coronary artery stenoses in prolonged rest angina: evidence of intracoronary thrombosis. J Am Coll Cardiol 1989; 14: 1429–35.

71. Sherman CT, Litvak F, Grundfest W, et al. Coronary angioscopy in patients with unstable angina. N Engl J Med 1986; 315: 913–9.

72. Ramee SR, White CJ, Collins TJ, Mesa JE, Murgo JP. Percutaneous angioscopy during coronary angioplasty using a steerable microangioscope. J Am Coll Cardiol 1991; 17: 100–5.

73. Uchida Y, Tomaru T, Nakamura F, Furuse A, Fujimori Y. Percutaneous coronary angioscopy in patients with ischemic heart disease. Am Heart J 1987; 1114: 1216–22.

74. Uchida Y. Percutaneous coronary angioscopy by means of a fiberscope with steerable guidewire. Am Heart J 1989; 117: 1153–5.

75. Ambrose JA, Winters SL, Stern A, et al. Angiographic morphology and the pathogenesis of unstable angina pectoris. J Am Coll Cardiol 1985; 5: 609–16.

76. Vetrovec GW, Cowley MJ, Overton H, Richardson DW. Intracoronary thrombus in syndromes of unstable angina myocardial ischemia. Am Heart J 1981; 102: 1202–8.

77. Mandelkorn JB, Wolf NM, Singh S, et al. Intracoronary thrombus in non-transmural myocardial infarction and in unstable angina pectoris. Am J Cardiol 1983; 52: 1–6.

78. Capone G, Wolf NM, Meyers B, Meister SG. Frequency of intracoronary filling defects by angiography in unstable angina pectoris at rest. Am J Cardiol 1985; 56: 403–6.

79. Gotoh K, Minamino T, Hatoh O, et al. The role of intracoronary thrombus in unstable angina: angiographic assessment and thrombolytic therapy during ongoing anginal attacks. Circulation 1988; 77: 526–34.

80. Badimon L, Badimon JJ, Galvez A, Chesebro JH, Fuster V. Influence of arterial damage and wall shear rate on platelet deposition. Ex vivo study in swine model. Arteriosclerosis 1986; 6: 312–20.

81. Badimon L, Badimon JJ, Turitto VT, Vallabhajosula S, Fuster V. Platelet thrombus formation on collagen type I. A model of deep vessel injury—influence of blood rheology, von Willebrand factor and blood coagulation. Circulation 1988; 78: 1431–42.

82. Badimon L, Badimon JJ. Mechanism of arterial thrombosis in non-parallel strealines: platelet grow at the apex of stenotic severely injured vessel wall. Experimental study in the pig model. J Clin Invest 1989; 84: 1134–44.

83. Lassila R, Badimon JJ, Vallabhajosula S, Badimon L. Dynamic monitoring of platelet deposition on severely damaged vessel wall in flowing blood. Effects of different stenosis on thrombus growth. Arteriosclerosis 1990; 10: 306–15.

84. Drake TA, Morrissey JH, Edgington TS. Selective cellular expression of tissue factor in human tissues: implications of hemostasis and thrombosis. Am J Pathol 1989; 134: 1087–97.

85. Wilcox JN, Smith SM, Schwartz SM, Gordon D. Localization of tissue factor in the normal vessel wall and atherosclerotic plaque. Proc Natl Acad Sci USA 1989; 86: 2839–43.

86. Holmes DR, Hartzler GO, Smith HC, Fuster V. Coronary artery thrombosis in patients with unstable angina. Br Heart J 1981; 45: 411–6.

87. Hirsh PD, Hillis LD, Campbell WB, Firth BG, Willerson JT. Release of prostaglandins and thromboxane into the coronary circulation in patients with ischemic heart disease. N Engl J Med 1981; 304: 685–91.

88. Fitzgerald DJ, Roy L, Catella F, FitzGerald GA. Platelet activation in unstable coronary disease. N Engl J Med 1986; 315: 983–9.

89. Hamm CW, Lorenz R, Bleifeld W, Kupper W, Weber W, Weber P. Biochemical evidence of platelet activation in patients with persistent unstable angina. J Am Coll Cardiol 1987; 9: 998–1004.

90. Van den Berg EK, Schmitz JM, Benedict CR, Malloy CR, Willerson JT, Dehmer GJ. Transcardiac serotonin concentration is increased in selected patients with limiting angina complex coronary lesion morphology. Circulation 1989; 79: 116–24.

91. Fuster V, Chesebro JH. Mechanisms of unstable angina. N Engl J Med 1986; 315: 1023–5.

92. Rentrop KP, Feit F, Blanke H, Sherman W, Thornton JC. Serial angiographic assessment of coronary artery obstruction and collateral flow in acute myocardial infarction. Circulation 1989; 80: 1166–75.

93. Van de Werf F, Arnold AER, and the European Cooperative Study Group for Recombinant Tissue-Type Plasminogen Activator (rt-PA). Effect of intravenous tissue plasminogen activator on infarct size, left ventricular function and survival in patients with acute myocardial infarction. Br Med J 1988; 297: 374–9.

94. Van Lierde, De Geest H, Verstraete M, et al. Angiographic assessment of the infarct-related residual coronary stenosis after spontaneous or therapeutic thrombolysis. J Am Coll Cardiol 1990; 16: 1545–9.

95. Fuster V, Stein B, Badimon L, Badimon JJ, Ambrose JA, Chesebro JH. Atheroscerotic plaque rupture and thrombosis: evolving concepts. Circulation 1990; 82(suppl II): 47–59.

96. Davies SW, Marchant B, Lyon JP, et al. Coronary lesion morphology in acute myocardial infarction: demonstration of early remodeling after streptokinase treatment. J Am Coll Cardiol 1990; 16: 1079–86.

97. Gulba DC, Barthels M, Westhoff-Bleck M, et al. Increased thrombin levels during acute myocardial infarction. Relevance for the success of therapy. Circulation 1991; 83: 937–44.

98. Badimon L, Badimon J, Lasilla R, Heras M, Chesebro JH, Fuster V. Thrombin inhibition by hirudin decreases platelet thrombus growth on areas of severe vessel wall injury. J Am Coll Cardiol 1989; 13: 145A.

99. Weitz JI, Hudoba M, Massel D, Maragamore J, Hirsh J. Clot-bound thrombin is protected from inhibition by heparin-antithrombin III but is susceptible to inactivation by antithrombin III-independent inhibitors. J Clin Invest 1990; 86: 385–91.

100. Fitzgerald DJ, Fitzgerald GA. Role of thrombin and thromboxane A_2 in reocclusion following coronary thrombolysis with tissue-type plasminogen activator. Proc Natl Acad Sci USA, 1989; 86: 7585.

101. Francis CW, Markham RE, Barlow GH, Florack TM, Dobrzynski DM, Marder VJ. Thrombin activity of fibrin thrombi and soluble plasmic derivatives. J Lab Clin Med 1983; 102: 220–30.

102. Hogg PJ, Jackson CM. Fibrin monomer protects thrombin from inactivation by heparin-antithrombin III: implications for heparin efficacy. Proc Natl Acad Sci USA 1989; 86: 3619–23.

103. Fitzgerald DJ, Catella F, Roy L, et al. Marked platelet activation in vivo after intravenous streptokinase in patients with acute myocardial infarction. Circulation 1988; 77: 142–50.

104. Eisenberg PR, Sherman LA, Jaffe AS. Paradoxic elevation of fibrinopeptide A after streptokinase: evidence for continued thrombosis despite intense fibrinolysis. J Am Coll Cardiol 1987; 10: 527–9.

105. Brown GB, Gallery CA, Badger RS, et al. Incomplete lysis of thrombus in the moderate underlying atherosclerosis le-

sion during intracoronary infusion of streptokinase for acute myocardial infarction: quantitative angiographic observation. Circulation 1986; 73: 653–61.

106. Serruys PW, Arnold AER, Brower RW, et al. Effects of continued rt-PA administration in acute myocardial infarction—A quantitative coronary angiography study of a randomized trial. Eur Heart J 1987; 8: 1172–81.

107. Waller BF, Rothbaum DA, Pinkerton CA, et al. Status of the myocardium and infarct-related coronary artery in 19 necropsy patients with acute recanalization using pharmacologic (streptokinase, r-tissue plasminogen activator), mechanical (percutaneous transluminal coronary angioplasty) or combined types of reperfusion therapy. J Am Coll Cardiol 1987; 9: 785–801.

108. Badger RS, Brown BG, Kennedy JW, et al. Usefulness of recanalization to luminal diameter of 0.6 millimeter or more with intracoronary streptokinase during acute myocardial infarction in predicting "normal" perfusion status, continued arterial patency and survival at one year. Am J Cardiol 1987; 59: 519–22.

109. Harrison DG, Ferguson DW, Collins SM, et al. Rethrombosis after reperfusion with streptokinase: importance of geometry of residual lesions. Circulation 1984; 69: 991–9.

110. Gash AK, Spann JF, Sherry S, et al. Factors influencing reocclusion after coronary thrombolysis for acute myocardial infarction. Am J Cardiol 1986; 57: 175–7.

111. De Guise P, Theroux P, Bonan R. Rethrombosis after successful thrombolysis and angioplasty in acute myocardial infarction. J Am Coll Cardiol 1988; 11(suppl A): 198.

112. Rowsell HC, Hegardt B, Downie HG, Mustard JF, Murphy EA. Adrenaline and experimental thrombosis. Br J Haematol 1966; 12: 66–73.

113. Haft JI, Fani K. Intravascular platelet aggregation in the heart induced by stress. Circulation 1973; 47: 353–8.

114. Mueller JE, Stone PH, Turi ZG, et al. The MILIS Study Group. Circadian variation in the frequency of onset of acute myocardial infarction. N Engl J Med 1985; 313: 1315–22.

115. Willich SN, Linderer T, Wegscheider K, et al. Increased morning incidence of myocardial infarction in the ISAM study: absence with prior β-adrenergic blockade. Circulation 1989; 80: 853–8.

116. Hjalmarson A, Gilpin E, Nicod P, Henning H, Ross J Jr. Circadian pattern of onset of symptoms in acute myocardial infarction differs among clinical subsets. Circulation 198; 78(suppl II): II-437.

117. Tofler GH, Brezinski D, Schafer AI, et al. Morning increase in platelet response to ADP and epinephrine: association with the time of increased risk of myocardial infarction and sudden cardiac death. N Engl J Med 1987; 316: 1514–8.

118. Levine PH. An acute effect of cigarette smoking on platelet function: a possible link between smoking and arterial thrombosis. Circulation 1973; 48: 619–23.

119. Fuster V, Chesebro JH, Frye RL, Elveback L. Platelet survival and the development of coronary artery disease in the young adult: effects of cigarette smoking, strong family history and medical therapy. Circulation 1981; 63: 546–51.

120. Bierenbaum ML, Fieischman AI, Stier A, Somol S, Wabon PB. Effects of cigarette smoking upon in vivo platelet function in man. Thromb Res 1978; 12: 1051–7.

121. Koch A, Hoffman K, Steck W, et al. Acute cardiovascular reactions after cigarette smoking. Atherosclerosis 1980; 35: 67–75.

122. Winniford MD, Wheelan KR, Kremers MS, et al. Smoking-induced coronary vasoconstriction in patients with atherosclerotic coronary artery disease: evidence for adrenergically mediated alterations in coronary artery tone. Circulation 1986; 73: 662–7.

123. Cullen JW, McKenna JW, Massey MM. International control of smoking and the US experience. Chest 1986; 89(suppl): 206–18.

124. Buhler FR, Vesanen K, Watters JT. Impact of smoking on heart attacks, strokes, blood pressure control, drug dose, and quality of life aspects in the International Prospective Primary Prevention Study in Hypertension. Am Heart J 1988; 115: 282–8.

125. Paul O. Background of the prevention of cardiovascular disease. II. Arteriosclerosis, hypertension and selected risk factors. Circulation 1989; 80: 206–14.

126. Hunt BJ. The relation between abnormal hemostatic function and the progression of coronary disease. Curr Op Cardiol 1990; 5: 758–65.

127. Badimon JJ, Badimon L, Turitto VT, Fuster V. Platelet deposition at high shear rates is enhanced by high plasma cholesterol levels. In vivo study in the rabbit model. Arteriosclerosis 1991; 11: 395–402.

128. Carvalho ACA, Colman RW, Lees RS. Platelet function in hyperlipoproteinemia. N Engl J Med 1974; 290: 434–8.

129. Stuart MJ, Gerrard JM, White JG. Effect of cholesterol on production of thromboxane B_2 by platelets in vitro. N Engl J Med 1980; 302: 6–10.

130. McCully KS. Vascular pathology of homocysteinemia: implications for the pathogenesis of arteriosclerosis. Am J Pathol 1969; 56: 111–28.

131. Boers GHJ, Smals AGH, Trijbels FJM, et al. Heterozygosity for homocystinuria in premature peripheral and cerebral occlusive arterial disease. N Engl J Med 1985; 313: 709–15.

132. Murphy-Chutorian DR, Wexman MP, Grieco AJ, et al. Methionine intolerance: a possible risk factor for coronary artery disease. J Am Coll Cardiol 1985; 6: 725–30.

133. Harker LA, Ross R, Slichter SJ, Scott C. Homocystine-induced arteriosclerosis: the role of endothelial cell injury and platelet response in its genesis. J Clin Invest 1976; 58: 731–41.

134. Berg K. A new serum system in man—the LP system. Acta Pathol Microbiol Scand 1963; 59: 369–82.

135. Dahlen GH, Guyton JR, Attar M, et al. Association of levels of lipoprotein Lp(a), plasma lipids, and other lipoproteins with coronary artery disease documented by angiography. Circulation 1986; 74: 758–65.

136. Seed M, Hoppichler F, Reaveley D, et al. Relation of serum lipoprotein(a) concentration and apolipoprotein(a) phenotype to CHD patients with familial hypercholesterolemia. N Engl J Med 1990; 332: 1494–9.

137. Armstrong VW, Cremer P, Eberle E, et al. The association between serum Lp(a) concentrations and angiographically assessed coronary atherosclerosis dependence on serum LDL levels. Atherosclerosis 1986; 62: 249–57.

138. McLean JW, Tomlinson JE, Kuang W-J, et al. cDNA sequence of human apolipoprotein(a) is homologous to plasminogen. Nature 1987; 330: 132–7.

139. Frank SL, Klisak I, Sparks RS. The apoprotein(a) gene resides on human chromosome 6q 26-27 in close proximity to the homologous gene for plasminogen. Hum Genet 1988; 79: 352–6.

140. Miles LA, Fless GM, Levine EG, Scanu AM, Plow EF. A potential basis for the thrombotic risks associated with lipoprotein(a). Nature 1989; 339: 301–3.

141. Hajjar KA, Gavish D, Breslow JL, Nachmann RL. Lipoprotein(a) modulation of endothelial surface fibrinolysis and its potential role in atherosclerosis. Nature 198; 339: 303–5.

142. Harpel PL, Gordon BR, Parker TS. Plasmin catalyzes binding of lipoprotein(a) to immobilized fibrinogen and fibrin. Proc Natl Acad Sci USA 1989; 56: 3847–51.

143. Edelberg JM, Gonzalez-Gronow M, Pizzo SV. Lipoprotein(a) inhibits streptokinesis-mediated activation of human plasminogen. Biochemistry 1989; 72: 374a.

144. Edelberg JM, Gonzalez-Gronow M, Pizzo SV. Lipoprotein(a) inhibition of plasminogen activation by tissue-type plasminogen activator. Thromb Res 1990; 57: 155–62.

145. Loscalzo J. Lipoprotein(a): a unique risk factor for atherothrombotic disease. Arteriosclerosis 1990; 10: 672–9.

146. Paramo JA, Colucci M, Collen D. Plasminogen activator inhibitor in blood of patients with coronary artery disease. Br Med J 1985; 291: 573–4.

147. Olofsson BO, Dahlen G, Nilsson TK. Evidence for increased levels of plasminogen activator inhibitor and tissue plasminogen activator in plasma of patients with angiographically verified coronary artery disease. Eur Heart J 1989; 10: 77–82.

148. Hamsten A, Wiman B, de Faire U, Blombäck M. Increased plasma levels of a rapid inhibitor of tissue plasminogen ac-

tivator in young survivors of myocardial infarction. N Engl J Med 1980; 303: 897–902.

149. Barbash GI, Hanoch H, Roth A, et al. Correlation of baseline plasminogen activator inhibitor activity with patency of the infarct artery after thrombolytic therapy in acute myocardial infarction. Am J Cardiol 1989; 64: 1231–5.

150. Oseroff A, Krishnamurti C, Hassett A, et al. Plasminogen activator and plasminogen activator inhibitor activities in men with coronary artery disease. J Lab Clin Med 1990; 113: 88–93.

151. Maseri A, L'Abbate A, Barodi G, et al. Coronary vasospasm as a possible cause of myocardial infarction: a conclusion derived from the study of "preinfarction" angina. N Engl J Med 1978; 299: 1271–7.

152. Little WC, Constantinescu M, Applegate RJ. Can coronary angiography predict the site of a subsequent myocardial infarction in patients with mild-to-moderate coronary artery disease? Circulation 1988; 78: 1156–66.

153. Ambrose JA, Tannenbaum MA, Alexopoulos D, et al. Angiographic progression of coronary artery disease and the development of myocardial infarction. J Am Coll Cardiol 1988; 12: 56–62.

154. Imparato AM, Riles TS, Gorstein F. The carotid bifurcation plaque: pathologic findings associated with cerebral ischemia. Stroke 1979; 10: 238–45.

155. O'Holleran LW, Kennelly MM, McClustan M, Johnson JM. Natural history of asyptomatic carotid plaque. Five year follow-up study. Am J Surg 1987; 154: 659–62.

156. Sterpetti AV, Schultz RD, Feldhaus RJ, et al. Ultrastructural features of carotid plaques and the risk of subsequent neurologic deficit. Surgery 1988; 104: 652–60.

157. Weinberger J, Ramos J, Ambrose JA, Fuster V. Morphologic and dynamic changes of atherosclerotic plaque at the carotid artery bifurcation. Sequential imaging by real time B mode ultrasonography. J Am Coll Cardiol 1988; 12: 1515–21.

158. Halperin J, Hart R. Atrial fibrillation and stroke. New ideas and persistent dilemmas. Stroke 1988; 19: 937–47.

159. Olsen TS, Skriver EB, Herning M. Cause of cerebral infarction in the carotid territory: its relation to the size and the location of the infarct and to the underlying vascular lesions. Stroke 1985; 16: 459–65.

160. Jorgensen L, Torvik A. Ischemic cerebrovascular diseases in an autopsy series. J Neurol Sci 1966; 3: 490–509.

161. Britton M, Gustafson C. Nonrheumatic atrial fibrillation as a risk factor for stroke. Stroke 1985; 16: 182–8.

162. Cerebral Embolism Task Force. Cardiogenic brain embolism. Arch Neurol 1986; 43: 71–84.

163. Foulkes MA, Wolf PA, Price TR. The stroke data bank: design, methods and baseline characteristics. Stroke 1988; 19: 547–54.

164. Rem JA, Hachinski VC, Boughner DR, Barnett HJM. Value of cardiac monitoring and echocardiography in TIA and stroke patients. Stroke 1985; 16: 950–6.

165. Fogelholm R, Melin J. Echocardiography in ischemic cerebral vascular disease. Br Med J 1987; 295: 305–6.

166. Criqui MH, Fronek A, Barrett-Connor E, Klauber MR, Gabriel S, Goodman D. The prevalence of peripheral arterial disease in a defined population. Circulation 1985; 71: 510–9.

167. Dormandy JA, Mahir SM. The natural history of peripheral atheromatous disease of legs. In: Greenhaigh RM, Jamiesen CW, Nicolaides AN, eds. Vascular surgery. Issues in current practice. London: Grune & Stratton, 1986:3–16.

168. Kannel WB, Skinner JJ Jr, Schwartz M, Shurtleff D. Intermittent claudication. Incidence in the Framingham study. Circulation 1970; 41: 875–88.

169. Kannel WB, McGee DL. Diabetes and cardiovascular disease. The Framingham study. JAMA 1979; 241: 2035–46.

170. Hertzer NR, Beren EG, Young JR, et al. Coronary artery disease in peripheral vascular patients. A classification of 1000 coronary angiograms and results of surgical management. Ann Surg 1984; 199: 223–30.

171. Jelnes R, Gaardsting O, Jensen KH, Baekgaard N, Tonnesen KH, Schroeder L. Fate in intermittent claudication. Outcome and risk factors. Br Med J 1986; 293: 1137–44.

172. Criqui MH, Coughlin SS, Fronek A. Noninvasively diagnosed peripheral arterial disease as a predictor of mortality: results from a prospective study. Circulation 1985; 72: 768–75.

173. Lassila R, Lepantalo M, Lindfors O. Peripheral arterial disease—natural outcome. Acta Med Scand 1986; 220: 295–304.

174. Stokes J III, Kannel WB, Wolf PA, Cuppler LA, D'Agostino RB. The relative importance of selected risk factors for various manifestations of cardiovascular disease among men and women from 35–64 years old. Thirty years of follow-up in the Framingham study. Circulation 1987; 75(suppl V)V: 65–72.

175. Sternby NH. Atherosclerosis, smoking and other risk factors. In: Gotto AM Jr, Smith LC, Allen B, eds. Atherosclerosis. V. New York: Springer-Verlag, 1980: 67–70.

176. Lassila R, Lepantalo M. Cigarette smoking and the outcome after lower limb arterial surgery. Acta Chir Scand 1988; 154: 635–41.

177. Humphries AW, Young JR. The severely ischemic leg. Curr Probl Surg 1970: 1–59.

178. Jonason T, Bergstrom R. Cessation of smoking in patients with intermittent claudication. Acta Med Scand 1987; 221: 253–62.

179. Greenhalgh RM, Laing SP, Cole PV, Taylor GW. Smoking and arterial reconstruction. Br J Surg 1981; 68: 605–17.

180. Johnson RC, Crissman RS, DiDio LJA. Endocardial alterations in myocardial infarction. Lab Invest 1979; 40: 183–93.

181. Hochman JS, Platia EB, Bulkley BH. Endocardial abnormalities in left ventricular aneurysm: a clinicopathologic study. Ann Intern Med 1984; 100: 29–35.

182. Roberts WC, Siegel RJ, McManus BM. Idiopathic dilated cardiomyopathy: analysis of 152 necropsy patients. Am J Cardiol 1967; 60: 1340–55.

183. Mikell FL, Asinger RW, Elsperger KJ. Regional stasis of blood in the dysfunctional left ventricle: echocardiographic detection and differentiation from early thrombosis. Circulation 1982; 66: 755–63.

184. Asinger RW, Mikell FL, Elsperger J, Hodges M. Incidence of left ventricular thrombosis after acute transmural myocardial infarction: serial evaluation by two-dimensional echocardiography. N Engl J Med 1981; 305: 297–302.

185. Weinreich DJ, Burke JF, Pauletto FJ. Left ventricular mural thrombi complicating acute myocardial infarction: long-term follow-up with serial echocardiography. Ann Intern Med 1984; 100: 789–94.

186. Shrestha NK, Moreno FL, Narcisco FV, Torres L, Calleja H. Two-dimensional echocardiographic diagnosis of left atrial thrombus in rheumatic heart disease: a clinicopathologic study. Circulation 1983; 67: 341–7.

187. Fulton RM, Duckett K. Plasma-fibrinogen and thromboemboli after myocardial infarction. Lancet 1976; 2: 1161–4.

188. Fuster V, Halperin JL. Left ventricular thrombi and cerebral embolism (editorial). N Engl J Med 1989; 320: 392–4.

189. Cabin HS, Roberts WC. Left ventricular aneurysm, intraaneurysmal thrombus and systemic embolus in coronary heart disease. Chest 1980; 77: 586–90.

190. Dewanjee MK, Fuster V, Rao SA, Forsham P, Kaye M. Noninvasive radioisotopic technique for detection of platelet deposition in mitral valve prostheses and quantification of visceral microembolism in dogs. Mayo Clin Proc 1983; 58: 307–14.

191. Acar J, Vahanian A, Fauchet M, Murdler O, Dorent R, Roger V. Detection of prosthetic valve thrombosis using Indium 111 platelet imaging (abstr). Eur Heart J 1989; 10(suppl): 261.

192. Chesebro JH, Adams PC, Fuster V. Antithrombotic therapy in patients with valvular heart disease and prosthetic heart valves. J Am Coll Cardiol 1986; 8(suppl B): 41–56.

193. Fuster V, Badimon L, Badimon JJ, Chesebro JH. Prevention of thromboembolism induced by prosthetic heart valves. Semin Thromb Hemost 1988; 14: 50–8.

194. Edmunds LH Jr. Thrombotic and bleeding complications of prosthetic heart valves. Ann Thorac Surg 1987; 44: 430–45.

195. Freiman DG. The structure of thrombi. In: Colman RW, Hirsh J, Marder VJ, Salzman EW, eds. Thrombosis and

hemostasis: basic principles and clinical practice. Philadelphia: JB Lippincott Co., 1982:766–80.

196. Hirsh J, Salzman EW. Pathogenesis of venous thromboembolism. In: Colman RW, Hirsh J, Marder VJ, Salzman EW, eds. Thrombosis and hemostasis: basic principles and clinical practice. Philadelphia: JB Lippincott Co., 1987:1199–207.

197. Kakkar VV, Flanc C, Howe CT, Clarke MB. Natural history of postoperative deep vein thrombosis. Lancet 1969; 2: 230–41.

198. Nicolaides AN, Kakkar VV, Field ES, Renney JTG. The origin of deep vein thrombosis: a venographic study. Br J Radiol 1971; 44: 653–66.

199. Stamatakis JD, Kakkar VV, Sagar S, et al. Femoral vein thrombosis and total hip replacement. Br Med J 1977; 2: 213–9.

200. Davies GS, Salzman EW. The pathogenesis of deep vein thrombosis. In: Joist HJ, Sherman LA, eds. Venous and arterial thrombosis. New York: Grune & Stratton, 1979:1.

3

INTERRELATIONSHIP BETWEEN ATHEROSCLEROSIS AND THROMBOSIS

NEVILLE WOOLF and MICHAEL J. DAVIES

THE BASIC PROCESS OF ATHEROSCLEROSIS

Atherosclerosis is a primarily intimal disease of large and medium sized arteries affecting principally the aorta, femoral, carotid, cerebral, coronary, and renal arteries. It is not a disease that is found in the smaller arteries lying within organs; thus the intracerebral and intramyocardial arteries measuring 100 to 500 microns in external diameter are spared, while the circle of Willis and the major epicardial coronary arteries are prime targets.

The intimal involvement is focal rather than diffuse, producing individual lesions known as plaques, best appreciated by examining the intimal surface of an artery opened longitudinally. The localization of the focal lesions (Fig. 3–1) is determined by hemodynamic forces acting on the endothelial surface, and areas of low wall shear rate are preferentially affected by early lesions with sparing of the flow divider areas at points of branching.[1–3]

The major constituents of all plaques, whatever their stage of development or size, are lipid, and the connective tissue matrix proteins, including collagen, elastin, and proteoglycans which are produced by smooth muscle cells. The lipid component of plaques may be contained within foam cells, largely of monocytic origin, or may be free within the tissue. The extracellular lipid component of plaques varies widely in amount, even within plaques of identical size in an individual.

A major limitation of all necropsy studies is that lesions can be observed at one moment in time only. Knowledge concerning the growth and progression of plaques in man can only be obtained indirectly from comparisons of the lesions present at necropsy in populations selected for different age. It is logical to assume that large plaques develop from smaller lesions, but it is far from certain that all small plaques progress.

Morphology of Atherosclerotic Lesions in Man

Examination of arteries from young subjects up to the age of 35 who died of nonvascular causes, usually homicide, suicide, or accidents, grouped into cohorts of five years allows the progression of human lesions to be inferred.[4,5] The first macroscopically recognizable atherosclerotic lesions are yellow dots or streaks, barely raised above the intimal surface, containing focal collections of lipid-filled foam cells. Such fatty streaks appear within the aorta and coronary arteries within the first year of life in a wide range of racial and geographic populations irrespective of the prevalence of clinically expressed ischemic heart disease in adults from that population.[6] Within the next ten years of life, plaques appear which contain, in addition to lipid-filled foam cells, a layer of smooth muscle cells just beneath the endothelium, and extracellular lipid. Both these factors mark progression to the formation of the raised plaque.[4]

Raised plaques are the archetypal expres-

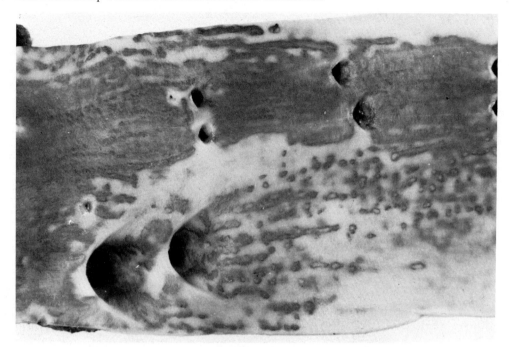

FIGURE 3–1. The thoracic aorta from a 19-year-old male. The specimen has been stained with oil red 0 and shows extensive fatty streaking. In relation to points of branching, lipid deposition is concentrated in the proximal portions of the ostia, where the wall shear rate is low. In contrast, the flow divider area is spared.

sion of atherosclerosis, since they may ultimately lead to clinical symptoms, either by chronically disturbing flow by virtue of their volume, or by causing an acute reduction in flow by the medium of thrombosis. When populations are compared, the number of raised plaques in the aorta, coronary, and cerebral arteries at necropsy mirrors the prevalence of cerebrovascular and ischemic heart disease.[6] Populations with factors known to be associated with an increased risk of ischemic heart disease, such as hypertension, cigarette smoking, or diabetes, have more plaques than control subjects.[5,7,8]

Raised fibrolipid plaques are far more heterogenous in composition than fatty streaks, there being great variation among plaques in the relative proportions of plaque volume which are made up of collagen and lipid. The archetypal microanatomy of a raised plaque is that the center, adjacent to the media, contains a mass of extracellular lipid (Fig. 3–2). The lipid is predominantly cholesterol, and its esters are thought to have been derived from plasma low-density lipoprotein (LDL). One mechanism by which such extracellular cholesterol is accumulated is via oxidation of intraintimal low-density lipoprotein followed by its ingestion by mac-

rophages, which bind modified apoprotein via their scavenger receptors.[9,10] This leads to the formation of lipid-filled "foam" cells within the intima. The subsequent death of these foam cells releases cholesterol into the intima. An alternative mechanism for extracellular cholesterol accumulation within the arterial intima envisages binding of low-density lipoprotein to proteoglycans, followed by local cleavage of the lipoprotein and deposition of its cholesterol ester moiety.[11] In some plaques the central core of lipid is crisscrossed by a lattice of collagen, while in others there is an actual cavity within the intima filled with cholesterol. It is to this latter state that the word lipid pool is most appropriately applied, and it is these plaques which extrude atheromatous "gruel" when squeezed in the autopsy room. The physicochemical nature of the lipid within the plaques suggests that it is semiliquid at body temperatures[12] and thus easily deformed with a consequent redistribution of mechanical stress to other parts of the arterial wall in systole. This redistribution is highly significant in relation to subsequent thrombosis.[13]

The lipid-rich core is separated from the lumen by a fibromuscular cap in which the smooth muscle cells can be seen to lie within

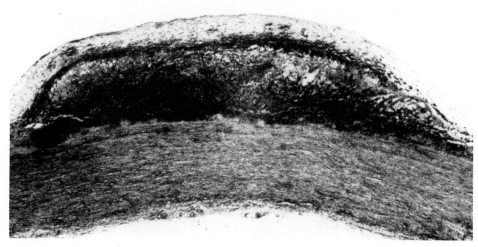

FIGURE 3–2. Frozen section of a human, aortic raised, fibrolipid lesion. The section has been stained with the fat-soluble dye oil red 0 and shows the presence of a massive lipid-rich basal pool covered by a relatively thin connective tissue cap (× 30).

lacunae between the collagen fibers. Lipid-filled macrophages cluster around the margins of the basal lipid core and may also infiltrate the cap. The surface of the plaque is covered by an endothelial layer which may or may not be intact. Very little is known of the relation between the different forms of raised plaque and whether lipid-rich and predominantly fibrous forms are separate from their initiation or evolve from each other with time.

The Progression of Atherosclerosis

The evidence so far available supports the view that there is a progression from fatty streaks to raised plaques; but by no means do all fatty streaks progress.[14] Clinical symptoms develop when a certain threshold is reached where (for example, in the coronary arteries) plaque size is sufficient to encroach significantly upon the lumen and thus limit flow. Angiographic studies of human atherosclerosis in the coronary arteries suggest that the progression of these obstructing lesions is not linear with time, but is instead intermittent and unpredictable.[15,16]

Angiography is, however, a poor method for assessing the size of atherosclerotic plaques, as distinct from the degree of narrowing of the lumen that they cause. Arteries containing plaques undergo a compensatory dilatation to accommodate the lesion and preserve the lumen dimensions and outline.

This compensatory mechanism is only exhausted when the volume of the plaque occupies more than 40 per cent of the original cross-sectional area of the lumen.[17] The media behind atherosclerotic plaques atrophies; thus, eccentrically situated plaques bulge outward rather than inward. The corollary of these facts is that an artery which is angiographically normal, or the lumen of which is slightly irregular in outline, can contain large plaques. Thus angiography can only indicate the progression of plaques that are already well established. The intermittent nature of the progression may well be explained by intermittent thrombosis and the reactions in the underlying vessel wall which such thrombi can cause. Thrombosis is also the complication of atherosclerosis which most often leads to acute clinical events such as infarction or stroke, and can be considered as the final stage of a progressive process. This chapter is concerned with the role that thrombosis may play in plaque initiation, in plaque growth, and in the final complications which lead to acute ischemic events.

THE INITIATION OF ATHEROSCLEROSIS

The initiation of atherosclerosis has been studied in animals with hyperlipidemia due to inherited defects in lipid metabolism, such as the Watanabe rabbit,[18] which lacks the low-density lipoprotein receptor; and the St.

Thomas' rabbit,[19] in which there is an over-production of very low-density lipoprotein (VLDL). Other models use high-fat diets.[20,21] The earliest observed morphological change in all these models is adhesion and migration of monocytes through the intact endothelial surface.[22] Subsequently, lipid-filled foam cells, largely of monocytic origin, accumulate and form the intimal fatty streak lesion. In some hyperlipidemic models, endothelial denudation occurs after some weeks (Fig. 3–3), and it is only then that platelet adhesion to exposed connective tissue matrix proteins begins. Thus there is no evidence for the involvement of growth factors released from activated platelets in plaque initiation. Such data do not imply that the endothelium is functionally normal; simply that denudation injury has not occurred. Platelet adhesion to an intact endothelial surface (i.e., one in which there is no exposure of subendothelial connective tissue matrix) has been observed only very rarely in animals exposed to graded doses of cigarette smoke[23] and in virally infected endothelial cells.

The optimum method of demonstrating endothelial continuity is scanning electron microscopy in vessels fixed by perfusion after flushing with heparin; such restraints limit the number of human studies, since obtaining suitable material is difficult. Limited studies on atherectomy specimens and in the coronary arteries taken from the explanted heart at transplantation confirm that the endothelium is intact over small fatty streaks, but denuded areas with platelet adhesion are common over larger, more complex plaques.[24]

The consensus view at present is that thrombosis, as expressed by platelet adhesion and aggregation, plays no part in plaque initiation. The only evidence discordant with

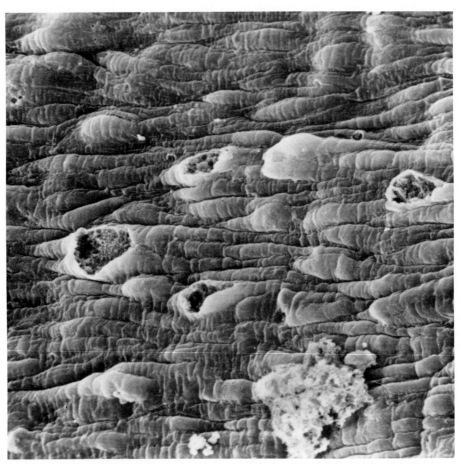

FIGURE 3–3. Cholesterol-fed rabbit: aortic fatty streak from a cholesterol-fed rabbit examined by scanning electron microscopy. It shows focal elevation of endothelial cells and some of these have undergone denudation revealing the underlying connective tissue matrix.

this view is that microthrombi were identified on apparently lesion-free segments of human arteries. Crawford and Levene[25] carefully selected areas of the aortic intima which were macroscopically free from lesions; the absence of any atherosclerotic plaque was confirmed histologically, but endothelial and subendothelial fibrin deposits were often noted. In another study,[26] macroscopically normal segments of human aorta were studied histologically and the degree of intimal edema graded from 0 to + + +. In 29 per cent of those segments with no edema, small microthrombi were found, while the percentage rose to 100 per cent when + + + edema was recorded. A homologous situation appears to exist in animal models; in the pig aorta, identification of focal increases in endothelial permeability by injection of Evans blue dye just before sacrifice has been followed by detailed histological analysis of these areas. Microthrombi were found over areas of intimal edema without there being other morphological evidence of an atherosclerotic lesion.[26] Chandler[27] reported studies of the proximal left anterior descending coronary artery in victims of accidental death ranging from 12 to 30 years of age. Microscopic mural thrombi were identified in seven of the nine cases, and in two of these the thrombi were not related to an established underlying plaque. The integrity of the endothelium underlying these microthrombi and overlying an area of intimal edema is not known. Microthrombi were, however, far more common over already established plaques. The study by Chandler does illustrate that thrombosis on a microscopic scale is far more common over established plaques as compared with "normal" intima; this process of microthrombosis begins at a relatively early age in the life of the subject (i.e., in the first two decades).

THROMBOSIS IN PLAQUE GROWTH

Plaque growth is mediated in large part by the proliferation of smooth muscle cells within the affected portion of intima, and in particular by the elaboration of extracellular connective tissue elements such as collagen, elastin, and proteoglycans, all of which the smooth muscle cells are capable of synthesizing.[28] Convincing experimental data now exist which suggest that one of the major factors stimulating this form of connective tissue proliferation is a series of interactions between platelets and the underlying artery wall mediated by growth factors. Of equal importance is the proposition that in man, mural thrombi containing both fibrin and platelets frequently occur in relation to established atherosclerotic plaques and may become incorporated into the substance of the artery wall. In such circumstances the degree of plaque thickening may be increased, partly by the bulk of the unorganized residuum of thrombus, and partly because of the brisk proliferative response which the presence of thrombus containing both platelets and fibrin can evoke in the arterial connective tissue.

The natural history of arterial mural thrombi has been studied in experimental models, and from these the reactions of the vessel wall subjacent to a thrombus have been studied and held to constitute an analogue of some of the processes which may be involved in plaque growth. In some models, lesions which were initially pure thrombus evolve into lesions very closely resembling atherosclerotic plaques.

EXPERIMENTAL PULMONARY EMBOLI

The earliest studies relate to experimental pulmonary emboli. Originally these were produced by the intravenous injection of fibrin or blood clots.[29] The introduction by Chandler[30] of a method by which platelet-rich "thrombi" were produced from plasma contained within rotating plastic loops provided more realistic emboli. Ardlie and Schwartz[31] studied the natural history of such platelet-rich pulmonary emboli in two groups of rabbits. The first was fed a normal stock diet, the second a cholesterol-enriched diet. The time elapsing between the injection of the emboli and sacrifice ranged from 1.5 hours to 18 weeks. In both groups of animals some evidence of endothelial covering of the retracted emboli was apparent by the third day and thought to be complete after a week. By four months many of the lesions seen were complex fibrolipid plaques, in which a dense connective tissue cap overlaid a basal, lipid-rich pool. This contrasts markedly with the fibrous plaques produced after embolization with pure fibrin clots. While stainable lipid was present in the lesions of animals receiving the stock diet, the amount of such lipid was greatly increased in those animals receiving the cholesterol-enriched diet. Calcification was also more common in the plaque-like lesions of those animals which had received the high-cholesterol diet. These results dispel the view that lesions arising on the basis of thrombus cannot contain significant amounts of lipid.

As a model system, pulmonary embolization has inherent weaknesses. Chief among these are that at some stage in their natural history, the emboli must, of necessity, be occlusive rather than mural and that the pressures in the pulmonary vascular bed differ considerably from those in systemic arteries.

EXPERIMENTAL MURAL THROMBOSIS IN SYSTEMIC ARTERIES

A wide variety of methods has been employed to induce mural thrombi in systemic arteries. These methods include intimal abrasion of the aorta under direct vision,[32] the use of a balloon catheter to denude the intima of its endothelial covering,[33,34] the insertion of a fine nylon filament,[35] and the insertion of indwelling polythene cannulae to produce repeated injury to the arterial intima.[36] All these methods produce loss of endothelium,

followed by adherence of platelets to the exposed subendothelial tissue (Fig. 3–4) and, in due time, by a striking degree of smooth muscle cell proliferation and elaboration of extracellular elements, most notably collagen and proteoglycans (Fig. 3–5). In direct abrasion with the aorta opened, or where an indwelling cannula has been inserted into the aorta, the resulting lesion, in the earlier stages of its natural history, is easily recognized as thrombus (Fig. 3–6). The use of a balloon catheter or a fine filament, however, as shown by scanning electron microscopy, is associated with a monolayer of platelets and white cells scattered over the raw area of the intima (Fig. 3–7). Nevertheless, despite the morphological disparity between all these expressions of different degrees of intimal injury, all are followed by localized fibromuscular hyperplasia—the degree of intimal injury is one determinant of the resulting proliferative response. Removal of a band of endothelial cells, 100 microns in width, by a fine nylon filament introduced into the rat aorta[35] is not associated with intimal thickening, but there is proliferation of the medial smooth muscle cells at the site.

Organization of Mural Thrombi

Within a few days of direct intimal abrasion (for example, in the pig aorta), light micro-

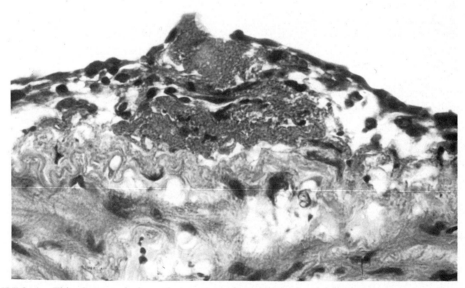

FIGURE 3–4. This photograph shows the presence of a small platelet-rich thrombus three days after intimal abrasion of the pig aorta. The internal elastic lamina is clearly intact showing that the damage was superficial. Some expansion of the intimal cell population is already apparent, though the precise differentiation of these new cells is not obvious at this stage. (H & E × 410.)

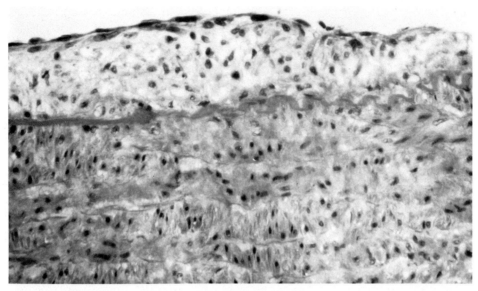

FIGURE 3–5. Fibromuscular intimal hyperplasia ten days postabrasion. This photograph shows obvious intimal hyperplasia in the pig aorta ten days after intimal abrasion. There is a single layer of surface cells which may or may not be endothelium, and a very considerable degree of expansion of the intimal connective tissue cell population. (H & E × 250.)

scopic and ultrastructural evidence of reen-dothelialization can be seen at the edges of the denuded areas of intima, and islands of flattened cells can be seen spread out over the surface of the thrombi.[37] Ten days after intimal injury, the remains of the thrombus (now greatly reduced in bulk) can be seen to have become incorporated within the substance of the vessel wall (Fig. 3–8). However, while on light microscopic examination the denuded area of intima appears to be fully covered by this stage, it is by no means certain

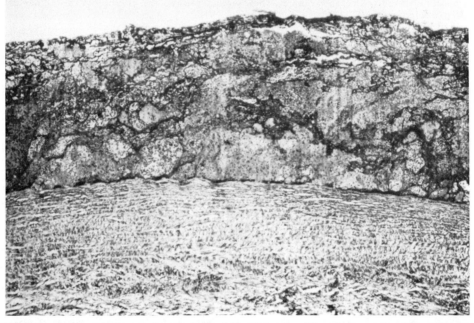

FIGURE 3–6. Sections of pig aorta four days after intimal abrasion. There is a large mural thrombus attached to the intima; this thrombus exceeds that of the media in thickness. The thrombus consists of a network of darkly staining fibrin admixed with pale staining platelets. (Picro-Mallory Stain × 24.)

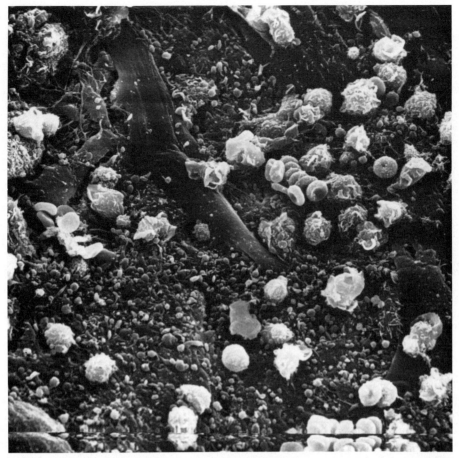

FIGURE 3–7. Rabbit aorta following balloon catheter injury. Numerous small areas of endothelial denudation are still present five weeks after injury. These areas of platelets and macrophages are adherent. (Scanning electron micrograph × 2,160.)

that this cellular covering is made up of normal endothelial cells. Scanning electron microscopic studies of areas of endothelial denudation produced by balloon catheter injury show that even after as long a postinjury period as five weeks, the new endothelium has an abnormal pattern. The new cells differ in size from one another and lack the regular arrangement so characteristic of the normal endothelial surface. Small raw areas and little "craters" can also be seen together with adherent large mononuclear phagocytes and small groups of platelets. One year after balloon-induced injury in the rat carotid artery,[38] the endothelium at the site was not fully regenerated and had ceased proliferating. Part of the luminal surface was lined by smooth muscle cells over which platelet adhesion was only marginally increased as compared with the adjacent endothelial cells. Thus, in arteries, a new steady state may be

produced in the absence of endothelium at the site of injury, although low-grade platelet adhesion may maintain smooth muscle proliferation.

In experimental mural thrombus in the pig aorta,[32] evidence of proliferation of mesenchymal cells within and around the thrombi can be seen within a comparatively short time. Within ten days from the time of injury the remains of the thrombus are separated from the luminal surface by several layers of cells, the histogenesis of which is far from clear.

The ultrastructural changes occurring in such organizing thrombi have been described, and one study[37] found that the early stages of organization of experimentally induced mural thrombi were characterized by the presence of at least two distinct cell populations. In view of the almost universal acceptance of the proposition that the smooth muscle cell in the post-thrombotic neointima

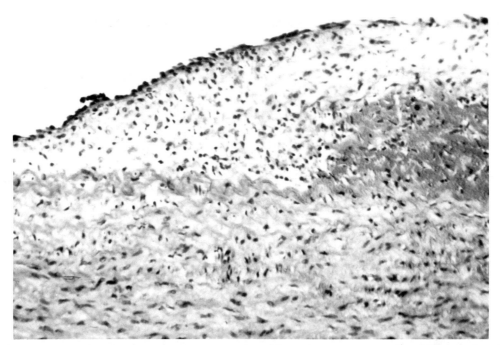

FIGURE 3–8. Buried thrombus ten days. A small plaque-like lesion is apparent even at this relatively early stage. The remains of the postabrasion thrombus are clearly visible within the depths of the neointima and this is covered by a cell-rich mass of connective tissue. The whole lesion bears, both in its shape and in the presence of a basal mass covered by a connective tissue cap, some resemblance to a spontaneous atherosclerotic plaque.

is always derived from the media, this study, in which a dissenting view of their origin is expressed, is worthy of consideration. One of the two cell types seen in the first few days after thrombus formation was clearly a mononuclear phagocyte, probably derived from the circulating blood. The second cell population comprised rather simple mesenchymal cells with haphazardly arranged intracytoplasmic fibrils. These were found lying along the luminal surface of the thrombus, but cells with identical ultrastructural features were found lying deeply within the substance of the thrombus at the same time after injury. Within a comparatively short time (three days after the stage just described), these relatively undifferentiated cells were replaced by cells that showed morphological features related to the acquisition of more specialized functions—notably, those associated with differentiation towards smooth muscle. At the same time, new vascular channels developed, which connected the depths of the thrombus with the main arterial lumen. However, before this linking of the arterial lumen and the substance of the thrombus was accomplished, small lumina appeared within the center of

some of the mesenchymal cell clumps, and in due time these came to be lined by new endothelial cells in no way different from those that appeared on the surface of the thrombus. Other members of this same cell population within the depths of the thrombus showed peripheral condensation of the intracytoplasmic filaments, developed fusiform dense bodies, and in some instances became bounded by basement membrane substance. These changes, all of which were accomplished within 10 to 12 days of injury (and hence, by implication, of thrombus formation) represent, in short, a considerable degree of differentiation towards smooth muscle.

Within three weeks of intimal injury and the consequent mural thrombosis there was a large population of easily recognizable smooth muscle cells which were concentrated in layers parallel to and just beneath the new luminal surface and overlying any thrombus which might still be (and often was) present. In the first few weeks, smooth muscle cells of this degree of maturity were certainly not seen to be invading the thrombus in its abluminal aspect. Within the first three days,[39] the medial smooth muscle immediately beneath the thrombus usually underwent necrosis with collapse of the elastic laminae one upon the other. These observations suggest that, in this model at least, the smooth muscle cell population of the neointima may not be derived from the underlying smooth muscle of the media by a process of colonization.

After three weeks there was a fibromuscular plaque at the site of injury (Fig. 3–9). In some instances, a fair amount of stainable lipid was present, most of which appeared to be within the smooth muscle cells of the neointima. These lesions did not appear to regress readily, and in some, the fibromuscular tissue proliferation resulted in the formation of large plaques. In some of these there was a central lipid pool containing foam cells and cholesterol clefts constituting a homologue, in morphological terms, of the human fibrolipid plaque.

That this rapid and marked degree of intimal proliferation is associated with the incorporation of thrombotic material can be shown by the identification of platelet antigens, first on the raw surface of the intima and covered a few days later by new endothelium and clearly within, rather than merely on, the artery wall. The bulk of the smooth muscle proliferation takes place on the luminal aspect of the newly endothelial-ized thrombus, and it is this that leads to the remains of the original thrombus being buried deeply within the thickened intima, often in close proximity to the internal elastic lamina.

Lipid Accumulation Within Post-thrombotic Experimentally Induced Plaques

In the pig, a single direct injury to the intima can result, in some instances, in a fibromuscular plaque with a central lipid-rich core. Similar lipid-containing intimal lesions form after experimental pulmonary embolization in the rabbit.[40] A single injury does not appear to produce this effect in the systemic arteries of normolipidemic rabbits,[41] but where the injury is repeated or continuous, then the full spectrum of atherosclerotic lesions as encountered in man may be seen. It is possible that the difference may be related to the actual bulk of fresh thrombus induced in these model systems. A single balloon catheter injury produces a thin "carpet" of platelets rather than a bulky thrombus,[42] whereas reinjury of a previously damaged artery results in the formation of a thrombus considerably larger than that pro-

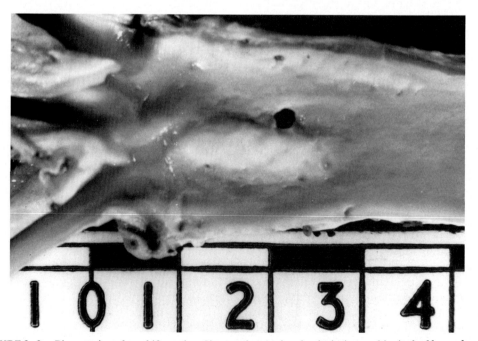

FIGURE 3–9. Pig aorta just above bifurcation. Six months previously, the intima at this site had been abraded with a gauze swab. At the site of injury there is now a large, white fibrous plaque.

duced by the first injury.[43] In experiments in which wires made of a magnesium-aluminium alloy were placed in the rabbit aorta,[44] lipid-laden macrophages could be identified in the thrombotic lesions up to three weeks from the time of the initial injury. After three weeks, extracellular lipid droplets appeared within the thickened intima and increased steadily thereafter, so that by two months a central lipid pool was well developed. The lipid composition of these post-thrombotic lesions showed a marked increase in both the free cholesterol and the cholesterol ester fraction.[45] Two weeks after insertion of the wire, the ester content of the thickened intima was six times greater than that of the normal intima. The fatty acid content of this ester showed an increase in the oleic:linoleic ratio, and C14-labeled oleic acid was preferentially incorporated into the cholesterol ester. Both these findings suggest that the ester content in some of the post-thrombotic lesions can be attributed, at least in part, to local synthesis within the artery wall.

The source of the lipid in post-thrombotic intimal lesions is uncertain. Duguid[46] suggested that the source of lipid might be the red cell membrane. However, foam cell accumulation occurs in the rabbit pulmonary embolization even if the emboli introduced were free from red cells.[31] The platelet, which is much richer in lipid than the red cell,[47] has also been canvassed as a major source of lipid in post-thrombotic and postembolic plaques. Certainly the morphological equivalent of foam cells can be found without difficulty in organizing thrombi, both in humans and in animals,[48] and similar foamy phagocytic cells can be seen after short-term culture of artificial thrombi prepared from platelet-rich plasma in rotating plastic loops. While this hypothesis is very attractive, chemical analyses of human plaques[49] suggest that the lipid profiles, when compared with those of platelets and, indeed, of thrombi, differ considerably. Woolf[50] showed that lipid present both in partly organized thrombi derived from human autopsy or operation samples, and in artificial in vitro thrombi prepared by the Chandler method in rotating plastic loops, was in the form of immunologically identifiable low-density lipoprotein. The antigen occurred in close spatial relation both to fibrin and platelets. Interestingly, it appeared to be present in greater amounts in spontaneously occurring human thrombi than in the "artificial thrombi," suggesting

that increments of low-density lipoprotein may be acquired during the natural history of the thrombi. The possibility that insudation and entrapment play a part in such accumulation of low-density lipoprotein is strengthened by the observation that mural thrombi which, presumably, were in contact with a passing stream of blood, consistently showed more fluorescence when treated with dye-coupled anti–low-density lipoprotein than did occlusive thrombi. Friedman and his colleagues[51] also imply that the lipid which accumulates in some post-thrombotic plaques is derived from the plasma. Their results differ from those described previously in that stainable lipid was found only in the plaques of rabbits which were hyperlipidemic at the time of injury. The stainable lipid in these lesions did not appear in those parts of the new intima which were in closest contact with the luminal blood, but in the deepest areas, either adjacent to or actually within the underlying media. In Friedman's view, the accumulation of lipid was due primarily to escape of a lipid-containing moiety of plasma from newly formed vessels within the post-thrombotic plaque, this egress of lipid owing to abnormal permeability of the new vessels. It is clear, therefore, that lipid can accumulate within experimentally induced post-thrombotic or postembolic plaques and that these can come to resemble, in some degree, spontaneous fibrolipid plaques as seen in human disease.

The Role of Platelets in the Initiation of Intimal Proliferation Following Injury

The important issue is whether the intimal hyperplasia that follows experimental mural thrombosis is caused by thrombus/vessel wall interaction or is simply a consequence of a direct injury to the endothelium and smooth muscle cells of the vessel wall. There are sources of growth factors other than platelets, including endothelium, macrophages and smooth muscle cells. The whole sequence of fibromuscular plaque formation, however, can occur in systemic arteries distal to an area of intimal abrasion where no intimal trauma has been applied. Similarly, pulmonary embolization by platelet-rich thrombi results in the formation of plaque-like lesions that may be rich in both lipid and connective tissue. Clearly, therefore, direct trauma is not a prerequisite of experimentally induced intimal smooth muscle cell proliferation.

THE RELATIONSHIP OF THE PLATELET COUNT TO MYOINTIMAL HYPERPLASIA

Predosing of rabbits with platelet antiserum to produce severe thrombocytopenia has been shown to largely inhibit the fibromuscular proliferation that follows denudation of arterial endothelium.[52,53] In the study carried out by Friedman and his colleagues, the mean platelet count was reduced from 36,000/cubic millimeter to 5,600/cubic millimeter by daily injections of highly specific sheep antirabbit platelet serum; 28 days after balloon catheter injury, the denuded intima in the control animals showed the usual brisk intimal reaction, the mean number of layers of intimal smooth muscle cells being 18.2. In contrast, the mean number of smooth muscle cell layers in the thrombocytopenic animals was 1.0. The inhibition of plaque formation following balloon catheter injury reported by these authors was related both to the degree of thrombocytopenia achieved and to the interval between the course of injections of platelet antiserum and traumatic injury of the aortic endothelium. Platelet counts of less than 7,000/cubic millimeter were necessary for the inhibition of intimal smooth muscle cell proliferation. Similarly, two to three days' treatment with serum platelet antiserum were necessary before the arterial injury if intimal hyperplasia were to be prevented. These results suggest that the postulated interaction between platelets and the arterial wall which results in the formation of a thickened neointima requires only a small number of intact platelets.

ANTIPLATELET DRUGS IN CHRONIC ENDOTHELIAL INJURY

Harker and his colleagues have devised a primate model of chronic endothelial injury by the experimental induction of homocystinemia. These studies, which were originally designed to elucidate the mechanisms involved in the progressive atherogenesis that is a feature of humans with homocystinemia, showed that long-term infusion of homocystine leads to the loss of up to 10 per cent of the aortic endothelium.[54] Platelet consumption was increased threefold in these animals, presumably indicating adhesion and aggregation of platelets over areas of endothelial denudation. After three months of homocystinemia, the animals were reported to have typical atherosclerotic plaques with 10 to 15 layers of smooth muscle cells, the usual connective tissue matrix constituents, and both intracellular and extracellular lipid. When these animals were given the phosphodiesterase inhibitor dipyridamole, both the increase in platelet consumption and the formation of a thickened neointima in the areas of endothelial cell loss were inhibited. The endothelial cell loss induced by homocystine infusions was in no way altered by the administration of dipyridamole, and it seems reasonable to assume, therefore, that interference with certain platelet functions by this drug, which inhibits both primary and secondary adenosine diphosphate-induced platelet aggregation and, in high concentrations, the platelet release reaction,[55] is the means by which the smooth muscle cell proliferation characteristic of neointima formation is inhibited. In the rat, when endothelial cells are removed by air drying of isolated segments of artery,[56] no correlation between the effects produced on platelet aggregability in vitro by aspirin, reserpine, and flurbiprofen, and those related to the putative effects of platelets on the subendothelial elements of the artery wall following endothelial denudation were found. When these drugs were given at a dose level sufficient to inhibit thrombin-induced platelet aggregation, there was no inhibition of myointimal thickening following endothelial removal. However, Karnovsky is quoted[57] as having found that dipyridamole did have an inhibiting effect of smooth muscle cell proliferation in his model, and this has been confirmed.[58] In another series of experiments, Clowes and Karnovsky[59] found that heparin in doses sufficient to prevent clotting markedly suppressed intimal smooth muscle cell proliferation following air-induced injury to the arterial endothelium, even though endothelial regeneration proceeded without any impairment. This heparin-related suppression of smooth muscle cell proliferation is of great interest because of the wide range of biological activities which this compound possesses. Clowes and Karnovsky suggest that heparin might act directly on smooth muscle cells. Alternatively, because of its charge, heparin might bind and inactivate platelet growth factor. It is possible that heparin might exert its effect indirectly through the clotting system, since thrombin and the other serine proteases activated at the denuded intimal surface might be mitogenic for smooth muscle cells,[60,61] or might generate smooth muscle cell mitogens from the adherent platelets.[62] In a similar model of intimal injury induced by air drying in the rat carotid artery defibrinogenation by Arvin, the size of the subsequent lesions[63] was also reduced, and later work showed that inhibition of fibrinolysis by oral administration of tranexamic acid enhanced lesion development. Plasminogen activator is expressed in the arterial wall after injury, and its inhibition may lead to persistence of fibrin, in turn invoking smooth muscle cell proliferation.[64]

DEFECTIVE PLATELET ADHESION AND ATHEROSCLEROSIS

The experimental data presented so far support the concept that platelet–vessel wall interaction can lead to local proliferation of smooth muscle cells and the extracellular connective tissue matrix characteristic of atherosclerotic plaques. For such interactions to take place, adhesion of platelets to exposed subendothelial elements, or perhaps to altered endothelial cells, is a prerequisite. If this is so, might a decrease in the adhesion of platelets influence atherogenesis? Von Willebrand's disease (vWd) constitutes a paradigm for this situation. Various anomalies of platelet function have been described in this bleeding disorder, such as impaired retention of platelets in glass bead filters and impaired ristocetin-induced platelet aggregation. Baumgartner and his colleagues have demonstrated impaired adhesion of platelets from patients suffering from von Willebrand's disease to the subendothelial surface of rabbit aorta.[65] These studies were performed by perfusing citrated blood (at arterial shear rates) through a chamber which contained segments of rabbit aorta from which the endothelium had been removed previously by means of balloon catheterization. The reduction of platelet adhesion with von Willebrand's disease blood has been recorded as ranging from 47 per cent[66] to 24 per cent.[67] The magnitude of this platelet adhesion defect is increased if the vessel segments in the perfusion chamber are first treated with alpha-chymotrypsin, or if the citrate content of the perfused blood is increased.[68] It is also strongly related to the shear rate at which the blood is perfused, being increased at high shear rates and decreased at lower ones.[67,69] In this system, a striking increase in adhesion was obtained if factor VIII was added to the citrated von Willebrand's disease blood before perfusion.[70]

For several years, a colony of pigs with von Willebrand's disease has been maintained.[71] These animals have all the hemostatic abnormalities found in the severe form of the disease in humans. When some of these pigs died from bleeding, the unexpected discovery was made that they showed negligible aortic atherosclerosis when compared with hemostatically normal pigs of the same age, prompting a series of elegant studies, both in the intact animal and in cell culture systems. In a study of the frequency of spontaneous lesions, the aortae of 11 pigs with the homozygous form of von Willebrand's disease were compared with those of 11 normal pigs of the same ages. Six of the controls showed multiple raised lesions. In contrast, none of the pigs with von Willebrand's disease had multiple plaques, and in only one of the animals was there a single plaque larger than 2 millimeters in diameter. However, in seven of the eleven von Willebrand's disease pigs, the portions of the aorta free from lesions showed extensive fatty infiltration after staining with Sudan IV, this change involving 5 to 30 per cent of the intimal surface. On histological examination, this accumulation of lipid within the intima was seen to be unaccompanied by any proliferation of intimal smooth muscle cells. When similar groups of animals were fed with a diet rich in tallow and cholesterol, a marked difference was found in the frequency of aortic lesions, the von Willebrand's disease pigs being affected to a lesser degree than the control. The differences were significant at the 1 per cent level. Despite this resistance to atherosclerosis, the intimal surfaces of the von Willebrand's disease pigs were not immune to injury, since the intravital injection of Evans' blue (prior to sacrifice) showed patchy dark blue staining of the luminal surface, and on scanning electron microscopy, these blue areas appeared grossly abnormal.

In normal animals, von Willebrand factor can be identified not only in plasma, but also in endothelial cells, platelets, and megakaryocytes. Its absence from the plasma, however, appears to be particularly significant in inhibiting atherogenesis in the von Willebrand's disease pig. This is suggested by the results obtained in a set of transplant experiments.[71] When normal porcine aorta segments were transplanted into the aortae of von Willebrand's disease pigs, the immunohistologically identifiable von Willebrand factor in the vasa vasorum was soon lost, and the transplanted segments were resistant to the formation of atherosclerotic plaques in the same way as the host artery. In contrast, when portions of aorta from vWd pigs were transplanted into normal pig aortae, the vasa acquired the von Willebrand factor, and atherosclerotic lesions developed in these segments. Fass[72] has reported some interesting studies, using cultured endothelial cells from normal and vWd pigs. The endothelial cells of normal pigs contain fibers which bind antibodies to von Willebrand factor in both immunofluorescent and peroxidase systems. The "von Willebrand endothelial cells" can also be seen to contain fibers when examined by scanning electron microscopy, but these fail to bind antibody to von Willebrand's disease factor. Platelets adhere to monolayers of endothelial cells from normal pigs when they are damaged, but fail to do so under similar circumstances when the cells are derived from vWd pigs. Interestingly, the platelet adhesion to damaged normal cells can be abolished by pretreatment with antibody to porcine von Willebrand factor. The resistance of the homozygous strain of von Willebrand's disease pigs to the induction of atherosclerosis has been confirmed.[73] However, when the coronary arteries of pigs heterozygous for von Willebrand's disease were injured with a balloon catheter, a brisk degree of intimal smooth muscle proliferation was observed. Such pigs (heterozygotes) have also been noted to develop atherosclerotic lesions without trauma to the intima.

Platelet Adhesion and Endothelial Damage in Spontaneous Atherosclerosis

In the pig model of smooth muscle cell proliferation described above, platelet adhesion has occurred secondary to a deliberately induced endothelial injury of various kinds. While models of this sort have much to tell us of the end results of interaction between platelets and connective tissue elements of the intima, it is right to question whether they have any counterpart in spontaneous atherogenesis in any species, including man. One species exists, the white carneau pigeon, which, independent of diet and other environmental circumstances, regularly develops atherosclerotic lesions in highly predictable areas and with a well-defined time course.[74] Over a period of three years, virtually all white carneau pigeons will develop atherosclerosis, and if they are allowed to survive for seven to eight years, 70 per cent of the birds will develop coronary atherosclerosis. Lewis and Kottke[75] have reported that the earliest morphological changes in the arteries of these species are an extensive "ruffling" of the luminal plasma membranes of the endothelial cells. This is followed by the appearance of pits and craters in the endothelium, leading to areas of endothelial denudation. These raw areas are regularly associated with the presence of adherent and sometimes aggregated platelets, which are attached to subendothelial fibrils and to altered endothelial cells. In addition to the platelets, a considerable number of macrophages are seen. These changes precede the accumulation of lipids and the onset of intimal smooth muscle cell proliferation, and constitute persuasive evidence of a role for the platelet in spontaneous as well as in experimental atherogenesis.

Interaction Between Platelets and Arterial Smooth Muscle Cells

If the adhesion of platelets to the injured artery wall is followed by localized smooth muscle cell proliferation, how is this brought about? Such insights as we possess at the moment were initiated by the studies of Russell Ross and his colleagues.[76] These workers have shown that media-derived, arterial smooth muscle cell cultures, grown in a medium containing allogeneic, cell-free, plasma-derived serum, remain for the most part quiescent, only about 3 per cent of the cells synthesizing DNA. However, if serum derived from whole blood which has been allowed to clot is added to the culture medium, the smooth muscle cell begins to proliferate quite rapidly. It has now been shown that the chief mitogenic effector of such "whole blood" serum is platelet-derived growth factor. This factor owes its release into the medium to the process of platelet adhesion and the subsequent platelet release reaction. Its relation to platelets can be demonstrated by adding an aliquot of purified platelets to culture media containing serum made from cell-free plasma. Mitogenic activity is conferred on this serum; the existence of a platelet-derived growth factor was confirmed by Kohler and Lipton,[77] who showed that freeze-thawing of a purified preparation of platelets provides a supernatant that is mitogenic for 3T3 cells in culture, and by Westermark and Wasteson,[78] who found that glial cells in culture were also stimulated to proliferate by a platelet growth factor. The mitogenic principle resides in the alpha-granules of the platelet[79] together with platelet factor 4 and alpha-thromboglobulin. Platelets which have no alpha-granules (as in the grey platelet syndrome) fail to stimulate the growth of arterial smooth muscle cells in culture.

After purification, the platelet growth factor is a dimer composed of two homologous polypeptide chains, A and B. One has a molecular weight of 28,000 daltons and appears to be the more active of the two, and the other has a molecular weight of 13,000 daltons. Both are highly cationic and resist inactivation, even by boiling. The effect of the growth factor on the smooth muscle cell is more complex and far reaching than that of a pure mitogen, since it rapidly (within three hours) increases endocytosis of, for example, horseradish peroxidase; it enhances protein synthesis, particularly of collagen, and, within two to three hours, it stimulates the synthesis of cholesterol by the cultured cells.[76] Ross and his co-workers[76] have suggested that the platelet growth factor has the capacity to recruit smooth muscle cells that are in G_0 (the prolonged postmitotic pause) to enter G_1 (postmitotic phase) and, thus, the reproductive cycle. It is thought that in vivo the intimal smooth muscle cells are normally in the quiescent state. The removal of endothelial cells and the consequent exposure of subendothelial tissue elements leads to platelet adhesion, aggregation, and release, with the production of an increase in smooth muscle cell turnover. An obligatory requirement for platelets in the smooth muscle proliferation that occurs after endothelial denudation is not, however, the entire story. In the balloon-injured rat carotid artery, smooth muscle proliferation continues after new recruitment of platelets over the denuded area has ceased.[38,80,81] After balloon injury of the

rat, carotid artery messenger ribonucleic acid for platelet-derived growth factor-A is expressed within the mesenchymal cells of a narrow zone in the intima immediately beneath the denuded area. These cells do not express either the A-chain receptor or platelet-derived growth factor-B. Throughout the intima, smooth muscle cells express the platelet-derived growth factor-B receptor. The results strongly suggest that autocrine stimulation of smooth muscle cells is occurring in the reparative phase after injury.[82] In an experimental model in which a suture is passed through the rat aorta and left in situ to produce thrombus within one week, mesenchymal cells expressing platelet-derived growth factor-A messenger ribonucleic acid, but not containing actin, appear. By three weeks the thrombus has been replaced by mesenchymal cells which now do not contain messenger ribonucleic acid for platelet-derived growth factor-A, but which have all the morphological features of smooth muscle cells and contain actin.[82] It can be concluded that either these mesenchymal cells are not derived from the media by migration, or that smooth muscle cells which migrate from the media may initially be modified with regard to the expression of contractile proteins. Platelet-derived growth factor is known to influence smooth muscle expression of actin.[83] Whatever the relation of the early mesenchymal cell to the smooth muscle cell, it is clear that platelet-derived growth factor derived from platelets is only a part of that potentially available in the vessel wall.

Other cell-derived factors exist that also appear to be capable of stimulating the growth of cells in culture. The rate of growth of 3T3 fibroblasts is increased when either endothelial cells or the medium in which endothelial cells have been cultured are added. The factor released into the culture medium by endothelial cells stimulates endothelial cell growth as well.[76] This factor is nondialyzable, sensitive to trypsin, and unlike the platelet growth factor, is completely destroyed by heating to 100° centigrade. Macrophages, according to the same authority, also secrete growth factors.

Mural Thrombi and their Contribution to Plaque Growth

Much of the resurgent interest in a possible role for the incorporation of mural thrombosis as a contributor to plaque growth stems from the studies of J. B. Duguid.[46] Duguid put forward the view that many of the lesions we now classify as atherosclerosis are in fact altered thrombi which, by the ordinary process of organization, have been transformed into fibrous thickenings. This, as Duguid himself pointed out, represents a partial return to the "encrustation" hypothesis enunciated by Rokinansky a century before.

IDENTIFICATION OF MURAL THROMBI AND THEIR RESIDUA IN ATHEROSCLEROTIC PLAQUES

It is possible in human plaques to identify transitions between recent mural thrombi, subendothelial deposits of thrombus, and the old remains of previously incorporated mural thrombi by the use of conventional histological techniques. Duguid's description[46] of the natural history of aortic mural thrombi was derived in just this way.

Duguid's observations were confirmed in a relatively short time by Heard,[84] who found similar features in stenosed renal arteries, by Morgan[85] in coronary arteries, and more recently, reemphasized in human coronary lesions.[86] Nearly 30 years ago, Crawford and Levene[25] carried out a study of the frequency and appearance of mural thrombi in the human aorta. In selecting blocks of artery for study, these workers avoided atherosclerotic plaques, and instead chose areas of aorta which appeared normal on naked-eye examination, but which when examined with a hand lens, showed some slight irregularity of the intimal surface. Of 99 such areas examined, 19 showed surface encrustations, ten showed superficial but definitely subendothelial deposits, and 24 showed fibrin situated deeply within the intima. In the same study, these workers also described the process of abluminal vascularization and organization of mural thrombi. Crawford and Levene's work found strong support in a series of papers by Movat, Haust, and More,[87] in which they make the point that the cells most active in the surface organization of mural thrombi are modified smooth muscle cells. The outstanding response of the artery wall to the presence of experimentally induced thrombi is proliferation of these same smooth muscle cells.

IMMUNOHISTOLOGICAL DEMONSTRATIONS OF FIBRIN IN THE HUMAN ARTERY WALL

All these studies depend essentially on the demonstration of thrombotic material on or within the arterial intima. While fibrin can be demonstrated in paraffin-embedded tissue sections by such methods as Mallory's phosphotungstic acid-hematoxylin stain or the picro-Mallory trichrome technique, it is, from the histological point of view, a substance which rapidly loses its specific staining characteristics with aging. The reactivity of fibrin with various staining reagents varies, depending on the circumstances of its formation and cross-linkage. Failure to show its presence within any single plaque by conventional histological methods probably has little validity and has led to an underrecording of the frequency with which fibrin is present in atherosclerotic lesions.

The need for more sensitive and reliable means for the identification of fibrin in the artery wall is largely met by the use of immunohistochemical methods on tissue sections. Antisera prepared in rabbits to human fibrin demonstrate fibrin or fibrinogen to be present even in aortic fatty streaks.[88] When a wide range of atherosclerotic lesions is examined for the presence of immunologically identifiable fibrinogen-related antigen, it becomes obvious that the antigen can be present within the thickened intima in two principal morphological forms. In the first of these, the antigen is diffusely distributed in the form of minute flecks of fluorescent material, so that at low magnification the whole of the thickened intima appears to exhibit apple-green fluorescence. In the second (Fig. 3–10), the antigen appears in the form of brilliantly fluorescent coarse aggregates of material which may exist as surface encrustations or, more frequently, lie at different levels within the plaque substance roughly parallel to the luminal surface. It has been suggested[89] that these widely disparate distribution patterns of the antifibrin-binding antigen represent the morphological expression of two distinct pathogenetic mechanisms; infiltration and binding of fibrinogen within the intima on the one hand, and incorporation of mural thrombus on the other. The demonstration of fibrin(ogen) in atherosclerotic plaques by such immunohistological techniques has been confirmed by a number of studies,[90] but in at least one study, the

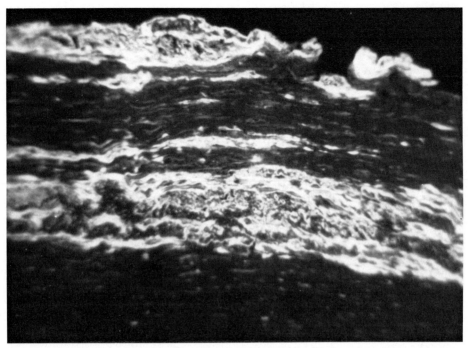

FIGURE 3–10. Frozen section of a human, aortic, raised fibrolipid plaque treated with a fluorescein-labeled antibody raised against human fibrin. There is a series of discrete bands of fibrin within the plaque cap at different levels. These bands represent the residua of previous episodes of thrombosis.

demonstration of fibrin within the artery wall is not regarded as representing the residuum of mural thrombus.[91]

The distribution of fibrinogen and its breakdown products in human atherosclerotic plaques has been reexamined by Bini and his colleagues[92] using a wide range of recently available monoclonal antibodies. Fibrin I is formed by thrombin cleavage at Aα 16-17 after release of fibrinopeptide A, fibrin II is formed by cleavage at both Aα 16-17 and Bβ 14-15 with release of fibrinopeptides A and B. Fragment D is a degradation product released by plasmin from fibrinogen; fragment DD is a degradation product of plasmin released from crosslinked fibrin II. When early lesions (that is, fatty streaks and small raised plaques) were examined, fibrinogen and fibrin I or II were present but not degradation products. In later plaques, fibrin I and II and both the degradation products produced by plasmin were present. The results suggest that conversion of insuded fibrinogen to fibrin and its subsequent degradation is a feature of plaque progression independent of the presence of surface thrombus formation. Fibrin or its degrada-

tion products may be a further factor stimulating smooth muscle proliferation in plaque growth. Studies of advanced aortic plaques taken from patients dying from myocardial infarction showed lower concentrations of fibrin degradation products and plasminogen than in equivalent plaques taken from control subjects. These data suggest a reduction of fibrinolytic activity within the plaques and therefore a persistence of fibrin.[93]

PLATELET ANTIGENS IN HUMAN ATHEROSCLEROTIC PLAQUES

The presence of fibrin within atherosclerotic plaques has been accepted by some as constituting prima facie evidence in favor of a contributory role for mural thrombosis in plaque growth. The crucial question, however, is whether the fibrin is derived from incorporated mural thrombus or from an infiltrating stream of fibrinogen. While this point is well taken insofar as the presence of fibrin is concerned, it would lose much of its validity if aggregates of platelets could be identified within the depths of atherosclerotic plaques, since their presence could not reasonably be ascribed to any mechanism other than the incorporation of thrombus.

The presence of platelet masses within atherosclerotic lesions was first convincingly demonstrated by Carstairs.[94] Approaching the problem histologically, he found that the platelet and fibrin components of recent thrombi could be differentially stained by the use of the Lendrum picro-Mallory method, provided that the blocks of tissue were fixed in formaldehyde-saline for the period of not less than 48 hours. If these conditions are met, the platelets stain a leaden blue color, while the strands of fibrin appear a clear bright red. If other fixatives such as Zenker's fluid are used, then the platelets and fibrin are both stained red and thus cannot be differentiated from each other.

Carstairs also described a method for the preparation of a highly specific antiplatelet serum which did not cross-react with fibrin.[95]

Relationship Between Platelet Antigens and Fibrin in Atherosclerosis Plaques

Binding of the fluoroscein-coupled human fibrin antisera occurs in two basic distribution patterns, the character of which gave rise to the suggestion that both infiltration and mural thrombosis might account for the presence of fibrin in atherosclerotic lesions. The presence of platelet masses constitutes unequivocal evidence of thrombus incorporation. With these considerations in mind, Woolf and Carstairs[96] sought to clarify the relationship, if any, between the different forms of antifibrin binding and the presence of platelet antigens in the same lesions. This assessment was made by studying sequential frozen sections of atherosclerotic plaques of different macroscopic type after treatment with both antifibrin and antiplatelet sera. The dual objective was to assess the relative frequency of the two types of antifibrin binding in relation to the macroscopic character of the lesions and the degree of correlation which existed between these patterns and the presence of clumps of platelet antigen.

Fatty streaks and small lipid plaques with no significant connective tissue cap showed a uniformly diffuse pattern of antifibrin binding, suggesting the presence of fibrinogen derived from the infiltration of plasma. No platelet antigens could be demonstrated in these lesions. In contrast, opaque fibrolipid plaques with a well-marked connective tissue cap showed the presence of the localized, banded pattern of antifibrin binding, suggesting the presence of polymerized fibrin in 38 out of 56 lesions. Platelet antigens (Fig. 3–11) could also be identified in just under half the lesions showing this pattern. From these results the inference was drawn that the presence of immunohistologically identifiable fibrin in the form of discrete band-like masses within fibrolipid plaques suggests that these accumulations represent the residuum of incorporated, incompletely organized thrombus. Similar findings have been reported by Hudson and McCaughey.[97]

That platelet antigens could be identified in only half the raised lesions to which incorporation of thrombus is deemed to have made a contribution raises a number of possibilities. The absence of identifiable platelet antigens from any single lesion could mean that platelets were never present in relation to that lesion, and that incorporation of mural thrombus played no part in its growth. Alternatively, platelets might be present at an earlier stage of the natural history of that lesion, but were no longer identifiable at necropsy. It is impossible from a study of human lesions to prove which of the hypotheses is correct, but some useful information relating to this has accrued from an experimental study in which mural thrombi were induced by light abrasion of the luminal surface of the pig aorta.[98] Within 30 days of the mural thrombi having been formed, fibromuscular plaques were present at the operation site. Sampling of the lesions at different times after operation showed that platelets are easily identifiable, first on (and later within) the intima, during the first three weeks after operation. Thereafter the number of lesions in which platelet antigens were identifiable fell off sharply, so that by six months platelet could be found in only 10 per cent of the lesions. Thus, in experimental situations, post-thrombotic fibromuscular plaques can be produced in which histological evidence of the original contribution by platelets is completely lacking.

FREQUENCY OF THROMBUS INCORPORATION IN HUMAN ATHEROSCLEROSIS

The frequency with which morphological features (either histological or immunohis-

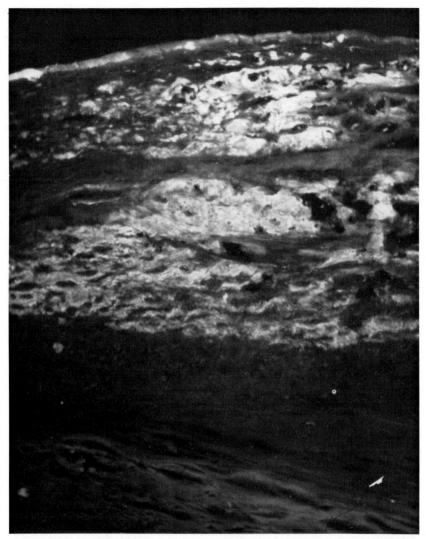

FIGURE 3–11. Frozen sections of a human, aortic, raised fibrolipid plaque treated with a fluorescein-labeled antihuman platelet serum. The plaque cap shows discrete bands of fluorescent material lying parallel to the vessel surface. These bands represent the residua of previous episodes of thrombosis, in a manner analogous to that seen in raised lesions treated with antifibrinogen antibodies. The thrombi have become incorporated within the plaque.

tochemical) occur, suggesting the presence of buried thrombus within atherosclerotic plaques, has been reviewed.[27] In the aorta there appears to be a fair degree of uniformity, as far as the proportion of all plaques is concerned (41 to 45 per cent), though there is a considerable degree of scatter when the proportion of cases in which buried thrombus can be found is considered.[99] It is possible that these differences may be related to differences in sampling, since the study which showed buried thrombus to be present in 89 per cent of aortae[99] was one in which every

intact nonulcerated raised lesion in each of 53 aortae was examined.

Studies have been carried out that attempt to relate the frequency with which "thrombotic" plaques could be found within a single vessel to the presence or absence of coronary heart disease in the patient.[99] In these studies, all the uncomplicated fibrolipid plaques in the aortae of 53 patients between 36 and 80 years of age were examined for the presence of the "banded" pattern of antifibrin binding. The 53 patients were divided into three groups: (a) those with no significant degree of coronary artery stenosis; (b) those with recent occlusion of the coronary arteries; and (c) those with histological evidence of old occlusion of the coronary arteries. The proportion of lesions expressed as a percentage of the number of plaques examined from each aorta, showing the localized or "banded" pattern of antifibrin binding was 24 per cent, 51 per cent, and 62 per cent, respectively. Not unexpectedly, a fairly wide scatter is present in each of these three groups. Despite this, a definite relationship is seen to exist between the presence of coronary artery occlusion whether recent or old, and a high frequency of aortic atherosclerotic plaques that show the banded pattern of antifibrin binding. The differences between the recent "occlusion" and "no stenosis" groups were found to be highly significant ($p < 0.001$). Similar results were obtained in a study of a much larger number of cases.[100] In this study, plaques in the coronary arteries, as well as those in the aorta, were examined for the presence of both fibrin and platelets. In the coronary artery plaques, evidence of incorporated thrombus was found in 71 per cent of the patients dying with coronary artery occlusion, and this figure must be interpreted in the light of the tissue blocks examined not having come from occluded segments of the coronary arteries. In those patients dying without evidence either of coronary artery occlusion or of significant degrees of arterial stenosis, "buried" residua of thrombus could be found in only 28 per cent.

The association between incorporated thrombus in raised lesions in the aorta and the presence of occlusive coronary artery disease is of considerable interest. Working from first principles, the increase in the frequency of incorporated thrombus could mean that the onset of the final occlusive episode in the coronary artery tree is preceded by a period in which there is an increased tendency for thrombi to form throughout the arterial system, and the observed differences between the aortic plaques of patients dying with recent coronary occlusion and those dying with old coronary artery occlusion could be taken as supporting this view. It is possible that such a period could be of relatively short duration, since animal studies at least[101] have shown that incorporation of thrombus can occur quite rapidly. It is equally possible that, in such patients, thrombolytic mechanisms might be impaired. The data also emphasize that thrombosis plays a major role in the intermittent growth of many plaques over long periods of time in an individual subject. Occasionally, one of the plaques in a carotid or coronary artery may undergo a sufficiently large episode of thrombosis that acute ischemic syndromes develop. Such acute clinical events mask the fact that many subclinical episodes of thrombosis will have occurred over many other plaques in that patient.

MORPHOLOGY OF THE ENDOTHELIAL SURFACE OVER ATHEROSCLEROTIC PLAQUES

Animal models of atherosclerosis permit the sequence of changes that occur in the endothelium over plaques to be studied, and also provide material that can be fixed by perfusion with gluteraldehyde for examination by scanning electron microscopy, which is the most appropriate method for showing endothelial surface integrity.

The first morphological change observed within 12 days of instituting high-lipid diets in primates is adhesion of monocytes to the intact endothelial surface followed by their migration into the intima.[21] By 12 weeks, sufficient monocytes have ingested lipid and accumulated within the intima to form visible fatty streaks. At this early stage an increased rate of endothelial cell replication is occurring, and it is postulated that there is desquamation of cells from the surface, but there is no exposure of the underlying connective tissue matrix to cause platelet adhesion.[102,103] The appearance of fibrolipid plaques in animal models is associated with a considerable increase in the number of monocytes on the endothelial surface, and by this stage (usually 3 to 4 months after the induction of hyperlipidemia), large clusters of lipid-filled macrophages form immediately beneath the endothelial surface. Over these aggregates of macrophages, focal defects in the endothelial surface appear (Fig. 3–3), and in some models, platelet adhesion is seen in these areas.[104,105] If similar endothelial denudation occurs over human fibrolipid plaques there would be a very close analogy with the experimental models of endothelial denudation produced by mechanical trauma; thus, all the data relating smooth muscle proliferation to platelet-derived growth factor may be equally relevant to human plaques.

The difficulty in the past has been to

acquire suitably prepared material in man to study the endothelium. Endarterectomy specimens are subject to such trauma in removal that artifactual denudation is inevitable; necropsy material has a deposit of protein and fibrin obscuring the endothelial surface. Explanted hearts removed from the recipients at the time of cardiac transplantation can, however, be perfused instantly, and provide ideal material for a study of endothelial integrity in human atherosclerotic arteries. Such studies[24] show that all the morphological features described in the endothelium of animal models are exactly replicated in man. Endothelial cells over atherosclerotic plaques of all types were irregularly arranged and varied in shape and size. Monocyte adhesion and migration occurred over all types of plaque. Simple fatty streaks had an intact endothelial covering, but over fibrolipid plaques, endothelial denudation ranging from loss of single cells (Fig. 3–12) to larger areas (Fig. 3–13) was common. Such endothelial defects were usually associated with a clustering of macrophages in the most superficial layers of the intima and with adhesion of platelets, undergoing shape change, to the exposed connective tissue (Fig. 3–14).

THROMBOSIS IN ACUTE ISCHEMIC SYNDROMES IN MAN

The clinical course of patients with coronary atherosclerosis is punctuated by acute episodes of myocardial infarction or unstable angina, and can be terminated by sudden death. In a similar manner, episodes of transient cerebral ischemia and stroke complicate carotid and cerebral atherosclerosis. There is abundant proof, both clinical and from necropsy, that these episodes are precipitated by thrombosis. Such a thrombus is much larger than the microscopic thrombi previously described as being implicated in plaque growth, and can be seen on angioscopy, or as a filling defect within the arterial lumen on angiography in life.

Acute Myocardial Infarction

Coronary thrombosis is now accepted almost everywhere as the factor which precip-

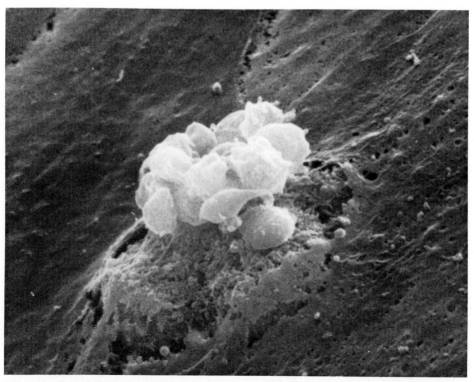

FIGURE 3–12. Scanning electron micrograph of human coronary artery plaque. This photograph shows a denuded area of intima where, apparently, a single endothelial cell has been lost. The raw surface is covered by a small mass of adherent and aggregated platelets which have clearly undergone shape change (× 3,570).

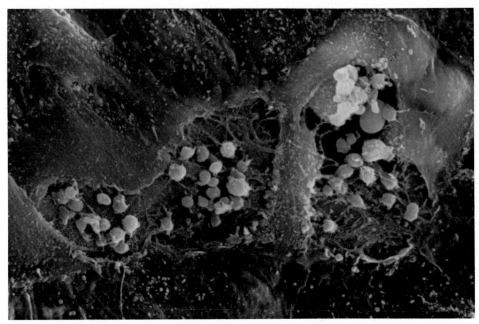

FIGURE 3–13. Scanning electron micrograph of human coronary artery plaque showing fairly extensive endothelial loss associated with the presence of adherent platelets which have undergone shape change (× 1,340).

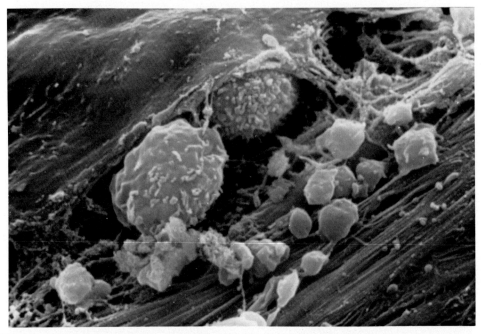

FIGURE 3–14. Scanning electron micrograph of human coronary artery plaque showing monocytes clustered under the edge of an endothelial cell adjacent to an area of denudation injury (× 5,300).

itates regional acute myocardial infarction. This view was not, and could not be, established from data derived from necropsies. Until the advent of angiography, during the early stages of acute infarction in living patients, there were controversies over the causal role of thrombosis.[106,107] The reasons for this historical controversy, which still lingers on amongst some pathologists, are worthy of some considerations.

Strictly speaking, the precise definition of acute myocardial infarction is that of necrosis consequent upon cessation or reduction in myocardial blood flow. Within this definition are encompassed a number of different types of necrosis whose pathophysiologies are very different. There is a range of morphological criteria allowing the identification of an area of myocardial necrosis both on macroscopic and light microscopic examination. The earliest objective change to appear is loss of intracellular enzymes, which can be demonstrated by simple histochemical techniques. Even with such a relatively sensitive method, nonviable cells cannot be identified morphologically until six to eight hours have elapsed from the time they suffered irreversible ischemic damage. Thus a patient may die within an hour or two of the onset of pain with a confident clinical diagnosis of acute infarction which cannot be verified morphologically.

When the patient has lived for a period of time exceeding six to eight hours following the onset of myocardial ischemia, and myocardial necrosis is sufficiently established for enzyme loss to have occurred in the necrotic area, staining of tissue slices of myocardium at necropsy for succinic dehydrogenase activity allows accurate delineation of the border between viable and nonviable tissue. Using this technique, infarcts can be divided into those which are regional (that is, anteroseptal, lateral, or posteroseptal, corresponding to major coronary arterial branches) or those which are more diffuse and cross the territories of two or more coronary arteries. Regional infarcts can be further divided into those which are confined to the subendocardial zone alone, or those which are transmural, extending to the epicardial surface. Coronary thrombosis is related almost exclusively to regional infarction. Pathological studies which included nonregional infarction and cases of sudden death without demonstrable infarction were those which found an inconsistent relation between in-

farction and thrombosis. A further difficulty was the pathological view that occlusive thrombi were relatively static; in reality, angiography in life shows thrombi to be very labile. It was not sufficiently appreciated that the state of blood flow in an artery some hours before death cannot be ascertained from its state at the moment of death. The apparent lack of total concordance between infarction and coronary thrombosis at necropsy led to a view that when thrombosis was present, it could be secondary to the infarction rather than vice versa.[108] All these matters have been resolved by consideration of pathological data obtained at necropsy in association with angiographic, angioscopic, and therapeutic information from living subjects with regional infarction.

REGIONAL TRANSMURAL MYOCARDIAL INFARCTION

Pathological studies in which subjects were selected specifically for the demonstrated presence of transmural regional infarction consistently record the following: first, morphological evidence of a major episode of thrombosis within the artery subtending the infarct; and second, an underlying atherosclerotic plaque which had undergone changes making it "unstable" or thrombogenic.[109–112] The majority of thrombi causing infarction develop due to cracking, splitting, fissuring, or rupture of an atherosclerotic plaque (see later). These pathological studies linking coronary thrombosis with regional transmural infarction have been complemented by data from coronary angiography in life during the development of infarction.[113–114] Within the first four hours of the onset of pain, there is a very high incidence (80 per cent plus) of the subtending artery being occluded, by 12 hours as many as 30 per cent of the arteries will have reopened spontaneously. This proportion becomes as high as 80 per cent if timely thrombolytic therapy is instituted. Following restoration of some antegrade flow, a residual lesion characterized by an area of stenosis with ragged overhanging edges often associated with an intraluminal filling defect appears. Such type II angiographic lesions are now known to be the hallmark of plaques undergoing fissuring and rupture.[111,115] The presence of plaque fissuring, which produces an intensely thrombogenic surface, is the major argument for thrombosis initiating infarction rather than being a secondary phenomenon owing to reduced flow. Injection of radiolabeled fibrinogen or platelets into subjects with established infarction, however, shows that intracoronary thrombosis continues for some time after infarction has occurred.[116,117] Detailed study of the thrombi at necropsy, however, shows that the proximal head of the thrombus is not labeled and thus precedes infarction, while it is the more distal propagated thrombus within the lumen which follows infarction.[107] There are sound theoretical grounds for the existence of a "vicious circle" where once some myocardial necrosis is established, perfusion of that area of myocardium falls due to plugging of the small vessels with polymorphs, endothelial swelling, and capillary collapse caused by tissue pressure. A reduction in the flow in the subtending artery encourages further thrombosis at the site of plaque fissuring. The onset of human infarction is probably always a "stuttering" phenomenon with multiple episodes of intermittent thrombotic occlusion occurring in the hours before the final occlusion. As emphasized above, part of the thrombus in the epicardial artery is indeed a postinfarction phenomenon.

Patients who die from acute transmural regional infarction show a much higher frequency of persistent occlusive coronary thrombosis at autopsy when compared with patients who survive to have coronary angiography in life after a regional transmural infarct. This suggests that the necropsy population is a selected one, and that persistent occlusion, particularly with distal propagation, carries a poor prognosis. This increase in risk of death is mediated by large infarct size, which in turn leads to infarct expansion, cardiogenic shock, and internal or external cardiac rupture.

REGIONAL SUBENDOCARDIAL INFARCTION

Pathological and angiographic studies of this form of infarction suggest that the subtending artery is more frequently patent than in transmural infarction, but that there is thrombosis on an unstable fissured plaque. One explanation is that antegrade flow is restored within the time needed for infarction to spread from the endocardium to the epicardium. This situation can be simulated

in dog models when a coronary artery is occluded and then reopened after a time interval of one to two hours. Another explanation is that previously established collateral flow protects the subepicardial zone.[118] In man, two facets of the pathology of nontransmural as compared with transmural regional infarction stand out. The first facet is that distal propagation of thrombus within the coronary artery is not present and the distal segment fills either by collaterals or by the maintenance or restoration of antegrade flow. The second is that many regional nontransmural infarcts appear to develop by the coalescence of many small foci of infarction of widely differing ages. Thus the pathological basis within the coronary artery of nontransmural infarction has considerable affinity with that of the crescendo form of unstable angina, and the final myocardial lesion may represent the additive effects of several ischemic episodes over several days. Preexisting high-grade stenosis favors nontransmural infarction because of the development of collaterals prior to the final episode of thrombotic occlusion. Conversely, the absence of previous stenosis favors the development of transmural infarction when thrombotic occlusion occurs.

Unstable Angina

The hallmark of the crescendo (type B) form of unstable angina[119] is intermittent myocardial ischemia at rest with a definite increased risk of sudden death and/or acute myocardial infarction in the near future. The mechanism of the ischemia is related to dynamic stenosis (i.e., the degree of obstruction to flow over a culprit lesion is varying rather than being fixed and static). Two main explanations—intermittent enhanced thrombosis at the site of the culprit lesion, and varying vasomotor tone either at an eccentrically situated culprit plaque or more distally—have been postulated as the mechanisms of dynamic stenosis. Neither of these processes is mutually exclusive, and in many patients both operate contiguously.

Angioscopic, angiographic, and pathological studies have all emphasized the role of thrombosis with type II stenosis as the culprit lesion in a high proportion of cases.[120-126] Well-documented cases of unstable angina exist, however, in which the culprit lesion is an eccentrically situated plaque preserving a segment of normal arterial wall capable of undergoing changes in vasomotor tone, and on which no thrombus was angiographically visible.[127] When there is an unstable plaque with overlying mural thrombus formation, distal embolization of platelet clumps into the myocardium leads to small microscopic foci of myocyte necrosis.[120,121] Pathological studies[120] have related the presence of such emboli with episodic rest pain immediately prior to death, and in vivo studies show that the presence of markers of platelet activation in the urine coincide with episodes of pain.[128,129] Therefore, unstable angina has much in common in its pathogenesis with transient cerebral ischemic attacks, which are due to platelet emboli from ulcerated plaques of atheroma in the carotid arteries.

In experimental situations, episodes of enhanced platelet adhesion to the endothelium within areas of high-grade eccentric stenosis is associated with intermittent increases in vasomotor tone.[130] In at least one human case of unstable angina owing to variable stenosis at an eccentric plaque without angiographic evidence of thrombosis, examination of the lesion which was excised at the time of inserting vein grafts showed microscopic mural thrombi to be present.[127]

Sudden Ischemic Death

Sudden ischemic death should be defined both in temporal and pathological terms as follows:

1. A subject who has previously been well and died within a short period of the onset of any symptom in the final episode. Short has been defined as intervals up to 24 hours, but most authorities would take intervals up to six hours, subdividing those with instantaneous death and those with less than one hour of symptoms.
2. At necropsy no cause of death other than coronary atherosclerosis is found.
3. The subject must have at least one segment of coronary artery stenosis in which the lumen is reduced by more than 50 per cent in diameter.

Within this rubric, both clinical and pathological studies show that there are two distinct entities differing in their pathology and pathophysiology.

On one hand, there is a group of patients who have evidence of a new acute ischemic event. The arterial pathology is that of a thrombus related to an unstable plaque comparable to that found in crescendo unstable angina.[131–133] The myocardial pathology ranges from tiny focal areas of myocardial necrosis due to platelet emboli, up to larger areas of early regional necrosis. Microscopically identifiable areas of necrosis are more common in those subjects who in retrospect have had prodromal pain prior to the final episode.[120]

On the other hand, there are subjects who have coronary atherosclerosis with stable high-grade stenosis but no evidence of thrombosis; the myocardium shows evidence of previous ischemic scarring often associated with significant left ventricular hypertrophy. The mechanism of death appears to be unrelated to acute ischemia, and is due to an arrhythmia arising in a myocardium prone to reentrant tachycardias. While there would be general agreement on the existence of these two groups, there is no agreement on their relative size, either from pathological studies at necropsy, or from clinical study of subjects who have survived an episode of out-of-hospital ventricular fibrillation. The reported frequency in survivors of those having new acute ischemia (and thus, by implication, had had thrombosis) ranges from 25 to 75 per cent. A large part of the discordance between these figures lies in case selection. A pathological study[134] comparing those subjects in whom a recent thrombus was present in the coronary arteries, with those without thrombus, found that factors such as presence of prodromal warning chest pain and no previous history of ischemic heart disease predicted for those with thrombus. Instantaneous death without prodromal pain in a subject known to have an old infarction predicted for those without new myocardial ischemia and without coronary thrombosis. Pathological studies have not in the past considered such selection factors. Subjects resuscitated from sudden ischemic "death" and studied electrophysiologically are also highly selected since such survivors represent no more than a 10 per cent cohort of those on whom resuscitation was attempted.

Local Factors Precipitating Thrombosis in Relation to Plaques

With very few exceptions, thrombosis does not occur in morphologically normal human arteries; an exception is thrombosis which may follow prolonged coronary vasoconstriction, one cause of which is cocaine abuse. Cerebral artery spasm in patients with intracerebral hemorrhage may lead to diffuse thrombosis in morphologically normal vessels. The vast majority of human arterial thrombi develop in relation to atherosclerotic plaques and come in a wide range of sizes. At one extreme there are ultramicroscopic thrombi demonstrable by scanning electron microscopy; next in scale are the microscopic thrombi found over many plaques. Both of these types of thrombi may well be contributory factors in plaque growth, but are far too small to be detected angiographically or to influence flow significantly by their size alone. At the other extreme are thrombi which are detectable as intraluminal filling defects and which are capable of producing a reduction in flow sufficient to cause acute ischemia in the myocardium or brain.

Reconstruction at necropsy of the plaques which underlie major human coronary thrombi, demonstrable by angiography and which had caused death, shows two distinct morphological patterns.[135] In 25 per cent there was an atheromatous plaque on which thrombus was superimposed as a result of superficial intimal injury (Fig. 3–15). The

basic structure of the underlying plaque itself did not show signs of recent change. Two factors were common to this form of thrombosis: high-grade stenosis at the site, which was often in one of the smaller epicardial arteries; and infiltration of the surface layers of the intima by numerous foam cells. This form of superficial thrombosis is likely to represent extensive endothelial denudation and is the extreme expression of the more focal endothelial denudation and microscopic thrombosis that occurs over many advanced fibrolipid plaques. This form of thrombosis is due to superficial intimal injury.

In contrast, three fourths of major coronary thrombi were related to plaques which had undergone deeper intimal injury with tears that extended from the lumen into the depths of the plaque itself (Fig. 3–16). Deep intimal injury differs from the more superficial form of intimal injury with thrombosis in two respects. First, the amount of collagen exposed is far greater, and tissue factor within the plaque[82] is exposed, providing a more major stimulus for thrombosis;[136] second, the thrombus forms initially within the soft interior of the plaque itself.[135] This intraintimal component of thrombus expands the volume of the plaque, and leads to a rapid increase in the degree of arterial narrowing. Intralu-

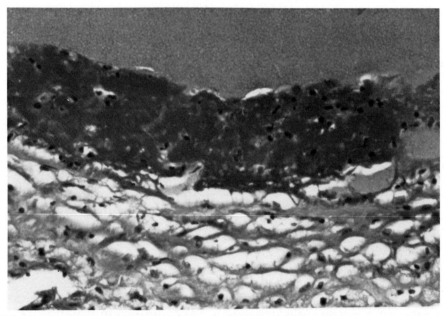

FIGURE 3–15. Superficial intimal injury. This photograph shows a small mural thrombus overlying a human coronary artery plaque. Note the absence of endothelium, the wide separation of collagen fibers, and the presence of large number of lipid-laden macrophages between these fibers. This is the archetypal appearance of superficial plaque injury leading to mural thrombosis (× 1,340).

FIGURE 3–16. Coronary artery from a patient dying suddenly. An intraluminal mass of platelets is seen to be continuous with the base of an ulcerated plaque. At one edge of the ulcerated area, the connective tissue plaque cap can be seen to have "hinged" upwards, the fissure having occurred at the junction between the plaque cap and the more normal part of the vessel wall. (H & E × 35.)

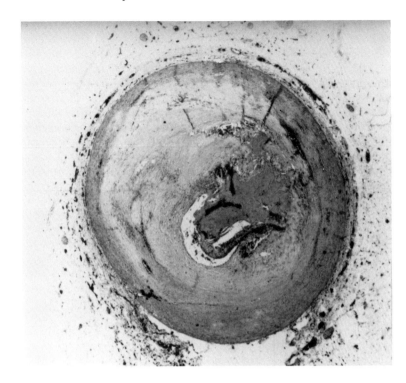

minal thrombus may or may not form subsequently over this site of tearing in the plaque cap.

The intimal tears range in size from cracks or fissures of microscopic dimensions, to tears visible to the naked eye measuring some millimeters in length. At the extreme end of the scale, the whole cap of a plaque measuring 2 centimeters in diameter may be removed leaving an "ulcer." Such extreme plaque disruption is more common in large arteries such as the aorta, femoral, or carotid arteries.

The process of plaque tearing or disruption going under the guise of many names which include cracking, splitting, tearing, fissuring, ulceration, or rupture has been recognized for many years by pathologists following the pioneer work of Constantinides.[137] Recent work showing that it can be recognized by its angiographic and angioscopic appearances in living patients has added considerable impetus to realizing the importance of plaque disruption in producing acute clinical symptoms. Postmortem angiography shows that plaques undergoing fissuring produce an eccentric stenosis with a ragged outline or overhanging edges;[111,115] intraluminal thrombus, if present, superimposes a filling defect within the lumen. These appearances have been designated as type II stenoses in contrast

to smooth type I stenoses. Type II coronary artery lesions have now been identified as being present in unstable angina,[122] transmural and nontransmural regional infarction,[125] and in subjects resuscitated from sudden ischemic "death."[138,139] Angioscopy of coronary arteries has allowed direct inspection of torn plaques in living subjects.[126]

By combining the information derived from necropsy and clinical studies, the stages by which thrombus formation occurs following disruption of a plaque can be understood.

Plaques which undergo disruption are most commonly those in which there is an eccentrically situated pool of extracellular lipid and debris encapsulated within the intima. This lipid in the intact plaque is separated from the lumen by a cap of fibromuscular tissue, and by the endothelium itself. The majority of tears through the plaque cap occur at its junction with the adjacent, more normal intima.[13] The tear allows blood to enter the lipid pool from the lumen, and thrombus forms within the plaque. The interior of the plaque is intensely thrombogenic owing to the large amount of types I and III collagen which is exposed. In addition, tissue factor produced by the macrophages is present within lipid-rich plaques.[140] The intraplaque thrombus is formed predominantly of platelets; to recruit such numbers there must be flow of blood into and out of the plaque for an appreciable period of time.

The second stage of the process leads to the formation of an intraluminal thrombus which protrudes from the site of plaque rupture into the arterial lumen (Figs. 3–16 and 3–17), but does not totally prevent antegrade blood flow. It is mural thrombi in this stage that have been identified by coronary angioscopy in patients with unstable angina.[126] The mural component of thrombus within the fissure itself consists of densely packed fibrin, although there is always a layer of platelets on the surface exposed to the lumen itself. Mural nonocclusive thrombi are associated in animal models with distal embolization of platelet clumps,[141] and there is abundant clinical and pathological evidence that the same is true in the cerebral and myocardial circulation of man.[120,121,142,143] Platelet microemboli within the myocardium are confined to regions downstream of a mural thrombus and are present in over 50

per cent of cases of unstable angina at necropsy. Such microemboli are associated with focal microscopic myocardial necrosis. In transient cerebral ischemic attacks, the "white bodies" seen within retinal arteries are platelet microemboli derived from ulcerated atherosclerotic plaques in the carotid artery.[143] Cholesterol crystals can also be washed out from the lipid pool when major plaque disruption has occurred. This process is not common in the coronary circulation, but cholesterol emboli are found frequently in the digital arteries of lower limbs amputated for atherosclerotic peripheral vascular disease.

A proportion of mural thrombi ultimately progresses to become occlusive (Fig. 3–18), at least for a period of time, and in the coronary arteries these are associated with acute regional infarction unless there is previously established collateral flow. Occlusive thrombi always have a major component of the intraluminal element which is more venous in type (i.e., has a loose network of fibrin containing red cells and a paucity of

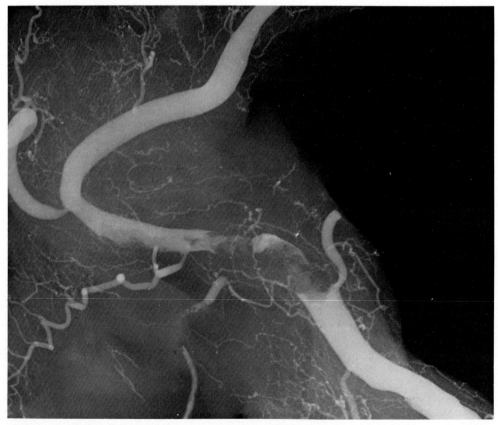

FIGURE 3–17. Postmortem human coronary angiogram. The coronary artery shows an area of high-grade stenosis with a ragged outline associated with an intraluminal filling defect due to thrombus.

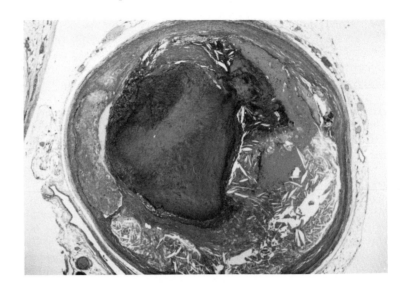

FIGURE 3–18. Transverse section through a coronary artery which contains an occlusive thrombus. The darkly staining thrombus has a typical dumbbell shape with the larger component being intraluminal and the remainder being intraintimal.

platelets). There is clear evidence, from studies using radiolabeled fibrinogen and platelets, that the intraluminal thrombus continues to propagate within the lumen after myocardial infarction has occurred, but the proximal nidus of the thrombus predates infarction.[144] The dynamic nature of this third stage of occluding thrombosis, which can wax and wane in size over short periods of time,[145] has not been appreciated in the past, particularly by pathologists, and was one factor which led to a decade of controversy over the presence or absence of coronary thrombosis in necropsy studies of acute infarction.

The structure of a major part of the intraluminal thrombus that forms in the final stage of occlusion in a human coronary artery makes it very susceptible to fibrinolysis, whether natural or therapeutic. Approximately 50 per cent of coronary arteries subtending infarcts are patent at three months,[146] while the studies of DeWood[113] and Stadius[114] show that in the early phase of infarction the majority of these vessels must have been totally occluded. While often angiographically patent in the sense that there is some antegrade flow, the arteries which supply the infarcted regions of myocardium do show residual high-grade stenosis. Where previous angiographic data are available, the sites at which these thrombi developed often did not show significant stenosis, while after the episode of thrombosis there was residual high-grade stenosis.[125] Thus, in these particular instances thrombosis can be seen to have been the major factor in plaque growth.

Angiograms carried out during the course of thrombolytic therapy in man for acute coronary thrombosis show initial rapid restoration of antegrade blood flow around the margins of a mass of thrombus projecting into the lumen.[147] With time there is a reduction in the size of this mass, but a resistant element of thrombus attached to a ragged stenosis representing the fissured plaque remains.[148] Lytic therapy is successful in restoring flow in 60 to 75 per cent of cases of arteries supplying acute myocardial infarcts. Successful lysis is probably associated with either superficial intimal injury or the lesser degrees of deep intimal injury. Unsuccessful lysis and a failure to achieve reperfusion is probably associated with major plaque fissures in which an intimal flap is raised, or where there is a very large intraplaque component of thrombus or where a plug of lipid is expressed into the arterial lumen.[149] Organization of unremoved fibrin by fibroblasts and capillaries leads either to chronic total obstruction or restoration of flow through a number of small tortuous channels within the original lumen;[150] a process known to pathologists as recanalization.

TEMPORAL SEQUENCE OF PLAQUE GROWTH IN HUMAN CORONARY ARTERIES

The predicted progress of atherosclerosis, were it based only upon the acquisition of lipid, and smooth muscle proliferation within the plaque, might be anticipated to be linear. The actual events as judged by angiography are episodic and unpredictable. Comparison of coronary angiograms taken at approximately yearly intervals shows some stenoses to progress, while others remain static. Progression at one site is totally unrelated to progression at other sites in an individual.

A study of 168 patients[151] who had coronary arteriography on three separate occasions showed that of patients who had progression in the first interval, only 32 had progression in the second interval. In only nine of these patients were the same segments of coronary artery involved. Conversely, of 102 patients who had no progression in the first interval, 37 progressed in the second interval. Although in general there was progression with time, the process was far from linear and predictable. Other studies have shown that new high-grade lesions causing over 50 per cent diameter stenosis in coronary arteries often appear in apparently normal segments of artery over short periods of time.[152] Angiograms cannot predict the future site of occlusive coronary thrombi.[153,154] The erratic and stepwise progression of coronary atherosclerosis is in keeping with the view that clinically silent episodes of intraplaque thrombosis or small surface thrombi precipitate plaque growth. Larger intraluminal thrombi can also cause sudden plaque growth, but are less frequently silent and recognized by virtue of the acute ischemic symptoms that they cause at the time.

Detailed analysis of the coronary arteries in control subjects who have died of nonvascular causes[133] shows that a recent plaque fissure with intraplaque, but not intraluminal thrombus formation, can be found in 8.7 per cent of subjects without hypertension and diabetes, and in 16.7 per cent of those subjects with these risk factors. The increase in the prevalence of fissures may indicate that subjects with hypertension have either more plaques at risk or a greater risk of an individual plaque undergoing fissuring.

Thus, fissuring is an important cause of plaque growth in any subject with atherosclerosis, and acts as an intermittent stimulus for intraluminal thrombosis. Whether intraluminal thrombosis does occur may depend on many factors. Some of these are local (that is, the magnitude of the fissure and the rate of blood flow over the lesion) and other factors are systemic (that is, the fibrinolytic or thrombogenic potential at the time). The risk of developing acute myocardial infarction is related to the plasma fibrinogen levels, the activated factor VII levels,[155] and the amount of plasminogen activator inhibitor-1 (PAI-1);[156] elevation of all of these factors will favor intraluminal thrombus formation when there is an episode of plaque fissuring.

Relation of Plaque Fissuring and Hemorrhage

Disruption and tearing open of the plaque cap leads inevitably to blood entering the interior of the plaque; the major result is the deposition of platelets, fibrin, and some red cells within the plaque itself. The process has been termed intraintimal or intraplaque thrombosis[111] because the platelet component is large and can have been accumulated only from flowing blood. The process has also aptly been termed dissecting intimal hemorrhage.[107]

There is a totally different phenomenon by which hemorrhage into the lipid pool of a plaque comes from new small blood vessels which enter the intima from across the media.[157] This form of hemorrhage is predominantly composed of red cells with virtually no fibrin or platelet component. Studies in which the whole plaque is reconstructed show that while this process is common in relation to large plaques, it is not related to intraluminal thrombus formation. Where platelets and fibrin are present within a plaque, serial sectioning will be consistently able to show a plaque cap tear either more proximally or more distally. The importance of studying plaque microanatomy by such reconstructions cannot be overemphasized.

Mechanisms of Plaque Fissuring

The majority of plaques which undergo fissuring and ulceration, whether they be coronary, carotid, or aortic, contain a large core of lipid in which part of the collagenous structure of the intima is broken down leading to a "pool" of pultaceous debris.[13,158] The soft nature of the core prevents it from carrying an equal share of the circumferential stress in systole, which must be redistributed, thus elevating and concentrating a mechanical load onto the fibrous cap of the plaque. The mechanical and biochemical properties of the fibromuscular cap tissue itself must be the other major determinant of the risk of plaques undergoing fissuring.

The cap tissue from aortic plaques which have undergone fissuring is very different from that derived from plaques which are intact:

I. Much less stress is required to reach fracture point in vitro in caps from fissured plaques as compared with those derived from intact plaques.

II. Caps from fissured plaques have:
 A. Less collagen.
 B. Less glycosaminoglycan.
 C. Fewer smooth muscle cells.
 D. More lipid-filled macrophages than caps from intact plaques.

These data suggest that the dynamic equilibrium between synthesis and breakdown of connective tissue matrix proteins, which are the main determinants of mechanical strength in the tissue, must be a major factor in the maintenance of plaque cap stability.

In connection with this area of potential interest, clearly needing further study is the relationship between smooth muscle cell proliferation and the accumulation of lipid-filled macrophages. The former constitutes the main repair mechanism within the arterial intima, while the latter through the secretory properties of activated macrophages may hold the key to connective tissue breakdown.

While the majority of plaque tears occur through the caps of lipid-rich plaques to enter the pultaceous core, a small minority are within more fibrous lesions either between layers of collagen or at the interface between plates of calcified tissue and collagen.[13] Such tears probably reflect dyshomogeneity in the mechanical properties of the tissue, in particular, an increase in stiffness enhancing shear local stress. The calcified plaques of older subjects may be more prone to such tears which are not related to large pools of lipid.

Atherosclerotic Cerebrovascular Disease

The terms stroke and cerebrovascular accident are imprecise in terms of pathology, reflecting the difficulty of distinguishing intracerebral hemorrhage from cerebral ischemic infarction in living patients. Computerized tomographic (CT) scanning has clarified the distinction. Cerebral hemorrhage has no direct link with atherosclerosis, and is owing to vascular changes in the smaller vessels mainly related to age and hypertension. Cerebral ischemic infarction is often related to atherosclerosis, although the cause-and-effect linkage is more complex than in the myocardium. Thrombotic occlusion of arteries in the circle of Willis may be due either to local atherosclerotic lesions or emboli. These emboli may arise from thrombus on atherosclerotic plaques in the aortic arch, carotid, or vertebral arteries, or may be unrelated to atherosclerosis, arising within the heart. Thrombi arising in situ within the cerebral arteries are caused by intimal injury to unstable plaques analogous to that which occurs in coronary arteries (see later). High-grade stenosis in segments of the cerebral arteries may be associated with areas of necrosis in the watershed territories between major arteries when hypotension occurs. Carotid atherosclerosis has one facet which is influenced by the large caliber of the vessel. Chronic ulceration of plaques (Fig. 3–19) occurs, leaving large areas of exposed thrombus which persist over long periods and form a nidus for chronic distal embolization. Within the coronary arteries, thrombi either occlude or resolve within a few days, reflecting the smaller lumen size.

Aortic Atherosclerosis and Lower Limb Vascular Disease

The segment of the aorta from the renal arteries to the bifurcation of the iliac arteries is consistently the site of the most severe degree of atherosclerosis. In Western populations, this segment of the aorta is covered by confluent plaques in most individuals over 50 years of age when examined at necropsy, even when there is little disease in the more proximal aorta. Symptoms are produced either by the formation of an aneurysm or by overlying mural thrombus forming a site for distal embolization. The reasons for aneurysm formation are uncertain. On one hand, it is known that the tunica media behind atherosclerotic plaques undergoes pressure or hypoxia-mediated atrophy and a loss of smooth muscle cells. Confluent atherosclerosis will thus lead to diffuse medial loss and potentiate aneurysm formation. On the other hand, they may be an active destruction of the media by infiltrating macrophages or an inflammatory immune reaction to lipids released within the plaques. Femoral

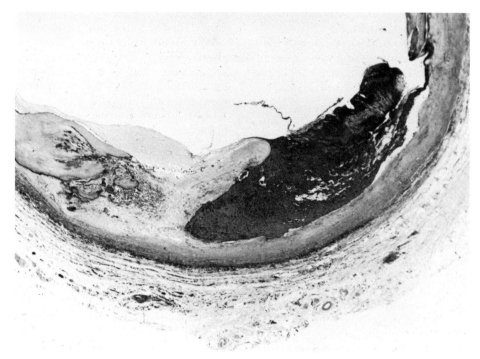

FIGURE 3–19. Carotid artery plaque fissure. There is a partly calcified carotid artery plaque which has undergone ulceration. The center of the plaque, formerly occupied by lipid, now contains a mass of darkly staining thrombus. The thrombus is covered by the residual portion of the plaque cap.

and iliac disease has close similarities to carotid disease in that either large areas of ulceration act as a focus for distal emboli or local obstruction develops.

RISK FACTORS FOR ATHEROSCLEROSIS RELATED TO THROMBOSIS

Classic epidemiological studies[160] have identified a number of risk factors associated with an increased risk of ischemic heart disease and stroke. How these factors are transmuted into the clinical expression of the disease is often obscure. Increased risk could be mediated by an increase in the amount of atherosclerotic "wall disease," by an increase in the likelihood of plaque instability (leading to thrombosis), or by an increase in the response of platelets and the clotting system to an unstable plaque. (See also Chapter 2.)

Cigarette Smoking and Atherosclerosis

The complexity of the problem is illustrated by one risk factor: cigarette smoking.

In the majority of multifactorial regression studies, smoking is identified as an independent risk factor for fatal or nonfatal events related to atherosclerosis[160] (see Chapter 2.) There is evidence from necropsy surveys of large numbers of aortas and coronary arteries that smokers have more raised plaques than nonsmokers.[5,161] Although smoking is a strong predictor of acute myocardial infarction, it is not a predictor of stable angina,[162] and the risk of death falls rapidly after smoking cessation, suggesting that the risk of clinical events is at least in part related to mechanisms other than a simple increase in severity of the basic atherosclerotic process.

Marked ultrastructural changes have been described in the endothelium of the umbilical vessels in infants born to mothers who smoked during pregnancy.[163] These took the form of numerous bleb-like protrusions from the surface of the intact endothelial cell; similar appearances are induced by cigarette smoking in a rat model[164] and in the latter prostacyclin (PGI_2) production by the aorta is reduced.[165] Thus, cigarette smoking is associated with structural and functional alterations in the endothelial cell which might potentiate plaque development. Enhancement of the thrombotic potential is suggested by the reduction in bleeding time after smoking two cigarettes, an effect preventable by aspirin,[166] (and the increased aggregation of platelets by adenosine diphosphate), an increase in factor VIII, ristocetin-agglutinating factor (RAG), an increase in plasma fibrinogen, and lower plasminogen and plasminogen activator levels.[167] Smokers also have higher levels of activated factor VII and fibrinogen as compared to nonsmokers, an effect which is reversed by smoking cessation.[168] Irrespective of other risk factors, these elevations of factor VII and fibrinogen are major risk factors for acute events in subjects with ischemic heart disease and must operate though enhancing the thrombotic response to any plaque instability.[168]

Cigarette Smoking and Platelet Function

The effect of cigarette smoking on platelet function clearly should not be disregarded. Platelet survival is significantly shorter during periods of smoking, and a single cigarette increased the platelets' response to a standard aggregating stimulus, and platelet aggregation has been found to be chronically increased in heavy smokers.[169,170] In adult rats exposed to fresh smoke, either in acute studies lasting about 30 minutes or in longer term studies, a series of morphological changes was produced regularly in the aortic endothelium. Many endothelial cells were swollen and showed the presence of bleb-like projections and microvillus-like processes on their luminal surface membrane.[164] Of even greater interest was the presence of microthrombi in the aortae of all the animals exposed to cigarette smoke. These occurred in the proximal portion of intercostal branches (the areas in which wall shear rates are lowest) and were found in 87 per cent of the 135 branches examined by scanning electron microscopy.

In a group of animals treated in an identical manner, there was a significant reduction of the ability of rings of aortic tissue to produce 6-keto-PGF$_1$ alpha as compared with controls which had been "sham smoked." An analogous series of studies was carried out of the effect of acute cigarette smoking on the interactions between human platelets and aortic endothelium.[171] This study made use of a modification of the Baumgartner technique,

the modification being the omission of any abrasion of the rabbit aortae which was used at the flow surface. When this nonabraded rabbit aorta was exposed for ten minutes to flowing blood from human volunteers before they had smoked, and the aorta examined with the scanning electron microscope, either no platelets at all or very few could be seen to adhere to the intact endothelial surface. Smoking of two medium-tar cigarettes resulted in the adherence of large numbers of platelets to the endothelium, and all of these platelets had undergone a shape change and hence, by implication, the release reaction. The mechanism of this change in platelet behavior is still unknown. It is not without interest that nicotine has been reported to inhibit prostacyclin production.[172] While an inhibition of the ability to produce prostacyclin was certainly seen in the aortae of animals exposed to smoke,[164] the administration of nicotine in a single dose did not produce a similar result, and it was only when nicotine was administered over a ten-day period by means of subcutaneous infusion pumps that any inhibitory effect on prostacyclin production could be noted.[165]

REFERENCES

1. Caro CG, Fitzgerald JM, Schroter RC. Atheroma and arterial wall shear. Observation, correlation and proposal of a shear dependent mass transfer mechanism for atherogenesis. Proc Soc Lond 1971; 177: 109–59.
2. Chien S. Significance of macrorheology and microrheology in atherogenesis. Ann NY Acad Sci 1976; 275: 10–27.
3. Zarins C, Giddens D, Bharadvaj B. Carotid bifurcation atherosclerosis: quantitation of plaque localization with flow velocity profiles and wall shear stress. Circ Res 1983; 53: 502–14.
4. Stary H. Evolution and progression of atherosclerotic lesions in coronary arteries of children and young adults. Arteriosclerosis 1989; 9: 1–19.
5. PDAY Research Group. Relationship of atherosclerosis in young men to serum lipoprotein cholesterol concentrations and smoking. A preliminary report from the pathological determinant of atherosclerosis in youth study. JAMA 1990; 264: 3018–24.
6. Deupree R, Fields R, McMahon C, Strong J. Atherosclerotic lesions and coronary heart disease. Key relationships in necropsied cases. Lab Invest 1973; 28: 252–62.
7. Robertson W, Strong J. Atherosclerosis in persons with hypertension and diabetes mellitus. Lab Invest 1968; 18: 538–51.
8. Strong J, Solberg L, Restrepo C. Atherosclerosis in persons with coronary heart disease. Lab Invest 1968; 18: 527–37.
9. Steinberg D, Parthasarathy S, Carew T, Khoo J, Witztum J. Beyond cholesterol. Modifications of low-density lipoprotein that increases its atherogenicity. N Engl J Med 1989; 320: 915–24.
10. Brown M, Goldstein J. Atherosclerosis. Scavenging for receptors. Nature 1990; 343: 508–9.
11. Guyton J, Klemp K. The lipid rich core region of human atherosclerotic fibrous plaques: prevalence of small lipid droplets and vesicles by electron microscopy. Am J Pathol 1989; 134: 705–17.

12. Lundberg B. Chemical composition and physical state of lipid deposits in atherosclerosis. Atherosclerosis 1985; 56: 93–110.

13. Richardson P, Davies M, Born G. Influence of plaque configuration and stress distribution on fissuring of coronary atherosclerotic plaques. Lancet 1989; ii: 941–4.

14. Freedman D, Newman WI, Tracy R. Black-white differences in aortic fatty streaks in adolescence and early adulthood: the Bogalusa heart study. Circulation 1988; 77: 856–64.

15. Bruschke A, Wijers T, Kolsters W, Landmann J. The anatomic evaluation of coronary artery disease demonstrated by coronary angiography in 256 non-operated patients. Circulation 1981; 63: 527–40.

16. Rafflenbeul W, Nellessen U, Galvao P, Kreft M, Peters S, Lichtlen P. Progression and regression of coronary artery disease as assessed with sequential coronary angiography. Z Kardiol 1984; 73: 33–40.

17. Glagov S, Weisenberd E, Zarins C, Stankunavicius R, Kolettis G. Compensatory enlargement of human atherosclerotic coronary arteries. N Engl J Med 1987; 316: 1371–5.

18. Rosenfeld M, Tsukada T, Gown A, Ross R. Fatty streak initiation in Watanabe heritable hyperlipemic and comparable hypercholesterolemic fat-fed rabbits. Arteriosclerosis 1987; 7: 9–23.

19. Seddon AM, Woolf N, Laville A, et al. Hereditary hyperlipidemia and atherosclerosis in the rabbit due to overproduction of lipoproteins. Preliminary report of arterial pathology. Arteriosclerosis 1987; 7: 113–24.

20. Faggiotto A, Ross R. Studies of hypercholesterolaemia in non-human primates. II. Fatty streak conversion to fibrous plaque. Arteriosclerosis 1984; 4: 341–56.

21. Faggiotto A, Ross R, Harker L. Studies of hypercholesterolaemia in the non-human primate. I. changes that lead to fatty streak formation. Arteriosclerosis 1984; 4: 323–40.

22. Scott R, Kim D, Schmee J, Thomas W. Atherosclerotic lesions in coronary arteries of hyperlipidemic swine. II. Endothelial cell kinetics and leukocyte adherence associated with early lesions. Atherosclerosis 1986; 62: 1–10.

23. Pittilo R, Clarke J, Harris D, et al. Cigarette smoking and platelet adhesion. Br J Haematol 1984; 58: 627–32.

24. Davies M, Woolf N, Rowles P, Pepper J. Morphology of the endothelium over atherosclerotic plaques in human coronary arteries. Br Heart J 1988; 60: 459–64.

25. Crawford T, Levene C. The incorporation of fibrin in the aortic intima. J Pathol Bacteriol 1952; 64: 523–6.

26. Jorgensen L, Packham M, Rowsell H, Mustard J. Deposition of formed elements of blood on the intima and signs of intimal injury in the aorta of rabbit, pig and man. Lab Invest 1972; 27: 341–50.

27. Chandler A. Mechanisms and frequency of thrombosis in the coronary circulation. Thromb Res 1974; 4: 3–23.

28. Wight T. Cell biology of arterial proteoglycans. Arteriosclerosis 1989; 9: 1–20.

29. Heptinstall R. The effects of high blood cholesterol on the pulmonary arterial changes produced in rabbits by the injection of blood clot. Br J Exp Pathol 1957; 38: 438–45.

30. Chandler A. In vitro thrombotic coagulation of the blood: a method for producing a thrombus. Lab Invest 1958; 7: 110–4.

31. Ardlie NG, Schwartz CJ. The organisation and fate of autologous pulmonary emboli in hypercholesterolaemic rabbits. J Path Bacteriol 1968; 95: 19–29.

32. Woolf N, Bradley J, Crawford T, Carstairs K. Experimental mural thrombosis in the pig aorta: the early natural history. Br J Exp Pathol 1968; 49: 257–64.

33. Baumgartner HR, Studer A. Folgen des Gefaesskatheter Ismus am nomo-und hypercholesterol inaemichsem. Patholog et Microbiol 1966; 29: 393–405.

34. Fingerle J, Johnson R, Clowes A, Majesky M, Reidy M. Role of platelets in smooth muscle cell proliferation and migration after vascular injury in rat carotid artery. Proc Natl Acad Sci USA 1989; 86: 8412–6.

35. Tada T, Reidy M. Endothelial regeneration IX. Arterial injury followed by rapid endothelial repair includes smooth muscle cell proliferation but not intimal thickening. Am J Pathol 1987; 129: 429–33.

36. Moore S. Thromboatherosclerosis in normolipemic rabbits:

37. Davies M, Ballantine S, Robertson W, Woolf N. The ultrastructure of organising experimental mural thrombi in the pig aorta. J Pathol 1975; 117: 75–81.

38. Clowes A, Clowes M, Reidy M. Kinetics of cellular proliferation after arterial injury. Lab Invest 1986; 54: 295–303.

39. Woolf N, Davies M, Bradley J. Medial changes following experimentally induced thrombosis in the pig aorta. J Pathol 1971; 105: 205–9.

40. Ardlie N, Schwartz C. A comparison of the organisation and fate of autologous pulmonary emboli and of artificial plasma thrombi in the anterior chamber of the eye in normocholesterolaemic rabbits. J Path Bacteriol 1968; 95: 1–18.

41. Moore S. Thrombosis and atherosclerosis. Thromb Diath Haemorrh 1974; 60: 205–13.

42. Baumgartner H, Muggli R. Adhesion and aggregation: Morphological demonstration and quantitation in vivo and in vitro. In: Gordon J, ed. Platelets in biology and pathology. Elsevier, North Holland: Biomedical Press, 1976: 23–60.

43. Stemerman M. Thrombogenesis of the rabbit arterial plaque. Am J Pathol 1973; 73: 7–26.

44. Mersereau W, Moore S, Fernandez H. Renal renin in experimental nephrosclerosis. J Pathol 1972; 108: 319–29.

45. Day A, Bell F, Moore S, Friedman R. Lipid composition and metabolism of thrombo-atherosclerotic lesions produced by continued endothelial damage in normal rabbits. Circ Res 1974; 34: 467–76.

46. Duguid J. The dynamics of atherosclerosis. Aberdeen: University Press, 1976: 48.

47. Barkhan P, Silver M, O'Keefe L. The lipids of human erythrocytes and platelets and their effect on thromboplastin formation. In: Johnson S, Morte R, Rebuck J, Horn R, eds. Blood platelets: Henry Ford Hospital international symposium. Boston: Little, Brown & Co, 1961: 303–18.

48. Poole J. Phagocytosis of platelets by monocytes in organising arterial thrombi. In: Luzio N, Paoletti R, eds. Adv Exp Med Biol 1967; 1: 484–7.

49. Smith E, Evans P, Downham M. Lipid in the aortic intima. The correlation of morphological and chemical characteristics. J Ath Res 1967; 7: 171–86.

50. Woolf N, Pilkington T, Carstairs K. The occurrence of lipoprotein in thrombi. J Path Bacteriol 1966; 91: 383–8.

51. Friedman M, Byers S, St.George S. Origin of lipid and cholesterol in experimental atherosclerosis. J Clin Invest 1962; 41: 828–41.

52. Moore S, Friedman R, Singal D, Blajchman M, Roberts R. Inhibition of injury-induced thromboatherosclerotic lesions by anti-platelet serum in rabbits. Thromb Haemost 1976; 35: 70–81.

53. Friedman R, Stemerman M, Wenz B, et al. The effect of thrombocytopenia in experimental arteriosclerotic lesion formation in rabbits. J Clin Invest 1977; 60: 1191–201.

54. Harker L, Ross R, Slichter S, Scott C. Homocystine induced atherosclerosis: the role of endothelial cell injury and platelet response in its genesis. J Clin Invest 1976; 58: 731–41.

55. Packham M, Mustard J. Non-steroidal anti-inflammatory drugs, pyrimido-pyrimidine compounds and tricyclic compounds: effect of platelet function. In: Hirsch J, Cade J, Gallus A, Schobaum E, eds. Platelets, drugs and thrombosis. London: Karger, 1975:111–123.

56. Clowes A, Karnovsky M. Failure of certain antiplatelet drugs to affect myointimal thickening following arterial endothelial injury in the rat. Lab Invest 1977; 36: 452–63.

57. Harker L, Ross R, Glomset J. Role of the platelet in atherogenesis. Ann NY Acad Sci 1976; 275: 321–9.

58. Ingerman-Wojenski CM, Silver MJ. Model system to study interaction of platelets with damaged arterial wall. II. Inhibition of smooth muscle proliferation by dipyridamole and APH-P719. Exp Mol Pathol 1988; 48: 116–34.

59. Clowes A, Karnovsky M. Suppression by heparin of smooth-muscle cell proliferation in injured arteries. Nature 1977; 265: 625–36.

60. Chen L, Buchanan J. Mitogenic activity of blood components. I. Thrombin and prothrombin. Proc Natl Acad Sci USA 1975; 72: 131–5.

61. Zetter B, Chen L, Sun T, Buchanan J. Thrombin enhances the mitogenic response of cultured fibroblasts to serum and other growth-promoting factors (abstr). J Cell Biol 1976; 70: 282.

62. Ross R, Glomset J. The pathogenesis of atherosclerosis. N Engl J Med 1976; 295: 420–5.

63. Van Pelt-Verkuil E, Van de Ree P, Emeis JJ. Defibrinogenation by Arvim reduces air drying produced arteriosclerosis in rat carotid artery. Thromb Haemost 1989; 61: 246–9.

64. Clowes AW, Clowes MM, Au YPT, Reidy MA, Belin D. Smooth muscle cells express urokinase during mitogenesis and tissue type plasminogen activator during migration in injured rat carotid artery. Circ Res 1990; 67: 61–7.

65. Weiss H, Tschopp T, Baumgartner H. Impaired interaction (adhesion-aggregation) of platelets with the subendothelium in storage pool disease and after aspirin ingestion—a comparison with von Willebrand's disease. N Engl J Med 1975; 293: 619–23.

66. Tschopp T, Weiss H, Baumgartner R. Decreased adhesion of platelets to subendothelium in von Willebrand's disease. J Lab Clin Med 1974; 83: 296–300.

67. Baumgartner H, Tschopp T, Weiss J. Shear rate dependence of platelet adhesion to collagenous surfaces in von Willebrand factor-depleted blood (abstr). Thromb Haemost 1977; 38: 50.

68. Weiss H, Baumgartner H, Tschopp T, Turitto V. A new method for identifying and classifying abnormalities of platelet function. Ann NY Acad Sci 1977; 283: 293–309.

69. Baumgartner H, Tschopp T, Weiss H. Defective adhesion of platelets to subendothelium in von Willebrand's disease and Bernard-Soulier syndrome. Thromb Haemost 1978; 39: 782–3.

70. Weiss H, Baumgartner H, Tschopp T, Turitto V, Cohen D. Correction by Factor VIII of the impaired platelet adhesion to subendothelium in von Willebrand's disease. Blood 1978; 51: 267–79.

71. Fuster V, Bowie E, Lewis J, Fass DN, Owen C Jr, Brown A. Resistance to arteriosclerosis in pigs with von Willebrand's disease: spontaneous and high-cholesterol diet-induced arteriosclerosis. J Clin Invest 1978; 61: 722–30.

72. Fass DN. Platelet responses to von Willebrand factor. In: Chandler A, Eurenius K, McMillan G, Nelson C, Schwartz C, Wessler S, eds. The thrombotic process in atherogenesis. New York: Plenum Press, 1977:392.

73. Griggs T. Induction of atherogenesis in heteroxygous von Willebrand pigs. In: Chandler A, Eurenius K, McMillan G, Nelson C, Schwartz C, Wessler S, eds. The thrombotic process in atherosclerosis. New York: Plenum Press, 1977:393.

74. Subbiah M, Unni K, Kottke B, Carlo I, Dinh D. Arterial and metabolic changes during the critical period of spontaneous sterol accumulation in pigeon aorta. Exp Mol Pathol 1976; 24: 287–301.

75. Lewis J, Kottke B. Endothelial damage and thrombocyte adhesion in pigeon atherosclerosis. Science 1977; 196: 1007–9.

76. Ross R. The pathogenesis of atherosclerosis—an update. N Engl J Med 1986; 8: 488–500.

77. Kohler N, Lipton A. Platelets as a source of fibroblast growth-promoting activity. Exp Cell Res 1974; 87: 297–301.

78. Westermark B, Wasteson A. A platelet factor stimulating human normal glial cells. Exp Cell Res 1976; 98: 170–4.

79. Witte L, Kaplan K, Nossel H, Lages B, Weiss H, Goodman D. Studies of the release from human platelets of the growth factor for cultured human arterial smooth muscle cells. Circ Res 1978; 42: 402–9.

80. Clowes A, Reidy M, Clowes M. Kinetics of cellular proliferation after arterial injury. I. Smooth muscle growth in the absence of endothelium. Lab Invest 1983; 49: 327–33.

81. Groves H, Kinlough-Rathbone R, Richardson M, Moore S, Mustard JF. Platelet interaction with damaged rabbit aorta. Lab Invest 1979; 40: 194–200.

82. Wilcox JN. Analysis of local gene expression in human atherosclerotic plaques by in-situ hybridisation. Trend Cardiovasc Med 1991; 1: 17–24.

83. Blank RS, Thompson MM, Owens GK. Cell cycle versus density dependence of smooth muscle alpha actin expres-sion in cultured rat aortic smooth muscle cells. J Cell Biol 1988; 107: 299–306.

84. Heard B. Mural thrombosis in renal artery and its relation to atherosclerosis. J Path Bacteriol 1949; 61: 635–7.

85. Morgan A. The pathogenesis of coronary occlusion. Vol 60. Oxford: Blackwell Scientific Publishing, 1956.

86. Roberts W. The coronary arteries and left ventricle in clinically isolated angina pectoris—a necropsy analysis. Am J Med 1979; 67: 792–9.

87. Haust M, More R, Movat H. The role of smooth muscle cells in the fibrogenesis of atherosclerosis. Am J Pathol 1960; 37: 377–9.

88. Woolf N, Crawford T. Fatty streaks in aortic intima studied by an immunohistochemical technique. J Path Bacteriol 1960; 80: 205–8.

89. Woolf N. The distribution of fibrin within the aortic intima: an immunohistochemical study. Am J Pathol 1961; 39: 521–32.

90. Walton K, Williamson N. Histological and immunofluorescent studies on the evolution of the human atheromatous plaque. J Atherosclerol Res 1968; 8: 599–624.

91. Kao V, Wissler R. A study of the immunohistochemical localisation of serum lipoproteins and other plasma proteins in human atherosclerotic lesions. Exp Mol Pathol 1965; 4: 465–79.

92. Bini A, Fenoglio J, Mesa-Tejada R, Kudryk B, Kaplan K. Identification and distribution of fibrinogen, fibrin and fibrin(ogen) degradation products in atherosclerosis. Use of monoclonal antibodies. Arteriosclerosis 1989; 9: 109–21.

93. Smith E, Ashall C. Fibrinolysis and plasminogen concentration in aortic intima in relation to death following myocardial infarction. Atherosclerosis 1985; 55: 171–86.

94. Carstairs K. The identification of platelets and platelet antigens in histological sections. J Path Bacteriol 1965; 90: 225–31.

95. Carstairs K, Woolf N, Crawford T. Immunohistochemical cross-reaction between platelets and fibrin. J Path Bacteriol 1964; 88: 537–40.

96. Woolf N, Carstairs K. Infiltration and thrombosis in atherogenesis—a study using immunofluorescent techniques. Am J Pathol 1967; 51: 373–86.

97. Hudson J, McCaughey W. Mural thrombosis and atherogenesis in coronary arteries and aorta. Atherosclerosis 1974; 19: 543–53.

98. Woolf N, Carstairs K. The survival time of platelets in experimental mural thrombi. J Pathol 1969; 97: 595–601.

99. Woolf N, Sacks MI, Davies MJ. Aortic plaque morphology in relation to coronary artery disease. Am J Pathol 1969; 57: 187–97.

100. Cottam D. Infiltration and thrombosis in atherosclerosis—an immunohistological study of the human aorta and coronary arteries. London: PhD thesis, 1971.

101. Woolf N, Bradley J, Crawford T, Carstairs K. Experimental mural thrombosis in the pig aorta: the early natural history. Br J Exp Pathol 1968; 49: 257–64.

102. Walker L, Reidy M, Bowyer D. Morphology and cell kinetics of fatty streak lesion formation in the hypercholesterolemic rabbit. Am J Pathol 1986; 125: 450–9.

103. Reidy M. A reassessment of endothelial injury and arterial lesion formation. Lab Invest 1985; 53: 513–20.

104. Schwartz C, Valente A, Sprague E, et al. Monocyte-macrophage participation in atherogenesis: inflammatory components of pathogenesis. Semin Thromb Hemost 1986; 12: 79–86.

105. Faggiotto A, Ross R. Studies in hypercholesterolaemia in non-human primates. II. Fatty streak conversion to fibrous plaque. Arteriosclerosis 1984; 4: 341–56.

106. Chapman I. The cause-effect relationship between recent coronary artery occlusion and acute myocardial infarction. Am Heart J 1974; 87: 267–71.

107. Davies M, Fulton W, Robertson W. The relationship of coronary thrombosis to ischaemic myocardial necrosis. J Pathol 1979; 127: 99–110.

108. Brosius FC, Roberts WC. Significance of coronary arterial thrombus in transmural acute myocardial infarction. A study of 54 necropsy patients. Circulation 1981; 63: 810–6.

109. Davies M, Woolf N, Robertson W. Pathology of acute myo-

cardial infarction with particular reference to occlusive coronary thrombi. Br Heart J 1976; 38: 659–64.

110. Horie T, Sekiguchi M, Hirosawa K. Coronary thrombosis in pathogenesis of acute myocardial infarction. Histopathological study of coronary arteries in 108 necropsied cases using serial section. Br Heart J 1978; 40: 153–61.

111. Davies M, Thomas A. Plaque fissuring—the cause of acute myocardial infarction, sudden ischaemic death and crescendo angina. Br Heart J 1985; 53: 363–73.

112. Falk E. Plaque rupture with severe pre-existing stenosis precipitating coronary thrombosis. Characteristics of coronary atherosclerotic plaque underlying fatal occlusive thrombi. Br Heart J 1983; 50: 127–31.

113. DeWood M, Spores J, Notske R, et al. Prevalence of total coronary occlusion during the early hours of transmural myocardial infarction. N Engl J Med 1980; 303: 897–902.

114. Stadius M, Maynard C, Fritz J. Coronary anatomy and left ventricular function in the first 12 hours of acute myocardial infarction: the Western Washington randomized intracoronary streptokinase trial. Circulation 1985; 72: 292–301.

115. Levin D, Fallon J. Significance of the angiographic morphology of localized coronary stenosis: histopathologic correlations. Circulation 1982; 66: 316–20.

116. Erhardt L, Unge G, Bowman G. Formation of coronary arterial thrombi in relation to onset of necrosis in acute myocardial infarction in man. Am Heart J 1976; 91: 592–8.

117. Henriksson P, Edhag O, Jansson B. A role for platelets in the process of infarct extension. N Engl J Med 1985; 313: 1660–1.

118. Piek JJ, Becker AE. Collateral blood supply to the myocardium at risk in human myocardial infarction: a quantitative postmortem assessment. J Am Coll Cardiol 1988; 11: 1290–6.

119. Braunwald E. Unstable angina, a classification. Circulation 1989; 80: 410–4.

120. Davies M, Thomas A, Knapman P, Hangartner R. Intramyocardial platelet aggregation in patients with unstable angina suffering sudden ischaemic cardiac death. Circulation 1986; 73: 418–27.

121. Falk E. Unstable angina with fatal outcome: dynamic coronary thrombosis leading to infarction and/or sudden death. Circulation 1985; 71: 699–708.

122. Fuster V, Badimon L, Cohen M, Ambrose J, Badimon J, Chesebro J. Insight into the pathogenesis of acute ischaemic syndromes. Circulation 1988; 77: 1213–20.

123. Ambrose J, Winters S, Arora R. Angiographic evolution of coronary artery morphology in unstable angina. JACC 1986; 7: 472–8.

124. Wilson R, Holida M, White C. Quantitative angiographic morphology of coronary stenoses leading to myocardial infarction or unstable angina. Circulation 1986; 73: 286–93.

125. Ambrose J, Tannenbaum M, Alexopoulos D, et al. Angiographic progression of coronary artery disease and the development of myocardial infarction. JACC 1988; 12: 56–62.

126. Forrester J, Litvak F, Grundfest W, Hickey A. A perspective of coronary disease seen through the arteries of a living man. Circulation 1987; 75: 505–13.

127. Lee G, Garcia J, Corso P, et al. Correlation of coronary angioscopic to angiographic findings in coronary artery disease. Am J Cardiol 1986; 58: 238–41.

128. Brown BG. Coronary vasospasm: observations linking the clinical spectrum of ischemic heart disease to the dynamic pathology of coronary atherosclerosis. Arch Intern Med 1981; 141: 716–22.

129. Fitzgerald D, Roy L, Catella F, Fitzgerald A. A platelet activation in unstable coronary disease. N Engl J Med 1986; 315: 983–9.

130. Lam JYT, Chesebro JH, Steele PM, Badimon L, Fuster V. Is vasospasm related to platelet deposition? Relationship in a porcine preparation of arterial injury in vivo. Circulation 1987; 75: 243–8.

131. Davies M, Thomas A. Thrombosis and acute coronary artery lesions in sudden cardiac ischaemic death. N Engl J Med 1984; 310: 1137–40.

132. Van-Dantiz JM, Becker AE. Sudden cardiac death and acute pathology of coronary arteries. Eur Heart J 1986; 7: 987–91.

133. El-Fawal MA, Berg GA, Wheatley DJ, Harland WA. Sud-

den coronary death in Glasgow: nature and frequency of acute coronary lesions. Br Heart J 1987; 57: 329–35.

134. Davies MJ, Bland JM, Hangartner JRW, Angelini A, Thomas AC. Factors influencing the presence or absence of acute coronary artery thrombi in sudden ischaemic death. Eur Heart J 1989; 10: 203–8.

135. Davies MJ. Macroscopic or microscopic view of coronary thrombi. Circulation 1990; 82: 1138–46.

136. Lam J, Chesebro J, Steele P, et al. Deep arterial injury during experimental angioplasty: relation to a positive indium-III-labelled platelet scintigram, quantitative platelet deposition and mural thrombosis. J Am Coll Cardiol 1986; 8: 1380–6.

137. Constantinides P. Plaque fissures in human coronary thrombosis. J Atherosclerol Res 1966; 6: 1–17.

138. Lo Y-SA, Cutler J, Blake K, Wright A, Kron J, Swerdlow C. Angiographic coronary morphology in survivors of cardiac arrest. Am Heart J 1988; 115: 781–5.

139. Stevenson W, Wiener I, Yeatman L, Wohlgelernter D, Weiss J. Complicated atherosclerotic lesions: a potential cause of ischaemic ventricular arrhythmias in cardiac arrest survivors who do not have inducible ventricular tachycardia? Am Heart J 1988; 116: 1–6.

140. Wilcox J, Smith K, Schwartz S, Gordon D. Localisation of tissue factor in the normal vessel wall and in the atherosclerotic plaque. Proc Natl Acad Sci USA 1989; 86: 2839–43.

141. Moore S, Belbeck L, Evans G, Pineau S. Effects of complete or partial occlusion of a coronary artery. Lab Invest 1981; 44: 151–7.

142. Fink R, Rooney P, Trowbridge J, Ross J. Coronary thrombosis and platelet/fibrin microemboli in death associated with acute myocardial infarction. Br Heart J 1988; 59: 196–200.

143. Imparato A, Riles T, Mintzer R, et al. The importance of hemorrhage in the relationship between gross morphologic characteristics and cerebral symptoms in 376 carotid artery plaques. Ann Surg 1983; 197: 195–203.

144. Fulton W, Sumner D. 125 I-labelled fibrinogen, autoradiography and stero-arteriography in identification of coronary thrombotic occlusion in fatal myocardial infarction. Br Heart J 1976; 38: 880.

145. Hackett D, Davies G, Chierchia S, Maseri A. Intermittent coronary occlusion in acute myocardial infarction. Value of combined thrombolytic and vasodilator therapy. N Engl J Med 1987; 317: 1055–9.

146. Bertrand M, Lefebvre J, Laisne C, Rousseau M, Carre A, Lekieffre J. Coronary arteriography in acute transmural myocardial infarction. Am Heart J 1979; 97: 61–9.

147. Brown B, Gallery C, Badger R, et al. Incomplete lysis of thrombus in the moderate underlying atherosclerotic lesions during intracoronary infarction: quantitative angiographic observations. Circulation 1986; 73: 653–61.

148. Isner J, Konstam M, Fortin R, Lefebvre M, Salem D. Delayed thrombolysis of streptokinase-resistant occlusive thrombus: documentation by pre- and post mortem coronary angiography. Am J Cardiol 1983; 52: 210–1.

149. Davies M. Successful and unsuccessful coronary thrombolysis. Br Heart J 1989; 61: 381–4.

150. Roberts W, Virmani R. Formation of new coronary arteries within a previously obstructed epicardial coronary artery (intra-arterial arteries). A mechanism for occurrence of angiographically normal coronary arteries after healing of acute myocardial infarction. Am J Cardiol 1984; 54: 1361–2.

151. Bruschke A, Kramer J, Bal E, Haque I, Detranto R, Goormastic M. The dynamics of progression of coronary atherosclerosis studied in 168 medically treated patients who underwent coronary arteriography three times. Am Heart J 1989; 117: 296–305.

152. Haft J, Haik B, Goldstein J, Brodyn N. Development of significant coronary artery lesions in areas of minimal disease. A common mechanism for coronary disease progression. Chest 1988; 94: 731–6.

153. Hackett D, Davies G, Maseri A. Pre-existing coronary stenoses in patients with first myocardial infarction are not necessarily severe. Eur Heart J 1988; 9: 1317–23.

154. Little W, Constantinescu M, Applegate R, et al. Can cor-

onary arteriography predict the site of subsequent myocardial infarction in a patient with mild to moderate coronary artery disease? Circulation 1988; 78: 1157–66.

155. Meade T, North W, Chakrabarti R. Haemostatic function and cardiovascular death: early results of a prospective study. Lancet 1980; i: 1050–4.

156. Meade T. Thrombogenic factors. In: Olson A, ed. Atherosclerosis biology and clinical science. Edinburgh, London, Melbourne, New York: Churchill-Livingstone, 1987: 453–5.

157. Barger AC, Beeuwkes R, Lainey LL, Silverman KJ. Hypothesis: vasa vasorium and neovascularisation of human coronary arteries: a possible role in the pathology of a atherosclerosis. N Engl J Med 1983; 310: 175–7.

158. Tracy R, Devaney K, Kissling G. Characteristics of the plaque under a coronary thrombus. Virchows Arch [A] 1985; 405: 411–27.

159. Tracy R, Kissling G. Comparisons of human populations for histologic features of atherosclerosis. Arch Pathol Lab Med 1988; 112: 1056–65.

160. Grundy S, Wilhelmsen L, Rose G, Campbell R, Assman G. Coronary heart disease in high-risk populations: lessons from Finland. Eur Heart J 1990; 5: 462.

161. Tracy R, Toca V, Strong J, Richards M. Relationship of raised atherosclerotic lesions to fatty streaks in cigarette smokers. Atherosclerosis 1981; 38: 347–57.

162. Hagman M, Wilhelmsen L, Wedel H, Pennert K. Risk factors of angina pectoris in a population study of Swedish men. J Chronic Dis 1987; 40: 265–75.

163. Asmussen I. Chromatin changes of endothelial cells in umbilical arteries in smokers. Clin Cardiol 1982; 5: 653–6.

164. Pittilo R, Mackie I, Rowles P, Machin S, Woolf N. Effects of cigarette smoking on the ultrastructure of rat thoracic aorta and its ability to produce prostacyclin. Thromb Haemost 1982; 148: 173–6.

165. Bull H, Pittlio R, Blow C. The effects of nicotine of PG12 production by rat endothelium. Thromb Haemost 1985; 54: 472–4.

166. Madsen H, Dyerberg J. Cigarette smoking and its effect on the platelet-vessel wall interaction. Scand J Clin Lab Invest 1984; 44: 203–6.

167. Belch J, McArdle B, Burns P, Lowe G, Forbes C. The effects of acute smoking on platelet behaviour fibrinolysis and haemorheology in habitual smokers. Thromb Haemost 1984; 51: 6–8.

168. Meade T, Brozovic M, Chakrabarti P. Haemostatic function and ischaemic heart disease: principal results of the Northwick Park study. Lancet 1986; 2: 533–7.

169. Levine P. An acute effect of cigarette smoking on platelet function: a possible link between smoking and arterial thrombosis. Circulation 1973; 48: 619–23.

170. Hawkins R. Smoking, platelets and thrombosis. Nature 1972; 236: 450–2.

171. Pittilo RM, Clarke JMF, Harris D, et al. Cigarette smoking and platelet adhesion. Br J Haematol 1984; 58: 627–32.

172. Wennmalm A. Effects of nicotine on cardiac prostaglandin and platelet thromboxane synthesis. Br J Pharmacol 1987; 64: 559–63.

4

CHARACTERISTICS ASSOCIATED WITH THE RISK OF ARTERIAL THROMBOSIS AND THE PRETHROMBOTIC STATE

THOMAS W. MEADE, G. J. MILLER, and ROBERT D. ROSENBERG

General recognition of the thrombotic component of clinically manifest ischemic heart disease (IHD) and also of ischemic stroke is comparatively recent. For a variety of reasons, the growing research endeavor that started after the Second World War and which was prompted by the increasing incidence of ischemic heart disease largely centered on atheroma and, because of its lipid content, the place of dietary fat and blood cholesterol levels. When interest did begin to focus on the role of thrombosis in the mid 1970s, it first had to contend with two major controversies. The first was whether thrombosis precedes or follows transmural myocardial infarction (MI). The issue was settled, as far as it then could be, by a consensus view of the evidence which concluded that thrombosis does precede and probably causes transmural myocardial infarction.[1] With the advent of thrombolytic therapy and the need to establish the rationale for its use and effects, angiography demonstrated the high frequency of total coronary occlusion during myocardial infarction,[2] and there is now no doubt about the significance of thrombosis in transmural myocardial infarction.[3] Thrombosis is probably also involved in subendocardial infarction, though the evidence on this point is less clear.[3] The second controversy, settled even more recently, was the place of thrombosis in sudden coronary death. Surprising though it may now seem,

reports in the mid 1970s of platelet thrombi and microemboli in the coronary vessels of those dying sudden vascular deaths[4] were often viewed with skepticism. It was not until the results of a series of particularly careful autopsy studies became available in the 1980s—the best example being the work of Davies and Thomas[5]—that the almost universal occurrence of at least a degree of thrombosis in sudden coronary death was recognized. The minority of events in which thrombosis is not apparently associated with plaque rupture (between 2 per cent[5] and about 25 per cent,[6] for example) are interesting in suggesting that characteristics of the circulating blood play a part in initiating some arterial thrombi, a central theme of this chapter. The observation that thrombi associated with sudden coronary death do not totally occlude the arterial lumen as often as those causing transmural myocardial infarction may be due to the intense fibrinolytic activity accompanying sudden death, with the consequence that thrombi initially responsible for the episode are at least partially lysed by the time of autopsy.[3,7]

On the epidemiological side, however, there had been much earlier recognition of a thrombotic component even though its detailed characteristics had not been fully clarified. Thus, it was Morris[8] who first drew attention to the involvement of a major process other than atherogenesis through his

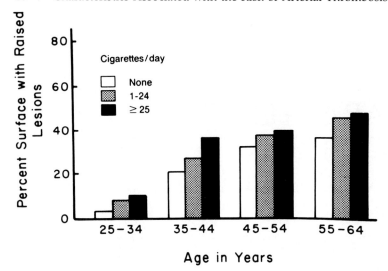

FIGURE 4–1. Percentage of coronary arteries affected by raised lesions in men at different ages according to previous smoking. (Reproduced with permission from McGill H. The cardiovascular pathology of smoking. Am Heart J 1988; 115: 250–7.)

analysis of postmortem findings at the London Hospital. There was no increase—if anything, a decrease—in the prevalence of advanced atheroma over a period during which mortality from ischemic heart disease had increased many times. Morris pointed out that the main epidemic had started just after the First World War and that some environmental change that had occurred about then might provide at least a partial explanation. One such possibility was the widespread adoption of cigarette smoking by men. If this was involved, it suggested a relatively short-term, acute affect rather than a longer-term influence. Another population-based study of the pathology of ischemic heart disease, the International Atherosclerosis Project, also provides an interesting indication of an acute process.[9,10] Figure 4–1 shows the percentage surface of coronary arteries affected by raised lesions in men at different ages according to the amount previously smoked. There is indeed a tendency toward greater involvement the larger the number of cigarettes. But as Table 4–1 shows,[11-14] the relative risk of death from ischemic heart disease in young smokers is several times that of nonsmokers

of the same age, and much more pronounced than the relationship between smoking and coronary atheroma. Once again, this contrast suggests the superimposition of another process to account for the clinical manifestations of ischemic heart disease, a conclusion also reached in an arteriographic study in women.[15] The rapid initial decline in the risk of ischemic heart disease in exsmokers[16] is another observation that implies modification of an acute process. Together, these findings suggest the involvement of a hemostatic component strongly influenced by cigarette smoking.

In 1953, Morris and his colleagues[17] began their series of publications showing the protective effect of physical activity at work against clinically manifest ischemic heart disease. In 1958, Morris and Crawford[18] complemented these findings with pathological data. The National Necropsy Survey was based on simple, standardized recordings from 206 (or 85 per cent) of the pathology departments in the British National Health Service, each of these departments contributing their findings in a total of 3,800 deaths from causes other than ischemic heart disease. Information was also obtained on the last occupation of the men in question and coded according to the level of physical activity involved. Figure 4–2 summarizes the clear results. There was no relationship between physical activity of occupation and atheroma of the coronary artery walls. There was some relationship between activity and coronary artery lumen occlusion. The strongest relationship was with large healed infarcts.

TABLE 4–1. Relative Risk of Ischemic Heart Disease Death in Young Male Smokers (Compared with 1.0)

Doll and Peto,[11] 1976	9.7
Weir and Dunn,[12] 1970	6.2
Kahn,[13] 1966	4.4
Hammond and Garfinkel,[14] 1969	2.8

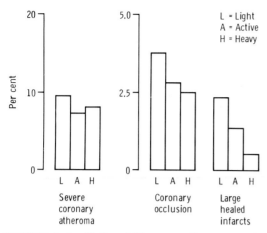

FIGURE 4–2. National Necropsy Survey results showing relationship between physical activity of work and different pathological manifestations of ischemic heart disease.

It is theoretically possible that men who had previously had infarcts tended to take up less physically demanding occupations before they died. However, if this were the explanation for the findings on infarcts, there would probably have been a similar relationship with coronary atheroma in view of the clear relationship between atheroma and infarction. In addition, there is increasing reason from other work[19] to believe not only that the relationship between physical activity and clinical disease is of causal significance, but that it operates through a short-term or antithrombotic effect. Thus, the findings of the National Necropsy Survey suggest that the effect of exercise, or of its absence, on occlusive episodes and infarction itself is mediated through some other pathway than atherogenesis.

HEMOSTATIC FUNCTION AND THROMBOSIS

Coronary artery thrombi are due to platelet aggregates and fibrin, in varying proportions. Most attention has so far been directed toward the contribution of platelets. Their very rapid adhesion to damaged endothelium and then to each other is central to arterial thrombosis. It is, however, fibrin which gives many developing thrombi their ultimate stability and volume. A recent biochemical (as distinct from morphological) study concluded that fibrin formation and platelet activation are probably equally important in the early hours

of myocardial infarction,[20] providing added reason for recognizing that the mechanical obstruction of the coronary artery is due to two main processes and that the most effective approach to antithrombotic therapy may involve platelet-active agents and anticoagulants used simultaneously.

Given a major thrombotic contribution, an obvious question for the clinician or epidemiologist is the extent to which those at risk of ischemic heart disease can be characterized on account of a thrombotic tendency. A major part of the answer depends on the results of studies which include measures of hemostatic function and relate these to the presence (prevalence) or subsequent onset (incidence) of ischemic heart disease. Examples of cross-sectional studies on hemostatic variables and ischemic heart disease are in Poller[21] and Meade.[22] However, this account mainly considers the evidence from prospective or incidence studies. Although they are usually quicker and cheaper, prevalence studies of hemostatic function and ischemic heart disease are subject to a number of substantial drawbacks. First, an association between a clotting factor activity level (for example) and the previous occurrence of a clinical episode of ischemic heart disease may be the result of the episode rather than having preceded it. This is a point of special importance in the case of fibrinogen, for example, the level of which may rise in response to a range of stimuli. Second, many prevalence studies have found weaker relationships than those later established in prospective studies. One reason may be the effect of a clinical episode on the measures in question, either because the episode itself has metabolic consequences on variables of potential interest or because those who have experienced them alter their dietary, smoking, and other habits. Third, more or less by definition, prevalence studies cannot include fatal episodes, the characteristics of which could differ from nonfatal episodes. Finally, many clinical cross-sectional studies have been too small, or cases and controls have been inadequately matched, for much confidence to be placed in their findings. This account will also concentrate on studies in those so far free of clinically manifest ischemic heart disease, since it is clear that in follow-up studies of recurrence in survivors of a previous episode, the main determinant of death (if not of further nonfatal episodes) is the extent of the initial infarction.[23]

Work on hemostatic function, thrombosis, and ischemic heart disease has identified two important preliminary considerations—one methodological, and the other conceptual.

Many components or measures of the hemostatic system are subject to high levels of variability—often much more than the variability in cholesterol, for example.[24,25] Laboratory variation is part of the explanation. But it is within-individual variation that makes it particularly difficult to characterize a person's true or habitual level. In evolutionary terms, this variability is to be expected of a system upon which changing demands may be made at quite short notice, as requirements for hemostasis vary either physiologically or in response to circumstances that might lead to injury. The main consequence of this variability is that larger numbers will be required to show a relationship with ischemic heart disease for a hemostatic variable that is subject to a high degree of variability than for a more stable measurement such as cholesterol. By the same token, any relationship between the hemostatic variable that does emerge, despite the variability, is likely to be a strong effect, a conclusion recognized in recent work on the "regression dilution effect."[26] Another consequence is the statistical disadvantage at which hemostatic variables may start in multiple regression analyses by comparison with less variable characteristics and the effect this may have on the demonstration of independent associations. In any case, the significance of statistical independence has been considerably exaggerated. A good example is the role of triglycerides, usually relegated to a position of secondary importance because levels are often not independently related to ischemic heart disease incidence, largely on account (it is now recognized) of within-person variation. But their biological role in modifying coagulability and fibrinolytic activity is now increasingly acknowledged.

The conceptual point arises from the view that there is unlikely to be any correlation between high clotting factor levels and ischemic heart disease. The epidemiologic studies cited below reveal a relationship of plasma factor VII activity and fibrinogen levels with the incidence of ischemic heart disease. Furthermore, the magnitude of differences in these studies between those who do or do not subsequently develop ischemic heart disease can (as with other variables) be related to the magnitude of this risk. Indeed, the effects of plasma factor VII activity and fibrinogen levels are at least as great as the effects of well-known characteristics such as blood pressure and the blood cholesterol. This observation, dealt with in more detail in later sections, is a major stimulus to the concept and definition of "hypercoagulability" and the "prethrombotic state."

This review considers the basic investigation, epidemiologic study, and practical implications of these concepts.

HYPERCOAGULABILITY

Attempts to link hemostatic variables with the development of ischemic heart disease implicitly assume that increased activity of coagulation proteins or platelets might serve as a marker of, or directly contribute to, the critical thrombotic component of this disease. It is epidemiologic studies of coagulation proteins that have so far been most rewarding with regard to this hypothesis, although the central role of platelets in thrombogenesis is acknowledged. The sections below summarize recent advances in our understanding of the in vivo function of the blood coagulation mechanism, and explore biochemical evidence for a hypercoagulable or prethrombotic state in humans. The information provided serves as a background for the subsequent discussion of the epidemiologic data.

The coagulation mechanism is composed of a series of linked proteolytic reactions[27] illustrated schematically in Figure 4-3. At each stage, a zymogen is converted to its corresponding serine protease, which activates the next zymogen in the cascade, ultimately leading to thrombin generation. This blood clotting enzyme is able to convert fibrinogen to fibrin and thereby initiate thrombus formation. In most steps, protein cofactors such as factors V and VIII are activated by blood clotting enzymes, bind different pairs of zymogen-serine proteases to cell surfaces, and accelerate generation of the next proteolytic enzyme within the pathway. Thus, the coagulation mechanism can be pictured as a series of reactions in which a zymogen, a cofactor and a converting enzyme interact to form a multimolecular complex on a natural surface. All the various reactants must be present if conversion of the zymogen is to take place at a significant rate. These transformations are suppressed if the converting

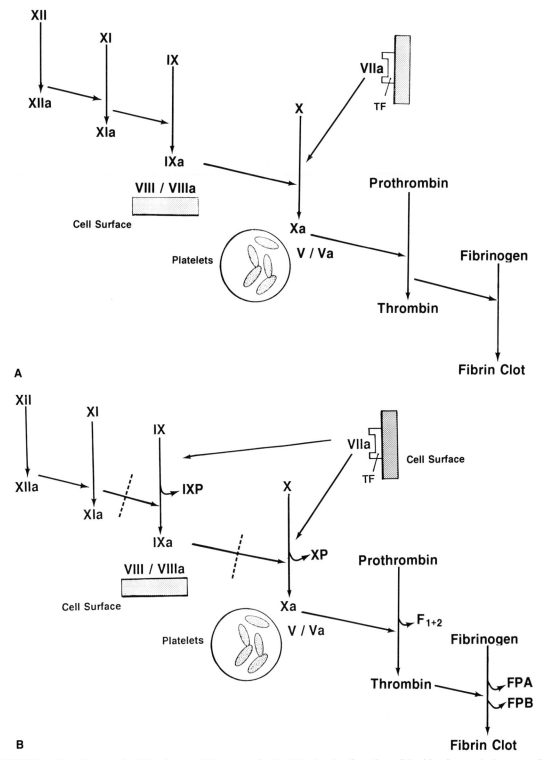

FIGURE 4–3.   The classical blood coagulation cascade (A). The in vivo function of the blood coagulation cascade (B). The dotted lines represent functional blocks which are removed during hemostasis/thrombosis.

enzyme is inhibited, the protein cofactor destroyed, or the surface receptors essential for the macromolecular complex sequestered.

The direct measurement of coagulation enzymes would be especially informative with regard to the detection of the hypercoagulable state in humans. Unfortunately, this approach has been unsuccessful because of the extremely short half-life of these enzymes within the circulation owing to natural anticoagulant mechanisms outlined below. However, the transition of zymogens to serine proteases at three separate stages in the coagulation mechanism occurs in concert with the release of an activation peptide, and thrombin-dependent production of fibrin also involves liberation of two small fragments of fibrinogen. The conversion of factor IX to activated factor IX leads to the formation of a serine protease with two polypeptide chains joined by a disulfide bridge. During this reaction, peptide bonds at arginine-145–alanine-146 and arginine-180–valine-181 are cleaved with the release of a highly glycosylated 35-amino-acid activation peptide with a molecular weight of 11,000 daltons.[28] The transformation of factor X to activated factor X also results in the generation of a serine protease with two chains joined by a single disulfide bridge. During this process, a peptide bond at arginine-194–isoleucine-195 is cleaved, which liberates a highly glycosylated 52-amino-acid peptide of molecular weight 14,000 daltons.[29] The transition of prothrombin to thrombin produces a serine protease with two peptide chains joined by a disulfide bridge. During this event, a peptide bond at arginine-273–threonine-274 is cleaved, which releases the nonthrombin half of the prothrombin (fragment F1+2) with a molecular weight of 31,000 daltons.[30,31] The thrombin-dependent conversion of fibrinogen to fibrin is marked by the cleavage of two sets of arginine-16–glycine-17 in the A-chain and arginine-14–glycine-15 bonds in the Bβ-chain with liberation of the 16-amino-acid fibrinopeptide A and the 14-amino-acid fibrinopeptide B.[32]

The plasma concentrations of factor IX activation peptide (F1Xp), factor X activation peptide (FXp), prothrombin activation peptide (F1+2), and fibrinopeptide A (FPA) can be accurately quantitated by radioimmunoassay and used to monitor the generation of specific blood clotting enzymes.[33–36] The various activation fragments exhibit half-lives within the circulation ranging from 5 to 90 minutes.[33–36] The normal levels of factor IX activation peptide, factor X activation peptide, prothrombin activation peptide, and fibrinopeptide A in individuals under the age of 45 years are approximately 66 picomoles/liter, 200 picomoles/liter, 1,500 picomoles/liter, and 1,200 picomoles/liter, respectively.[33–36] The basal plasma concentrations of these peptides indicate continuous procoagulant activity within the hemostatic mechanism, albeit at an extremely low flux. This basal activity may well have more to do with the process of vascular repair than hemostasis per se, which is only required when the vessel wall endothelial lining has been breeched.

The development of peptide activation assays has allowed examination of the basal in vivo functioning of the blood coagulation mechanism (Fig. 4–3). This has been accomplished by measuring the concentrations of the activation peptides in patients with congenital deficiencies of factors VII, VIII, and IX prior to and immediately after normalization with purified or recombinant proteins.[34,35,37] These studies demonstrate that the factor VII-tissue factor pathway is also mainly responsible for the activation of factor IX with minimal contribution from contact phase reactions of the intrinsic pathway (factor XII-factor XI). The latter observation confirms the suspicions of previous investigators who studied these reactions in purified systems.[38,39] The high levels of activated factor IX produced by the factor VII-tissue factor pathway are, surprisingly, not able to convert factor X to activated factor X. This conclusion is documented by infusion of purified factor IX into individuals deficient in this protein, which normalizes the plasma concentrations of factor IX activation peptide, but has no effect on the plasma levels of factor X activation peptide or prothrombin activation peptide.[37] These results are reinforced by infusion of purified factor VIII into patients deficient in this cofactor, which does not alter the levels of factor X activation peptide or prothrombin activation peptide.[37] However, it is possible that the activated factor IX generated by the factor VII-tissue factor pathway could produce circulating activated factor VII in a reaction which is independent of tissue factor or activated factor VIII (see below).

Thus, the factor VII-tissue factor pathway serves as the major driving force to establish the basal activity of the coagulation mechanism. The intrinsic pathway is dormant (with regard to thrombin generation), which appears to be due to the inability of activated factor IX produced by the factor VII-tissue factor pathway to act on factor X because of the absence of circulating activated factor VIII or activated platelets. It is surmised that vessel wall injury raises thrombin concentrations above basal levels via the factor VII-tissue pathway, which then converts small amounts of factor VIII to activated factor VIII and possibly activates platelets with resultant amplifications of thrombin production by the action of existing activated factor IX on factor X. In this scenario, the generation of activated factor XI by the contact phase reactions may play a secondary role in augmenting plasma concentrations of activated factor IX produced by the factor VII-tissue factor pathway. We suspect that the intrinsic cascade amplification outlined above is essential to generate sufficient thrombin to create the normal hemostatic plug, but may also be involved in pathologic situations to produce arterial thrombi (see below).

The coagulation mechanism has been described as a cascade or "waterfall" in which each molecule of enzyme activates many molecules of its zymogen substrate at each stage, so that the system functions as a biochemical amplifier.[40,41] Careful comparison of the plasma concentrations of activation peptides corrected for their half-lives in the circulation reveal that these linked zymogen transitions are tightly controlled during basal levels of activity and at the point of thrombosis with much less overall step-to-step amplification than previously suspected. Indeed, the blood coagulation cascade should be conceptualized as a set of zymogen conversion events which are individually regulated by several potent natural anticoagulant mechanisms.[42] The heparan sulfate-antithrombin III mechanism of the blood vessel wall is responsible for the neutralization of circulating activated factor XI, activated factor IX, activated factor X, and thrombin.[43,44] The protein C-thrombomodulin mechanism of the blood vessel wall captures thrombin, which then generates activated protein C that destroys activated cofactors VIII and V, employed in the production of activated factor X and thrombin, respectively.[45] The fibrinolytic system is able to prevent fibrin deposition by transforming fibrin-1 (removal of fibrinopeptide A) to a fragment of fibrinogen via a plasmin-dependent cleavage of the Bβ-chain, which suppresses conversion to insoluble fibrin-II (removal of fibrinopeptide B).[46] The basal functioning of these natural anticoagulant mechanisms has been documented as outlined for the procoagulant side of the coagulation mechanism by the measurement of thrombin-antithrombin complex, protein C activation peptide, and fibrinopeptide A/Bβ1-42 cleavage products.[47–49]

The hypercoagulable state exists between the extremes of normal basal coagulation system function and the augmented generation of serine proteases which takes place during thrombus formation. This prethrombotic state is operationally defined by small elevations of serine protease generation and fibrin deposition as measured by peptide activation assays which show that coagulation system activity is exceeding the inhibitory threshold of the natural anticoagulant mechanisms. The above model suggests that it should be possible to detect an imbalance between the procoagulant and natural anticoagulant mechanisms, which would eventually lead to thrombotic phenomena. To examine this hypothesis, biochemical alterations of the coagulation mechanism were sought in patients with protein C deficiency.[50] Specific assays for prothrombin activation peptide, protein C activation peptide, and fibrinopeptide A were utilized to examine 23 asymptomatic individuals with this disorder. The mean concentrations of prothrombin activation peptide were significantly elevated by about twofold, and the mean levels of protein C activation peptide were significantly decreased by about twofold, whereas the mean concentrations of fibrinopeptide A were minimally changed when compared to an age-matched control group. The metabolic behavior of prothrombin activation peptide was similar in the protein C-deficient group, with elevated levels of this marker as compared to normal individuals. Identical results have been obtained in a more limited number of kindreds with protein S deficiency.[50] Based upon these data, it would appear that our model of hypercoagulability might have validity in more complex acquired prethrombotic states.

The known association of ischemic heart disease with age prompted an evaluation of coagulation activity perturbations induced by the aging process.[51] The levels of prothrombin activation peptide, factor IX activation peptide, factor X activation peptide, and fibrinopeptide A were quantitated in 199 healthy males between the ages of 42 and 80.[51] The population was constructed by

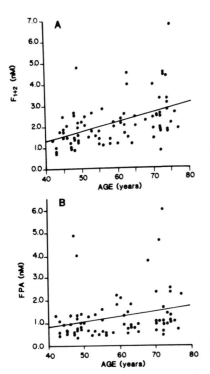

FIGURE 4–4. Concentration of prothrombin activation peptide (A) and fibrinopeptide A (B) as a function of age in 82 Normative Aging Study participants. Lines represent the best linear squares fit of the data.

carefully screening the medical records of a normative aging study to exclude those individuals who had developed coexistent medical conditions which might cause alterations in coagulation system activity. None of the individuals examined exhibited an immunochemical deficiency of circulating natural anticoagulant proteins. The results showed a highly significant correlation between elevated levels of the activation peptides and increasing age as illustrated in Figure 4–4. These data appear to be due to an increasing number of individuals within each advancing age group who exhibit markedly augmented values of the markers. The elevated concentrations of these activation peptides are not due to decreased clearance as judged by metabolic studies of radiolabeled fragments. It is also of interest to note the existence of a remarkably tight correlation between the concentrations of factor IX activation peptide and factor X activation peptide with a significantly lesser correlation between the levels of these two markers and those of prothrombin activation peptide and fibrinopeptide A (Bauer KA, Rosenberg RD, unpublished

findings). These observations are interpreted to indicate that certain males over the age of 45 years exhibit increased activity of the factor VII-tissue factor pathway with augmented levels of activated factors IX and X which are variably manifest as more extensive conversion of prothrombin to thrombin with detectable elevation of fibrinogen to fibrin generation. Thus, these results suggest that many apparently normal individuals exhibit a biochemical defect with increasing age which denotes the presence of an acquired prethrombotic state.

The coagulation abnormalities outlined above can be visualized as early changes in the exposure of tissue factor and/or the extent of conversion of factor VII to activated factor VII. The production of thrombin and fibrin in these individuals appears to be variably suppressed by the natural anticoagulant mechanisms as outlined above. Thus, a subset of these individuals might also exhibit significant reductions in the function of the heparan sulfate-antithrombin III, or thrombomodulin-protein C mechanisms. These alterations might be due to decreased synthesis of anticoagulantly active heparan sulfate or thrombomodulin by endothelial cells or a variety of other molecular defects. The above abnormalities would allow the augmented activity of the factor VII-tissue factor pathway to generate increased levels of thrombin and fibrin. Thus, some men over the age of 45 years may exhibit enhanced activity of different stages of the coagulation cascade, which is poised to respond to events such as coronary artery plaque fissure with sufficient production of free thrombin to ignite the dormant intrinsic pathway and lead to a thrombotic event.

The hypercoagulable state outlined above has been delineated with the activation peptide assays. Prior investigators have utilized more classical assay techniques to define the prethrombotic state. The biochemical abnormalities uncovered by the activation peptide assays suggest that classical coagulation assays might detect elevated levels of factor VII activity in hypercoagulable individuals. Particular attention is focused on this coagulation protein for reasons provided below. Factor VII is produced by the liver as a single-chain zymogen which can be cleaved to a two-chain species without release of an activation peptide upon exposure to activated factors XII, IX, X, and thrombin.[52,53] Current biochemical data indicate that activated factor VII is able to activate factors IX and X when coupled with tissue factor, but significant controversy exists about the ability of the zymogen to carry out the same reactions, albeit at a greatly reduced level.[54-56] Thus, elevated plasma levels of factor VII activity in hypercoagulable individuals would most likely be due to increased conversion of factor VII to activated factor VII. The increased production of prothrombin activation peptide which occurs during the hypercoagulable state might also induce augmented levels of factor VII as well as other vitamin K-dependent coagulation factors, which could further elevate the apparent plasma levels of factor VII activity.[57] If the plasma levels of factor VII activity and the concentrations of activation peptides reflect the same underlying biochemical changes which define the prethrombotic state, the two abnormalities would be positively correlated. Studies are currently underway to test this possibility. Finally, it should also be acknowledged that elevated plasma concentrations of fibrinogen might also play a role in the hypercoagulable state, since they might be expected to generate a larger thrombus for equivalent amounts of thrombin generated.

The importance of the hypercoagulable state in ischemic heart disease is presently at an interesting transitional stage with regard to clinical and epidemiologic studies. The past investigations have utilized classical coagulation assays to show strong associations of plasma factor VII activity and levels of fibrinogen with cardiovascular disease as outlined below. The application of activation peptide assays now provides a technique for more directly assessing the relationship between coagulation system activity and ischemic heart disease as well as monitoring preventive anticoagulant therapy.

EPIDEMIOLOGIC EVIDENCE

There is still no generally accepted measure of platelet function that has been shown to be associated with the later onset of ischemic heart disease in those so far free of clinical disease, though the results of a recent study[58] support the conclusions of others in suggesting that spontaneous platelet aggregation may well be associated with recurrence.

The levels of factor VII activity and of plasma fibrinogen are the two aspects of the hemostatic system that have so far been particularly highlighted by the results of prospective studies. Factor VII coagulant activity was measured in the Northwick Park Heart Study by a semiautomated one-stage bioassay.[59] The test plasma is diluted 1 in 40, and its activity assessed by the addition of equal (0.1 milliliter) volumes of a factor VII-deficient substrate plasma, a 1 in 32 dilution of a commercial rabbit brain thromboplastin as the source of tissue factor (Diagen) and M/40 $CaCl_2$. The time from addition of the calcium-thromboplastin mixture to the formation of fibrin clot is measured at 37° centigrade with a coagulometer (Amelung KC 10). It is important to note that the Northwick Park assay is distinctive in that the factor VII-deficient substrate plasma is prepared from an absorbed bovine plasma to which has been added a human concentrate of factors IX, X, and prothrombin with less than 0.5 per cent factor VII activity per 1 milliliter of reconstituted concentrate. Many other laboratories employ instead a human factor VII-deficient substrate plasma.

Precisely what aspect of factor VII in the test plasma this bioassay measures is still not entirely clear, because of the uncertainty that exists as to whether single-chain factor VII possesses any intrinsic serine protein activity when coupled with tissue factor[54-56] and the absence of an assay that can distinguish factor VII from activated factor VII in vivo. However, the finding of a diurnal variation in factor VII activity in the absence of any similar variation in factor VII antigen concentration suggests that elevated levels in factor VII activity are more likely to reflect increased generation of activated factor VII from VII in vivo,[60] although an elevation in single-chain factor VII concentration cannot be excluded as a cause of a high factor VII activity on bioassay.

Northwick Park Heart Study (NPHS)

In 1980, Meade et al.[61] showed preliminary results suggesting that high levels of factor VII coagulant activity and of plasma fibrinogen, and possibly also of factor VIII activity, were associated with mortality from cardiovascular disease, principally ischemic heart disease. The main results of Northwick Park Heart Study[62] are summarized in Figure 4–

5. They are based on 143 deaths from all causes, of which 68 were due to ischemic heart disease, and on nonfatal episodes of myocardial infarction. High levels of factor VII coagulant activity and of fibrinogen were associated with mortality from all causes. The use of deaths from all causes has the advantage that it does not depend on opinions about the cause of death. At the same time, ischemic heart disease is the commonest cause in men in the age group concerned and, if high clotting factor levels are strongly asso-

ciated with ischemic heart disease, this should be evident in analyses based on total mortality. The relationships of factor VII coagulant activity and fibrinogen with the incidence specifically of ischemic heart disease within five years of recruitment were, if anything, stronger than for cholesterol, though the latter relationship—as expected—was also demonstrated. There were no clear relationships between factor VII coagulant activity or fibrinogen and the incidence of cancer, the commonest nonvascular cause of serious

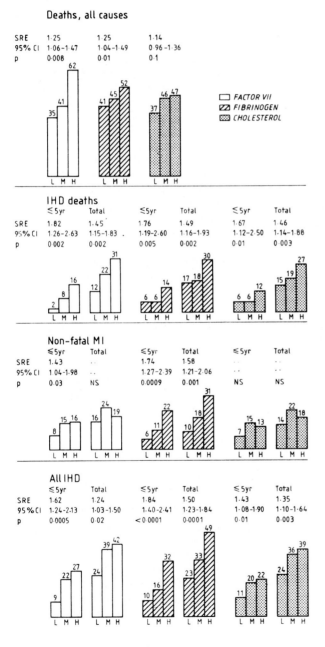

FIGURE 4–5. **Main results of the Northwick Park Heart Study. Numbers of events within five years and for total follow-up period by low (L), middle (M), and high (H) thirds of distributions. Standardized regression effects (SRE) show increases in risk of ischemic heart disease for a standard deviation increase in the variable concerned; for example, SRE of 1.50 indicates that for a standard deviation rise, risk increases by 50 per cent. (Reproduced with permission from the Lancet 1986; 2: 533–7.)**

TABLE 4–2. Mean Fibrinogen Levels (grams/liter) at Entry to Goteborg Study According to Subsequent Outcome

Ischemic Heart Disease	Stroke	Deaths From Other Causes	No Event
N = 92	N = 37	N = 60	N = 608
3.56*	3.70*	3.37	3.30

*$p < 0.01$.

illness and death, so that the findings do appear to be specific for vascular disease.

Goteborg Study

In 1984, Wilhelmsen et al.[63] showed a relationship, in a study of 792 men born in 1913, between high fibrinogen levels and the incidence of both ischemic heart disease and, in particular, stroke. Their findings are summarized in Table 4–2. For stroke, the data suggested an interaction between fibrinogen and systolic blood pressure (men with high levels of both being at considerably greater risk than might have been expected from the sum of the two effects separately, though the relatively small number of events on which this analysis is based need to be taken into account).

Leigh Study

In 1985, Stone and Thorp[66] reported an association between high fibrinogen levels and ischemic heart disease incidence in a group of 297 men aged between 40 and 69 who were followed for up to 20 years. The relationship was stronger than for cholesterol, blood pressure, or cigarette smoking. In this study, too, there was suggestive evidence of an interaction between fibrinogen

and blood pressure. Thus, men whose systolic blood pressure and plasma fibrinogen levels fell in the top third of the respective distributions experienced 12 times the incidence of ischemic heart disease compared with those both of whose levels fell in the low third.

Framingham Study

In 1985, Kannel et al.[65] reported an association between high fibrinogen levels and the incidence of cardiovascular disease in 554 men and 761 women aged between 45 and 79 who had not previously experienced a cardiovascular event (cardiovascular disease being defined as the sum of ischemic heart disease, stroke, heart failure, and peripheral arterial disease). Subsequent publications[66,67] established a clear relationship between fibrinogen and the incidence of ischemic heart disease in both men and women and between fibrinogen and stroke in men but not in women and also suggested (Table 4–3) that the effects of simultaneously high levels of fibrinogen and blood pressure may be of particular importance.

Caerphilly Study

The results of this study[68] also show a strong relationship between not only fibrinogen, but also viscosity and the incidence of ischemic heart disease.

No prospective study besides Northwick Park Heart Study has so far published main results on factor VII coagulant activity, but together with the Northwick Park Heart Study results on factor VII coagulant activity, these studies as a whole suggest that the biochemical disturbance leading to ischemic heart disease lies at least as much in the

TABLE 4–3. Cardiovascular Disease by Fibrinogen and Hypertensive Status: Framingham Study Subjects 45 to 79 Years of Age, 12-Year Rate per 1,000

Fibrinogen (grams/liter)	Normotensive		Mild Hypertension		Definite Hypertension	
	Men	Women	Men	Women	Men	Women
<2.65	2.27	1.53	4.21	1.92	5.39	3.78
2.65–3.11	2.61	1.54	5.19	2.40	4.10	2.82
>3.12	4.67	2.18	5.38	3.78	7.08	5.43

TABLE 4–4. Dutch Hemophiliacs: Ratios of Observed to Expected Deaths

Neoplasm	2.5
Lung cancer	8.6
Accidents	2.6
Renal failure	30.0
Stroke	5.0
Ischemic heart disease	0.2

coagulation system as in the metabolism of cholesterol.

However, factor VII coagulant activity and the fibrinogen level are almost certainly not the only components of the coagulation system involved in the onset of ischemic heart disease. Although considerably weaker than for factor VII coagulant activity and fibrinogen, there were also suggestive associations in Northwick Park Heart Study between high factor VIII levels and poor fibrinolytic activity with incidence,[61,62] and impaired fibrinolytic activity may also influence the recurrence of myocardial infarction.[69] In the case of factor VIII, supporting evidence comes from studies showing a lower than expected incidence of ischemic heart disease in hemophiliacs and exemplified in Table 4–4 by the results of a Dutch study.[70] The higher than expected mortality from stroke and accidents is due to bleeding. The increased mortality from renal disease may partly be due to the greater prevalence of hypertension in hemophiliacs. The precise explanation for the increased mortality from malignant disease is not (so far) clear. By contrast, the very much lower than expected mortality from ischemic heart disease is obvious. Some caution is necessary in interpreting these and other findings,[71] since the high mortality of hemophiliacs from other causes introduces the concept of "competing risks" as a possible reason for lower mortality from IHD. However, the very considerable reduction in ischemic heart disease in the Dutch study, coupled with the suggestive if inconclusive Northwick Park Heart Study findings, indicate that the possible contribution of factor VIII to ischemic heart disease should at least not be overlooked.

The potential defense mechanisms against thrombosis include antithrombin III and the vitamin K-dependent anticoagulatory factors, protein C and protein S. Intuitively, it is low levels that seem likely to be associated with increased risk. This is certainly true for the inherited thrombophilias leading to venous thrombosis. However, some of the relationships of antithrombotic factors to the risk of arterial thrombosis and thus of ischemic heart disease seem paradoxical. In the case of antithrombin III, for example, vegetarians with a lower than average risk of ischemic heart disease nevertheless have significantly lower levels than nonvegetarians.[72] Two studies[73,74] have reported significantly higher antithrombin III levels in postmenopausal women than in premenopausal women of the same age, the incidence of ischemic heart disease being higher in the former. Levels may also be higher in diabetics than in nondiabetics,[75] the increased risk of ischemic heart disease in the former being well known. Yue et al.[76] found a gradient of rising antithrombin III values from those at low risk of ischemic heart disease via those at intermediate risk or with chronic ischemic heart disease to those with acute myocardial infarction. Findings at recruitment to the Northwick Park Heart Study[22] also suggested higher rather than lower values in those who had previously experienced ischemic heart disease. By contrast, others[77–79] have reported lower levels in those with a past history of infarction or other manifestations of arterial disease. These apparently contradictory findings could be partly explained by postulating that antithrombin III levels, for example, tend not to be elevated in those who are at low risk of arterial disease and who do not therefore need to make an antithrombotic response. In those at high risk, on the other hand, antithrombin III levels may be low or high. Inability to increase antithrombin III levels in some may directly contribute to subsequent events in which high procoagulatory clotting factor levels are involved, while levels in others may rise as a compensatory defense mechanism. While the studies summarized are compatible with an explanation of this kind, they have so far all been cross-sectional, so that it has not been possible to relate antithrombin III levels to later clinical events. Northwick Park Heart Study data[80] do suggest that both low and high levels may be associated with increased risk.[91]

However, association does not necessarily imply causation. Besides prospective studies, other types of evidence also have to be considered in establishing whether levels of factor VII coagulant activity, fibrinogen, and perhaps other hemostatic variables are associated with the subsequent incidence of ischemic heart disease because they are causally involved or simply because they are markers of some other process. The results of randomized controlled trials are particularly valuable in this context, providing as they do, unbiased evidence on the consequences of altering clotting factor activities.

CLINICAL TRIALS

It is part of the mythology of oral anticoagulants that they are ineffective after myocardial infarction. However, even before the most recent evidence, this assertion was demonstrably incorrect. Thus, overviews of the evidence from long-term trials[81] and of short-term trials[82] established a 20 per cent reduction in mortality attributable to oral anticoagulants after infarction. This observation, and a larger reduction in recurrent nonfatal events, was confirmed in the Dutch Sixty Plus trial[83] and, very recently, in the WARIS trial.[84] Warfarin reduces the activity levels of the other procoagulatory clotting factors besides factor VII, (that is, II, IX, and X) and also of the anticoagulatory factors, protein C and protein S. It is therefore not possible to explain the effects of warfarin solely in terms of factor VII coagulant activity, though it is reasonable to conclude that lowering the general level of coagulability prevents recurrent episodes. There is also evidence on the effects of raising factor VII coagulant activity, summarized in Table 4–5. This is based on a randomized comparison of estrogens and surgery for the treatment of carcinoma of the prostate.[85,86] The increase in factor VII coagulant activity owing to estrogens parallels the obvious increase in thromboembolic events in those treated in this way. Again, other procoagulatory clotting factors may

have been affected and, as Table 4–5 also shows, there is little doubt that antithrombin III levels were lowered by estrogen treatment. While, once more, it is therefore not possible conclusively to identify factor VII coagulant activity as the reason for the increased incidence of thromboembolism, it may be involved, and the result provides further evidence that the onset of thromboembolic episodes is at least partly determined by the general level of coagulability. There are two sources of trial evidence involving fibrinogen. One is the World Health Organization clofibrate trial.[87] This trial was based on the relationship between cholesterol (not fibrinogen) and ischemic heart disease, and was carried out in men with hyperlipidemia, based on the cholesterol-lowering property of clofibrate. There was a significant reduction (about 20 per cent) in the incidence of myocardial infarction attributable to clofibrate, but there was also an increase in deaths from a variety of causes for reasons which are still unclear but which preclude the general use of clofibrate. However, it is clear that clofibrate also lowers fibrinogen levels.[88] Furthermore, the beneficial effect of clofibrate against infarction appears to have been confined, as Table 4–6 shows, to heavy smokers who were also hypertensive. The heavy smokers will have had high fibrinogen levels. Besides suggesting that the effect of clofibrate may have been to reduce the risk of myocardial infarction through its effect on fibrinogen, this analysis is also interesting in supporting the suggestion of an interaction between blood pressure and fibrinogen, already referred to, since it was in those at risk on both accounts that the benefit of treatment was mostly seen. The other source of evidence is a series of studies[89] in both man and animals showing that ancrod, a defibrinating agent, reduces thrombosis and improves clinical function in immune kidney disease.

CIGARETTE SMOKING, DIET, AND OTHER CHARACTERISTICS

Another useful if more circumstantial component of the epidemiological evidence is the extent to which levels of the clotting factors associated with ischemic heart disease alter according to personal and environmental characteristics associated with the disease. This evidence is summarized in Table 4–7, which shows with a high degree of consis-

TABLE 4–5. Major Cardiovascular Events (at One Year) and Coagulation Changes (at Six Weeks) in Trial of Estrogens in Prostatic Carcinoma

	ESTROGENS (N = 53)	ORCHIDECTOMY (N = 47)
Events	13	0
Factor VII coagulant activity	+51 per cent	+11 per cent
Antithrombin III	−12 per cent	+3 per cent

TABLE 4–6. Heart Attacks per 1,000 per Annum in World Health Organization Clofibrate Trial

| | NONSMOKERS | | SMOKERS | | | |
| | | | <20/day | | >20/day | |
	Active	Placebo	Active	Placebo	Active	Placebo
Normotensive	3.4	3.5	6.2	9.6	9.6	9.1
Hypertensive	3.9	6.0	12.1	14.3	8.7	*18.3

*$p < 0.01$.

tency that factor VII coagulant activity and/or fibrinogen levels rise or fall in association with characteristics which respectively raise or lower the risk of ischemic heart disease. In the case of factor VII coagulant activity, it is worth noting that the effect of oral contraceptives depends on the estrogen dose,[90] which is also related to the risk of thromboembolic episodes in oral contraceptive users.[91] Probably of greatest interest are the relationships of cigarette smoking with fibrinogen, and dietary fat intake with factor VII coagulant activity.

Cigarette Smoking

Uniformly, all the large scale studies already referred to (and other, smaller studies) have found the highest fibrinogen levels in smokers, intermediate levels in exsmokers, and the lowest levels in nonsmokers.[92] There is a dose-response relationship between the number of cigarettes smoked and the fibrinogen level.[93] Finally, starting or resuming smoking is associated with an increase in fibrinogen, while stopping is accompanied by a decrease.[94] Figure 4–6, from data at entry to the Northwick Park Heart Study, shows a rapid initial decline in fibrinogen on stopping, but levels remain above those for nonsmokers for up to five and perhaps ten years after discontinuation—a time course that closely mirrors the decline in the risk of ischemic heart disease itself after smoking cessation.[16] This effect has also been shown prospectively.[94] Thus, over the six-year follow-up period in the Northwick Park Heart Study, fibrinogen levels rose (over and above the increase with age) in those who started or resumed smoking, while they fell in those who discontinued. The relatively rapid initial fall in fibrinogen after discontinuation (Fig. 4–6) is one of the reasons for questioning the frequent assertion that high fibrinogen levels associated with the incidence of ischemic heart disease only reflect the extent of underlying atheroma (although the association would still be useful even if this were

TABLE 4–7. General Epidemiological Characteristics of Factor VII Coagulant Activity and Fibrinogen

FACTOR VII COAGULANT ACTIVITY	FIBRINOGEN
Higher Levels	
Increasing age	Increasing age
Obesity	Obesity
Oral contraceptive use	Oral contraceptive use
Menopause	Menopause
Diabetes	Diabetes
"Imprudent" diet	Smoking
	Low employment grade
Lower Levels	
Black ethnic group	Moderate alcohol intake
Vegetarians	

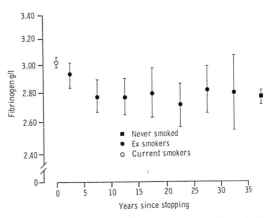

FIGURE 4–6. Plasma fibrinogen (age adjusted) by time since stopping smoking in exsmokers and in current and nonsmokers (log scale; bars show 95 per cent confidence intervals). (Reproduced with permission from the Lancet 1987; 2: 986–8.)

the explanation). Given the very great difficulty of achieving the regression of atheroma other than by exceptionally intensive methods, it is unlikely that the fall in fibrinogen soon after discontinuation is due to a reduction in atheroma. The extent to which fibrinogen levels are genetically determined (see below) also represents a component of high fibrinogen levels that cannot be explained as a response to atheroma. Bearing in mind the strong relationship between fibrinogen levels and the risk of ischemic heart disease or stroke, the fall in fibrinogen in exsmokers is enough to account for a large part of the decline in their risk of ischemic heart disease and strengthens the conclusion that much of the relationship between cigarette smoking and ischemic heart disease is mediated through the fibrinogen level. It is, however, important to remember that high levels are associated with an increased risk of ischemic heart disease in nonsmokers[62] as well as in smokers.

Dietary Fat Intake

Experimental studies in healthy adults have shown a significant positive association between day-to-day variation in total fat intake and factor VII coagulant activity.[95] Indeed, the influence of fat consumption on factor VII coagulant activity is sufficiently rapid for an association to exist between the diurnal variation in plasma triglyceride concentration induced by the meal pattern, and the diurnal fluctuation in factor VII coagulant activity.[60] The diurnal rhythm in factor VII coagulant activity lags behind that in plasma triglyceride by approximately two to three hours. The link between total fat intake and subsequent factor VII coagulant activity is probably the postprandial chylomicronemia, the large lipoprotein particles inducing a rise in factor VII coagulant activity. By contrast, no association appears to exist between diurnal fluctuations in factor VII antigen concentration and plasma triglyceride.[60]

The association between factor VII coagulant activity and total dietary fat intake can be observed in the general community. The demonstration of such a relation is handicapped of course by the difficulty in measurement of fat intake in the habitual diet, a problem that has thwarted most attempts to show an association between fat intake and serum cholesterol concentration within communities. Nevertheless, a significant positive correlation with factor VII coagulant activity has been demonstrated in middle-aged men when fat intake was expressed relative to body size (since it is overconsumption rather than absolute intake that is important for factor VII coagulant activity).[96]

Two experimental studies, one of seven days' duration[60] and one of 14 days,[97] examined the effects of dietary fat composition on factor VII coagulant activity.[96] Unlike total fat intake, the ratio of polyunsaturated fatty acid to saturated fatty acid in the diet (P/S ratio) had no demonstrable effect on factor VII coagulant activity.

Many clinical conditions in which there is a hyperlipidemia are associated with an increased factor VII coagulant activity, for example, the primary hyperlipoproteinemias,[98,99] pregnancy,[100] and diabetes mellitus.[75] Reduction of plasma lipid levels, particularly triglyceride, is associated with a decrease in factor VII coagulant activity.[101] When plasma lipid concentrations tend to be low, as in vegetarians, factor VII coagulant activity is also reduced.[72]

Genetic Contribution

A series of studies using molecular techniques[102–104] and path analysis[105] have now begun to explain the genetic contribution to both factor VII coagulant activity and fibrinogen. In the case of the latter, the greater the extent to which environmental determinants such as cigarette smoking and the genetic contribution explain high fibrinogen levels, the less that can be attributed to nonspecific chronic- or acute-phase influences such as atheroma, though high levels due to these may also be involved not simply as indices of vessel wall damage, but, through effects on atheroma,[106] viscosity,[107] platelet aggregation,[108] and fibrin formation,[109] in the causation of thrombosis as well.

PRACTICAL IMPLICATIONS

The risk of ischemic heart disease can be modified either through changes in lifestyle or pharmacologically.

Lifestyle changes can be encouraged by central policies affecting dietary habits or tobacco advertising, for example, and directed at populations as a whole or they can be adopted through individual choice. They have almost certainly been responsible for much of the decline in ischemic heart disease incidence in many countries over the last 25 years. But their acceptance and implementation takes time. Many find the recommended changes difficult or impossible to adhere to, and in some of those who do take them up, they are ineffective. There is thus always likely to be a case for pharmacological intervention. Before considering this in further detail, however, there are some lessons for prevention through lifestyle changes that are emerging from the recognition of the thrombotic component in ischemic heart disease and its characteristics. While this new information alters no general principles, it does in some respects enable their sharper application. First, the independent relationship between high fibrinogen levels and the risk of ischemic heart disease is sufficiently strong to warrant the addition of the fibrinogen level to the definition of the "high-risk profile." Second, the similarity of the time course for the fall in fibrinogen and in the risk of ischemic heart disease itself in exsmokers emphasizes the importance of not overlooking the considerable period of time during which an exsmoker remains at increased risk or the thrombotic contribution to this risk. Turning to diet, the very rapid effect of changes in fat intake on coagulability provides a sound basis for the adoption of dietary measures at any age, and argues strongly against any remaining belief that these will only succeed if they are adopted in early life (though doing so then may well influence atherogenesis as well). The potential value of fish oils on platelet activity carries the same implication.

Where pharmacological measures for primary prevention are necessary, it is of course with the modification of platelet aggregation and fibrin formation that antithrombotic measures are concerned. The value of aspirin in primary prevention is still rather uncertain, the trial in American doctors[110] suggesting a reduction in the incidence of myocardial infarction of 44 per cent, but no effect on death from all vascular causes, while the trial in British doctors[111] shows no apparent benefit against myocardial infarction. An overview of the two trials suggests a significant reduction of 32 per cent,[112] although there is marginally significant heterogeneity between the two trials in this respect, and an increase of 18 percent in nonfatal stroke, which is not,

however, significant, but contrasts with the obvious reduction in stroke owing to aspirin in the secondary prevention trials. There is, therefore, a need for further information from primary prevention trials of aspirin, including the effects of aspirin doses in the range of 40 to 80 milligrams/day. A fairly consistent finding in secondary prevention trials has so far been a somewhat greater benefit due to oral anticoagulants than aspirin, though this conclusion is mainly based on indirect comparisons. Thus, the reduction in mortality attributable to anticoagulants is, at 20 per cent or more somewhat greater than the typical figures of 15 to 20 per cent for aspirin. Similarly, anticoagulants reduce recurrent myocardial infarction between a third and a half compared with a reduction of 25 or 30 percent in the case of aspirin. If there truly is a more than marginal advantage of anticoagulants over aspirin, the greater complexity of anticoagulant treatment should not automatically rule it out in what is, after all, a common condition in which even small differences in effectiveness may be reflected in many lives saved and events avoided. A second consideration for the potential value of anticoagulants is the growing conviction that their benefit may perhaps be achieved at much lower than conventional levels of anticoagulation. There would also be less bleeding and less need for monitoring. In addition, there is also the real possibility that the simultaneous modification of platelet function and fibrin formation may be more effective than the modification of either process on its own. The most striking demonstration of this possibility comes from the ISIS-2 trial[113] in which the combination of aspirin and streptokinase was more effective than either active agent on its own, though each also reduced cardiovascular mortality. The case for establishing the potential value of low-intensity oral anticoagulation in primary prevention is strengthened by the relationship between factor VII activity and the incidence of ischemic heart disease,[62] bearing in mind that factor VII is one of the vitamin K-dependent clotting factors whose activity is reduced by warfarin. Accordingly, the separate and combined effects of 75 milligrams aspirin and/or warfarin achieving an international normalized ratio of about 1.5 are currently being investigated by the Thrombosis Prevention Trial[114,115] which, unlike the American and British doctors' trials, is based on men at considerably increased risk of ischemic heart disease. The encouraging results of the RISC trial[116] in unstable angina provide a further strong incentive to the evaluation of 75 milligrams aspirin in primary prevention.

REFERENCES

1. Chandler AB, Chapman I, Erhardt LR, et al. Coronary thrombosis in myocardial infarction. Report of a workshop on the role of coronary thrombosis in the pathogenesis of acute myocardial infarction. Am J Cardiol 1974; 34: 823–33.
2. DeWood MA, Spores J, Notske R, et al. Prevalence of total coronary occlusion during the early hours of transmural myocardial infarction, N Engl J Med 1980; 303: 897–901.
3. Davies MJ. Thrombosis in acute myocardial infarction and sudden death. In: Thrombosis and platelets in myocardial ischemia. Mehta JL, Conti CR, Brest AN, eds. Philadelphia: FA Davis Co., 1987: 151–9.
4. Haerem JW. Mural platelet microthrombi and major acute lesions of main epicardial arteries in sudden coronary death. Atherosclerosis 1974; 19: 529–41.
5. Davies MJ, Thomas A. Thrombosis and acute coronary-artery lesions in sudden cardiac ischemic death. N Engl J Med 1984; 310: 1137–40.
6. El Fawal MA, Berg GA, Wheatley DJ, Harland WA. Sudden coronary death in Glasgow: nature and frequency of acute coronary lesions. Br Heart J 1987; 57: 329–35.
7. Meade TW, Howarth DJ, Stirling Y. Fibrinopeptide A and sudden coronary death. Lancet 1984; 2: 607–9.
8. Morris JN. Recent history of coronary disease. Lancet 1951; 1: 1–7, 69–73.
9. Strong JP, Richards ML. Cigarette smoking and atherosclerosis in autopsied men. Atherosclerosis 1976; 23: 451–76.
10. McGill HC. The cardiovascular pathology of smoking. Am Heart J 1988; 115: 250–7.
11. Doll R, Peto R. Mortality in relation to smoking 20 years' observations on male British doctors. Br Med J 1976; 1525–36.
12. Weir JM, Dunn JE. Smoking and mortality a prospective study. Cancer 1970; 25: 105–12.
13. Kahn HA. The Dorn study of smoking and mortality among U S veterans: report on eight and one-half years of observation. In: Haenzel W, ed. Epidemiological approaches to the study of cancer and other chronic diseases. National Cancer Institute Monograph No 19. US Department of Health, Education and Welfare, Public Health Service, National Institutes of Health, National Cancer Institute, 1966: 1–125.
14. Hammond EC, Garfinkel L. Coronary heart disease, stroke and aortic aneurysm. Factors in the etiology. Arch Environ Health 1969; 19: 167–82.
15. Freedman DS, Gruchow HW, Walker JA, et al. Cigarette smoking and non-fatal myocardial infarction in women: is the relation independent of coronary artery disease? Br Heart J 1989; 62: 273–80.
16. Cook DG, Shaper AG, Pocock SJ, Kussick SJ. Giving up smoking and the risk of heart attacks. Lancet 1986; 2: 1376–80.
17. Morris JN, Heady JA, Raffle PAB, Roberts CG, Parks JW. Coronary heart disease and physical activity of work. Lancet 1953; 2: 1053–7, 1111–20.
18. Morris JN, Crawford MD. Coronary heart disease and physical activity of work. Evidence of a national necropsy survey. Br Med J 1958; 2: 1485–96.
19. Morris JN, Clayton DG, Everitt MG, et al. Exercise in leisure time: coronary attack and death rates. Br Heart J 1990; 63: 325–34.
20. Rapold HJ, Haeberli A, Kuemmerli H, Weiss M, Baur HR, Straub WP. Fibrin formation and platelet activation in patients with myocardial infarction and normal coronary arteries. Eur Heart J 1989; 10: 323–33.
21. Poller L. Thrombosis and factor VII activity. J Clin Pathol 1957; 10: 348–50.
22. Meade TW. Epidemiology of atheroma, thrombosis and ischaemic heart disease. In: Haemostasis and thrombosis. 2nd edition. Bloom AL, Thomas DP, eds. New York: Churchill Livingstone, 1987: 697–720.
23. Haines AP, Howarth D, North WRS, et al. Haemostatic variables and the outcome of myocardial infarction. Thromb Haemost 1983; 50: 800–3.
24. Meade TW, North WRS, Chakrabarti R, Haines AP, Stirling Y. Population-based distributions of haemostatic variables. Br Med Bull 1977; 33: 283–8.
25. Thompson SG, Martin JC, Meade TW. Sources of variability in coagulation factor assays. Thromb Haemost 1987; 58: 1073–77.
26. MacMahon S, Peto R, Cutler J, et al. Blood pressure, stroke, and coronary heart disease. Part 1, prolonged differences in blood pressure: prospective observational studies corrected for the regression dilution bias. Lancet 1990; 335: 765–74.
27. Furie B, Curie BC. The molecular basis of blood coagulation. In: Hoffman R, Benz EJ Jr, Shattil SJ, Furie B, Cohen HJ, eds., Hematology: Basic Principles and Practices. New York: Churchill Livingstone, 1991.
28. Di Scipio RG, Kurachi K, Davie EW. Activation of human factor IX (Christmas factor). J Clin Invest 1978; 61: 1528–38.
29. Di Scipio RG, Hermodson MA, Davie EW. Activation of human factor X (Stuart factor) by a protease from Russell's viper venom. Biochemistry 1977; 16: 5253–60.
30. Stenn KA, Blout ER. Mechanism of bovine prothrombin activation by an insoluble preparation of bovine factor Xa. Biochemistry 1972; 11: 4502–15.
31. Esmon CT, Jackson CM. The conversion of prothrombin to thrombin. J Biol Chem 1974; 249: 7782–90.
32. Crabtree GR. The molecular biology of fibrinogen. In: Stamatoyannopoulos G, Nienhuis AW, Leder P, Majerus PW, eds., The molecular basis of blood diseases. Philadelphia: WB Saunders Co., 1987.
33. Teitel JM, Bauer KA, Lau HK, Rosenberg RD. Studies of the prothrombin blood activation pathway utilizing radioimmunoassay for the F2/F1+2 fragment and thrombin-antithrombin complex. Blood 1982; 59: 1086–97.
34. Bauer KA, Kass BL, ten Cate H, Bednarek MA, Hawiger JJ, Rosenberg RD. Detection of factor X activation in humans. Blood 1989; 74: 2007–15.
35. Bauer KA, Kass BL, ten Cate H, Bednarek MA, Hawiger JJ, Rosenberg RD. Factor IX is activated in vivo by the tissue factor mechanism. Blood 1990; 76: 731–6.
36. Nossel HL, Yudelman I, Canfield RE, et al. Measurement of fibrinopeptide A in human blood. J Clin Invest 1974; 54: 43–53.
37. Bauer KA, Mannucci PM, Barzegar S, et al. The factor IXa-factor VIII/VIIIa-phospholipid complex does not contribute to the basal activation of the common coagulation pathway in vivo. Submitted.
38. Josso F, Prou-Wartelle O. Interaction of tissue factor and factor VII at the earliest phase of coagulation. Thromb Diath Haemorr 1965; 17(suppl).
39. Osterud B, Rapaport SI. Activation of factor IX by the reaction product of tissue factor and factor VII: additional pathway for initiating blood coagulation. Proc Natl Acad Sci USA 1977; 74: 5260–4.
40. Macfarlane RG. An enzyme cascade in the blood clotting mechanism, and its function as a biochemical amplifier. Nature 1964; 202: 498–9.
41. Davie EW, Ratnoff OD. Waterfall sequence for intrinsic blood clotting. Science 1964; 145: 1310–2.
42. Rosenberg RD. The biochemistry and pathophysiology of the prethrombotic state. Annu Rev Med 1987; 38: 493–508.
43. Marcum JA, Atha DH, Fritze LMS, Nawroth P, Stern D, Rosenberg RD. Cloned bovine aortic endothelial cells synthesize anticoagulantly active heparin sulfate proteoglycan. J Biol Chem 1986; 261: 7507–17.
44. Marcum JA, McKenney JB, Rosenberg RD. Acceleration of thrombin-antithrombin complex formation in rat hindquarter via naturally occurring heparin-like molecules bound to the endothelium. J Clin Invest 1984; 74: 341–50.

45. Esmon NL, Owen WG, Esmon CT. Isolation of a membrane bound cofactor for thrombin-catalyzed activation of protein C. J Biol Chem 1982; 257: 859–64.

46. Nossel HL. Relative proteolysis of the fibrinogen B beta chain by thrombin and plasmin as a determinant of thrombosis. Nature 1981; 291: 165–7.

47. Lau H, Rosenberg RD. The isolation and characterization of a specific antibody population directed against the thrombin-antithrombin complex. J Biol Chem 1980; 255: 5885–93.

48. Bauer KA, Kass BL, Beeler DL, Rosenberg RD. The detection of protein C activation in humans. J Clin Invest 1984; 74: 2033–41.

49. Owen J, Kvam D, Nossell HL, Kaplan KL, Kernoff PBA. Thrombin and plasmin activity and platelet activation in the development of venous thrombosis. Blood 1983; 61: 476–82.

50. Bauer KA, Brockmans AW, Bertina RM, et al. Hemostatic enzyme generation in the blood of patients with hereditary protein C deficiency. Blood 1988; 71: 1418–26.

51. Bauer KA, Weiss LM, Sparrow D, Vokonas PS, Rosenberg RD. Aging associated changes in indices of thrombin generation and protein C activation in humans. J Clin Invest 1987; 80: 1527–34.

52. Zur M, Radcliffe RD, Oberdick J, Nemerson Y. The dual role of factor VII in blood coagulation. J Biol Chem 1982; 257: 5623–31.

53. Bach R, Oberdick J, Nemerson Y. Immunoaffinity purification of bovine factor VII. Blood 1984; 63: 393–8.

54. Rao LVM, Rapaport SI, Bajaj SP. Activation of human factor VII in the initiation of tissue factor-dependent coagulation. Blood 1986; 68: 685–91.

55. Williams EB, Krishnaswamy S, Mann KG. Zymogen/enzyme discrimination using peptide chloromethyl ketones. J Biol Chem 1989; 264: 7536–45.

56. Wildgoose P, Berkner KL, Kisiel W. Synthesis, purification and characterization of an Arg 152-Glu site-directed mutant of recombinant human blood clotting factor VII. Biochemistry 1990; 29: 3413–20.

57. Mitropoulos KA, Esnouf MP. The prothrombin activation peptide regulates synthesis of the vitamin K-dependent proteins in the rabbit. Thromb Res 1990; 57: 541–9.

58. Trip MD, Cats VM, van Capelle FJL, Vreeken J. Platelet hyperreactivity and prognosis in survivors of myocardial infarction. N Engl J Med 1990; 322: 1549–54.

59. Brozovic M, Stirling Y, Harricks C, North WRS, Meade TW. Factor VII in an industrial population. Br J Haematol 1974; 28: 381–91.

60. Miller GJ, Martin JC, Mitropoulos KA, et al. Plasma factor VII is activated by postprandial triglyceridaemia, irrespective of dietary fat composition. Atherosclerosis 1991; 86: 163–71.

61. Meade TW, North WRS, Chakrabarti R, Stirling Y, Haines AP, Thompson SG. Haemostatic function and cardiovascular death: early results of a prospective study. Lancet 1980; 1: 1050–4.

62. Meade TW, Mellows S, Brozovic M, et al. Haemostatic function and ischaemic heart disease: principal results of the Northwick Park Heart Study. Lancet 1986; 2: 533–7.

63. Wilhelmsen L, Svardsudd K, Korsan-Bengtsen K, Welin L, Tibblin G. Fibrinogen as a risk factor for stroke and myocardial infarction. N Engl J Med 1984; 311: 501–5.

64. Stone MC, Thorp JM. Plasma fibrinogen—a major coronary risk factor. J R Coll Gen Pract 1985; 35: 565–9.

65. Kannel WB, Castelli WP, Meeks SL. Fibrinogen and cardiovascular disease. Abstract of paper for 34th Annual Scientific Session of the American College of Cardiology, March 1985, Anaheim, California.

66. Kannel WB, Wolf PA, Castelli WP, D'Agostino RB. Fibrinogen and risk of cardiovascular disease. JAMA 1987; 258: 1183–6.

67. Kannel WB. Hypertension and other risk factors in coronary heart disease. Am Heart J 1987; 114: 918–25.

68. Yarnell JWG, Baker IA, Sweetnam PM, et al. Fibrinogen, viscosity, and white blood cell count are major risk factors for ischemic heart disease. The Caerphilly and Speedwell Collaborative Heart Disease Studies. Circulation 1991; 83: 836–44.

69. Hamsten A, de Faire U, Wallius G, et al. Plasminogen activator inhibitor in plasma: risk factor for recurrent myocardial infarction. Lancet 1987; 2: 3–9.

70. Rosendaal FR, Varekamp I, Smit C, et al. Mortality and causes of death in Dutch haemophiliacs, 1973–86. Br J Haematol 1989; 71: 71–6.

71. Rosendaal FR, Briet E, Stibb J, et al. Haemophilia protects against ischaemic heart disease: a study of risk factors. Br J Haematol 1990; 75: 525–30.

72. Haines AP, Chakrabarti R, Fisher D, Meade TW, North WRS, Stirling Y. Haemostatic variables in vegetarians and non-vegetarians. Thromb Res 1980; 19: 139–48.

73. Meade TW, Dyer S, Howarth DJ, Imeson JD, Stirling Y. Antithrombin III and procoagulant activity: sex differences and effects of the menopause. Br J Haematol 1990; 74: 77–81.

74. Meilahn E, Kuller LH, Kiss JE, Matthews KA, Lewis JH. Coagulation parameters among pre- and post-menopausal women. Am J Epidemiol 1988; 128: 908.

75. Fuller JH, Keen H, Jarrett RJ, et al. Haemostatic variables associated with diabetes and its complications. Br Med J 1979; 2: 964–6.

76. Yue R, Gertler M, Starr T, Koutrouby R. Alterations of plasma antithrombin III levels in ischemic heart disease. Thromb Haemost 1976; 35: 598–606.

77. Banerjee R, Sahni A, Kumar V, Arya M. Antithrombin III deficiency in maturity onset diabetes mellitus and atherosclerosis. Thromb Diath Haemorrh 1974; 31: 339–45.

78. O'Brien J, Etherington M, Jamieson S, Lawford P, Lincoln S, Alkjaersig N. Blood changes in atherosclerosis and long after myocardial infarction and venous thrombosis. Thromb Diath Haemorr 1975; 34: 493–97.

79. Innerfield I, Goldfischer J, Reichter-Reiss H, Greenberg J. Serum antithrombins in coronary artery disease. Am J Clin Pathol 1976; 65: 64–68.

80. Meade TW, Cooper J, Miller GJ, Howarth D, Stirling Y. Antithrombin III and arterial disease: an unexpected relationship. Lancet 1991; (in press).

81. International Anticoag Review Group. Collaborative analysis of long-term anticoagulant administration after acute myocardial infarction. Lancet 1970; 1: 203–9.

82. Chalmers TV, Matta RJ, Smith H, Kunzler A-M. Evidence favoring the use of anticoagulants in the hospital phase of acute myocardial infarction. N Engl J Med 1977; 297: 1091–6.

83. Sixty-Plus Reinfarction Study Research Group. A double-blind trial to assess long-term oral anticoagulant therapy in elderly patients after myocardial infarction. Lancet 1980; 2: 989–94.

84. Smith P, Arnesen H, Holme I. The effect of warfarin on mortality and reinfarction after myocardial infarction. N Engl J Med 1990; 323: 147–52.

85. Henriksson P, Edhag O. Orchidectomy versus oestrogen for prostatic cancer: cardiovascular effects. Br Med J 1986; 2: 413–5.

86. Henriksson P, Blomback M, Bratt G, Edhag O, Eriksson A. Activators and inhibitors of coagulation and fibrinolysis in patients with prostatic cancer treated with oestrogen or orchidectomy. Thromb Res 1986; 44: 783–91.

87. Co-operative trial in the primary prevention of ischemic heart disease using clofibrate. Br Heart J 1978; 40: 1069–1118.

88. Green KG, Heady A, Oliver MF. Blood pressure, cigarette smoking and heart attack in the WHO co-operative trial of clofibrate. Int J Epidemiol 1989; 18: 355–60.

89. Becker GJ. Ancrod in glomerulonephritis. Q J Med 1988; 69: 849–50.

90. Meade TW, Chakrabarti R, Haines AP, Howarth DJ, North WRS, Stirling Y. Haemostatic, lipid and blood-pressure profiles of women on oral contraceptive containing 50μg or 30μg oestrogen. Lancet 1977; 2: 948–51.

91. Meade TW, Greenberg G, Thompson SG. Progestogens and cardiovascular reactions associated with oral contraceptives and a comparison of the safety of 50- and 30μg oestrogen preparations. Br Med J 1980; 1: 1157–61.

92. Meade TW, Imeson JD, Stirling Y. The epidemiology of haemostatic and other variables in coronary disease. In: Thrombosis and Haemostasis 1987. Verstraete M, Ver-

mylen J, Lijnen R, Arnount J, eds. Leuven University Press, 1987; 37–60.

93. Wilkes HC, Kelleher C, Meade TW. Smoking and plasma fibrinogen (letter). Lancet 1988; 1: 307–8.

94. Meade TW, Imeson J, Stirling Y. Effects of changes in smoking and other characteristics on clotting factors and the risk of ischaemic heart disease. Lancet 1987; 2: 986–8.

95. Miller GJ, Martin JC, Webster J, et al. Association between dietary fat intake and plasma factor VII coagulant activity—a predictor of cardiovascular mortality. Atherosclerosis 1986; 60: 269–71.

96. Miller GJ, Cruickshank JK, Ellis LJ, et al. Fat consumption and factor VII coagulant activity in middle-aged men. An association between a dietary and thrombogenic coronary risk factor. Atherosclerosis 1989; 78: 19–24.

97. Marckmann P, Sandstrom B, Jespersen J. Effects of total fat content and fatty acid composition in diet on factor VII coagulant activity and blood lipids. Atherosclerosis 1990; 80: 227–33.

98. Constantino M, Merskey C, Kudzma DJ, Zucker MB. Increased activity of vitamin K-dependent clotting factors in human hyperlipoproteinaemia-association with cholesterol and triglyceride levels. Thromb Haemost 1977; 38: 465–74.

99. Carvallo de Sousa J, Bruckert E, Giral P, et al. Plasma factor VII, triglyceride concentration and fibrin degradation products in primary hyperlipidaemia: a clinical and laboratory study. Haemostasis 1989; 19: 83–90.

100. Stirling Y, Woolf L, North WRS, Seghatchian MJ, Meade TW. Haemostasis in normal pregnancy. Thromb Haemost 1984; 52: 176–82.

101. Simpson HCR, Mann JI, Meade TW, Chakrabarti R, Stirling Y, Woolf L. Hypertriglyceridaemia and hypercoagulability. Lancet 1983; 1: 786–90.

102. Humphries SE, Cook M, Dubowitz M, Stirling Y, Meade TW. Role of genetic variation at the fibrinogen locus in determination of plasma fibrinogen concentrations. Lancet 1987; 1: 1452–5.

103. Thomas AE, Green FR, Kelleher CH, et al. Variation in the promoter region of the β fibrinogen gene is associated with plasma fibrinogen levels in smokers and non-smokers. Thromb Haemost 1991; 65: 487–90.

104. Green FR, Kelleher CK, Wilkes HC, Temple A, Meade TW, Humphries SE. A common genetic polymorphism associated with lower coagulation factor VII levels in healthy individuals. Arteriosclerosis and Thrombosis 1991; 11: 540–546.

105. Hamsten A, Iselius L, de Faire U, Blomback M. Genetic and cultural inheritance of plasma fibrinogen concentration. Lancet 1987; 2: 988–90.

106. Thompson WD, Smith EB et al. Atherosclerosis and the coagulation system: J Pathol 1989; 159: 97–106.

107. Lowe GDO. Blood rheology in arterial disease. Clin Sci 1986; 71: 137–46.

108. Meade TW, Vickers MV, Thompson SG, Stirling Y, Haines AP, Miller GJ. Epidemiological characteristics of platelet aggregability. Br Med J 1985; 290: 428–32.

109. Gurewich V, Lipinski B, Hyde E, et al. The effect of the fibrinogen concentration and the leukocyte count on intravascular fibrin deposition from soluble fibrin monomer complexes. Thromb Haemost 1976; 36: 605–14.

110. Physicians' Health Study Research Group. Final report on the aspirin component of the ongoing Physicians' Health Study. N Engl J Med 1989; 321: 129–35.

111. Peto R, Gray R, Collins R, et al. Randomized trial of prophylactic daily aspirin in British male doctors. Br Med J 1988; 296: 313–16.

112. Hennekens CH, Buring JE, Sandercock P, Collins R, Peto R. Aspirin and other antiplatelet agents in the secondary and primary prevention of cardiovascular disease. Circulation 1989; 80: 749–56.

113. ISIS-2 (Second International Study of Infarct Survival) Collaborative Group. Random trial of intravenous streptokinase, oral aspirin, both, or neither among 17 187 cases of suspected acute myocardial infarction: ISIS-2. Lancet 1988; 2: 349–60.

114. Meade TW, Wilkes HC, Stirling Y, Brennan PJ, Kelleher C, Browne W. Randomized controlled trial of low dose warfarin in the primary prevention of ischaemic heart disease in men at high risk: design and pilot study. Eur Heart J 1988; 9: 836–43.

115. Meade TW. Low-dose warfarin and low-dose aspirin in the primary prevention of ischemic heart disease. Am J Cardiol 1990; 65: 7c–11c.

116. RISC Group. Risk of myocardial infarction and death during treatment with low dose aspirin and intravenous heparin in men with unstable coronary artery disease. Lancet 1990; 336: 827–30.

5

CLINICAL PHARMACOLOGY OF PLATELET INHIBITORS

BERNARDO STEIN and VALENTIN FUSTER

Platelets are fragments of membrane-enclosed megakariocytic cytoplasm that interact with the coagulation and fibrinolytic systems in the maintenance of hemostasis. Platelets do not interact with intact endothelium but rapidly adhere to damaged vascular tissue. Under appropriate stimulation, platelets release the contents of their intracytoplasmic granules, produce thromboxane A_2, and undergo conformational changes that result in the exposure of their membrane receptors to adhesive macromolecules. These reactions, in turn, lead to the recruitment of additional platelets and the formation of aggregates at sites of vessel wall injury.

In addition, platelets provide a surface for the localization and interaction among various coagulation factors, thus ultimately increasing the rate of conversion of prothrombin to thrombin. Thrombin plays a fundamental role in the pathogenesis of thromboembolic disorders through several mechanisms. It initiates potent positive feedback mechanisms on the coagulation cascade resulting in the generation of more procoagulant factors, it catalyzes the conversion of fibrinogen to fibrin, which provides support to the growing platelet–thrombus mass, and it is a direct and powerful activator of platelets. Therefore, platelets and the coagulation system are intimately interrelated in the pathogenesis of thrombosis (Fig. 5–1).

Delivery and activation of platelets at the site of vascular injury are dependent on both shear rate and degree of vessel wall injury. Low shear rate occurs predominantly within the venous system and cardiac chambers; these conditions of slow blood flow favor the activation of clotting mechanisms and the

development of thrombi composed mainly of erythrocytes within a fibrin lattice ("red" thrombi). Conventional anticoagulants such as heparin or warfarin are usually effective in preventing the development of these thrombotic processes, because they interfere with the generation of thrombin and fibrin. In contrast, thrombi that develop in areas of rapid blood flow where shear rate is increased, such as in areas of ulcerated plaques, stenoses, or bends within the arterial system, have a different pathogenesis and histologic appearance.[1] The high shear rate present in the arterial system promotes contact between blood elements and the vessel wall and favors platelet activation.[2] These thrombi are formed predominantly by platelets ("white" thrombi), but a fibrin network is necessary to provide stability to the growing platelet mass. In the immediate vicinity distal to stenoses, where shear rate is lower, the thrombus is composed mainly of fibrin, erythrocytes, and leukocytes.[1]

The degree of vessel injury directly influences the process of thrombus formation. Superficial injury is usually associated with transient and limited deposition of platelets, whereas deep injury exposes collagen and other elements of the vessel wall, leading to marked platelet activation and aggregation, and potentially resulting in persistent thrombotic vessel occlusion.[3] Platelet-rich thrombi may be more resistant to the available anticoagulant and thrombolytic agents, but responsive to inhibitors of platelet metabolism.

These concepts are relevant to the pathogenesis of different cardiovascular disorders, and their understanding may permit a more rational approach to their management.

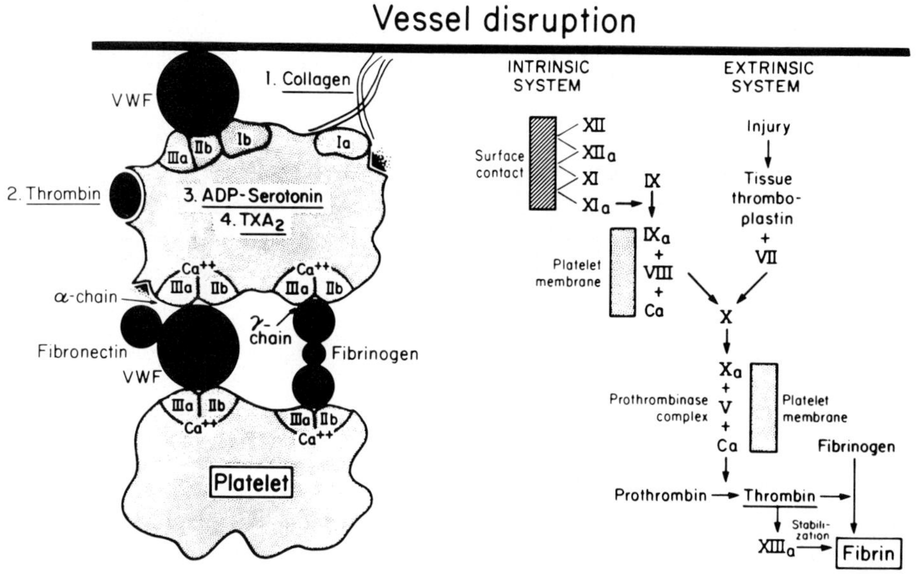

Vessel disruption

FIGURE 5–1. (*Left*) Schematic representation of the interaction among platelet membrane receptors (glycoproteins Ia, Ib, and IIb-IIIa), adhesive macromolecules (von Willebrand factor [VWF], fibrinogen, fibronectin), and the disrupted vessel wall. Numbers indicate the different pathways of platelet activation dependent on (*1*) collagen, (*2*) thrombin, (*3*) adenosine diphosphate (ADP) and serotonin, and (*4*) thromboxane A$_2$ (TXA$_2$). (*Right*) The intrinsic, extrinsic, and common pathways of the coagulation sequence. Note the interaction among clotting factors and the platelet membrane. CA = calcium. (From Stein B, et al. Platelet inhibitor agents in cardiovascular disease: an update. J Am Coll Cardiol 1989; 14: 813–36, by permission of the American College of Cardiology.)

Given the central role of platelets in thromboembolic processes, the possibility of inhibiting their function with different pharmacologic agents has generated enormous interest in the medical and pharmaceutical communities for the last two decades. Although some of the effects of salicylate-containing plants have been known for thousands of years, it was not until the end of last century when aspirin became available, thanks to the pioneering efforts of Hoffman and Dreser.[4] By the early 1900s, aspirin was known for its analgesic, anti-inflammatory, and antipyretic effects. However, many years had to elapse before its antithrombotic effects were recognized. In the late 1960s, aspirin was found to have platelet inhibitory effects. In 1971, Vane and colleagues discovered that aspirin and aspirin-like drugs inhibited the enzyme that generates prostaglandins.[5] During the next decade, however, the beneficial effects of platelet inhibition with aspirin were questioned. This skepticism resulted from the lack of clear understanding of the role of thrombosis in the pathogenesis of myocardial infarction and the disappointing effects of aspirin and other platelet inhibitors in the secondary prevention of coronary disease.

The decade of the 1980s has witnessed the emergence of a renewed interest on platelet inhibitors, which resulted from a better understanding of the role of platelets and thrombosis in the pathogenesis of coronary disease. In addition, information from better designed trials of aspirin in patients with cardiovascular and cerebrovascular disease have lent further support to the use of antiplatelet therapy in unstable angina, acute myocardial infarction, chronic coronary disease, coronary revascularization procedures, and cerebrovascular ischemia. Moreover, the role of platelet inhibition for primary prevention of coronary disease and for prevention of stroke in patients with atrial fibrillation is currently evolving.

Platelets are not the only elements that participate in the pathogenesis of thrombosis and embolism. These result from interactions among platelets, the coagulation system, endogenous inhibitors of thrombosis, and the fibrinolytic system. In this review we will focus on salient pharmacologic and clinical aspects of platelet inhibitor therapy for patients with cardiovascular disorders, and on some of the recent developments and future research directions in this field. The pharmacology of anticoagulants and thrombolytic agents is discussed in other sections (see Chapters 6 and 10).

PHARMACOLOGY OF PLATELET INHIBITOR DRUGS

Agents that interfere with platelet metabolism and function have the potential of reducing thrombotic and embolic complications in patients with various disorders involving the arterial system and in those with prosthetic cardiovascular devices. The ideal platelet inhibitor should be effective when administered orally, relatively inexpensive, have adequate antithrombotic properties, sustained action, and be devoid of toxic side effects, particularly bleeding.[6] Although not ideal, aspirin is clearly the most widely used antiplatelet agent. Other available drugs include dipyridamole, ticlopidine, sulfinpyrazone, fish oils, prostaglandins, and dextran. Several other compounds that are undergo-

ing intensive research include inhibitors of thromboxane A_2 and serotonin, inhibitors of thrombin, and monoclonal antibodies directed against platelet membrane receptors or adhesive glycoproteins.

In this section we will review briefly the pharmacologic properties of available drugs and experimental compounds that: (a) inhibit the arachidonic acid pathway; (b) increase platelet cyclic adenosine monophosphate (cAMP); (c) inhibit thrombin; (d) block platelet membrane receptors; and (e) inhibit platelets through other mechanisms (Fig. 5–2).

Inhibitors of the Arachidonic Acid Pathway

CYCLOOXYGENASE INHIBITORS: ASPIRIN

The major antithrombotic effect of aspirin is associated with its ability to inhibit platelet thromboxane A_2 synthesis.[7] At physiologic shear rates, aspirin has no effect on platelet

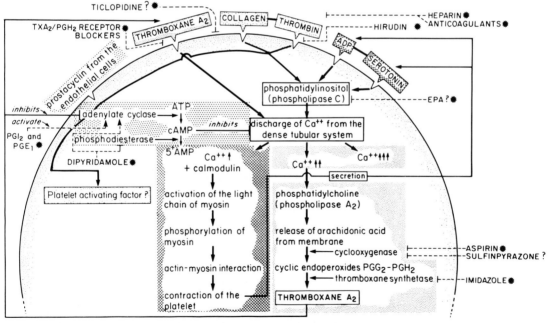

FIGURE 5–2. Mechanisms of platelet activation and presumed sites of action of various platelet inhibitors. Platelet agonists lead to the mobilization of calcium (Ca^{++}), which functions as a mediator of platelet activation through metabolic pathways dependent on adenosine diphosphate (ADP), thromboxane A_2 (TXA_2), thrombin, and collagen. Cyclic adenosine monophosphate (cAMP) inhibits calcium mobilization from the dense tubular system. *Asterisk* (*) indicates a platelet inhibitor. *Dashed line* indicates a presumed site of drug action. ATP = adenosine triphosphate; EPA = eicosapentaenoic acid; PGE_1 = prostaglandin E_1; PGH_2 = prostaglandin H_2; PGI_2 = prostaglandin I_2. (Reproduced from Stein B, et al. Platelet inhibitor agents in cardiovascular disease: an update. J Am Coll Cardiol 1989; 14: 813–36, by permission of the American College of Cardiology.)

adhesion and, therefore, does not prevent formation of the initial layer of platelets on the damaged endothelium or subendothelium. Likewise, it does not inhibit the release of serotonin, adenosine diphosphate (ADP), or platelet-derived growth factor from the platelet granules.[8] Because aspirin does not affect the release of platelet-derived growth factor, it cannot be expected to inhibit atherogenesis or the proliferative response of smooth muscle cells after vascular injury.[9] Aspirin inhibits the secondary wave of aggregation induced by adenosine diphosphate, epinephrine, and low doses of collagen. However, thrombin and high concentrations of collagen can cause a full aggregation response even in the presence of aspirin.[10] This is clinically relevant because high local concentrations of thrombin and collagen are likely to be exposed to and stimulate platelets during atherosclerotic plaque rupture in the acute coronary syndromes, despite treatment with aspirin.

Because aspirin irreversibly acetylates the serine residue at the active site of the enzyme cyclooxygenase, and platelets are unable to generate new enzyme, the inhibition of cyclooxygenase lasts for the lifetime of the cell. It has been shown that single doses of 6 to 100 milligrams of aspirin result in a linear inhibition of thromboxane B_2 production, ranging from 12 to 95 per cent after 24 hours.[11] A single dose of 300 milligrams is sufficient to almost completely suppress thromboxane A_2 synthesis for 48 hours, suggesting that megakaryocytes are also affected.

In the platelet, cyclooxygenase is responsible for the transformation of arachidonic acid to thromboxane A_2; and in the vascular wall, for the conversion of arachidonic acid to prostacyclin and prostaglandin E_1.[7] Thromboxane A_2 has proaggregatory and vasoconstrictive properties, whereas prostacyclin opposes the action of thromboxane A_2 through its antiaggregatory and vasodilative effects.

The differential effects of various doses of aspirin on platelet and vessel wall prostanoid synthesis have been extensively debated. Early studies[12,13] suggested that platelet cyclooxygenase was more sensitive to the effects of aspirin than vessel wall cyclooxygenase, because endothelial cells were able to synthesize new enzyme. This theoretical advantage led to the recommendation of low-dose aspirin (300 milligrams/day or less) in clinical practice. However, more recent studies comparing the effects of aspirin on arterial and venous biopsy samples[14] or on blood from skin bleeding time wounds,[15] found a significant reduction in the synthesis of both thromboxane and prostacyclin. It is currently accepted that even very low doses of aspirin (35 milligrams/day), affect both platelet thromboxane A_2 and endothelial prostacyclin formation.[15]

Aspirin is rapidly absorbed in the stomach and upper small intestine, reaching appreciable plasma levels in 20 minutes and platelet inhibition in approximately 60 minutes. The antiplatelet effect lasts for the life of the platelet (nine to ten days). The clinical benefit of aspirin appears similar at a wide dosage range that varies from as low as 75 milligrams to as high as 1,500 milligrams/day. High aspirin doses do not appear more efficacious than lower ones,[16,17] but are clearly associated with increased gastrointestinal side effects including erosive gastritis or ulceration, bleeding, epigastric distress, nausea, vomiting, and constipation. Therefore, lower aspirin doses (75 to 325 milligrams/day) are currently recommended.

Absorption from enteric-coated tablets is sometimes incomplete, but may produce less gastrointestinal irritation. Preparations containing alkali or buffer may also be better tolerated. Aspirin does not cause a generalized bleeding diathesis, except when given to patients with an underlying bleeding abnormality, or when used in high doses (more than 500 milligrams/day) in combination with anticoagulants.

A number of large clinical trials have recently confirmed the beneficial effects of aspirin in patients with different cardiovascular disorders. Aspirin has demonstrated its usefulness in several trials in patients with unstable angina, in doses ranging from 75 to 1,300 milligrams/day (Table 5–1).[18–21] A recent study[21] in men with unstable angina or non-Q wave myocardial infarction showed that low-dose aspirin (75 milligrams/day) markedly reduced the risk of myocardial infarction or death by 69 per cent. Heparin alone was not found effective, but the use of the combination of aspirin and heparin for the first five days of the trial produced maximal benefit (risk reduction, 75 per cent) (Fig. 5–3).

For patients with acute myocardial infarction, the landmark Second International Study of Infarct Survival (ISIS-2),[22] which included more than 17,000 patients, dem-

TABLE 5–1. Platelet Inhibitor Therapy in Unstable Angina (See also Chapter 13)

TRIAL	NUMBER OF PATIENTS	FOLLOW-UP	DRUG (MILLIGRAMS/DAY)	REDUCTION DEATH + MI (%)	P VALUE
Lewis[18]	1,266	12 weeks	Aspirin (324)	51	<.001
Cairns[19]	555	18 months	Aspirin (1,300)	51	<.01
			Sulfinpyrazone (800)	(−6)	NS
Théroux[20]	479	6 days	Aspirin (650)	72	<.01
			Heparin (24,000 U)	89	<.001
			Aspirin (650) + heparin (24,000 U)	88	.001
RISC[21]	796	3 months	Aspirin (75)	58	<.005
			Heparin (20,000 U)	5	NS
			Aspirin (75) + heparin (20,000 U)	68	<.0005
Balsano[93]	652	6 months	Ticlopidine (500)	53	<.01

MI = Myocardial infarction; NS = nonsignificant.

onstrated that aspirin alone (160 milligrams/day) reduced vascular mortality at five weeks by 21 per cent, and that this benefit was maintained at the 15-month follow-up. When aspirin was combined with streptokinase, a 40 per cent mortality reduction was seen (Fig. 5–4). Aspirin was found to reduce reinfarction and stroke by approximately one-half in this group of patients. (See Chapters 14 and 16.)

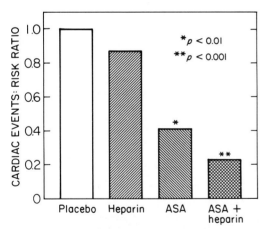

FIGURE 5–3. Efficacy of low-dose aspirin (ASA) (75 milligrams/day) and of the combination of aspirin and intravenous heparin in reducing the risk of myocardial infarction and death in patients with unstable angina or non-Q wave myocardial infarction. Note that the combination of aspirin plus heparin was more effective than either agent alone during the first five days of the trial. A rebound increase in ischemic events was seen after discontinuation of heparin (see text). (Data derived from Walentin et al. The RISC Group. Risk of myocardial infarction and death during treatment with low dose aspirin and intravenous heparin in men with unstable coronary artery disease. Lancet 1990; 336: 827–30.)

This impressive benefit from aspirin in patients with acute ischemic syndromes cannot be expected when this drug is used for patients with stable coronary disease, given the lower incidence and the multifactorial origin of clinical endpoints in the latter group. No single study of aspirin for secondary prevention of myocardial infarction has provided definitive results. However, the results of an extensive overview of available clinical trials[23] that included more than 18,000 patients suggest that platelet inhibitor therapy reduced cardiovascular mortality by 13 per cent, nonfatal reinfarction by 31 per cent, and nonfatal stroke by 42 per cent. In addition, aspirin, at a dose of 325 milligrams on alternate days, was effective for primary prevention of myocardial infarction in asymptomatic men albeit at a slight increase in the risk of hemorrhagic stroke, according to the United States Physician's Health Study.[24] Recent studies[25,26] have also found this drug useful in the treatment of patients with stable coronary disease.

Aspirin, with or without dipyridamole, has been found clearly effective for prevention of acute occlusion and myocardial infarction in patients undergoing percutaneous transluminal coronary angioplasty[27–31] (Table 5–2). Its important antithrombotic role has also been documented in aortocoronary saphenous vein graft surgery,[17,32–34] particularly when treatment was started before or immediately after surgery (Table 5–3). The Veterans Administration Study[17] showed that a single daily dose of 325 milligrams of aspirin was as effective as aspirin given three times a day. A recently published trial[34] demonstrated that aspirin, at a dose of 324 milligrams/day started within one hour after sur-

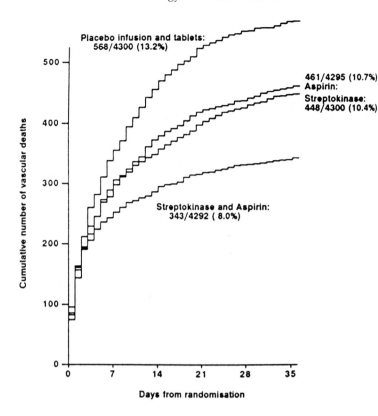

FIGURE 5–4. Cumulative vascular mortality within 35 days after a suspected acute myocardial infarction. The odds reduction in mortality were 23 per cent for aspirin alone, 25 per cent for streptokinase alone, and 42 per cent for the combination of streptokinase and aspirin. (From the ISIS-2 Collaborative Group. Randomized trial of intravenous streptokinase, oral aspirin, both, or neither among 17,187 cases of suspected acute myocardial infarction: ISIS = 2. Lancet 1988; 2: 349–60, with permission.)

TABLE 5–2. Trials of Antiplatelet Agents for Prevention of Acute Complications During Coronary Angioplasty (See also Chapter 21)

TRIAL	NUMBER OF PATIENTS	DRUG (DOSE) (MONTH/DAY)	ACUTE COMPLICATIONS (%)	RESULTS
White[27]	333	Aspirin (650) + dipyridamole (225)	5.0	Reduction in occlusion
		Ticlopidine (750)	2.0	or dissection
		Placebo	14.0	($p < 0.005$)
Schwartz[28]	376	Aspirin (990) + dipyridamole (225)	1.6	Reduction in acute MI
		Placebo	6.9	($p = 0.01$)*
Chesebro[29]	207	Aspirin (975) + dipyridamole (225)	11.0	Beneficial trend
		Placebo	20.0	($p = 0.07$)†
Bertrand[94]	266	Ticlopidine (500)	5.1	Reduction in acute
		Placebo	16.2	occlusion ($p < 0.01$)
Barnathan[30]	220	Aspirin (NR)	1.8	Reduction in thrombotic
		Aspirin + dipyridamole (NR)	0	occlusion or CABG
		None	10.7	($p = 0.005$)
Kent[31]	500	Aspirin (65)	1.3	Reduction in MI or
		None	6.5	CABG ($p < 0.001$)

* Primary endpoint was effect of therapy on restenosis.
† Reduction in coronary occlusion, infarction, repeat angioplasty, or urgent surgery.
MI = myocardial infarction; CABG = coronary artery bypass graft surgery
NR - dose not reported.

TABLE 5–3. Trials of Platelet Inhibitors in Coronary Artery Surgery: Early Initiation of Therapy (<48 hours) (See also Chapter 20)

TRIAL	NUMBER OF PATIENTS	DRUG (MILLIGRAMS/DAY)	FOLLOW-UP	VEIN GRAFT PATENCY (%)		P VALUE
				Rx	CONTROL	
Mayer[152]	174	Aspirin (1,300) + dipyridamole (100)	3–6 months	92	77	< 0.02
Chesebro[32,155]	407	Aspirin (975) + dipyridamole (225)*	8 days	97	90	< 0.0001
			12 months	89	75	< 0.0001
Baur[102]	255	Sulfinpyrazone (800)	1–2 months	96	91	< 0.025
Lorenz[153]	60	Aspirin (100)	4 months	90	68	0.012
Rajah[154]	125	Aspirin (990)* + dipyridamole (225)*	6 months	92	75	< 0.01
Limet[96]	173	Ticlopidine (500)	10 days	93	87	< 0.05
			6 months	85	76	< 0.02
			12 months	84	74	< 0.01
Goldman[17]	555	Aspirin (325)	9 days	94	85	<0. 01
		Aspirin (975)		92		<0.05
		Aspirin (975) + dipyridamole (225)*		92		<0.05
		Sulfinpyrazone (801)*		90		NS
Goldman[156]		Aspirin groups	12 months	84	77	< 0.03
		Sulfinpyrazone		82		NS
Sanz[33]	1,112	Aspirin (150)	10 days	86	82	0.058
		Aspirin (150) + dipyridamole (225)*		87		< 0.02
Cavaghan[34]	237	Aspirin (324)	7 days	98	94	0.004
			12 months	94	88	0.01

* Preoperative initiation of therapy.
NS = not signficant; Rx = treatment.

gery, was very effective in reducing early (one week) and late (one year) graft occlusion rates, and also reduced the rate of progression to total occlusion of grafts that were patent on early angiography. A nonsignificant increase in early reoperation rate, however, was seen in aspirin-treated patients.

Low-dose aspirin therapy has also demonstrated benefit in reducing the incidence of stroke in patients with transient ischemic attacks[16] and in those with nonvalvular atrial fibrillation.[35] Based on data derived from clinical trials, the currently recommended dose of aspirin for antithrombotic treatment is 75 to 325 milligrams/day.

The search for more effective aspirin formulations has generated considerable interest. Pedersen and FitzGerald[36] demonstrated a reduction in thromboxane B_2 formation by 20 milligrams of oral aspirin, before any aspirin was detected in the systemic circulation. These investigators suggested that slow administration of very low doses of aspirin may inhibit platelets circulating in the portal system (presystemic inhibition), without impairing the endothelial production of prostacyclin because of reduced systemic bioa-

vailability of the drug. In another study,[37] Cerletti et al. showed that after the administration of 325 milligrams of enteric-coated aspirin, thromboxane B_2 generation was reduced shortly after ingestion but before any aspirin was detected in the peripheral circulation, demonstrating a presystemic inhibitory effect of this enteric-coated aspirin preparation. However, no difference in inhibition of vascular prostacyclin generation was seen when enteric-coated aspirin was compared to regular aspirin.[37] Therefore, enteric-coated aspirin, at a dose of 325 milligram, did not produce a "selective" inhibition of platelet cyclooxygenase.

In a more recent study,[38] Clarke et al. showed that, whereas low-dose aspirin (160 milligrams/day or 325 milligrams on alternate days) inhibited both platelet and endothelial prostaglandin synthesis, a controlled-release, low-dose (75 milligram) aspirin preparation completely inhibited platelet thromboxane A_2 generation without affecting systemic vascular wall prostacyclin production. This interesting concept is currently being tested in several clinical trials. If this "selective" inhibition of cyclooxygenase can be proved clinically relevant, a controlled-release low-dose aspirin may become the optimal aspirin regimen for antithrombotic therapy.

The nonsteroidal anti-inflammatory drugs inhibit cyclooxygenase in a reversible fashion, and thus have a reduced effect on platelet function and a shorter duration of action. An experimental study[39] suggested that ibuprofen reduces platelet deposition and mural thrombosis after deep arterial injury. However, the antithrombotic properties of these compounds have not been adequately tested in clinical trials and its use can not be recommended. In addition, one of these agents, indomethacin, was found to increase vascular resistance and exacerbate ischemia in patients with coronary artery disease.[40]

DRUGS THAT AFFECT PLATELET MEMBRANE PHOSPHOLIPIDS: OMEGA-3 FATTY ACIDS

Ingestion of a diet rich in omega-3 fatty acids may prevent or delay atherosclerosis and thrombosis. Both eicosapentaenoic acid ($20:5\omega3$) and docosahexaenoic acid ($22:6\omega3$) are present in high concentration in saltwater fish and may account for the lower incidence of coronary disease in populations that include fish in their diet.[41-43] These polyunsaturated fatty acids become incorporated into the platelet membrane between one and four weeks after administration and result in decreased aggregation responses.[44] Eicosapentaenoic acid competes with arachidonic acid for platelet cyclooxygenase. This leads to the formation of two endoperoxidases (prostaglandins G_3 and H_3) and of thromboxane A_3, which have minimal biologic activity. In endothelial cells, production of prostacyclin is not markedly inhibited and prostaglandin I_3 is produced, which retains platelet inhibitory properties.[45] The net result is a shift in the hemostatic balance toward an antiaggregatory and vasodilative state.

Fish oils were shown experimentally to suppress thromboxane production and accelerate the response to thrombolysis in a canine model of coronary thrombosis.[46] In addition to their interference with platelet metabolism, omega-3 fatty acids have multiple other effects including reduced production of leukotriene B_4, platelet-derived growth factor, interleukin-1, tumor necrosis factor, and fibrinogen.[47] They also reduce blood pressure, blood viscosity, triglycerides and very low-density lipoprotein levels, and increase the actions of endothelium-derived relaxing factor.[47] Whether these actions of fish oils result in antiatherogenic and antithrombotic effects in human trials, remains to be determined.

The use of omega-3 fatty acids in patients undergoing angioplasty has generated a great deal of interest; however, five clinical trials[48-52] have yielded conflicting results (Table 5-4). In a carefully conducted trial,[48] Dehmer et al. treated patients with high-dose fish oils for seven days before angioplasty and evaluated the effects of therapy on platelet fatty acid concentration. Restenosis rates per dilated lesion were reduced from 36 per cent to only 16 per cent, restenosis occurred in 46 per cent of controls and in 19 per cent of treated patients. Even though two additional studies,[51,52] using mostly nonangiographic definitions of restenosis, disclosed some beneficial effects from therapy, the other two studies[49,50] that relied on angiographic follow-up failed to show any benefit from fish oils. In addition, gastrointestinal side effects are common with the high doses used in these studies, which limits patient compliance. Given available conflicting data, no firm recommendations can be given. There is

TABLE 5–4. Use of Omega-3 Fatty Acids for Prevention of Restenosis after Coronary Angioplasty
(See Chapter 21)

STUDY	NUMBER OF PATIENTS	DOSE (GRAM/DAY)	PRETREATMENT (DAYS)	METHOD OF FOLLOW-UP	RESTENOSIS (%)		P VALUE
					Rx	CONTROL	
Dehmer[48]	82	3.2	7	Angiography	19	46	0.007
Grigg[49]	108	3.0	1	Angiography	34	33	NS
Reis[50]	186	6.0	5	Angiograph	34	23	NS
Milner[51]	194	4.5	0	Clinical	22	35	< 0.04
Slack[52]	162	2.4	0	Clinical	35	39	NS*

* For patients with single vessel angioplasty, treatment reduced restenosis from 33 per cent to 16 per cent ($p < 0.05$).
NS = not significant; Rx = treatment.

some evidence, however, that for selected patients, pretreatment with large doses of omega-3 fatty acids before angioplasty may be beneficial.

There are no other prospective controlled human trials of fish oils for prevention of atherosclerosis and thrombosis. Although fish consumption may decrease the incidence of coronary heart disease,[42,43] administration of pharmacologic doses of omega-3 fatty acids can be associated with potentially adverse events such as increased bleeding diathesis and reduced inflammatory and immune responses.[53] Thus, whereas a diet that includes fish appears sensible, pharmacologic doses of fish oils cannot be presently recommended for primary prevention of cardiovascular disease.

Drugs That Increase Platelet Cyclic Adenosine Monophosphate

DIPYRIDAMOLE

Dipyridamole is a pyrimidopyrimidine compound with antithrombotic and vasodilating properties. Although the exact mechanism of action remains unknown, in vitro studies have disclosed three mechanisms by which intracellular platelet cyclic adenosine monophosphate is increased. At high concentrations, dipyridamole inhibits phosphodiesterase, which reduces breakdown of cyclic adenosine monophosphate; it also activates the enzyme adenylate cyclase by a prostacyclin-mediated effect on the platelet membrane. At more physiologic concentrations, dipyridamole increases plasma adenosine levels by inhibiting its uptake from vascular endothelium and erythrocytes,[54] thereby enhancing platelet adenylate cyclase activity.

Although aspirin was shown to potentiate the antithrombotic effects of dipyridamole on arteriovenous cannulae in the baboon model,[26] there is conflicting evidence regarding the pharmacokinetic interactions between these two agents in humans. More importantly, there are no convincing data indicating that such interaction leads to a synergistic antithrombotic effect.[55] Dipyridamole does not reduce platelet aggregation or mural thrombosis in animal models of arterial stenosis[56] or injury.[57] In contrast, there is some evidence supporting an effect on prosthetic surfaces. Animal studies have shown that dipyridamole reduces platelet deposition and improves patency of artificial grafts.[58,59]

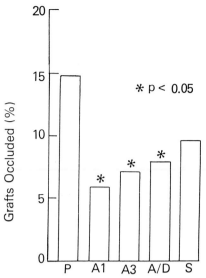

FIGURE 5–5. Occluded vein grafts (percentage) within 60 days after bypass surgery in different treatment groups. Only the aspirin-containing regimens improved graft patency (by cluster analysis). P = placebo; A1 = aspirin (325 milligrams/day); A3 = aspirin (325 milligrams three times/day); A/D = aspirin plus dipyridamole (325 and 75 milligrams three times/day, respectively); S = sulfinpyrazone (267 milligrams three times/day). (Reproduced from Goldman, et al. Improvement in early saphenous vein graph patency after coronary artery bypass surgery with antiplatelet therapy: results of a Veterans Administration cooperative study. Circulation 1988; 77: 1324–32, by permission of the American Heart Association, Inc.)

In humans, dipyridamole prolongs the shortened platelet survival times associated with prosthetic heart valves and prosthetic grafts.[60,61] In addition, platelet activation associated with cardiopulmonary bypass is reduced, as is early postoperative blood loss.[62] In a recent randomized trial of patients with coronary bypass surgery,[63] dipyridamole increased significantly vein graft blood flow during surgery. However, graft patency rates were only marginally better in treated patients compared to controls.

In accordance with experimental evidence, dipyridamole has a limited effect on biologic surfaces in humans. With the exception of one study[64] in patients with peripheral vascular disease, most clinical trials in survivors of myocardial infarction or stroke (and in those undergoing coronary angioplasty or bypass surgery)[17,65–69] have not been able to document an advantage of the combination of aspirin and dipyridamole over aspirin alone (Fig. 5–5).

Because dipyridamole, as opposed to aspirin, does not increase perioperative bleeding in patients undergoing coronary bypass surgery, its use for two days before surgery has been recommended.[32] Whether this is necessary, remains unknown. More importantly, antiplatelet therapy should be started in the immediate postoperative period.[34] Whereas one study[17] found no advantage of adding dipyridamole to aspirin, a more recent and larger trial[33] disclosed a small advantage from combined therapy. In this study of 1,112 patients, early graft occlusion rates were 18 per cent in the placebo group, 12.9 per cent in the aspirin plus dipyridamole group ($p = 0.017$), and 14 per cent in the aspirin-treated patients ($p = 0.058$)[33] (Table 5–3).

As mentioned before, the antithrombotic effects of dipyridamole are more evident on prosthetic surfaces. Patients with prosthetic mechanical heart valves are at continuous risk of thromboembolism despite adequate anticoagulation. For patients at the highest risk, the addition of a platelet inhibitor to the anticoagulant regimen has been advocated[70–76] (Table 5–5). Most studies have shown that adding dipyridamole reduces the incidence of embolism, without increasing the risk of bleeding. Aspirin was also found effective in some trials, but its use at doses of 500 milligrams/day or higher carries a substantial risk of gastrointestinal hemorrhage.[74]

Absorption of dipyridamole is variable and greatly reduced when gastric pH is above 4. Its main side effects are headache, epigastric discomfort, and nausea, which occur in up to 10 per cent of patients, is dose-related, and often subsides with continued use. Dipyridamole does not exacerbate gastroduodenal ulcers and does not increase the bleeding, even when combined with an anticoagulant.[74]

PROSTAGLANDINS E_1 AND I_2

These prostaglandins increase the concentration of cyclic adenosine monophosphate in platelets and thus are potent inhibitors of platelet metabolism. They are also powerful systemic vasodilators. Intravenous prostaglandin E_1 is commonly used in neonates with congenital heart disease, who are dependent on the persistence of a patent ductus arteriosus until surgical correction can be done. In addition, it has been used in some patients with acute myocardial infarction complicated by left ventricular dysfunction for its beneficial hemodynamic effects.[77]

Prostacyclin (prostaglandin I_2) is a potent, naturally occurring platelet inhibitor. Its clinical use has been limited by its instability and its propensity to cause significant systemic hypotension at doses required for platelet inhibition. Its pharamacologic effects disappear within 30 minutes after infusion. Prostacyclin has been shown to limit platelet interaction with artificial surfaces, preserve the platelet count during extracorporeal circulation, and enhance the efficacy of heparin, perhaps by limiting the release of platelet factor 4, which neutralizes heparin.[78,79] Al-

TABLE 5–5. Trials of Platelet Inhibitors Added to Anticoagulants in Patients with Mechanical Valve Prostheses (See also Chapter 11)

TRIAL	NUMBER OF PATIENTS	DRUG (MILLIGRAMS/DAY)	EMBOLIC EVENTS (%)	RESULTS
Sullivan[70]	84	Anticoagulants + placebo	14	Reduction in embolism
	79	Anticoagulants + dipyridamole (400)	1	($p < 0.01$)
Kasahara[71]	39	Anticoagulants	21	Reduction in embolism
	40	Anticoagulants + dipyridamole (400)	5	($p < 0.05$)
PACTE[72]	154	Anticoagulants	5	No benefit
	136	Anticoagulants + dipyridamole (375)	3	
Rajah[73]	87	Anticoagulants	13	Reduction in embolism
	78	Anticoagulants + dipyridamole (225–400)	4	($p < 0.05$)
Chesebro[74]	183	Anticoagulants	4	Favorable trend for
	181	Anticoagulants + dipyridamole (400)	1	dipyridamole; no
	170	Anticoagulants + aspirin (500)	4	benefit from aspirin*
Altman[75]	65	Anticoagulants	20	Reduction in embolism
	57	Anticoagulants + aspirin (500)	5	($p < 0.05$)
Dale[76]	73	Anticoagulants + placebo	12	Reduction in embolism
	75	Anticoagulants + aspirin (1,000)	2	($p < 0.0.1$)

* Significant increase in gastrointestinal hemorrhage with aspirin.
PACTE = prevention des accidents Thromboemboliques Systemiques Recherche Groupe.

though prostacyclin has been used alone in extracorporeal circuits, its use should probably be restricted to situations in which heparin use must be limited.[10]

Whereas animal studies have shown prostacyclin to have a beneficial effect in models of myocardial ischemia, the results from small human trials have been controversial.[80] More recent studies[81–83] in patients with stable and unstable angina or acute myocardial infarction showed that, despite favorable effects on platelet aggregation and systemic hemodynamics, prostacyclin administration does not improve clinical outcome. In fact, one study[83] suggested that the potent vasodilatory effects of prostacyclin may lead to subendocardial to subepicardial "steal" and result in aggravation of ischemia in patients with severe coronary occlusions.

A few trials[84,85] have suggested that these prostanoids improve the results of intracoronary thrombolysis in acute myocardial infarction. However, recent experimental[86] and clinical[87] studies with iloprost, a stable prostacyclin analogue, showed that these prostanoids increase the hepatic degradation of tissue plasminogen activator, and thus may reduce its thrombolytic activity. Similarly, controversy has surrounded the use of these agents in patients undergoing coronary angioplasty. One study[88] showed that ciprostene, another stable analogue of prostacyclin, produced a trend toward lower restenosis rate and a significant reduction in ischemic events within six months after angioplasty. In contrast, short-term prostacyclin infusion was not shown to affect restenosis rates in another study,[89] although it reduced the incidence of acute vessel closure. Given these conflicting data, further animal and clinical research appears necessary before recommendations can be made.

Other Platelet Inhibitors

TICLOPIDINE

Ticlopidine, one of the most potent antiplatelet agents available, has been approved recently for clinical use by the Food and Drug Administration. It is chemically unrelated to other platelet inhibitors and does not inhibit prostaglandin synthesis or cyclic adenosine monophosphate degradation. Ticlopidine may act on the platelet membrane to alter its reactivity and may block the interaction of fibrinogen and von Willebrand factor with platelets.[90] It mainly inhibits adenosine diphosphate-induced platelet aggregation, even at high agonist concentrations.[91] Platelet aggregation induced by low concentrations of thrombin, collagen, thromboxane A_2, and platelet activating factor is also inhibited, but high agonist concentrations may overcome these effects.[91] Ticlopidine prolongs the bleeding time.

Optimal efficacy is reached only after several days of onset of therapy; the inhibition of platelet function may persist for more than 72 hours after discontinuation of the drug, with return to baseline values after four to ten days.[91,92] The ex vivo inhibition of adenosine diphosphate-induced aggregation appears proportional to the dose administered, reaching a maximum effect at a dose of 500 milligrams/day.[92] The ability to inhibit thromboxane A_2-induced aggregation without impairing prostacyclin synthesis may give ticlopidine an advantage over aspirin.

Clinical evaluation is now underway. In the Italian Study of Ticlopidine in Unstable Angina,[93] 652 patients were randomly allocated to receive ticlopidine (250 milligram twice daily) or placebo and followed for six months. Ticlopidine reduced myocardial infarction rate, vascular mortality, and total coronary events by approximately 50 per cent (Table 5–1). In two other studies,[27,94] ticlopidine (500 to 750 milligrams/day) markedly reduced the incidence of abrupt thrombotic occlusion and ischemic complications in patients undergoing coronary angioplasty (Table 5–2). Unfortunately, it was found ineffective in reducing the rate of restenosis after angioplasty.[94,95]

In a well-designed, placebo-controlled trial of patients undergoing bypass surgery,[96] ticlopidine (250 milligrams twice daily) was started on the second postoperative day and continued for one year. The drug reduced significantly the graft occlusion rates on day ten (7.1 versus 13.4 per cent), day 180 (15 versus 24 per cent), and day 360 (15.9 versus 26.1 per cent) (Fig. 5–6). Treatment was fairly well tolerated. Neutropenia was observed in seven patients on ticlopidine and three on placebo. Severe neutropenia was reversible in all cases.

Two large trials of patients with cerebrovascular disease were recently published.[97,98] Hass et al.[97] randomized 3,069 patients with transient or mild persistent cerebral or retinal ischemia to aspirin (1,300 milligrams/day) or ticlopidine (500 milligrams/day). At the end of three years, the rate of nonfatal stroke or

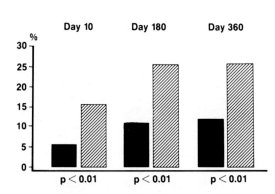

FIGURE 5–6. Reduction in the occlusion rate of individual saphenous vein grafts by ticlopidine (250 milligrams twice/day) at different time intervals after aortocoronary bypass surgery. (From Limet R, et al. Prevention of aorta-coronary bypass graft occlusion. J Thorac Cardiovasc Surg 1987; 94: 773–83, with permission.)

death was 17 per cent in the ticlopidine group and 19 per cent in the aspirin group (12 per cent risk reduction, $p = 0.048$). Ticlopidine was also more effective than aspirin in reducing the rates of fatal and nonfatal stroke in both sexes. However, side effects were more common in the ticlopidine group, including diarrhea (20 per cent), rash (12 per cent) and severe but reversible neutropenia (0.9 per cent).

In the Canadian American Ticlopidine Study (CATS),[98] Gent et al. randomly allocated 1,072 patients with a recent thromboembolic stroke to ticlopidine (250 milligrams twice daily) or placebo. This agent reduced incidence of stroke or vascular death by 24 and 40 per cent, by intention-to-treat and efficacy analysis, respectively. It was effective for both men and women. Side effects included rash, diarrhea, and neutropenia, which promptly resolved upon discontinuation of the drug.

In summary, the recently approved potent platelet inhibitor agent, ticlopidine, is effective in a variety of clinical disorders including unstable angina, coronary angioplasty, coronary bypass surgery, and cerebrovascular disease. Its widespread acceptance by the medical community will depend on several issues such as cost, safety, and relative efficacy when compared with aspirin. It may be particularly useful for patients intolerant to aspirin.

SULFINPYRAZONE

This agent is structurally related to phenylbutazone, but has minimal anti-inflammatory activity. In contrast to aspirin, it is a competitive inhibitor of platelet cyclooxygenase, but the exact mechanism of action remains unknown.[55] It inhibits platelet adhesion to collagen, reduces thrombus formation on subendothelium, and may protect the endothelium from chemical injury.[55,99] Sulfinpyrazone produces a dose-dependent inhibition in experimental thromboembolism in artificial cannulae,[55] reduces thrombosis of arteriovenous cannulae, and normalizes platelet survival in patients with artificial heart valves.

Like dipyridamole, the overall beneficial effects of sulfinpyrazone have been more consistent on prosthetic than on biologic surfaces. Its clinical benefits have been variable. Some benefit was seen when given to patients after myocardial infarction[100,101] or aortocoronary bypass surgery.[17,102] However, no benefit was evident in patients with unstable angina[19] or stroke.[103]

The drug is well absorbed orally, reaching plasma peak concentrations in one to two hours. It is strongly protein bound and, therefore, may displace other protein-bound drugs such as warfarin and the sulfonylureas, causing potentiation of their effects. Other side effects include exacerbation of peptic ulcer, renal insufficiency, and precipitation of uric acid stones.

DEXTRAN

Intravenous infusion of dextran results in prolongation of the bleeding time. Its mechanism of antiplatelet activity is unclear. It may involve some alteration of platelet membrane function or interference with factor VIII-von Willebrand factor complex.[104] Despite antithrombotic activity demonstrated experimentally, no beneficial effect was found in patients undergoing coronary angioplasty.[105] Dextran infusions are currently being used before and immediately after placement of intravascular coronary stents, for prevention of acute thrombotic occlusion. Its potential side effects include volume overload and anaphylactoid reactions.

Thrombin Inhibitors

Because thrombin is a powerful platelet activator, and because thrombin-mediated platelet–thrombus formation appears to be an important process in the development of vascular occlusion after arterial injury, interventions that inhibit the action of thrombin have triggered extensive research. Pharmacologic agents that inhibit thrombin can be divided into two broad categories: those that act via the natural coagulation inhibitor antithrombin III and those with a mechanism of action independent of antithrombin III. Although a complete discussion of this subject is beyond the scope of this review, salient aspects of these therapeutic modalities will be briefly mentioned.

ANTITHROMBIN III-DEPENDENT THROMBIN INHIBITORS: HEPARIN

Heparin has played an essential role in the management of patients with different cardiovascular disorders. It not only inhibits the formation of fibrin, but through its antithrombin effects, may interfere with the processes of platelet activation and aggregation. The clinical pharmacology of heparin is reviewed in Chapter 6. A few of its pharmacologic properties are mentioned in this section, only for purpose of comparison with other antithrombin III-independent inhibitors.

Heparin is a naturally occurring sulfated glycosaminoglycan; its anticoagulant activity is mediated predominantly through two intermediate cofactors, antithrombin III and heparin cofactor II. During the coagulation process in the adult, antithrombin III is involved in the neutralization of approximately 65 per cent of thrombin formed, whereas cofactor II binds only 10 per cent, the remainder being neutralized by alpha$_2$-macroglobulin. In the presence of heparin, however, the proportion of thrombin neutralized by antithrombin III increases considerably, and only a small proportion becomes bound to other cofactors. The interaction of heparin with antithrombin III leads to a conformational change in the inhibitor that greatly accelerates its interaction with coagulation proteases, particularly thrombin and activated factors IX and X. Because thrombin exerts a positive feedback action on the coagulation cascade that would rapidly result in the generation of large concentrations of thrombin, the inhibition of the first traces of thrombin may be important in preventing activation of factors V and VIII, hence reducing prothrombinase generation. The absence or deficiency of antithrombin III renders heparin useless or ineffective for antithrombotic therapy.

Heparin is a heterogeneous mixture of polysaccharide molecules with molecular weights ranging from 3,000 to 40,000 daltons. The effects of heparin on platelets are complex and occasionally contradictory, partly because of the variability among different commercially available preparations.[106,107] It can be fractionated either on the basis of molecular weight or affinity for antithrombin III. Low molecular weight fractions (5,000 to 7,000 daltons) effectively catalyze the inactivation of activated factor X by antithrombin III, but do not prolong the activated partial thromboplastin time or the thrombin time as standard heparin does.[106,108] Therefore, low molecular weight heparins are able to inhibit activated factor X activity while producing less interference with the coagulation cascade. This may lead to a more favorable ratio of antithrombotic activity to hemorrhagic risk compared to standard heparin, as has been demonstrated experimentally.[109]

In addition, low molecular weight heparin is less active than high molecular weight fractions in inducing platelet aggregation with secondary thrombocytopenia and prolongation of bleeding time.[106,108] Because low molecular weight heparins with a high ratio of anti-Xa to antithrombin activity develop the same antithrombotic effect as standard heparin in platelet-dependent thrombosis with less impairment in hemostatic function,[109] these agents may provide useful antiplatelet therapy with less risk of bleeding. Clinical investigations are currently underway.

ANTITHROMBIN III-INDEPENDENT THROMBIN INHIBITORS

This group of thrombin inhibitors exert their antithrombotic activity either by directly binding to thrombin or by inhibiting a cofactor that is essential for thrombin formation. Their mechanism of action is independent of antithrombin III. Experience with these agents is largely experimental, although preclinical dose-finding studies are currently being conducted.

Hirudin. Hirudin, a 65 amino acid polypeptide initially isolated from the salivary gland of the medicinal leech, is the most potent and selective inhibitor of thrombin known.[110] It has a molecular weight of approximately 7,000 daltons and through deoxyribonucleic acid (DNA) recombinant technology, has become available in sufficient quantities for animal and human testing. Because of the high affinity for thrombin, relatively low concentrations of hirudin are able to neutralize this coagulation enzyme. In the hirudin–thrombin complex, all proteolytic functions of the enzyme are blocked. Thus, hirudin prevents not only fibrin formation but the thrombin-catalyzed hemostatic reactions, such as activation of factors V, VIII, XIII, and the thrombin-induced platelet reactions.[110] Because of its high affinity for the thrombin receptor, hirudin can displace thrombin from its binding site on platelets.[111] Whereas platelet factor 4 is the naturally occurring inhibitor of heparin, there is no natural inhibitor of hirudin. Thus, the dose of hirudin administered is the only limiting factor for thrombin blockade.

According to its high antithrombin activity, hirudin is most effective in experimental stasis-induced venous thrombosis and in disseminated intravascular coagulation.[110] Because of the importance of platelets in models of arterial or vascular graft thrombosis and the high affinity of thrombin for platelets, higher hirudin concentrations are necessary for the inhibition of the thrombin–platelet reaction than of the thrombin–fibrinogen reaction.

Hirudin has been shown to prevent thrombosis in a porcine model of carotid angioplasty, producing a more significant reduction in platelet deposition and thrombus

formation than therapeutic or even high (250 units/kilogram) doses of heparin[112] (Fig. 5–7). In addition, it markedly enhances thrombolysis by tissue plasminogen activator in the same animal model of deep arterial injury and occlussive platelet-rich thrombosis.[113]

These observations have clinical relevance in the context of coronary thrombolysis. Thrombin bound to a fibrin clot remains active and poorly accessible to the heparin-antithrombin III complex. During fibrinolysis, thrombin becomes exposed at the surface of the residual clot and may account for the thrombotic reocclusion that commonly occurs after thrombolysis. Recent in vitro[114,115] and in vivo studies[116,117] found that hirudin, in contrast to heparin, neutralizes both free and fibrin-bound thrombin, and prevents more efficiently the activation of coagulation during thrombolysis. In a recent experiment,[118] hirudin was more effective than platelet receptor antibodies in accelerating thrombolysis and preventing reocclusion after infusion of tissue plasminogen activator.

The superiority of hirudin over heparin is probably related to several factors. First, fibrin-bound thrombin is poorly accessible to the large heparin-antithrombin III complex, but is neutralized by hirudin. Second, natural inhibitors of heparin such as platelet factor 4 and fibrin II monomer are present at the

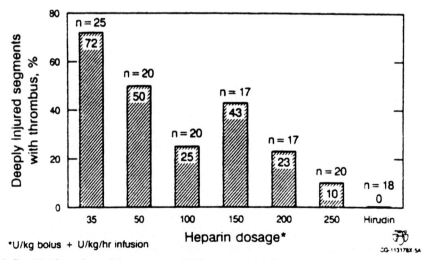

FIGURE 5–7. Number of arterial segments with deep arterial injury that had mural thrombus. *n* Value at the top of the bar is the number of segments with deep injury in each group. The height of the bars represents the percentage with thrombus. There was a reduction in thrombus formation from 72 per cent in the lowest heparin group to 10 per cent in the highest heparin group. No thrombus was seen in the hirudin-treated animals. (From Heras M, et al. Effects of thrombin inhibition on the development of acute platelet thrombus deposition during angioplasty in pigs. Circulation 1989; 79: 657–65, by permission of the American Heart Association, Inc.)

site of vascular injury, whereas hirudin lacks natural inhibitors. Third, heparin, but not hirudin, requires endogenous cofactors for its activity. Fourth, at the same degree of antihemostatic effect, hirudin has a much greater thrombin inhibitor effect than heparin. Preclinical, dose-finding studies of recombinant hirudin in humans have already begun.

Synthetic Thrombin Inhibitors. Multiple synthetic thrombin-inhibitor peptides have been tested over the last ten years. One of these compounds, D-phenylalanyl-L-prolyl-L-arginyl-chloromethyl ketone (PPACK), was shown to be a potent irreversible inhibitor of thrombin.[119] The covalent PPACK–thrombin complex binds and inactivates the high-affinity functional thrombin receptor in platelets. In the baboon model of prosthetic vascular grafting,[119] a continuous infusion of PPACK into the graft abolished platelet deposition on the graft, platelet hemostatic plug formation, and vascular graft occlusion. In addition, it prevented thrombin-induced platelet aggregation and thrombin-induced blood clotting. In contrast, anticoagulant levels of heparin were ineffective in this model. The investigators concluded that thrombin is the principal mediator of platelet-dependent high-flow thrombosis and occlusion, and that synthetic antithrombins may prove effective for both arterial and venous thrombosis by simultaneously inhibiting platelet activation and fibrin formation.[119]

Further investigations have confirmed the ability of PPACK to reduce platelet deposition and abolish thrombosis in a platelet-dependent, heparin-resistant model of endovascular stent implantation.[120] In addition, in vitro studies[115] showed that antithrombin III-independent inhibitors such as hirudin derivatives or PPACK were effective in inactivating clot-bound thrombin, whereas heparin was not.

Another synthetic competitive thrombin inhibitor, argatroban, has been studied by several groups. Argatroban abolished cyclic flow variations due to platelet aggregate formation in a canine model of coronary thrombosis,[121] suggesting that thrombin is an important mediator of this process. In another model of vascular injury,[122] argatroban was found clearly superior to heparin in preventing platelet deposition and thrombosis. In a canine preparation of coronary thrombosis with superimposed high-grade stenosis,[123] argatroban accelerated coronary thrombolysis with tissue-type plasminogen activator and, combined with aspirin, prevented reocclusion. In addition, these effects were achieved with less prolongation of the bleeding time than observed with a potent antiplatelet glycoprotein receptor.

The pharmacodynamic and pharmacokinetic effects of argatroban are being examined in humans. In a recent study,[124] argatroban was shown to produce a dose-dependant prolongation of coagulation parameters, that returned to baseline one hour after discontinuation of the drug. Argatroban did not increase the bleeding time when given alone and did not further prolong the bleeding time when given in combination with aspirin. These preliminary findings suggest that the combination of aspirin and an antithrombin III-independent thrombin inhibitor such as argatroban may prove effective for prevention of arterial thrombosis.[124]

Activated Protein C. Activated protein C is a natural, vitamin K-dependent anticoagulant, generated by the catalytic complex of thrombin and thrombomodulin. It inhibits thrombin formation by means of enzymatic cleavage and destruction of coagulation activated factors V and VIII, thus providing negative feedback regulation of coagulation. The activity of human activated protein C was investigated in a prosthetic vascular graft preparation in primates.[125,126] Infusion of activated protein C resulted in a reduction of platelet deposition on the graft by 40 to 70 per cent and maintenance of graft patency. Activated protein C inhibited blood clotting, as measured by the activated partial thromboplastin time, without affecting hemostatic plug formation by the template bleeding time.

These experiments suggest that activated protein C effectively inhibits thrombus formation without impairing primary hemostasis. Activated protein C combined with urokinase was recently shown to reduce platelet-dependent thrombus formation compared to urokinase alone in a vascular graft animal model.[127] This effect was achieved without impairing normal hemostatic mechanisms. Therefore, administration of human activated protein C in the clinical setting may be effective and less likely to cause bleeding than administration of other available platelet antagonists or thrombin inhibitors.

Because arterial thrombosis still occurs despite treatment with conventional antiplatelet agents plus heparin, considerable interest has tioned inhibitors of thrombin, may be effective in the short-term management of patients at very high risk of thrombotic occlusion. However, long-term therapy is hazardous because of the increased risk of bleeding.

REFERENCES

1. Davies MJ, Thomas T. The pathological basis and microanatomy of occlusive coronary thrombus formation in human coronary arteries. Philos Trans R Soc Lond 1981; 294: 225–9.
2. Goldsmith HL, Turitto VT. Rheological aspects of thrombosis and haemostasis: basic principles and applications. Thromb Haemost 1986; 55: 415–35.
3. Badimon L, Badimon JJ, Galvez A, Chesebro JH, Fuster V. Influence of arterial wall damage and wall shear rate on platelet deposition: ex vivo study in a swine model. Arteriosclerosis 1986; 6: 312–20.
4. Vane JR, Flower RJ, Botting RM. History of aspirin and its mechanisms of action. Stroke 1990: 21(suppl IV): IV-12–23.
5. Vane JR. Inhibition of prostaglandin synthesis as a mechanism of action for aspirin-like drugs. Nature New Biol 1971; 231: 232–5.
6. Harker LA. Antithrombotic therapy. In: Williams WJ, Beutler E, Erslev AJ, Lichtman MA, eds. Hematology. New York: McGraw-Hill, 1990: 1569–81.
7. Moncada S, Vane JR. Arachidonic acid metabolites and the interactions between platelets and blood vessel walls. N Engl J Med 1979; 300: 1142–7.
8. Tschopp TB. Aspirin inhibits platelet aggregation, but not adhesion to collagen fibrils: and assessment of platelet adhesion and deposited platelet mass by morphometry and 51-Cr-labeling. Thromb Res 1977; 11: 619–32.
9. Clowes AW, Karnovsky MJ. Failure of certain antiplatelet drugs to affect myointimal thickening following arterial endothelial injury in the rat. Lab Invest 1977; 36: 452–64.
10. Oates JA, FitzGerald GA, Branch RA, Jackson EK, Knapp HR, Roberts LJ II. Clinical implications of prostaglandin and thromboxane A formation. N Engl J Med 1988; 319: 689–98.
11. Patrignani P, Filabozzi P, Patrono C. Selective cumulative inhibition of platelet thromboxane production by low-dose aspirin in healthy subjects. J Clin Invest 1982; 69: 1366–72.
12. Buchanan MR, Dejana E, Cazenave JP, Richardson M, Mustard JF, Hirsh J. Differences in inhibition of PGI production by aspirin in rabbit artery and vein segments. Thromb Res 1980; 20: 447–60.
13. Jaffe EA, Weksler BB. Recovery of endothelial cell prostacyclin production after inhibition by low doses of aspirin. J Clin Invest 1979; 63: 532–5.
14. Weksler BB, Pett SB, Richter RC, et al. Differential inhibition by aspirin of vascular and platelet prostaglandin synthesis in atherosclerotic patients. N Engl J Med 1983; 308: 800–5.
15. Kyrle PA, Eichler HG, Jager U, Lechner K. Inhibition of prostacyclin and thromboxane A generation by low-dose aspirin at the site of plug formation in man in vivo. Circulation 1987; 75: 1025–9.
16. UK-TIA Study Group. United Kingdom Transient Ischemic Attack (UK-TIA) Aspirin Trial: interim results. Br Med J 1988; 296: 316–20.
17. Goldman S, Copeland J, Moritz T, et al. Improvement in early saphenous vein graft patency after coronary artery bypass surgery with antiplatelet therapy: results of a Veterans Administration cooperative study. Circulation 1988; 77: 1324–32.
18. Lewis HD, Davis JW, Archibald DG, et al. Protective effects of aspirin against acute myocardial infarction and death in men with unstable angina: results of a Veterans Administration cooperative study. N Engl J Med 1983; 309: 396–403.
19. Cairns JA, Gent M, Singer J, et al. Aspirin, sulfinpyrazone,

20. Théroux P, Ouimet H, McCans J, et al. Aspirin, heparin, or both to treat acute unstable angina. N Engl J Med 1988; 319: 1105–11.
21. The RISC Group. Risk of myocardial infarction and death during treatment with low dose aspirin and intravenous heparin in men with unstable coronary artery disease. Lancet 1990; 336: 827–30.
22. ISIS-2 (Second International Study of Infarct Survival) Collaborative Group. Randomized trial of intravenous streptokinase, oral aspirin, both, or neither among 17,187 cases of suspected acute myocardial infarction: ISIS-2. Lancet 1988; 2: 349–60.
23. Antiplatelet Trialists' Collaboration. Secondary prevention of vascular disease by prolonged antiplatelet treatment. Br Med J 1988; 296: 320–31.
24. The Steering Committee of the Physicians' Health Study Research Group. Final report on the aspirin component of the ongoing Physicians' Health Study. N Engl J Med 1989; 321: 129–35.
25. Chesebro JH, Webster MWI, Smith HC, et al. Antiplatelet therapy in coronary disease progression: reduced infarction and new lesion formation (abstr). Circulation 1989; 80(suppl II): II-266.
26. Ridker PM, Manson JE, Gaziano JM, Buring JE, Hennekens CH. Low dose aspirin therapy for chronic stable angina (abstr). Circulation 1990; 82(suppl III): III-200.
27. White CW, Chaitman B, Lassar TA, et al. Antiplatelet agents are effective in reducing the immediate complications of PTCA: results from the ticlopidine multicenter trial (abstr). Circulation 1987; 76(suppl IV): IV-400.
28. Schwartz L, Bourassa MG, Lesperance J, et al. Aspirin and dipyridamole in the prevention of restenosis after percutaneous transluminal coronary angioplasty. N Engl J Med 1988; 318: 1714–9.
29. Chesebro JH, Webster MWI, Reeder GS, et al. Coronary angioplasty: antiplatelet therapy reduces acute complications but not restenosis (abstr). Circulation 1989; 80(suppl II): II-64.
30. Barnathan ES, Schwartz JS, Taylor L, et al. Aspirin and dipyridamole in the prevention of acute coronary thrombosis complicating coronary angioplasty. Circulation 1987; 76: 125–34.
31. Kent KM, Ewels CJ, Kehoe MK, Lavelle P, Krucoff MV. Effect of aspirin on complications during transluminal coronary angioplasty (abstr). J Am Coll Cardiol 1988; 11(suppl A): 132A.
32. Chesebro JH, Clements IP, Fuster V, et al. A platelet inhibitor-drug trial in coronary-artery bypass operations: benefit of perioperative dipyridamole and aspirin therapy on early postoperative vein-graft patency. N Engl J Med 1982; 307: 73–8.
33. Sanz G, Pajaron A, Alegria E, et al. Prevention of early aortocoronary bypass occlusion by low-dose aspirin and dipyridamole. Circulation 1990; 82: 765–73.
34. Gravahan TP, Gebski V, Baron DW. Immediate postoperative aspirin improves vein graft patency early and late after coronary artery bypass graft surgery. A placebo-controlled, randomized study. Circulation 1991; 83: 1526–33.
35. Preliminary report of the Stroke Prevention in Atrial Fibrillation Study. N Engl J Med 1990; 322: 863–8.
36. Pedersen AK, FitzGerald GA. Dose-related kinetics of aspirin. Presystemic acetylation of platelet cyclooxygenase. N Engl J Med 1985; 311: 1206–11.
37. Cerletti C, Marchi S, Lauri D, et al. Pharmacokinetics of enteric-coated aspirin and inhibition of platelet thromboxane A_2 and vascular prostacyclin generation in humans. Clin Pharmacol Ther 1987; 42: 175–80.
38. Clarke R, Mayo G, Price P, FitzGerald GA. Preservation of systemic vascular prostacyclin despite maximal presystemic platelet cyclooxygenase inhibition by controlled release low dose aspirin (abstr). Circulation 1990; 82(suppl III): III-602.
39. Nishizawa EE, Wynalda DJ. Inhibitory effect of ibuprofen (Motrin) on platelet function. Thromb Res 1981; 21: 347–56.
40. Friedman PL, Brown EJ, Gunther S, et al. Coronary va-

soconstrictor effect of indomethacin in patients with coronary artery disease. N Engl J Med 1981; 305: 1171–5.

41. Bang HO, Dyerberg J, Hjorne N. The composition of food consumed by Greenland Eskimos. Acta Med Scand 1976; 200: 69–73.

42. Kromhout D, Bosschieter EB, Coulander CDL. The inverse relation between fish consumption and 20-year mortality from coronary heart disease. N Engl J Med 1985; 312: 1205–9.

43. Shekelle RB, Missel L, Paul O, Shyrock AM, Stamler J. Fish consumption and mortality from coronary heart disease (letter). N Engl J Med 1985; 313: 820.

44. Dyerberg J, Bang HO. Haemostatic function and platelet polyunsaturated fatty acids in Eskimos. Lancet 1979; 2: 433–5.

45. Von Schacky C. Prophylaxis of atherosclerosis with marine omega-3 fatty acids: a comprehensive strategy. Ann Intern Med 1987; 107: 890–9.

46. Braden GA, Knapp HR, Fitzgerald DJ, FitzGerald GA. Dietary fish oil accelerates the response to coronary thrombolysis with tissue-type plasminogen activator. Evidence for a modest platelet inhibitory effect in vivo. Circulation 1990; 82: 178–87.

47. Leaf A. Cardiovascular effects of fish oils. Beyond the platelet. Circulation 1990; 82: 624–8.

48. Dehmer GJ, Popma JJ, van den Berg EK, et al. Reduction in the rate of early restenosis after coronary angioplasty by a diet supplemented with n-3 fatty acids. N Engl J Med 1988; 319: 733–40.

49. Grigg LE, Kay TWH, Valentine PA, et al. Determinants of restenosis and lack of effect of dietary supplementation with eicosapentaenoic acid on the incidence of coronary restenosis after angioplasty. J Am Coll Cardiol 1989; 13: 665–72.

50. Reis GJ, Boucher TM, Sipperly ME, et al. Randomised trial of fish oil for prevention of restenosis after coronary angioplasty. Lancet 1989; 2: 177–81.

51. Milner MR, Gallin RA, Leffingwell A, et al. Usefulness of fish oil supplements in preventing clinical evidence of restenosis after percutaneous transluminal coronary angioplasty. Am J Cardiol 1989; 64: 294–9.

52. Slack JD, Pinkerton CA, Vantaseel J, et al. Can oral fish oil supplement minimize re-stenosis after transluminal coronary angioplasty? (abstr). J Am Coll Cardiol 1987; 9(suppl A): 64A.

53. Leaf A, Weber PC. Cardiovascular effects of n-3 fatty acids. N Engl J Med 1988; 318: 549–57.

54. Gresele P, Arnout J, Deckmyn H, Vermylen J. Mechanisms of the antiplatelet action of dipyridamole in whole blood: modulation of adenosine concentration and activity. Thromb Haemost 1986; 55: 12–8.

55. FitzGerald GA. Dipyridamole. N Engl J Med 1987; 316: 1247–57.

56. Folts JD, Rowe GG. Dipyridamole alone or with low dose aspirin does not inhibit thrombus formation in stenosed canine coronary arteries nor does it protect against renewal of thrombus formation by epinephrine. J Vasc Med Biol 1989; 4: 225.

57. Steele PM, Chesebro JH, Fuster V. The natural history of arterial balloon angioplasty in pigs and intervention with platelet-inhibitor therapy: implications for clinical trials (abstr). Clin Res 1984; 32: 209A.

58. Hanson SR, Harker LA, Bjornsson TD. Effect of platelet-modifying drugs on arterial thromboembolism in baboons: aspirin potentiates the antithrombotic actions of dipyridamole and sulfinpyrazone by mechanism(s) independent of platelet cyclooxygenase inhibition. J Clin Invest 1985; 75: 1591–9.

59. Fujitani RM, Nordestgaard AG, Marcus CS, Wilson SE. Perioperative suppression of platelet adherence to small-diameter polytetrafluoroethylene grafts. J Surg Res 1988; 44: 455–60.

60. Harker LA, Slichter SJ. Studies of platelet and fibrinogen kinetics in patients with prosthetic heart valves. N Engl J Med 1970; 283: 534–7.

61. Harker LA, Slichter SJ. Platelet and fibrinogen consumption in man. N Engl J Med 1972; 287: 999–1005.

62. Theo KH, Christakis GT, Weisel RD, et al. Dipyridamole preserved platelets and reduced blood loss after cardiopulmonary bypass. J Thorac Cardiovasc Surg 1988; 96: 332–41.

63. Ekestrom SA, Gunnes S, Brodin UB. Effect of dipyridamole (Persantin) on blood flow and patency of aortocoronary vein bypass grafts. Scand J Thorac Cardiovasc Surg 1990; 24: 191–6.

64. Hess H, Mietaschk A, Deichsel G. Drug-induced inhibition of platelet function delays progression of peripheral occlussive arterial disease: a prospective double-blind arteriographically controlled trial. Lancet 1985; 1: 415–9.

65. The Persantin-Aspirin Reinfarction Study Group. Persantine and aspirin in coronary heart disease. Circulation 1980; 62: 449–61.

66. Bousser MG, Eschwege E, Haugenau M, et al. "AICLA" controlled trial of aspirin and dipyridamole in the secondary prevention of atherothrombotic cerebral ischemia. Stroke 1983; 14: 5–14.

67. American-Canadian Cooperative Study Group. Persantine-aspirin trial in cerebral ischemia. Part II: Endpoint results. Stroke 1985; 16: 406–15.

68. Brown BG, Cukingnan RA, DeRouen T, et al. Improved graft patency in patients treated with platelet-inhibiting therapy after coronary bypass surgery. Circulation 1985; 72: 138–46.

69. Lembo JN, Black AJ, Roubin GS, et al. Effect of pretreatment with aspirin versus aspirin plus dipyridamole on frequency and type of acute complications of percutaneous transluminal coronary angioplasty. Am J Cardiol 1990; 65: 422–6.

70. Sullivan JM, Harken DE, Gorlin R. Pharmacologic control of thromboembolic complications of cardiac-valve replacement. N Engl J Med 1971; 284: 1391–4.

71. Kasahara T. Clinical effect of dipyridamole ingestion after prosthetic heart valve replacement—especially on the blood coagulation system. Nippon Kyobu Geka Gakkai Zasshi 1977; 25: 1007–21.

72. Groupe de Recherche PACTE. Prevention des accidents thromboemboliques systemiques chez les porteurs de prosthesis valvulaires artificielles: essai cooperatif controle du dipyridamole. Arch Mal Coeur 1978; 9: 915–69.

73. Rajah SM, Sreeharan N, Joseph A, et al. A prospective trial of dipyridamole and warfarin on heart valve patients (abstr). Acta Therapeutica 1980; 6(suppl 93): 54.

74. Chesebro JH, Fuster V, Elveback LR, et al. Trial of combined warfarin plus dipyridamole or aspirin in prosthetic heart valve replacement: danger of aspirin compared with dipyridamole. Am J Cardiol 1983; 51: 1537–41.

75. Altman R, Boullon F, Rouvier J, et al. Aspirin and prophylaxis of thromboembolic complications in patients with substitute heart valves. J Thorac Cardiovasc Surg 1976; 72: 127–9.

76. Dale J, Myhre E, Storstein O, et al. Prevention of arterial thromboembolism with acetylsalicylic acid: a controlled clinical study in patients with aortic ball valves. Am Heart J 1977; 94: 101–11.

77. Popat KD, Pitt B. Hemodynamic effect of prostaglandin E_1 infusion in patients with acute myocardial infarction and left ventricular failure. Am Heart J 1982; 103: 485–9.

78. Coppe D, Sobel M, Seavans L, Levine F, Salzman E. Preservation of platelet function and number by prostacyclin during cardiopulmonary bypass. J Thorac Cardiovasc Surg 1981; 81: 274–8.

79. Smith MC, Danviriyasup K, Crow JW, et al. Prostacyclin substitution for heparin in long-term hemodialysis. Am J Med 1982; 73: 669–78.

80. Pitt B, Shea MJ, Romson JL, Lucchesi BR. Prostaglandins and prostaglandin inhibitors in ischemic heart disease. Ann Intern Med 1983; 99: 83–92.

81. Théroux P, Latour J-G, Diodati J, et al. Hemodynamic, platelet and clinical responses to prostacyclin in unstable angina pectoris. Am J Cardiol 1990; 65: 1084–9.

82. Armstrong PW, Langevin LM, Watts DG. Randomized trial of prostacyclin infusion in acute myocardial infarction. Am J Cardiol 1988; 61: 455–7.

83. Bugiardini R, Galvani M, Ferrini D, et al. Myocardial ischemia during intravenous prostacyclin administration: hemodynamic findings and precautionary measures. Am Heart J 1987; 113: 234–40.

6

HEPARINS AND ORAL ANTICOAGULANTS

MARC VERSTRAETE and STANFORD WESSLER

HEPARIN

Twenty years elapsed between the chance discovery of heparin by a medical student (1916) and its first therapeutic use (1937). Since then considerable progress has been made in the purification, chemistry, and mode of action of heparin.

Chemistry

Heparin consists of a simple chain constructed of repeating disaccharide units, all of which contain glucosamine and uronic acid; the latter may be glucuronic acid or iduronic acid (Fig. 6–1). The iduronic acid residues and possibly the glucuronic acid residues are sulfated to varying degrees (one to three sulfate groups per disaccharide unit), mainly at the C-2 position. The glucosamine moieties are ester sulfated to a variable extent at the C-3 and the C-6 position. The sulfur content is about 10 per cent, and because of the large number of acid groups, heparin is a strong acid. A combination of chemical properties determines its anticoagulant activity: free carboxyl groups, 3-0-sulfate ester groups from hexuronic acid, sulfamino groups on glucosamine and incomplete conversion of glucuronic acid to iduronic acid.[1–4]

The biosynthesis of heparin is initiated by attachment of a carbohydrate-protein linkage region to the serine residues of a specific polypeptide chain;[1] the complex series of events that modify this core protein into the final product are not completely understood. Macromolecular heparin consists of a core protein of unknown size with variable numbers of mucopolysaccharide chains of molecular weight 30,000 to 100,000 daltons.

Heparin exerts the main part of its anticoagulant action via a plasma protein called antithrombin III. Heparin induces a conformational change in the antithrombin III molecule accelerating its binding to the serine proteases of the coagulation system. Preparation of heparin fragments by chemical or enzymatic degradation have led to the isolation of a polysaccharide sequence required for the heparin-antithrombin III interaction. The antithrombin III binding domain has been identified as a pentasaccharide sequence[3,5,6] (Fig. 6–2). Disruption of a single disulfide bridge in antithrombin III leads to a reduced affinity for heparin and a corresponding loss of inhibitory activity in the presence of heparin. This indicates that heparin and thrombin bind at different sites of the antithrombin III molecule. Seven arginine residues thought to be required for heparin binding are located near the amino terminal part of antithrombin III. This labile alpha-helix is widely separated from the protease binding domain in the carboxyl terminal end.

Pharmacology

MODE OF ACTION

The anticoagulant activity of heparin is primarily related to its ability to accelerate the formation of a molecular complex between antithrombin III and the serine proteases of the coagulation system, thereby blocking the enzymatic activity of coagulation

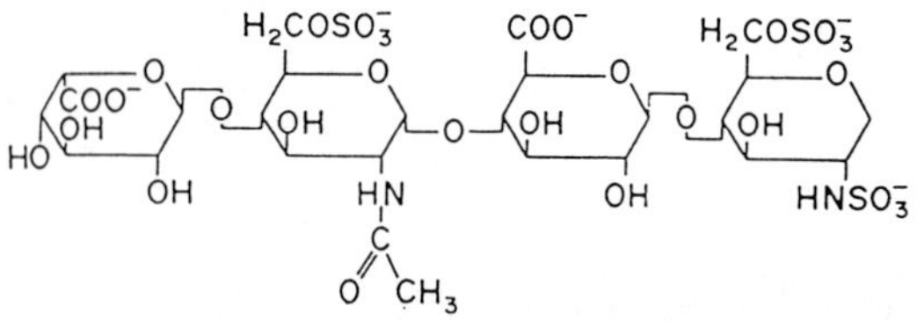

FIGURE 6–1. Heparin, or more specifically, glycosaminoglycuronan sulphate esters, consist of a chain of alternating glucuronic acid and N-acetylglucosamine moieties to the proteoglycan. The terrasaccharide sequence, L-iduronic acid, sulphated N-acetyl D-glucosamine, D-glucuronic acid, N-disulphated D-glucosamine is shown, which represents the antithrombin III binding domain. (From Verstraete M, Vermylen J. Thrombosis. New York: Pergamon Press, 1984, with permission.)

factors. The term antithrombin III is a misnomer for several reasons, as this protein inhibits not only thrombin but also the activated forms of numerous coagulation factors (XII, XI, IX, and X) as well as of plasmin and kallikrein (Fig. 6–3). However, the in-

hibition of thrombin and activated factor X is particularly important and clinically relevant (See also Chapter 8).

Thrombin and antithrombin III form an extremely tightly bound complex, but at a relatively slow rate. A unique aspect of this interaction is an enormous enhancement (a 1,000-fold acceleration) by high-affinity heparin.[7,8] This acceleration is due to an allosteric alteration in the position of the critical arginine residue, so that this amino acid moiety of antithrombin III is more readily available for interaction with thrombin. There is still uncertainty as to the site on antithrombin which binds to heparin. Strong clues come from studies of human variants of antithrombin that have altered heparin affinity and were shown to have a loss of the arginine 47 and proline 41. Taken together, there is strong evidence that these are key residues in the binding of heparin to antithrombin.

The active center of thrombin (serine) reacts with the reactive arginine site of heparin-antithrombin III. During this catalytic

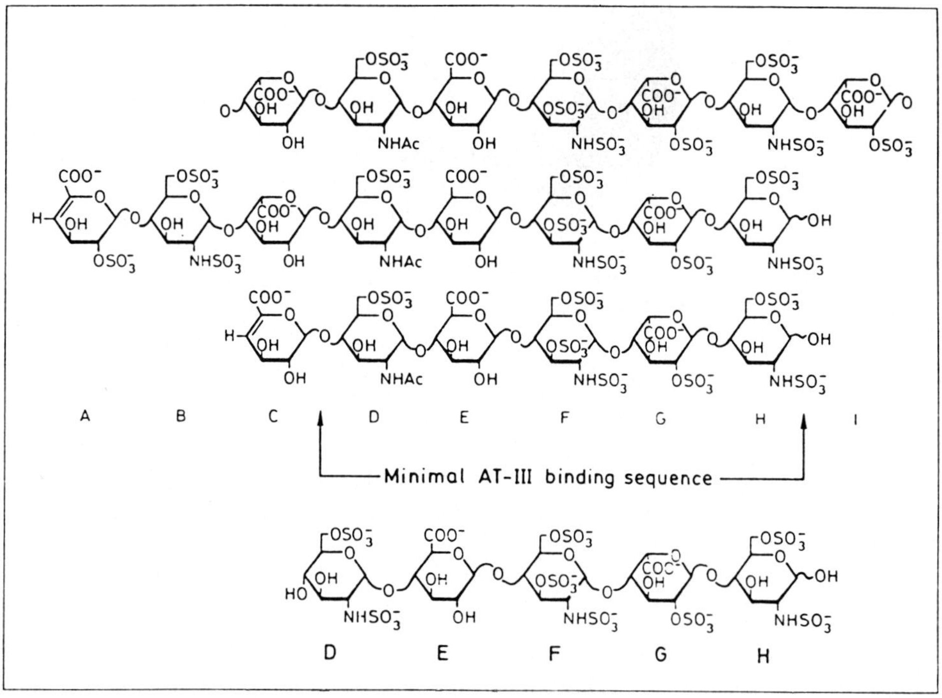

FIGURE 6–2. Pentasaccharide sequence responsible for binding of low molecular weight heparin to antithrombin III. This sequence (DEFGH) was first characterized through structural studies of oligosaccharides obtained from different preparations of heparin or CY 216 (octasaccharide and hexasaccharide shown on the middle lines were obtained after enzymatic cleavage of heparin). It was then synthesized. Most remarkable is the central 3-0-sulfated glucosamine unit (F). A synthetic pentasaccharide lacking the 3-0-sulfate is completely devoid of affinity for antithrombin III thus proving the critical role of this group. (From Choay et al. Structural studies on a biologically active hexasaccharide obtained from heparin. Ann NY Acad Sci 1981; 370: 644–9, with permission.)

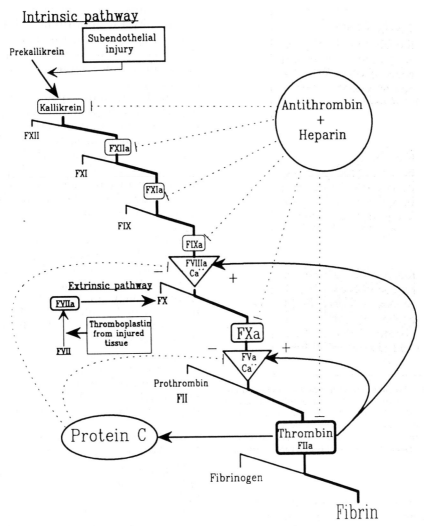

Intrinsic pathway

Extrinsic pathway

FIGURE 6–3. The coagulation cascade with its sequence of amplifying proteolytic reactions. Thrombin-mediated positive and negative (via protein C) feedback loops are shown. Broken lines denote inhibitory activity. (From Matzsch T. Low molecular weight heparin. Animal experiments and clinical studies. Doctoral Dissertation, Malmö 1990, with permission.

interaction the 1:1 stoichiometry of the enzyme-inhibitor reaction is unaffected. Once the inhibition reaction is completed, heparin is released from the antithrombin III-thrombin complex and can be utilized again. The remaining antithrombin III-thrombin complexes are removed by the reticuloendothelial system. There is evidence that a three-way complex is required in which heparin, antithrombin III, and thrombin bind to each other for maximal heparin-enhanced inhibition of thrombin by antithrombin (Fig. 6–4). At least 16 to 20 monosaccharide units per heparin molecule (circa 4,800 daltons) are necessary for full expression of the potential ability of antithrombin to inhibit thrombin. The bind-

ing of thrombin to heparin is of an electrostatic nature and strongly depends on the length of the heparin molecule: the longer the molecule, the greater is the ability of thrombin to diffuse along the heparin chain into the antithrombin III molecule which is also bound to heparin. In this "sliding" model, an increase in chain length of heparin results in an increased reaction rate because of a higher probability of interaction between thrombin and heparin in solution.[9,10] The inhibition of activated factor X is due to the formation of a binary complex between antithrombin III and activated factor X, in which heparin binds and activates antithrombin III but does not bind activated factor X

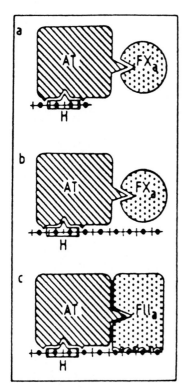

FIGURE 6–4. Mechanism of interaction between antithrombi (AT), factor Xa (FXa), thrombin (FIIa) and heparin molecules (H) of different molecular weight (chain length of 8 and 18 monosaccharides). (From Holmer E. Heparin and its low molecular weight derivatives. Doctoral Dissertation, Stockholm 1987, with permission.)

(Fig. 6–4). Small heparin molecules result in activated factor X inactivation, provided they contain the antithrombin III binding domain, but may be too small to form a complex with antithrombin III and thrombin (which would result in inhibition of thrombin action by ternary complex formation). Small heparin fractions will thus selectively inhibit activated factor X.

HEPARIN FRACTIONS WITH HIGH OR LOW AFFINITY FOR ANTITHROMBIN III

In pharmaceutical grade heparin (average molecular weight 12,000 to 15,000 daltons), most anticoagulant activity is accounted for by a small functional fraction of the molecules, those with high affinity to antithrombin III. The remaining molecules have only a very limited anticoagulant effect, but may still increase bleeding in experimental animals,[11] inhibit the activation of prothrombin by activated factor X,[12,13] or potentiate the action of high-affinity, low molecular weight frac-

tions.[14] Furthermore, heparin molecules with low affinity for antithrombin III appear to inhibit hyperplasia of vascular smooth muscle,[15] can activate lipoprotein lipase,[16] suppress aldosterone secretion, and induce platelet aggregation.

At higher than therapeutic concentrations, heparin and heparin-like mucopolysaccharides have an additional effect by catalyzing the inhibition of thrombin by another plasma protein, heparin cofactor II.[17]

After parenteral injection, heparin is also found in vascular endothelial cells. In vitro experiments have also shown that human endothelial cells in culture have saturable binding sites for heparin. Endothelial cells bind selectively those chains of heparin that have a higher molecular weight, more charge density (degree of sulfation), and greater anticoagulant (anti-IIa and anti-Xa) activity.[18] Approximately 25 per cent of the bound heparin can be internalized by endothelial cells before heparin is depolymerized.[18] It should be made clear that high- and low-affinity heparin are two types of heparin that have either bound or not bound, respectively, to an antithrombin III column. The molecular weights of both heparins approximate that of standard unfractionated heparin.

LOW MOLECULAR WEIGHT VERSUS HIGH MOLECULAR WEIGHT HEPARIN

Heparins of low molecular weight may be either fractions or fragments with a mean molecular weight range between less than 3,000 and about 9,000 daltons. Heparin fractions represent material that has been harvested by gel filtration or solvent extraction from what is already present in naturally occurring mixtures of glycosaminoglycans, but this is a low-yield procedure. Fragments are produced by partial hydrolytic cleavage of heparin molecules and isolated by a variety of techniques, including gel and ultrafiltration, solvent extraction, enzymatic or thermal depolymerization (Fig. 6–5).

Heparins of low molecular weight that have been tested clinically are most often produced from standard heparin of pharmacopeial quality by solvent or nitrous acid polymerization. Although these heparins may have a similar mean molecular weight, they may have different characteristics.

Fragments below 16 to 20 monosaccharides units per heparin molecule (molecular weight less than 5,000 daltons), while containing the specific pentasaccharide sequence essential for binding to antithrombin III, are not long

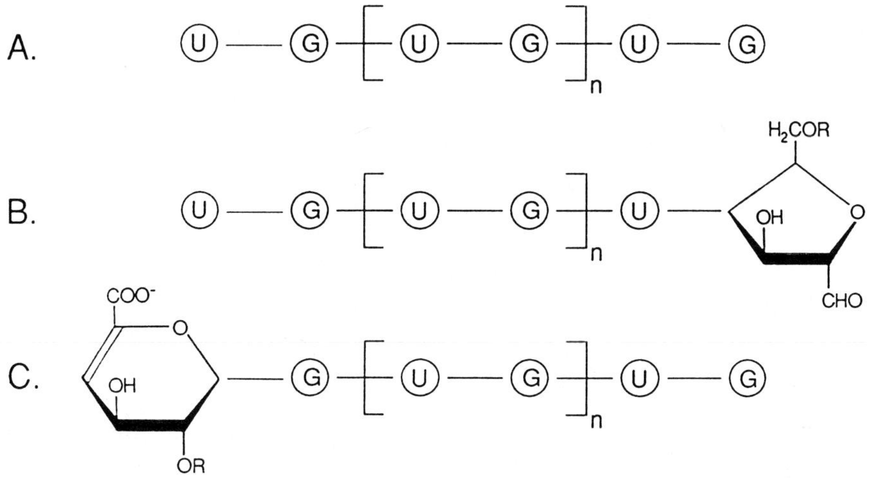

A. (U)—(G)⎡(U)—(G)⎤(U)—(G)
             ⎣   ⎦ₙ

B. (U)—(G)⎡(U)—(G)⎤(U)— [pentose ring structure with H₂COR, OH, O, CHO]
             ⎣   ⎦ₙ

C. [uronic acid ring structure with COO⁻, O, OH, OR]—(G)⎡(U)—(G)⎤(U)—(G)
                                                          ⎣   ⎦ₙ

FIGURE 6–5. Schematic representation of structures of low molecular weight heparin obtained by different manufacturing techniques. A, Enrichment. B, Depolymerization by nitrous acid. C, Depolymerization by β-elimination, enzymatic or chemical. U = uronic acid; G = glucosamine. (From Holmer E. Heparin and its low molecular weight derivatives. Doctoral Dissertation, Stockholm 1987, with permission.)

enough to permit binding to thrombin; they therefore inhibit only activated factor X.[2] Even a synthetic pentasaccharide of only 5 monosaccharides units (molecular weight of approximately 1,700 daltons) contains the domain that binds to antithrombin III (but not heparin cofactor II) and possesses a high specific activity in vitro against activated factor X but little activity against thrombin.[3,19] Heparin preparations weighing more than 5,000 daltons maintain their inhibitory property against activated factor X, but with increasing chain length, gain a progressively stronger inhibitory capacity against thrombin. The unexpected discovery that heparins of low molecular weight prolong moderately the clotting time (indicating no thrombin inhibition) but are still capable of potentiating the inhibition of activated factor X, raised the hope of dissociating the antithrombotic property (anti-Xa) from the anticoagulant property (inhibition of thrombin), which then would avoid the hemorrhage-inducing effect of unfractionated heparin. The rationale for this assumption is that it would be of importance to inhibit the cascade system, with its multiplying effect, at as early a stage as possible without altering normal hemostasis (Fig. 6–6). With low molecular weight heparins, the latter conditions could be fulfilled due to their limited inhibition of thrombin, which would allow the local accumulation of this substance for normal hemostasis. It has been shown in animal experiments that anti-Xa activity is a prerequisite, although not

sufficient in itself, for a thrombosis-preventing effect. Heparin molecules, large enough to retain some thrombin-blocking action are indeed also necessary. The lack of correlation between blood levels as measured by anti-Xa assay and impairment of stasis thrombosis in animals described some years ago[4,11,20,21] has recently been confirmed.[22] It appears that inhibition of thrombin is a more effective way of preventing thrombosis, and the catalysis of thrombin inhibition provides a more reliable in vitro index for estimating possible antithrombotic effects of glycosaminoglycans.

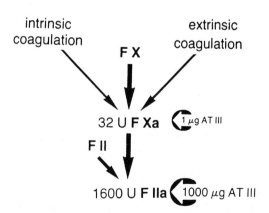

FIGURE 6–6. Simplified graph of the amplification mechanism of the blood coagulation cascade. (From Haas S et al. An objective evaluation of the clinical potential of low molecular weight heparin in the prevention of thromboembolism. Sem Thromb Haemost 1989;15:424–34, with permission).

It is possible that activated factor X can be "protected" from the inhibitory action of the heparin-antithrombin III complex in prothrombinase by binding to phospholipid, platelets, or tissue factor. Some other factors, possibly a molecular weight-dependent vascular wall interaction or a heparin-binding protein such as placental protein 5 may also contribute to the antithrombotic effect of glucosaminoglycans.[11,20,21] These findings refute the hypothesis that the antithrombotic properties of low molecular weight heparins are mainly due to their ability to catalyze the inhibition of activated factor X. Moreover, at a very early stage of its development, Thomas and co-workers[20] did question whether low molecular weight heparin would be associated with a lower incidence of hemorrhagic side effects than unfractionated heparin, a point which until now has not been unequivocally proven in clinical trials comparing low molecular weight heparins with subcutaneous unfractionated heparin.

Low molecular weight heparins interact less with platelets than high molecular weight heparin. It is logical that larger heparins would have greater affinity than smaller ones of equivalent sulfation, as the larger species would present more negatively charged areas for binding to positively charged regions on the platelet surface; a secondary factor may be the balance of sugar moieties. Reduced bleeding in animals may therefore be more related to a decreased effect on platelets than to the reduced antithrombin property of low molecular weight heparin; alternative explanations have been suggested such as the release of lipase enzymes or the presence of a low-affinity heparin fragment.

Pharmacokinetics

PHARMACOKINETICS AND SOME OTHER PROPERTIES OF UNFRACTIONATED HEPARIN

For years, the anticoagulant activity of intravenously administered unfractionated heparin has been described as disappearing following a single exponential curve, admittedly with a large range of half-life values (between 23 and 360 minutes). However, according to more recent findings, heparin follows nonlinear kinetics; the disappearance of the anticoagulant activity of heparin is compatible with a model based on the combination of a saturable mechanism (most

probably rapid uptake by the endothelium and desulfation by mononuclear phagocytes)[18] and a linear (that is, unsaturable) mechanism (most probably elimination by the kidney).[23] The faster disappearance of the thrombin inhibitor activity (anti-IIa activity) than the anti-Xa activity on the initial clearance phase also suggests an earlier elimination mechanism of large molecules having a high anti-IIa/anti-Xa ratio.

PHARMACOKINETICS AND SOME OTHER PROPERTIES OF LOW MOLECULAR WEIGHT HEPARIN

The term "low molecular weight heparins" (LMW heparins) is applied to all fractions or fragments of heparin of a mean molecular weight less than 6,000 daltons. However, these preparations still differ in molecular size, in their affinity for antithrombin III, and in many other characteristics. It is therefore necessary to examine every new heparin fraction or fragment in order to establish its specific properties. Low molecular weight heparins have in common a lower affinity for endothelial cells than unfractionated heparin (Table 6–1).

In conclusion, it appears that all low molecular weight heparins are readily absorbed from subcutaneous tissue and are less bound to endothelium than unfractionated heparin. Their bioavailability is thus increased and biological half-life is almost twice as long as that of the unfractionated varieties. Low molecular weight heparins do not cross the placenta, although after enoxaparin, circulating anti-Xa activity was found in the fetal blood of pregnant sheep but not in women during the first or second trimester of pregnancy. The same holds for Novo LHN-1. Whether low molecular weight heparins release endogenous tissue-plasminogen activator and thus contribute to a faster lysis of an existing thrombus is a matter of dispute (Table 6–2).

Dosage and Administration

Heparin is not absorbed when given by mouth and must be given parenterally. Absorption from intramuscular sites is variable and may delay the recognition of major hemorrhage in the hip or back, especially if the intramuscular injections are given in the buttock. This route of administration has been abandoned. Intravenous heparin may be given by continuous infusion or by intermit-

TABLE 6–1. Characteristics of Low Molecular Weight Heparins*

	MEAN MOLECULAR WEIGHT	ANTI-XA (UNITS/MILLIGRAM)	ANTI-IIA (UNITS/MILLIGRAM)	ANTI-XA CLEARANCE (HALF-LIFE IN MIN)		BIOAVAILABILITY (%)
				Intravenous	*Subcutaneous*	
CY-216	4,500	85 (200 Institut Choay Units)	50		214	98
Enoxaparin	3,500–5,500	90–110	20–40	180	360	91
Kabi-2165	4,000–6,000	160	40	120	240	87
Novo LHN-1	4,900	86	44	116	110	
OP 2123	3,500–5,000	90	50			90
Sandoz CH-8140	4,500–8,000	80	40			

* Specific activities are expressed with reference to the First International Standard for low molecular weight heparins.

tent injection (Fig. 6–7). Major bleeding is less frequent with continuous infusion which is effective for prevention of thromboembolism. Moreover, continuous infusion reduces the dosage of the drug, and the accelerated clearance of heparin seen in patients with pulmonary embolism makes it difficult to attain adequate concentrations for any duration with usual intermittent regimens. It is uncertain how intense the anticoagulant effect of heparin must be to prevent thrombosis in man. In rabbits, venous thrombus extension is prevented by heparin levels between 0.3 and 0.5 international units/milliliter. The relationship of the degree of effect to bleeding complications is also uncertain.

When given by continuous intravenous infusion, standard dosage is a loading dose of 5,000 international units (sometimes 10,000 international units) given as a bolus, followed by 15 to 20 international units/kilogram/hour in normal saline or 5 per cent dextrose and administered with an automatic infusion pump over the first 24 hours. Subsequently, the rate of the infusion is regulated to keep

the activated partial thromboplastin time (APTT) at approximately twice the baseline level.

Given by intravenous route and intermittently, the usual dose of standard unfractionated heparin is 10,000 international units at six-hour intervals or 15,000 units at eight-hour intervals, while others recommend 5,000 to 10,000 international units heparin intravenously every four hours. In the experience of most investigators, failure to monitor the appropriate coagulation parameters increases the risk of major bleeding. There is a wide variation between individuals in the anticoagulant response to a given dose of heparin or in the dose required to produce a particular anticoagulant response. The wide variation in clearance of heparin between individuals and in different types of patients also suggests the desirability of monitoring therapy so that dosage can be adjusted appropriately.

Concentrated aqueous unfractionated heparin usually contains between 20,000 and 25,000 units/milliliter and is given subcuta-

TABLE 6–2. Difference of Low Molecular Weight Heparins to Unfractionated Heparin

	LOW MOLECULAR WEIGHT HEPARINS	UNFRACTIONATED HEPARIN
Faxtor Xa to anti-IIa ratio	+ + +	+
Absorption from subcutaneous tissue	+ + +	+
Binding to endothelium	+	+ + +
Half-life	Longer	Shorter
Effect of lipoprotein lipase	+	+ +
Increases fibrinolytic potential	+ +	+
Interaction with platelets	+	+ +
Transplacental passage	−	+
Antigenicity	+	+ +
Protamine neutralization	+	+ +

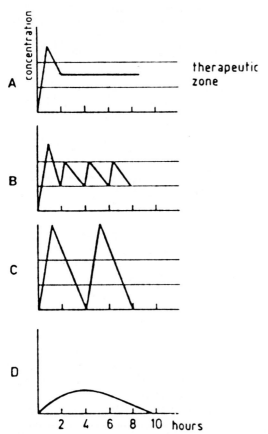

FIGURE 6–7. Blood concentration of heparin after: A, bolus injection followed by continuous intravenous infusion; B and C, intermittent intravenous injections; D, subcutaneous injection. (From Verstraete M, Vermylen J. Thrombosis. New York: Pergamon Press, 1984, with permission.)

neously in a skin fold raised from the abdominal wall. The "full" dose of this slow-release heparin is 20,000 to 30,000 international units per 24 hours, administered in one or two injections. In the "low-dose" regimen, 5,000 international units of concentrated heparin are given subcutaneously at 8- or 12-hour intervals for the prophylaxis of deep vein thrombosis. In most cases it causes only slight, if any, prolongation of clotting times and no clinically significant bleeding, except in a few cases after major orthopedic surgery when 5,000 units are required every eight hours.

The various low molecular weight heparins each have a distinct profile of their pharmacological effects in both the in vitro and in vivo tests and thus different antithrombotic/bleeding properties. Due to their individual polycomponent nature this is still the case if these agents are potency standardized against the World Health Organization (WHO) endorsed low molecular weight heparin standard.[24] No overall recommended dose for the prevention and treatment of thromboembolic disorders can therefore be given, and presently recommended doses for each commercialized low molecular weight heparin are less well established than for standard unfractionated heparin.

The recommended dose of Fraxiparin is for prophylaxis 7,500 anti-Xa Institut Choay units two hours before surgery and subsequently once daily. In patients at high thrombotic risk, 100 anti-Xa Institut Choay Units/kilogram are recommended 12 hours before surgery and once daily the first three days, and subsequently 150 anti-Xa units/kilogram/day (Table 6–3). For treatment of deep vein thrombosis, two subcutaneous doses of 225 anti-Xa Institut Choay Units/kilogram are given at 12-hour intervals. The prophylaxis with Fragmin is started two to four hours before surgery with 2,500 anti-Xa units followed by the same dose once daily. In patients at high thrombotic risk 2,500 anti-Xa units two to four hours before surgery and 2,500 anti-Xa units in the evening after the operation followed by 5,000 anti-Xa units once daily from the first operative day is recommended. Alternatively, 5,000 anti-Xa units is given in the evening of the day before the operation followed by 5,000 units in the evening in the postoperative period. For treatment of deep vein thrombosis, 100 to 120 anti-Xa units/kilogram every 12 hours are administered subcutaneously the first day, and the dose thereafter adapted to obtain 0.5 to 1 anti-Xa unit/ml four hours after subcutaneous injection. Enoxaparin contains 90 to 110 anti-Xa units/milligram and for subcutaneous prophylaxis, a single daily dose of 20 milligrams (0.2 milliliters) started two hours before surgery in moderate-risk patients, and of 40 milligrams (0.4 milliliters) started 12 hours before surgery in patients at high thrombotic risk are adequate. The dose of Fluxum is 4,000 anti-Xa units (moderate thrombotic risk) or 8,000 anti-Xa units administered in a single daily subcutaneous injection. With low molecular weight heparin Sandoz, one subcutaneous injection of 1,500 activated partial thromboplastin time units is adequate in patients at moderate antithrombotic risk, and the protection can be increased by addition of 0.5 dihydroergotamine (Embolex). Heparin-dihydroergotamine prepa-

TABLE 6–3. Prevention of Postoperative Deep Vein Thrombosis

AGENT	RECOMMENDED DAILY DOSE (ONE SUBCUTANEOUS INJECTION PER DAY)	DOSE IN ANTI-XA UNITS*
Patients at medium thrombotic risk		
Enoxaparin (Clexane)	20 milligrams (0.2 milliliter)	2,000
CY-216 (Fraxiparine)	7,500 anti-Xa Institut Choay units (0.3 milliliter) (36 milligrams)	3,100
Kabi-2165 (Fragmin)	2,500 anti-Xa units (0.25 milliliter) (18 milligrams)	2,500
Novo LHN-1 (Logiparin)	3,500 anti-Xa units	3,500
Patients at high thrombotic risk (e.g., orthopedic surgery)		
Enoxaparin (Clexane)	40 milligrams (0.4 milliliter); first injection 12 hour before surgery	4,000
CY-216 (Fraxiparine)	150 anti-Xa Institut Choay units kilograms†	3,000
Kabi-2165 (Fragmin)	5,000 anti-Xa units (0.5 milliliter); first injection 12 hr before surgery	4,500
Novo LHN-1 (Logiparin)	50 anti-Xa units/kilograms body weight	50 units/kilogram body weight

* With reference to the First International Standard for low molecular weight heparins.
† Body weight 70 kilograms.

rations have a small but demonstrable risk of arterial coronary spasm, and the benefit of adding dihydroergotamine is therefore debatable.

Precautions and Adverse Effects

BLEEDING

Bleeding is the most frequent complication of heparin and is a direct result of its therapeutic action. Spontaneous bleeding is most likely to occur in subjects older than 60 years of age ($\times$ 3), in the presence of underlying morbidity ($\times$ 4), in chronic drinkers ($\times$ 7), in women ($\times$ 2), and in patients with a blood urea nitrogen (BUN) over 50 milligrams per 100 milliliters ($\times$ 1.5). Postoperative or post-traumatic bleeding is more common than spontaneous bleeding.

The primary experimental findings that low molecular weight heparin produces less bleeding for an equivalent antithrombotic effect than unfractionated heparin has still to be established in humans. There appears to be a relationship between the risk of bleeding and anti-Xa level measurements ex vivo, but no clear relationship with the dose of low molecular weight heparin administered.[25] Unfortunately, it is still not known exactly which molecules in low molecular weight heparin are responsible for the antithrombotic effect, nor whether the hemorrhagic effects can be ascribed to the same molecules.

THROMBOCYTOPENIA

There is considerable confusion about the heparin-platelet interactions often lumped together as "heparin-induced thrombocytopenia."[26] A nonidiosyncratic interaction, which is usually immediate in onset, should be distinguished from a delayed idiosyncratic heparin-platelet interaction resulting in thrombocytopenia alone or in combination with acute arterial thrombosis.

The acute nonidiosyncratic heparin-platelet interaction is a heparin-induced platelet aggregation which may result in a transient drop in the platelet count and prolongation of the bleeding time. This reaction depends on the characteristics of the heparin preparation (particularly on the presence of high molecular weight heparin fractions) and varies considerably among individuals. There is considerable evidence that low molecular weight heparins do not significantly enhance platelet aggregation.

The idiosyncratic heparin-induced thrombocytopenia, complicated or not with arterial thrombosis, occurs between days 7 and 11 of treatment and is more frequent with bovine lung unfractionated heparin (versus porcine gut) and after previous exposure to heparin; in the latter case, thrombocytopenia also develops sooner, suggesting an anamnestic response. Heparin may act as a hapten and induce an immune response against the platelet-heparin complex. This would explain why the delayed idiosyncratic heparin-induced thrombocytopenia is not dose dependent and can also occur after subcutaneous injections and even from heparin flushes. There is no evidence supporting, or refuting, the possibility that low molecular weight heparins are less antigenic than unfractionated heparin, or that they do not interact with platelet IgG Fc receptor.

An analogue of heparin, pentosan polysulfate, a low molecular weight sulfated polysaccharide and low molecular weight heparin may also induce thrombocytopenia and arterial thrombosis.

If heparin can injure the platelets, it is surprising that spontaneous bleeding so rarely develops despite the presence of heparin and occasional very low platelet counts. An interesting hypothesis is that heparin-dependent antibodies bind to platelets as well as to endothelial cells; the platelet-endothelial cell interaction may trigger the release of procoagulants from the vessel wall, predisposing to thrombosis.

Antibody-induced platelet aggregation is not a passive agglutination but an active process requiring metabolic energy which is prostaglandin- and adenosine diphosphate-dependent. This explains why aspirin combined with dipyridamole can in most cases suppress the in vitro aggregation induced by the serum of affected patients. Management of idiosyncratic thrombocytopenia demands immediate discontinuation of heparin. Some investigators recommend switching the type of heparin (from a bovine lung to an intestinal mucosal preparation or to a low molecular weight heparin), especially when in vitro platelet aggregation studies between patients' platelets and the heparin preparation are to be used. Aspirin combined with dipyridamole may be helpful. Fibrinolytic treatment has been instituted successfully in cases of occlusive thrombosis. When urgent surgery is required in patients with idiosyncratic thrombocytopenia, use of plasmapheresis and high-dose gamma globulin can be considered.

HEPARIN-INDUCED OSTEOPOROSIS

Long-term treatment with heparin can cause osteoporosis; this complication is suspected to be related to the dosage of heparin rather than to duration of treatment. Decreased synthesis and increased resorption of bone is a possible mechanism.[27] Reduction of mineral bone has also been observed with low molecular weight heparin, to the same degree as with unfractionated heparin. It is therefore less likely that the osteoporotic effect is related to the size of the heparin molecule.

HEPARIN-INDUCED SKIN NECROSIS

Hypersensitivity reactions to unfractionated or low molecular weight heparins continue to be reported; they may induce a global cardiovascular collapse, be limited to necrosis of the skin overlying the injection sites, or cause distant cutaneous necrosis, without any site of predilection. Histological examination suggests an Arthus-type reaction, with the formation of antigen-antibody complexes, with or without deposition of aggregated platelets. It is interesting to note that intradermal tests with different brands of heparin give positive delayed reaction responses; however, patch tests using only the antimicrobial preservative chlorbutal as used in commercial heparin preparations produce no response, apparently disproving an earlier hypothesis that this preservative was responsible for skin lesions.

EFFECT OF HEPARIN ON LIPOPROTEIN LIPASE

The marked appearance of lipolytic activity in plasma immediately following injection of unfractionated heparin is due to the release of hepatic triglyceride lipase and lipoprotein lipase, probably by displacement from tissue sites, for example, the endothelial surface. The release of these enzymes causes rapid clearance of lipoproteins and leads to increased plasma levels of free fatty acids which may be associated with cardiac arrhythmia.[28] The lipoprotein lipase catabolism of serum lipoproteins yields lipid remnants that are processed rapidly by the liver and at extrahepatic sites. Patients with dysbetalipoproteinuria (type III hyperlipidemia) are unable to catabolize these lipid remnants, and their accumulation can cause serious hyperlipidemia (that is, such patients constitute a special risk group). With Fragmin[29] and with Fraxiparine[30] the lipolytic activity was considerably less than with unfractionated heparin, apparently as a result of more rapid clearance. However, Enoxaparin appears to retain the full capabilities of unfractionated heparin to induce both hepatic lipase and lipoprotein lipase.

SUPPRESSIVE EFFECT OF HEPARIN ON ALDOSTERONE PRODUCTION

The suppressive effect of full-dose heparin (20,000 international units/day or more) on adrenal aldosterone production, with resultant hyperkalemia, is well known; a similar inhibitory effect is also obtained with low-dose heparin. Hospitalized patients with congestive heart failure or acute myocardial infarction commonly receive digitalis, diuretics, and low-dose heparin. The likelihood of heparin-induced hyperkalemia may be particularly increased when potassium-sparing diuretics and converting enzyme inhibitors are used in patients with chronic renal insufficiency.[31] After heparin is discontinued, these patients may be at risk of hypokalemia and cardiac arrhythmia from enhanced kaliuresis; in addition, sodium retention and worsening congestive heart failure may result from diminished natriuresis.

Interference with Diagnostic Test

Heparin preparations of bovine or porcine origin can, independent of the route of administration, induce a reversible increase in serum aminotransferases. A twofold increase of gamma-glutamyl transpeptidase with maximal values after seven days treatment has also been observed without an increase in serum levels of alkaline phosphatase or thrombocytopenia.[32] A progressive return to normal enzyme concentrations follows three days after maximal values have been reached; enzyme concentrations may normalize after drug withdrawal or even despite its continuation. The cause of transiently increased transaminases associated with heparin therapy is probably subcellular damage in the liver.

Contraindications

Anticoagulant drugs, including heparin, should not be used in unreliable outpatients, or patients in whom there is a definite risk of hemorrhage that cannot be avoided by careful adjustment of dosage, particularly when the bleeding could occur in certain tissues (for example, eyes, brain, central nervous system). Uncontrolled arterial hypertension is an absolute contraindication. The presence of a congenital or acquired hemostatic defect (for example, thrombocytopenia, declining platelet counts during heparin administration) obviously contraindicates the initiation or further continuation of heparin treatment. Attention must be given to electrolyte balance during and after treatment

with heparin, particularly if this drug is used with other drugs influencing the kalemia.

Monitoring of Therapy

The response of all antithrombotic drugs can be measured reasonably well; during administration of oral anticoagulants the prothrombin time is used (see Chapter 9). Some form of monitoring is desirable with continuous infusion of heparin (for example, thrombin clotting time or, preferably, activated partial thromboplastin time), particularly in patients with significant hepatic or renal dysfunction. However, monitoring is not essential for short-term intravenous administration (for example, before heart catheterization). A simple test such as the activated partial thromboplastin time is beset by pitfalls, since the result of the test largely depends on the cleanliness of blood sampling, the time interval from blood drawing to assay, the numbers of platelets in plasma, and the sensitivity of the commercial partial thromboplastin used. The desired prolongation factor may thus vary from laboratory to laboratory. In general, a prolongation of activated partial thromboplastin time of twice the control value corresponds to a heparin concentration of 0.2 to 0.4 international units/milliliter plasma. This is the concentration that prevents extension of experimental thrombi. A more intensive anticoagulation is required in patients with malignant disease and in patients with pulmonary embolism. It should be noted that the dosage requirement may change after the first two to three days of treatment, but thereafter the dose response in any patient is usually stable. The thrombin clotting time of plasma (therapeutic range 0.2 to 0.4 international units heparin/milliliter) was found to be more closely related to the measurement of heparin using a chromogenic substrate.[33] However, there is not always a good relationship between the results of blood tests and the prevention of bleeding or recurrent thromboembolism. The major therapeutic usefulness of laboratory control is to insure the presence of at least some anticoagulant effect at all times during treatment. Coagulation must be inhibited continuously to prevent fibrin deposition or impede extension of the thrombus.

For prophylaxis, monitoring of subcutaneously administered unfractionated heparin and of low molecular weight heparin is not necessary in patients at moderate risk, and a fixed dose is most often effective. In patients at high thrombotic risk (for example, those undergoing orthopedic surgery, after fracture or in urinary surgery, patients with cancer), prophylaxis is more effective if based on the results of in vitro coagulation tests. A simple set of laboratory screening tests for hemostatic competence is recommended (platelet count, activated partial thromboplastin time, prothrombin time) before initiation of prophylaxis with heparin because of the hazards of this drug in patients with a hemostatic defect.

ORAL ANTICOAGULANTS

There are two types of vitamin K antagonists: coumarins (dicumarol, warfarin, acenocoumarol, phenprocoumon) and indanediones (phenindione) (Fig. 6–8). The latter group has an excess of nonhemorrhagic toxicity. Among coumarins, the most popular in the United States is warfarin. This compound, therefore, will be utilized in this section as the prototypical oral anticoagulant.

Chemistry

Two comprehensive reviews of the mechanism of action of coumarin compounds and their effect on coagulation have been published.[34,35] Warfarin acts as an anticoagulant by inhibiting carboxylation of glutamic acid to gamma-carboxyglutamic acid residues. The presence of gamma-carboxyglutamic acids imparts two essential properties to the vitamin K-dependent clotting zymogens: the proteins bind Ca^{2+} in the physiologic range and also bind to a negatively charged phospholipid surface in the presence of Ca^{2+}. In man, the noncarboxylated proteins are released into the circulation. Thus, warfarin alters the synthesis of six vitamin K-dependent zymogens; factors II, VII, IX, X, protein C, and protein S (Fig. 6–9). These six vitamin K-dependent proteins involved in the coagulation sequence have now been isolated, characterized, and identified by biochemical function.

The essential chemical characteristic for anticoagulant activity of the coumarin type of vitamin K antagonist is an intact 4-hydroxycoumarin nucleus with a substituent in the 3 position. Warfarin sodium, as well as other coumarins, has an asymmetric carbon atom in the substituent group at the 3 position of the coumarin nucleus, which means that the clinically available preparations are racemic mixtures composed of two optical isomers.[36]

A second postulated mechanism for warfarin's antithrombotic action in humans is the

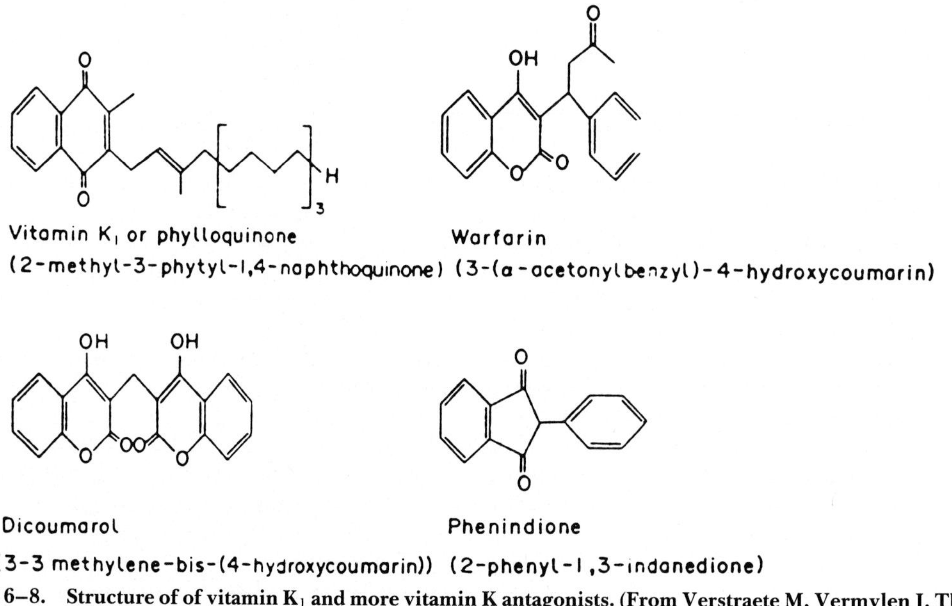

Vitamin K_1 or phylloquinone
(2-methyl-3-phytyl-1,4-naphthoquinone)

Warfarin
(3-(α-acetonylbenzyl)-4-hydroxycoumarin)

Dicoumarol
(3-3 methylene-bis-(4-hydroxycoumarin))

Phenindione
(2-phenyl-1,3-indanedione)

FIGURE 6–8.   Structure of of vitamin K_1 and more vitamin K antagonists. (From Verstraete M, Vermylen J. Thrombosis. New York: Pergamon Press, 1984, with permission.)

Blood coagulation mechanism

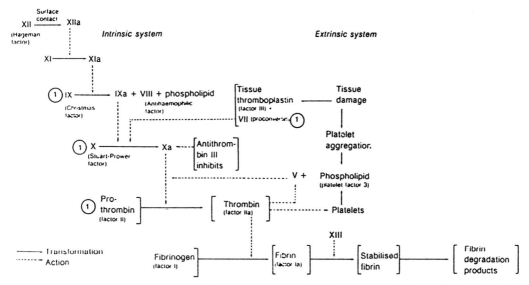

FIGURE 6–9. Diagrammatic and simplified representation of the human coagulation mechanism. Coumarin and indanedione anticoagulants reduce the activity of vitamin K-dependent coagulation factors II, VII, IX, and X. (From Verstraete M. Chapter XXIII, Haemotologic disorders. In: Speight TM, ed., Avery's Drug Treatment. Auckland: Adis Press, 1987, with permission.)

release of certain proteins that are deficient in gamma-carboxyglutamic acid.[37] Experimentally, at least one such protein can decrease the rate at which prothrombin is activated in vitro,[38] thereby retarding thrombin production. Whether such action is antithrombotic has not been established.

Warfarin also increases the rate at which plasma inhibits clotting proteases, as measured by the rate of activated factor X inhibition.[39,40] Thrombosis-prone families have been described who have had an isolated defect in this inhibitory rate.[41]

It is not yet known whether the lack of gamma-carboxyglutamic acid affects the activities of proteins C and S. However, the warfarin-induced depression of protein C, protein S, or both could counterbalance the anticoagulant action of the drug, initially producing a potentially thrombotic state.

The mechanism of action of warfarin is now well understood, at least with respect to the carboxylation of coagulation proteins in the liver. However, the mechanism that directs the carboxylase toward a specific glutamic acid residue is unclear. In particular, in contrast to certain other post-translational modifications of proteins, such as glycosylation, the target residues are not contained within a "consensus sequence." Recently,

however, sequence data on the complementary deoxyribonucleic acid (cDNA) for several Gla-containing proteins have indicated the presence of a "propeptide" region between the amino terminus of the mature protein and the leader peptide sequence.[42–44] Thus, the regulation of carboxylation may be accomplished by a region on each gene that directs the enzymatic machinery, but that is not itself translated into the secreted protein.

Pharmacology

Absorption of warfarin is rapid and complete with peak blood levels in two to four hours. The biologic half-life varies around 36 hours. The high degree of binding of warfarin to plasma albumin explains its clinical pharmacology: the prolonged half-life and biologic effect, the absence of warfarin in red blood cells or cerebrospinal fluid, and the lack of unchanged warfarin in stool or urine.[36] Thus, warfarin is administered therapeutically at time intervals of 24 hours, which is shorter than its half-life of 36 hours. This practice permits a patient to reach a steady state with respect to warfarin dose and prothrombin time.

Warfarin is hydroxylated to an inactive

compound. Thus, although warfarin passes the placental barrier, it appears in the milk of nursing mothers in an inactive form. Direct testing has shown no unchanging drug in maternal milk.[36] Accordingly, contrary to the current opinion of many, warfarin given postpartum to nursing mothers poses no hazard to the full-term infant.[45]

Dose: Monitoring and Administration

Modifications of the Quick prothrombin time are the most widely used tests to monitor warfarin therapy. The lack of standardization of the prothrombin time assay, particularly of the nature and reproducibility of the thromboplastic reagent, has led to striking discrepancies, which have been further compounded by the variety of ways in which the data are expressed for clinical use. This variability has led not only to confusion among clinicians, but also to different intensities of treatment. Thus, the same coagulation defect acceptable as therapeutic at one institution might be considered as almost homeopathic at another, or interpreted as a dangerous overdose at a third. To decrease the problems related to lack of standardization, a system of reporting results based on thromboplastin standards has been developed. One primary standard, the World Health Organization international reference thromboplastin, and three secondary standards, a rabbit brain, a human brain, and an ox brain (Thrombotest) preparation, have been calibrated against each other and assigned international normalized ratios (INR).[46,47] With this accomplished, any commercial thromboplastin reagent can be calibrated against a related reference standard, and the calibration curve employed to translate a given reporting method to the international normalized ratios. A table can be presented with prothrombin time ratio ranges obtained using rabbit thromboplastin (US range) and the equivalent international normalized ratio range.

Blood for prothrombin time determinations should be collected in polypropylene or properly siliconized glass syringes and test tubes. If it is collected in regular glass containers or in some commercially prepared siliconized glass containers, marked shortening of the prothrombin time may occur with time, leading to erroneously large increases in warfarin dosages.[48] The effect of glass on the prothrombin time may be minimized if specimens are transferred within one hour to appropriate plastic containers.

Currently recommended doses for both primary and secondary prophylaxis in cardiovascular states such as prosthetic heart valves, atrial fibrillation, myocardial infarction, stroke, and venous thromboembolism are reported elsewhere (see corresponding chapters). These levels are, however, being reexamined by clinical trials (see Chapter 9). In addition, much of the old and new trial data will be subjected to meta-analysis. It should be recalled that one of the early uses of this methodology was effectively applied to measure the benefit of oral anticoagulants on the course of acute myocardial infarction.[49] The advantages as well as the caveats, as recently defined, should be helpful to clinicians in interpreting future meta-analysis of anticoagulant therapy.[50] As trial data are accumulated, prothrombin time ratios below 1.3, for the prevention of at least some cardiovascular states, may prove effective. If regimens of 1 milligram/day of warfarin, for example, were to prove effective, monitoring prothrombin times might no longer be required.

Precautions and Adverse Effects

HEMORRHAGE

Since the primary hazard in using anticoagulants is hemorrhage, the hemostatic competence of the patient must be established before or, in emergencies, as soon as possible after institution of therapy. It is through the history, including current drug use, physical examination, and several readily available laboratory tests, that hemostatic competence is defined. Such competence can be determined with minimum effort, time, and cost by ascertaining that the patient does not have a tendency to bleed easily; has never hemorrhaged excessively when cut, bruised, or subjected to dental procedures or surgery; that bleeding is not occurring from any site at the time of examination; and that the hematocrit, platelet count, partial thromboplastin time, prothrombin time, and bleeding time, as well as urine analysis and stool examination for gross or occult hemorrhage, are normal.

For patients on long-term warfarin therapy, it is important to appreciate that bleeding may occur at unusual sites. Hemorrhage into the bowel lumen, intestinal wall, mesentery, rectus muscle, or from the corpus luteum may simulate an acute abdominal crisis. Similar considerations apply to genitourinary bleeding that may mimic a renal tumor. Hematomas may cause carpal tunnel compression and, rarely, pericardial, adrenal, or retroperitoneal hemorrhage. Maintaining long-term patients at a prothrombin time ratio at the lower end of the 1.5 to 2.0 range should minimize hemorrhage, as has been found in Europe.

When to search for the cause of an episode of spontaneous bleeding, such as from the genitourinary or gastrointestinal tracts, can best be decided if the prothrombin time is obtained within 24 hours of hemorrhage. Experience has shown that when the prothrombin time ratio is in the range of 1.5 to 2.0, the likelihood of finding a localized bleeding lesion is significantly greater than if the prothrombin time ratio is in excess of 2.5. It is in the former situation that further efforts to identify the bleeding source should be undertaken promptly.

Among patients with diabetes who require long-term warfarin therapy, the question often arises whether anticoagulation represents a risk of vitreous or retinal hemorrhage, particularly among patients with advanced retinopathy. Not only are there no data to support such concerns, but trials of anticoagulants initiated to treat retinal venous occlusion complicated by retinal hemorrhage have not been associated with any enhancement of existing ocular bleeding.[51]

AGE AND SEX

It has not been established that either age or sex, per se, represents an increased risk of hemorrhage, provided that the patient is hemostatically competent, anticoagulant regimens are prudent, and prothrombin times are appropriately monitored.

FERTILITY, TERATOGENICITY, AND PREGNANCY

Fertile women receiving warfarin must be warned of the risks of teratogenicity if they become pregnant.[52] When pregnancy is an immediate possibility, consideration should be given to substituting heparin for the oral anticoagulant. Specific warfarin-induced embryopathies occur in the 6th to 12th week of pregnancy, and central nervous system and ocular fetal anomalies may occur at any time during pregnancy.[53] If the patient has been alerted to notify her physician that her menstrual period is late by only a few days, there is a human B-chorionic gonadotropin radioimmunoassay specific for detecting pregnancy from the 14th postconception day. Even if menses are delayed by one to two weeks, there is still time to discontinue warfarin therapy and markedly diminish, if not avoid, the likelihood of teratogenesis. If pregnancy is recognized too late, termination might be considered. Sonography provides no assistance in making this decision. If anticoagulants are indicated in a confirmed pregnancy, heparin is the drug of choice (see Chapter 26). Because of the risk of heparin-associated osteoporosis, however, the patient should be switched post partum to warfarin, which poses no hazard to the breast feeding infant.[45]

BLOOD PRESSURE

Blood pressures significantly in excess of 160 systolic and 90 diastolic incur the risk of cerebral hemorrhage, and all reasonable efforts should be undertaken to reduce such elevations toward these benchmark values. In this regard, it should be appreciated that cerebral hemorrhage in hypertensive patients does not correlate well with the absolute level of blood pressure, that isolated systolic hypertension may pose an even greater threat of cerebral hemorrhage than diastolic hypertension, and that the former often proves more difficult to manage. Having acknowledged these facts, it may still be appropriate, on a benefit-to-risk basis, to utilize anticoagulant prophylaxis in some patients at high risk of cerebral embolism in whom hypertension cannot be totally eliminated despite optimal therapy. For these patients, physicians would be well advised to consider utilizing the lowest reasonable therapeutic range for warfarin, because there is a correlation between cerebral hemorrhage and the intensity of anticoagulation.

Since hypertension is a risk factor for cerebral hemorrhage among patients with cerebral vascular disease, two additional observations are warranted: (a) transient elevations of blood pressure may accompany acute cerebral infarction, and (b) normotensive individuals may develop hypertension months to years after initiation of warfarin prophylaxis. These observations not only provide additional reasons for delaying the administration of anticoagulation after acute cerebral infarction, but also stress the importance of periodic evaluation, especially in the elderly, so if hypertension develops, attention can be initiated to treat it effectively.

DIET

There are no food restrictions as such for patients receiving warfarin. The public, however, receives advice about pharmaceuticals in lay publications. There are statements in this literature that patients maintained on oral anticoagulants should avoid excessive consumption of foods rich in vitamin K because the compound promotes clotting. Listed among such foods are leafy green vegetables, asparagus, bacon, broccoli, Brussels sprouts, and beef liver. Physicians should advise patients that these foods are entirely safe in and of themselves, and should not be restricted because they are taking warfarin. The point, rather, is that any major change in diet, as with the addition or deletion of other drugs, should be reported to the patient's physician so that drug can be adjusted on the basis of more frequent determinations of the prothrombin time.

WARFARIN RESISTANCE

There are rare patients who are congenitally resistant to coumarin therapy.[54] Some of these individuals may require 75 milligrams/day of warfarin. In such situations, heparin remains an alternative choice.

WARFARIN NECROSIS

Coumarin-induced necrosis of the skin and subcutaneous tissues is a rare but striking complication of warfarin therapy and is not to be confused with simple hemorrhage. The lesion appears within three to ten days of drug administration, usually in the lower half of the body. It occurs particularly in women and in areas of abundant subcutaneous fat, such as the buttocks, breasts, thighs, and abdomen. Beginning as an erythematous patch, frank hemorrhagic necrosis may develop within 24 hours. No explanation for this toxic reactions has been established, although it may be related to protein C depression in many instances. When coumarin-induced necrosis occurs, warfarin should be discontinued. If further anticoagulant therapy is indicated, heparin should be substituted for warfarin, although heparin-associated skin necrosis has also been reported (see Heparin). In any event it is incumbent on physicians to examine each patient ade-

quately during the first days of therapy for evidence of local erythema, particularly in adipose and dependent regions, and to consider options as recently described.[55]

DRUG-DRUG INTERACTIONS

(See Chapter 7).

CONCURRENT USE OF ASPIRIN AND OTHER ANTIPLATELET DRUGS

Stated simply, aspirin and anticoagulant therapy, in their usual dosage, should not be administered concurrently because of the increased risk of bleeding. This observation confronts physicians with a special dilemma, because aspirin, aside from its several nonvascular indications, has been approved by the Food and Drug Administration (FDA) for transient ischemic attacks (TIAs), unstable angina, and secondary myocardial infarction. A review of the available evidence suggests that in patients with transient ischemic attacks, aspirin should take precedence over warfarin for the first six months following the onset of transient ischemic attack. If there has been a prior embolic stroke, atrial fibrillation, or a failure of aspirin to prevent further transient ischemic attacks, then warfarin should be considered in place of aspirin. Among patients with unstable angina, aspirin should also take precedence over warfarin for the first six months unless an acute myocardial infarction supervenes, in which case anticoagulants should be administered. For the prevention of secondary myocardial infarction, however, the value of aspirin is less clear, and if, for example, atrial fibrillation is present, warfarin is preferable. These statements concerning aspirin and warfarin may well be modified as more trial data become available. Regimens of "very low-dose" aspirin plus "very low-dose" warfarin have been reported. Whether this will result in improved efficacy without hemorrhage will require further trials.

In regard to other antiplatelet agents, dipyridamole has a potential antithrombotic role only when added to warfarin for patients with prosthetic heart valves.[56] However, platelet antiaggregants alone or in any combination are not a substitute for warfarin among these patients.

The nonsteroidal, anti-inflammatory drugs that have mild antiplatelet action may be used in conjunction with warfarin without incurring an *increased* risk of bleeding. The intrinsic risk of hemorrhage from these drugs, of course, remains. Calcium channel blockers that minimally impair platelet aggregation do not apparently increase the risk of hemorrhage from warfarin.

FALLS IN THE ELDERLY

Falls among the elderly in the absence of anticoagulants are a major health hazard. A total of 11,600 individuals were killed by falls in the United States in 1984, and 58 per cent of those falls occurred in people older than 75 years of age.[57] One half of the fatalities were from concussion or cerebral hemorrhage. The remainder of the deaths resulted from pulmonary embolism, bronchopneumonia, or respiratory failure. For example, osteoporosis was responsible for 1.2 million fractures in the United States, more than a quarter of a million of which were hip fractures. By extreme old age, one of every three women and one of every six men will have had a hip fracture. These are fatal in 12 to 20 per cent of cases.[58] Several analyses have been published indicating that falls among the elderly appear to result from the accumulated effect of multiple specific disabilities, some of which are remedial.[59] Particular steps that families of patients or patients themselves can take to minimize the likelihood of falling have been published.[60,61]

The unanswered question is whether a low-dose warfarin regimen would in fact facilitate the development or aggravate the degree of a cerebral hemorrhage secondary to a fall. Each physician must resolve this dilemma based on his or her evaluation of the likelihood of a major head injury from a fall against the likelihood of a cerebral embolism. For example, if the patient does not fall frequently and could be helped to avoid falling, he should be anticoagulated if a prosthetic heart valve or atrial fibrillation is present. Part of the periodic reevaluation that involves blood pressure determination should also include evaluation of the likelihood that the patient will fall. Tests to determine the risk of a fall have also been published.[60] Ironically, low-dose warfarin may be desirable prophylaxis, if the fall results in a hip fracture instead of a cerebral hemorrhage. Lethal pulmonary embolism is not a rare complication of a hip fracture, and warfarin in low doses may prevent this untoward outcome.

OVERLAPPING HEPARIN AND WARFARIN

When patients are being switched from heparin to warfarin, conventional wisdom used to dictate that the drugs should be overlapped for two days because of the one- to two-day delay in the peak prothrombin time response. Further eludication of the pharmacological nature of both compounds provides additional support for maintaining this overlap and, perhaps, even increasing its duration.

Although heparin administration frequently depresses the plasma concentration of antithrombin III, the effect of that depression is debatable during heparin therapy because the consequent decrease in the antithrombin III concentration will be more than offset by the increased reaction rate induced by the drug. When heparin therapy is terminated in the absence of other antithrombotic agents, however, patients with a heparin-induced decrease in antithrombin III can be considered to be in a potentially hypercoagulable state for approximately three days until the plasma antithrombin III level has returned to normal. This is a second reason for overlapping the anticoagulants for at least that period of time.

In addition, the warfarin-induced depression of protein C occurs within the first 12 to 24 hours of drug administration at about the same rate as factor VII depression. The depression of protein C while factors X, IX, and II are still near normal levels may also represent a thrombotic risk and is further reason for overlapping the use of the two drugs for several days.

Finally, in view of work in animals indicating that warfarin has a delayed, additive, antithrombotic effect six days after administration,[40] some physicians may wish to extend the period of overlap to five to six days—an approach that has anecdotal support in clinical reports. If such an extended overlap is planned, it rarely prolongs the hospital stay.

INTERVAL SURGERY

For minor surgery such as tooth extraction, interruption of warfarin therapy is rarely necessary. In contrast, guidelines have been less clearly defined for patients facing major elective general surgery who are already on a maintenance dose of warfarin. One choice is to discontinue the drug for four days before operation and for one to two days postoperatively before resuming oral anticoagulation. A second alternative is to discontinue warfarin four days before operation, substituting a low-dose heparin regimen in the perioperative period and then reinstituting warfarin prophylaxis. Finally, there is the option of limiting the prothrombin time ratio to or slightly below 1.5 prior to surgery and maintaining this intensity in the perioperative and immediate postoperative period. Published trial data do not identify the extent of the hemorrhagic risk, if any, with this third alternative. Whether the risk is as low as starting warfarin on the day before or the day of operation has not been established. Nevertheless, some knowledgeable investigators believe that it is safe to continue the preoperative warfarin regimen through the surgical procedure, provided the prothrombin time is not excessively prolonged.

REBOUND PHENOMENON

It is difficult to establish whether a rebound thrombotic effect occurs when warfarin is discontinued. First, the discontinuance of therapy may possibly return the patient to the clinical status responsible for the initial thrombotic episode. Second, warfarin-induced alterations in clotting factors become normal over a period of hours or days, even when the drug is discontinued abruptly. Data from patients in whom warfarin was abruptly discontinued are conflicting, with most of the thrombotic episodes occurring after the vitamin K-dependent proteins returned to normal levels. Conversely, clotting studies have indicated a slight temporary increase in prothrombin above control levels right after the cessation of therapy. The transitory depression of protein C, S, or both upon drug withdrawal produces a potentially hypercoagulable state. It is certainly true that patients who are congenitally deficient in protein C or S are prone to thrombosis. However, depressed levels of these coagulation proteins due to warfarin administration have yet to be correlated with the development of clinical thrombosis promptly after the discontinuance of warfarin therapy.

Contraindications

Oral anticoagulants should not be employed in patients with the following conditions: pregnancy; a hemorrhagic diathesis; hypertension with a diastolic pressure persistently greater than 105 torr; cerebrovascular hemorrhage; major trauma; active ulceration or overt bleeding from the gastrointestinal, genitourinary, or respiratory tracts; inadequate laboratory facilities; or unsatisfactory cooperation of the patient with the therapeutic regimen.

For other, though less stringent, contraindications, the risk must be weighed against the benefit of prophylaxis.

These relative contraindications include a fertile woman, use of platelet-suppressive agents, renal and liver disease, and thyrotoxicosis treated with radioactive iodine because of the possibility of gland hemorrhage. Caution is recommended in the use of warfarin in vasculitis, bacterial endocarditis, and pericarditis complicating acute myocardial infarction because of the danger of hemopericardium. Adequate preparation before administration of oral anticoagulants may reduce the hazard of bleeding in disorders such as malnutrition, vitamin C and K deficiencies, ulcerative colitis, sprue, steatorrhea, and pancreatitis.

Antidotes

The natural vitamin K_1 (Mephyton, Aquamephyton, Konakion), in doses of 0.5 to 10 milligrams effectively reverses a moderately excessive anticoagulant effect. Some correction of the prothrombin time is noted within six hours, full correction usually within 24 hours. If the patient is to remain on warfarin, the dose of vitamin K_1 preferably should be limited to 0.5 to 1 milligram. Higher amounts, up to 10 milligrams may be indicated if the patient is not to be maintained on therapy after the hemorrhage is controlled. Large doses of vitamin K_1 may subsequently make the patient resistant to warfarin for many days, preventing effective anticoagulant therapy for that time period. Vitamin K_1 may be administered intravenously, subcutaneously, or orally. The water-soluble vitamin K_1 derivatives are distinctly less effective than is the natural vitamin.

An immediate reversal of the clotting defect can be achieved by transfusion of blood, plasma, or plasma concentrates rich in the vitamin K-dependent clotting factors. Because these factors are relatively stable, they remain fully potent in ordinary ACD-banked blood or banked or lyophilized plasma. Three units, or 15 milliliters/kilogram, of blood or plasma should suffice for an initial effect, providing time for concomitant vitamin K_1 administration to exert its action.

In patients with limited cardiac reserve, the recommended values of blood or plasma may precipitate pulmonary edema unless significant blood loss has occurred. Plasma concentrates rich in factors II, VII, IX, and X will obviate the hazard of hypervolemia, but may carry with them the risk of thrombosis and hepatitis.

Comparable Antithrombotic Activities of Heparin and Warfarin

Clinically, it would be helpful to have available alternative antithrombotic drugs of equivalent prophylactic efficacy and bleeding risk for specific patients or groups of patients with specific conditions, of which pregnancy is one example. Data obtained from clinical trials and animal models[62,63] indicate that 20,000 units of heparin per 24 hours may be equivalent to warfarin doses, resulting in prothrombin time ratios of 1.2 to 1.3. These anticoagulant levels have comparable bleeding risks.

REFERENCES

1. Lindahl U, Höök M, Backström G, et al. Structure and biosynthesis of heparin-like polysaccharides. Fed Proc 1977; 36: 19–24.
2. Choay J, Lormeau JC, Petitou M, Sinay P, Fareed J. Structural studies on a biologically active hexasaccharide obtained from heparin. Ann NY Acad Sci 1981; 370: 644–9.
3. Choay J, Petitou M, Lormeau JC, Sinaij P, Casu B, Gatti G. Structure activity relationships in heparin: a synthetic pentasaccharide with high affinity for antithrombin III and eliciting high anti factor Xa activity. Biochem Biophys Res Commun 1983; 116: 492–9.
4. Walenga JM, Petitou M, Samama M, Fareed J, Choay J. Importance of a 3-0-sulfate group in a heparin pentasaccharide for antithrombotic activity. Thromb Res 1988; 52: 553–63.
5. Lindhardt RJ, Grant A, Cooney CL, Langer R. Differential anticoagulant activity of heparin fragment prepared using microbial heparinase. J Biol Chem 1982; 257: 7310–3.
6. Lindahl U, Backström G, Thunberg L. The antithrombin-binding sequence in heparin. J Biol Chem 1983; 258: 9826–30.
7. Jordan RE, Oosta GM, Gardner WT, Rosenberg RD. The kinetics of hemostatic enzyme-antithrombin interactions in the presence of low molecular weight heparin. J Biol Chem 1980; 255: 10081–90.
8. Rosenberg RD, Damus PS. The purification and mechanism of action of human antithrombin-heparin cofactor. J Biol Chem 1973; 248: 6490–505.
9. Pletcher CH, Nelsestuen GL. Two-substrate reaction model for the heparin-catalyzed bovine antithrombin/protease reaction. J Biol Chem 1983; 258: 1086–91.
10. Hoylaerts M, Owen WG, Collen D. Involvement of heparin chain length in the heparin-catalyzed inhibition of thrombin by antithrombin III. J Biol Chem 1984; 259: 5670–7.
11. Ockelford P, Carter CJ, Cerskus A, Smith CA, Hirsh J. Comparison of the in vivo haemorrhagic and antithrombotic effects of a low antithrombin III affinity heparin fraction. Thromb Res 1982; 27: 679–90.
12. Walker FJ, Esmon CT. Interactions between heparin and factor Xa, inhibition of prothrombin activation. Biochim Biophys Acta 1979; 585: 405–15.
13. Ofosu FA, Blajchman MA, Hirsh J. The inhibition by heparin of the intrinsic pathway activation of factor X in the absence of antithrombin III. Thromb Res 1980; 20: 391–403.
14. Barrowcliffe TW, Merton RE, Havercroft SJ, Thunberg U, Thomas DP. Low affinity heparin potentiates the action of high affinity heparin oligosaccharides. Thromb Res 1984; 34: 124–33.
15. Rosenberg RD, Reilly C, Fritze L. Atherogenic regulation by heparin-like molecules. Ann NY Acad Sci 1985; 454: 270–9.
16. Bengtsson-Olivecrona G, Olivecrona T. Binding of active and inactive forms of lipoprotein lipase to heparin: effects of pH. Biochem J 1985; 226: 409–13.
17. Tollefsen DM, Blank MK. Detection of a new heparin-dependent inhibitor of thrombin in human plasma. J Clin Invest 1981; 68: 589–96.
18. Barzu T, Molho P, Tobelem G, Petitou M, Caen J. Binding and endocytosis of heparin by human endothelial cells in culture. Biochim Biophys Acta 1985; 845: 196–203.
19. Petitou M, Duchaussoy P, Lederman I, et al. Synthesis of heparin fragments: a methyl α-pentoside with high affinity for antithrombin III. Carbohydrate Res 1987; 67: 67–75.
20. Holmer E, Mattson C, Nilsson S. Anticoagulant and antithrombotic effects of heparin and low molecular weight heparin fragments in rabbits. Thromb Res 1982; 25: 475–85.
21. Thomas DP, Merton RE, Barrowcliffe TW, Thunberg L, Lindahl U. Effects of heparin oligosaccharides with high affinity for antithrombin III in experimental venous thrombosis. Thromb Haemostas 1982; 47: 244–8.
22. Thomas DP, Merton RE, Gray E, Barrowcliffe TW. The relative antithrombotic effectiveness of heparin, a low molecular weight heparin, and a pentasaccharide fragment in an animal model. Thromb Haemost 1989; 61: 204–7.
23. Boneu B, Caranobe C, Gabaig AM, et al. Evidence for a saturable mechanism of disappearance of standard heparin in rabbits. Thromb Res 1987; 46: 835–44.
24. Fareed J, Walenga PM, Rancanelli A, et al. Biochemical and pharmacological studies on unfractionated and low molecular weight heparins. In: Breddin K, Fareed J, Samama M, eds. Fraxiparine. Analytical and structural data, pharmacology, clinical trials. Stuttgart: Schattauer Verlag, 1989: 41–68.
25. Levine MN, Hirsh J. An overview of clinical trials with low molecular weight heparin fractions. Acta Chir Scand 1988; 543 (suppl): 73–9.
26. Carreras LO. Thrombosis and thrombocytopenia induced by heparin. In: Verstraete M, Machin S, eds. Clinical usage of heparin. Present and future trends. Scand J Haematol 1980; 25(suppl 36): 64–80.
27. Mätzsch T, Bergqvist D, Hedner U, Østergaard P. Heparin-induced osteoporosis in rats. Thromb Haemost 1986; 56: 293–4.
28. Tansey MJB, Opie LH. Relation between plasma free fatty acids and arrhythmias within the first twelve hours of acute myocardial infarction. Lancet 1983; i: 419–22.
29. Persson E, Nördenström J, Nilsson-Ehle P, Hagenfeldt L. Lipolytic and anticoagulant activities of a low molecular weight fragment of heparin. Eur J Clin Invest 1985; 15: 215–20.
30. Kakkar VV, Djazaseri B, Fok J, Fletscher M, Scully MF, Westwick J. Low molecular weight heparin and prevention of postoperative deep vein thrombosis. Br Med J 1982; 284: 375–9.
31. Durand D, Ader JL, Rey JP, et al. Inducing hyperkalemia by converting enzyme inhibitors and heparin. Kidney Int 1988; 34 (Suppl 25): S196–7.
32. Lambert M, Laterre PF, Leroy Ch, Lavenne E, Coche E, Moriau M. Modifications of liver enzymes during heparin therapy. Acta Clin Belg 1986; 41: 307–10.
33. Bounameaux H, Marbet GA, Lämmle B, Eichlisberger R, Duckert F. Monitoring of heparin treatment. Comparison of thrombin time, activated partial thromboplastin time, and plasma heparin concentration, and analysis of the behaviour of antithrombin III. Am J Clin Pathol 1980; 74: 68–73.
34. Stenflo J, Suttie JW. Vitamin K-dependent formation of γ-carboxyglutamic acid. Ann Rev Biochim 1977; 46: 157–72.
35. Suttie JW, Jackson CM. Prothrombin structure, activation, and biosynthesis. Physiol Rev 1977; 57: 1–70.
36. O'Reilly RA, Aggeler PM. Determinants of the response to

oral anticoagulant drugs in man. Pharmacol Rev 1970; 22: 35–96.

37. Hemker HC, Veltkamp JJ, Loeliger EA. Kinetic aspects of the interaction of blood clotting enzymes. III. Demonstration of an inhibitor of prothrombin conversion in vitamin K deficiency. Thromb Diath Haemorrh 1968; 19: 346–63.

38. Hemker HC, Muller AD. Kinetic aspects of the interaction of blood-clotting enzymes. VI. Localization of the site of blood-coagulation inhibition by the protein induced by vitamin K absence (PIVKA). Thromb Diath Haemorrh 1968; 20: 78–87.

39. Ødegård OR, Teien AN. Antithrombin III, heparin cofactor and antifactor Xa in a clinical material. Thromb Res 1976; 8: 173–8.

40. Wessler S, Gitel SN, Bank H, Martinowitz U, Stephenson RC. An assay of the antithrombotic action of warfarin: its correlation with the inhibition of stasis thrombosis in rabbits. Thromb Haemost 1978; 40: 486–98.

41. Sørensen PJ, Dyerberg J, Stofferson E, Jensen MK. Familial functional antithrombin III deficiency. Scand J Haematol 1980; 24: 105–9.

42. Long GL, Belagaje RM, MacGilivrary RTA. Cloning and sequencing of liver DNA coding for bovine protein C. Proc Natl Acad Sci USA 1984; 81: 5653.

43. Pan LC, Price PA. The propeptide of rat bone gamma-carboxyglutamic acid protein shares homology with other vitamin K-dependent protein precursors. Proc Natl Acad Sci USA 1985; 82: 6109–13.

44. Suttie JW, Hoskins JA, Engelke J, et al. Vitamin K-dependent carboxylase: possible role of the "propeptide" as an intracellular recognition site (gamma-carboxyglutamic acid/protein C). Proc Natl Acad Sci USA 1987; 84: 634–7.

45. Fries K, König FE, Reich TH. Einfluss der Marcoumar-Therapie bei voll gestillten Kindern. Schweiz Med Wochenschr 1957; 87: 615–7.

46. Hermans J, van den Besselaar, Loeliger EA, van der Velde EA. A collaborative calibration study of reference materials for thromboplastins. Thromb Haemost 1983; 50: 712–7.

47. Koepke JA, Triplett DA. Standardization of the prothrombin time—finally. Arch Pathol Lab Med 1985; 109: 800–1.

48. Palmer RN, Kessler CM, Gralnick HR. Warfarin anticoagulation: difficulties in interpretation of the prothrombin time. Thromb Res 1982; 25: 125–30.

49. Chalmers TC, Matta RJ, Smith H Jr, et al. Evidence favoring the use of anticoagulants in the hospital phase of acute myocardial infarction. N Engl J Med 1977; 207: 1091–6.

50. Goodman SN. Have you ever meta-analysis you didn't like? Ann Int Med 1991; 114: 244–6.

51. Kienast J, Vermylen J, Verstraete M, et al. Venous thromboses in particular organs. J Am Coll Cardiol 1986; 8: 137B–45B.

52. Salazar E, Zajarias A, Gutierrez N, Itube I. The problem of cardiac valve prostheses, anticoagulants and pregnancy. Circulation 1984; 70 (suppl I): I-169–77.

53. Hall JG, Pauli RM, Wilson KM. Maternal and fetal sequelae of anticoagulation during pregnancy. Am J Med 1980; 68: 122–40.

54. O'Reilly RA. Vitamin K in hereditary resistance to oral anticoagulant drugs. Am J Physiol 1971; 22: 1237–30.

55. Comp PC, Elrod JP, Karzenski S. Warfarin-induced necrosis. Semin Thromb Hemost 1990; 16: 293–8.

56. Chesebro JH, Fuster F, Elveback LR, et al. Trial of combined warfarin plus dipyridamole or aspirin therapy in prosthetic heart valve replacement: danger of aspirin compared to dipyridamle. Am J Cardiol 1983; 51: 1537–41.

57. National Safety Council Accident Facts. Chicago: National Safety Council, 1985: 83.

58. Cummings SR, Kelsey JL, Nevitt K, et al. Epidemiology of osteoporosis and osteoporotic fractures. Epidemiol Rev 1985; 7: 178–208.

59. Tinetti ME, Williams TF, Mayewski R. Fall risk index for elderly patients based on number of chronic disabilities. Am J Med 1986; 80: 429–34.

60. Allen D. Falls—big worry for the elderly. Family Safety 1979; 38: 23.

61. Perszcynski M. Why people fall. Am J Nurs 1965; 65: 86–8.

62. Hull R, Delmore T, Carter C, et al. Adjusted subcutaneous heparin versus warfarin sodium in the long-term treatment of venous thrombosis. N Engl J Med 1982; 306: 189–4.

63. Gitel SN, Wessler S. Dose dependent antithrombotic effect of warfarin in rabbits. Blood 1983; 61: 435–8.

7

DRUG INTERFERENCE WITH HEPARIN AND ORAL ANTICOAGULANTS

MARC VERSTRAETE and STANFORD WESSLER

DRUG INTERACTIONS WITH ORAL ANTICOAGULANTS

The effects of interaction between drugs are well known in the case of oral coumarin anticoagulants because the pharmacological effect is easily and routinely checked by measuring the "prothrombin time," and also because the patient becomes aware of prolonged bleeding in cases of excessive enhancement of the activity of the coumarin anticoagulant. Apart from the effect of pathophysiological conditions (for example, liver disease, congestive heart failure, renal dysfunction) which in themselves can alter the response to oral anticoagulants, other determinants which make a clinically important interaction more likely to occur have not been well defined. A change in concurrent therapy in a patient on a stable anticoagulant regimen can, however, be important. Drugs which are capable of altering oral anticoagulant response can be used concurrently, provided the dosage of the anticoagulant has been modified appropriately. Thus, in an already stable regimen, barbiturates taken regularly as anticonvulsants do not affect anticoagulant control, but barbiturates used occasionally as hypnotics can affect anticoagulant control. Introduction of hypnotic drugs such as barbiturates and dichlorphenazone, which in some patients can significantly induce drug metabolizing enzymes in the hepatic endoplasmatic reticulum, may increase over a period of some days the rate of metabolism of coumarins and thus lead to a marked increase in anticoagulant dose requirements to regain

the desired level of anticoagulation.[1,2] Sudden withdrawal of the inducing drug (for example, at the time of or shortly after discharge from hospital) without corresponding reduction of the dose of anticoagulant can have disastrous effects. Such interactions are difficult to recognize because the enhanced anticoagulant effect develops gradually over a period of some days or weeks and the interindividual variation in effect is marked.

In practice, although the potential for interaction is considerable, clinically harmful interactions are not that common, and predictable effects are largely confined to a few drugs such as phenylbutazone, oxyphenbutazone, clofibrate, allopurinol, cimetidine, and danazol (potentiate anticoagulant effect), and barbiturates, rifampicin, aminoglutethimide, and cholestyramine (antagonize anticoagulant effect) (Table 7–1). Nevertheless, several fatalities have resulted from severe bleeding,[3–5] and conversely, many patients taking potentially interacting drugs may not achieve desirable anticoagulant control if seen only irregularly.

Some coumarin anticoagulants (dicoumarol) can affect the metabolism of other drugs such as phenytoin, tolbutamide, and chlorpropamide. Phenindione has only rarely been implicated in clinically important interactions with other drugs, but it is also much less used.

In Table 7–1, drugs are listed which are expected to or may potentiate the effect of oral anticoagulants as well as drugs which antagonize or may antagonize the effect induced by oral anticoagulants. A few drugs

141

TABLE 7–1. Drug Interactions with Oral Anticoagulants

DRUGS EXPECTED TO POTENTIATE ORAL ANTICOAGULANTS	
Alcohol abuse only	Fenofibrate
Allopurinol	Feprazone
Amiodarone	Glucagon
Anabolic steroids	Ketoprofen
Aspirin and its	Mefenamic acid
analogues (in large	Mercaptopurine
doses)	Methotrexate
Azapropazone	Metronidazole
Bezafibrate	Naproxen
Chloramphenicol	Neomycin
Chlorpromazine	Oxymetholone
Cimetidine	Oxyphenbutazone
Clofibrate	Phenylbutazone
Clofibric acid	Phenyramidol
Co-trimoxazole	Quinidine
Cyclophosphamide	Salicylates (see aspirin)
Danazol	Sulfinpyrazone
Dextrothyroxine	Tamoxifen
Disulfiram	Thyroxine
Ethycrinic acid	

DRUGS WHICH MAY POTENTIATE ORAL ANTICOAGULANTS	
Aminoglycosides:	Indomethacin
Amikacin	Intraconazole
Gentamycin	Isoxicamum
Kanamycin	Ketoconazole
Neomycin	Liquid paraffin
Streptomycin	Mefenamic acid
Tobramycin	Methotrexate
Aminoglutethimide	Methylphenidate
Aminosalicylic acid	Metoclopramide
Amoxicillin	Metronidazole
Ampicillin (oral)	Miconazole
Azapropazone	Monoamine oxidase
Butyrophenones	inhibitors
Cephalosporins:	Nalidixic acid
Cephaloridine	Oxalamine
Cephamandole	Paracetamol—high
Cephazolin	doses for several
Latamoxef	weeks (in
Chloral hydrate and	dextropropoxyphene)
related compounds	particularly in
Chlorpropamide	combination with
Chlortetracycline	propoxyphene
Corticosteroids	Penicillin G in large
Cyclophosphamide	doses intravenously
Cycloserine	Phenformin
Dextropropoxyphene	Piroxicam
Diazoxide	Propylthiouracil
Dichloralphenazone	Quinine salts
Diflunisal	Rifampicin
Disopyramide	Streptotriad
Erythromycin	Sulfonamides (long
Fenclofenac	acting)
Fenoprofen calcium	Sulindac
Floctafenine	Tetracyclines
Fluconazole	Tolbutamide
Flufenamic acid	Triclofos sodium
Flurbiprofen	Tricyclic antidepressants
Gemfibrozil	Vaccination against
Glucagon	influenza
Ibuprofen	

Continued

TABLE 7–1. Drug Interactions with Oral Anticoagulants *continued*

DRUGS WHICH DEFINITELY ANTAGONIZE ANTICOAGULANT THERAPY (MARKED EFFECT)	
Aminoglutethimide	Mercaptopurine
Barbiturates	Phenytoin
Carbamazepine	Rifampicin
Cholestyramine	Vitamin K_1 and K_2 (diet
Colestipol	and nutritional
Glutethimide	products)

DRUGS WHICH MAY ANTAGONIZE ANTICOAGULANT THERAPY (OF SLIGHT OR DOUBTFUL SIGNIFICANCE)	
Antacids	Haloperidol
Antihistaminics	Methaqualone
Dichloralphenazone	Phenazone
Contraceptives (oral)	Primidone
Cyclophosphamides	Spironolactone
Griseofulvin (Fulvin)	

DRUGS POTENTIATED BY ORAL ANTICOAGULANTS	
Chlorpropamide	Tolbutamide
Phenytoin	

are also potentiated by oral anticoagulants.[3,6–23]

Mechanisms of Interaction and Time Course of Interaction Effect

There are many possible mechanisms for interaction[24] (Fig. 7–1). These include either interference with clotting factor synthesis (for example, ?anabolic steroids, ?quinidine), alteration of vitamin K availability (cephalosporins and other oral broad-spectrum antibiotics, ion exchange resins, colestipol, oil laxatives) or interference with the rate of decay of clotting factors (for example, thyroid drugs), and pharmacokinetic mechanisms such as interference with absorption (for example, cholestyramine, alkalinizing agents, antacids), acceleration of coumarin metabolism due to enzyme induction (for example, barbiturates, rifampicin, carbamazepine), or inhibition of coumarin metabolism (biotransformation) (for example, phenylbutazone, metronidazole, co-trimoxazole, sulphinpyrazone, cimetidine, amiodarone, chloramphenicol, erythromycine). In the case of the latter (inhibition of drug metabolism), the interaction with warfarin observed with drugs such as phenylbutazone, metronidazole, co-trimoxazole, and sulphinpyrazone is known to

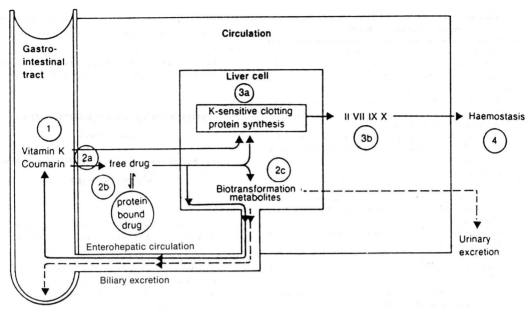

FIGURE 7–1. Possible sites of drug interactions with action of oral coumarin anticoagulants. (*1*) Vitamin K bioavailability; (*2a*) coumarin absorption; (*2b*) coumarin binding to plasma albumin (note: displacement of a coumarin from its binding sites results in only a transient increase in the concentration of unbound drug; (*2c*) coumarin metabolism; (*3a*) prothrombin-complex synthesis; (*3b*) prothrombin-complex catabolism; (*4*) hemostasis (From Verstraete M, Boogaerts MA. In: Speight TM, ed., Avery's Drug Treatment. Auckland: Adis Press, 1987, with permission.)

have a stereoselective basis. These drugs have been reported to selectively inhibit the metabolism of the more potent S(−) enantiomer of warfarin while having no effect on (or in some cases even inducing) the metabolism of the less active (R+) enantiomer. The net effect is an increased anticoagulant response to a single dose of racemic warfarin; this may occur despite no apparent change in the racemic warfarin half-life.[8] In some cases, more than one mechanism is probably involved, such as decreased binding and inhibition of metabolism (for example, phenylbutazone).

The time course of onset and also the extent of the interaction effect vary considerably among patients and depend on the mechanism involved with the specific drug, its dose, and duration of administration.[3,8]

Avoiding Interactions

Adverse clinical events due to interactions with coumarin anticoagulants can be prevented by following a few simple rules:[3]

1. Before prescribing, know all medications the patient is taking and instruct him or her not to change or add to their intake of medication, either physician-prescribed or self-prescribed, without first communicating with their doctor.

2. Drug therapy should always be kept as simple as possible and restricted to those drugs genuinely indicated and of proven benefit.

3. Occasional use of predictably interacting drugs should be avoided and alternatives prescribed (see Table 7–1).

4. Changes of drug therapy should be kept to a minimum. If changes are necessary and involve known interacting drugs, some alteration in coumarin dosage can be anticipated, but dose adjustment should only be made on the basis of results of close monitoring of anticoagulant control over a period of some weeks after the change. The time course and extent of interaction can vary considerably among individual patients.

5. The prothrombin time should be checked every three weeks.

6. A secretary or a person in charge should quickly transmit to the physician (or to the patient) the result of the prothrombin time and the recommended dose of oral anticoagulant.

The use of "fingerstick" may be useful in the

TABLE 7–2.   Rules for Patients on Oral Anticoagulant Therapy*

1. Take your anticoagulant tablets before your evening meal and remind yourself that you have done so by crossing out on the form the number indicating how many you have taken.
2. Never change the dose without consulting us.
3. Avoid aspirin (acetylsalicylic acid) or commercial compounds containing it.
4. Be moderate in drinking alcoholic beverages. Eat fruit and vegetables regularly. Notify the Centre before making any appreciable change in dietary habits (e.g., high-bran diet).
5. If your doctor prescribes some other medicine(s), tell him that you are on oral anticoagulant therapy. Inform the Centre about any drugs you start to take or stop taking.
6. If you injure yourself or notice signs of internal bleeding (reddish urine, black tarry stools), get in touch with the Centre immediately (day or night).
7. If you have to make an appointment to have a tooth pulled, be sure to come to the Centre the day before. Your blood will be checked, and you will be given the correct amount of vitamin K_1 to protect you against unusual bleeding.
8. If you have to undergo an operation, be sure to inform the Centre well in advance, because special measures must be taken to make certain that the wound will heal normally.
9. If you are ever admitted to a hospital, inform the Centre or have someone do this for you. Inform the hospital staff that you are on anticoagulant therapy.
10. If you stop taking the tablets and thus terminate the anticoagulant prophylaxis, please ask your doctor for written notification and bring it with you when you come to the Centre for the last time.
11. It is important to notify the Centre of any change in your address, telephone number, health insurance, and other personal data.
12. Please inform the Centre in advance if you plan to go away on a trip or vacation.

* From the Dutch Thrombosis Center, with permission.

future for the easier assessment of prothrombin times.

A leaflet describing rules for patients on long-term anticoagulant therapy has been prepared by Dutch Thrombosis Centers and this is printed on the back of the daily-dosage calendar as a constant reminder (Table 7–2).[4]

So-Called Warfarin Resistance

Patients receiving liquid food preparations may develop an acquired coumarin resistance due to the vitamin K_1 content of the food, which amounts to more than 1.5 milligram/1,000 kilogram (6.3 milligram/1,000 kilocalories).[25–28] The same holds for some liquid nutrition preparations available in health food stores and used in hypoalimentation or weight-reduction programs (Table 7–3).[29] It seems also that avocado antagonizes warfarin, although its content in vitamin K is low.[30]

DRUG INTERFERENCE WITH HEPARIN

The Heparin Action Influenced by Other Drugs

A large number of drugs inhibit platelet aggregation, and these agents, if given simultaneously with heparin, should be used cautiously. This is particularly true for aspirin, ticlopidine, and nonsteroidal anti-inflammatory compounds; some of the latter are available in the United States without a prescription (Table 7–4).

Because of the formation of relatively insoluble complexes, heparin should not be mixed in the infusion fluid with most antibiotics (for example, penicillin, tetracycline, erythromycin) and a number of psychotropic drugs (for example, chlordiazepoxide, chlorpromazine). It is wise not to mix heparin with fat emulsions, in order to avoid the risk of flocculation. Also, the mixing of dobutamine hydrochloride and heparin causes precipitation.

Propyleneglycol-induced heparin resistance during nitroglycerin (glyceryl trinitrate) infusion has been reported at doses used in coronary care units.[31] The prolongation of coagulation tests is decreased by approximately 50 per cent. It is important to note that most commercial nitroglycerin preparations are diluted in alcohol and propyleneglycol, and under intensive care conditions this interaction could be clinically significant.

Effect of Heparin on the Action of Other Drugs

Reduction of digitoxin binding to plasma proteins has been reported after administration of heparin.[32] The artifactual increase of as much as 50 per cent in total thyroxine (T_4), estimated by a competitive protein-binding assay, and of as much as 30 per cent in triiodothyronine (T_3) resin uptake are in all probability the results of rapid and continuing lipolytic hydrolysis of triglycerides after blood has been drawn. Thyroid function tests

TABLE 7–3. The Vitamin K Content of Some Common Foods and Beverages

<1.0 MICROGRAMS/ 100 GRAMS	1–10 MICROGRAMS/ 100 GRAMS	10–50 MICROGRAMS/ 100 GRAMS	50–100 MICROGRAMS/ 100 GRAMS	>100 MICROGRAMS/ 100 GRAMS
Canned pears	Peanut oil	Sunflower oil	Olive oil	Soya bean oil
Banana	Corn oil	Sesame oil	Liver (beef)	Rape seed oil
Orange	Safflower oil	"Vegetable" oil	Cauliflower	Broccoli
Apple (no peel)	Apple (with peel)	Pumpkin	Asparagus	Cabbage
Potatoes	Blueberries	Mustard	Watercress	Spinach
Onions	Cranberries	Cheese		Lettuce
Black tea	Tomatoes	Butter		Brussels sprouts
Orange juice	Sweet potatoes	Liver (pork,		Turnip greens
Apple juice	Squash	chicken)		Kale
Grapefruit juice	Whole wheat flour	Eggs		Chewing tobacco
Cranberry juice	Milk	Green beans		
Lemonade	Corn	Peas		
Ginger ale	Carrots	Oats		
Cola	Peaches			
Vinegar	Corn flakes cereal			
Lemon extract	Rice Krispies cereal			
Vanilla extract				
Almond extract				
Brewed coffee				
Honey				
Salt				
Sugar				
Peanut butter				
Graham crackers				
White flour				
Egg white				
White rice				
Brown rice				
White pasta				
Chicken breast				
Lean pork				
Lean ground beef				

TABLE 7–4. Drug Interference with Heparin

1. The risk of bleeding increases when full-dose heparin is combined with aspirin, ticlopidine, or nonsteroidal anti-inflammatory compounds.
2. Heparin should not be mixed in the infusion fluid with most antibiotics, some psychotropic drugs, and fat emulsions.
3. Blood for thyroid function should be taken before or a sufficient time after heparin treatment.
4. Heparin increases the concentration of free diazepam.

should therefore always be performed in blood samples taken before (or a sufficient time after) heparin treatment.[33]

Heparin increases the concentration of free diazepam and of its active metabolite (N-desmethyldiazepam). The clinical relevance of this effect is not clear, but could be of importance when heparin is used in some surgical situations.[34]

There is evidence that intravenous administration of tobramycin or gentamicin via the device used for the infusion of heparin reduces the antibacterial action of these antibiotics.[35]

REFERENCES

1. Breckenridge A, Orme M, Davis DS. Kinetics of warfarin absorption in man. Clin Pharmacol Ther 1973; 14: 955–61.
2. Breckenridge A. Oral anticoagulant drugs. Semin Haematol 1978; 15: 19–26.
3. Koch-Weser J, Sellers EM. Drug interactions with coumarin anticoagulants. N Engl J Med 1971; 285: 547–58.
4. Loeliger EA, Van Dijk-Wierda CA, Van Den Besselaer AMHP, Broekmans AW, Roos J. Anticoagulant control and the risk of bleeding. In: Meade TW, ed. Anticoagulants and myocardial infarction: a reappraisal. Chichester: John Wiley and Sons, 1984: 135–77.
5. Wintzen AR, de Jonghe H, Loeliger EA, Bots GTAM. The risk of intracerebral hemorrhage during oral anticoagulant treatment: a population study. Ann Neurol 1984; 16: 553–8.
6. MacLeod SM, Sellers EM. Pharmacodynamic and pharmacokinetic drug interactions with coumarin anticoagulants. Drugs 1976; 11: 461–70.
7. The British Society for Haematology. The guidelines on oral anticoagulation. 2nd Ed. J Clin Pathol 1990; 43: 177–83.
8. Serlin MJ, Breckenridge AM. Drug interactions with warfarin. Drugs 1983; 25: 610–20.
9. Loeliger EA. Drugs affecting blood coagulation and hae-

mostasis. In: Dukes MNG, Ellis J, eds. Side effect of drugs. Annual 8. Amsterdam, New York, Oxford: Elsevier, 1984: 327–32.

10. Loeliger EA. Drugs affecting blood coagulation and haemostasis. In: Dukes MNG, Beeley L, eds. Side effects of drugs. Annual 9. Amsterdam, New York, Oxford: Elsevier, 1985: 302–10.

11. Verstraete M, Broekmans AW. Drugs affecting blood coagulation and haemostasis. In: Dukes MNG, Beeley L, eds. Side effects of drugs. Annual 10. Amsterdam, New York, Oxford: Elsevier, 1986: 310–22.

12. Verstraete M, Broekmans AW. Drugs affecting blood coagulation and haemostasis. In: Dukes MNG, Beeley L, eds. Side effects of drugs. Annual 11. Amsterdam, New York, Oxford: Elsevier, 1987: 316–20.

13. Verstraete M, Vermylen J. Drugs affecting blood coagulation and haemostasis. In: Dukes MNG, Beeley L, eds. Side effects of drugs. Annual 12. Amsterdam, New York, Oxford: Elsevier, 1988: 309–15.

14. Loeliger EA, Broekmans AW. Drugs affecting blood coagulation and haemostasis. In: Dukes MNG, Meyler S, eds. Side effects of drugs. Amsterdam, New York, Oxford: Elsevier, 1988: 733–75.

15. Sax MJ, Sawyer WT. Warfarin interactions with cimetidine and randidine: a critical analysis of the literature. Adv Ther 1988; 5: 153–67.

16. Almog S, Martinowitz U, Halkin M, Bank HZ, Farbel Z. Complex interaction of rifampicin and warfarin. South Med J 1988; 81: 1304–6.

17. Weifert RT, Lorentz S, Towsend RJ, Cook CE, Klauber MR, Jagger PI. Effect of erythromycin in patients receiving long-term warfarin therapy. Clin Pharmacol 1989; 8: 210–4.

17. Tenni P, Lalich DL, Byrne MJ. Life-threatening interaction between tamoxifin and warfarin. Br Med J 1989; 298: 93–5.

19. O'Donnell D. Antibiotic-induced potentiation of oral anticoagulant agents. Med J Aust 1989; 150: 163–4.

20. Caraco Y, Chajek-Shaul T. Incidence and clinical significance of amiodarone and acenocoumarol interaction. Thromb Haemost 1989; 62: 906–8.

21. Shulman S, Henricksson K. Interaction of ibuprofen and warfarin on primary haemostasis. Br J Rheumatol 1989; 28: 46–9.

22. Yeh J, Soo SC, Summerton C, Richardson C. Potentiation of action of warfarin by itraconazole. Br Med J 1990; 301: 669.

23. Vermylen J, Vanhove PH, Verstraete M. Drugs affecting blood coagulation and haemostasis. In: Dukes MNG, Beeley L, eds. Side effect of drugs. Annual 14. Amsterdam, New York, Oxford: Elsevier, 1990: 309–13.

24. Speight TM. Avery's drug treatment. Principles and practice of clinical pharmacology and therapeutics. 3rd ed. ADIS Press, 1987: 977.

25. Broekmans AW, Mulder CJ. Coumarine-resistentie en vitamine K_1. Ned Tijdschr Geneeskd 1981; 125: 1974–5.

26. Watson AJM, Pegg M, Green JR. Enteral feeds may antagonise warfarin. Br Med J 1984; 288: 357–61.

27. Kalra PA, Cooklin M, Wood G, O'Shea GM, Holmes AM. Dietary modification as cause of anticoagulant instability. Lancet 1988; ii: 803–5.

28. Sadowski JA, Bovill EG, Mann KG. Warfarin and the metabolism and function of vitamin K. In: Poller L, ed. Blood coagulation. Recent advances (NR 6). New York: Churchill Livingstone, 1991: 93–118.

29. Michaelson R, Kempin SJ, Navia B, et al. Inhibition of the hypoprothrombinemic effect of warfarin (coumadin) by Ensure Plus, a dietary supplement. Clin Bull 1980; 10: 171–2.

30. Blickstein D, Shaklai M, Inbal A. Warfarin antagonism by avocado. Lancet 1991; 337: 914–5.

31. Col J, Col-Debeys C, Lavenne-Pardonge E, et al. Propylene-glycol-induced heparin resistance during nitroglycerin infusion. Am Heart J 1985; 110: 171–3.

32. Lohman JJHM, Hooymans PM, Koten MLP, et al. Effect on digitoxin protein binding. Clin Pharmacol Ther 1985; 37: 55–60.

33. Wilkens TA, Midgley JEM, Giles AF. Treatment with heparin and results for free thyroxin. An in vivo or an in vitro effect? Clin Chem 1980; 28: 2441–2.

34. Routledge PA, Kitchell BB, Bjornsson TD, Skinner T, Linnoila M, Shand DG. Diazepam and N-desmethyldiazepam redistribution after heparin. Clin Pharmacol Ther 1980; 27: 528–32.

35. Yourassowski E, De Broe M, Vanderlinden MP, Monsieur R. The influence of heparin on the bactericidal activity rate of gentamicin. Pathol Biol 1974; 22: 389–90.

8

OPTIMAL THERAPEUTIC RANGES FOR UNFRACTIONATED HEPARIN AND LOW MOLECULAR WEIGHT HEPARINS

JACK HIRSH

HEPARIN
(See also Chapter 6)

Commercial heparin is heterogeneous with molecular weights ranging from 3,000 to 30,000 (mean 15,000) daltons. Only about one third of heparin binds to antithrombin III (AT III) and this fraction is responsible for most of its anticoagulant effect.[1,2] The remaining two thirds of the heparin has minimal anticoagulant activity at therapeutic concentrations, but at high concentrations (greater than usually obtained clinically) it catalyzes the antithrombin effect of a second plasma protein cofactor named heparin cofactor II (HC-II).[3]

Heparin binds to platelets in vitro, and depending on the experimental conditions, can either induce or inhibit platelet aggregation.[4,5] High molecular weight heparin fractions with low affinity for antithrombin III have a greater effect on platelet function than low molecular weight (LMW) heparin fractions with high affinity for antithrombin III.[6] Heparin prolongs the bleeding time in man[7] and enhances blood loss from the microcirculation in rabbits.[8-10] The interaction of heparin with platelets[8] and endothelial cells[9] may contribute to heparin-induced bleeding by a mechanism which is independent of its anticoagulant effect.[10]

In addition to its anticoagulant effects, heparin increases vessel wall permeability,[9] and suppresses the proliferation of vascular smooth muscle cells[11] through binding sites which are independent of its anticoagulant activity.[12]

Heparin/antithrombin III inactivates a number of coagulation enzymes including thrombin, activated factors X, XII, XI, and IX;[13] of these, thrombin and activated factor X are most responsive to inhibition, and human thrombin is more responsive to inhibition by heparin/antithrombin III complex than activated factor X by about one order of magnitude.[3,13] For inhibition of thrombin, heparin must bind to both the coagulation enzyme and antithrombin III, but binding to the enzyme is not required for the inhibition of activated factor X (fXa).[14] Molecules of heparin with fewer than 18 saccharides are unable to bind to thrombin and antithrombin III simultaneously and, therefore, cannot catalyze thrombin inhibition. In contrast, very small heparin fragments (containing as few as six saccharides) which contain the high-affinity pentasaccharide sequence are able to catalyze the inhibition of activated factor X by antithrombin III.[15-18] The reaction most responsive to the inhibitory effect of heparin on coagulation is the inhibition of thrombin-induced activation of factor V and factor VIII.[19-21]

Administration and Pharmacokinetics

Heparin is poorly absorbed from the gastrointestinal tract and is administrated by intravenous or subcutaneous injection. When heparin is added to plasma in vitro, or when it is administered in vivo, it binds to many plasma proteins including vitronectin,[22] histidine-rich glycoprotein,[23] and fibronectin, which limits its access to antithrombin III and results in a variable loss of recovered anticoagulant activity. The recovery of fixed concentrations of heparin to the plasma of sick hospitalized patients and patients with venous thrombosis is considerably less (50 per cent of expected) than in healthy controls.[24] The addition of heparin with no affinity to antithrombin III results in an unmasking of heparin in the patient plasma, probably because the no-affinity heparin displaces the anticoagulantly active heparin from binding proteins, and so makes it available for binding to antithrombin III.[24] The pharmacokinetics of heparin are not completely understood, and data are limited to studies in experimental animals and healthy volunteers.[25-28] The volume of distribution and/or clearance of heparin in sick patients with thromboembolism could differ from healthy controls, and these differences could account for the variability in anticoagulant response in patients with thrombosis. After an intravenous injection into healthy volunteers, there is a rapid phase of elimination owing to equilibration, followed by a more gradual disappearance best explained as a combination of a saturable and a first order mechanism of clearance.[25,26] The saturable phase of clearance is much more rapid than the nonsaturable phase which follows first order kinetics. Because of these kinetics, the anticoagulant response to heparin at therapeutic doses is not linear, but the anticoagulant effect increases disproportionally both in its intensity and duration with increasing dose.[25,26] Thus, the apparent biological half-life of heparin increases from approximately 30 minutes with an intravenous bolus of 25 units/kilogram, to 60 minutes with an intravenous bolus of 100 units/kilogram, to 150 minutes with a bolus of 400 units/kilogram (Table 8–1).[27,28]

TABLE 8–1. Effect of Heparin Dosage on Apparent Biological Half-Life

DOSE OF HEPARIN UNITS/ KILOGRAM (70 KILOGRAMS)	HALF-LIFE (MINUTES)	AUTHOR
25 (1,750)	30	Bjornsson[28]
75 (5,250)	60	Bjornsson[28]
100 (7,000)	56	Olsson[27]
400 (28,000)	152	Olsson[27]

The saturable phase of heparin clearance is thought to be the result of heparin binding to receptors on endothelial cells and macrophages where it is internalized, depolymerized, and metabolized into smaller and less sulfated forms.[25] The interaction of heparin with endothelial cells in vivo also results in the displacement of platelet factor 4, a heparin neutralizing protein[29] which is capable of inactivating circulating heparin. Results of animal experiments indicate that the capacity of the cellular mechanism to clear heparin is restored rapidly after heparin disappears from the blood.[25] A plausible explanation for these findings is that heparin bound to cell surface receptors is internalized, thereby freeing up cell surface receptors to bind more circulating heparin and so providing a renewable site for rapid removal of subsaturating concentrations of heparin from the plasma. When heparin is administered in progressively increasing doses which exceed the saturating concentration, an increased proportion is cleared by the slower nonsaturable (possibly renal) mechanism. This proposed mechanism of heparin clearance explains why at a steady state, low doses of heparin do not produce measurable heparin levels[26] and why with increasing doses over a dose range of 0 to 30,000 units of heparin/ 24 hours by continuous infusion, the recovered anticoagulant effect of heparin does not increase in a linear manner with dose but rather increases disproportionally with increasing dose. This proposed mechanism also provides an explanation for the poor bioavailability of even moderate doses of heparin (20,000 units/24 hours) administered by subcutaneous injection. Thus, as heparin gradually enters the blood system from subcutaneous depots, it binds cell surface receptors and is internalized at a speed which exceeds its rate of entry into the circulation. Even at relatively high doses administered subcutaneously, the plasma recovery of heparin is reduced. Thus, studies in patients with venous thrombosis have shown that at doses of 30,000 units/24 hours (after 5,000 units intravenous bolus), the recovered anticoagulant effect of heparin administered by subcutaneous injection (in two divided doses) is significantly less than when administered by the continuous intravenous route.[30] Even when administered in a dose of 35,000 units/24 hours, the plasma recovery of heparin is significantly less when administered by the subcutaneous route (12 hourly) than when administered intravenously.[31]

In summary, the proposed model of pharmacokinetics of heparin provides an explanation for some of the puzzling observations associated with heparin usage. Thus, the marked variability in dosage requirements among patients treated with heparin can be explained in part by differences in the concentrations of heparin binding proteins and, in part, by the variability in heparin clearance among patients. Since some heparin binding proteins are acute phase reactions, heparin binding to these might explain the resistance to heparin seen in sick patients with inflammatory and malignant disorders. The poor bioavailability of low doses of heparin is also contributed to by its rapid clearance by a renewable cellular clearance mechanism which is not fully saturated even at doses of 10,000 to 15,000 units/24 hours administered for six hours by continuous infusion.[26] The bioavailability of heparin administered by the subcutaneous route is reduced (compared to intravenous administration) because the gradual entry of heparin into the circulation does not keep pace with the clearance of heparin from the plasma by the saturable clearance mechanism. This also explains the delay in reaching steady-state heparin levels when heparin is administered by subcutaneous injection 12 hourly even at a dose of 30,000 to 35,000 units/24 hours,[30,31] and why the dosage requirement for subcutaneous heparin to achieve therapeutic heparin concentrations (0.2 to 0.4 units/milliliter by protamine titration) is approximately 10 to 15 per cent higher than when heparin is administered by intravenous infusion.[31]

The elimination of heparin from plasma is accelerated in clinical and experimental acute pulmonary embolism[32,33] by a mechanism which is poorly understood. There is no evidence that the pharmacokinetics or the anticoagulant properties of heparins derived from porcine or bovine sources, or prepared as sodium or calcium salts are different. There are reports that intravenous nitroglycerine may increase heparin dosage requirements acutely,[34,35] but interaction was not seen in a randomized crossover study using relatively low doses of nitroglycerin.[36] This potential interaction deserves further study.[37]

The anticoagulant effect of heparin is modified by platelets, fibrin, vascular surfaces, and plasma proteins. Platelets inhibit the anticoagulant effect of heparin by binding activated factor X and protecting it from inactivation by the heparin/antithrombin III complex[38,39] and by secreting the heparin-neutralizing protein, platelet factor 4.[40] Fibrin binds thrombin and protects it from inactivation by heparin/antithrombin III complex.[41,42] In plasma, much higher concentrations of heparin are needed to inactivate fibrin-bound thrombin than free thrombin.[41] In contrast, fibrin-bound thrombin is not protected from inactivation by antithrombin III-independent thrombin inhibitors such as hirudin or hirudin fragments,[41] an observation which might explain why heparin is less effective than hirudin in preventing the formation of experimental arterial thrombosis[43] and in preventing the extension of experimental venous thrombosis.[44] The relative resistance of fibrin-bound thrombin to inhibition by heparin could also explain why higher concentrations of heparin are required to prevent extension of venous thrombosis than to prevent its formation[45] and why heparin fails to inhibit thrombin activity in some patients after successful coronary thrombolysis.[46–48] Thrombin bound to subendothelial surfaces is also protected from inactivation by heparin,[49] possibly through mechanisms which are similar to those that protect fibrin-bound thrombin.

Monitoring Heparin Treatment

Heparin therapy is usually monitored to maintain its anticoagulant effect within a defined range in order to limit recurrence and extension of thrombosis while minimizing the risk of bleeding. This range is commonly referred to as the therapeutic range. The concept of a therapeutic range for the control of heparin therapy has been validated by studies in animals and by results from clinical trials in patients with venous thrombosis[30,50] and acute myocardial infarction.[51-53] The need for monitoring heparin therapy adds to the expense and complexity of heparin treatment because the dosage requirements differ among patients and can differ within patients during their course of treatment. The causes for this variability are unknown, but are likely to be contributed to by variations in levels of heparin-binding proteins (which compete with antithrombin III for heparin binding), the proportion of the administered dose cleared by the more rapid saturable phase of clearance, and the concentration of coagulation factors which affect the relationship between heparin levels and anticoagulant response (see later). Heparin monitoring was performed initially by the whole blood clotting time. A whole blood clotting time (WBCT) of twice control was selected as the therapeutic range based on studies in the 1950s by Wessler examining the effect of heparin on experimental jugular vein thrombi in rabbits.[54] Because of its imprecision and inconvenience, the whole blood clotting time was replaced by activated partial thromboplastin time (APTT).[55-58] In comparative in vitro studies on heparinized blood, a whole blood clotting time of two to three times control was found to be equivalent to an activated partial thromboplastin time ratio (patients activated partial thromboplastin time/mean laboratory activated partial thromboplastin time) of 1.5 to 2.5.[59] Unfortunately, because of the lack of standardization, the activated partial thromboplastin time in its present form is far from ideal as a test for monitoring heparin therapy because its responsiveness (sensitivity) to heparin varies considerably among different activated partial thromboplastin time reagents[59] and even among different batches of the same brand of activated partial thromboplastin time reagent.[60] Various technical factors influence the responsiveness of activated partial thromboplastin time reagent to heparin including: (a) the type of contact activator (reagents using ellagic acid are less sensitive than kaolin-derived reagents);[61] (b) the buffering capacity and the phospholipid composition of the reagent;[62] and (c) the method of clot detection including the use of automated procedures.[63] As a consequence of this variability, it is inappropriate to compare the results obtained when heparin is monitored by different activated partial thromboplastin time reagents.[60] The situation is complicated further because the relationship between the activated partial thromboplastin time result and heparin levels obtained on control plasma when increasing doses of heparin is added in vitro may not reflect the relationship obtained when heparin is added in vitro to plasma of patients with thrombosis, and does not correspond to the relationship obtained on ex vivo samples when the activated partial thromboplastin time and heparin assays are performed on plasma obtained from patients who are being treated with heparin.[64,65] Standardization can be obtained within laboratories by establishing a relationship between the activated partial thromboplastin time ratio and heparin levels on plasma obtained from heparinized patients over a wide range of values and by comparing each new batch of reagent with the previous batch. If the curves describing the relationship between the heparin level and the activated partial thromboplastin time results obtained with the new batch and previous batch are parallel over the therapeutic range, a correction factor can be applied to avoid the confusion of changing the therapeutic range of the activated partial thromboplastin time ratio every time the batch of activated partial thromboplastin time reagent is changed. At the Hamilton District Laboratory Program, which serves the hospitals affiliated with McMaster University, we purchase a new batch of reagent from the same manufacturer every two years and have had to standardize each new reagent against the expiring batch to avoid confusing the clinicians by changing the recommended therapeutic range every time a new batch is obtained.

Dosing Considerations

The mean dose of heparin required to produce an activated partial thromboplastin time of 1.5 to 2.5 times control (heparin level by protamine titration of 0.2 to 0.4 units/milliliter) and by anti-Xa assay of 0.35 to 0.7 units/milliliter is approximately 32,000 units/24 hours when heparin is administered by continuous intravenous infusion, and 35,000 units/24 hours when it is administered by subcutaneous injection 12 hourly. For continuous intravenous infusion, the heparin effect should be measured six hours after the bolus injection and then six hourly until a stable dose response is obtained.[66] For subcutaneous heparin, the heparin effect should be measured daily six hours after injection. Approximately 30 per cent of patients with thrombosis require higher doses of heparin to achieve an activated partial thromboplastin time result in the therapeutic range. The mechanism of heparin resistance in these patients is not fully understood. In some (approximately a third of heparin resistant patients), the circulating heparin level is in the therapeutic range but the activated partial thromboplastin time is below the therapeutic range. These patients have circulating procoagulants which shorten the pretreatment of the activated partial thromboplastin time and inhibit its prolongation by heparin. Preliminary results of a randomized study suggest that it is safe to monitor these patients by heparin assay. The remaining two thirds of patients are truly heparin resistant. Some have high concentrations of heparin-binding proteins which compete with antithrombin III for binding, while others may have an increased rate of heparin clearance.

Clinical Use of Heparin

Heparin is effective in the prevention and treatment of venous thrombosis and pulmonary embolism, in the prevention of mural thrombosis after myocardial infarction, in the treatment of patients with unstable angina and acute myocardial infarct, and in the prevention of coronary artery rethrombosis after thrombolysis.

As noted above, the anticoagulant response to heparin varies widely among patients with thromboembolic disease, and the clinical efficacy of heparin is optimized if the anticoagulant effect is maintained in a therapeutic range.[30,67] For these reasons, heparin treatment is usually monitored to maintain the activated partial thromboplastin time test equivalent to a heparin level of 0.2 to 0.4 U/ml by protamine titration or an anti-Xa level of 0.35 to 0.7 units/milliliter. For many activated partial thromboplastin time reagents this is equivalent to a ratio (test/lab control activated partial thromboplastin time) of 1.5 to 2.5, referred to as the therapeutic range. The recommended therapeutic range[30,50] is supported by evidence from animal studies[68] and by subgroup analysis of prospective cohort studies of the treatment of deep vein thrombosis, of the prevention of mural thrombosis after myocardial infarction, and in the prevention of recurrent ischemia following coronary thrombolysis (Table 8–2).[52,53] The heparin regimens which have been shown to be effective in trials of venous and arterial thrombosis are summarized in Table 8–3.

LOW MOLECULAR WEIGHT HEPARINS
(See also Chapter 6)

Interest in low molecular weight heparins (LMWHs) as potential antithrombotic agents was stimulated by two observations in the mid 1970s and early 1980s. The first was the finding by Johnson and associates[69] and Andersson and associates,[2] that low molecular weight heparin fractions prepared from standard unfractionated heparin (SH) progressively lose their ability to prolong the activated partial thromboplastin time while retaining their ability to inhibit activated factor X. The second was the observation that low molecular weight heparins produce less bleeding

TABLE 8–2. Relationship Between Failure to Reach Lower Limit of Therapeutic Range and Thromboembolic Events from Subgroup Analysis of Prospective Studies

STUDY	TYPE OF PATIENTS	OUTCOME	NUMBER	RELATIVE RISK
Hull, et al.[30]	DVT	Recurrent VTE	115	15.0
Basu, et al.[50]	DVT	Recurrent VTE	157	10.7
Turpie, et al.[51]	AMI	LVMT	112	22.2*
Kaplan, et al.[52]	AMI	Recurrent MI/AP	75	6.0†
Camilleri, et al.[53]	AMI	Recurrent MI/AP	70	13.3

* Estimated by assuming a normal distribution of the reported heparin levels.
† Kaplan used a partial thromboplastin time measurement and reported the relative risk associated with partial thromboplastin time values less than 50 seconds compared with partial thromboplastin time values of more than 100 seconds.
DVT = deep vein thrombosis, AMI = acute myocardial infarction, LVMT = left ventricular mural thrombosis, AP = angina pectoris.

TABLE 8–3. Clinical Use of Heparin

CONDITION	RECOMMENDATIONS
Venous thromboembolism	
Prophylaxis of DVT + PE	5,000 units SC 12 hourly or 8 hourly or adjusted low-dose heparin*
Treatment of DVT	5,000 units IV bolus followed by 30,000 to 35,000 units/24 hours by IV infusion or 35,000 to 40,000 units/24 hours SC adjusted to maintain APTT at 1.5 to 2.5 times control†
Coronary heart disease	
Unstable angina and acute myocardial infarction (including post-thrombolytic therapy)	5,000 units IV bolus followed by 24,000 units/24 hours IV infusion adjusted to maintain APTT at 1.5 to 2.5 times control†

* 3,500 units heparin SC 8 hourly adjusted to an APTT in upper normal range.
† Equivalent to heparin level of 0.2 to 0.4 units/milliliter by protamine titration or an anti-Xa level of 0.35 to 0.7 units/milliliter
SC = subcutaneous, IV = intravenous, APTT = activated partial thromboplastin time, DVT = deep vein thrombosis, PE = pulmonary embolism.

in experimental models for an equivalent antithrombotic effect than the standard unfractionated heparins from which they are derived.[70]

The clinical effectiveness and safety of low molecular weight heparin has now been demonstrated. Low molecular weight heparins are effective when used for the prevention or treatment of venous thrombosis, have better bioavailability and a longer plasma half-life than standard unfractionated heparin, and are more effective than standard low-dose heparin in preventing venous thrombosis after hip surgery or stroke, and for equal efficacy, produce less bleeding than standard unfractionated heparins in animal models and in patients after hip surgery.

Production of Low Molecular Weight Heparins

The low molecular weight heparins in clinical use are produced from standard unfractionated heparin by depolymerization into low molecular weight fragments with mean molecular weight −5,000 (Table 8–1).[71] All of these low molecular weight heparins contain the unique pentasaccharide required for binding to antithrombin III, but in lower proportions than the standard unfractionated heparin from which they have been derived. Two heparinoids are also being evaluated clinically. These are dermatan sulfate and lomoparan (ORG 10172), which is a mixture of heparan sulfate, dermatan sulfate, and chondroitin sulfate.

Depolymerization invariably leads to partial loss of the original catalytic activity, with the ability to catalyze thrombin inhibition decreasing more rapidly than the ability to catalyze activated factor X inhibition.[71] Nonetheless, low molecular weight heparins probably achieve their antithrombotic and anticoagulant effects by the same mechanisms as standard unfractionated heparin (see later).[71–73]

Anticoagulant Effects and Low Molecular Weight Heparins

Like heparin, low molecular weight heparins increase the rate at which antithrombin III forms inactive complexes with coagulation enzymes.[74] After complexing with these coagulation enzymes, antithrombin III is cleaved at the reactive bond.[75–78] Low molecular weight heparins catalyze thrombin inhibition less efficiently than standard unfractionated heparin; the difference between the catalytic action of heparin on activated factor X and thrombin inhibition is inversely proportional to the molecular weight of the glycosaminoglycans. Low molecular weight heparin also catalyzes activated factor X inhibition slightly less efficiently than standard unfractionated heparin. The slightly greater activity of high molecular weight heparin for activated factor X inhibition may reflect the presence of two antithrombin-binding sites in these long polysaccharide chains,[79,80] or some other unknown mechanism(s). At least 18 saccharide units are required by heparin molecules to inactivate thrombin. The requirement for an additional sequence of 13 saccharide units over and above the unique pentasaccharide sequence to obtain acceleration of the antithrombin-thrombin reaction reflects the need for the glycosaminoglycan to bind to the thrombin molecule by nonspecific electrostatic interaction while the inhibition of the enzyme by antithrombin III is facilitated by the conformational change induced in antithrombin by binding to the high affinity pentasaccharide.[15,81-83] A chemically synthesized high-affinity pentasaccharide containing only the antithrombin-binding sequence of heparin accelerates the inhibition of activated factor X by antithrombin to nearly the same extent as standard unfractionated heparin.[84]

Low molecular weight heparins also prolong the activated partial thromboplastin time to a lesser extent than standard unfractionated heparin.[85-87] Some studies suggest that low molecular weight heparins catalyze activated factor X inhibition within the prothrombinase complex less efficiently than standard unfractionated heparin,[87] while others have reported that some low molecular weight heparins are more effective than standard unfractionated heparin in inhibiting thrombin formation in platelet-rich plasma (see later).[88] Low molecular weight heparins of a chain length less than 18 saccharide units are resistant to neutralization with platelet factor 4, becoming progressively more resistant to neutralization with decreasing molecular size.[16] Similarly, the neutralizing activity of protamine sulfate is influenced by the heparin chain length, since anti-Xa activity of low molecular weight heparins is not completely neutralized by protamine.

The mean molecular weight of most commercial low molecular weight heparins ranges from 4,000 to 6,000 (13 to 20 saccharide units) daltons. Since the molecular weight distribution of low molecular weight heparins differs among the different commercial preparations, and a variable proportion of these preparations is made up of fragments of 18 or more oligosaccharide units, these fragments are able to catalyze the inhibition of thrombin (FrIIa) by antithrombin III. As a consequence of this heterogeneity in molecular size distribution, the various commercial low molecular weight heparins have different ratios of anti-IIa to anti-Xa activity and, therefore, have different profiles of anticoagulant activity. Thus, if the ratio of anti-Xa:anti-IIa activity of standard unfractionated heparin is defined as 1:1, then the ratio of activities of the various low molecular weight heparins varies between 4:1 and 2:1.

Because of their different profiles of anti-IIa:anti-Xa activity, it is difficult to compare the anticoagulant potencies of the various low molecular weight heparins. An attempt has been made to overcome the problem by the development of an international low molecular weight heparin standard.[89,90] This standard has a specific activity of 168 international units anti-Xa/milligram and 68 international units anti-IIa/milligram (ratio anti-Xa/anti-IIa of 2.6). The international standard has shortcomings because its anti-Xa:anti-IIa ratio is not identical to all low molecular weight heparins,[91,92] nevertheless, it provides the most practical means of verifying the stated potency of batches of low molecular weight heparins.

Recent investigations indicate that despite their different profiles of anti-Xa to anti-IIa activity, like heparin, many low molecular weight heparins achieve their main anticoagulant effects in whole blood and plasma by inactivating activating factor II. Thus, using different experimental conditions, Beguin and Hemker,[88] and Ofosu and associates[71,73,87] monitored the concentrations of thrombin and activated factor X in clotting plasma and made the following observations: (a) in nonheparinized plasma, peak thrombin activity appears earlier than peak activated factor X activity, suggesting that only traces of activated factor X (too low to be detected by the assay system) are necessary to allow enough thrombin to form to activate factor V and factor VIII to produce an explosive burst of thrombin activity; (b) it is necessary to almost completely inhibit activated factor X in order to reduce thrombin formation through inhibition of prothrombinase; (c) the appearance of thrombin activity is delayed and the peak level of thrombin activity reduced by heparin and by the low molecular weight heparins tested; (d) most low molecular weight heparins are not different from standard unfractionated heparin in their relative abilities to inhibit thrombin activity and anti-Xa activity, although the low molecular weight heparin enoxaparin, has a greater ability to inhibit prothrombinase than standard unfractionated heparin; (e) that low molecular weight heparins are more effective than standard unfractionated heparin in inhibiting peak thrombin activity in platelet-rich plasma, possibly because low molecular weight heparins are less susceptible to inhibition by platelet factor 4 released from activated platelets; and (f) that it is possible to totally inhibit thrombin activity in recalcified plasma by low molecular weight heparins despite high residual concentrations of activated factor X activity.

Antithrombotic Effects of Low Molecular Weight Heparins in Experimental Animal Models

The antithrombotic effect of low molecular weight heparin, and heparinoids have been evaluated in experimental models of venous thrombosis. In these models, activation of blood coagulation is induced by the injection of serum, activated factor X, thrombin, or tissue factor.[70,93–95] Heparin, low molecular weight heparins, and dermatan sulfate are all effective in inhibiting thrombosis. On a weight-for-weight basis, standard unfractionated heparin is the most effective glycosaminoglycan, while low molecular weight heparins with a mean molecular weight of approximately 5,000 daltons are more effective than dermatan sulfate or heparan sulfate. When compared on a weight basis, unfractionated heparin is approximately twice as effective in preventing experimental venous thrombosis as the low molecular weight heparins. The effectiveness of these glycosaminoglycans as antithrombotic agents has also been investigated in experiments designed to simulate with a therapeutic model their ability to inhibit accretion of radioactive fibrin onto experimental jugular vein thrombi. On a weight-for-weight basis, standard unfractionated heparin is the most effective glycosaminoglycan. Low molecular weight heparins are more effective than dermatan sulfate or the heparinoid ORG 10172.[96,97]

Hemorrhagic Effects of Low Molecular Weight Heparins in Experimental Animal Models

A number of investigators have reported that low molecular weight heparin fractions are less hemorrhagic than standard unfractionated heparin for an equivalent antithrombotic activity,[70,93,98,99] while other investigators[100,101] have found that equivalent antithrombotic doses of some low molecular weight heparin fractions have similar hemorrhagic effects to standard unfractionated heparin. Differences in the degree of sulfation of the various low molecular weight

heparins may have contributed to the variations in hemorrhagic effects reported.[95] There is evidence that differences between the effects of standard unfractionated heparin and low molecular weight heparins on platelet aggregation may be responsible for the differences in the hemorrhagic properties of these glycosaminoglycans. Salzman and associates[6] were the first to report that low molecular weight heparin gave less enhancement of adenosine diphosphate-induced platelet aggregation than standard unfractionated heparin, and similar results have been reported by others. Our group reported marked differences on the effects of standard unfractionated heparin and a variety of low molecular weight heparins on collagen-induced platelet aggregation ex vivo at concentrations of the glycosaminoglycans which induced hemorrhagic effects. A good correlation was found between inhibition of platelet aggregation and bleeding induced by these glycosaminoglycans[8,95,102] suggesting that the observed association is causal. Another potential mechanism for the differences in hemorrhagic effects between standard unfractionated heparin and low molecular weight heparin have been suggested by Blajchman and associates.[9] These investigators reported that doses of standard unfractionated heparin which increase the bleeding time in rabbits also increase vessel permeability. In contrast to standard unfractionated heparin, similar doses of low molecular weight heparins had a markedly lesser effect on vascular permeability.[9] In their model, dermatan sulfate reduced the increased permeability produced by heparin.

Pharmacokinetics

The pharmacokinetics and bioavailability of low molecular weight heparins and standard unfractionated heparin are very different, possibly because of differences in their binding characteristics to plasma proteins and endothelial cells.

Low molecular weight heparins exhibit much less binding to plasma proteins and endothelial cells than standard unfractionated heparin and, therefore, have much better bioavailability at low doses, and a longer plasma half-life which is dose independent. Unlike standard unfractionated heparin, most of the administered low molecular weight heparin is excreted in the urine un-

TABLE 8–4. Plasma Half-Life of Low Molecular Weight Heparins and Standard Unfractionated Heparin*

| TYPE OF HEPARIN | DOSE | HALF-LIFE IN MINUTES | |
		Intravenous Administration	Subcutaneous Administration
Enoxaparin	25 milligrams	180	
	30 milligrams	129	
	40 milligrams		275
	60 milligrams	135	330
	75 milligrams		360
Standard unfractionated heparin	5,000 units	51	180
	5,000 units	35	177
KABI 2165	40 units/kilogram	126	
	60 units/kilogram	139	
Standard unfractionated heparin	5,000 units	57	
Fraxiparin	7,500 units		201
	18,750 units		214
Standard unfractionated heparin	5,000 units		141
LMN, NOVO	2,500–5,000 units		110

* Adapted from Bara L, Samama M, Acta Chir Scand 1990; 556:57–61, with permission.

changed and in an active form. The pharmacokinetics of low molecular weight heparin have been studied in man using measurements of biological and amidiolytic anti-Xa and anti-IIa activities. The half-life of anti-Xa activity is between three and four hours following intravenous injection (Table 8–4).[103–107]

Low molecular weight heparins are cleared principally by the renal route through a non–dose-dependent mechanism. Boneu and associates[25] observed that the biological half-life of low molecular weight heparin is prolonged in renal failure.

Clinical Potential of Low Molecular Weight Heparins

A number of different low molecular weight heparins have been approved for use in Europe and have been evaluated in North America. Because of their longer half-life than standard unfractionated heparin, low molecular weight heparins are effective in preventing venous thrombosis when administered by subcutaneous injection once daily. There is also increasing evidence that a number of low molecular weight heparins are effective for the treatment of venous thrombosis when using weight-adjusted dose regimens without laboratory monitoring.

The picture on safety of low molecular weight heparins, relative to placebo and standard unfractionated heparin was blurred initially by the early studies which reported a high incidence of bleeding with a number of low molecular weight heparins when they were administered in higher doses than are currently recommended. However, recent studies have shown that when used in more appropriate doses which are highly effective in preventing thrombosis, low molecular weight heparins are not associated with an increased risk of perioperative bleeding, even in patients who undergo hip surgery, and one recent study has shown that a low molecular weight heparin produced less bleeding than standard heparin for an equivalent antithrombotic effect.[108]

Primary Prophylaxis

Low molecular weight heparins have been evaluated for their ability to prevent venous thrombosis in general surgical patients, in medical patients (including stroke), and in patients who have undergone major orthopedic surgical procedures. In general surgical patients, low molecular weight heparins administered as a once daily dose subcutaneously have proven to be at least as effective as standard unfractionated heparin administered three times daily by subcutaneous injection.[109–114] Bleeding has been minimal with both forms of heparin. Studies in medical patients, although more limited, indicate that low molecular weight heparins are very effective in reducing the incidence of venous thrombosis in patients suffering from stroke,[11,79–119] and a recent study has shown that low molecular weight heparin is more effective than standard low-dose heparin.[119] Most clinical experience with low molecular weight heparins has been obtained following major orthopedic surgical procedures. Low molecular weight heparins are highly effective in reducing the incidence of venous thrombosis associated with elective total hip replacement,[108,120–127] spinal surgery,[128] surgery for hip fracture, and major knee surgery.[129] In these studies, low molecular weight heparins have proven to be more effective than placebo, standard low-dose heparin (5,000 units subcutaneously 8 hourly), dextran, and warfarin, and of equal efficacy to an adjusted-dose heparin regimen in which heparin is monitored to maintain the activated partial thromboplastin time in the upper normal range. Compared with placebo, the risk reduction with low molecular weight heparins is approximately 70 per cent in hip[120] and major knee surgery.[129] Compared to standard unfractionated heparin 5,000 subcutaneously 8 hourly, the risk reduction with low molecular weight heparins is approximately 50 per cent in hip surgery[122] and 70 per cent in stroke.[119] Low molecular weight heparins did not increase the incidence of clinically important bleeding in any of the placebo-controlled studies when used in currently recommended dosages. The dosage regimens that are recommended for prophylaxis with the different low molecular weight heparins are summarized in Table 8–5.

Treatment of Established Venous Thrombosis

Low molecular weight heparins have been compared to standard unfractionated heparin for the treatment of venous thrombosis in a number of relatively small studies. In all of these, the primary outcome measure was the change in thrombus size as determined by a second venogram performed approximately one week after starting treatment.[130–135] Low molecular weight heparins proved to be as least as effective as standard unfractionated heparin. The recommended dosage regimens for low molecular weight heparins are summarized in Table 8–5; these regimens are subject to change as more experience is obtained for this indication. Recent reports in small numbers of patients suggest that it might be feasible to administer out-of-hospital low molecular weight heparins for treatment of established deep vein thrombosis in selected patients.[136,137] The out-of-hospital use of low molecular weight heparins is facilitated by their longer plasma half-life (than standard unfractionated heparin) and a more predictable dose response than standard unfractionated heparin, possibly owing to their relative lack of binding to plasma and platelet proteins and to endothelial cells.

REFERENCES

1. Lam LH, Silbert JE, Rosenberg RD. The separation of active and inactive forms of heparin. Biochem Biophys Res Commun 1976; 69: 570–7.
2. Andersson LO, Barrowcliffe TW, Holmer E, Johnson EA, Sims GEC. Anticoagulant properties of heparin fractionated by affinity chromatography on matrix-bound antithrombin III and by gel filtration. Thromb Res 1976; 9: 575–83.
3. Ofosu FA, Modi GJ, Hirsh J, Buchanan M, Blajchman MA.

TABLE 8–5. Dosages of Low Molecular Weight Heparins Used in Clinical Studies

Type of LMWH	Prophylaxis DVT General Surgery	Prophylaxis DVT Orth. Surgery	Treatment of DVT
Enoxaparine (Lovenox)	20 milligrams OD SC	40 milligrams OD SC or 30 milligrams BID SC*	90 mg BID SC
Tedelparine (Fragmine)	2,500 international units OD SC	2,500 IU BID SC	120 anti-Xa IV/ kilogram BID SC
Logiparine	1,500 APTT units SC OD	35 international units/kilogram	—
Fraxiparine	7,500 units/IC OD SC	—	450 units anti-Xa IC/ kilogram OD SC

* Starting 12 to 24 hours postoperatively.
DVT = deep vein thrombosis, LMWH = low molecular weight heparin, SC = subcutaneous administration, OD = once daily, IC = between meals, BID = twice daily, APTT = activated partial thromboplastin time; IV = intravenously.

Mechanisms for inhibition of the generation of thrombin activity by sulfated polysaccharides. Ann NY Acad Sci 1986; 485: 41–55.

4. Eika C. Inhibition of thrombin-induced aggregation of human platelets in heparin. Scand J Haematol 1971; 8: 216–22.

5. Kelton JG, Hirsh J. Bleeding associated with antithrombotic therapy. Semin Hematol 1980; 17: 259–91.

6. Salzman EW, Rosenberg RD, Smith MH, Lindon JN, Favreau L. Effect of heparin and heparin fractions on platelet aggregation. J Clin Invest 1980; 65: 64–73.

7. Heiden D, Mielke CH, Rodvien R. Impairment by heparin of primary haemostasis and platelet (14C)5-hydroxytryptamine release. Br J Haematol 1977; 36: 427–36.

8. Fernandez F, Nguyen P, Van Ryn J, Ofosu FA, Hirsh J, Buchanan MR. Hemorrhagic doses of heparin and other glycosaminoglycans induce a platelet defect. Thromb Res 1986; 43: 491–5.

9. Blajchman MA, Young E, Ofosu FA. Effects of unfractionated heparin, dermatan sulfate and low molecular weight heparin on vessel wall permeability in rabbits. Ann NY Acad Sci 1989; 556: 245–53.

10. Ockelford PA, Carter CJ, Cerskus A, Smith CA, Hirsh J. Comparison of the in vivo hemorrhagic and antithrombotic effects of a low antithrombin III affinity heparin fraction. Thromb Res 1982; 27: 679–90.

11. Clowes AW, Karnovsky MJ. Suppression by heparin of smooth muscle cell proliferation in injured arteries. Nature 1977; 265: 625–6.

12. Castellot JJ, Favreau LV, Karnovsky MJ, Rosenberg RD. Inhibition of vascular smooth muscle cell growth by endothelial cell-derived heparin. Possible role of a platelet endoglycosidase. J Biol Chem 1982; 257: 11256–60.

13. Rosenberg RD. The heparin-antithrombin system: a natural anticoagulant mechanism. In: Colman RW, Hirsh J, Marder VJ, Salzman EW, eds. Hemostasis and thrombosis: basic principles and clinical practice. 2nd ed. Philadelphia: JB Lippincott Co, 1987:1373–92.

14. Casu B, Oreste P, Torri G, et al. The structure of heparin oligosaccharide fragments with high anti-(factor Xa) activity containing the minimal antithrombin III-binding sequence. Biochem J 1981; 197: 599–609.

15. Lindahl U, Thunberg L, Backstrom G, et al. Extension and structural variability of the antithrombin binding sequence in heparin. J Biol Chem 1984; 259: 12368–76.

16. Lane DA, Denton J, Flynn AM, et al. Anticoagulant activities of heparin oligosaccharides and their neutralization by platelet factor 4. Biochem J 1984; 218: 725–32.

17. Oosta GM, Gardner WT, Beeler DL, Rosenberg RD. Multiple functional domains of the heparin molecule. Proc Natl Acad Sci USA 1981; 78: 829–33.

18. Nesheim ME. A simple rate law that describes the kinetics of the heparin-catalyzed reaction between antithrombin III and thrombin. J Biol Chem 1983; 258: 14708–17.

19. Ofosu FA, Sie P, Modi GJ, et al. The inhibition of thrombin-dependent feedback reactions is critical to the expression of anticoagulant effects of heparin. Biochem J 1987; 243: 579–88.

20. Ofosu FA, Hirsh J, Esmon CT, et al. Unfractionated heparin inhibits thrombin-catalyzed amplification reactions of coagulation more efficiently than those catalyzed by factor Xa. Biochem J 1989; 257: 143–50.

21. Beguin S, Lindhout T, Hemker HC. The mode of action of heparin in plasma. Thromb Haemost 1988; 60: 457–62.

22. Preissner KT, Muller-Berghaus G. Neutralization and binding of heparin by S-protein/vitronectin in the inhibition of factor Xa by antithrombin III. J Biol Chem 1987; 262: 12247–53.

23. Lijnen HR, Hoylaerts M, Collen D. Heparin binding properties of human histidine-rich glycoprotein. Mechanism and role in the neutralization of heparin in plasma. J Biol Chem 1983; 258: 3803–8.

24. Young E, Petrowski P, Hirsh J. Glycosaminoglycans displace anticoagulantly-active heparin from plasma protein binding sites (abstr). Thromb Haemost 1991;65:933. Abst. #844.

25. Boneu B, Caranobe C, Cadroy Y, et al. Pharmacokinetic studies of standard unfractionated heparin, and low molecular weight heparins in the rabbit. Semin Thromb Hemost 1988; 14: 18–27.

26. De Swart CAM, Nijmeyer B, Roelofs JMM, Sixma JJ. Kinetics of intravenously administered heparin in normal humans. Blood 1982; 60: 1251–8.

27. Olsson P, Lagergren H, Ek S. The elimination from plasma of intravenous heparin. An experimental study on dogs and humans. Acta Med Scand 1963; 173: 619–30.

28. Bjornsson TO, Wolfram BS, Kitchell BB. Heparin kinetics determined by three assay methods. Clin Pharmacol Ther 1982; 31: 104–13.

29. Dawes J, Smith RC, Pepper DS. The release, distribution and clearance of human B-thromboglobulin and platelet factor 4. Thromb Res 1978; 12: 851–61.

30. Hull RD, Raskob GE, Hirsh J, et al. Continuous intravenous heparin compared with intermittent subcutaneous heparin in the initial treatment of proximal-vein thrombosis. N Engl J Med 1986; 315: 1109–14.

31. Pini M, Pattacini C, Quintavalla R, et al. Subcutaneous vs intravenous heparin in the treatment of deep venous thrombosis—A randomized clinical trial. Thromb Haemost 1990; 64: 222–6.

32. Hirsh J, van Aken WG, Gallus AS, Dollery CT, Cade JF, Yung WG. Heparin kinetics in venous thrombosis and pulmonary embolism. Circulation 1976; 53: 691–5.

33. Chui HM, van Aken WG, Hirsh J, Regoeczi E, Horner AA. Increased heparin clearance in experimental pulmonary embolism. J Lab Clin Med 1977; 90: 204–15.

34. Habbab MA, Haft JI. Heparin resistance induced by intravenous nitroglycerin. Circulation 1986; 74(suppl II): 321.

35. Pizzulli L, Nitsch J, Luderitz B. Inhibition of the heparin effect by nitroglycerin. Doutsche Med Wochenschrift 1988; 133: 1837–40.

36. Bode V, Welzel D, Franz G, Polensky U. Absence of drug interaction between heparin and nitroglycerin: randomized placebo-controlled crossover study. Arch Intern Med 1990; 150: 2117–9.

37. Becker RC, Corrao JM, Bovill EG, et al. Intravenous nitroglycerin-induced heparin resistance: a qualitative antithrombin III abnormality. Am Heart J 1990; 119: 1254–61.

38. Marciniak E. Factor X_a inactivation by antithrombin III: evidence for biological stabilization of factor X_a by factor V-phospholipid complex. Br J Haematol 1973; 24: 391–400.

39. Walker FJ, Esmon CT. The effects of phospholipid and factor V_a on the inhibition of factor X_a by antithrombin III. Biochem Biophys Res Comm 1979; 90: 641–7.

40. Holt JC, Niewiarowski S. Biochemistry of α-granule proteins. Semin Hematol 1985; 22: 151–63.

41. Weitz JI, Hudoba M, Massel D, Maraganore J, Hirsh J. Clot-bound thrombin is protected from inhibition by heparin-antithrombin III but is susceptible to inactivation by antithrombin III independent inhibitors. J Clin Invest 1990; 86: 385–91.

42. Hogg PJ, Jackson CM. Fibrin monomer protects thrombin from inactivation by heparin-antithrombin III: implications for heparin efficacy. Proc Nat Acad Sci USA 1989; 86: 3619–23.

43. Heras M, Chesebro JH, Penny WJ, et al. Effects of thrombin inhibition on the development of acute platelet-thrombus deposition during angioplasty in pigs. Heparin versus recombinant hirudin, a specific thrombin inhibitor. Circulation 1989; 79: 657–65.

44. Agnelli G, Pascucci C, Cosmi B, Nenci GG. The comparative effects of recombinant hirudin (CGP 39393) and standard heparin on thrombus growth in rabbits. Thromb Haemost 1990; 63: 204–7.

45. Hirsh J, Ofosu FA, Levine MN. The development of low molecular weight heparins for clinical use. In: Verstraete M, Vermylen J, Lijnen R, Amout J, eds. Brussels: Thrombosis XIth Congress Haemostasis, 1987:325–48.

46. Eisenberg PR, Sherman L, Rich M, et al. Importance of continued activation of thrombin reflected by fibrinopeptide A to the efficacy of thrombolysis. J Am Coll Cardiol 1986; 7: 1255–62.

47. Owen J, Friedman KD, Grossman BA, Wilkins C, Berke AD, Powers ER. Thrombolytic therapy with tissue plasminogen activator or streptokinase induces transient thrombin activity. Blood 1988; 72: 616–20.

48. Rapold JH, Kuemmerli H, Weiss M, et al. Monitoring of fibrin generation during thrombolytic therapy of acute myocardial infarction with recombinant tissue-type plasminogen activator. Circulation 1989; 79: 980–9.

49. Bar-Shavit R, Eldor A, Vlodavsky I. Binding of thrombin to subendothelial extracellular matrix. Protection and expression of functional properties. J Clin Invest 1989; 84: 1096–2004.

50. Basu D, Gallus A, Hirsh J, Cade JF. A prospective study of the value of monitoring heparin treatment with the activated partial thromboplastin time. N Engl J Med 1972; 287: 324–7.

51. Turpie AGG, Robinson JG, Doyle DJ, et al. Comparison of high-dose with low-dose subcutaneous heparin to prevent left ventricular mural thrombosis in patients with acute transmural anterior myocardial infarction. N Engl J Med 1989; 320: 352–94.

52. Kaplan K, Davison R, Parker M, et al. Role of heparin after intravenous thrombolytic therapy for acute myocardial infarction. Am J Cardiol 1987; 59: 241–4.

53. Camilleri JF, Bonnet JL, Bouvier JL, et al. Thrombolyse intraveineuse dans l'infarctus du myocarde. Influence de la qualite de l'anticoagulation sur le taux de recidives precoces d'angor ou d'infarctus. Arch Mal Coeur 1988; 81: 1037–41.

54. Wessler S, Morris LE. Studies in intravascular coagulation. IV. The effect of heparin and dicoumarol on serum-induced venous thrombosis. Circulation 1956; 12: 563–6.

55. Soloway HB, Cornett BM, Grayson JW. Comparison of various activated partial thromboplastin reagents in the laboratory control of heparin therapy. Am J Clin Pathol 1973; 59: 587–90.

56. Spector I, Corn M. Control of heparin therapy with activated partial thromboplastin times. JAMA 1967; 201: 75–7.

57. Struver GP, Bittner DL. The partial thromboplastin time (cephalin time) in anticoagulant therapy. Am J Clin Pathol 1962; 38: 473–81.

58. Zucker S, Charache MH. Control of heparin therapy. Sensitivity of the activated partial thromboplastin time for monitoring the antithrombotic effects of heparin. J Lab Clin Med 1969; 73: 320–6.

59. Shapiro GA, Huntzinger SW, Wilson JE. Variations among commercial activated partial thromboplastin time reagents in response to heparin. Am J Clin Pathol 1977; 67: 477–80.

60. Shojania A, Tetreault J, Turnbull G. The variations between heparin sensitivity of different lots of activated partial thromboplastin time reagent produced by the same manufacturer. Am J Clin Pathol 1988; 89: 29–33.

61. Barrowcliffe TW, Gray E. Studies of phospholipid reagents used in coagulation. II. Factors influencing their sensitivity to heparin. Thromb Haemost 1981; 46(2): 634–7.

62. Stevenson KJ, Daston AC, Curry A, Thomson JM, Poller L. The reliability of activated partial thromboplastin time methods and the relationship to lipid composition and ultrastructure. Thromb Haemost 1986; 55(2): 250–258.

63. van den Besselaar AMHP, Meeuwisse-Braun J, Jansen-Gruter R, Bertina RM. Monitoring heparin therapy by the activated partial thromboplastin time—the effect of preanalytical conditions. Thromb Haemost 1987; 57: 226–231.

64. Triplett DA, Harms CS, Koepke JA. The effect of heparin on the activated partial thromboplastin time. Am J Clin Pathol 1978; 70: 556–9.

65. van den Besselaar AMHP, Meeuwise-Braun J, Bertina RM. Monitoring heparin therapy: relationships between the activated partial thromboplastin time and heparin assays based on ex-vivo heparin samples. Thromb Haemost 1990; 63: 16–23.

66. Cruickshank MK, Levine MN, Hirsh J, Roberts RS, Siguenza M. A standard heparin nomogram for the management of heparin therapy. Arch Intern Med 1991; 151: 333–7.

67. Levine MN, Hirsh J. Hemorrhagic complications of anticoagulant therapy. Semin Thromb Hemost 1986; 12: 39–57.

68. Chiu HM, Hirsh J, Yung WL, Rogocczi E, Gent M. Relationship between the anticoagulant and antithrombotic effects of heparin in experimental venous thrombosis. Blood 1977; 49: 171–84.

69. Johnson EA, Kirkwood TBL, Stirling Y, et al. Four heparin preparations: anti-Xa potentiating effect of heparin after subcutaneous injection. Thromb Haemost 1976; 35: 586.

70. Carter CJ, Kelton JG, Hirsh J, Cerskus AL, Santos AV, Gent M. The relationship between the hemorrhagic and antithrombotic properties of low molecular weight heparins and heparin. Blood 1982; 59: 1239–45.

71. Ofosu FA, Barrowcliffe TW. Mechanisms of action of low molecular weight heparins and heparinoids. In: Hirsh J, ed. Antithrombotic therapy. Bailliere's clinical haematology, Vol 3. London: Bailliere Tindall Ltd, 1990; 3: 505–529.

72. Ofosu FA. In vitro and ex-vivo activities of CY216: comparison with other low molecular weight heparins. Haemostasis 1990; 20(suppl 1): 180–192.

73. Ofosu FA, Choay J, Anvari N, Smith LM, Blajchman MA. Inhibition of factor X and factor V activation by dermatan sulfate and the synthetic pentassacharide with high affinity to antithrombin III. Eur J Biochem 1990; 193: 485–493.

74. Rosenberg RD, Damus PS. The purification and mechanism of action of human antithrombin-heparin cofactor. J Biol Chem 1973; 248: 6490–505.

75. Bjork I, Fish WW. Production in vitro and properties of a modified form of bovine antithrombin, cleaved at the active site by thrombin. J Biol Chem 1982; 257: 9487–93.

76. Bjork I, Jackson CM, Jornvall H, et al. The active site of antithrombin: release of the same proteolytically cleaved form of the inhibitor from complexes with Factor IX, Factor X and thrombin. J Biol Chem 1982; 257: 2406–11.

77. Jornvall H, Fish WW, Bjork I. The thrombin cleavage site in bovine antithrombin. FEBS Lett 1979; 106(2): 358–62.

78. Marciniak E. Thrombin-induced proteolysis of human antithrombin III: an outstanding contribution of heparin. Br J Haematol 1981; 48: 325–36.

79. Rosenberg RD, Jordon RE, Favreau LV, Lam LH. Highly active heparin species with multiple binding sites for antithrombin. Biochem Biophys Res Commun 1979; 86: 1319–24.

80. Jordan RE, Favreau LV, Braswell EH, Rosenberg RD. Heparin with two binding sites for antithrombin or platelet factor 4. J Biol Chem 1982; 257: 400–6.

81. Nordenman B, Bjork I. Binding of low affinity and high-affinity heparin to antithrombin. Ultraviolet difference spectroscopy and circular dichroism studies. Biochemistry 1978; 17: 3339–44.

82. Olson ST, Srinivasan KR, Bjork I, et al. Binding of high affinity heparin to antithrombin III: stopped flow kinetic studies of the binding interaction. J Biol Chem 1981; 256: 11073–9.

83. Villanueva GB, Danishefsky I. Evidence for a heparin-induced conformational change on antithrombin III. Biochem Biophys Res Commun 1977; 74: 803–9.

84. Petitou M. Synthetic heparin fragments: new and efficient tools for the study of heparin and its interactions. Nouv Rev Fr Hematol 1984; 26: 221–6.

85. Barrowcliffe TW, Merton RE, Gray E, Thomas DP. Heparin and bleeding: an association with lipase release. Thromb Haemost 1988; 60: 434–6.

86. Barrowcliffe TW, Thomas DP. Low molecular weight heparins: antithrombotic and haemorrhagic effects and standardization. Acta Chir Scand 1988; 543: 57–64.

87. Ofosu FA, Smith LM, Anvari N, Blajchman MA. An approach to assigning in vitro potency to unfractionated and low molecular weight heparins based on the inhibition of prothrombin activation and catalysis of thrombin inhibition. Thromb Haemost 1988; 60: 193–8.

88. Beguin S, Mardiguian J, Lindhout T, Hemker HC. The mode of action of low molecular weight heparin preparation (PK 10169) and two of its major components on thrombin generation in plasma. Thromb Haemost 1989; 61: 30–4.

89. Bara L, Samama MM. The need for standardization of low molecular weight heparin (LMWH). Thromb Haemost 1986; 56: 418.

90. Barrowcliffe TW, Curtis AD, Johnson EA, et al. An international standard for low molecular weight heparin. Thromb Haemost 1988; 60: 1–7.

91. Fareed J, Hoppensteadt DA, Walenga JM, et al. Validity of the newly established low molecular weight heparin standard in cross referencing low molecular weight heparins. Haemostasis 1988; 3(suppl): 33–47.

92. Hemker HC. A standard for low molecular weight heparin? Haemostasis 1989; 1: 1–4.

93. Cade JF, Buchanan MR, Boneu B, et al. A comparison of the antithrombotic and hemorrhagic effects of low molecular weight heparin fractions. Thromb Res 1984; 35: 613–25.

94. Ockelford PA, Carter CJ, Mitchell L, Hirsh J. Discordance between the anti-Xa activity and antithrombotic activity of an ultra-low molecular weight heparin fraction. Thromb Res 1982; 28: 401–9.

95. Van Ryn-McKenna J, Ofosu FA, Hirsh J, Buchanan M. Antithrombotic and bleeding effects of glycosaminoglycans with different degrees of sulfation. Br J Haematol 1989; 71: 265–9.

96. Boneu B, Buchanan MR, Cade JF, et al. Effects of heparin, its low molecular weight fractions and other glycosaminoglycans on thrombus growth in vivo. Thromb Res 1985; 40: 81–9.

97. Van Ryn-McKenna J, Gray E, Weber E, et al. Effects of sulphated polysaccharides on inhibition of thrombus formation initiated by different stimuli. Thromb Haemost 1989; 61: 7–9.

98. Andriuolli G, Mastacch R, Barbanti M, Sarret M. Comparison of the antithrombotic and hemorrhagic effects of heparin and a new low molecular weight heparin in rats. Haemostasis 1985; 15: 324–30.

99. Esquivel CO, Bergqvist D, Bjork CG, Nilsson B. Comparison between commercial heparin, low molecular weight heparin and pentosan polysulfate on hemostasis and platelets in vivo. Thromb Res 1982; 28: 389–399.

100. Diness Y, Nielson JI, Pedersen PC, Wolfbrandt KH, Ostergaard PB. A comparison of the antithrombotic and hemorrhagic effects of low molecular weight heparin (PHN-1) and conventional heparin. Thromb Haemost 1986; 55: 410–4.

101. Pangrazzi J, Abbadini M, Zameta M, et al. Antithrombotic and bleeding effects of a low molecular weight heparin fraction. Biochem Pharmacol 1985; 34: 3305–8.

102. Fernandez F, Van Ryn J, Ofosu FA, Hirsh J, Buchanan MR. The hemorrhagic and antithrombotic effects of dermatan sulfate. Br J Haematol 1986; 64: 309–17.

103. Bratt G, Toprnebohm E, Widlund L, et al. Low molecular weight heparin (KABI 2165, FRAGMIN): pharmacokinetics after intravenous and subcutaneous administration in human volunteers. Thromb Res 1986; 42: 613–20.

104. Matzch T, Bergqvist D, Hedner U, et al. Effect of an enzymatically depolymerized heparin as compared with conventional heparin in healthy volunteers. Thromb Haemost 1987; 57: 97–101.

105. Bara L, Samama MM. Pharmacokinetics of low molecular weight heparins. Acta Clin Scand 1988; 543(suppl): 65–72.

106. Bara L, Billaud E, Gramond G, et al. Comparative pharmacokinetics of low molecular weight heparin (PK 10169) and unfractionated heparin after intravenous and subcutaneous administration. Thromb Res 1985; 39: 631–6.

107. Frydman AM, Bara L, Le Roux Y, et al. The antithrombotic activity and pharmacokinetics of enoxaparine, a low molecular weight heparin, in humans given single subcutaneous doses of 20 to 80 mg. J Clin Pharmacol 1988; 28: 609–18.

108. Levine MN, Hirsh J, Gent M, et al. A randomized trial comparing enoxaparine low molecular weight heparin with standard unfractionated heparin in patients undergoing elective hip surgery. Ann Intern Med 1991; 114: 545–51.

109. Kakkar VV, Murray WJG. Efficacy and safety of low molecular weight heparin (CY216) in preventing postoperative venous thromboembolism: a co-operative study. Br J Surg 1985; 72: 786–91.

110. European Fraxiparin Study Group. Comparison of a low molecular weight heparin and unfractionated heparin for the prevention of deep vein thrombosis in patients undergoing abdominal surgery. Br J Surg 1988; 75: 1058–63.

111. Koller M, Schoch U, Buchmann P, et al. Low molecular weight heparin (KABI 2165) as thromboprophylaxis in elective visceral surgery. A randomized double-blind study versus unfractionated heparin. Thromb Haemost 1986; 56: 243–6.

112. Bergqvist D, Burmark US, Frisell J, et al. Low molecular weight heparin once daily compared with conventional low dose heparin twice daily. A prospective double bind multicentre trial on prevention of postoperative thrombosis. Br J Surg 1986; 3: 204–8.

113. Caen JP. A randomized double-blind study between a low molecular weight heparin Kabi 2165 and standard heparin in the prevention of deep vein thrombosis in general surgery. Thromb Haemost 1988; 59: 216–20.

114. Bergqvist D, Matzsch T, Burmark US, et al. Low molecular weight heparin given the evening before surgery compared with conventional low dose heparin in prevention of thrombosis. Br J Surg 1989; 75: 888–91.

115. Fricker J-P, Vergnes Y, Schach A, et al. Low dose heparin versus low molecular weight heparin (Kabi 2165, Fragmin®) in the prophylaxis of thromboembolic complications of abdominal oncological surgery. Eur J Clin Invest 1988; 18: 561–7.

116. Samama M, Bernard P, Bonnardot VP, et al. Low molecular weight heparin (enoxaparine) compared with unfractionated heparin thrice a day in prevention of postoperative thrombosis. Br J Surg 1988; 75: 128–31.

117. Prins MH, den Ottolander GJH, Gelsema R, et al. Deep vein prophylaxis with a low molecular weight heparin (Kabi 2165) in stroke patients. Thromb Haemost 1987; 1(suppl): 418a.

118. Turpie AGG, Levine MN, Hirsh J, et al. A double-blind randomized trial of ORG 10172 low molecular weight heparinoid in the prevention of deep vein thrombosis in thrombotic stroke. Lancet 1987; 1: 523–6.

119. Turpie AGG, Levine MN, Powers P, et al. A double blind randomized trial of ORG 10172 low molecular weight heparinoid versus unfractionated heparin in the prevention of deep vein thrombosis in patients with thrombotic stroke. Thromb Haemost 1991; 65: 753. Abst. #303.

120. Turpie AGG, Levine MN, Hirsh J, et al. A randomized controlled trial of low molecular weight heparin (enoxaparine) to prevent deep vein thrombosis in patients undergoing elective hip surgery. N Engl J Med 1986; 315: 925–9.

121. Hoek J, Nurmohamed MT, ten Cate H, et al. Prevention of deep vein thrombosis (DVT) following total hip replacement by a low molecular weight heparinoid (ORG 10172). Thromb Haemost 1989; 62(1): 520–#1637.

122. Planes A, Vochelle N, Mazas F, et al. Prevention of postoperative venous thrombosis: a randomized trial comparing unfractionated heparin with low molecular weight heparin in patients undergoing total hip replacement. Thromb Haemost 1988; 60: 407–10.

123. Estoppey D, Hochreiter J, Breyer HG, et al. ORG 10172 (Lomoparan) versus heparin-DHE in prevention of thromboembolism in total hip replacement—a multicentre trial. Thromb Haemost 1989; 62(1): 356–#1107.

124. Leyvraz PF, Postel M. Prevention of post-operative deep vein thrombosis (DVT) in elective total hip replacement (THR) by LMW heparin (CY 216). A controlled, randomized, collaborative trial. XIIth Congress of the International Society on Thrombosis and Haemostasis Staellite Symposium (Tokyo), In Press, 1991.

125. Dechavanne M, Ville D, Berruyer M, et al. Randomized trial of a low-molecular weight heparin (Kabi 2165) versus adjusted-dose subcutaneous standard heparin in the prophylaxis of deep-vein thrombosis after elective hip surgery. Haemostasis 1989; 19: 5–12.

126. Barre J, Pfiser G, Potron G, et al. Efficacite et tolerance comparee du KABI 2165 et de l'heparine standard dans la prevention des thromboses veineuses profondes au cours des protheses totales de hanche. J des Maladies Vasc 1987; 12: 90–5.

127. Lassen MR. A comparison of antithrombotic efficacy of enoxaparin with dextran 70 in hip arthroplasties. Arch Intern Med (In Press) 1991.

128. Green D, Lee MY, Lim AC, et al. Prevention of thromboembolism after spinal cord injury using low-molecular-weight heparin. Ann Intern Med 1990; 113: 571–4.

129. Leclerc J, Desjardins L, Geerts W, Jobin F, Delorme F. A randomized trial of enoxaparin for the prevention of deep vein thrombosis (DVT) after major knee surgery. Blood 1990; 76(10): 511–#2043.

130. Bratt G, Tornebohm E, Granqvist S, et al. A comparison between low molecular weight heparin (KABI 2165) and

standard heparin in the intravenous treatment of deep venous thrombosis. Thromb Haemost 1985; 54: 813–7.

131. Duroux P. Treatment of proximal deep vein thrombosis of the lower limb by CY216 (LMWH) versus unfractionated heparin (UFH). Thromb Haemost 1987; 1(suppl): 437a.

132. Faivre R, Neuhart E, Kieffer Y, et al. Subcutaneous administration of a low molecular weight heparin (CY222) compared with subcutaneous administration of standard heparin in patients with acute deep vein thrombosis. Thromb Haemost 1987; 1(suppl): 430a.

133. Holm HA, Ly B, Handeland GF, et al. Subcutaneous heparin treatment of deep vein thrombosis: a comparison of unfractionated and low molecular weight heparin. Haemostasis 1986; 16(12): 30–7.

134. Levine MN, Hirsh J. Clinical use of low molecular weight heparins and heparinoids. Semin Thromb Haemost 1988; 14: 116–25.

135. Vogel C, Machulik M. Efficacy and safety of a low molecular weight heparin (LMW-heparin Sandoz) in patients with deep vein thrombosis. Thromb Haemost 1987; 1(suppl): 427a.

136. Vitoux JF, Fiessinger JN, Roncato M, et al. Long term treatment of acute deep venous thrombosis with low molecular weight heparin derivative. JAMA 1988; 259: 1180–1.

137. Bakker M, Dekker PJ, Knot EA, et al. Home treatment for deep venous thrombosis with low molecular weight heparin. Lancet 1988; 2: 1142.

9

OPTIMAL THERAPEUTIC RANGES FOR ORAL ANTICOAGULATION

LEON POLLER and JACK HIRSH

Oral anticoagulants are still the most widely used drugs for prophylaxis and treatment of venous and arterial thrombosis. Recent randomized controlled trials[1-7] have confirmed their efficacy in these situations. In latter years strenuous efforts have also been made to improve the safety of anticoagulant treatment based on lower-dose warfarin regimens which have been facilitated by moves to standardize the performance and reporting of the prothrombin time test.[8,9]

PHARMACOLOGY OF WARFARIN

Oral anticoagulants act by interfering with the cyclic interconversion of vitamin K and its 2;3-epoxide (vitamin K epoxide). Warfarin (a 4-hydroxycoumarin compound) is the most widely used compound because its onset and duration of action is a good compromise between the rapid-acting and slow-acting drugs. Warfarin gives rapid induction with reasonable stability of effect. Pharmacological and dosage observations relate only to warfarin; but the mode of action, pharmacodynamics, laboratory monitoring, optimal therapeutic ranges, clinical efficacy, and safety aspects will refer to all vitamin K antagonist oral anticoagulants. Vitamin K is an essential cofactor for the post-translational carboxylation of glutamate resides on the N-terminal regions of vitamin K-dependent proteins to gamma-carboxyglutamates (Gla). This reaction is catalyzed by a vitamin K-dependent carboxylase requiring the reduced form of quinone vitamin K (vitamin KH_2 or hydro-

quinone), molecular oxygen, and carbon dioxide. In this way gamma-carboxyglutamic acid residues are formed and the hydroquinone is oxidized to vitamin K epoxide (Fig. 9–1). Vitamin K epoxide is recycled to vitamin K by vitamin K epoxide reductase, and the vitamin K is then reduced to hydroquinone by vitamin K epoxide reductase. Warfarin, by inhibiting vitamin K epoxide reductase and vitamin K reductase, leads to the accumulation of vitamin K epoxide in the liver and plasma and depletion of hydroquinone. Decrease in hydroquinone limits the gamma-carboxylation of the vitamin K-dependent coagulant proteins (prothrombin, factor VII, factor IX, and factor X), and of the coagulation inhibitors proteins C and S. As a result of the process of gamma-carboxylation, these vitamin K-dependent proteins acquire metal binding properties so that in the presence of calcium ions they undergo a conformational change which is necessary for calcium dependent complexing of vitamin K-dependent protein to their cofactors on phospholipid surfaces. Normal vitamin K-dependent coagulation proteins normally contain 10 to 13 gamma-carboxyglutamate residues within their amino terminal. Molecules with less than six gamma-carboxyglutamate residues have about 2 per cent of normal activity, while those with nine gamma-carboxyglutamate residues have 70 per cent of normal activity.[10] Doses of vitamin K used to reverse warfarin overdosage, or dietary intake of large amounts of vitamin K overcome the inhibiting effects of warfarin by generating active hydroquinone cofactor via the warfarin

161

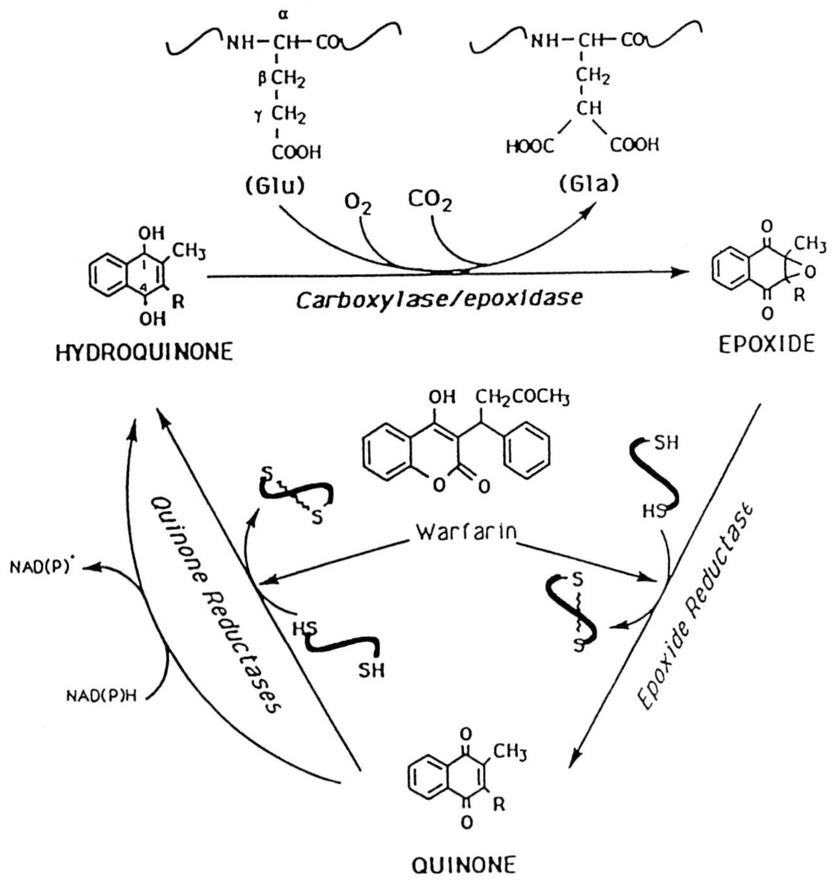

FIGURE 9–1. Schematic representation of the vitamin K cycle. (From Sadowski JA et al. Warfarin and the metabolism function of vitamin K. In: Poller L, ed. Recent Advances in Blood Coagulation No. 5. Edinburgh: Churchill Livingstone; 1991:93–118, with permission.)

insensitive pyridine nucleotide-dependent pathway (for a review of pharmacology of warfarin, see Sadowski et al.[11]).

Although warfarin can be administered by injection, it is normally only given orally. Racemic warfarin is a mixture of roughly equal amounts of two optically active isomers, the R and S forms. It is rapidly and extensively absorbed from the gastrointestinal tract and reaches maximal blood concentrations in healthy volunteers in 90 minutes.[12] It has a half-life of 36 to 42 hours, circulates bound to plasma proteins, and is rapidly accumulating in the liver, principally in microsomes. The R and S isomers are metabolized by different pathways.[13] The R-warfarin is metabolized primarily by reduction of the acetenyl sidechain into warfarin alcohols excreted in the urine, and the S-warfarin is metabolized by oxidation to 7-hydroxy-S-warfarin eliminated in the bile. In stabilized patients there is a direct relationship between the dose of warfarin and its anticoagulant response within individuals, but a marked variation among subjects. Variations in response also occur in the same patient during an extended course of therapy due to many causes including drug interactions, intercurrent illness, and dietary vitamin K intake. These can produce major practical problems in monitoring. In many instances the causes of change in dose response cannot be identified. Changes in receptor affinity, vitamin K availability, levels of vitamin K-dependent coagulation factors, pharmacokinetics of warfarin, and other factors affect the pharmacodynamics of warfarin. Other important causes for variable response include poor patient compliance and poor communication between patient and physician.

Hereditary resistance to warfarin has been described in rats and humans.[14] Warfarin-resistant patients required warfarin 5 to 20 times the average dose to achieve the desired anticoagulant effect; the plasma warfarin levels also had to be much higher than average. Warfarin resistance is thought to be caused by an altered affinity of the receptor for the drug. Subjects receiving long-term oral anticoagulation may be affected by fluctuating levels of dietary vitamin K. This is obtained predominantly from phylloquinone in vegetables.[15] Diets rich in green vegetables (for example, weight reduction regimens) and nutritional fluid supplements rich in vitamin K reduce the anticoagulant response to warfarin, whereas vitamin K absorption is impaired in fat malabsorption states which potentiate the effects of warfarin. Impaired hepatic function also increases the response to warfarin as do hypermetabolic states produced by fever or hyperthyroidism. An increase of synthesis of vitamin K-dependent clotting factors may cause mild warfarin resistance during pregnancy or when heart failure hepatic congestion is reversed.

THE THERAPEUTIC RANGE FOR THE CONTROL OF ORAL ANTICOAGULANT THERAPY

A number of different tests have been employed for laboratory monitoring of anticoagulant therapy, but the test by far the most widely used is the one-stage prothrombin time (PT) introduced by Quick in 1935. This test, which measures the reductions by warfarin of factors II, VII, and X, is performed by adding calcium and thromboplastin to citrated plasma. The term thromboplastin describes a lipoprotein extract of human or animal tissue that contains both tissue factor and the phospholipid necessary to promote the activation of factor X by factor VII.

The interpretation of prothrombin time results has been complicated because the routine thromboplastin reagents of commercial or local origin are manufactured by different methods, and thus vary in their responsiveness to reduction of vitamin K-dependent clotting factors.[16] An identical prothrombin time result with different reagents may mask a very different level of anticoagulant effect. In particular, this has caused problems in North America. When oral anticoagulant treatment was first introduced in the early 1940s, thromboplastin reagents were manually prepared from human brain by individual hospital labora-

tories and resembled the human thromboplastin which was distributed later throughout the United Kingdom in the 1960s. This was more responsive to the warfarin-induced defect than commercial thromboplastin reagents adapted for use in North America in the 1950s and 1960s. Wright, on behalf of the American Heart Association had recommended that the targeted therapeutic range for oral anticoagulants should be equivalent to a prothrombin time ratio of 2.0 to 2.5.[17] The same target prothrombin ratios were maintained for the next 30 years, thus increasing the intensity of anticoagulation used in North America with the introduction of less responsive reagents. Poller and Taberner[18] showed (Fig. 9–2) that the dosage of warfarin in the United States and Canada has been higher than that recommended by the British Society for Haematology.[16] Although the difference in responsiveness between commercial thromboplastins and possible dose implications were documented,[19,20] most clinicians in North America and in most other countries did not recognize the reason. The evidence from recent clinical trials comparing different levels of intensity of anticoagulation indicates that the unsuspected increase in anticoagulant dosage was of a sufficient magnitude to lead to an increase in clinically important bleeding.[3,21]

The higher incidence of anticoagulant-induced hemorrhage than in the United Kingdom and the Netherlands reported from North America and elsewhere since the early 1960s had suggested that the intensity of anticoagulation varied greatly in different countries. The international survey of dosage was performed at representative centers in countries in Europe, Asia, North America, and Australia.[18] The aim was to assess dosage in equivalent treated groups. Information was requested on the mean anticoagulant dosage of 20 serial stabilized patients in routine practice. Seventy-four centers from 23 countries participated in the survey. Warfarin was the only anticoagulant drug used in sufficient numbers for comparative data. The mean daily dosage ranged from 2.45 to 8.76 milligrams. All the North American centers were amongst those prescribing the highest doses. Much of the discrepancy could be attributed to the type of tissue extract thromboplastin employed in the prothrombin time test. The rabbit preparations referred to in Figure 9–2 were less responsive thrombo-

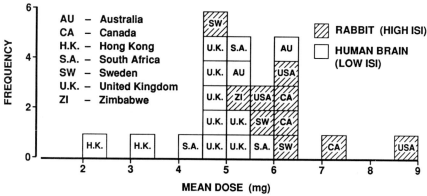

FIGURE 9–2. Mean warfarin doses in different geographical locations relevant to type of thromboplastin in prothrombin time test used in laboratory monitoring. High international sensitivity index = >2.0. Low international sensitivity index = <2.0.

plastins associated with higher mean warfarin doses.

To resolve these dosage problems, a scheme of prothrombin time standardization for anticoagulant control based on international reference preparations (IRP) for thromboplastin and a uniform method of reporting results termed international normalized ratios (INR) was introduced by the World Health Organization in 1983. The international normalized ratio is the ratio result which it is calculated would have been obtained if the primary international reference preparations had been used in the prothrombin time test instead of the local reagent. International normalized ratios are derived from the international sensitivity index (ISI) for each thromboplastin. This is obtained by testing normal and coumarin-treated patients' plasmas with the local reagent and the international reference preparations in parallel and comparing their responsiveness. The logarithm of the prothrombin time results with the two thromboplastins are plotted, and an orthogonal regression line is drawn. The reference international reference preparations is always on the x axis and the test reagent on the y axis. The international sensitivity index is derived from the slope of the resultant orthogonal regression line compared with that of the primary international reference preparations which is by definition 1.0. International normalized ratios may then be obtained from the calculation,

$$INR = Ratio^{ISI}.$$

The accompanying nomogram (Fig. 9–3) avoids the need for such calculations.

As well as facilitating uniform warfarin therapy on a world scale, international normalized ratios also provide greater safety in treatment by permitting accurate segmentation of the blanket therapeutic scale previously used according to clinical condition. International normalized ratios have demonstrated that lower-dose warfarin administration could be employed with relative safety in North America and other countries where poorly responsive thromboplastins (international sensitivity index > 2.0) and high-intensity dosage have been the norm (Tables 9–1 and 9–2).

Three groups have made recommendations on the optimum therapeutic ranges in international normalized ratios according to the clinical indications. The British Society for Haematology (BSH) in 1984 was the first, and these were slightly revised in 1990.[16] The second was from a group which met in Leuven in 1984,[22] and the third set came from two meetings of the American College of Chest Physicians/National Heart Lung and Blood Institute (ACCP/NHLBI).[9] The three sets of recommendations which are presented in Table 9–1 show a large measure of conformity.

PREVENTION OF DEEP VEIN THROMBOSIS AFTER SURGERY

A number of studies have demonstrated that oral anticoagulants are effective in preventing deep vein thrombosis in major surgery and after hip operations. (See also Chapter 24.)

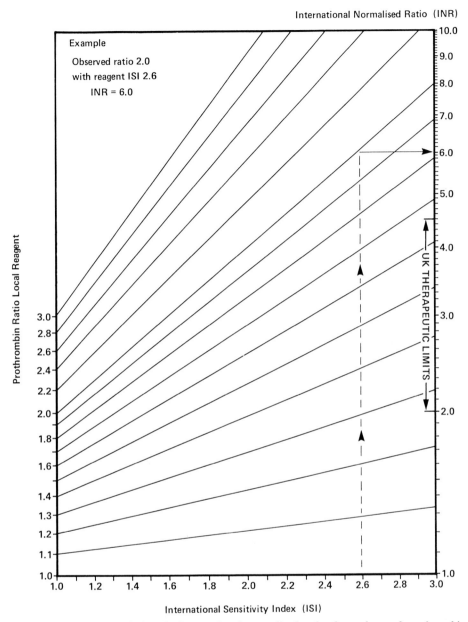

FIGURE 9–3. Nomogram to derive the international normalized ratios from observed prothrombin ratio and international sensitivity index of thromboplastin.

Major Gynecological Surgery

The three groups have made recommendations on low-dose warfarin for deep vein thrombosis prophylaxis in gynecological procedures. All three sets of recommendations entail much lower dose warfarin than the traditional high-dose North American regimens. The American College of Chest Physicians/National Heart Lung and Blood In-

stitute 2.0 to 3.0, International normalized ratio range is slightly more intense and is based on the success with lower-dose warfarin treatment group in the two intensities of treatment study.[3] The Leuven group's therapeutic interval of 1.5 to 2.5 is marginally less intense than the British Society for Haematology range of 2.0 to 2.5 international normalized ratio. The 1.5 lower limit now has the support of a prospective randomized

TABLE 9–1. Therapeutic Recommendations in International Normalized Ratios by Three Representative Groups

	BRITISH SOCIETY FOR HAEMATOLOGY[16]	LEUVEN CONFERENCE[22]	AMERICAN COLLEGE OF CHEST PHYSICIANS/ NATIONAL HEART LUNG AND BLOOD INSTITUTE CONSENSUS[9]
Prophylaxis of postoperative deep vein thrombosis (general surgery)	2.0–2.5	1.5–2.5	2.0–3.0
Prophylaxis of postoperative deep vein thrombosis in hip surgery and fractures	2.0–3.0	2.0–3.0	2.0–3.0
Myocardial infarction prevention of venous thromboembolism	2.0–3.0	2.0–3.0	2.0–3.0
Treatment of venous thrombosis	2.0–3.0	2.0–4.0	2.0–3.0
Treatment of pulmonary embolism	2.0–3.0	2.0–4.0	2.0–3.0
Transient ischemic attacks	2.0–3.0		
Tissue heart valves	2.0–3.0	?	2.0–3.0
Atrial fibrillation	2.0–3.0	?	2.0–3.0
Valvular heart disease	2.0–3.0	?	2.0–3.0
Recurrent deep vein thrombosis and pulmonary embolism	3.0–4.5	2.0–4.0	2.0–3.0
Arterial disease including myocardial infarction	3.0–4.5	3.0–4.5	2.0–3.0
Mechanical prosthetic valves	3.0–4.5	3.0–4.5	3.0–4.5
Recurrent systemic embolism	3.0–4.5	3.0–4.0	3.0–4.5

TABLE 9–2. Prevention of Deep Vein Thrombosis in Major Gynecological Surgery

LEVEL I STUDIES	ORAL ANTICOAGULANT	INTERNATIONAL NORMALIZED RATIO RANGE	UNTREATED CONTROL	LOW-DOSE HEPARIN GROUP	DEEP VEIN THROMBOSIS DIAGNOSIS
Taberner et al. (1978)[1] (five days preoperative induction)		2.0–2.5 Preoperative 2.0–4.0 Postoperative			[125]I fibrinogen scanning
Total number	48		48	49	
Deep vein thrombosis incidence	3		11	3	
Vroonhoven et al. (1974)[25] (induction postoperative)		2.4 Postoperative			[125]I fibrinogen scanning
Total number	50		—	50	
Deep vein thrombosis incidence	9		—	1	
Poller et al. (1987)[23] (induction five days preoperative)		1.5–2.5 Preoperative 2.0–3.0 Postoperative		Minidose warfarin	[125]I fibrinogen scanning, impedence plethysmography, and ultrasound
Total number	35	1.05 Mini-dose	37	32 mg/day	
Deep vein thrombosis incidence	1		11	3	

TABLE 9–3. Warfarin Deep Vein Thrombosis Prophylaxis in Hip Surgery

	TIME OF INDUCTION	WARFARIN (NUMBER)	PROTHROMBIN TIME RATIO	INTERNATIONAL NORMALIZED RATIOS	DEEP VEIN THROMBOSIS/ PULMONARY EMBOLISM	CONTROL (NUMBER)	DEEP VEIN THROMBOSIS/ PULMONARY EMBOLISM
Powers et al. (1989)[6]	Postoperative	65		2.0–2.7	13 (20 per cent)	63	29 (46 per cent)
Francis et al. (1983)[25]	Preoperative	53	1.3–1.5	2.0–2.6	11 (21 per cent)	57	30 (53 per cent)

study[23] in prevention of deep vein thrombosis. Table 9–2 gives the studies from which these recommendations are derived.

A fixed minidose warfarin (1 milligram/day) regimen also reduced deep vein thrombosis in this group, although the series was small and the significant benefit remains to be confirmed in other studies.[23] An advantage is that minidose treatment does not prolong the prothrombin time or activated partial thromboplastin time on the day of surgery and appears to cause no additional bleeding. The results support the view that comparatively low doses of warfarin may be sufficient to prevent deep vein thrombosis in the moderate-risk situations. Fixed minidose fixed warfarin (1 milligram/day) regimen has also been shown to prevent thrombotic blocking of central venous lines.[24]

Prophylaxis of Deep Vein Thrombosis in Hip Surgery

Elective and emergency hip operations are associated with a very high incidence of deep vein thrombosis (40 to 70 per cent venographically proved deep vein thrombosis with 1 to 5 per cent pulmonary embolism). Studies by Francis et al.[26] and Powers et al.,[6] have indicated that the incidence can be more than halved by warfarin at moderately low-intensity dosage (approximately, international normalized ratios 2.0 to 2.7) (Table 9–3). The main concerns of surgeons have been the

fear of bleeding with oral anticoagulation and the need for laboratory monitoring, although Sevitt[27] showed that the danger of bleeding was not high with good laboratory control even when the oral anticoagulant prophylaxis was commenced before operation.

Warfarin, however, has not proved popular in hip surgery—Brenkel and Clancy[28] in a questionnaire survey of United Kingdom orthopedic surgeons found that only 8 per cent ever used the drug. It is of considerable interest, therefore, that in the McMaster study[6] where warfarin was only commenced after operation for hip fracture that the incidence of deep vein thrombosis was greatly reduced. In general, warfarin is reserved for select groups of patients with a previous deep vein thrombosis or undergoing major orthopedic procedures.

TREATMENT OF ESTABLISHED DEEP VEIN THROMBOSIS AND PULMONARY EMBOLISM

Oral anticoagulation following intravenous heparin has been the conventional approach to treatment for deep vein thrombosis. With previous trials having no adequate randomized untreated group, the main data (Table 9–4) comes indirectly from investigations reported by Hull et al.[2,3] In the first study, after initial heparin, patients with established deep vein thrombosis were randomized to

TABLE 9–4. Treatment of Deep Vein Thrombosis (Randomized Studies)

LEVEL I	NUMBER	RATIO	INTERNATIONAL NORMALIZED RATIOS	INCIDENCE OF HEMORRHAGE	RECURRENCE OF VENOUS THROMBOSIS	DEEP VEIN THROMBOSIS DIAGNOSIS
Hull et al (1979)[2]						
Warfarin	33	1.5–2.0	2.4–4.6	21 per cent	0 per cent	[125]Ifibrinogen scanning
Subcutaneous heparin	35	—	—		25.7 per cent	IPG and venography
Hull et al. (1982)[3]						
Simplastin control	49	1.5–2.0	2.4–4.6	22.4 per cent	2.0 per cent	[125]I fibrinogen scanning
Manchester comparative reagent control	47	2.0–2.5	2–2.5	4.3 per cent	2.1 per cent	IPG and venography
Lagerstedt et al. (1985)[28]						
Oral anticoagulant	23	—	2.5–4.2	0 per cent	0 per cent	^{99m}Tc-plasmin venography
Controls	28	—		0 per cent	29 per cent	

receive subcutaneous low-dose heparin or moderate-intensity warfarin (international normalized ratios 2.4 to 4.6). Nine of thirty-five patients receiving heparin for 12 weeks, but none of 33 receiving warfarin, had recurrences. The latter resulted, however, in a high incidence of bleeding (in 21 per cent).

A further randomized trial was then undertaken by the McMaster team[3] to decide whether hemorrhagic complications could be reduced by treatment with "low-dose" warfarin (that is, the conventional dosage used in the United Kingdom). Two intensities of treatment were studied (that is, moderate-dose international normalized ratios 2.4 to 4.6, approximately) as in the previous study based on control with a poorly responsive North American thromboplastin in the prothrombin time, and "low-dose" treatment (international normalized ratios 2.0 to 2.5), based on Manchester comparative reagent. Protection from rethrombosis was equal in the two groups, but with lower-dosage warfarin, bleeding was reduced to less than a fifth.

The benefit of oral anticoagulation given for three months in calf vein thrombosis was demonstrated in a study by Lagerstedt et al. from Denmark.[29] (See also Chapter 25.)

MYOCARDIAL INFARCTION

In venous thrombosis, the value of warfarin may be unequivocal, but this is not the case in arterial disease, particularly in myocardial infarction. Initial claims made in the 1940s and 1950s lacked scientific basis. New studies begun in the 1960s were undermined by problems of laboratory control, with a resulting tendency to undertreatment. A summary of the main studies in myocardial infarction is given in Table 9–5. Approximate international normalized ratio values are given for these studies. In most instances this is possible because the local control system had been checked against the standardized thromboplastin Manchester reagent, a batch of which in 1969 was designated as a reference reagent, the British comparative thromboplastin.[30] This had an international sensitivity index value of 1.08. International normalized ratio values are in some cases only approximate in these, but are nevertheless a reasonable approximation. The British Medical Research Council (MRC) study (1969)[31] unintentionally substituted too low a target anticoagulant level of 1.8 international normalized ratio (approximately) in place of the 2.0 to 3.0 international normalized ratio of the earlier successful low-dose Medical Research Council long-term study (1964).[32] The dose of the anticoagulant phenindione per patient was significantly less compared with the earlier study. In this report, as well as in the United States Veterans'[33] and the Danish study,[34] which used relatively low-dose oral anticoagulation, there was significant reduction in stroke and pulmonary embolism, but only slight reduction in mortality and recurrence of myocardial infarction. An analysis of pooled data from seven

TABLE 9–5. Myocardial Infarction

		TREATMENT		SIGNIFICANT REDUCTION IN		
STUDY	Year	Level	International Normalized Ratios	Mortality	Recurrence	Embolism
			Long Term			
Medical Research Council	1959*	Low	2.0–2.5	–	+	+
	1964*	Low				
United States Veteran's[33]	1973	Low	2.0–2.5	?	–	–
Sixty Plus Reinfarction[4]	1981	Moderate	2.7–4.5	+	+	+
Smith et al[7]	1990	Moderate	2.8–4.8	+	+	+
			Short Term			
Hilden et al.[34]	1962*	Minimal	1.2–1.5	–	–	+
Medical Research Council[31]	1969*	Minimal	1.6–2.0	–	–	+
United States Veteran's[33]	1973	Low	2.0–2.5	–	–	+
Drapkin and Merskey[37]	1972	Low	2.0–2.5	+	–	–

* Based on comparisons with British comparative thromboplastin.

randomized trials published between 1964 and 1980 reported that long-term treatment during a one- to six-year period significantly reduces the combined endpoints of mortality and nonfatal reinfarction by approximately 20 per cent.[35]

The "Sixty Plus" Reinfarction Study of the Netherlands Thrombosis Service[4] challenged the practice of withholding anticoagulants from patients with myocardial infarction. In this "stopping" trial, with moderate-dose treatment (target range of 2.7 to 4.5 international normalized ratio) there was a significant reduction in mortality and of recurrent myocardial infarction in those maintained on oral anticoagulation. Investigators from Norway, whose long-term study was reported recently[7] showed significant reduction in both mortality and morbidity from warfarin compared with placebo. The study involved 1,214 patients with a moderate-dose warfarin treatment range of 2.8 to 4.8 international normalized ratio. There were 94 deaths on warfarin and 123 on placebo on an intention-to-treat basis (a 24 per cent reduction 95 per cent confidence interval). Recurrent myocardial infarctions were 82 with warfarin and 124 with placebo, respectively. Indirect support for the efficacy of oral anticoagulants in patients with coronary artery disease comes from a randomized trial of patients with peripheral arterial disease.[36] (See also Chapters 12 and 14.)

VALVULAR HEART DISEASE

The second American College of Chest Physicians/National Heart Lung and Blood Institute Consensus Conference[9] strongly recommended that patients at risk for thromboembolism from rheumatic mitral valve disease be given moderate-dose warfarin at an international normalized ratio of 3.0 to 4.5 for one year, after which time the international normalized ratio should be reduced to low-dose 2.0 to 3.0 international normalized ratios recommended by the British Society for Haematology[16] and Leuven groups.[22] (See Chapter 11.)

PROSTHETIC HEART VALVES

Patients with a mitral mechanical prosthetic valve generally require life-long anticoagulants. The three consensus groups agree on a moderate-intensity warfarin regimen (international normalized ratio of 3.0 to 4.5) and that patients with bioprosthetic valves in the mitral position should be treated for the first three months only after valve insertion with a "low dose" of warfarin (international normalized ratio of 2.0 to 3.0).

A clinical trial has been performed in patients with mechanical prosthetic heart valves who were treated with warfarin for six months and then randomized to receive warfarin (of uncertain intensity), or one of two aspirin-containing antiplatelet drug regimens.[38] The incidence of thromboembolic complications in the warfarin group was significantly less than either of the two antiplatelet drug groups (relative risk reduction 60 to 79 per cent). The incidence of bleeding was highest in the warfarin group.

Turpie et al.[5] showed that low-intensity warfarin with Manchester reagent control gave the same protection from thromboembolism as moderately intense treatment (international normalized ratio 3.0 to 4.5) with a North American type thromboplastin, but bleeding was significantly less with the Manchester reagent (Table 9–6).

In a further randomized study from Saudi Arabia,[39] two levels of treatment based on

TABLE 9–6. Prosthetic Heart Valves: Different Intensities of Anticoagulation

STUDY	VALVE TYPE	INTERNATIONAL NORMALIZED RATIOS		THROMBOEMBOLISM		BLEEDING	
		Lower Dose	*Higher Dose*	*Lower Dose*	*Higher Dose*	*Lower Dose*	*Higher Dose*
Turpie et al. (1988)[5]	Tissue	2.0–2.5	3.0–4.5	1.2 per cent	1.2 per cent	5.7 per cent	20.6 per cent
Saour et al. (1990)[39]	Mechanical	1.9–3.6	7.4–10.8	1.4 per cent	1.3 per cent	21.3 per cent	42.4 per cent

laboratory control with a relatively unresponsive thromboplastin (international sensitivity index = 2.3) were given. One group received relatively low-intensity warfarin approximating to 1.9 to 3.6 international normalized ratio, and the other group received traditional North American high-dose warfarin (international normalized ratio 7.4 to 10.8). No gain in prevention of embolism resulted in the excessively treated group, but there was greatly increased hemorrhage.

A study is now needed in mechanical valves to determine whether lower doses of warfarin would be effective and still prevent embolism. The less thrombogenic types of mechanical valves might be studied first. (See Chapter 11.)

ATRIAL FIBRILLATION

Three randomized trials have recently been published, all of which included an untreated control group and also an aspirin group in the two reports by Petersen et al.,[40] and the Stroke Prevention Study[41] (Table 9–7). In the Danish study,[40] patients with chronic nonrheumatic atrial fibrillation were randomized to received a moderate-dose warfarin regime (international normalized ratio range of 2.4 to 4.2). The yearly incidence of thromboembolism was 2 per cent on warfarin and significantly less than the 5.5 per cent in randomized aspirin and placebo groups. The two other studies, the Stroke Prevention in Atrial Fibrillation (AF) Study[41] and the Boston Study,[42] showed a low- to moderate-dose warfarin regimen approach was successful. Their control reagents were not standard-

ized, and the international normalized ratio can only be regarded as an approximation. The stated international normalized ratio of the Stroke Prevention Study does not correspond to any international sensitivity index equivalents for 1.3 to 1.8 ratio prolongation. Assuming an international sensitivity index value between 1.8 and 2.6 at the various centers, the international normalized ratio equivalents are marked with an asterisk in Table 9–7. Similarly, there was no standardization of international sensitivity index of the thromboplastins in the Boston Study, and the stated 1.5 to 2.7 international normalized ratio equivalents of the 1.2 to 1.5 prothrombin ratio target range are listed also in Table 9–7.

In both studies, however, it is clear that the treatment was of intermediate intensity, but not sufficiently well defined in international normalized ratio terms to discount the 2.0 to 3.0 international normalized ratio recommendations for atrial fibrillation of the British Society for Haematology[16] and the American College of Chest Physicians/National Heart Lung and Blood Institute.[9] (See Chapter 12.)

PRIMARY INTERVENTION STUDIES

An even lower-dose warfarin study with a target of international normalized ratio of 1.6 is being used in a large United Kingdom multicenter primary prevention study in healthy adult males with high levels of fibrinogen or factor VII coagulant activity, which are major risk factors for ischemic heart

TABLE 9–7. Atrial Fibrillation

	WARFARIN VERSUS PLACEBO TREATMENT				STROKES (n)	
	Warfarin	*Placebo*	*Inclusion (per cent)*	*Stated INR Range*	*Warfarin*	*Placebo*
Petersen et al. 1989[40]	335	336	37	2.4–4.2	5	21
*Stroke Prevention Study 1990[41]	580 +aspirin	656	47	2.0–3.5*	7	18
†Boston BAATAF Study[42]	212	208		1.5–2.7†	2	13

			*		†
Stated INR Range			2.0–3.5		1.5–2.7
but if thromboplastin ISI is	1.8	≡	1.6–2.9		1.4–2.0
	2.0	≡	1.7–3.25		1.4–2.25
	2.3	≡	1.8–3.9		1.5–2.55
	2.6	≡	2.0–4.6		1.6–2.9

disease.[43] A fixed warfarin 1 milligram/day regimen also seems to be effective in reducing the elevated levels of factor VII coagulant activity in healthy adult males detected in a population screening program.[44] (See Chapter 4.)

ADVERSE EFFECTS

Bleeding is the main complication of oral anticoagulant therapy. The risk of bleeding is influenced by the intensity of anticoagulant therapy (Table 9–8), by the patient's underlying clinical disorder,[45] and by the concomitant use of aspirin. The risk of major bleeding has been reported to be increased in association with age over 65 years, a history of stroke or gastrointestinal bleeding, atrial fibrillation, and the presence of serious co-morbid conditions such as renal insufficiency or anemia. Bleeding which occurs when the international normalized ratio is less than 3.0 may be associated with an obvious underlying cause[3] or an occult gastrointestinal or renal lesion.

The most important nonhemorrhagic side effect of warfarin is skin necrosis. This uncommon complication is usually observed on the third to eighth day of therapy[45] and is caused by extensive thrombosis of the venules and capillaries within the subcutaneous fat. An association has been reported between warfarin-induced skin necrosis and protein C-deficiency,[46,47] and less commonly, protein S-deficiency, but this complication can also occur in individuals without deficiency of either of these natural coagulation inhibitors.

The pathogenesis is unknown. A role for protein C-deficiency seems probable and is supported by the similarity of the lesions to those seen in neonatal purpura fulminans which complicates homozygous protein C-deficiency. The reason for the unusual localization of the lesions remains a mystery. (See Chapter 9.)

PREGNANCY

Oral anticoagulants cross the placenta and can produce a characteristic embryopathy, central nervous system abnormalities, or fetal bleeding.[48] Warfarin embryopathy, which includes nasal hypoplasia, frontal bossing, and/or stippled epiphyses, has only been reported with first-trimester warfarin exposure, but central nervous system abnormalities have been reported with warfarin exposure during any trimester. In a review of 970 pregnancies associated with oral anticoagulant therapy, there were 45 cases of warfarin embryopathy and 26 cases of central nervous system abnormalities. Since most of these reports came from descriptive studies, these rates may not be reliable. The most concrete evidence of increased risk of fetopathic effects from oral anticoagulants used in pregnancy comes from a small prospective study in 72 pregnancies in patients with valvular heart disease.[49] Warfarin embryopathy was reported in 28.6 per cent of infants exposed to warfarin between the sixth and twelfth weeks of gestation, although the intensity of anticoagulation, presumably high-dose, is not stated. No cases of warfarin embryopathy occurred in the 19

TABLE 9–8. Bleeding and Intensity of Anticoagulant Therapy

STUDY	PATIENT (NUMBER)	ANTICOAGULANT DURATION	THERAPEUTIC RANGE (INTERNATIONAL NORMALIZED RATIOS)	TOTAL PER CENT OF BLEEDING	P VALUE
Hull et al. (1982) (86)[3]					
Deep vein thrombosis	96	3 months	2.4–4.6* versus 2.0–1.5	22.4 versus 4.3	0.015
Turpie et al. (1988) (97)[5]					
Prosthetic heart valves (tissue)	210	3 months	3.0–4.5† versus 2.0–2.5	13.9 versus 5.9	<0.002
Saour et al. (1989) (98)[44]					
Prosthetic heart valves (mechanical)	247	3.47 years	7.4–10.8 versus 1.9–3.6	42.4 versus 21.3	<0.002

* Based on prothrombin time ratio of 1.5 to 1.85 with Simplastin.
† Based on prothrombin time ratio of 1.5 to 2.0 with Dade thromboplastin.

patients in whom heparin was substituted for warfarin between the sixth and twelfth weeks of gestation. No central nervous system abnormalities were reported.

Warfarin should not normally be used in the first trimester of pregnancy: if possible, it should also be avoided throughout the entire pregnancy. Heparin is preferred when anticoagulants are indicated in pregnancy. Contrary to earlier reports, there is convincing evidence that warfarin does not induce an anticoagulant effect in the breast-fed infant when the drug is administered to a nursing mother. (See Chapter 26.)

CONCLUSION

Great progress has been made in the development of more effective and safer oral anticoagulant regimens. These improvements have arisen from the firmer basis for the treatment provided by recent randomized trials and the wider tendency to administer warfarin in lower doses to improve the benefit:risk ratio. The latter has been facilitated by improvement in laboratory monitoring from the application of the international normalized ratio system of prothrombin time standardization. International normalized ratios have also permitted segmentation of the previous blanket therapeutic range to tailor requirements for specific clinical states thus providing greater margins of safety in dosage.

REFERENCES

1. Taberner DA, Poller L, Burslem RW, Jones JB. Oral anticoagulants controlled by British Comparative Thromboplastin versus low dose heparin in prophylaxis of deep vein thrombosis. Br Med J 1978; 1: 272–4.
2. Hull R, Delmore T, Carter C, et al. Warfarin sodium versus low dose heparin in the long term treatment of venous thrombosis. N Engl J Med 1979; 301: 855–8.
3. Hull R, Hirsh J, Carter C, et al. Different intensities of oral anticoagulant therapy in the treatment of proximal vein thrombosis. N Engl J Med 1982; 307: 1676–81.
4. Report of the Sixty Plus Reinfarction Study Research Group. A double blind trial to assess long term oral anticoagulant therapy in elderly patients after myocardial infarction. Lancet 1980; 2: 989–94.
5. Turpie AGG, Gunstensen J, Hirsh J, et al. Randomized comparison of two intensities of oral anticoagulant therapy after tissue heart valve replacement. Lancet 1988; 1: 1242–5.
6. Powers PJ, Gent M, Jay KM, et al. A randomized trial of less intense post operative warfarin or aspirin therapy in the prevention of venous thromboembolism after surgery for fractured hip. Arch Int Med 1989; 149: 771–4.
7. Smith P, Arnesen H, Holme I. The effect of warfarin on mortality and reinfarction after acute myocardial infarction. N Engl J Med 1990; 323: 147–152.
8. Poller L. Progress in laboratory control of anticoagulant treatment. In: Poller L, ed. Recent advances in blood coagulation. London: Churchill Livingstone, 1969:137–55.
9. Hirsh J, Poller L, Deykin D, et al. Optimal therapeutic range for oral anticoagulants. Chest 1989; 95: S5–11.
10. Malhotra OP. Dicoumarol induced 9-gamma carboxy glutamic acid prothrombin. Isolation and comparison with 6-, 7-, 8- and 10-gamma carboxy glutamic acid isomers. Biochem J 1991, in press.
11. Sadowski JA, Bovill EG, Mann KG. Warfarin and the metabolism of vitamin K. In: Poller L, ed. Recent advances in blood coagulation—5. Edinburgh: Churchill Livingstone, 1991:93–118.
12. Breckenridge AM. Oral anticoagulant drugs: pharmacokinetic aspects. Semin Hematol 1978; 15: 19–26.
13. O'Reilly RA. Vitamin K and other oral anticoagulant drugs. Annu Rev Med 1976; 27: 245–61.
14. O'Reilly RA, Aggeler PM, Hoag MS, et al. Hereditary transmission of exceptional resistance to coumarin anticoagulant drugs. N Engl J Med 1983; 308: 1229–30.
15. Suttie JW, Muhah-Schendel LL, Shah DV, Lyle BJ, Greger JL. Vitamin K deficiency from dietary vitamin K restriction in humans. Am J Clin Nutr 1988; 47: 475–80.
16. British Society for Haematology. Guidelines on oral anticoagulation. 2nd ed. J Clin Pathol 1990; 43: 177–83.
17. Wright IS. Recent developments in antithrombotic therapy. Ann Intern Med 1969; 71(4): 823–31.
18. Poller L, Taberner DA. Dosage and control of oral anticoagulants—an international survey. Br J Haematol 1982; 51: 479–85.
19. Poller L. The effect of the use of different tissue extracts on one stage prothrombin times. Acta Haematol 1964; 32: 292–8.
20. Zucker S, Cathey MH, Sox PJ, Haljec EC. Standardisation of laboratory tests for controlling anticoagulant therapy. Am J Clin Pathol 1970; 53: 348–54.
21. Hirsh J, Levine M. Confusion over the therapeutic range for monitoring oral anticoagulant therapy in North America. Thromb Haemost 1988; 59(2): 129–32.
22. Loeliger EA, Poller L, Samama M, et al. Questions and answers on prothrombin time standardisation in oral anticoagulant control. Thromb Haemost 1985; 54: 515–8.
23. Poller L, McKernan A, Thomson JM. Fixed minidose warfarin: a new approach to prophylaxis against venous thrombosis after major surgery. Br Med J 1987; 295: 1309–12.
24. Bern MM, Lokich JJ, Wallach SR, et al. Very low doses of warfarin can prevent thrombosis in central venous catheters. Ann Intern Med 1990; 112(6): 234–8.
25. Vroonhoven TJMV, van Zijl J, Muller H. Low-dose subcutaneous heparin versus oral anticoagulants in the prevention of postoperative deep-venous thrombosis. Lancet 1974; 1: 375–7.
26. Francis CW, Marder VJ, McCollister C, et al. Two step warfarin therapy. JAMA 1983; 249: 374–8.
27. Sevitt S, Gallagher NG. Prevention of venous thrombosis and pulmonary embolism in injured patients: a trial of anticoagulant prophylaxis with phenindione in middle-aged and elderly patients with fractured necks of femur. Lancet 1959; 2: 981–6.
28. Brenkel IJ, Clancy MJ. Total hip replacement and antithrombotic prophylaxis. Br J Hosp Med 1990; 42: 282–4.
29. Lagerstedt CI, Fagher BO, Albrechtsson U, et al. Need for long-term anticoagulant treatment in symptomatic calf-vein thrombosis. Lancet 1985; 2: 515–8.
30. Poller L. The British Comparative Thromboplastin. The use of the national thromboplastin reagent for uniformity of laboratory control of oral anticoagulants and expression of results. Association of Clinical Pathologists Broadsheet 1970: No. 71.
31. Medical Research Council. Assessment of short term anticoagulant administration after cardiac infarction. Br Med J 1969; 1: 335–42.
32. Medical Research Council. Second report of the working party on anticoagulant therapy after myocardial infarction. Br Med J 1964; 2: 837–43.
33. US Veterans Administration Co-operative Study. Anticoagulants in myocardial infarction. JAMA 1973; 225: 724–6.

34. Hilden T, Iversen K, Raaschou F. Anticoagulants in myocardial infarction. Lancet 1961; 2: 327–31.
35. Resnikov L, Chediak J, Hirsh J, Lewis HD Jr. Antithrombotic agents in coronary artery disease. Chest 1989; 95(2): 52S–72S.
36. Kretschmer G, Wenzl E, Schemper M, et al. Influence of postoperative anticoagulant treatment of patient survival after femoropopliteal vein bypass surgery. Lancet 1988; 1: 797–8.
37. Drapkin A, Merskey C. Anticoagulant therapy after acute myocardial infarction. JAMA 1972; 222: 541–3.
38. Mok CK, Boey J, Wang R, et al. Warfarin versus dipyridamole-aspirin and pentoxifylline-aspirin for the prevention of prosthetic heart valve thromboembolism: a prospective clinical trial. Circulation 1985; 72(5): 1059–63.
39. Saour JN, Sieck JO, Maimo AR, Gallus AS. Trial of different intensities of anticoagulation in patients with prosthetic heart valves. N Engl J Med 1990; 322: 428–31.
40. Petersen P, Boysen G, Godtfredsen E, et al. Placebo controlled randomised trial of warfarin and aspirin for prevention of thromboembolic complications in atrial fibrillation. Lancet 1989; 1: 175–8.
41. Stroke Prevention in Atrial Fibrillation Study Group Investigators. Preliminary report of the Stroke Prevention in Atrial Fibrillation Study. N Engl J Med 1990; 322: 863–8.
42. Boston Area Anticoagulant Trial for Atrial Fibrillation Investigators. The effect of low dose warfarin on the risk of stroke with non-rheumatic atrial fibrillation. N Engl J Med 1990; 323: 1506–11.
43. Meade TW. Epidemiology of atheroma, thrombosis and ischaemic heart disease. In: Bloom AL, Thomas DP, eds. Haemostasis and thrombosis. 2nd ed. Edinburgh: Churchill Livingstone, 1987:697–720.
44. Poller L, MacCallum PK, Thomson JM, Kerns W. Reduction of factor VII coagulant activity (VIIC), a risk factor for ischaemic heart disease, by fixed dose warfarin: a double blind crossover study. Br Heart J 1990; 63: 231–3.
45. Levine MN, Raskob G, Hirsh J. Hemorrhagic complications of long term anticoagulant therapy. Chest 1989; 95(suppl 2): 26S–36S.
46. Samama M, Horellou MH, Soria J, et al. Successful progressive anticoagulation in a severe protein C deficiency and previous skin necrosis at the initiation of oral anticoagulation treatment. Thromb Haemost 1984; 51: 332–3.
47. Broekmans AW, Bertina RM, Loeliger EA, et al. Protein C and the development of skin necrosis during anticoagulation therapy. Thromb Haemost 1983; 49: 244–51.
48. Hall JAG, Pauli RM, Wilson KM. Maternal and fetal sequelae of anticoagulation during pregnancy. Am J Med 1980; 68: 122–40.
49. Iturbe Alessio I, del Carmen Fonseca M, Mutchinik O, et al. Risks of anticoagulant therapy in pregnant women with artificial heart valves. N Engl J Med 1986; 315: 1390–3.

10

THROMBOLYTIC AGENTS

MARC VERSTRAETE and DÉSIRÉ COLLEN

The fibrinolytic system comprises an inactive proenzyme, plasminogen, which can be converted to the active enzyme, plasmin, that degrades fibrin into soluble fibrin degradation products. Two immunologically distinct types of physiologic plasminogen activators have been identified: tissue-type plasminogen activator (t-PA) and urokinase-type plasminogen activator (u-PA). Inhibition of the fibrinolytic system may occur at the level of plasminogen activators, by plasminogen activator inhibitors (PAI-1 and PAI-2), or at the level of plasmin, mainly by alpha$_2$-antiplasmin. Regulation and control of the fibrinolytic system depend on specific molecular interactions between its main components. Plasminogen activation may also be induced by an "intrinsic" pathway involving several proteins such as factor XII, high molecular weight kininogen (HMWK), and prekallikrein. The various physiologic pathways of activation of the fibrinolytic system are shown schematically in Figure 10–1.

MAIN COMPONENTS OF THE FIBRINOLYTIC SYSTEM

The fibrinolytic system, schematically represented in Figure 10–1, contains a proenzyme, plasminogen, which can be converted to the active enzyme plasmin by the action of several different types of plasminogen activators. Plasmin is a serine protease which digests fibrin to soluble degradation products. Natural inhibition of the fibrinolytic system occurs both at the level of the plasminogen activators and also at the level of plasmin.

Plasminogen

Human plasminogen is a single-chain glycoprotein with a molecular weight of 92,000 daltons, containing 790 amino acids and five homologous triple-loop structures, or "kringles" (Fig. 10–2). The normal plasma concentration is about 1.5 to 2 micromoles. Native plasminogen has NH$_2$-terminal glutamic acid (Glu-plasminogen) but is easily converted by limited plasmic digestion to modified forms with NH$_2$-terminal lysine, valine, or methionine, commonly designated Lys-plasminogen. This conversion occurs by hydrolysis of the arginine-67–methionine-68, lysine-76–lysine-77, or lysine-77–valine-78 peptide bonds. The hydrodynamic properties of both types have been reviewed elsewhere.

A 2.7 kb insert of a complementary deoxyribonucleic acid (cDNA) clone for human plasminogen containing the complete coding region has been sequenced. The amino acid sequence predicted from this complementary deoxyribonucleic acid is close to the published protein sequence and differs in only four amide assignments (Glx, Asx) and in the presence of an extra isoleucine at position 85, yielding a total of 791 amino acids for human plasminogen. The plasminogen gene was mapped to the long arm of chromosome 6 at band q26 or 27.

Plasminogen is converted to plasmin by cleavage of a single arginine–valine peptide bond corresponding to the arginine-560–valine-561 bond. The two-chain plasmin molecule is composed of a heavy chain, or A-chain, originating from the NH$_2$-terminal part of plasminogen and a light chain, or B-chain, constituting the carboxyl group-terminal part. The B-chain was found to contain an active site similar to that of trypsin, composed of histidine-602, aspargine-645, and serine-740. Investigation of the activation pathways of plasminogen with the use of monoclonal antibodies specific for Lys-plasminogen has revealed that activation of Glu-

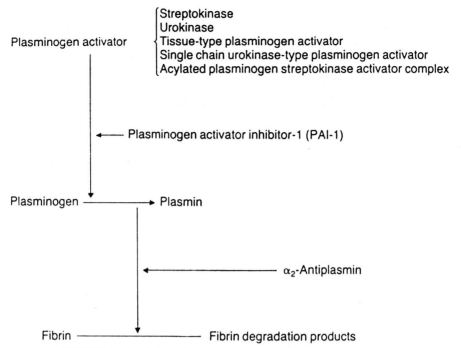

FIGURE 10–1. Schematic representation of the fibrinolytic system.

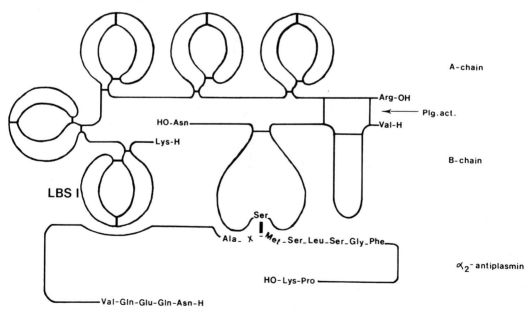

FIGURE 10–2. Schematic representation of the structure of the plasminogen molecule and the interaction between plasmin and alpha₂-antiplasmin. Plg.act indicates where the plasminogen molecule is cleaved by activators. The heavy or A-chain originates from the aminoterminal part of the molecule; the light or B-chain constitutes the carboxyl group-terminal part; the latter contains the active serine site.

plasminogen in human plasma occurs by direct cleavage of the arginine-560–valine-561 peptide bond without generation of Lys-plasminogen intermediates.

The plasminogen molecule contains structures called lysine binding sites, which are located in the plasmin A-chain. These lysine binding sites mediate its interaction with fibrin and with alpha$_2$-antiplasmin. Therefore, it has been suggested that the lysine binding sites play a crucial role in the regulation of fibrinolysis.

Alpha$_2$-Antiplasmin

Alpha$_2$-antiplasmin is a glycoprotein of the serine protease inhibitor (Serpin) superfamily, composed of 452 amino acids with arginine-364–methionine-365 as the reactive site. Alpha$_2$-Antiplasmin reacts very rapidly with plasmin, first to form a reversible but inactive complex, which is then slowly converted into an irreversible complex (Fig. 10–2). The rapidity of the first step of the reaction is dependent on the presence of free lysine binding sites and a free active center in the plasmin molecule.

Plasminogen Activator Inhibitor

Plasminogen activator inhibitor-1 (PAI-1) is a fast acting inhibitor of tissue-type plasminogen activator and urokinase, occurring at very low concentration in the blood, but which may be significantly increased in several disease states including venous thromboembolism and ischemic heart disease. It is a serpin, composed of 379 amino acids with arginine-346–methionine-347 as the reactive site.

Plasminogen Activators

Plasminogen activators are serine proteases with a high specificity for plasminogen, which hydrolyze the arginine-560–valine-561 peptide bond, yielding the active enzyme plasmin. They are described in the section Agents Activating Plasminogen Indirectly.

Thrombolytic agents include: (a) proteolytic enzymes acting directly on fibrin (for example, plasmin and Aspergillus protease [brinase]), and (b) drugs capable of activating plasminogen, either indirectly (streptokinase) or directly (for example, single-chain urokinase-type plasminogen activator or saruplase, two-chain urokinase-type plasminogen activator or urokinase and tissue-type plasminogen activator) and thereby enhancing enzymatic fibrinolysis. Only streptokinase, urokinase, saruplase, and tissue-type plasminogen activator have been shown to be effective and safe in hastening lysis of thrombi from both the venous and arterial circulations in patients.

AGENTS WITH A DIRECT PROTEOLYTIC ACTIVITY ON FIBRIN

Plasmin

The first commercial preparation of thrombolytic agents were mixtures of plasmin and streptokinase (Ortho: Actase; Merck, Sharp and Dohme: Thrombolysin). Because of the high antiplasmin titres in circulating plasma these products had a limited proteolytic activity which was primarily attributable to the plasminogen activating potential of the streptokinase component of these preparations.[1]

Brinase

Brinase is a proteolytic enzyme preparation which is obtained by submerged cultivation of the microorganism *Aspergillus oryzae*. The final enzyme preparation is composed of two enzymatically active components: a serine protease which represents about 98 per cent of the total enzymatic activity, and a metalloprotease with zinc in its active center. Brinase is rapidly inhibited by endogenous alpha$_1$-antitrypsin and alpha$_2$-macroglobulin; inhibition was found to be complete within 30 seconds.[2] The alpha$_2$-macroglobulin protease complex retains part of the activity of the free enzyme.

Brinase lyses fibrin and fibrinogen directly, without activating the plasminogen-plasmin system. The thrombolytic properties of brinase have primarily been established in experimental animals.[3–5] The initial clinical studies could not be extended because the production of clinical grade brinase was discontinued.

AGENTS ACTIVATING
PLASMINOGEN INDIRECTLY

Streptokinase

PHYSICOCHEMICAL PROPERTIES

Streptokinase is produced by several strains of hemolytic streptococci. It consists of a single polypeptide chain with a molecular weight of 47,000 to 50,000 daltons and contains 414 amino acids.[6] The region comprising amino acids 1 to 230 shows some homology with trypsin-like serine proteinases but lacks an active-site serine residue. Streptokinase has no peptidase or amidase activity and is not inhibited by active-site titrants such as diisopropyl fluorophosphate.

MECHANISM OF PLASMINOGEN ACTIVATION

Streptokinase activates plasminogen to plasmin indirectly, following a three-step mechanism.[7] In the first step, streptokinase forms an equimolar complex with plasminogen, which undergoes a conformational change resulting in the exposure of an active site in the plasminogen moiety. In the second step, this active site catalyzes the activation of plasminogen to plasmin. In a third step, plasminogen-streptokinase molecules are converted to plasmin-streptokinase complex.[8] The presence of an active site in the plasminogen-streptokinase complex was demonstrated by reaction with an active-site titrant, thereby blocking its conversion to the plasmin-streptokinase complex.[7,9] The plasminogen activating potential of the plasminogen-streptokinase complex is two- to threefold higher than that of the plasmin-streptokinase complex.[10] The activation of Glu-plasminogen by the plasminogen-streptokinase complex is enhanced 6.5-fold in the presence of fibrin and twofold in the presence of fibrinogen.[11,12] The plasminogen-streptokinase complex is not inhibited by plasma protease inhibitors, and hydrolyzes the chromogenic plasmin substrate D-Val-Leu-Lys-p-nitroanilide. These phenomena are the basis of the spectrophotometric determination of plasminogen in plasma after addition of excess streptokinase.

Conversion of the equimolar plasminogen-streptokinase complex to the plasmin-streptokinase complex occurs rapidly by proteolytic cleavage of both the plasminogen and the streptokinase moieties. In plasminogen, the arginine-560–valine-561 and the lysine-77–lysine-78 peptide bonds are cleaved,[13,14] while four modified forms of streptokinase differing in molecular weight by 4,000 to 5,000 daltons have been observed, depending on the species origin of the plasminogen.[15] With human plasminogen, a major proteolytic derivative with molecular weight of 36,000 daltons is generated.[16] The plasmin-streptokinase complex can also be formed by mixing plasmin and streptokinase, which react with a rate constant of $3 \times 5 \times 10^7$ moles/second.[17] The complex has a dissociation constant of 5×10^{-11} moles; these data indicate that the complex is strong and that it is extremely rapidly formed. The active-site residues in the plasmin-streptokinase complex are the same as those in the plasmin molecule. The main differences in the enzymatic properties of plasmin and the plasmin-streptokinase complex are found in their interaction with plasminogen and with alpha$_2$-antiplasmin. Plasmin, in contrast to its complex with streptokinase, is unable to activate plasminogen, while the plasmin(ogen)-streptokinase complex is virtually not inhibited by alpha$_2$-antiplasmin, which inhibits plasmin very rapidly.

Apart from its effects on fibrin within the thrombus, plasmin also degrades plasma proteins involved in the maintenance of blood coagulation. Since streptokinase ultimately activates plasmin, it is associated with a "systemic fibrinolytic state," characterized by plasminogen activation in plasma (hyperplasminemia), diminished alpha$_2$-antiplasmin, and breakdown of fibrinogen, factor V, and factor VIII.

PHARMACOKINETIC PROPERTIES

Streptokinase disappears from the circulation with a biphasic pattern: initial clearance half-life of 4 minutes and terminal clearance half-life of 30 minutes.[18] The level of antistreptokinase antibodies, which may result from previous infections with beta-hemolytic streptococci, varies largely amongst individuals. Approximately 350,000 units of streptokinase are required to neutralize the circulating antibodies in 95 per cent of a healthy population, with individual requirements ranging between 25,000 and 3 million units.[19] Since streptokinase is inactivated by interaction with antibodies, sufficient streptokinase must be infused to neutralize the antibodies. A few days after streptokinase administration, the antistreptokinase titer rises rapidly to 50 to 100 times the preinfusion value and remains high for four to six months, during which period renewed thrombolytic treatment with streptokinase or compounds containing streptokinase are impracticable.

DOSAGE OF STREPTOKINASE

The dosage of streptokinase at which systemic fibrinolysis occurs is dependent mainly on the plasma levels of antistreptococcal antibodies (from prior streptococcal infection) and antiplasmin, and hence is variable among individuals.

An initial dose must be given which is adequate to neutralize their effect; the streptokinase-antibody complex thus formed is rapidly cleared from the circulation. The initial dose for an individual patient can be determined by either the streptokinase resistance test (if laboratory facilities are available or time permits), or a standard initial intravenous dose ranging from 500,000 units to 750,000 units can be given over a period of 10 to 30 minutes, followed by a continuous intravenous maintenance dose of 100,000 units hourly for one or more days. Such a fixed dosage regimen produces a satisfactory thrombolytic effect in the vast majority of patients.[19,20] Moreover, laboratory control is simplified and thrombolytic treatment can be started without delay. In the last ten years, high-dose (1.5 million units), short-term (15 to 20 minute infusion) systemic streptokinase treatment is routinely used with great success in patients with acute myocardial infarction. Local infusion of streptokinase in the immediate vicinity of a thrombus requires 2,000 units streptokinase/minute over 60 to 120 minutes and is applied in occlusions of pulmonary and limb arteries.

ADVERSE EFFECTS OF STREPTOKINASE

Transient hypertension and bradycardia may occur during streptokinase therapy and appears to be related to histamine or/and bradykinin release. In the larger, detailed trials, incidences as high as 10 per cent have been reported.[21] While a hypotensive episode may be dramatic, it is usually halted by cessation of infusion. The more rapidly streptokinase is infused, the more likely a hypotensive reaction will occur; therefore, the intravenous infusion should not exceed 1,000 units/kilogram/minute. The incidence of hypotension does not seem to be affected by premedication with steroids.

Like other foreign proteins, streptokinase is antigenic in humans and thus is able to provoke serious anaphylactic reactions (urticaria, bronchospasm, angioedema). In practice, however, major allergic reactions are rare. Shivering, pyrexia, or rashes appear in 10 per cent of patients during or shortly after streptokinase infusion. There have also been isolated reports of serum sickness-type illnesses after streptokinase thrombolysis.

Streptokinase infusion, if repeated between five days and six months following the initial infusion, may be clinically ineffective as a result of a high titer of circulating antibodies. In a recent study, it was found that three months after streptokinase treatment, neutralization titres were such that 1.5 million units of streptokinase would have been fully neutralized.[22] At four to eight months, 18 of 20 patients had neutralization titres such that at least 50 per cent of a dose of 1.5 million units of streptokinase would have been neutralized. After eight months, neutralization titres ranged from 0.4 to 2.0 million units in 40 per cent of the patients.

Hemorrhage is the most common complication of streptokinase. Minor bleeding (not requiring transfusion) occurs in 3 to 4 per cent of patients.[21] These are usually related to puncture or injection sites, but microscopic hematuria and blood-streaked sputum or vomit are also noted. Significant or major bleeding (requiring transfusion) occurs in 0.4 to 10 per cent of all patients.[21] Anticoagulant and/or aspirin treatment may also enhance the frequency of bleeding, as do invasive catheter approaches. The most serious complication is cerebral bleeding, which is reported at an incidence of 0.1 to 0.2 per cent, while ischemic stroke during streptokinase treatment of myocardial infarction occurs in 0.8 per cent. In large trials there is an excess of "early" hemorrhagic or other strokes on the day of streptokinase treatment or the day after. However, there are fewer strokes thereafter, rendering the overall risk of stroke similar in streptokinase and placebo-treated patients.[21] One can therefore conclude that in view of the placebo-related incidence of cerebrovascular events, there does not appear to be a clinically significant extra risk of stroke during streptokinase therapy.

Anisoylated Plasminogen Streptokinase Activator Complex (APSAC)

Anisoylated plasminogen-streptokinase activator complex was constructed with the intention to control the enzymatic activity of the plasmin(ogen)-streptokinase complex by a specific reversible chemical protection of its catalytic center (that is, by insertion of a p-anisoyl group). This approach should prevent premature neutralization of the agent in the bloodstream and enable its activation to proceed in a controlled and sustained manner.[23]

PHYSICOCHEMICAL PROPERTIES

Anisoylated human plasminogen-streptokinase activator complex (APSAC, anistreplase, or Eminase) is an equimolar noncovalent complex between human lysine-plasminogen and streptokinase (Fig. 10–3). The catalytic center is located at the caraboxylic-terminal region of plasminogen, whereas the lysine-binding site is comprised within the aminoterminal region of the molecule. Specific acylation of the catalytic center is achieved by the use of a reversible acylating agent, p-amidinophenyl-p'-anisate-HCl. The cationic amidino group is positioned to interact with the anionic carboxyl group of asparagine-734 within the catalytic center of plasminogen. The anisoyl head is located at a position near the serine-740 residue of the active center, so that the required acyl-transfer can take place.[23]

PHARMACOKINETIC PROPERTIES

Streptokinase slowly dissociates from the plasminogen-streptokinase complex with a rate constant of less than 10^{-4}/second.[24] The deacylation rate constant of anistreplase on the other hand, is greater than 10^{-4}/second,[25] which means that the activity of the complex will be controlled by the deacylation rate rather than by dissociation. The deacylation half-life of anistreplase in human plasma and in whole blood was claimed to be 105 to 120 minutes,[26] although it was previously reported to be 40 minutes in buffer.[23] In healthy volunteers, an apparent clearance half-life of 70 minutes was found for anistreplase, as compared to 25 minutes for the plasminogen-streptokinase complex formed upon administration of streptokinase alone.[18] In patients with acute myocardial infarction treated with anistreplase, half-lives of 90 to 112 minutes were reported for the plasma clearance of fibrinolytic activity.[27] This reversible blocking of the catalytic site by acylation delays the formation of the fibrinolytic enzyme plasmin, but has no influence on the lysine-binding sites involved in binding the complex to fibrin, although the affinity of plasminogen for fibrin is very weak. Deacylation commences immediately after dissolving the lyophilized material, and proceeds gradually after intravenous injection. Deacylation uncovers the catalytic center, which converts plasminogen to plasmin. This deacylation of the complex, however, does occur both in the circulation and at the fibrin surface, and the

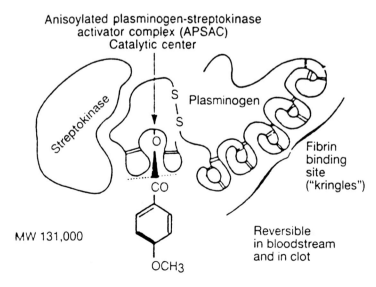

Anisoylated plasminogen-streptokinase activator complex (APSAC)
Catalytic center

Streptokinase

S
S

Plasminogen

O

CO

Fibrin binding site ("kringles")

MW 131,000

OCH3

Reversible in bloodstream and in clot

FIGURE 10–3. Schematic representation of the molecular configuration of anistreplase or anisoylated plasminogen streptokinase activator complex. (Reproduced from McIintock DK, Bell PH. The mechanism or activation of human plasminogen by streptokinases. Biochem Biophys Res Commun 1971; 53:694–702, with permission.)

fibrin-specificity of thrombolysis by anistreplase is, at best, only marginal.

DOSAGE OF ANISTREPLASE

The recommended standard dose in acute myocardial infarction is 30 Units anistreplase (1 milligram = international unit and 30 milligrams contain approximately 1.25 million units streptokinase) to be given as a bolus injection. In aggregate, comparative studies indicate that the efficacy for coronary thrombolysis (angiographic patency) of anistreplase is comparable or somewhat higher than that of intravenous streptokinase, but lower than that of intracoronary streptokinase.[28]

ADVERSE EFFECTS

In comparative trials of anistreplase (30 Units) versus intravenously infused streptokinase (1.5 × 10[6] international unit over 60 minutes), the same fall in fibrinogen concentrations and the same incidence of adverse events were noted in the two treatment groups.[29–31]

As anistreplase contains considerable amounts of streptokinase, it causes immunization, and the antibody titre may increase up to 60-fold after two or three weeks, and may still be very high three months later.[18,22] Repeat administration should not be considered in the first 6 to 12 months.

AGENTS CAPABLE OF ACTIVATING PLASMINOGEN DIRECTLY

Urokinase

PHYSICOCHEMICAL PROPERTIES

Urokinase is a trypsin-like enzyme composed of two polypeptide chains (molecular weight 20,000 and 34,000 daltons). This naturally occurring plasminogen activator is excreted in human urine, from which it can be extracted; urokinase may also be isolated from tissue cultures of human embryonic kidney cells. It may occur in two molecular forms designated S_1 (33,000 daltons, low molecular weight urokinase) and S_2 (55,000 daltons, high molecular weight urokinase), the former being a proteolytic degradation product of the latter[33] (Fig. 10–4). The complete primary structure of high molecular weight urokinase has been elucidated;[34] the light chain contains 158 amino acids and the heavy chain 253. The interchain disulfide bond Cysteine-194–Cysteine-222 was shown to be require for the activity of urokinase.[35] The catalytic center is located in the carboxyl group-terminal chain and is composed of asparagine-255, histidine-204, and serine-356. The NH$_2$-terminal chain contains a growth factor domain and one kringle domain. A low molecular weight two-chain urokinase-type plasminogen activator (molecular weight 33,000 daltons) can be generated with plasmin by hydrolysis of the lysine-135 to lysine-136 peptide bond following previous cleavage of the lysine-158–isoleucine-159 peptide bond.[36]

MECHANISM OF PLASMINOGEN ACTIVATION

Urokinase activates plasminogen directly, following Michaelis-Menten kinetics. This double-chain molecule has no specific activity for fibrin, and activates fibrin-bound and circulating plasminogen relatively indiscriminately. Extensive plasminogen activation and depletion of alpha$_2$-antiplasmin may occur following treatment with urokinase, leading to degradation of several plasma proteins including fibrinogen, factor V, and factor VIII. The half-life of urokinase is approximately 15 minutes.

DOSE OF UROKINASE

During over a decade, an initial intravenous dose of 4,000 units/kilogram body weight over 10 minutes followed by the same maintenance dose per kilogram hourly was recommended for the treatment of acute major pulmonary embolism. At present, a bolus dose in the right atrium of 15,000 units/kilogram body weight has been recommended in this indication and an intravenous infusion of 3 million units of urokinase (1 million units over 10 minutes and 2 million units over the next 110 minute) is presently being tested.

In acute myocardial infarction the dose of urokinase is 2 million units given as a bolus, or 3 million units administered over 90 minutes.

ADVERSE EFFECTS OF UROKINASE

Purified urokinase preparations are non-antigenic, nonpyrogenic, and their proper use is most often associated with a milder coagulation defect than that with streptokinase, but with a similar incidence of bleeding to that shown for streptokinase-treated patients. As the level of inhibitors in plasma is relatively constant, a fixed dosage regimen can readily be used.

Single-Chain Urokinase-Type Plasminogen Activator

PHYSICOCHEMICAL PROPERTIES

Single-chain urokinase-type plasminogen activator (scu-PA, pro-urokinase, saruplase) is synthesized by a variety of cells including endothelial cells and mononuclear cells. It is a single-chain glycoprotein with a molecular weight of 55,000 daltons containing 411 amino acids (Fig. 10–4).[37] Saruplase is the native zymogenic precursor of urokinase. Limited hydrolysis by plasmin or kallikrein of the lysine-158–isoleucine-159 peptide bond converts the molecule to two-chain urokinase-type plasminogen activator (Fig. 10–5). Specific hydrolysis of the glutamic acid-143–leucine-144 peptide bond in saruplase by an unidentified protease yields a low molecular weight saruplase with a molecular weight of 33,000 (saruplase-32k).[38] Thrombin cleaves the arginine-156–phenylalanine-157 peptide bond in saruplase, resulting in an active two-chain urokinase-type plasminogen activator molecule.[39]

MECHANISM OF PLASMINOGEN ACTIVATION

Saruplase does not have a specific affinity for fibrin.[40] In purified systems, saruplase

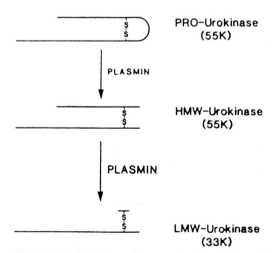

FIGURE 10–4. Schematic representation of the primary structure of single-chain urokinase-type plasminogen activator. The arrow indicates cleavage site for plasmin. The active-site residues are indicated with an asterisk.

has some intrinsic plasminogen activating potential, however, which is less than or equal to 1 per cent of that of two-chain urokinase-type plasminogen activator.[40] Conversion of saruplase to two-chain urokinase-type plasminogen activator in the vicinity of a fibrin clot apparently constitutes a significant positive feedback mechanism for clot lysis in human plasma in vitro.[41,42] This conversion may, however, play a less important role in in vivo thrombolysis, owing to preferential fibrin-associated activation of plasminogen by saruplase.

Recombinant saruplase is under clinical investigation in patients with acute myocardial infarction. Therapeutic doses range between 40 and 80 milligrams, infused over one hour.[43] These doses were found to cause a clear systemic activation of the fibrinolytic system and fibrinogen degradation. This may be due, at least in part, to conversion of saruplase to two-chain urokinase type plasminogen activator in the circulation.

Low molecular weight (saruplase-33k), purified form the conditioned medium of a human lung adenocarcinoma cell line[38] or prepared by recombinant deoxyribonucleic acid technology[49] had a fibrinolytic capacity in a rabbit jugular vein thrombosis model comparable to that of wild type recombinant saruplase.[49] The relative fibrin specificity of saruplase, as compared to two-chain urokinase-type plasminogen activator, was maintained at thrombolytic doses. Provided this relative fibrin specificity also holds for patients with thromboembolic disease, saruplase-33k might be a practical alternative molecule for the large-scale production of a relative fibrin-specific thrombolytic agent by recombinant deoxyribonucleic acid technology.

DOSE OF SARUPLASE

There is still limited clinical experience with recombinant saruplase. The generic name for full-length unglycosylated human recombinant saruplase obtained rom *Escherichia coli* is saruplase. With a preparation containing 160,000 units/milligram, the dose used successfully in patients with acute myocardial infarction was 20 milligrams given as a bolus, and 60 milligrams in the next 60 minutes, immediately followed by an intravenous heparin infusion (20 international units/kilogram/hour) for 72 hours.[43]

ADVERSE EFFECTS OF SARUPLASE

In a direct double-blind comparison between intravenous saruplase (80 milligrams

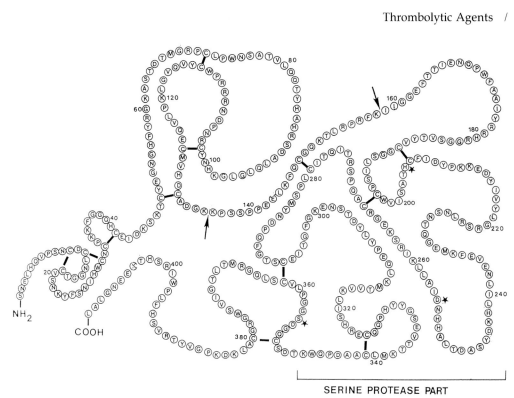

SERINE PROTEASE PART

FIGURE 10–5. Diagram represents the single-chain structure of saruplase, its proteolytic conversion at bond 158–159 to the two-chain high molecular weight form by trace amounts of plasmin, and its degradation by large amounts of plasmin to the low molecular weight form at bond 143–144. The active site residues are indicated with an asterisk. The black bars represent disulphide bonds.

over 60 minutes) and streptokinase (1.5 million international units over 60 minutes) in 401 patients with acute myocardial infarction, a somewhat smaller reduction in circulating fibrinogen levels was observed in patients treated with saruplase. There were significantly less bleeding episodes in the saruplase group versus the streptokinase group (14 versus 25 per cent), and less transfusion requirement (4 versus 11 per cent).[43]

Tissue-Type Plasminogen Activator

The plasminogen activator found in blood is synthesized and secreted by endothelial cells and is now called tissue-type plasminogen activator (t-PA). Antigen levels of tissue-type plasminogen activator in normal plasma are about 5 nanograms/milliliter. Tissue-type plasminogen activator has been purified from the tissue culture fluid of stable human melanoma cell lines in sufficient amounts to study its biochemical and biological properties;[50] it is presently produced for clinical use by recombinant deoxyribonucleic acid technology.[51]

PHYSICOCHEMICAL PROPERTIES

Tissue-type plasminogen activator is a serine proteinase with a molecular weight of about 70,000 daltons, consisting of a single polypeptide chain of 527 amino acids with serine as the NH_2-terminal amino acid (Fig. 10–6). The complete primary structure has been deduced from the complementary deoxyribonucleic acid sequence.[51] It was subsequently shown that native tissue-type plasminogen activator contains an NH_2-terminal extension of three amino acids (Gly-Ala-Arg).[52] Plasmin (but also kallikrein and activated factor X) converts tissue-type plasminogen activator to a two-chain molecule by hydrolysis of the arginine-275–isoleucine-276 peptide bond (using a numbering system based on a total of 527 amino acids). The NH_2-terminal region (heavy chain) is composed of multiple structural-functional domains, including a "finger-like" domain (F) homologous to the finger domains in fibronectin,[53] an "epidermal growth factor-like domain" (E) homologous to that of urokinase, protein C and coagulation factors IX and X, and two disulphide bonded triple loop struc-

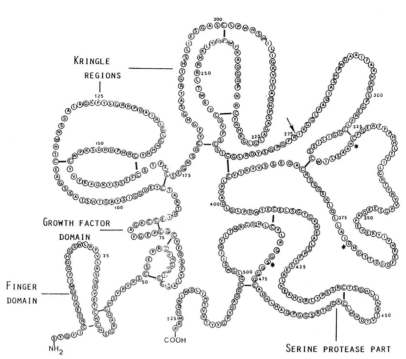

FIGURE 10–6. Schematic representation of the primary structure of tissue-type plasminogen activator. The arrow indicates the cleavage site for plasmin converting single-chain t-PA to two-chain t-PA. The active-site residues are indicated with an asterisk. Black bars indicate disulphide bonds.

tures commonly called "kringles" (K_1 and K_2), homologous to the kringle regions in plasminogen[51] and apolipoprotein (a). The carboxyl group-terminal region (light chain), comprising residues 276 to 527, is homologous to other serine proteinases and contains the catalytic site, which is composed of histidine-322, asparagine-371, and serine-478.[51]

The assembly of the tissue-type plasminogen activator gene is an example of the "exon shuffling" principle; the different structural domains on the heavy chain are encoded by a single exon or by two adjacent exons.[54] Because of the striking correlation between the intron-exon distribution of the gene and the domain structure of the protein,[55] it was suggested that these domains would be autonomous, structural, and/or functional entities ("modules").[53,56] These structural domains of tissue-type plasminogen activator are involved in most of its functions and interactions, including its enzymatic activity, binding to fibrin, stimulation of plasminogen activation by fibrin, binding to receptors, and inhibition by plasminogen activator inhibitors. The validity of the "exon-shuffling" concept for tissue-type plasminogen activator has been investigated by the construction of

mutants with precise domain deletions, insertions, or substitutions, and the evaluation of the fibrin affinity, the fibrin specificity and the pharmacokinetic and thrombolytic properties of such mutants. The relevance of this approach for a better understanding of the structure-function relationships in tissue-type plasminogen activator and for the development of new thrombolytic agents will be discussed.

FIBRIN AFFINITY OF TISSUE-TYPE PLASMINOGEN ACTIVATOR

The structures involved in the fibrin binding of tissue-type plasminogen activator are fully comprised within the NH_2-terminal (heavy) chain, as evidenced by the intact fibrin affinity of the heavy chain isolated after mild reduction of two-chain tissue-type plasminogen activator.[57,58] Evidence obtained with domain deletion mutants of tissue-type plasminogen activator indicated that its affinity for fibrin is mediated via the finger domain and mainly via the second kringle domain.[59] A lysine-binding site is involved in the interaction of the kringle-2 domain but not of the finger domain with fibrin. Gething et al.[60] have suggested, however, that the kringle-1 and kringle-2 domains of tissue-type plasminogen activator would be equivalent in their affinity for fibrin, although the kringle-1 domain does not contain a lysine-binding site.[59] The presence of a weaker lysine-binding site in kringle-2 similar to the aminohexyl-site in plasminogen has also been suggested.[61] This aminohexyl-site would interact with internal lysine residues in the fibrin matrix, whereas the lysine-binding site would interact with carboxyl group-terminal lysine residues.[54]

It has been suggested that in the process of fibrinolysis, binding of tissue-type plasminogen activator to intact fibrin would initially be mediated by the F domain. Subsequently, upon partial fibrin digestion by plasmin, increased binding of tissue-type plasminogen activator to newly exposed carboxyl group-terminal lysine residues would occur via the lysine-binding site in the kringle-2 domain. Because of its aminohexyl site, the kringle-2 domain may also play a role in the initial binding to intact fibrin.[61] During degradation of fibrin(ogen) by plasmin, the new tissue-type plasminogen activator binding sites with markedly lower dissociation constants (two to four orders of magnitude) are formed, but the increased binding of tissue-type plasminogen activator does not involve a lysine-binding site.[62] Deletion mutants of alteplase, lacking one or more of the structural domains in the heavy chain, have recently been used to identify the domains involved in the augmented binding of tissue-type plasminogen activator to fibrin after limited plasmic digestion.[63] These studies indicated that the increased binding can be attributed partially to the lysine-binding site in kringle-2, and partially to the F domain.

Some authors have not found a difference between the fibrin binding properties of single-chain and two-chain tissue-type plasminogen activator,[62] whereas another study reported a significant difference.[65] Recent findings have suggested that the fibrin-binding properties of tissue-type plasminogen activator may change considerably by plasmin-induced conversion from a single-chain to a two-chain molecule,[66] resulting in enhanced binding of two-chain tissue-type plasminogen activator to a large number of low-affinity binding sites on fibrin. It has also been reported that cross-linking of fibrin by activated factor XIII may result in masking of high-affinity binding sites for tissue-type plasminogen activator that are present in noncross-linked fibrin.[66] It is not clear whether the relative resistance of older fibrin clots to lysis may be related to crosslinking of the clot.

Binding of tissue-type plasminogen activator to fibrin thus appears to be a dynamic interaction, which may be modulated during fibrinolysis by partial degradation of fibrin and by conversion of single-chain to two-chain tissue-type plasminogen activator.

MECHANISM OF PLASMINOGEN ACTIVATION

The structures required for the enzymatic activity of tissue-type plasminogen activator are fully comprised within the carboxyl group-terminal (B)chain, as evidenced by the intact activity of the isolated B-chain, separated chemically[58,67,68] or prepared by recombinant deoxyribonucleic acid technology.[59,69] This carboxyl group-terminal region contains the catalytic triad composed of histidine-322, asparagine-370, and serine-478.[51]

In the absence of fibrin, tissue-type plasminogen activator is a poor plasminogen activator, mainly because of a low affinity for its substrate.[70] Single-chain tissue-type plasminogen activator is less active towards low molecular weight substrates and inhibitors,[71] but its activity towards plasminogen was shown to be comparable to that of the two-chain form.[72] The intrinsic enzymatic activity of single-chain tissue-type plasminogen activator was confirmed by the construction of alteplase mutants in which the plasmic cleavage site of conversion to two-chain tissue-type plasminogen activator was destroyed by site-specific mutagenesis of arginine-275 to glutamic acid or to all other amino acids.[65,62] Such mutants were demonstrated to have lower activity than two-chain tissue-type plasminogen activator in the absence of fibrin, but full plasminogen activating activity in the presence of fibrin.[65] Inhibition by plasminogen activator inhibitor-1 was also comparable for the wild-type and mutant tissue-type plasminogen activator. In contrast to other zymogen precursors of serine proteinases, the single-chain form of tissue-type plasminogen activator thus appears to be an active enzyme.

In the presence of fibrin, tissue-type plasminogen activator is a potent plasminogen activator, mainly due to a strongly enhanced affinity for its substrate.[70] The isolated proteinase part of two-chain tissue-type plasminogen activator, which is fully active, is not stimulated by fibrin, indicating that the structures involved in the fibrin-stimulation are also localized in the NH_2-terminal region.[58,69] The kinetic data suggest that the fibrin stimulation of plasminogen activation by tissue-type plasminogen activator occurs by sequential ordered addition of tissue-type plasminogen activator and plasminogen to fibrin, producing a thermodynamically more stable cyclic ternary complex.[70] This may imply that the fibrin affinity of tissue-type plasminogen activator and the fibrin stimulation of plasminogen activation are causally related, and that both properties would evolve in parallel.

CLEARANCE OF TISSUE-TYPE PLASMINOGEN ACTIVATOR

Tissue-type plasminogen activator has a short in vivo half-life: in patients with acute myocardial infarction the initial clearance half-life of single-chain alteplase was found to be four minutes and the terminal clearance half-life about 46 minutes.[74] Animal experiments have indicated that rapid clearance of tissue-type plasminogen activator (initial half-life one to four minutes in rabbits and mice)[56,75] occurs via the heavy chain and almost exclusively via liver hepatocytes. Although a receptor for tissue-type plasminogen activator has not yet been identified, the rapid uptake probably involves receptor-mediated endocytosis and lysosomal degradation.

Two different recognition systems for removal of tissue-type plasminogen activator have been characterized, a protein-mediated pathway via hepatocytes, and a carbohydrate-mediated pathway via endothelial cells in the liver.[77] Recently, studies with alteplase deletion mutants suggested that interaction of tissue-type plasminogen activator with hepatocytes would primarily involve kringle-1 and in addition would occur via the F and E domains, whereas binding to endothelial cells would occur mainly via the F and E domain.[78]

REACTIVITY OF TISSUE-TYPE PLASMINOGEN ACTIVATOR WITH PLASMINOGEN ACTIVATOR INHIBITOR-1

Plasminogen activator inhibitor-1 is a serpin (serine protease inhibitor); it neutralizes very rapidly single-chain, two-chain tissue-type plasminogen activator and urokinase.[79] To design mutants of tissue-type plasminogen activator that are resistant to inhibition by plasminogen activator inhibitor-1 Sambrook et al.[80] and Madison et al.[81] have

modeled the interactions between the active site of tissue-type plasminogen activator and plasminogen activator inhibitor-1 based on the known three-dimensional structure of the trypsin-trypsin inhibitor complex. They have identified specific amino aids (residues lysine-296–histidine–arginine–arginine–serine–proline–glycine-302 and arginine-304) in tissue-type plasminogen activator which make contact with plasminogen activator inhibitor-1 but not with the substrate plasminogen. Mutants of the alteplase obtained by site-specific mutagenesis in this region were shown to be fully active towards substrates, but to display significant resistance to inhibition by plasminogen activator inhibitor-1. In view of the large excess of tissue-type plasminogen activator over plasminogen activator inhibitor-1 achieved during thrombolytic therapy, resistance of tissue-type plasminogen activator mutants to plasminogen activator inhibitor-1 may not directly constitute a significant advantage over wild-type tissue-type plasminogen activator. High plasminogen activator inhibitor-1 levels may, however, contribute to the occurrence of reocclusion, and plasminogen activator inhibitor-1-resistant mutants of alteplase may be useful for maintenance infusion after initial thrombolysis.

DOSE OF ALTEPLASE

For the treatment of acute myocardial infarction, the recommended dose of alteplase (Activase, Actilyse) is 100 milligrams administered as 60 milligrams in the first hour (of which six to ten milligrams is administered as a bolus over the first one to two minutes), 20 milligrams over the second hour, and 20 milligrams over the third hour. More recently it was proposed to give the same total dose of 100 milligrams but "front loaded," commencing with a bolus of 15 milligrams, followed by 50 milligrams in the next 30 minutes, and the remaining 35 milligrams in the following 60 minutes.[83] At present, the dose of 15 milligrams intravenous bolus of alteplase, followed by 0.75 milligrams/kilogram over 30 minutes (not to exceed 50 milligrams), and then 0.05 milligrams/kilogram over 60 minutes (not to exceed 35 milligrams) is being tested in a large scale trial (GUSTO). Whichever the dose regimen given, it is important to co-administer intravenous heparin during and after alteplase treatment.

For catheter-directed local thrombolysis with alteplase in patients with recent peripheral arterial occlusion, the dose of 0.05 to 0.10 milligrams/kilogram/hour over an eight-hour period is usually recommended.

Duteplase

Duteplase is the generic name for recombinant tissue-type plasminogen activator, produced in its two-chain form by the Burroughs-Wellcome company. It also differs from recombinant human alteplase due to a substitution of a methionine for a valine in position 245 in the amino acid sequence, and is therefore a variant of the naturally occurring human tissue-type plasminogen activator. The specific activity of duteplase is approximately 300,000 units/milligram protein, but different production lots may have specific activities which vary as much as ± 100,000.[84] For this reason, the dosage of duteplase is given in megaunits/kilogram body weight (0.6 to 1.0 megaunits/kilogram over four hours).[85,86]

ADVERSE EFFECTS

Bleeding complications are the most common and feared side effects with any thrombolytic agent, including alteplase. The reported rates of bleeding during treatment with any thrombolytic agent depend on the methods of data collection, which can be very elaborate in trials on a limited number of patients, or limited in megatrials that include thousands of patients. Valid conclusions can only be obtained by direct comparisons between drugs in a given trial. In a recent large trial directly comparing alteplase and streptokinase, the reported incidence of cerebral bleeding (confirmed by computed tomographic scan and necropsy) was similar for the two thrombolytic agents, but overall, significantly more strokes were reported in the alteplase group.[83] For both agents there was an excess of strokes in patients above 70 years of age (greater than 70 years: 2.7 per cent alteplase; 1.6 per cent streptokinase; less than or equal to 70 years: 0.9 per cent alteplase; 0.8 per cent streptokinase). Significantly more major bleeds occurred in patients allocated to streptokinase. However, the total number of bleeds (minor plus major) was significantly higher with alteplase (4.2 versus 3.3 per cent). More allergic reactions (0.2 versus 1.7 per cent) and hypotension (1.7 versus 3.8 per cent) were seen with streptokinase.

To avoid bleeding and other complications, the relative and absolute contraindications to thrombolysis should be carefully observed.

REFERENCES

1. Sawyer WD, Alkjaersig N, Fletcher AP. Thrombolytic therapy. Arch Intern Med 1961; 107: 274–83.
2. Kiessling H, Frisch EP. Determination of the enzymatic activity of brinase and of the brinase inhibitor capacity by the azocollagen assay. Thromb Res 1988; 50: 249–52.
3. Roschlaw WHE, Fisher AM. Thrombolytic therapy with local perfusion of CA-7 (fibrinolytic enzyme from Aspergillus oriyzae) in the drug. Angiology 1966; 17: 670–82.
4. Frish EP. Clinical pharmacology of the thrombolytic enzyme preparation brinase. Semin Thromb Hemost 1989; 15: 341–6.
5. Frish EP, Blombäck M. Blood coagulation studies in patients treated with brinase. In: Davidson JF, ed. Progress in chemical fibrinolysis and thrombolysis. Vol. IV. Edinburgh: Churchill Livingstone, 1979: 184–7.
6. Jackson KW, Tang J. Complete amino acid sequence of streptokinase and its homology with serine proteases. Biochemistry 1982; 21: 6620–5.
7. Reddy KNN. Mechanism of activation of human plasminogen by streptokinase. In: Kline DL, Reddy KNN, eds. Fibrinolysis. Boca Raton: CRC Press, 1980: 71–94.
8. Summaria L, Wohl RC, Boreisha IG, Robbins KC. A virgin enzyme derived from human plasminogen. Specific cleavage of the arginyl-560-valyl peptide bond in the diisopropyphosphinyl virgin enzyme by plasminogen activators. Biochemistry 1982; 21: 2056–9.
9. McClintock DK, Bell PH. The mechanism of activation of human plasminogen by streptokinases. Biochem Biophys Res Commun 1971; 53: 695–702.
10. Markus G, DePasquale JL, Wissler FC. Quantitative determination of the binding of E-aminocaproic acid to native plasminogen. J Biol Chem 1978; 253: 727–32.
11. Fears R, Hibbs MJ, Smith RAG. Kinetic studies on the interaction of streptokinase and other plasminogen activators with plasminogen and fibrin. Biochem J 1985; 229: 555–8.
12. Camiolo SM, Markus G, Evers JL, Hobika GH. Augmentation of streptokinase activator activity by fibrinogen or fibrin. Thromb Res 1980; 17: 697–706.
13. McClintock DK, Englert ME, Dziobkowski C, Snedeker EH, Bell PH. Two distinct pathways of the streptokinase-mediated activation of highly purified human plasminogen. Biochemistry 1974; 13: 5334–44.
14. Bajaj SP, Castellino FJ. Activation of human plasminogen by equimolar levels of streptokinase. J Biol Chem 1977; 252: 492–8.
15. Reddy KNN. Kinetics of active center formation in dog plasminogen by streptokinase and activity of a modified streptokinase. J Biol Chem 1976; 251: 6624–9.
16. Siefring GE Jr, Castellino FJ. Interaction of streptokinase with plasminogen. Isolation and characterization of a streptokinase degradation product. J Biol Chem 1976; 251: 3913–20.
17. Cederholm-Williams SA, De Cock F, Lijnen HR, Collen D. Kinetics of the reactions between streptokinase, plasmin and α₂-antiplasmin. Eur J Biochem 1979; 100: 125–32.
18. Staniforth DH, Smith RAG, Hibbs M. Streptokinase and anisoylated streptokinase plasminogen complex. Their action on haemostasis in human volunteers. Eur J Clin Pharmacol 1983; 24: 751–6.
19. Verstraete M, Vermylen J, Amery A, Vermylen C. Thrombolytic therapy with streptokinase using a standard dosing scheme. Br Med J 1966; 5485: 454–6.
20. Hirsh J, O'Sullivan EF, Martin M. Evaluation of a standard dosage schedule with streptokinase. Blood 1970; 35: 341–9.
21. Goa KL, Henwood JM, Stolz JF, Langley MS, Clissold SP. Intravenous streptokinase. A reappraisal of its therapeutic use in acute myocardial infarction. Drugs 1990; 39: 693–719.
22. Jalihal S, Morris GK. Antistreptokinase titers after intravenous streptokinase. Lancet 1990; 1: 184–5.

23. Smith RAG, Dupe RJ, English PD, Green J, Fibrinolysis with acyl-enzymes: a new approach to thrombolytic therapy. Nature 1981; 290: 505–8.

24. Toerngren S. Optimal regimen of low-dose heparin prophylaxis in gastrointestinal surgery. Acta Chir Scand 1979; 145: 87–93.

25. Esmail AF, Dupe RJ, English PD, Smith RAG. Pharmacokinetic and pharmacodynamic comparisons of acylated streptokinase-plasminogen complexes with different deacylation rate constants. Haemostasis 1984; 14: 84.

26. Ferres H, Hibbs M, Smith RAG. Deacylation studies in vitro on anisoylated plasminogen streptokinase activator complex. Drugs 1987; 33 (suppl 3): 80–2.

27. Nunn B, Esmail A, Fears R, Ferres H, Strandring R. Pharmacokinetic properties of anisoylated plasminogen streptokinase activator complex and other thrombolytic agents in animals and in humans. Drugs 1987; 33: 88–92.

28. Verstraete M. Thrombolytic treatment in acute myocardial infarction. Circulation 1990; 82 (suppl II): II96–109.

29. Monnier P, Sigwart U, Vincent A, et al. Anisoylated plasminogen streptokinase activator complex versus streptokinase in acute myocardial infarction. Preliminary results of a randomised study. Drugs 1987; 33 (suppl 3): 175–8.

30. Monassier JP, Hanssen M. Haematological effects of anisoylated plasminogen activator complex and streptokinase in patients with acute myocardial infarction: interim report of the IRS II study. Drugs 1987; 33 (suppl 3): 247–52.

31. Hoffmann JJML, Bonnier JJRM, de Swart JBRM, Custers P, Vijgen M. Systemic effects of anisoylated plasminogen streptokinase activator complex and streptokinase therapy in acute myocardial infarction: coagulation aspects of the Dutch Invasive Reperfusion Study. Drugs 1987; 33 (suppl 3): 242–6.

32. Prowse CV, Hornsey V, Ruckley CV, Boulton FE. A comparison of acylated streptokinase-plasminogen complex and streptokinase in healthy volunteers. Thromb Haemost 1982; 47: 132–5.

33. White WF, Barlow GH, Mozen MM. The isolation and characterization of plasminogen activators (urokinase) from human urine. Biochemistry 1966; 5: 2160–9.

34. Guenzler WA, Steffens GJ, Oetting F, Kim SMA, Frankus E, Flohé L. The primary structure of high molecular mass urokinase from human urine. The complete amino acid sequence of the A chain. Hoppe-Seyler's Z Physiol Chem 1982; 363: 1155–65.

35. Miwa N, Sawada T, Suzuki A. Conformational changes in human urokinase induced by a specific reduction of disulfide bond in Cys194-Cys222 associated with exhibition of enzymatic activity. Biochim Biophys Acta 1984; 791: 1–8.

36. Steffens GJ, Guenzler WA, Oetting F, Frankus E, Flohé L. The complete amino acid sequence of low molecular mass urokinase from human urine. Hoppe-Seyler's Z Physiol Chem 1982; 363: 1043–58.

37. Holmes WE, Pennica D, Blaber M, et al. Cloning and expression of the gene for pro-urokinase in Escherichia coli. Biotechnology 1985; 3: 923–9.

38. Stump DC, Lijnen HR, Collen D. Purification and characterization of single-chain urokinase-type plasminogen activator from human cell cultures. J Biol Chem 1986; 261: 1274–8.

39. Ichinose A, Fujikawa K, Suyama T. The activation of pro-urokinase by plasma kallikrein and its inactivation by thrombin. J Biol Chem 1986; 261: 3486–9.

40. Lijnen HR, Zamarron C, Blaber M, Winkler ME, Collen D. Activation of plasminogen by pro-urokinase. I. Mechanism. J Biol Chem 1986; 261: 1253–8.

41. Lijnen HR, Van Hoef B, De Cock F, Collen D. The mechanism of plasminogen activation and fibrin dissolution by single chain urokinase-type plasminogen activator in a plasma milieu in vitro. Blood 1989; 73: 1864–72.

42. Declerck PJ, Lijnen HR, Verstreken M, Moreau H, Collen D. A monoclonal antibody specific for two-chain urokinase-type plasminogen activator. Application to the study of the mechanism of clot lysis with single-chain urokinase-type plasminogen activator in plasma. Blood 1990; 75: 1794–1800.

43. PRIMI Trial Study Group. Randomised double-blind trial of recombinant pro-urokinase against streptokinase in acute myocardial infarction. Lancet 1989; 1: 863–8.

44. Nelles L, Lijnen HR, Collen D, Holmes WE. Characterization of a fusion protein consisting of amino acids 1 to 263 of tissue-type plasminogen activator and amino acids 144 to 411 of urokinase-type plasminogen activator. J Biol Chem 1987; 262: 10855–62.

45. Lijnen HR, Nelles L, Van Hoef B, Demarsin E, Collen D. Structural and functional characterization of mutants of recombinant single-chain urokinase-type plasminogen activator obtained by site-specific mutagenesis of Lys[158], Ils[159] and Ile[160]. Eur J Biochem 1988; 177: 575–82.

46. Gurewich V, Pannell R, Broeze RJ, Mao J. Characterization of the intrinsic fibrinolytic properties of pro-urokinase through a study of plasmin-resistant mutant forms produced by site-specific mutagenesis of lysine 158. J Clin Invest 1988; 82: 1956–62.

47. Collen D, Mao J, Stassen JM, et al. Thrombolytic properties of Lys[158] mutants of recombinant single chain urokinase-type plasminogen activator in rabbits with jugular vein thrombosis. J Vasc Med Biol 1989; 1: 46–9.

48. Fujitani R, Furuichi M, Okamura H, Komiya M, Karasawa T, Tokemoto H. Thrombolytic properties of recombinant single chain urokinase type plasminogen activator and its mutants (abstract 1730). Thromb Haemost 1989; 62: 544.

49. Lijnen HR, Nelles L, Holmes WE, Collen D. Biochemical and thrombolytic properties of a low molecular weight form (comprising Leu144 through Leu411) of recombinant single-chain urokinase-type plasminogen activator. J Biol Chem 1988; 263: 5594–8.

50. Collen D, Rijken DC, Van Damme J, Billiau A. Purification of human tissue-type plasminogen activator in centigram quantities from human melanoma cell culture fluid and its conditioning for use in vivo. Thromb Haemost 1983; 48: 294–6.

51. Pennica D, Nedwin E, Hayflick JS, et al. Human tumour necrosis factor: precursor structure, expression and homology to lymphotoxin. Nature 1984; 312: 724–9.

52. Joernvall H, Pohl G, Bergsdorf N, Wallén P. Differential proteolysis and evidence for a residue exchange in tissue plasminogen activator suggest possible association between two types of protein microheterogeneity. FEBS Lett 1983; 156: 47–50.

53. Banyai L, Varadi A, Patthy L. Common evolutionary origin of the fibrin-binding structures of fibronectin and tissue-type plasminogen activator. FEBS Lett 1983; 163: 37–41.

54. Patthy L. Evolution of the proteases of blood coagulation and fibrinolysis by assembly from modules. Cell 1985; 41: 657–63.

55. Ny T, Elgh F, Lund B. The structure of the human tissue-type plasminogen activator gene: correlation of intron and exon structures to functional and structural domains. Proc Natl Acad Sci USA 1984; 81: 5355–9.

56. Pannekoek H, de Vries C, van Zonneveld AJ. Mutants of human tissue-type plasminogen activator (t-PA): structural aspects and functional properties. Fibrinolysis 1988; 2: 123–32.

57. Rijken DC, Groeneveld E. Isolation and functional characterization of the heavy and light chains of human tissue-type plasminogen activator. J Biol Chem 1986; 261: 3098–102.

58. Holvoet P. Ontwikkelen van nieuwe laboratoriumtechnieken gebaseerd op monoclonale antistoffen voor de diagnose van diepe veneuze thrombose en voor de evaluatie van de systemische effecten van thrombolytische behandeling met weefsel-type plasminogeenactivator. Verh K Acad Geneesk Belg 1986; XLVIII: 377–99.

59. van Zonneveld AJ, Chang GTG, van den Berg J, et al. Quantification of tissue-type plasminogen activator (t-PA) mRNA in human endothelial-cell cultures by hybridization with a t-PA cDNA probe. Biochem J 1986; 235: 385–90.

60. Gething MJ, Adler B, Boose JA, et al. Variants of human tissue-type plasminogen activator that lack specific structural domains of the heavy chain. EMBO J 1988; 7: 2731–40.

61. Verheijen JH, Caspers MPM, de Munk GAW, Enger-Valk BE, Chang GTG, Pouwels PH. Sites in tissue-type plasminogen activator involved in the interaction with fibrin, plasminogen and low molecular weight ligands. Thromb Haemost 1987; 58: 491–8.

62. Higgins DL, Vehar GA. Interaction of one-chain and two-

chain tissue plasminogen activator with intact and plasmin-degraded fibrin. Biochemistry 1987; 26: 7786–91.

63. de Vries C, Veerman H, Pannekoek H. Identification of the domains of tissue-type plasminogen activator involved in the augmented binding to fibrin after limited digestion with plasmin. J Biol Chem 1989; 264: 12604–10.

64. Rijken DC, Hoylaerts M, Collen D. Fibrinolytic properties of one-chain and two-chain human extrinsic (tissue-type) plasminogen activator. J Biol Chem 1982; 257: 2920–5.

65. Tate KM, Higgins DL, Holmes WE, Winkler ME, Heyneker HL, Vehar GA. Functional role of proteolytic cleavage at Arginine-275 of human tissue plasminogen activator as assessed by site-directed mutagenesis. Biochemistry 1987; 26: 338–43.

66. Husain SS, Hasan AAK, Budzynski AZ. Differences between binding of one-chain and two-chain tissue plasminogen activators to non-cross-linked and cross-linked fibrin clots. Blood 1989; 74: 999–1006.

67. Rijken DC, Emeis JJ. Clearance of the heavy and light polypeptide chains of human tissue plasminogen activator in rats. Biochem J 1986; 238: 643–6.

68. Rijken DC, Groeneveld E. Isolation and functional characterization of the heavy and light chains of human tissue-type plasminogen activator. J Biol Chem 1986; 261: 3098–102.

69. Verheijen JH, Caspers MPM, Chang GTG, De Munk GAW, Pouwels PH, Enger-Valk BE. Involvement of finger domain and kringle 2 domain of tissue-type plasminogen activator in fibrin binding and stimulation of activity by fibrin. EMBO J 1986; 5: 3525–30.

70. Hoylaerts M, Rijken DC, Lijnen HR, Collen D. Kinetics of the activation of plasminogen by human tissue plasminogen activator. Role of fibrin. J Biol Chem 1982; 257: 2912–19.

71. Wallén P, Bergsdorf N, Rånby M. Purification and identification of two structural variants of porcine tissue plasminogen activator by affinity adsorption on fibrin. Biochim Biophys Acta 1982; 719: 318–28.

72. Rijken DC, Van Hinsberg VWM, Sens EHC. Quantitation of tissue-type plasminogen activator in human endothelial cell cultures by use of an enzyme immunoassay. Thromb Res 1984; 33: 145–53.

73. Boose JA, Kuismanen E, Gerard R, Sambrook J, Gething MJ. The single-chain form of tissue-type plasminogen activator has catalytic activity: studies with a mutant enzyme that lacks the cleavage site. Biochemistry 1989; 28: 635–43.

74. Garabedian HD, Gold HK, Leinbach RC, et al. Comparative properties of two clinical preparations of recombinant human tissue-type plasminogen activator in patients with acute myocardial infarction. J Am Coll Cardiol 1987; 9: 599–607.

75. Korninger C, Stassen JM, Collen D. Turnover of human extrinsic (tissue-type) plasminogen activator in rabbits. Thromb Haemost 1981; 46: 658–61.

76. Fuchs HE, Berger H, Pizzo SV. Catabolism of human tissue plasminogen activator in mice. Blood 1985; 65: 539–44.

77. Kuiper J, Otter M, Rijken DC, van Berkel TJC. Characterization of the interaction in vivo of tissue-type plasminogen activator with liver cells. J Biol Chem 1988; 263: 18220–4.

78. Chen SA, Foster DL, Keyt BA, et al. Correlation of hepatocyte uptake with in vivo clearance of recombinant tissue-type plasminogen activator and identification of the domains responsible for clearance (abstr 1040). Thromb Haemost 1989; 62: 337.

79. Kruithof EKO, Tran-Thang C, Ransijn A, Bachmann F. Demonstration of a fast-acting inhibitor of plasminogen activators in human plasma. Blood 1984; 64: 907–13.

80. Sambrook J, Hanahan D, Rodgers L, Gething MJ. Expression of human tissue-type plasminogen activator from lytic viral vectors and in established cell lines. Mol Biol Med 1986; 3: 459–81.

81. Madison EL, Goldsmith EJ, Gerard RD, Gething MJH, Sambrook JF, Bassel-Duby RS. Amino acid residues that affect interaction of tissue-type plasminogen activator with plasminogen activator inhibitor 1. Proc Natl Acad Sci USA 1990; 87: 3530–3.

82. Neuhaus KL, Feuerer W, Jeep-Tebbe S, Nierderer W, Vogt A, Tebbe U. Improved thrombolysis with a modified regimen of recombinant tissue-type plasminogen activator. J Am Coll Cardiol 1989; 14: 1366–9.

83. The International Study Group. In-hospital mortality and clinical cause of 20,891 patients with suspected acute myocardial infarction randomised between alteplase and streptokinase with or without heparin. Lancet 1990; 336: 71–5.

84. Christodoulides M, Boucher DW. The potency of tissue-type plasminogen activator (TPA) determined with chromogen and clot lysis assay. Biologicals 1990; 18: 103–11.

85. Grines CL, for the Burroughs Wellcome Study Group. Efficacy and safety of weight adjusted dosing of a new tissue plasminogen activator preparation in acute myocardial infarction (abstr). Circulation 1988; 78 (suppl II): 127.

86. Grines CL, Nissen SE, Booth DC, et al. A new thrombolytic regimen for acute myocardial infarction using combination half dose tissue-type plasminogen activator with full dose streptokinase: a pilot study. J Am Coll Cardiol 1989; 14: 573–80.

11

VALVULAR HEART DISEASE AND PROSTHETIC HEART VALVES

JAMES H. CHESEBRO and VALENTIN FUSTER

Pathogenesis and Risk

As in other cardiovascular problems, antithrombotic therapy in patients with valvular heart disease and prosthetic heart valves is based on pathogenesis and risk (see Chapter 23).[1] Higher risk problems may require different therapy. The pathogenesis involves intracavitary mural thrombi in cardiac chambers, changes in rheology of blood flow with stasis activating the coagulation system or turbulent flow activating platelets, and differing substrates for thrombosis which include calcified or deendothelialized valve leaflets (which may expose subendothelial collagen), heterotopic or xenotopic valvular tissue, or prosthetic materials such as the sewing rings common to all prosthetic valves (attracts acute platelet deposition immediately after valve replacement[2]) or the prosthetic structures of the valve which may vary in thrombogenicity. Prolene suture material appears to be the least thrombogenic of five different materials.[3] The most highly thrombogenic substrate is thrombus itself, especially if acute embolism has exposed a fresh surface of the inner thrombus which contains thrombin adsorbed to fibrin.[4,5] Thus, a recent thromboembolism always signifies a high risk of recurrent thromboembolism.

Definition of Thromboembolism

Thromboembolism is a clinical diagnosis; it is clinically manifest less frequently than the pathologic incidence (in part due to size of emboli and the organ involved), and 80 to 90 per cent of the time is manifested in the brain or eye.[6,7] The definition of thromboembolism to the brain or eye is a temporary or permanent neurologic deficit of sudden onset with focal motor weakness or visual deficit. Emboli may also involve the limbs, heart, kidneys, splanchnic bed, or spleen. Thromboemboli to the limbs are diagnosed by the presence of ischemic pain, paresthesias, pallor, and pulselessness. The presumed diagnosis of coronary emboli may be made on the basis of a myocardial infarction occurring in a patient under the age of 40, or in the presence of previously documented normal coronary arteries by angiography. The effects of thromboemboli may be categorized as: (a) minor or transient, (b) major with permanent residua, or (c) fatal. Unfortunately, these data have not often been recorded in published studies, but improvement has been occurring in quality peer-reviewed journals. Because a permanent neurologic deficit occurs in approximately half of thromboemboli to the brain, and because some studies only record a permanent deficit as an embolic event (and disregard reversible ischemic neurologic deficit [RIND] or transient ischemic attack [TIA]), the incidence of thromboemboli may be as much as 50 per cent underestimated. Frequency and regularity of follow-up may also influence the identification of thromboembolic events. Patient questionnaires will also underestimate events compared with questionnaires plus interviews of the patient. Thus the incidence of thromboembolism may be difficult to measure and compare from study to study because of different or uncertain definitions of events, different methods of follow-up, and variable reporting of linearized or actuarial rates.

Principles for Antithrombotic Therapy

As an example, Table 11–1 outlines clinical indications for anticoagulation in patients with valvular heart disease. In addition, the international normalized ratio (INR) for the standardization of prothrombin times is of great importance for achieving appropriate level of the anticoagulation (see Chapter 9).[47] The nomogram designed by Poller[47] is extremely useful in converting the observed prothrombin time ratio for different thromboplastins (which have different sensitivity) to the international normalized ratio.

The therapeutic range for oral anticoagulation differs depending upon the thromboembolic risk and pathogenesis (based mainly on thrombogenicity of the substrate).[1] Thus patients at high risk with valvular heart disease (those with previous thromboembolism) should have an international normalized ratio of 3.0 to 4.5 or the prothrombin time prolonged to 1.5 to 1.8 times control for the average North American thromboplastin. For all other patients with valvular heart disease who are at medium risk, an international normalized ratio of 2.0 to 3.0 or prothrombin time ratio of 1.3 to 1.5 times control is optimal.[1,53]

Clinical recommendations for the use of antithrombotic therapy can be classified into five levels as previously described.[48]

Level I studies are randomized trials with a low false-positive or alpha error in which a convincing and statistically significant benefit for treatment is found with a 95 per cent confidence interval for the difference well away from zero (such as a previous prospective randomized trial in aortocoronary bypass graft operation where the difference between treatment and placebo was highly significant, $p = 10^{-6}$ or 95 per cent confidence interval 16 to 35 per cent, which is well away from zero[49]). In addition, level I trials should have a low false-negative or beta error with a high power or 95 per cent confidence interval which excludes any practical possibility of therapy being beneficial in a sufficiently large trial (such as the lack of benefit of sulfinpyrazone in patients with unstable angina in the trial by Cairns et al.[50] (which excluded any practical possibility that sulfinpyrazone could halve the risk of myocardial infarction and cardiac death).

Level II studies are also randomized trials, but have a high false-positive or alpha error, a high false-negative or beta error (low power, such as five of the six trials with aspirin therapy after myocardial infarction that showed positive but statistically insignificant trends favoring aspirin), or both errors.

Level III studies are nonrandomized comparisons between patients (concurrent cohorts) who did and who did not receive antithrombotic therapy. Most of the studies in valvular heart disease and prosthetic heart valves are in this category.

Level IV studies are also nonrandomized comparisons between patients who did and who did not receive antithrombotic therapy. However, the groups are not concurrent in time, but consist of a treatment group which is current and a control group which is historical or from a different time period. Most of the studies in patients with mitral valve disease are in this category.

Level V studies are case series without controls.

Grade A, B, or C recommendations are derived from level I to V studies. *Grade A recommendations* are supported by at least one and preferably more than one level I randomized trial. *Grade B recommendations* are

---

TABLE 11–1. Valvular Heart Disease: Indications for Anticoagulation*

Medium Risk†

1. Atrial fibrillation (chronic or paroxysmal) in mitral regurgitation or after anticoagulation for one year in mitral stenosis
2. Sinus rhythm with a very large left atrium (>55 millimeters by M-mode echocardiography)
3. Presence of heart failure or severe left ventricular dysfunction

High Risk‡

4. Atrial fibrillation (chronic or paroxysmal) in mitral stenosis during the first year of anticoagulation
5. History of previous systemic embolism

* Modified from Chesebro JH, et al. Antithrombotic therapy in patients with valvular heart disease and prosthetic heart valves. J Am Coll Cardiol 1986; 8:41B–56B, with permission.
† International normalized ratio = 2.0 to 3.0.[47] Prothrombin time 1.3 to 1.5 times control for usual North American thromboplastins.
‡ International normalized ratio = 3.0 to 4.5[17] (prothrombin time to 1.5 to 1.8 times control).

supported by at least one level II randomized trial. *Grade C recommendations* are only supported by level III, IV, or V studies. Thus, although studies in valvular heart disease are grade C recommendations supported by level III or IV studies, these are supported by an extremely high risk of thromboembolism in mitral stenosis being reduced to a very low risk of thromboembolism (less than 1 per cent per year) in patients on adequate anticoagulation and by recent grade A recommendations in nonvalvular atrial fibrillation where there is a level I study[41] and two level II studies[51,52] documenting the significant reduction in stroke by warfarin compared to placebo.

Reporting of Thromboembolism

Reporting of thromboembolism has improved since criteria for high quality were outlined and discussed.[91] A greater proportion of the ten criteria are addressed, but some of the last three or four criteria are less well adhered to. These factors facilitate a comparison of studies at different centers and include:

1. *Adequacy of follow-up.* This includes proportion of patients and duration of follow-up.
2. *Proportion of patients responding to specific questions.* This should also include frequency of follow-up, whether it was by questionnaire only or direct patient contact as well.
3. *Specific definition of thromboembolism.* Succinct definitions were given earlier and are discussed in more detail elsewhere.[23,91]
4. *Categorization of thromboembolism.* (a) Minor or transient, (b) major or associated with a permanent neurologic deficit, myocardial infarction, or reoperation (or other significant therapeutic modality), or (c) lethal. Emboli to the retina or brain cause a residual deficit in about half the cases and are lethal in about 10 per cent.[6]
5. *Actuarial rate.* The incidence of thromboembolism or bleeding at a specific point in time should be provided in either tabular or graphic form or in the text. Data for at least four to five years of follow-up or beyond are preferable.
6. *Linearized rate.* This should be given or calculable as per cent of events per year or events per 100 patient years.
7. *Valve thrombosis.* This should be listed separately from thromboembolic events since it is often lethal and is also an indication of the durability of the valve.
8. *Duration of anticoagulation.* The proportion of patients who received anticoagulation for specified time intervals should be stated.
9. *Adequacy of control.* Prothrombin times need to be standardized to the international normalized ratio in order to compare prothrombin times from different laboratories using thromboplastins of different sensitivity. The international sensitivity index of the thromboplastin should be stated, and the international normalized ratio of the targeted therapeutic range.
10. *Analysis of affect of anticoagulation.* Adequacy of anticoagulation should be compared with the incidence of thromboembolism. The proportion of prothrombin times within the defined therapeutic range, the proportion to low, and the proportion to high should be given for each group of patients. In addition, the prothrombin time at the time of thromboembolic or bleeding event should also be reported. The incidence of thromboembolism in patients who have a given proportion of prothrombin times in range is useful to report. The different intensities of anticoagulation and variability about the mean probably accounts for the great range in incidence of thromboembolism in reports of the same valve type. Recent data of more than 20,000 prothrombin times in more than 180 patients with a prosthetic valve for 5 to over 20 years are showing that increased variability of prothrombin times adds to the risk of thromboembolism.
11. *Bleeding events.* Bleeding events should be defined and reported as in 5, 6, and 10, so as to give an appreciation for the incidence of bleeding and the relation to adequacy of anticoagulation. A major bleeding event is usually defined as an intracranial bleed or one that results in death or requires hospitalization or a blood transfusion.

VALVULAR HEART DISEASE

Incidence of Thromboembolism

In patients with valvular heart disease, the incidence of thromboembolism depends on the valve involved, the degree of left ventricular dysfunction, left atrial size, atrial fibrillation, and history of previous thromboembolism.[8-15]

Mitral Stenosis

This is the most common form of valvular disease causing thromboembolism. Associated mitral regurgitation may also be present. Thrombi are localized to either the left atrial appendage or the left atrial wall with about equal frequency. Thromboembolism is the presenting symptom in more than 10 per cent of patients with mitral stenosis and may occur with all degrees of stenosis. A conservative incidence of thromboembolic events is more than 2 to 5 per cent per year with up to 16 per cent being fatal.[8,9,14,16–21] Atrial fibrillation increases the risk of thromboembolism by 5- to 18-fold and thus to a severe level.[8,9,11,15,22]

Mitral Regurgitation

The incidence of thromboembolism is 1 to 3 per cent per year, is less common than with mitral stenosis, but is higher in those with severe regurgitation or in those with associated mitral stenosis. It is especially associated with atrial fibrillation and reduced left ventricular function. With the latter three risks, the incidence is more than 4 per cent of patients per year and involving at least 14 to 18 per cent of patients.[8,9,19] In 65 patients with severe mitral regurgitation followed for at least ten years at the Mayo Clinic, thromboembolism occurred in 2.9 per cent of patients per year.[23] Thus patients with significant mitral regurgitation have at least a medium risk of thromboembolism and require anticoagulation for its prevention.

Mitral Valve Prolapse

This is extremely common and occurs in 2 to 6 per cent of the general population when diagnosed by auscultatory and echocardiographic criteria.[24–26] Up to 17 per cent of young women may have mitral valve prolapse.[25] Although the relation between cerebral ischemia and mitral valve prolapse was proposed more than 15 years ago,[27] it is difficult to establish a causal relation between valvular disease and cerebral ischemia in the individual patient. More common causes of cerebral ischemia must be excluded before implicating mitral valve prolapse, especially in the elderly patient.[28]

Patients with redundant mitral valve leaflets have the highest frequency of complications as shown in a long-term follow-up of 237 patients with mitral valve prolapse documented by echocardiography.[26] Cerebral emboli occurred in ten patients, of which two had predisposing factors (infective endocarditis in one and left ventricular aneurysm with thrombus in another). In the remaining eight patients, six had atrial fibrillation with left atrial enlargement; only two patients had no atrial fibrillation or other predisposing causes (one with and one without redundant mitral valve leaflets).

Valvular thrombi are the most likely source of cerebral emboli in patients with mitral valve prolapse.[24,27,29] Another source is left atrial thrombi in those with paroxysmal or chronic atrial fibrillation. Fortunately, massive cerebral infarction is uncommon in the absence of atrial fibrillation. Most cerebral emboli in patients with mitral valve prolapse are transient ischemic attacks or small strokes.[30,31]

Aortic Valve Disease

Thromboembolism is much less frequent than in mitral valve disease and is most often associated with other risks such as coexistent mitral valve disease, atrial fibrillation, or endocarditis.[32–34] The precise incidence is less certain. In 68 patients with significant aortic regurgitation followed at the Mayo Clinic, the incidence of thromboembolism was 0.8 per cent per year and occurred in 4.4 per cent of patients followed at least ten years.[23]

In aortic stenosis, most emboli are calcareous, observed in the retinal arteries on funduscopic examinations, and may be clinically silent.[35,36] The first indication of calcific aortic stenosis may uncommonly be an embolus. The risk of embolism is not increased with the severity of valvular stenosis. Emboli may be dislodged during cardiac catheterization or at surgery unless great care is taken. Platelet–fibrin thrombi may be seen on disrupted valvular endothelium in pathologic specimens.[37] In aortic valve disease transient monocular blindness or retinal artery occlusion occurs more frequently than brain infarction. These clinical observations suggest that relatively small emboli are associated with calcific aortic stenosis.[28]

RISK FACTORS FOR SYSTEMIC EMBOLISM

Atrial Fibrillation. Lone atrial fibrillation in the absence of cardiopulmonary disease or hypertension (even under treatment) in persons under age 60 accounts for only 2–3 per cent of those with atrial fibrillation and does not increase significantly the risk of thromboembulism. Atrial fibrillation is the most important risk factor and marker for thromboembolism is chronic or paroxysmal atrial fibrillation.[8–11,15,19,23,38,39] The frequency of atrial fibrillation greatly increases with age, regardless of gender.[40] Atrial fibrillation unrelated to valvular disease (nonvalvular atrial fibrillation) starts at a mean age of 64 years, affects 2 to 5 per cent of the general population over the age of 60, and is associated with a 5 to 7 per cent yearly risk of thromboembolism (see Chapter 12).[15] In patients with valvular disease, atrial fibrillation is nearly always associated with mitral valve disease. Thromboembolism often occurs early after the onset of atrial fibrillation. In one study, 33 per cent of thromboemboli occurred within the first month and 66 per cent within 12 months of the onset of atrial fibrillation.[8] Patients with paroxysmal atrial fibrillation are at equal risk of thromboembolism as those with chronic atrial fibrillation, even in patients without valvular disease.[15,41] Atrial fibrillation greatly increases the risk of thromboembolism in patients with valvular disease. Thus it is critical to constantly look for atrial fibrillation by history or telephone monitoring and even anticipate it in those with a large left atrium.

Left Atrial Size. Patients with mitral valve disease have the most profound left atrial enlargement. However, after atrial fibrillation is established in mitral valve disease, the degree of enlargement as assessed by M-mode echocardiography is not an independent risk factor for thromboembolism.[38] In nonvalvular atrial fibrillation, a retrospective study suggests that left atrial enlargement may increase the risk of stroke,[12] and so data from a prospective study (Stroke Prevention in Atrial Fibrillation [SPAF] Study) finds left ventricular dysfunction to be a stronger factor than left atrial size in patients with established atrial fibrillation (Stroke Prevention in Atrial Fibrillation Investigators, personal communication, 1991). Thus left atrial enlargement in patients *with sinus rhythm* may indirectly lead to thromboembolism because of the predisposition to atrial fibrillation. This is why prophylactic anticoagulation may be started in patients with a very large left atrium.

Previous Embolism. This, especially if recent, is a strong risk factor for subsequent thromboembolism, probably because residual thrombus is a highly thrombogenic substrate.[4,5] The incidence of recurrent embolism in patients with valvular heart disease is approximately 10 per cent per year, and overall, occurs in 30 to 75 per cent of patients.[8,10,20,43–45] Most recurrent thromboemboli occur within the first six months after the initial event.[8,20] Mortality from recurrent emboli in patients with mitral stenosis may be as high as 42 per cent.[8,18] Thus, therapy in such patients should be designed as a high-risk category with a higher level of anticoagulation.[1]

Other Factors. In nonvalvular atrial fibrillation hypertension (even under treatment) and heart failure are strong clinical risk factors for thromboembolism (SPAF Investigators, personal communication, 1991). Symptoms due to valvular disease or functional class do not predict the likelihood of thromboembolism.[9,19] Nor does mitral valvotomy with relief of symptoms eliminate the risk of recurrent embolism.[9,17] Low cardiac output is an important risk factor for thromboembolism and may in part be related to left ventricular dysfunction or a very large left atrium.[1,8,9,13,38] Although age appears to be an independent risk factor, this may be related to the higher incidence of atherosclerosis and atrial fibrillation in the older age group.[40] In mitral valve disease the initial thromboembolism is most common during the fourth decade of life, and at least 38 per cent of patients will have had an embolism by the seventh decade[46] unless prophylactic therapy is started.

RECOMMENDATIONS FOR ANTITHROMBOTIC THERAPY

Mitral Valve Disease. Patients who are at risk for thromboembolism (Table 11–1) should be anticoagulated. Decisions for therapy are made somewhat easier by the recent trials in atrial fibrillation documenting the need for therapy in all patients with paroxysmal or chronic atrial fibrillation, even those without valvular heart disease.[41,51,52] The older patient with more marked disease is also at greater risk, partly because of the risk factors listed in Table 11–1, but also because of concomitant atherosclerotic vascular disease.[15] Thus, a medium-risk patient with a thromboembolic event while on low-dose anticoagulation requires the level of anticoagulation recommended for high-risk patients.

Patients with valvular disease with no risk factors for thromboembolism have no greater risk for thromboembolism than from severe hemorrhage secondary to anticoagulant therapy.[54] Thus, anticoagulant therapy is not appropriate in these low-risk patients. Although platelet inhibitor therapy with sulfinpyrazone has been reported to reduce systemic embolism,[55] concomitant anticoagulant therapy was used in two thirds of the patients, thus sulfinpyrazone was not adequately tested alone.

Mitral Valve Prolapse. The incidence of thromboembolism is extremely small, thus prophylactic therapy is not warranted unless risk factors are present (Table 11–1). After a mild or transient embolic event, initial treatment with oral anticoagulation is warranted for three to six months. If risks in Table 11–1 are not present, this may empirically be followed by a platelet inhibitor such as aspirin (80 to 325 milligrams/day). If present, anticoagulation is indicated. As previously mentioned, valvular thrombi are probably the most frequent cause of systemic embolism in these patients and such emboli are usually small. If the thromboembolism is large or recurs during antiplatelet therapy, the search for other causes and the use of long-term anticoagulant therapy is warranted.

Aortic Valve Disease. There are a few patients with aortic valve disease who have risk factors for thromboembolism (Table 11–1) and require oral anticoagulation. Most emboli in these patients are calcarious. Such emboli are not preventable, and if proven to originate from the aortic valve (which may be difficult), replacement may be justified for recurrent embolism. It is possible that turbulent flow may disrupt valvular endothelium even across a mildly abnormal aortic valve (or in a bicuspid valve) and stimulate platelet deposition.[37] Thus some neurologic symptoms in patients with aortic stenosis may be from platelet emboli and warrant a trial of platelet inhibitor therapy. However, this hypothesis is untested. There are no data to support the routine use of platelet inhibitor therapy in these patients.

PROSTHETIC HEART VALVES

Incidence and Mechanisms

Patients with prosthetic heart valve replacement have a medium to high and long-term risk of thromboembolism.[1,6,7] The proportion of patients free of thromboembolism decreases throughout the first and second decades after operation in spite of administration of oral anticoagulants. In the long-term follow-up of Starr-Edwards prosthetic valves, only 66 per cent had no thromboembolism at ten years and only 58 per cent no thromboembolism at 15 years after operation.[6]

Pathogenesis Involves Platelets and Coagulation

Factors of perioperative injury, stasis or turbulent flow, and thrombogenicity (valvular materials and coagulation) contribute to valvular thrombus and thromboembolism (Table 11–2). Thrombosis begins during operation. The damaged perivalvular tissue and prosthetic materials lead to contact activation of the coagulation cascade with thrombin generation and platelet activation as soon as blood begins flowing across the valve.[56–59] Thrombin may also be formed on platelet membranes (via the prothrombin activator complex which accelerates thrombin generation by 278,000 times) after their adhesion and activation by a prosthetic surface. Thrombin is the most sensitive activator of platelets in the arterial circulation and also promotes fibrin-thrombus generation. It takes five times greater levels of thrombin inhibition to prevent platelet thrombi compared with fibrin thrombi.[58] Thus, inhibition of both coagulation and platelets may be necessary to maximize antithrombotic effects with prosthetic heart valves. Since specific thrombin inhibition can totally prevent experimental arterial thrombus after deep injury and limit platelet deposition to a single layer, this type of therapy may be promising in the future.[59]

In addition, both mechanical and bioprosthetic valves contain a Dacron sewing ring which may activate both the coagulation cascade and platelets. Indium-III-labeled platelets may be used experimentally with scintigraphy to image platelet deposition on this ring within the first 24 hours after operation when either a mechanical or a bioprosthetic valve is placed in the animal.[2,56] Platelet-rich thrombi may be additionally stabilized by fibrin, which adsorbs thrombin and may further activate platelets. Stasis and decreased blood flow (as in the left atrium during atrial fibrillation or during low cardiac

TABLE 11–2. Prosthetic Heart Valves and Systemic Embolism Pathophysiology and Risk Stratification

	Thrombi			Emboli
Type	Injury*	Flow†	Coagulation‡	*100 patient-years§* *No anticoagulation(anticoagulation)*
Mitral mechanical	+ +	+ +	+	5(2.5)
Aortic mechanical	+ +	+	+	4(2)
Mitral bioprosthesis	+	+	0	2(1)
Aortic bioprosthesis	+	0	0	1(0.5)

* Suture-prosthesis (early).
† Atrial fibrillation (left atrium size), design of prosthesis (thrombosis-emboli).
‡ Adequacy anticoagulation, previous thromboembolism, others.
§ Collection methods and analysis (that is, prospective, timing, source).

output states with left ventricular dysfunction) may also promote additional fibrin formation. This early thrombus formation translates into increased thromboembolic risk early after prosthetic heart valve replacement.[60–66]

A shortened platelet survival indicates an increased risk of thromboembolism and is frequently present in patients with prosthetic heart valve replacement.[67–69] The amount of decrease in platelet survival depends on the surface area of the prosthetic valve. The aortic valve has a smaller surface area than the mitral. A shortened platelet survival correlates with increased risk of thromboembolism since this reflects ongoing platelet aggregation and deaggregation which may culminate in a clinical event.[67,69] Platelet inhibitor therapy which corrects a shortened platelet survival appears to predict the effectiveness of this therapy in preventing thromboembolism and is the reason that dipyridamole at 400 milligrams/day was chosen as adjunctive therapy to anticoagulation.[67–69]

Fibrinopeptide A is marker of in vivo thrombin formation as reflected by the conversion of fibrinogen to fibrin by thrombin. Elevated levels reflect ongoing conversion of fibrinogen to fibrin by thrombin and incomplete inhibition of coagulation. Since a five times greater level of thrombin inhibition is required to inhibit the formation of platelet thrombi compared to fibrin thrombi,[58,59] inhibition of elevated levels of fibrinopeptide A does not necessarily reflect inhibition of platelet activity and the formation of platelet thrombi. The level of oral anticoagulation is inversely related to fibrinopeptide A levels in patients with mechanical and bioprosthetic heart valves. Fibrinopeptide A levels remain elevated above the normal for healthy sub-

jects in patients with mechanical prosthetic heart valves receiving oral anticoagulation with the prothrombin time at the optimal therapeutic level with the international normalized ratio 3.0 to 4.5.[70] Patients with bioprosthetic heart valves in the mitral position treated with oral anticoagulation to the same international normalized ratio have lower levels of fibrinopeptide A which do not significantly differ from normal. However, lower levels of anticoagulation in patients with bioprosthetic heart valves leads to abnormally elevated levels of fibrinopeptide A.[70] This suggests an incomplete antithrombotic effect of our currently recommended levels of anticoagulation in patients with mechanical and bioprosthetic heart valves, but studies of clinical outcome and risk of thromboembolism in conjunction with fibrinopeptide A levels have not been done. The incomplete effect against fibrinopeptide A is of even greater concern when it is realized that a greater level of thrombin inhibition is required to prevent platelet thrombi.[58,59,70]

Risk Factors for Thromboembolism

There is a cumulative increase in risk of thromboembolism directly with time after operation. In addition, there are patient factors and valve factors which contribute to this risk (Table 11–3).

Valve Location. Patients with aortic valve replacement have the lowest risk of thromboembolism. Mitral valve replacement has a higher risk, and double valve replacement has a similar or higher risk. This increased risk may be in part related to the surface area of the prosthetic heart valve as well as

TABLE 11–3. Risk Factors for Thromboembolism in Patients With Prosthetic Heart Valves*

Cumulative incidence increases directly with time after operation
Patient factors
    Valve location†
    Adequacy of anticoagulation (level and variability)
    Atrial fibrillation
    Sinus rhythm with large left atrium (>50 millimeters)
    Previous thromboembolism
    Left ventricular dysfunction
    Year of operation (today, operation is performed earlier in course of disease)
Valve factors
    Design: less turbulence and stasis
    Materials: less thrombogenic

* Modified from Chesebro JH, et al. Antithrombotic therapy in patients with valvular heart disease and prosthetic heart valves. J Am Coll Cardiol 1986; 8:41B–56B, with permission.
† Aortic, mitral, or combined valve replacement.

TABLE 11–5. Starr-Edwards Prosthesis: Systemic Embolism and Adequacy of Anticoagulation*†

	PER CENT EVENTS (PATIENT-YEARS)	
ANTICOAGULATION	**MVR**	**AVR**
Adequate†	6.4	6.5
Inadequate	14.2	8.5
p Value	<0.01	NS

* From Fuster V, et al. Systemic thromboembolism in mitral and aortic Starr-Edwards prostheses: a 10–19 year follow-up. Circulation 1982; 66(suppl I):I-157–61, with permission from the American Heart Association, Inc.
† Rabbit brain thromboplastin ratio of 1.5 to 2.5 (international normalized ratio = 3.0 to 7.5); inadequate if less than the lower ratio.
AVR = aortic valve replacement; MVR = mitral valve replacement; NS = not significant.

to more advanced heart disease in those with double valve replacement. Thus there is a greater potential for left ventricular dysfunction and atrial fibrillation following double valve replacement.

Adequacy of Anticoagulation. Optimal anticoagulation is probably the most important factor in the prevention of thromboembolism.[6,71–75] This also has a theoretical basis in the inverse relationship between fibrinopeptide A (reflecting thrombin activity) and the level of anticoagulation.[70] Previously, adequacy of anticoagulation was defined as

a prothrombin time ratio of 1.5 to 2.5 times control (international normalized ratio 3.0 to 7.5) and by the proportion of prothrombin times within this therapeutic range. In observing over 12,000 prothrombin times and the relationship to thromboembolism or bleeding (Table 11–4), we observed that patients who had thromboembolism had a significantly greater proportion of prothrombin times less than 1.5 times control overall (41 per cent) compared with those without thromboembolism (30 per cent overall), and over half the time had a prothrombin time less than 1.5 times control at the time of the thromboembolic event. Likewise, patients who had a major bleeding episode had a significantly greater proportion of prothrombin times (11 per cent) more than 2.5 times

TABLE 11–4. Clinical Events Versus Adequacy of Prothrombin Time*†

	THROMBOEMBOLISM	BLEEDING
EVENT	*Per cent Patients with Low Prothrombin time (less than 1.5 times control)*	*Per cent of Patients with High Prothrombin Time (more than 2.5 times control)*
No	30	4
Yes (overall)	41	11
Yes (at time of event)	54	38

* Derived from Chesebro JH, et al. Trial of combined warfarin plus dipyridamole or aspirin therapy in prosthetic heart valve replacement: danger of aspirin compared with dipyridamole. Am J Cardiol 1983; 51: 1537–41, with permission.
† Therapeutic prothrombin time (PT) is defined as 1.5 to 2.5 times control.

TABLE 11–6. Platelet Inhibitors Alone for Mechanical Prosthetic Heart Valves

STUDY	**DRUG**	**THROMBO-EMBOLISM (%/YEAR)**
Dale et al. (1977)[133]	Acetylsalicylic acid (100 milligrams/day)	15
Salazar et al. (1984)[187]	Acetylsalicylic acid (1000 milligrams/day)	29 pregnancy
Chaux et al. (1984)[109]	Acetylsalicylic acid (975 milligrams/day) Dipyridamole (275 milligrams/day)	7
Mok et al.[193] (1985)	Acetylsalicylic acid (1000 milligrams/day) Dipyridamole (275 milligrams/day)	7

control compared with those who had no bleeding event (4 per cent of prothrombin times above 2.5 times control), and 38 per cent of patients had a prothrombin time above 2.5 times control at the time of the event.[75]

In another study anticoagulation was de-fined as adequate if the prothrombin times were (on the average) above or equal to 1.5 times control value for the preceding year. Using these criteria, adequacy of anticoagulation reflected the incidence of thromboembolism in mitral valve replacement when adequate anticoagulation versus inadequate

TABLE 11–7. Thromboembolism in Mechanical Valve Replacement

		AVR/MVR			
		%/Year			
STUDY	Pt (No)	TE	Thromb	Bleed	YEARS OF OPERATION
Starr-Edwards valve					
Murphy[91] (1983)	467/342	2.0/3.4	<0.1/<0.1	2.4/1.4	1973–1977
Perier[88,92] (1985/1984)	100/100	2.4/4.3	0.5/0.1	1.4/1.1	1974–1978
Fessatidis, Hackett[93,94] (1987)	327/279	1.6§/1.2§	0/0	0.7/0.3	
AVR + MVR	46	5.6	0	0.4	1974–1983
Schoevaerdts[95] (1988)	—/549	—/3.1	—/0	—/1.1	1965–1985
Cobanoglu[96] (1988)	707/—	2.8/—	0/—	2.0/—	1965–1986
Bjork-Shiley valve					
Murphy[91] (1983)	110/105	1.2/2.2	0.5/1.6	2.0/2.2	1973–1977
Perier[88,92] (1985/1984)	100/100	2.0/4.6	0.2/1.1	2.4/1.1	1974–1977
Horstkotte[97] (1983)	393/442	1.9/2.8*	0.2/0.3	1.8/2.9	1974–1982
Marshall[98] (1983)	—/357	—/3.7	—/0.7	—/0.3	1973–1978
Cohen[83,99] (1984/1985)	294/178†	1.9/4.6	0.3/0.5	1.2/1.7	1982–1983
Harjula[100] (1986)	—/176	—/2.5	—/0.4	—/0.5	1973–1982
Bloomfield[101] (1986)	100/122	1.4/5.0	—	1.5/1.5	1975–1979
Borkon[102] (1987)	266/—	1.4/—	0.2/—	6.2/—	1976–1981
Lindblom[103,104] (1987/ 1988)	1573/	1.0*/2.2*	0.1/0.6	1.4/1.2	1969–1983
Thulin[105] (1988)	214/163	3.4/5.0	0/0	—/—	1982–1985
Milano[106] (1989)	147/	1.0/	0.1/	1.3/	1970–1985
Fessatidis[107] (1989)	—/331	—/0.4§	—/0	—/0.1	1973–1985
St. Jude valve					
Horstkotte[97] (1983)	147/167	0.73/0.93§	0/0	2.6/2.8	1978–1980
Douglas[108] (1985)	67/—	2.8/—	—	7.9	1979–1981
Chaux[109]	73/90	1.3/2.3	0.3/0	—	1978–1982
AVR + MVR	25	3.7	—	—	
(antiplatelet Rx only) (1984)	12	6.5	—	—	
Baudet[110]	471/95	0.34/0.45‡	0/0	0.65	1978–1983
(if no ACRx) (1985)	65/10	6.1/16.7	6.2/5.6	—	
Kinsley[111] (1986)	335/330	2.5/2.7	0.1/0.8	—	1980–1984
AVR + MVR	126	1.7	0.4	—	same
Nakano[112] (1987)	140/244	0.7/2.0	0.3/0.2	—	1978–1984
Montalescot[113] (1989)	49/—	0.93/—	—/0	3.3/—	1978–1981
Arom[114] (1989)	469/340	1.1/1.8	—/0.1	0.6	1977–1987
AVR + MVR	75	1.6	—	—	
Omniscience valve (AV/MV)					
Callaghan[115] (1987)	76/102	3.1	0.6	2.6	1979–1985
Carrier[116] (1987)	33/72	3.0	0.8	3.4	1980–1984
Lillehei-Kastor valve					
Stewart[117] (1988)	273/—	1.5/—	0.2/—	2.0/—	1975–1984

* Excludes transient cerebral ischemic attacks.
† Mitral valve replacement (102 Bjork-Shiley, 34 Beall, and 42 Harken valves).
‡ Thromboembolism undefined.
§ PT 2.5 to 4.0 times control ("standardized British corrected") in anticoagulation clinics.

ACRx = oral anticoagulant therapy; AVR/MVR = aortic valve replacement/mitral valve replacement (the values in each column compare the number of per cent of cases in each group); bleed = bleeding episodes; No/ = number; Pt = patient; Rx = therapy; TE = thromboembolism; Thromb = thrombosis of valve.

anticoagulation was considered. However, there was only a trend but not a significant relationship between the adequacy of anticoagulation and the incidence of thromboembolism after aortic valve replacement (see Table 11–5). The lack of difference for patients with aortic valve replacement may reflect the high flow across the aortic valve, which can predispose to thrombi consisting predominantly of platelets compared with fibrin thrombi that appears to be more prominent after mitral valve replacement. The extreme of inadequate anticoagulation is the use of no anticoagulation; combined aspirin and dipyridamole may be better than aspirin alone in patients temporarily unable to take anticoagulants (Table 11–6). Observational studies after mechanical aortic valve replacement have shown an extremely high risk of thromboembolism in the absence of anticoagulation, documenting the need for oral anticoagulation after all mechanical prosthetic valve replacements (Table 11–7).

A recent study suggests that the variability in prothrombin times is probably as important as the intensity,[76] since a high and equal number of emboli (4.0 and 3.0 per cent per year in the moderate- and high-intensity groups, respectively) occurred whether the target prothrombin time ratio was 1.5 ± 0.2 (international normalized ratio 2.65) or 2.5 ± 0.2 (international normalized ratio 9); 19 of the 33 emboli occurred when the prothrombin time ratio was less than 1.5 (approximately half in each group). Preliminary unpublished data from our group suggests that increased variability, especially into the long range, in prothrombin times confirms an increased risk of thromboembolism in patients with prosthetic heart valves.

Only recently have a small number of studies begun to record the intended goal of prothrombin times in reports of thromboemboli and bleeding after prosthetic heart valve replacement (Tables 11–4 and 11–8). The intensity and variability of the prothrombin times are probably the major factors in the frequency of thromboembolism and will need to be recorded in future reports of prosthetic heart valves and the treatment of other thromboembolic problems. The intensity of prothrombin times with low variability may have accounted for the lower rates of thromboemboli in the studies by Fessatidis (Table 11–4) and Vallejo (Table 11–5).

Atrial Fibrillation

During valve replacement in the 1960s, this was not an independent risk factor for thromboembolism since nearly all patients with mitral valve replacement had atrial fibrillation owing to deferral of the operation until the later stages of the disease.[6,71,73] The risk of thromboembolism has been increased by atrial fibrillation in more recent studies.[76,77] Thromboembolism from bioprosthetic valves may occur more often in patients with atrial fibrillation.[65,78–82] Thus, because even paroxysmal atrial fibrillation increases the risk of stroke,[41,51,52] it is important to observe for this during follow-up after valve replacement. Patients with atrial fibrillation for less than one year before operation are more likely to convert to sinus rhythm after operation, especially after hospital discharge. Up to one third of patients with atrial fibrillation before operation may convert to sinus rhythm after operation.[83] Atrial fibrillation increases

TABLE 11–8. Thromboembolism in Medtronic Hall Mechanical Valve and Targeted International Normalized Ratios

			AVR/MVR			
				%/Year		
STUDY	Pt (No)	Targeted INR	TE	Throm	Bleed	YEARS OF OPERATION
Butchart[118] (1988)	255/460	2.5–3.5	1.6/3.2	0/0	0.7	1979–1987
MVR + AVR	137	2.5–3.5	3.4	0	same	
Antunes[119] (1988)	257/386	poor compliance (third world)	3.5/3.1	1.1/1.1	1.0/0.5	1980–1984
Vallejo[120] (1990)	117/143	3.0–4.5	0.7/1.5	0/0.1	0.39	1981–1986

INR = international normalized ratio; AVR/MXR = aortic valve replacement/mitral valve replacement (the values in each column compare the number of per cent of cases in each group); Pt = patient; No = number; TE = thromboembolism; Thromb = thrombosis of valve; Bleed = bleeding episodes.

with age and thus should be closely looked for in patients over age 60, including those with aortic valve replacement. After aortic valve replacement, as many as 60 per cent of patients over age 70 may have at least transient atrial fibrillation.[84] In mitral valve disease, earlier operation may be justified to restore sinus rhythm and prevent or delay chronic atrial fibrillation, especially if valve reconstruction is undertaken.[85-88] Patients with a large left atrium are at high risk of developing atrial fibrillation and thus should be anticoagulated.

Previous Thromboembolism. This indicates a high risk for subsequent thromboembolism, as previously noted. Thus all patients with this history should be anticoagulated after valve replacement regardless of type of valve or after mitral valve repair.

Left Ventricular Dysfunction. Patients with a dilated, poorly functioning left ventricle are at risk of thromboembolism even without valve replacement and thus require anticoagulation.[13]

Year of Operation. An older year of operation (especially before 1980) usually places patients at a higher risk of thromboembolism, since patients today undergo operation at an earlier stage of their disease,[90] usually have better left ventricular function, a smaller left atrium, and a lower incidence of atrial fibrillation.

Valve Design and Materials. Older valves created greater turbulent flow and regions of enhanced platelet activation. Older valves also used more thrombogenic materials. Today, valves are designed for less turbulent flow. Although materials are less thrombogenic, none of the mechanical valves can be used without anticoagulation.

Mechanical Prosthetic Cardiac Valves

Incidence of Thromboembolism. Reports of mechanical valve replacement are summarized in Table 11–7 for different valve types. The Starr-Edwards valve has the longest track record and very low rates of valve thrombosis. Even when more recent models are considered, it has as low a rate of thromboembolism as most other mechanical valves. The St. Jude valve appears to have the lowest rate of thromboembolism overall, but is not immune from valve thrombosis, especially when anticoagulants are not used. The Starr-Edwards, St. Jude, and Medtronic Hall valve

(Table 11–7) appear to have the lowest rates of valve thrombosis. The Björk-Shiley appears to have the highest risk of thrombosis.

The greatest difference in rates of thromboembolism appear to be related to the intensity and variability of anticoagulation, but this was seldom properly assessed. Only in recent studies has a targeted range for anticoagulation been stated (Table 11–8). Reliable means for carrying out targeted goals for anticoagulation need to be implemented whether it be via anticoagulation clinics or a nurse or secretary specifically assigned to making sure the patient has prothrombin times at least every three to four weeks (and contacts the physician with the results so that optimal control can be maintained). The importance of appropriately high levels of anticoagulation, close monitoring, and positive encouragement of reliable patients is suggested by the studies of Fessatidis and colleagues[93,94,107] (Table 11–7), and by the lower rate of thromboembolism for higher (and probably less variable) levels of anticoagulation achieved for the same valve type (Table 11–8). Randomized prospective trials comparing mechanical prosthetic heart valves (Table 11–9) may help define in vivo thrombogenicity of different valves. However, detailed information concerning the adequacy of anticoagulation within valve groups was not included in the reports cited in Table 11–9.

In our prospective study[7] of mechanical prosthetic valve replacement from 1979 to 1981 that involved mainly Starr-Edwards and Björk-Shiley valves and a small number of St. Jude valves, the incidence of thromboembolism was low (1.2 to 1.8 per cent per year) and did not differ among any of these valve types. The highest rates of thromboembolism occur during the first year after operation when there is probably more variability in anticoagulation, and fresh tissue injury at the valve excision site and prosthetic surfaces are exposed to flowing blood. Thus the greatest protection from thromboembolism is required during the first year. In addition, anticoagulation is essential for chronic prevention of thromboembolism and valve thrombosis. Platelet inhibitor therapy alone is not effective enough[109,110] and should only be used temporarily if anticoagulation needs to be interrupted.

Prospective Intervention Trials. Because oral anticoagulation cannot completely prevent thromboembolism in patients with me-

TABLE 11–9. THROMBOEMBOLISM IN TRIALS OF MECHANICAL CARDIAC VALVES

STUDY	VALVE	PT (NO)	%/YEAR			YEARS OF OPERATION
			TE	*Thromb*	*Bleed*	
Randomized prospective studies						
Mikaeloff[121]	BS-MV	—/178	4.3	0.4	2.4	1979–1981
(1989)	SJM-MV	—/179	2.3	0.4	1.6	1979–1983
	SE-MV	65	5.3	0	1.6	1982–1983
	BS	160	1.3		—	1982–1987
Kuntze[122]	MHV	148	3.4		—	
	EDV	88	5.1		—	
Vogt[123]	BS	84	1.4	0	2.2	1981–1983
(1990)	SJM	94	2.0	0	1.7	
Nonrandomized, concomitant patients, same center						
Cortina[124]	BS	—/51	—/1.1	—/0	—/	1980–1983
(1986)	MHV	—/152	—/2.2	—/0.4	—/	
	OmS	—/65	—/4.5	—/3.1	—/	

BS = Björk-Shiley; SJM = St. Jude Medical; SE = Starr-Edwards; MHV = Medtronic Hall valve; EDV = Edwards Duromedics valve; OmS = Omniscience valve; Pt = Patient; No = number; TE = thromboembolism; Thromb = thrombosis of valve; Bleed = bleeding episodes; MV = mitral valve.

chanical heart valves (Tables 11–7 through 11–9), prospective randomized trials of oral anticoagulation with and without platelet inhibition have been conducted. Dipyridamole has been approved by the United States Food and Drug Administration for the prevention of thromboembolism in conjunction with oral anticoagulation in patients with mechanical prosthetic heart valves. Dipyridamole has its best antiplatelet effect against prosthetic surfaces.[125,126] Dipyridamole decreased the incidence of thromboembolism in mechanical prosthetic heart valves when added to oral anticoagulation compared to anticoagulation alone in five trials (one level I study[127] and four level II studies[7,128–130]) (Table 11–10). Although the level I study by Sullivan et al. has been criticized for not reporting levels of anticoagulation in both groups, over 4,000 prothrombin times were subsequently collected for both groups and showed comparable levels of anticoagulation in each group.[131] A dipyridamole dosage of 300 to 400 milligrams/day or 5 to 6 milligrams/kilograms/day was chosen in these studies because this dosage maximally prolonged a

TABLE 11–10. Antithrombotic Therapy in Patients With Mechanical Prosthetic Heart Valves*

STUDY	METHODS	FOLLOW-UP (YEAR)	TREATMENT GROUP	DOSE (MG/DAY)	PATIENT (NUMBER)	THROMBOEMBOLIC EVENTS (%/YEAR)
Sullivan[127]	Prospective, randomized	1	A/C + placebo		84	14
			A/C + D	400	79	1
Kasahara[128]	Prospective, randomized	1 to 3 (mean 30 mo)	A/C		39	21
			A/C + D	400	40	5
Groupe PACTE[129]	Prospective, randomized	1	A/C		154	5
			A/C + D	375	136	3
Rajah[130]	Prospective, randomized	1 to 2	A/C		87	13
			A/C + D	300	78	4
Dale[133]	Prospective, randomized, blind	1	A/C + placebo		38	9
			A/C + ASA	1,000	39	2
			ASA	1,000	77	15
Altman[134]	Prospective, randomized	2	A/C		65	20
			A/C + ASA	500	57	5

* Reproduced from Fuster V, Chesebro JH. Antithrombotic therapy: role of platelet inhibitor drugs; management of arterial thromboembolic and atherosclerotic disease. Mayo Clin Proc 1981; 56: 265–73, by permission of the Mayo Foundation.
A/C = anticoagulant; ASA = acetylsalicylic acid (aspirin); D = dipyridamole.

shortened platelet survival in patients with prosthetic heart valve replacement.[67,132] Aspirin was added to oral anticoagulation in two trials[133,134] and reduced thromboembolism. However, the incidence of gastrointestinal bleeding was significantly increased with an aspirin dosage of 1 gram/day,[133] and the incidence of melena was increased in the other trial.[134] Aspirin, 250 milligrams twice daily combined with warfarin, also significantly increased gastrointestinal bleeding and should be avoided.[7] However, it appears that aspirin 80 milligrams/day combined with warfarin may be useful and safe for high-risk cardiovascular problems, especially where the thrombogenic substrate is biologic rather than prosthetic material.[1] Additional studies with low-dose aspirin are in progress.

BIOPROSTHETIC CARDIAC VALVES

Incidence of Thromboembolism. Thromboembolism after bioprosthetic valve replacement may be less frequent than after mechanical valve replacement in patients with similar degrees of anticoagulation (Tables 11–7 and 11–11). However, the incidence is extremely variable and may depend on the patient selection and severity of underlying disease (risk factors for thromboembolism) and the intensity and variability of anticoagulation used early after valve replacement when the risk of thromboembolism is ex-

TABLE 11–11. Thromboembolism in Bioprosthetic Valve Replacement

STUDY	Pt (No)	Chronic ACRx (%)	%/Year			YEAR OF OPERATION
			TE	Throm	Bleed	
Porcine valve						
Marshall[98] (1983)	—/96	13*	—/4.4	—/0.3	—/0.3	1974–1978
Perier[87,92] (1985/1989)	100/253	21*/75*	0.6/1.0	0/0.2	0.1/0.3	1974–1979
MV repair	100	50*	0.6	0	—/0.3	1974–1977
Gonzales-Lavin[135] (1984)	—/206	51*	—/4.6	—/0	—/2.5	1974–1982
Douglas[108] (1985)	120/—	16*†	1.9/—	0/—	2.4/—	1979–1981
Jamieson[136] (1984)	155/154	10/45*†	1.1/1.7	0/0	0.1	1976–1983
Cohen[83,99] (1984/1985)	663/528	AF	1.7/2.4	0.1/0	0.2/0.4	1972–1983
Zussa[137] (1985)	287/506	AF*	0.5/3.2	0.3	0.8	1974–1980
Louagie[138] (1986)	88/38	100‡,AF	3.8/2.7	0	1.2	1977–1984
Bortolotti[139] (1987)	71	90	1.3	0	1.3	1970–1983
AVR + MVR						
Kimose[140] (1989)	—/188	100	0.5	0	1.2	1976–1986
Magilligan[141] (1989)	492/554	—	0.7	0	—	1971–1987
Second Generation						
Jamieson[142] (1988)	546/225	36‡/52§‡	2.8/2.4	0.0	0.3/1.2	1981–1985
AVR + MVR	95	AF*	1.7	0	1.1	same
Bovine pericardial valve						
Gonzales-Lavin[135] (1985)	—/322	0*	—/0.4	—/0	—/0.6	1974–1982
Brais[143] (1985)	292/140	5‖	1.4/4.0	0	—	1977–1983
Reul[144] (1985)	1,427/982	30/63	1.4/2.8	—/—	—/—	1978–1983
AVR + MVR	258	70	2.0	—/—	—/—	
Revuelta[145] (1986)	239/—	AF§	1.1	0.1		1977–1984
Xiaodong[146] (1988)	55/381	AF	0.41	0	—	1976–1985
Daeven[147] (1988)	220/121	171§/61§	0.6/2.2	0	—	1980–1985
AVR + MVR	63	49§	1.8	0		same
Second Generation						
Revuelta[148] (1988)	89/27	36(AF)§	1.2	0	—	1982–1986
Homograft Aortic Valve						
Matsuki[149] (1988)	555/—	—	0.34/0	—	—	1964–1986

* Short-term oral anticoagulant therapy in all for two to six months.
† Additional 47 per cent received antiplatelet agents.
‡ This percentage received anticoagulant or platelet inhibitor therapy.
§ Short-term oral AC or antiplatelet Rx × three months.
‖ In remainder, five to seven days, "minimal heparinization," then aspirin 975 mg + dipyridamole 150 mg/day.
AF = Chronic anticoagulant therapy if atrial fibrillation, large left atrium, intracardiac thrombus. AVR/MVR = atrial valve replacement/mitral valve replacement; Pt = patient; No = number; TE = thromboembolism; Throm = thrombosis or valve; ACRx = oral anticoagulant activity.

tremely high. Previous[60-65] and more recent[66,150] studies have documented that the highest risk of thromboembolism is within the first three months after operation. In a randomized prospective trial of two different intensities of oral anticoagulation (international normalized ratio 2.5 to 4.0 versus 2.0 to 2.25) for the first three months after operation, the incidence of thromboemboli was high and similar in both groups (12.1 per cent per three months in the standard or higher intensity group and 12.8 per cent per three months in the lower intensity group).[150] Oral anticoagulation was started when patients were able to take medications by mouth. Only low-dose subcutaneous heparin (5,000 units every 12 hours) was used early after operation for up to seven days. No antiplatelet therapy was used.

By contrast, when subcutaneous heparin is started six hours after operation to prolong the activated partial thromboplastin time (APTT) to just beyond the upper limit of normal until the chest tubes are removed, and then the heparin is increased to prolong the activated partial thromboplastin time to 1.5 to 2 times control, and immediately followed by oral anticoagulation, the incidence of thromboembolism is extremely low after both aortic and mitral valve replacement in studies by Perier and colleagues (Table 11–11).[87,92,151] In a retrospective review we found a similar very high incidence of thromboembolism during the first three months (which was highest during the first ten days) and a lower incidence during the next 4 to 12 years of 1.8 per cent per year for aortic valve replacement (whether or not patients remained on oral anticoagulation) and for mitral valve patients 1.2 per cent per year if on oral anticoagulation and 4.3 per cent per year if not anticoagulated ($p < 0.05$).[66] These studies suggest that more intense antithrombotic therapy is required very early (for three months) after operation and that chronic antithrombotic therapy should be continued thereafter.

No prospective randomized intervention trials for the prevention of thromboembolism have been done in patients with bioprosthetic heart valves. One level IV study involved young patients (mean age 44) who had mitral valve replacement with a porcine bioprosthesis and had atrial fibrillation; one group had valve replacement between 1975 and 1979; were treated with 1 gram aspirin per day starting on the second postoperative day,

and had an incidence of thromboemboli of 1.3 per cent per year; the second group had valve replacement after 1979, were treated with 0.5 gram aspirin every other day starting on the first postoperative day, and had an incidence of thromboembolism of 0.3 per cent per year. There was no control group. Thus aspirin alone may be effective, but requires further study. Aspirin alone was better than placebo in the Stroke Prevention in Atrial Fibrillation (SPAF) Study where enteric coated aspirin at 325 milligrams/day significantly reduced stroke from 6.3 per cent per year to 3.2 per cent per year in patients with no significant valvular disease.[41]

Thus it appears that valve location (aortic or mitral), adequacy of antithrombotic therapy, observation before or beyond the first three months after operation, and the presence of atrial fibrillation are all significant influences upon the risk of thromboembolism after bioprosthetic valve replacement. These factors and the previous studies all provide knowledge of the pathogenesis and risk of thromboembolism and provide valuable information for the current recommendations which follow.

CURRENT RECOMMENDATIONS

Recommendations for antithrombotic therapy for prosthetic valve replacement are outlined in Table 11–12. Because platelet–thrombus deposition (predominantly on the sewing ring) begins as soon as blood flows through the prosthetic valve and can be imaged within hours after operation by indium-III-platelet scintigraphy,[2,56] antithrombotic therapy would ideally be started before operation and continued early after operation, but such studies have not yet been performed. Warfarin should be started within 24 to 48 hours after operation and administered at a dose sufficient to prolong the international normalized ratio to 3.0 to 4.5) (prothrombin time to 1.5 to 1.8 times control for the average North American thromboplastin). Warfarin should be continued indefinitely to prolong the international normalized ratio to 3.0 to 4.5.

Therapy which needs testing in terms of benefit (antithrombic) versus risk (hemorrhage) includes aspirin 160 milligrams down the nasogastric tube plus subcutaneous heparin 12,500 units starting six hours after operation in all patients for all types of prosthetic valves (it takes approximately 48 to 60 hours to reach therapeutic levels to maintain

TABLE 11–12. Antithrombotic Therapy for Prosthetic Heart Valves: Current Recommendations

IN ALL PATIENTS, BEGIN HD WARFARIN STARTING 24 TO 48 HOURS AFTER OPERATION
(MAY START DOWN NASOGASTRIC TUBE). INR TO 3.0 TO 4.5.

Valve	Situation	Therapy
Mechanical	Routine	HD warfarin†
	High risk*	HD warfarin† + D 400 milligrams/day
		If intolerant to D, HD warfarin† + Sulf 800 milligrams/day
	ACRx problems (bleeding)	1) ↓ LD warfarin§ + D 400 milligrams/day
		2) D 400 mg/day + Sulf 800 milligram/day (?ASA)
	Recurrent embolism	Consider reoperation
Bioprosthetic	AVR routine − NSR	HD warfarin for 3 months, then ASA 80 milligrams/day
	MVR routine − NSR	HD warfarin† for 3 mo, then ASA 80 milligrams/day
	If AF or LA >50 millimeters	LD warfarin‡ long-term
	If LA thrombus or previous TE	HD warfarin† long-term

* High risk includes patients with mechanical prosthetic valve implanted before 1980, previous thromboembolism, poor compliance, high variability in prothrombin times (INR <3.0 more than 40 per cent of time), or patient population with an incidence of thromboembolism >2.0 per cent/year on warfarin alone.

† High risk, thus higher dose (HD) warfarin to prolong INR to 3.0 to 4.5 (prothrombin time to 1.5 to 1.8 times control for usual North American thromboplastin with ISI of 2.2 to 2.6).

‡ Medium risk, thus lower dose (LD) warfarin to prolong INR to 2.0 to 3.0, (prothrombin time to 1.2 to 1.5 times control). ACRx = anticoagulant therapy; AF = atrial fibrillation; ASA = aspirin; AVR = aortic valve replacement; D = dipyridamole; LA = left atrium; MVR = mitral valve replacement; NSR = normal sinus rhythm; Sulf = sulfinpyrazine; TE = thromboembolism; INR = international normalized ratio; ISI = international sensitivity index.

the activated partial thromboplastin time at 1.5 to 2.0, the upper limit of normal). Then subcutaneous heparin, 12,500 units every 12 hours, would be continued (adjusting to maintain the activated partial thromboplastin time at 1.5 to 2 times the upper limit of normal) until the time of hospital dismissal or until the prothrombin time has been in range with oral anticoagulation for approximately three to five days.

Patients with Mechanical Prosthetic Heart Valves. All patients should receive oral anticoagulants. Patients at high risk of thromboembolism (valve implanted before 1980, previous thromboembolism, anticoagulation decreased or stopped due to bleeding, poor patient compliance, high variability in prothrombin times, patient population with an incidence of thromboembolism more than 2.0 per cent per year on warfarin alone) should have supplemental antithrombotic therapy with dipyridamole. There is a lower risk of thromboembolism when dipyridamole is added to anticoagulation (Table 11–10). The dipyridamole dosage 350 to 400 milligrams/day or 5 to 6 milligrams/kilograms/day (for example, 75 milligrams three times daily with meals and 150 milligrams at bedtime) and should be added to warfarin therapy (grade A recommendation) in high-risk patients.

Approximately 5 to 10 per cent of patients have intolerance to dipyridamole due to gas-

trointestinal upset or headache.[7] The former may be diminished by administering therapy concomitantly with food or in a sustained release form (available in Europe and some other countries). The vasodilator effects (headaches) may also be diminished by slowing the absorption with food or slightly lowering the dose to see if symptoms are diminished. In an emergency, the vasodilator effects (such as angina from an overdose of dipyridamole) can be reversed immediately with intravenous aminophylline (50 to 100 milligrams infused over one to two minutes).[152]

In high-risk patients who remain intolerant of dipyridamole in spite of these measures, an alternative therapy is the addition of sulfinpyrazone (800 milligrams/day) to warfarin therapy. This is a grade C recommendation and is based on one level III study.[69] Sulfinpyrazone has not been used in a randomized prospective trial. The study was uncontrolled and suggested that sulfinpyrazone was effective in certain patients, mainly those in whom it prolongs the shortened platelet survival. Sulfinpyrazone may prolong the prothrombin time in patients on warfarin (see Chapter 27); thus, it should be checked more frequently after initiating this therapy. In patients with recurrent thromboemboli or who have significant vascular problems (biologic tissue exposure to blood) which increase risk of thromboemboli, low-dose aspirin (80 milligrams/day) may also be used. For antipyrexia or analgesia, acetaminophen, sodium salicylate or salsalate should be used rather than larger doses of aspirin.

In patients who have bleeding during anticoagulation when the prothrombin time is not beyond twice control (international normalized ratio less than or equal to 4.5), we recommend evaluation for a secondary cause of bleeding (such as an underlying tumor or a low platelet count) and lower doses of warfarin, international normalized ratio 2.0 to 3.0, (prothrombin time 1.3 to 1.5 times control), in combination with dipyridamole. Bleeding is also more frequent after the initiation of anticoagulation since underlying lesions such as tumors may be revealed by the secondary bleed.

For patients unable to tolerate anticoagulation, we recommend a trial of dipyridamole (400 milligrams/day as outlined) combined with sulfinpyrazone at 200 milligrams four times daily as empiric but temporary therapy. These two platelet inhibitors are the most effective against thrombosis on prosthetic materials. This therapy is not recommended indefinitely because antiplatelet therapy is not effective in the long term in patients with mechanical prosthetic cardiac valves (Tables 11–6 and 11–7). A patient who has recurrent thromboembolism while on adequate antithrombotic therapy with warfarin plus platelet inhibition should be seriously considered as a candidate for another valve replacement.

Bioprosthetic Cardiac Valve Replacement. Warfarin should be administered within 24 to 48 hours after operation at a dose to prolong the international normalized ratio to 3.0 to 4.5 (prothrombin time to 1.5 to 1.8 times control for usual North American thromboplastin with international sensitivity index of 2.2 to 2.6) for three months. Patients at high risk (previous thromboembolism or left atrial thrombus) should be continued on this dose of warfarin indefinitely. Patients with paroxysmal or chronic atrial fibrillation, a large left atrium (more than 50 millimeters by M-mode echocardiography), or left ventricular dysfunction (ejection function less than 30 per cent or fractional shortening less than 25 per cent by echocardiography) should be continued on warfarin to prolong the international normalized ratio to 2.0 to 3.0. For patients with aortic or mitral valve replacement without the latter risk factors, aspirin (80 milligrams/day) may be continued indefinitely (grade C recommendation) as

empiric therapy from one level IV study.[153] Aspirin combined with warfarin may be needed for the first 10 to 90 days after operation and in patients who have associated aortocoronary bypass grafts, but additional studies are needed. Prospective randomized controlled trials are needed to determine the optimal antithrombotic therapy.

Prothrombin times should be monitored at least every three to four weeks in patients who are stable and receiving therapy with warfarin. More frequent monitoring should be done whenever the prothrombin time is above or below the therapeutic range or whenever the patient's condition or therapy changes (Table 11–13) (see Chapter 27). Many drugs can alter the prothrombin time (see partial list in Chapter 27). Whenever any medication is added or deleted, always recheck the prothrombin time one week later. Close monitoring of therapy is important since increased variability appears related to increased risk of thromboembolism and probably bleeding. On the average, in a routine practice, 30 per cent of prothrombin times may be too low, and 5 to 10 per cent may be too high.[7] Patients should avoid extremes in diet and try to keep green vegetable intake at a steady level since ingestion of vitamin K-containing food such as broccoli, lettuce, or other green vegetables can lower or normalize the prothrombin time.[154]

Diagnosis and Treatment of Prosthetic Valve Thrombosis. Acute prosthetic valvular thrombosis is usually a medical emergency which carries a high risk of mortality unless diagnosed early and treated promptly. Thus, suspicion of the problem should be high, and urgent diagnosis is required. Mechanical prosthetic valvular thrombosis may occur at any time and is associated with inadequate anticoagulation in more than 50 to 70 per cent of patients.[155–167] Bioprosthetic valve thrombosis is uncommon, may occur especially during the early months after operation, and appears preventable by therapy with warfarin (international normalized ratio 3.0 to 4.5) for three months.[83,87,92,98,137,145,151]

Symptoms vary from insidious and mild to abrupt circulatory failure. Any new or worsening symptoms require a thorough evaluation to exclude valve obstruction. Usual symptoms are new onset and progressive dyspnea, often for more than one week. New onset angina may occur in half of patients. Acute myocardial infarction is unusual.[164] Many

TABLE 11–13. Patient Conditions Can Change Warfarin Dosage

DECREASE DOSE	INCREASE DOSE
↓ Oral intake (postop)	↑ Vitamin K Intake
↓ Vitamin K stores (recent A/C, NPO, antibiotics)	Leafy green vegetables (broccoli, lettuce, spinach)
Liver disease	
Hepatic congestion	
Renal disease (↓ or Δ albumin)	Green beans
Malignancy, sepsis	Cauliflower
Diarrhea, steatorrhea	Liver
Hypermetabolism (hyperthyroidism, fever)	Hypometabolism (hypothyroidism)
Hereditary ↓ vitamin K clotting factors	Hereditary resistance

A/C = anticoagulant therapy; NPO = nothing orally; postop = postoperatively; ↓ = decrease; ↑ = increase; Δ = changes.

patients present in acute pulmonary edema or severe heart failure.[155–161]

On physical examination most patients have pulmonary rales and may have signs of right heart failure such as edema, hepatomegaly, and elevated jugular venous pressure. A new murmur is present in 90 per cent of these patients. Abnormal (absent or decreased) opening or closing clicks are present in 60 per cent.

Rapid diagnosis is necessary and can be accomplished using Doppler echocardiography to measure transvalvular flow velocities for calculation of pressure gradients, and measurements of pressure half-time to estimate valve area. These same techniques may substitute for cardiac catheterization and may also be used to monitor progress of thrombolysis if this therapy is chosen.[159] Fluoroscopy, phonocardiography, and two-dimensional echocardiography are of limited value.[157,159] However, some have found biplane cinefluoroscopy valuable for simple rapid diagnosis of reduced disc/leaflet motion in patients with radiopaque disc valves.[157,161]

Treatment is usually urgent valve replacement or debridement with a mortality risk of 8 to 50 per cent. This risk is mainly related to preoperative functional class (18 per cent for class IV and 5 per cent for classes I to III).[156–158,160,161] In patients with tricuspid valve thrombosis or those at high surgical risk for left-sided valve replacement, thrombolysis of valvular thrombus may be considered.[155,159]

For mitral or aortic valve thrombosis, duration of thrombolytic therapy has ranged from 5 to 95 hours, with success in 82 per cent and emboli in 18 per cent.[155,163] Streptokinase and urokinase have been used most frequently. Streptokinase is often administered as a loading dose of 250,000 to 500,000 international units intravenously over 30 minutes followed by an infusion of 100,000 international units/hour for 9 to 96 hours or 150,000 international units/hour for 10 hours.[155,159,162,163,166] Urokinase may also be used in doses recommended for pulmonary embolism, 4,500 international units/kilogram/hour intravenous infusion over 12 to 24 hours without a loading dose.[155] Tricuspid valve thrombosis has also been treated with a single intravenous dose of streptokinase (750,000 international units) over 20 minutes or recombinant tissue plasminogen activator (150 milligrams altephase intravenously over eight hours ± an additional 50 milligrams intravenously over the next eight hours, or 70 milligrams intravenously over five hours, or 10 milligrams bolus plus 40 milligrams intravenously over two hours along with simultaneous heparin.[168–174] Because thrombolytic agents activate thrombin and platelets, simultaneous heparin infusion should be administered for five to seven days, maintaining the activated partial thromboplastin time at 1.5 to 2 times control before switching to warfarin to maintain the international normalized ratio at 3.0 to 4.5. Doppler echocardiography is an excellent method for monitoring progress and outcome of thrombolysis.

SPECIAL SITUATIONS

Patients with prosthetic cardiac valve replacement may develop four situations which could require alteration of their antithrombotic therapy.

Non Cardiac Surgery. Discontinuation of anticoagulation for five to ten days appears to carry a low risk for patients undergoing a noncardiac operation.[174] In order to minimize risk, we recommend stopping warfarin four to five days before operation, continuing dipyridamole (400 milligrams/day, or starting it if it is not being administered), and starting a heparin infusion (to maintain the activated partial thromboplastin time at twice control) when the prothrombin time decreases to less than 1.5 times control (international normalized ratio 3.0). The heparin infusion should be continued until four to five hours before operation. Subcutaneous heparin (15,000 units/day given in two or three divided doses) should be continued during and early after the operation, except in patients undergoing brain or intraocular operations. The heparin therapy should be increased as soon as possible to 12,500 units twice daily (and titrated to an activated partial thromboplastin time of twice control 6 to 12 hours after a dose), and warfarin therapy should be restarted as soon as possible after operation.

Prosthetic Valve Endocarditis. Patients with prosthetic valve endocarditis who are not receiving anticoagulant therapy have a 50 per cent risk of thromboembolism to the brain.[175-177] Anticoagulant therapy can probably decrease the incidence of thromboembolism by six- to ninefold, as suggested by three nonrandomized clinical studies.[175,176,178] Hemorrhage into the brain occurred in 14 per cent of these patients, but the overall risk appears to be considerably lower with anticoagulation. Thus, we advise continuing therapeutic anticoagulation for the patient with prosthetic valve endocarditis as long as there is no clinical or laboratory evidence of intracranial hemorrhage or gastrointestinal bleeding. Patients should be switched to a heparin infusion therapy (αPTT 1.5–2.0 × control) in the hospital for versatility in case emergency operation is required or significant bleeding occurs.

Anticoagulation After a Thromboembolic Event. The optimal time to start anticoagulation after a thromboembolic event to the brain has been controversial. A second embolism may occur early after the first event; thus immediate anticoagulation appears advisable. However, caution is advised because anecdotal reports and experimental studies suggest that immediate anticoagulation, especially in patients with a large embolic brain infarct, can result in secondary hemorrhages with increased morbidity. Data from 15 prospective and retrospective level V studies[28] suggest that approximately 12 per cent of patients (range 0 to 22) with aseptic embolism to the brain from a cardiac source experience a second embolic event within two weeks. Early recurrence is evenly distributed over the initial two weeks at about 1 per cent per day.

Recurrent thromboembolism appears to be decreased by immediate anticoagulation with heparin. In patients receiving anticoagulation, there was a reduction in early recurrent embolism within 14 days to about one third of that in patients who did not receive anticoagulants in six level III and level IV studies.[28] A level II randomized trial[179] of 45 patients showed that patients who received anticoagulants had a lower recurrence rate of thromboembolism. However, another randomized study showed the opposite effect.[180] There are large variations in the reported risk of cerebral hemorrhage after anticoagulating for embolic stroke. The risk of hemorrhages ranges from 0 to 24 per cent.[28] Details of intensity of anticoagulation are lacking for an analysis of risk.

A large brain infarct appears to place patients at a higher risk of hemorrhage when anticoagulated immediately after an embolic stroke. Spontaneous hemorrhagic transformation may be delayed for several days but occurs most frequently within 48 hours.[28,181] A national conference on antithrombotic therapy has made recommendations concerning this delicate problem.[28]

Immediate anticoagulation of small to moderate sized embolic strokes appears advisable if a computed tomographic scan of the head performed within 24 to 48 hours of the stroke does not indicate hemorrhage and if acute hypertension (greater than or equal to 180/100 mm Mg) is not present. The same principles apply for continuation of anticoagulant therapy in patients with a prosthetic heart valve who have an embolic stroke during long-term anticoagulant therapy. Patients with a large embolic infarct appear to be at special risk for delayed hemorrhagic transformation; thus anticoagulation is usually postponed for five to seven days before restarting or initiating anticoagulation. This allows time to document that a repeat computed tomographic scan of the head does not show hemorrhagic transformation. An infusion of heparin is preferable to large boluses to avoid large swings in anticoagulation and activated partial thromboplastin times beyond 2.0 times the upper limit of normal. A therapeutic range of 1.5 to 2.0 times control is recommended for the activated partial thromboplastin time.

Antithrombotic Therapy During Pregnancy. Anticoagulant therapy in general during pregnancy is discussed in detail in Chapter 26. For women with a prosthetic cardiac valve and of childbearing age, education concerning pregnancy and anticoagulation is critical. Pregnancy should be well planned. Warfarin should be stopped as soon as possible after conception to avoid the teratogenic risk of warfarin that is especially prominent during the first trimester. Women who receive warfarin therapy at the time of conception and during the first trimester have a high fetal wastage. This wastage may be higher than 80 per cent in women with multiple prosthetic heart valves.[182] Exposure after the first trimester may also predispose to congenital anomalies. The major anomalies include nasal hypoplasia, stippling of bones (chondrodysplasia punctata or Conradi's syndrome), mental retardation, optic atrophy, microcephaly, and spasticity or hypotonia.[182–186] Coumarin derivatives cross the placental barrier, anticoagulate the fetus, and can lead to hemorrhagic complications, especially at the time of delivery.

Anticoagulation should be switched from warfarin to subcutaneous heparin at the time of suspected conception such as with flattening of the temperature curve at the time of anticipated ovulation, or at the time of a positive test for human chorionic gonadotropin which can detect pregnancy five days before the missed menstrual period.

Administration of subcutaneous heparin should be continued throughout the first trimester. Some advocate continuation throughout the entire pregnancy to try to minimize any possible risk of congenital anomaly. Heparin therapy should be started at a minimum dose of 12,500 units every 12 hours following a bolus of 5,000 units intravenously to saturate intravascular binding sites and adjusted upward as necessary to maintain the activated partial thromboplastin times within 1.5 to 2.5 times control when drawn 6 to 12 hours after the previous dose. This appears to maintain good antithrombotic protection against thromboembolism.[188] A tuberculin syringe with a 25-gauge needle and heparin in a concentration of 20,000 or 40,000 units/milliliter are convenient for repeated injection in the abdominal region with continued rotation of sites over the entire abdominal wall. A dose of 5,000 units of heparin every 12 hours is not sufficient for the prevention of thromboembolism in patients with prosthetic heart valves.[186,189] Subcutaneous heparin should be continued

through the first trimester, at which time oral anticoagulation can be restarted and continued through week 37 or until one to two weeks before anticipated delivery. At that time the patient should be switched to a heparin infusion, which is continued until the induction of labor. At labor the patient is switched to low-dose subcutaneous heparin, 5,000 units every eight hours. Fortunately, heparin does not cross the placental barrier. Warfarin therapy should be restarted immediately after delivery. Nursing mothers can use warfarin because only an inactive metabolite of warfarin is found in breast milk, and this does not change the prothrombin time of the infant.[190,191] To be certain that there is not an unusual situation, the infant should have a prothrombin time checked on one occasion after the nursing mother is on warfarin therapy and has been nursing the infant regularly.

A bioprosthetic heart valve is preferred for women of childbearing age who wish to bear children, because many do not require long-term anticoagulant therapy (that is, assuming they have no other risk factors for thromboembolism). However, the risk of bioprosthetic calcification in women under age 35, and short durability of the bioprosthetic valve (10 to 15 years) has to be kept in mind. Platelet inhibitor drugs should be avoided as a routine during pregnancy because aspirin may cause premature closure of the ductus arteriosus. Dipyridamole and sulfinpyrazone have indeterminant effects on the fetus and are not approved for use during pregnancy. Maternal and fetal outcomes during pregnancy of women with prosthetic heart valves have been variable in reports.[187,188,192] However, careful planning of conception and antithrombotic therapy appears extremely valuable for minimizing the risk to both mother and infant.

REFERENCES

1. Stein B, Fuster V, Halperin JL, Chesebro JH. Antithrombotic therapy in cardiac disease. An emerging approach based on pathogenesis and risk. Circulation 1989; 80: 1501–13.
2. Dewanjee MK, Fuster V, Rao SA, Forshaw PL, Kaye MP. Noninvasive radioisotopic technique for detection of platelet deposition in mitral valve prostheses and quantitation of visceral microembolism in dogs. Mayo Clin Proc 1983; 58: 307–14.
3. Dahlke H, Dociu N, Thurau K. Thrombogenicity of different suture materials as revealed by scanning electron microscopy. J Biomed Mater Res 1980; 14: 251–68.
4. Badimon L, Lassila R, Badimon J, Vallabahajosula S, Ches-

ebro JH, Fuster V. Residual thrombus is more thrombogenic than severely damaged vessel wall (abstr). Circulation 1988; 78(suppl II): II–119.

5. Liu CY, Nossel HL, Kaplan KL. The binding of thrombin to fibrin. J Biol Chem 1979; 254: 10421–5.

6. Fuster V, Pumphrey CW, McGoon MD, Chesebro JH, Pluth JR, McGoon DC. Systemic thromboembolism in mitral and aortic Starr-Edwards prostheses: a 10–19 year follow-up. Circulation 1982; 66(suppl I): I-157–61.

7. Chesebro JH, Fuster V, Elevback LR, et al. Trial of combined warfarin plus dipyridamole or aspirin therapy in prosthetic heart valve replacement: danger of aspirin compared with dipyridamole. Am J Cardiol 1983; 51: 1537–41.

8. Szekely P. Systemic embolism and anticoagulant prophylaxis in rheumatic heart disease. Br Med J 1964; 1: 1209–12.

9. Coulshed N, Epstein EJ, McKendrick CS, Galloway RW, Walker E. Systemic embolism in mitral valve disease. Br Heart J 1979; 32: 26–34.

10. Fleming HA, Bailey SM. Mitral valve disease, systemic embolism and anticoagulants. Postgrad Med J 1971; 47: 599–604.

11. Wolf PA, Dawber TR, Thomas HE Jr, et al. Epidemiologic assessment of chronic atrial fibrillation and risk of stroke: the Framingham Study. Neurology 1978; 28: 973–7.

12. Caplan LR, D'Crux I, Hier DB, Reddy H, Shah S. Atrial size, atrial fibrillation, and stroke. Ann Neurol 1986; 19: 158–161.

13. Fuster V, Gersh BJ, Giuliani ER, et al. The natural history of idiopathic dilated cardiomyopathy. Am J Cardiol 1981; 47: 525–31.

14. Pumphrey CW, Fuster V, Chesebro JH. Systemic thromboembolism in valvular heart disease and prosthetic heart valves. Mod Concepts Cardiovasc Dis 1982; 51: 131–6.

15. Chesebro JH, Fuster V, Halperin JL. Atrial fibrillation—risk marker for stroke. N Engl J Med 1990; 323: 1556–8.

16. Askey JM, Berstein S. The management of rheumatic heart disease in relation to systemic arterial embolism. Prog Cardiovasc Dis 1960; 3: 220–32.

17. Deveral PB, Olley PM, Smith DR, Watson DA, Whitaker W. Incidence of systemic embolism before and after mitral valvotomy. Thorax 1968; 23: 530–6.

18. Abernathy WS, Willis PW. Thromboembolic complications of rheumatic heart disease. Cardiovasc Clin 1973; 5: 131–75.

19. Nielson GH, Galea EG, Hossack KF. Thromboembolic complications of mitral valve disease. Aust NZ J Med 1978; 8: 372–6.

20. Easton JD, Sherman DG. Management of cerebral embolism of cardiac origin. Stroke 1980; 11: 433–42.

21. Hart RG, Miller VT. Cerebral infarction in young adults: a practical approach. Stroke 1983; 14: 110–4.

22. Wolf PA, Abbott RD, Kannel WB. Atrial fibrillation: a major contributor to stroke in the elderly: the Framingham Study. Arch Intern Med 1987; 147: 1561–4.

23. Chesebro JH, Adams PC, Fuster V. Antithrombotic therapy in patients with valvular heart disease and prosthetic heart valves. J Am Coll Cardiol 1986; 8: 41B–56B.

24. Barnett JH, Boughner DR, Taylor DW, et al. Further evidence relating mitral-valve prolapse to cerebral ischemic events. N Engl J Med 1980; 302: 139–44.

25. Savage DD, Garrison RJ, Devereaux RB, et al. Mitral valve prolapse in the general population. I. Epidemiologic features: the Framingham Study. Am Heart J 1983; 106: 571–6.

26. Nishimura RA, McGoon MD, Shub C, Miller FA, Ilstrup DM, Tajik AJ. Echocardiographically documented mitral-valve prolapse: long-term follow-up of 237 patients. N Engl J Med 1985; 313: 1305–9.

27. Barnett HJM, Jones MW, Boughner DR, Kostuk WJ. Cerebral ischemic events associated with prolapsing mitral valve. Arch Neurol 1976; 33: 777–82.

28. Sherman DG, Dyken ML, Fisher M, Harrison MJG, Hart RG. Antithrombotic therapy for cerebrovascular disorders. Chest 1989; 95(suppl): 140S–55S.

29. Barnett HJ. Heart in ischemic stroke—a changing emphasis. Neurol Clin 1983; 1: 291–315.

30. Schnee MA, Bucal AA. Fatal embolism in mitral valve prolapse. Chest 1983; 83: 285–7.

31. Jackson AC, Boughner DR, Barnett HJ. Mitral valve prolapse and cerebral ischemic events in young patients. Neurology 1984; 24: 384–7.

32. Dry BTJ, Willius FA. Calcareous disease of the aortic valve: a study of 228 cases. Am Heart J 1939; 17: 138–57.

33. Kumpe CW, Bean WB. Aortic stenosis: a study of the clinical and pathologic aspects of 107 proved cases. Medicine 1948; 27: 139–85.

34. Rotman M, Morris JJ Jr, Behar VS, et al. Aortic valvular disease. Comparison of types and their medical and surgical management. Am J Med 1971; 51: 241–57.

35. Holley KE, Bahn RC, McGoon DC, Mankin HT. Spontaneous calcific embolization associated with calcific aortic stenosis. Circulation 1963; 27: 197–202.

36. Brockmeier LB, Adolph RJ, Gustin BW, Holmes JC, Sacks JG. Calcium emboli to the retinal artery in calcific aortic stenosis. Am Heart J 1981; 101: 32–7.

37. Stein PD, Sabbah HN, Pitha JV. Continuing disease process of calcific aortic stenosis. Role of microthrombi and turbulent flow. Am J Cardiol 1977; 39: 159–63.

38. Sherrid MV, Clark RD, Cohn K. Echocardiographic analysis of left atrial size before and after operation in mitral valve disease. Am J Cardiol 1979; 43: 171–8.

39. Rogers PH, Sherry S. Current status of antithrombotic therapy in cardiovascular disease. Prog Cardiovasc Dis 1976; 19: 235–53.

40. Kannel WB, Abbott RD, Savage DD, et al. Epidemiologic features of chronic atrial fibrillation. N Engl J Med 1982; 306: 1018–22.

41. Stroke Prevention in Atrial Fibrillation Study Group Investigators. Preliminary report of the SPAF Study. N Engl J Med 1990; 322: 863–8.

43. Daley R, Mattingly TW, Holt CL, et al. Systemic arterial embolism in rheumatic heart disease. Am Heart J 1951; 42: 566–81.

44. Carter AB. Prognosis of cerebral embolism. Lancet 1965; ii: 514–9.

45. Darling RC, Austen WG, Linton RR. Atrial embolism. Surg Gynecol Obstet 1967; 124: 106–14.

46. Casella L, Abelmann WH, Ellis LB. Patients with mitral stenosis and systemic emboli. Arch Intern Med 1964; 114: 773–81.

47. Poller L. Simple nanogram for the derivation of international normalised ratios for the standardisation of prothrombin time. Thromb Haemost 1988; 60: 18–20.

48. Sackett DL. Rules of evidence and clinical recommendations on the use of antithrombotic agents. Chest 1986; 89(suppl 2): 2S–3S.

49. Chesebro JH, Fuster V, Elveback LR, et al. Effect of dipyridamole and aspirin on late vein-graft patency after coronary bypass operation. N Engl J Med 1984; 310: 209–14.

50. Cairns JA, Gent M, Singer J, et al. Aspirin, sulfinpyrazone, or both, in unstable angina: results of a Canadian multicenter trial. N Engl J Med 1985; 313: 1369–75.

51. Petersen P, Boysen G, Godtfredsen J, Andersen ED, Andersen B. Placebo controlled, randomized trial of warfarin and aspirin for prevention of thromboembolic complications in chronic atrial fibrillation: the Copenhagen AFASAK Study. Lancet 1989; 1: 175–9.

52. Boston Area Anticoagulation Trial for Atrial Fibrillation Investigators. The effect of low-dose warfarin on the risk of stroke in patients with nonrheumatic atrial fibrillation. N Engl J Med 1990; 323: 1505–11.

53. Dalen JE, Hirsh J. Second ACCP conference on antithrombotic therapy. Chest 1989; 95(suppl): 1S–169S.

54. Levine MN, Raskob G, Hirsh J. Hemorrhagic complications of long-term anticoagulant therapy. Chest 1989; 95(suppl): 26S–36S.

55. Steele P, Rainwater J. Favorable effect of sulfinpyrazone on thromboembolism in patients with rheumatic heart disease. Circulation 1980; 62: 462–5.

56. Dewanjee MK, Trastek VF, Tago M, Kaye MP. Radioisotopic techniques for noninvasive detection of platelet deposition in bovine tissue mitral-valve prostheses and in vitro quantification of visceral microembolism in dogs. Invest Radiol 1984; 6: 535–42.

57. Forbes CD, Prentice CRM. Thrombus formation and artificial surfaces. Br Med Bull 1978; 34: 201–7.

58. Markwardt F, Kaiser B, Nowak G. Studies on antithrombotic effects of recombinant hirudin. Thromb Res 1989; 54: 377–88.

59. Heras M, Chesebro JH, Webster MWI, et al. Hirudin, heparin, and placebo during deep arterial injury in the pig: the in vivo role of thrombin in platelet-mediated thrombosis. Circulation 1990; 82: 1476–84.

60. Pipkin RD, Buch WS, Fogarty TS. Evaluation of aortic valve replacement with a porcine xenograft without long-term anticoagulants. J Thorac Cardiovasc Surg 1976; 71: 179–86.

61. Stinson EB, Griepp RB, Oyer PE, Shumway NE. Long-term experience with porcine aortic valve xenografts. J Thorac Cardiovasc Surg 1977; 73: 54–63.

62. Ionescu MI, Pakrashi BC, Mary DAS, Bartek IT, Woolner GH, McGoon DC. Long-term evaluation of tissue valves. J Thorac Cardiovasc Surg 1974; 68: 361–79.

63. Cevese PG. Long-term results of 212 xenograft valve replacement. J Cardiovas Surg 1975; 16: 639–42.

64. Davila JC, Magilligan DJ, Lewis JW. Is the Hancock porcine valve the best cardiac valve substitute today? Ann Thorac Surg 1978; 26: 303–16.

65. Edmiston WA, Harrison EC, Duwick GF, Parnassus W, Lau FYK. Thromboembolism in mitral porcine valve recipients. Am J Cardiol 1978; 41: 508–11.

66. Heras M, Chesebro JH, Grill DE, Penny W, Bailey K, Orszulak TA. Chronic risk of thromboembolism after bioprosthetic valve replacement (abstr). Eur Heart J 1989; 10(suppl C): 260.

67. Harker LA, Slichter SJ. Studies of platelet and fibrinogen kinetics in patients with prosthetic heart valves. N Engl J Med 1970; 283: 1302–5.

68. Weily HS, Genton E. Altered platelet function in patients with prosthetic mitral valves: effects of sulfinpyrazone therapy. Circulation 1970; 42: 967–72.

69. Steele P, Rainwater J, Vogel R. Platelet suppressant therapy in patients with prosthetic cardiac valves: relationship of clinical effectiveness to alteration of platelet survival time. Circulation 1979; 60: 910–3.

70. Pengo V, Peruzzi P, Baca M, et al. The optimal therapeutic range for oral anticoagulant treatment as suggested by fibrinopeptide A (FpA) levels in patients with heart valve prosthesis. Eur J Clin Invest 1989; 19: 181–4.

71. Friedli B, Aerichide N, Grondin P, Campeau L. Thromboembolic complications of heart valve replacement. Am Heart J 1971; 81: 702–8.

72. Gadboys HL, Litwak RS, Niemetz J, Wisch N. Role of anticoagulants in preventing embolization from prosthetic heart valves. JAMA 1967; 202: 134–8.

73. Cleland J, Molloy PJ. Thromboembolic complications of the cloth-covered Starr-Edwards prostheses no. 2300 aortic and no. 6300 mitral. Thorax 1973; 28: 41–7.

74. Barnhorst DA, Oxman HA, Connolly DC, et al. Long-term follow up of isolated replacement of the aortic or mitral valve with the Starr-Edwards prosthesis. Am J Cardiol 1975; 35: 228–33.

75. Saour JN, Sieck JO, Mamo LAR, Gallus AS. Trial of different intensities of anticoagulation in patients with prosthetic heart valves. N Engl J Med 1990; 322: 428–32.

76. Björk VO, Henze A. Ten years' experience with the Björk-Shiley tilting disk valve. J Thorac Cardiovasc Surg 1979; 78: 331–42.

76a. Huber KC, Gersh BJ, Bailey KR, Hodge DO, Chesebro JH. Variability in anticoagulation control predicts thromboembolism: a 23 year population based study. (abstr). Circulation 1991; 84(suppl IV), in press.

77. Dale J, Myhre E. Can acetylsalicylic acid alone prevent arterial thromboembolism? A pilot study in patients with aortic ball valve prosthesis. Acta Med Scand 1981; 645(suppl): 73–8.

78. Cohn LH, Koster JK, Meed RBB, Collins JJ. Long-term follow up of the Hancock bioprosthetic heart valve (abstr). Circulation 1979; 60(suppl I): 1–87.

79. Hetzer R, Hill JD, Kerth WJ, et al. Thromboembolic complications after mitral valve replacement with Hancock xenograft. J Thorac Cardiovasc Surg 1978; 75: 651–8.

80. Oyer PE, Stinson ER, Griepp RB, Shumway NE. Valve replacement with the Starr-Edwards and Hancock prostheses. Ann Surg 1977; 186: 301–9.

81. Lakier JB, Khaja R, Magilligan DJ Jr, Goldstein S. Porcine xenograft valves: long-term (60–90 month) follow-up. Circulation 1980; 62: 313–8.

82. Anderson ET, Hancock EWL. Long-term follow-up of aortic valve replacement with the mesh aortic homograft. J Thorac Cardiovasc Surg 1976; 72: 150–6.

83. Cohn LH, Alfred EN, Cohn LA, et al. Early and late risk of mitral valve replacement: a 12 year concomitant comparison of the porcine bioprosthetic and prosthetic disc mitral valves. J Thorac Cardiovasc Surg 1985; 90: 872–81.

84. Douglas P, Hirshfeld JW, Edmunds LH. Clinical correlates of post-operative atrial fibrillation (abstr). Circulation 1984; 70(suppl II): II–165.

85. Cohn LH, Alfred EN, Cohn LA, DiSesa VJ, Shemin RJ, Collins JJ Jr. Long-term results of open mitral valve reconstruction for mitral stenosis. Am J Cardiol 1985; 55: 731–4.

86. Carpentier A, Chauvaud S, Fabiani JN, et al. Reconstructive surgery of mitral valve incompetence. J Thorac Cardiovasc Surg 1980; 79: 338–48.

87. Perier P, Deloche A, Chauvaud S, et al. Comparative evaluation of mitral valve repair and replacement with Starr, Björk, and porcine valve prostheses. Circulation 1984; 70(suppl I): I-187–92.

88. Spencer FC, Colvin SB, Culliford AT, Isom OW. Experiences with the Carpentier techniques of mitral valve reconstruction in 103 patients (1980–1985). J Thorac Cardiovasc Surg 1985; 90: 341–50.

89. Macmanus Q, Grunkemeier GL, Lambert LE, Teply JF, Harlan BJ, Starr A. Year of operation as a risk factor in the late results of valve replacement. J Thorac Cardiovasc Surg 1980; 80: 834–41.

90. McGoon DC. The risk of thromboembolism following valvular operations: how does one know? J Thorac Cardiovasc Surg 1984; 88: 782–6.

91. Murphy DA, Levine FH, Buckley MJ, et al. Mechanical valves: a comparative analysis of the Starr-Edwards and Björk-Shiley prostheses. J Thorac Cardiovasc Surg 1983; 86: 746–52.

92. Perier P, Bessou JP, Swanson JS, et al. Comparative evaluation of aortic valve replacement with Starr, Björk, and porcine valve prostheses. Circulation 1985; 72(suppl II): II-140–5.

93. Hackett D, Fessatidis I, Saphsford R, Oakley C. Ten year clinical evaluation of Starr-Edwards 2400 and 1260 aortic valve prostheses. Br Heart J 1987; 57: 356–63.

94. Fessatidis I, Hackett D, Oakley CM, Sapsford RN, Bentall HH. Ten-year clinical evaluation of isolated mitral valve and double-valve replacement with the Starr-Edwards prosthesis. Ann Thorac Surg 1987; 43: 368–72.

95. Schoevaerdts JC, el Gariani A, Lichtsteiner M, Jaumin P, Ponlot R, Chalant CH-H. Twenty years' experience with the Model 6120 Starr-Edwards valve in the mitral position. J Thorac Cardiovasc Surg 1987; 94: 375–82.

96. Cobanoglu A, Fessler CL, Guvendik L, Grunkemeier G, Starr A. Aortic valve replacement with the Starr-Edwards prosthesis: a comparison of the first and second decades of follow-up. Ann Thorac Surg 1988; 45: 248–52.

97. Horstkotte D, Körfer R, Seipel L, Bircks W, Loogen F. Late complications in patients with Björk-Shiley and St. Jude medical heart valve replacement. Circulation 1983; 68(suppl II): II-175–84.

98. Marshall WG, Kouchoukos NT, Karp RB, Williams JB. Late results after mitral valve replacement with the Björk-Shiley and porcine prostheses. J Thorac Cardiovasc Surg 1983; 85: 902–10.

99. Cohn LH, Allred EN, DiSesa VJ, Sawtelle K, Shemin RJ, Collins JJ Jr. Early and late risk of aortic valve replacement: a 12 year concomitant comparison of the porcine bioprosthetic and tilting disc prosthetic aortic valves. J Thorac Cardiovasc Surg 1984; 88: 695–705.

100. Harjula A, Mattila S, Maamies T, et al. Long-term follow-up of Björk-Shiley mitral valve replacement. 10 years' experience. Scand J Thorac Cardiovasc Surg 1986; 20: 79–84.

101. Bloomfield P, Kitchin AH, Wheatley DJ, Walbaum PR,

Lutz W, Miller HC. A prospective evaluation of the Björk-Shiley Hancock, and Carpentier-Edwards heart valve prostheses. Circulation 1986; 73: 1213–22.

102. Borkon AM, Soule LM, Baughman KL, et al. Comparative analysis of mechanical and bioprosthetic valves after aortic valve replacement. J Thorac Cardiovasc Surg 1987; 94: 20–33.

103. Lindblom D. Long-term clinical results after aortic valve replacement with the Björk-Shiley prosthesis. J Thorac Cardiovasc Surg 1988; 95: 658–67.

104. Lindblom D. Long-term clinical results after mitral valve replacement with the Björk-Shiley prosthesis. J Thorac Cardiovasc Surg 1988; 95: 321–33.

105. Thulin LI, Bain WH, Huysmans HH, et al. Heart valve replacement with the Björk-Shiley monostrut valve: early results of a multicenter clinical investigation. Ann Thorac Surg 1988; 45: 164–70.

106. Milano AD, Bortollotti U, Mazzucco A, Guerra F, Magni A, Gallucci V. Aortic valve replacement with the Hancock standard, Björk-Shiley, and Lillehei-Kaster prostheses. A comparison based on follow-up from 1 to 15 years. J Thorac Cardiovasc Surg 1989; 98: 37–47.

107. Fessatidis JT, Vassiliadis KE, Monro JL, Ross JK, Shore DF, Drury PJ. Thirteen years evaluation of the Björk-Shiley isolated mitral valve prosthesis. The Wessex experience. J Cardiovasc Surg 1989; 30: 957–65.

108. Douglas PS, Hirshfeld JW, Edie RN, et al. Clinical comparison of St. Jude and porcine aortic valve prostheses. Circulation 1985; 72(suppl II): II-135–9.

109. Chaux A, Czer LSC, Matloff JM, et al. The St. Jude Medical bileaflet valve prosthesis: a 5 year experience. J Thorac Cardiovasc Surg 1984; 88: 706–17.

110. Baudet EM, Oca CC, Roques XF, et al. A 5½ year experience with the St. Jude Medical cardiac valve prosthesis: early and late results of 737 valve replacements in 671 patients. J Thorac Cardiovasc Surg 1985; 90: 137–44.

111. Kinsley RH, Antunes MJ, Colsen PR. St. Jude Medical valve replacement. J Thorac Cardiovasc Surg 1986; 92: 349–60.

112. Nakano K, Imamura E, Hashimoto A, et al. Six-year experience with the St. Jude Medical prosthesis: early and late results of 540 valves in 462 patients. Jpn Circ J 1987; 51: 275–83.

113. Montalescot G, Thomas D, Drobinski G, et al. Clinical and ultrasound results after aortic valve replacement: intermediate-term follow-up with the St. Jude Medical prosthesis. Am Heart J 1989; 118: 104–13.

114. Arom KV, Nicoloff DM, Kersten TE, Northrup WF III, Lindsay WG, Emery RW. Ten years' experience with the St. Jude Medical valve prosthesis. Ann Thorac Surg 1989; 27: 831–7.

115. Callaghan JC, Coles J, Damle A. Six year clinical study of use of the omniscience valve prosthesis in 219 patients. J Am Coll Cardiol 1987; 9: 240–6.

116. Carrier M, Martineau J-P, Bonan R, Pelletier LC. Clinical and hemodynamic assessment of the Omniscience prosthetic heart valve. J Thorac Cardiovasc Surg 1987; 93: 300–7.

117. Stewart S, Cianciotta D, Hicks GL, DeWeese JA. The Lillehei-Kaster aortic valve prosthesis. Long-term results in 273 patients with 1253 patient-years of follow-up. J Thorac Cardiovasc Surg 1988; 95: 1023–30.

118. Butchart EG, Lewis PA, Grunkemeier GL, Kulatilake N, Breckenridge IM. Low risk of thrombosis and serious embolic events despite low-intensity anticoagulation. Experience with 1,004 Medtronic Hall valves. Circulation 1988; 78(suppl I): I-66–77.

119. Antunes MJ, Wessels A, Sadowski RG, et al. Medtronic Hall valve replacement in a third-world population group. A review of the performance of 1000 prostheses. J Thorac Cardiovasc Surg 1988; 95: 980–93.

120. Vallejo JL, Gonzales-Santos JM, Albertos J, et al. Eight years' experience with the Medtronic-Hall valve prosthesis. Ann Thorac Surg 1990; 50: 429–36.

121. Mikaeloff PH, Jegadan O, Ferrini M, Coll-Mazzei J, Bonnefoy JY, Rumolo A. Prospective randomized study of St. Jude Medical versus Björk-Shiley or Starr-Edwards 6120 valve prostheses in the mitral position. Three hundred and fifty-seven patients operated on from 1979 to December 1983. J Cardiovasc Surg 1989; 30: 666–975.

122. Kuntze CEE, Ebels T, Eijgelaar A, van der Heide JNH. Rates of thromboembolism with three different mechanical heart valve prostheses: randomised study. Lancet 1989; 1 (8637): 514–7.

123. Vogt S, Hoffmann A, Roth J, et al. Heart valve replacement with the Björk-Shiley and St. Jude Medical prostheses: a randomized comparison in 178 patients. Eur Heart J 1990; 11: 583–91.

124. Cortina JM, Martinell J, Artiz V, Fraile J, Rabago G. Comparative clinical results with Omniscience (STM1), Medtronic-Hall, and Björk-Shiley convexo-concave (70 degrees) prostheses in mitral valve replacement. J Thorac Cardiovasc Surg 1986; 91: 174–83.

125. Nuutinen LS, Pihlajaniemi R, Saarela E, Karkola P, Hollmen A. The effect of dipyridamole on the thrombocyte count and bleeding tendency in open-heart surgery. J Thorac Cardiovasc Surg 1977; 74: 295–8.

126. Pumphrey CW, Fuster V, Dewanjee MK, Chesebro JH, Vlietstra RE, Kaye MP. Comparison of antithrombotic action of calcium antagonist drugs with dipyridamole in dogs. Am J Cardiol 1983; 51: 591–5.

127. Sullivan JM, Harken DE, Gorlin R. Pharmacologic control of thromboembolic complications of cardiac-valve replacement. N Engl J Med 1971; 284: 1391–4.

128. Kasahara T. Clinical effect of dipyridamole ingestion after prosthetic heart valve replacement—especially on the blood coagulation system. J Jpn Assoc Thorac Surg 1977; 25: 1007–21.

129. Groupe de Recherche PACTE. Prevention des accidents thromboemboliques systémiques chez les porteurs de prothésis valvulaires artificielles: essai cooperatif controlé du dipyridamole. Coeur 1978; 9: 915–69.

130. Rajah SM, Sreeharan N, Joseph A, et al. A prospective trial of dipyridamole and warfarin in heart valve patients (abstr). Acta Therapeutica 1980; 6(suppl 93): 54.

131. Ranhosky A. Dipyridamole. N Engl J Med 1987; 317: 1734.

132. Fuster V, Chesebro JH. Antithrombotic therapy: current concepts of thrombogenesis: role of platelets. Mayo Clin Proc 1981; 56: 102–12.

133. Dale J, Myhre E, Storstein O, et al. Prevention of arterial thromboembolism with acetylsalicylic acid: a controlled clinical study in patients with aortic ball valves. Am Heart J 1977; 94: 101–11.

134. Altman R, Boullon F, Rouvier J, et al. Aspirin and prophylaxis of thromboembolic complications in patients with substitute heart valves. J Thorac Cardiovasc Surg 1976; 72: 127–9.

135. Gonzalez-Lavin L, Tandon AP, Chi S, et al. The risk of thromboembolism and hemorrhage following mitral valve replacment: a comparative analysis between the porcine xenograft valve and Ionescu-Shiley bovine pericardial valve. J Thorac Cardiovasc Surg 1984; 87: 340–51.

136. Jamieson WRE, Pelletier C, Janusz MT, Chaitman BR, Tyers GFO, Miyagishima RT. Five-year evaluation of the Carpentier-Edwards porcine bioprosthesis. J Thorac Cardiovasc Surg 1984; 88: 324–33.

137. Zussa C, Ottino G, diSumma M, et al. Porcine cardiac bioprostheses: evaluation of long-term results in 990 patients. Ann Thorac Surg 1985; 39: 243–50.

138. Louagie Y, Muteba P, Marchandise B, Kremer R, Schoevaerdts JC, Chalant CH. Experience with selective use of the Carpentier-Edwards bioprosthesis. Thorac Cardiovasc Surg 1986; 34: 77–81.

139. Bortolotti U, Milano A, Thiene G, et al. Long-term durability of the Hancock porcine bioprosthesis following combined mitral and aortic valve replacement: an 11-year experience. Ann Thorac Surg 1987; 44: 139–44.

140. Kimose HH, Lund O, Ljungström. Isolated mitral valve replacement with Carpentier-Edwards bioprosthesis: independent risk factors for long-term survival and prosthesis failure. Thorac Cardiovasc Surg 1989; 37: 135–42.

141. Magillian DJ, Lewis JW, Stein P, Alam M. The porcine bioprosthetic heart valve: experience at 15 years. Ann Thorac Surg 1989; 48: 324–30.

142. Jamieson WRE, Munro AI, Miyagishima RT, et al. The Car-

pentier-Edwards supraannular porcine bioprosthesis. J Thorac Cardiovasc Surg 1988; 96: 652–66.

143. Brais MP, Bedard JP, Goldstein W, Koshal A, Keon WJ. Ionescu-Shiley pericardial xenografts: follow-up of up to 6 years. Ann Thorac Surg 1985; 39: 105–11.

144. Reul GJ, Cooley DA, Duncan JM, et al. Valve failure with the Ionescu-Shiley bovine pericardial bioprosthesis: analysis of 2680 patients. J Vasc Surg 1985; 2: 192–204.

145. Revuelta JM, Duran CM. Performance of the Ionescu-Shiley pericardial valve in the aortic position: 100 months clinical experience. Thorac Cardiovasc Surg 1986; 24: 247–51.

146. Xiaodong Z, Jiaqiang G, Yingchun C, Chengjun T, Ganxing X. Ten-year experience with pericardial xenograft valves. J Thorac Cardiovasc Surg 1988; 95: 572–6.

147. Daenen W, Noyez L, Lesaffre E, Goffin Y, Stalpaert G. The Ionescu-Shiley pericardial valve results in 473 patients. Ann Thorac Surg 1988; 46: 536–41.

148. Revuelta JM, Bernal JM, Gutierrez JA, Gaite L, Alonso C, Duran CMG. Mitroflow heart valve: 5.5 years clinical experience. Thorac Cardiovasc Surg 1988; 36: 262–5.

149. Matsuki O, Robles A, Gibbs S, Bodnar E, Ross DN. Long-term performance of 555 aortic homografts in the aortic position. Ann Thorac Surg 1988; 46: 187–91.

150. Turpie AGG, Gunstensen J, Hirsh J, Nelson H, Gent M. Randomized comparison of two intensities of oral anticoagulant therapy after tissue heart valve replacement. Lancet 1988; 1: 1242–5.

151. Perier P, Deloche A, Chauvaud S, et al. A 10-year comparison of mitral valve replacement with Carpentier-Edwards and Hancock Porcine Bioprostheses. Ann Thorac Surg 1989; 48: 54–9.

152. Gould KL. Noninvasive assessment of coronary stenoses by myocardial perfusion imaging during pharmacologic coronary vasodilation. 1. Physiologic basis and experimental validation. Am J Cardiol 1978; 41: 267–78.

153. Nunez L, Aguado G, Larrea JL, Celemin D, Oliver J. Prevention of thromboembolism using aspirin after mitral valve replacement with porcine bioprosthesis. Ann Thorac Surg 1984; 37: 84–7.

154. Kempin SJ. Warfarin resistance caused by broccoli. N Engl J Med 1983; 308: 1229–30.

155. Lorient Roudaut M-F, Ledain L, Roudaut R, Besse P, Boisseau MR. Thrombolytic treatment of acute thrombotic obstruction with disk valve prostheses: experience with 26 cases. Semin Thromb Hemost 1987; 13: 201–5.

156. Deviri E, Sareli P, Wisenbaugh T, Cronje SL. Obstruction of mechanical heart valve prostheses: clinical aspects and surgical management. J Am Coll Cardiol 1991; 17: 646–50.

157. Kontos GJ, Schaff HV, Orszulak TA, Puga FJ, Pluth JR, Danielson GK. Thrombotic obstruction of disc valves: clinical recognition and surgical management. Ann Thorac Surg 1989; 48: 60–5.

158. Massad M, Fahl M, Slim M, et al. Thrombosed Björk-Shiley standard disc mitral valve prosthesis. J Cardiovasc Surg 1989; 30: 976–80.

159. Zoghbi WA, Desir RM, Rosen L, Lawrie GM, Pratt CM, Quinones MA. Doppler echocardiography: application to the assessment of successful thrombolysis of prosthetic valve thrombosis. J Am Soc Echo 1989; 2: 98–101.

160. Montero CG, Mula N, Brugos R, Pradas R, Figuera D. Thrombectomy of the Björk-Shiley prosthetic valves revisited: long-term results. Ann Thorac Surg 1989; 48: 824–8.

161. Balram A, Kaul U, Rao R, et al. Thrombotic obstruction of Björk-Shiley valves—diagnostic and surgical considerations. Int J Cardiol 1984; 6: 61–9.

162. Tyagi S, Gambhir DS, Khalilullah M. Thrombolytic therapy for a thrombosed Björk-Shiley mitral valve prosthesis. Indian Heart J 1988; 40: 507–8.

163. Graver LM, Gelber PM, Tyras DH. The risks and benefits of thrombolytic therapy in acute aortic and mitral prosthetic valve dysfunction: report of a case and review of the literature. Ann Thorac Surg 1988; 46: 85–8.

164. Quintanilla MA, Haque AK. Thrombotic obstruction of prosthetic aortic valve presenting as acute myocardial infarction. Am Heart J 1989; 117(6): 1378–9.

165. Tapanainen J, Ikäheimo M, Jouppila P, Kortelainen M-L, Salmela P. Thrombosis in a mechanical aortic valve prosthesis during subcutaneous heparin therapy in pregnancy;

a case report. Eur J Obstet Gynecol Reprod Biol 1990; 36: 175–7.

166. Witchitz S, Veyrat C, Moisson P, Scheinman N, Rozenstajn L. Fibrinolytic treatment of thrombus on prosthetic heart valves. Br Heart J 1980; 44: 545–54.

167. Minami K, Horstkotte D, Schulte HD, Bircks W. Thrombosis of two St. Jude Medical prostheses in one patient after triple valve replacement. Eur J Cardio-thoracic Surg 1988; 2: 48–52.

168. Mosseri M, Galoon E, Gotsman MS, Rosenheck S, Milgarter E. Successful treatment of an immobile and thrombosed prosthetic tricuspid valve by fibrinolysis with a single dose of streptokinase. Isr J Med Sci 1988; 24: 114–6.

169. Cambier P, Mombaerts P, De Geest H, Collen D, Van de Werf F. Treatment of prosthetic tricuspid valve thrombosis with recombinant tissue-type plasminogen activator. Eur Heart J 1987; 8: 906–9.

170. Prieto Palomino MA, Ruiz de Elvira MJ, Sanchez Llorente F, et al. Successful thrombolysis on a mechanical tricuspid prosthesis. Eur Heart J 1989; 10: 1115–7.

171. Tischler MD, Lee RT, Kirshenbaum JM. Successful treatment of prosthetic tricuspid valve thrombosis with short-course recombinant tissue-type plasminogen activator. Am Heart J 1990; 120: 975–7.

172. Matsuda M, Matsuda Y, Okuda F, et al. Thrombolysis of tricuspid Björk-Shiley prosthesis with tissue-type plasminogen activator. Jpn Circ J 1988; 52: 583–7.

173. Cohen ML, Barzilai B, Gutierrez F, Jaffe AS, Eisenberg P. Treatment of prosthetic tricuspid valve thrombosis with low-dose tissue plasminogen activator. Am Heart J 1990; 120: 978–80.

174. Tinker JH, Tarhan S. Discontinuing anticoagulant therapy in surgical patients with cardiac valve prostheses: observations in 180 operations. JAMA 1978; 234: 738–9.

175. Garvey GJ, Neu HC. Infective endocarditis—an evolving disease. A review of endocarditis at the Columbia-Presbyterian Medical Center 1968–1973. Medicine 1978; 57: 105–27.

176. Wilson WR, Geraci JE, Danielson GK, et al. Anticoagulant therapy and central nervous system complications in patients with prosthetic valve endocarditis. Circulation 1978; 57: 1004–7.

177. Block PC, DeSanctis RW, Weinberg AN, Austen WG. Prosthetic valve endocarditis. J Thorac Cardiovasc Surg 1970; 60: 540–8.

178. Karchmer AW, Dismukes WE, Buckley MJ, Austen WG. Late prosthetic valve endocarditis: clinical features influencing therapy. Am J Med 1978; 64: 199–206.

179. Cerebral Embolism Study Group. Immediate anticoagulation of embolic stroke: a randomized trial. Stroke 1983; 14: 668–76.

180. Lodder J, van der Lugt PJ. Evaluation of the risk of immediate anticoagulant treatment in patients with embolic stroke of cardiac origin. Stroke 1983; 14: 42–6.

181. Cerebral Embolism Study Group. Immediate anticoagulation of embolic stroke: brain hemorrhage and management options. Stroke 1983; 14: 42–6.

182. Lutz DJ, Noller KL, Spittel JA, Danielson GK, Fish CR. Pregnancy and its complications following cardiac valve prostheses. Am J Obstet Gynecol 1978; 131: 460–6.

183. Bloomfield DK. Fetal deaths and malformations associated with the use of coumarin derivatives in pregnancy: a critical review. Am J Obstet Gynecol 1970; 107: 883–8.

184. Becker MH, Genieser NB, Finegold M, Miranda D, Spackman T. Chondrodysplasia punctata. Is maternal warfarin therapy a factor? Am J Dis Child 1975; 129: 356–9.

185. Shaul WL, Hall JG. Multiple congenital anomalies associated with oral anticoagulants. Am J Obstet Gynecol 1977; 127: 191–8.

186. Iturbe-Alessio I, Fonseca MDC, Mutchinik O, Santos MA, Zajaraias A, Salazar E. Risks of anticoagulant therapy in pregnant women with artificial heart valves. N Engl J Med 1986; 315: 1390–3.

187. Salazar E, Zajaria A, Gutierrez N, Iturbe I. The problem of cardiac valve prostheses, anticoagulants, and pregnancy. Circulation 1984; 70(suppl I): I-169–77.

188. Sareli P, England MJ, Berk MR, et al. Maternal and fetal sequelae of anticoagulation during pregnancy in patients

with mechanical heart valve prostheses. Am J Cardiol 1989; 63: 1462–5.

189. Wang RYC, Lee PK, Chow JSF, Chen WWC. Efficacy of low-dose, subcutaneously administered heparin in treatment of pregnant women with artificial heart valves. Med J Aust 1983; 2: 126–8.

190. Baty JD, Breckenridge A, Lewis PJ, et al. May mothers taking warfarin breast feed their infants. Br J Clin Pharmacol 1976; 3: 969.

191. O'Reilly RA, Aggeler PM. Determinants of the response to

oral anticoagulant drugs in man. Pharmacol Rev 1970; 22: 35–96.

192. Vitali E, Donatelli F, Quaini E, Groppeli G, Pellegrini A. Pregnancy in patients with mechanical prosthetic heart valves: our experience regarding 98 pregnancies in 57 patients. J Cardiovasc Surg 1986; 27: 221–7.

193. Mok CK, Boey J, Wang et al. Warfarin vs dipyridamole-aspirin and pentoxifylline-aspirin for the prevention of prosthetic heart valve thromboembolism: a prospective randomized clinical trial. Circulation 1985; 72: 1059–83.

12

THROMBOSIS IN THE CARDIAC CHAMBERS:
Ventricular Dysfunction and Atrial Fibrillation

JONATHAN L. HALPERIN and PALLE PETERSEN

CARDIOGENIC THROMBOEMBOLISM— EPIDEMIOLOGICAL PERSPECTIVE

Cardiogenic cerebral embolism is the mechanism responsible for nearly 100,000 strokes each year among North Americans, and perhaps a million or more worldwide. These thrombotic episodes derive from a diversity of cardiac disorders (Fig. 12–1). There is a history of atrial fibrillation in just under half the cases, valvular heart disease in a quarter, and left ventricular mural thrombi in almost a third.[1,2]

Epidemiologic studies have estimated the risk of stroke and systemic embolism associated with atrial fibrillation as five to six events per 100 patient-years, at least five times the rate among comparable patients without this cardiac rhythm disturbance, and accumulating to a 35 per cent lifetime risk of stroke for patients with atrial fibrillation. The risk appears related to age, such that among stroke victims over 85 years of age, a history of atrial fibrillation can be found in nearly half.[3–5]

Sixty per cent of the emboli of left ventricular origin are associated with acute myocardial infarction; the remainder occur in patients with chronic ventricular dysfunction resulting from coronary disease, hypertension, or other forms of dilated cardiomyopathy.[6,7] Each year, over a million survivors of myocardial infarction face a risk of stroke that is over 5 per cent within the first few weeks for those with large anterior infarcts. In addition, within the even larger population of patients with chronic left ventricular dysfunction, the potential for cerebral emboli is persistent.

Cardioembolic stroke is usually associated with substantial functional disability and yet is often unheralded by warning signs of transient cerebral ischemia. This makes a preventive strategy for defined high-risk groups the only sensible clinical approach. The additional incidence of subclinical "silent" strokes is not known, and this mechanism may take an uncounted toll on cognitive function, perhaps contributing to the problem of multi-infarct dementia among the elderly.[4–6]

PATHOGENESIS OF INTRACARDIAC THROMBI

The pathogenesis of intracavitary mural thrombosis may be outlined along the lines established over a century ago by pathologist Rudolph Virchow, who defined a triad of precipitating factors: endothelial injury, a zone of circulatory stasis, and a hypercoagulable state.[8] In addition, the clinical significance derives from the potential for systemic embolism, which also depends upon dynamic forces of the circulation. In the first few days following acute myocardial infarction, leukocytic infiltration separates endothelial cells

215

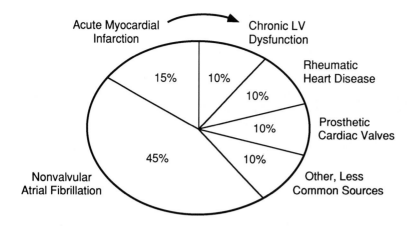

FIGURE 12–1. Sources of cerebral embolism.

from their basal lamina.[9] The resulting exposure of subendothelial tissue to intracavitary blood serves as the nidus for thrombus development. Specific endocardial abnormalities have also been identified histologically in surgical and postmortem specimens from patients with left ventricular aneurysms,[9] and at necropsy in patients with idiopathic dilated cardiomyopathy.[10]

Experimental[12] as well as clinical studies[13,14] have emphasized the importance of wall-motion abnormalities in the development of left ventricular mural thrombi, and it seems clear that stasis of blood in regions of akinesia or dyskinesia is the essential factor. Similarly, stasis is important in the development of atrial thrombi[15] when effective mechanical atrial activity is impaired, as occurs in atrial fibrillation, atrial enlargement, mitral stenosis, and cardiac failure. Stasis is tantamount to conditions of low shear rate, and activation of the coagulation system plays the predominant pathogenetic role in the development of intracavitary thrombi. One study of patients with acute myocardial infarction found a significantly greater incidence of thromboembolism in cases of elevated serum fibrinogen levels,[16] and similar findings have been reported among patients with chronic atrial fibrillation,[17] suggesting a hypercoagulable tendency in this condition. Although this limb of Virchow's triad remains controversial, it is conceivable that a systemic procoagulant tendency arises during the acute stage of myocardial infarction and predisposes to thromboembolic events. More relevant is experimental evidence which suggests that the surface of a fresh thrombus is itself highly thrombogenic, producing at least a local (if not a systemic) hypercoagulable

state,[18] and this may be heightened in the milieu of endocardial injury.

Both platelet activation and activation of the coagulation cascade leading to fibrin deposition have been implicated in the process of intravascular thrombus formation. During the process of mural thrombosis in the cardiac chambers, fibrin and thrombin accumulate to a greater degree, and thrombin is even more powerful than collagen as an activator of platelet aggregation. Since platelets and the coagulation system are closely interrelated in the genesis of left ventricular mural thrombosis, a potential role exists for both platelet inhibitor and anticoagulant medication for the prevention of these thrombi and the embolic phenomena they can produce.

MECHANISMS RESPONSIBLE FOR EMBOLISM

The problems of thromboembolism originating from the cardiac chambers prompt consideration of the balance between the effects of regional injury, stasis, and procoagulant factors, all of which favor thrombus formation, and dynamic forces of the circulation, which are responsible for the migration of thrombotic material into the systemic circulation. In patients with atrial fibrillation, thrombi are most frequently detected at postmortem examination in the left atrial appendage. Just as in cases of left ventricular aneurysm, stasis favors thrombus formation within this circulatory cul-de-sac, but isolation from dynamic circulatory forces protects against embolic migration.[7,19] In diffusely dilated cardiomyopathy, however, mural thrombus is not isolated from the circulation, and the embolic risk is higher.[20] Thus, factors leading to thrombus formation are not the same as those which produce systemic embolism, and this paradox must not be neglected in the selection of therapeutic options.

CLINICAL STRATIFICATION OF THROMBOEMBOLIC RISK

Atrial Fibrillation

RHEUMATIC VALVULAR HEART DISEASE

Some patients with atrial fibrillation—those, for example, with rheumatic valvular heart disease or prosthetic heart valves—face a particular danger of stroke and systemic embolism. These patients carry at least an 8 to 10 per cent per year risk of ischemic thromboembolic events, at least ten times that of patients in normal sinus rhythm in the Framingham Heart Study,[21] and enough to justify in the minds of most clinicians the hemorrhagic risks associated with maintenance anticoagulant therapy with an agent such as warfarin, even in the absence of randomized trials.[22]

RECENT THROMBOEMBOLISM

Among those with nonvalvular atrial fibrillation, the risk appears greatest when stroke or systemic embolism has occurred within the previous two years—in such cases the risk of recurrent stroke is even greater than 10 per cent per year.[23–25] The mechanism responsible for this incremental risk is not clear, but may be related either to the potential for the surface of freshly formed thrombus to stimulate additional coagulation,[7,16] or to the association of other clinical factors, such as hypertension or atherosclerotic vascular disease, which may contribute to ischemic events in these patients.

THYROTOXICOSIS

Several reports have suggested that patients with atrial fibrillation in the setting of thyrotoxicosis, often associated with decompensated congestive heart failure, are also at particularly high risk (averaging 14 per cent over varying periods of observation),[26–28] though the exact mechanism underlying this enhanced embolic potential is not clear.[28–30] The notion of increased thromboembolic risk in thyrotoxic atrial fibrillation has been challenged on the basis of comparison between these patients and those with thyrotoxicosis in sinus rhythm; a logistic regression analysis found only age an independent predictor of cerebral ischemic events.[30] In that study, however, 13 per cent of patients with atrial fibrillation had ischemic cerebrovascular events (6.4 per cent per year), compared with 3 per cent of those with normal sinus rhythm (1.7 per cent per year). When transient ischemic attacks are discounted, the increased risk of stroke in patients with atrial fibrillation did reach statistical significance ($p = 0.03$).[30] It remains controversial whether patients with atrial fibrillation associated with thyrotoxicosis are at higher risk of thromboembolic cerebrovascular events than those in whom this dysrhythmia accompanies other forms of organic heart disease,[31] but consensus has emerged that thyrotoxic patients with atrial fibrillation should be treated with anticoagulant medication unless a contraindication to such therapy stands in the way, at least until an euthyroid state has been restored and congestive heart failure has been corrected.

LONE ATRIAL FIBRILLATION

On the other end of the spectrum of risk are patients younger than 60 years of age with "lone" atrial fibrillation in the absence of clinical history, symptoms, signs, or echocardiographic evidence of associated cardiopulmonary disease. These patients represented between 2.7 and 11.4 per cent of cases of atrial fibrillation in the Framingham Heart Study.[32] Kopecki reported the findings of a cohort study involving 99 such patients extending over nearly 15 years in Olmstead County, Minnesota, in which the incidence of stroke was 0.4 per cent per year and the mortality rate was 0.1 per cent per year, not significantly greater than rates in patients with normal sinus rhythm.[33] Since lone atrial fibrillation is associated with such a low risk of stroke, it appears that the rhythm disturbance itself is not the cause of stroke, but rather represents a marker of associated cardiovascular pathology, which is the true source of cerebral ischemia. Older age, hypertension, and congestive heart failure are among the factors which substantially increase the stroke risk in the presence of atrial fibrillation.[32]

NONVALVULAR ATRIAL FIBRILLATION WITH CARDIAC DISEASE

Between these extremes are a large number of patients with nonvalvular atrial fibrillation at intermediate risk of thromboembolism, which appears, based upon both older epidemiologic data and more recently available results of randomized trials, to average about 5 per cent per year. The range of risk is relatively wide (at least 3 per cent and perhaps more than 8 per cent per year), reflecting the clinical diversity of this patient population, and partially accounting for the controversy about anticoagulant therapy, particularly when this is contemplated for an extended period of time. It has long been suspected that within this broad range of patients with atrial fibrillation, subgroups at relatively greater or lesser risk might be defined on the basis of clinical or echocardiographic features. Duration since the onset of atrial fibrillation, for example, has been suspected to relate to embolic risk.[34] Differences in rates of thromboembolic events have also been cited on the basis of the constant or paroxysmal character of atrial fibrillation,[35] and the presence or absence of hypertension, congestive heart failure, or mitral regurgitation.[4] Enlargement of the left atrium, seemingly a correlate of stasis within the atrial appendage, has not been validated as a particular marker of stroke risk,[36–38] but recent studies have supported the view that associated left ventricular dysfunction may contribute an important element of risk.[20,39]

Left Ventricular Dysfunction

In patients with very localized forms of chronic left ventricular dysfunction following ventricular aneurysm formation beyond three months after myocardial infarction, thrombi can be identified in almost half the cases by echocardiography or other imaging techniques, but the incidence of systemic embolism is substantially lower, no more than one event per 100 patient-years.[40] On the other hand, when left ventricular systolic function is more diffusely reduced as occurs in dilated cardiomyopathy, the risk of cerebral embolism is greater, in the range of 3 to 4 per cent per year.[20] This points again to the balance between the effect of regional circulatory stasis, which favors thrombus formation within the aneurysmal cavity, and the isolation from the dynamic forces of the circulation, which protects against embolic migration. In contrast, protrusion and mobility of the thrombotic mass within the ventricular chamber are associated with much greater embolic potential.[41]

MECHANISMS OF STROKE

The etiologies of ischemic stroke in patients with nonvalvular atrial fibrillation are diverse, ranging from emboli derived from distant stasis-related thrombi in the left atrium or left ventricle, to thrombotic complications of associated cerebrovascular disease.[1,4,39] Abnormal endocardial tissue surfaces including myxomatous or fibrotic mitral valve leaflets, mitral annular dilatation or calcification, damaged chordae tendineae, or other lesions may stimulate platelet aggregation as well as the coagulation system. Alterations in hemostatic function have also been identified in patients with nonvalvular atrial fibrillation whether or not they have sustained prior ischemic stroke. Specifically, higher plasma concentrations of von Willebrand factor, coagulation factor VIIIc, fibrinogen, the fibrinolytic product D-dimer, beta-thromboglobulin, and platelet factor 4, the platelet component released upon platelet adhesion, were found in one study comparing these measurements with those in age- and gender-matched patients with prior stroke and sinus rhythm as well as with healthy control subjects.[42] These biochemical changes may be either a cause or effect of ongoing thrombosis in patients with atrial fibrillation, and their correlation with morphologic evidence of thrombus formation or with clinical thromboembolic risk remains to be established.

Beyond these primary thrombotic mechanisms, coexisting atherosclerotic lesions in the aorta, extracranial, or intracranial arteries may reduce cerebral perfusion by direct obstruction or as a result of thrombus formation provoked by exposure of lipid material and subintimal vascular collagen.[43] The prevalence of atherosclerotic disease of the carotid arteries is twice as great in patients with atrial fibrillation as in age-matched controls,[44] but only one in four patients with atrial fibrillation and stroke has significant carotid disease apparent on ultrasound examination.[45] Clinical estimates of the incidence of cardiogenic embolism as the etiology of stroke in patients with atrial fibrillation vary widely and are difficult to verify, but are generally in excess of 50 per cent.[4,46,47]

Systemic emboli in patients with atrial fibrillation are suspected to originate as thrombi formed within the left atrial cavity or appendage.[14] To the extent that stasis-related thrombi are responsible for ischemic stroke in patients with atrial fibrillation, administration of anticoagulant medication such as warfarin represents a logical preventive approach. The presence of endothelial lesions within the heart or blood vessels which might be a nidus for thrombus formation raises the likelihood of a response to platelet inhibitors such as aspirin.[43] The differential responses to warfarin and aspirin in recent clinical trials of antithrombotic therapy in patients with nonvalvular atrial fibrillation may reflect, in part, the relative predominance of these etiologic properties.

Patients with chronic left ventricular dysfunction often have a history of atherosclerosis, hypertension, or other disorders independently associated with disease of the extracranial or intracranial cerebral vasculature. Ischemic cerebrovascular disease and intracranial hemorrhage account for an uncertain proportion of strokes in patients with potential sources of cardiogenic thromboembolism. In clinical practice, determination of the etiology of any given stroke is often difficult, though certain angiographic features and the appearance of computed tomographic (CT) scans and magnetic resonance images (MRI) may be characteristic. Diagnosis is often based in large measure upon the perceived embolic risk attributed to the nature of coexisting heart disease as well as upon the identification of carotid or vertebrobasilar artery lesions, which may also respond favorably to antithrombotic medication.

Asymptomatic Cerebral Infarction

Clinical stroke in patients with atrial fibrillation is typically associated with substantial acute neurological deficit and often with lasting functional disability. A number of studies have suggested additionally that episodes of cerebral infarction may occur without symptoms. These clinically silent events are usually identified as small subcortical hypodense zones on computerized cerebral tomography, though cortical infarction or large deep areas of infarction have been reported in up to 10 per cent of patients.[48] Histopathologic confirmation of the ischemic nature of these infarcts is lacking, and there is as yet no proof

that they are due to cardiogenic thromboembolism, though this seems a likely etiology. A series of studies in Denmark found minor cerebral infarcts in 48 per cent of 29 patients with chronic atrial fibrillation present for at least one year,[49] but a lower rate among patients with paroxysmal atrial fibrillation.[50] Another study in Japan found the incidence of silent infarction 58 per cent in patients with chronic and 38 per cent with paroxysmal atrial fibrillation.[51] Interpretation of these data is hampered by uncertainty about the prevalence of asymptomatic cerebral infarction in older persons without atrial fibrillation, though the prevalence of evidence of prior silent stroke in acute stroke patients is reportedly 10 to 11 per cent.[52,53]

Extracerebral Systemic Embolism

While at least 75 per cent of symptomatic arterial emboli of cardiac origin involve the central nervous system, other regions of the systemic circulation are not spared, particularly the abdominal viscera and the extremities. Emboli to multiple sites occurs in approximately one fifth of cases of rheumatic heart disease,[54] and a similar pattern is likely in patients with other conditions predisposing to thromboembolism derived from the cardiac chambers.

DETECTION OF INTRACARDIAC THROMBI

Role of Echocardiography

ATRIAL FIBRILLATION

Aside from the identification of mitral stenosis, specific echocardiographic features of patients with atrial fibrillation which predict greater or lesser thromboembolic risk have not been established. Most studies have focused upon the diameter of the left atrium in the anteroposterior dimension, as measured by M-mode echocardiography. Enlargement of the left atrium appears related to thromboembolic risk in patients with prosthetic heart valves,[55] but this relationship has not been confirmed for patients with rheumatic heart disease or nonvalvular atrial fibrillation.[55,56] The left atrium appears to enlarge progressively as the duration and persistence of atrial fibrillation increases.[37,38,57–60] Any relationship between left atrial size and stroke risk in patients with atrial fibrillation may be difficult to interpret in view of a recent report which suggests that left atrial diameter as determined from the M-mode echocardiogram may be an independent predictor of stroke risk among the elderly, even after adjustment for such factors as age, blood pressure, and atrial fibrillation.[61]

Transesophageal echocardiography more frequently identifies potential sources of cerebral embolism in patients with acute brain infarction than transthoracic echocardiography,[62] and this is particularly true for detection of thrombi in the left atrial appendage. This technique also appears more sensitive for detection of spontaneous echo contrast ("smoke sign"), which is associated with circulatory stasis and thrombus formation.[63,64] Atherosclerotic lesions of the proximal aorta are relatively frequently discovered by transesophageal ultrasound imaging, sometimes accompanied by the appearance of mobile echodensities protruding into the aortic lumen—representing potentially additional sources of atheroembolism and thromboembolism.

LEFT VENTRICULAR THROMBI

Two-dimensional echocardiography is the most widely accepted means of detecting left ventricular thrombi, and yet the sensitivity and specificity of this method have not been clearly established. The coefficient of correlation with autopsy series has been reported in the range of 0.85, but these analyses tend to overrepresent larger infarcts and may not apply to thrombi which develop clinically in less catastrophic cases.[13,65] The sensitivity and specificity of echocardiography for detection of left ventricular thrombi are reported to range from 92 to 95 per cent and from 80 to 88 per cent, respectively.[66,67] There is no consensus regarding echocardiographic criteria by which left ventricular mural thrombi may be defined, but those proposed by Asinger are most widely cited.[12] These include detection of an echo-dense mass within the left ventricular cavity on at least two views distinguished from adjacent endocardium in a region of asynergy. The order of resolution with two-dimensional transthoracic echocardiography techniques reflects a mass of thrombus beyond the threshold sufficient to inflict extensive embolic—and usually cerebral—tissue damage.

About one fourth of left ventricular thrombi are identified within the first 24 hours after acute myocardial infarction, 50 per cent are detected within the first two to three days, 75 per cent within the first six days, and the remainder generally appear by the end of two weeks.[18,41,68,69] Early echocardiographic appearance of ventricular intracavitary thrombus is associated with worse prognosis than those which develop later in the course, perhaps owing to the greater extent of myocardial damage in the early cases.[69,70] Protrusion and mobility of the thrombotic mass has been associated with increased embolic risk.[41,71] Spontaneous resolution occurs at a rate of 20 to 30 per cent per year, and this process can be accelerated with anticoagulant therapy.[40,69,71–73]

Spontaneous echo contrast, seen most often in dilated cardiac chambers with reduced blood flow, appears to reflect red cell or platelet aggregation within areas of blood stasis in the ventricular cavity adjacent to a thrombogenic mural surface, and may be an early sign of thrombus development.[74,75] Left ventricular spatial flow patterns identified by Doppler echocardiography exhibit some predictive capacity for thrombus formation,[76,77] but remain abnormal even beyond three months after acute myocardial infarction. Although transesophageal echocardiography is superior to transthoracic imaging for the detection of left atrial thrombi, this technique has not been validated for the diagnosis of left ventricular thrombi.

Other Imaging Techniques

Contrast ventriculography appears to have a lower sensitivity and specificity than echocardiography for the detection of left ventricular mural thrombi, and carries the risk of inducing embolism by mechanical dislodgement of thrombotic material. Indium-111-labeled platelet scintigraphy requires a latency of 48 to 72 hours for detection of intracardiac thrombi and, like "ultra-fast" gated cardiac computed tomography and magnetic resonance imaging, the method has been investigated in a relatively small number of cases.[78] This technique entails a latency of several days before sufficient platelet accumulation occurs on the surface of a ventricular thrombus to permit imaging, but false-positive results appear less frequent than with echocardiographic imaging, and it has been hypothesized that the method may identify thrombotically active masses prone to embolism.[79] The diagnostic accuracy and clinical usefulness of computerized tomography and magnetic resonance imaging for detection of ventricular thrombi in patients with myocardial infarction is emerging, but there has as yet been no satisfactory demonstration of the superiority of these methods for selection of patients requiring more intensive forms of antithrombotic therapy.[80]

ANTITHROMBOTIC THERAPY FOR PREVENTION OF CARDIOGENIC THROMBOEMBOLISM

Atrial Fibrillation

Before the availability of data from recently reported randomized trials, a consensus of the American College of Chest Physicians and the National Heart, Lung and Blood Institute issued a recommendation for long-term anticoagulant therapy aimed at prolonging prothrombin time (PT) to 1.5 to 2.0 times control (standard international normalized ratio of prothrombin suppression [INR] 3.0 to 4.5) in patients with a history of systemic embolism in the previous two years.[22,23] Other patients at substantial risk of embolism are those with atrial fibrillation associated with mitral stenosis or prosthetic heart valves. Data from numerous nonrandomized and uncontrolled trials suggested that anticoagulation reduces the rates of embolism and death in patients with rheumatic valvular disease by 25 per cent.[22] Based on known embolic risk and on results of clinical trials,[22,29] chronic anticoagulation to prolong prothrombin time to 1.3 to 1.5 times control (international normalized ratio 2.0 to 3.0) was recommended for these patients. At the lower end of the spectrum of embolic risk in pa-

tients with atrial fibrillation are those without evidence of associated organic heart disease. The natural history of lone atrial fibrillation suggests that for patients under the age of 60 years with atrial fibrillation but no evidence of organic heart disease, the hazards of chronic anticoagulation outweigh its potential benefits.[33]

In a retrospective study of a less restrictive population of patients with nonvalvular atrial fibrillation at the Montreal Heart Institute, those not given anticoagulant medication had an incidence of systemic embolism of 5.5 per cent per year, whereas anticoagulated patients had a significantly lower embolic rate of 0.7 per cent per year.[81] Until recently, however, there were no data available from randomized trials to balance the benefits of antithrombotic therapy against attendant hemorrhagic risks.

CLINICAL TRIALS OF PROPHYLACTIC ANTITHROMBOTIC MEDICATION

Over the past several years, no fewer than six prospective trials aimed at the primary prevention of stroke and systemic embolism in patients with atrial fibrillation have been undertaken, and results from four have been reported.[82–85] While these share certain features, there are sufficient differences in the demographics of the populations investigated, specific trial designs, and results to leave some issues still in dispute. Salient features of those studies from which results are available are summarized in Tables 12–1, 12–2, and 12–3.

The Copenhagen Atrial Fibrillation-Aspirin-Anticoagulation (AFASAK) study[82] involved 1,007 patients with constant atrial fibrillation randomly assigned to therapy with warfarin (prothrombin time prolonged to an international normalized ratio of 2.8 to 4.2), aspirin (75 milligrams/day), or placebo, followed on treatment a mean of 11 months by

TABLE 12–1. Randomized Trials of Antithrombotic Therapy in Nonvalvular Atrial Fibrillation: Design

	AFASAK[82]	SPAF[83]	BAATAF[84]	CAFA[85]
Input/output	Output	Both	Both	Both
Constant/input	Constant	Both	Both	Both
PTR	1.7	1.5	1.3	1.3
Dose ASA (milligrams/day)	75	325	?	—
Blind	Partial	Partial	No	Yes

PTR = prothrombin time ratio; ASA = acetylsalicylic acid (aspirin).

TABLE 12–2. Randomized Trials of Antithrombotic Therapy in Nonvalvular Atrial Fibrillation: Patient Features

	AFASAK[82]	SPAF[83]	BAATAF[84]	CAFA[85]
Number	1007	1330	420	378
Follow-up (years)	1.2	1.3	2.2	1.3
Age (years)	74	67	68	68
Male (%)	54	71	72	75
CHF (%)	52	19	26	22
Prior MI (%)	8	8	12	13
Hypertension (%)	32	52	51	39
LA diameter (millimeters)	49	46	41	46

CHF = congestive heart failure; MI = myocardial infarction; LA = left atrium.

a single investigator with primary endpoint events including stroke (both ischemic and hemorrhagic), transient cerebral ischemia, and systemic embolism. The mean patient age was 74 years, and the prevalence of congestive heart failure (51 per cent) was greater than in the other trials.[83–85] The proportion of women was more evenly balanced with men than in the other trials, noteworthy because the Framingham Heart Study found no difference in the incidence of atrial fibrillation on the basis of gender. Although 38 per cent of patients assigned to anticoagulant therapy were withdrawn, warfarin seemed protective ($p < 0.05$) while aspirin did not. Of 57 primary events, 25 occurred among those given placebo, 21 in the aspirin group and 11 in those assigned to warfarin, three occurred during periods of subtherapeutic anticoagulation and six after anticoagulant medication was withdrawn (Fig. 12–2).[31] The incidence of events increased with the duration of atrial fibrillation. Only one patient with a primary event had active thyrotoxicosis at the time of enrollment in the study. The dimension of the left atrium, determined by M-mode echocardiography at the time of patient enrollment, did not correlate with thromboembolic risk, but a history of myocardial infarction appeared to represent a significant risk factor for development of a primary event during follow-up for a maximum of two years.[86]

In the United States, the Stroke Prevention in Atrial Fibrillation (SPAF) study[83,87] randomized 1,244 patients with either intermittent (34 per cent) or constant atrial fibrillation who were candidates for anticoagulation (group I) to receive warfarin (international normalized ratio 1.7 to 4.5), aspirin (325 milligram/day,) or placebo, and those ineligible for warfarin (group II) to receive either aspirin or placebo. Only the aspirin and placebo arms were blinded. The mean age in

TABLE 12–3. Randomized Trials of Antithrombotic Therapy in Nonvalvular Atrial Fibrillation: Outcome*

	AFASAK[82]	SPAF[83]	BAATAF[84]	CAFA[85]
Control				
Event rate	6.0	6.3	3.0†	4.6
Warfarin				
Event rate	2.6	2.3	0.4	3.0
Per cent reduction	57	67	86	35
Aspirin				
Event rate	5.0	3.6	—	—
Per cent reduction	17	42		
Control mortality				
(Per cent per year)	6.1	6.5	6.0†	3.3
Warfarin bleeding				
Risk‡		0.8		1.2

* Intention-to-treat analysis.
† Not placebo-controlled; values refer to control group, nearly half of which used aspirin for unspecified periods.
‡ Major hemorrhage, variably defined, but generally implying central nervous system involvement, hospitalization, transfusion, surgery, or death.

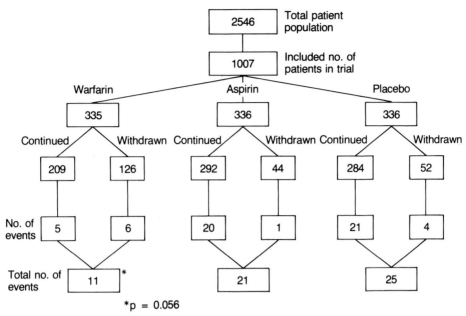

FIGURE 12–2. Intention-to-treat distribution of thromboembolic events in the Copenhagen AFASAK study. (From Peterson P. Thromboembolic complications in atrial fibrillation. Stroke 1990; 21: 4–13, with permission.)

this study was 67 years, and only 10.9 per cent of patients assigned to warfarin were withdrawn. The primary events were ischemic stroke and systemic embolism. Patients were followed a mean of 1.13 years when placebo administration was terminated because the event rate with active therapy (1.6 per cent per year) was less than with placebo (8.3 per cent per year) in group I (risk reduction 81 per cent). An insufficient number of events were observed in the active treatment arms of group I to detect a difference between warfarin and aspirin, and the results with warfarin were not initially reported separately from those in group I assigned to aspirin. Nevertheless, even if all events in group I occurred among patients assigned to one active therapy or the other, the resulting 61-per cent (p = 0.02, 95 per cent confidence interval 17 per cent to 82 per cent) reduction in primary events with the less effective agent would support a beneficial effect of that therapy compared with placebo. Among all 517 patients given aspirin, the rate of primary events was 3.2 per cent per year, compared with 6.3 per cent per year in those given placebo (groups I and II combined; risk reduction 49 per cent; 95 per cent confidence interval 15 to 69 per cent; $p < 0.02$). Aspirin appeared particularly

effective in those 75 years or younger (p = 0.0042), with reduction in risk of stroke or systemic embolism of 65 per cent (95 per cent confidence interval 34 to 81 per cent) for event rates of 2.2 per cent per year in those treated with aspirin and 6.2 per cent per year with placebo. Conversely, the benefit of aspirin seemed to evaporate in patients over the age of 75 years—for the limited number of patients over 75 years (n = 238) the rate of stroke was identical in patients assigned to aspirin and placebo, each 7.4 per cent per year (Fig. 12–3).

In the Boston Area Anticoagulation Trial for Atrial Fibrillation (BAATAF)[84] 420 patients (35 per cent with paroxysmal rather than constant atrial fibrillation) were randomly assigned to warfarin (international normalized ratio 1.5 to 2.7) or control groups. Aspirin was permitted in the control group, and reportedly taken by 46 per cent. Follow-up extended over a mean of 2.2 years, and the primary endpoint event was ischemic stroke. The incidence of stroke was very low in the group given warfarin (0.41 per cent per year) compared with the control group (3.0 per cent per year; risk reduction 86 per cent). The mortality rate was also lower in patients assigned to warfarin (2.3 per cent per year) than to the control group (6.0 per

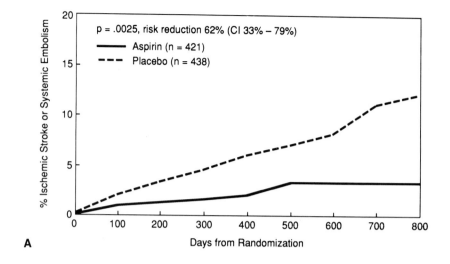

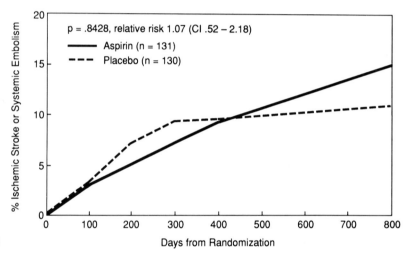

FIGURE 12–3. Ischemic stroke and systemic embolism in relation among patients assigned to aspirin (325 milligrams/day) or placebo in the Stroke Prevention in Atrial Fibrillation (SPAF) study. (A) Patients age 75 years or younger Stroke Prevention in Atrial Fibrillation Study Group Investigators.

cent per year), particularly for death attributed to noncardiac causes. The mean age was 68, and only 10 per cent of warfarin patients stopped therapy. Twenty six per cent of patients had a history of congestive heart failure, and 13 per cent had previously sustained myocardial infarction, with prevalence similar to those in the Stroke Prevention in Atrial Fibrillation study.[83] Mitral annular calcification (present in 30 per cent of patients) and age were significantly related to stroke risk.

The results of the Canadian Atrial Fibrillation Anticoagulation (CAFA) study have been reported only in preliminary form;[85] the trial was terminated before statistically

meaningful endpoints were reached because of convincing results in other trials favoring antithrombotic therapy. Of all the published studies, however, this was the only one to incorporate a double-blind design for administration of warfarin, and as such is of particular value as it avoids potential bias in event detection.

In none of these studies was the incidence of major hemorrhagic complications significantly increased with anticoagulant therapy, even though the average patient age was nearly 70 years (Tables 12–1, 12–2, and 12–3). Taken together, these trials confirm observations in epidemiologic studies that the risk of ischemic stroke in patients with nonvalvular atrial fibrillation is about 5 per cent per year, approximately five to seven times that of the general population of comparable age and gender. Each study provides support for the view that anticoagulation with warfarin is effective in comparatively low intensity (international normalized ratio 1.5 to 4.5) for reducing the risk of stroke in patients with nonvalvular atrial fibrillation by about 3 per cent per year. This benefit offsets the increased risk of bleeding sufficiently severe to require hospitalization, transfusion, or surgery (about 1 to 2 per cent per year). Aspirin is also effective in reducing the incidence of ischemic stroke in patients with atrial fibrillation, but the results of the two studies which included aspirin arms differed on the basis of aspirin dose and patient population. Secondary analysis of data from the Stroke Prevention in Atrial Fibrillation study[83] suggested reduced aspirin efficacy in older patients, which might account, in part, for the minimal beneficial effect of aspirin in the Copenhagen Atrial Fibrillation-Aspirin-Anticoagulation study.[82] The lower incidence of stroke in the control group of the Boston Area Anticoagulation Trial for Atrial Fibrillation study[84] than in the Stroke Prevention in Atrial Fibrillation and Copenhagen Atrial Fibrillation-Aspirin-Anticoagulation studies may be due to the use of aspirin in nearly half the patients.

Because ischemic stroke in patients with atrial fibrillation may involve any of a number of mechanisms, the disparate antithrombotic actions of aspirin (platelet inhibitor) and warfarin (anticoagulant) may prevent strokes of entirely different etiologies. Indeed, the relative efficacy of warfarin and aspirin for prevention of disabling ischemic cerebral events in patients with atrial fibrillation remains an unsettled issue and a priority for continued research. At this point, however, it seems reasonable to conclude that most patients with nonrheumatic cardiac disease associated with atrial fibrillation who can safely tolerate these antithrombotic medications should be given either aspirin or warfarin to prevent stroke and systemic embolism. Aspirin may be slightly less efficacious, particularly in the elderly.

ANTICOAGULATION AT THE TIME OF CARDIOVERSION

The notion that risk of stroke should be greater proximate to chemical or electrical attempts to restore sinus rhythm in patients with atrial fibrillation is fraught with conjecture, particularly since spontaneous termination of episodes of atrial fibrillation among patients in whom fibrillation is paroxysmal is not associated with increased risk.[34] Nevertheless, several reports cite an unexpectedly high incidence of stroke within the first several days following successful electrical reversion to sinus rhythm by direct-current countershock, and suggest that the risk may be lowered by anticoagulant therapy (Table 12–4).[88] It is difficult to interpret these reports, however, because of the relatively high incidence of rheumatic heart disease subtending atrial fibrillation in many of the cases studied. In the largest study, 437 patients with a variety of atrial arrhythmias (58 per cent of whom had underlying rheumatic heart disease) underwent electrical cardioversion procedures with or without anticoagulant medication depending upon the practice of referring physicians. Those receiving anticoagulants had presumed embolic events at a rate of 0.8 incidents per 100 successful conversions, compared with 5.3 per cent in those not anticoagulated ($p = 0.016$), despite greater prevalence of rheumatic heart disease, congestive heart failure, prior embolism, and cardiac enlargement among those receiving anticoagulants.[89,90] Half of the thromboembolic events occurred in patients with nonrheumatic cardiac disorders. This study is mentioned not so much for its implications regarding therapy, which involved long-term rather than short-term anticoagulation, but because it illustrates the limitations imposed by nonrandomized design and other issues.[91]

Undoubtedly, a heightened awareness of danger may contribute to event detection under these circumstances, or patients at greater intrinsic risk of thromboembolism (such as those with left ventricular dysfunction) may more frequently be candidates for cardioversion. Just as there should be no difference in rates of thromboembolism associated with spontaneous, chemical, or electrical means of cardioversion, the risk of stroke at the time of cardioversion is most likely linked with the intrinsic cardiovascular factors which contribute to risk on a chronic basis. More aggressive use of anticoagulant medication may be justified for a period of three to four weeks prior to cardioversion (assumed time for thrombus, if present, to become organized) and another three to four weeks after cardioversion because of the reduced cumulative danger of hemorrhage

TABLE 12–4. Embolic Risk During Cardioversion of Atrial Fibrillation

Trial	Number of Patients	(%) with RHD	Method of Conversion	A/C Therapy	Incidence of Embolism* n	%	Comments
Sokolow (1956)[122]	177	53	Quinidine	In few pts	2	(1.3)	A/C given to pts with prior embolism
Goldman (1960)[123]	400	?	Quinidine	No	6	(1.5)	
Lown (1963)[124]	50	94	Electrical	In some pts	1	(1.7)	A/C given to pts with mitral stenosis
Killip (1963)[125]	62	Most	Electrical	In 45%	0		
Freeman (1963)[126]	100	11	Quinidine	Yes	0		
Rokseth (1963)[127]	274	52	Quinidine	Yes	2	(1.6)	Additional pulmonary embolus occurred
Morris (1964)[128]	70	66	Electrical	In 6%	3	(3.4)	Embolic events in pts not on A/C
Oram (1964)[129]	100	65	Electrical	In some pts	2	(1.9)	A/C used in pts at highest embolic risk
Hurst (1964)[130]	121	27	Electrical	No	2	(1.3)	
Morris (1966)[131]	108	62	Electrical	In some pts	4	(2.5)	Embolic events in pts with RHD on no A/C
Korsgren (1965)[132]	138	58	Electrical	Yes	0		No emboli even in pts with prior embolism
Halmos (1966)[133]	175	80	Electrical	No	1	(0.4)	
Selzer (1966)[134]	189	3	Electrical	No	4	(2.1)	
Lown (1967)[135]	350	70	Electrical	In 29%	3	(0.9)	Embolic events in pts not on A/C
Resnekov (1967)[136]	204	50	Electrical	In some pts	2	(0.6)	Additional embolus in pt post-infarction
Hall (1968)[137]	142	68	Electrical	In 39%	1	(0.8)	Embolic event in pt not on A/C
Radford (1968)[138]	156	56	Electrical	In 17%	0		Only pts with prior emboli received A/C
Aberg (1968)[139]	207	58	Electrical	In most pts	2	(0.7)	Embolus in pt with low A/C dosage
Bjerkelund (1969)[89]	437	58	Electrical	Yes	2	(1.1)	A/C reduced embolic incidence by 86% (p = 0.012)
				No	11	(5.6)	
McCarthy (1969)[140]	149	44	Electrical	In some pts	2	(1.6)	Embolic events in pts not on A/C
Henry (1976)[141]	37	65	Electrical	In some pts	3	(5.6)	Emboli in pts with HCM, despite A/C
Roy (1986)[81]	152	?	Electrical	In 72%	2	(1.3)	Emboli in atrial flutter pts not on A/C

* Calculated per successful cardioversion attempts.
HCM = hypertrophic cardiomyopathy; RHD = rheumatic heart disease; A/C = anticoagulants; pts = patients.

when the intensity of anticoagulation is closely controlled over a relatively short period of time. The need for therapy past cardioversion is based upon the latency of the onset of cerebral ischemic symptoms in some patients, which has been attributed to delayed activation of left atrial contractile function which retards the embolic propulsion of thrombus across the mitral orifice and into the circulation.[92–94]

Left Ventricular Thromboembolism

ACUTE MYOCARDIAL INFARCTION

Epidemiology of Ventricular Thromboembolism. Without antithrombotic therapy, left ventricular mural thrombi develop in 20 per cent of cases of acute myocardial infarction, 40 per cent of anterior infarcts, and 60 per cent of those large anterior infarcts which involve the ventricular apex and produce

TABLE 12–5. Prevalences of Mural Thrombus Formation and Systemic Embolism in Patients With Acute Myocardial Infarction and Chronic Forms of Left Ventricular Dysfunction

DISORDER	MURAL THROMBI (%)	STROKE AND EMBOLISM (EVENTS PER 100 PATIENT-YEARS)
Acute Myocardial Infarction		
All	10–20	1–3
Anterior	30–40	2–6
Large apical	60–70	10–20
Inferior	<5	<1
Chronic Ventricular Aneurysm	50	1
Dilated Cardiomyopathy		
Diffuse	30	3–4
Segmental	15	3

peak serum creatine kinase concentrations greater than 2,000 units/liter in the absence of thrombolytic reperfusion. Autopsy studies after fatal myocardial infarction, representing the largest infarcts, have found the incidence of mural thrombi in the range of 40 to 70 per cent when anticoagulant therapy was not given,[12,13,69,95] but this incidence is substantially reduced, to 22 to 24 per cent by anticoagulant treatment.[96,97] While more than one third of patients with acute anterior myocardial infarction develop left ventricular thrombi, this complication occurs in less than 5 per cent of those with inferior infarction (Table 12–5).[79]

In the setting of acute myocardial infarction, over 90 per cent of ventricular thrombi occur when apical akinesis or hypokinesis enlarges the zone of intraventricular stasis. A propensity to thrombus formation probably begins at the onset of myocardial necrosis, when endocardial inflammation creates a thrombogenic surface.[9] Experimental data also support the view that intervention with antithrombotic medication should be initiated as early as possible in patients at greatest risk.[98] Although thrombi most often develop within the first ten days,[99] the tendency to coagulation along the endocardial surface persists over a period of one to three months, during which the risk of thrombosis remains related to the amount of myocardium damaged.[13]

Stroke attributed to cerebral embolism occurs in 1 to 3 per cent of all patients with acute myocardial infarction, 2 to 6 per cent of those with anterior infarcts, and 10 to 20 per cent of those with the large anteroapical infarcts cited above.[66] Cerebral embolism occurs clinically in about 10 per cent of patients with echocardiographically evident mural thrombi associated with acute myocardial infarction. The incidence of embolism is highest during the period of active thrombus formation in the first one to three months, yet the embolic risk remains substantial even beyond the acute phase in patients with persistent myocardial dysfunction, congestive heart failure, or atrial fibrillation (Table 12–5).

In terms of survival, the significance of echocardiographic detection of mural thrombus in patients with acute myocardial infarction is still controversial. Most studies suggest that prognosis for survival of patients developing left ventricular mural thrombi in the course of acute myocardial infarction is less favorable than for those who do not have this echocardiographic finding.[69,70] This has been attributed to larger infarct size in patients with thrombus development, and the association with anterior rather than inferior infarction site, and it is not clear whether mural thrombus formation constitutes an independent risk factor for mortality.[100]

In one recent study,[101] the prognosis for survival was actually better in patients with evidence of thrombus formation, and the risk of stroke was no greater than in those without thrombi, leading the authors to conclude that such thrombi may offer a protective effect (by preventing myocardial rupture) and that antithrombotic medication may not be needed. Early in-hospital mortality was greater in patients without thrombi than in those in whom thrombi occurred. Nearly half the early deaths occurred within three days of admission, yet detectable thrombotic masses did not usually develop before the sixth day, so patients at highest risk may not have survived long enough for ventricular thrombi to form. Although thrombi remained echocardiographically apparent one year after myocardial infarction in over one third of patients in whom the diagnosis was initially made, and at two years 24 per cent still had evidence of thrombi, no early or late embolic events were identified in these cases. The implied benignity of the echocardiographic finding of left ventricular thrombus formation after myocardial infarction in this

TABLE 12–6. Prevention of Systemic and Pulmonary Embolism by Short-Term Anticoagulation

TRIAL	NUMBER OF PATIENTS	SYSTEMIC EMBOLISM (%)			PULMONARY EMBOLISM (%)		
		AC	Control	Red	AC	Control	Red
MRC[106]	1,427	1.3	3.4	62*	2.2	5.6	61*
BMH[107]	1,136	1.7	2.3	26	3.8	6.1	38
VACT[96]	999	0.8	5.4	85*	2.0	4.8	58*

* Denotes a statistically significant difference ($p < 0.01$).

AC = Anticoagulant group; Red = Reduction; MRC = Medical Research Council Trial; BMH = Bronx Municipal Hospital Study; VACT = Veterans Administration Cooperative Trial.

study may reflect the limited number of cases of large anterior infarction studied.[102]

A considerable body of evidence supports the view that patients in whom left ventricular thrombi are detected echocardiographically early after acute myocardial infarction are at greater risk of systemic arterial embolism.[13,41,68,99,103–105] One study indicates that this risk persists well beyond the acute phase following infarction.[69] Features, visible echocardiographically, which increase the probability of embolism include protrusion and mobility of intracavitary thrombi as determined in multiple views.[41,71,99] A relatively large, prospective assessment[99] found an adjacent zone of hyperkinesis an additional risk factor for systemic embolism which, if validated, would lend additional credence to the

notion that it is the combination of regions of stasis and motion within the cardiac chambers that predispose to thromboembolism.

Prevention of Ventricular Thrombus Formation. Because stasis predominantly activates the coagulation system leading more to fibrin formation than platelet aggregation in the pathogenesis of ventricular thrombi, anticoagulant drugs have long been the principal therapeutic agents. Over the past 20 years, three large trials involving patients with acute inferior and anterior myocardial infarctions concluded that initial treatment with heparin followed by administration of an oral anticoagulant reduced the occurrence of cerebral embolism from 3 per cent to 1 per cent when compared with no anticoagulation (Table 12–6). Differences were statistically

TABLE 12–7. Randomized Trials of Anticoagulant Therapy in Acute Anterior Myocardial Infarction for Prevention of Left Ventricular Thrombosis

STUDY	NUMBER OF PATIENTS	ANTITHROMBOTIC REGIMEN	PATIENTS WITH LEFT VENTRICULAR THROMBI (%)		Results
			Treatment	Control	
Nordrehaug[108]	53	IV heparin (400 units/kilogram/day) followed by warfarin versus placebo	0	26	Positive ($p < 0.01$)
Davis[109]	52	IV heparin (1,000 units/hour) followed by warfarin versus low-dose A/C	56	56	Negative
Gueret[110]	46	IV heparin (1,000 units/hour) followed by SQ heparin versus no A/C	38	52	No significant difference
Arvan[111]	30	IV heparin (1,000–3,000 units/hour) followed by warfarin versus no A/C	31	35	Negative
Turpie[112]	183	High-dose SQ heparin (12,500 units) versus low-dose (5,000 units) every 12 hours	11	32	Positive ($p = 0.0004$)
SCATI[113]	200	SQ heparin (12,500 units) every 12 hours versus no A/C	18	36	Positive ($p < 0.01$)*

* Some patients admitted within six hours of onset of infarction received intravenous streptokinase.

IV = intravenous; SQ = subcutaneous; A/C = anticoagulation.

significant in two of the studies, with a concordant trend in the third.[96,106,107] Within the past decade, six randomized studies involving patients with acute myocardial infarction have addressed the relationship of echocardiographically detected left ventricular thrombi and cerebral embolism (Table 12–7).[106–113] In aggregate, thrombus formation was reduced by more than 50 per cent with anticoagulation; individually, however, each trial had insufficient sample size to detect significant differences in embolism.

Regarding the intensity of anticoagulation for prevention of left ventricular mural thrombus formation in patients with acute myocardial infarction, Turpie et al.[112] described a randomized prospective trial involving 221 patients with acute anterior myocardial infarction who did not receive thrombolytic agents in the acute phase, where subcutaneous administration of calcium heparin in a dose of 12,500 units every 12 hours offered greater benefit for prevention of left ventricular mural thrombi during the first ten days than the lower dosage of 5,000 units every 12 hours conventionally given for prevention of venous thrombosis. Thrombi were detected echocardiographically in 11 per cent of the group given the higher heparin dose, compared with 32 per cent of those receiving the lower dose ($p = 0.0004$). This beneficial effect correlated strongly with plasma heparin activity. The overall incidence of nonhemorrhagic stroke in the early period following infarction was just under 1 per cent in those initially treated with high-dose heparin, and close to 4 per cent in the low-dose group ($p = 0.17$), but insufficient event rates may have been the reason there was no significant difference in embolic complications. Hemorrhagic complications were equally frequent in both treatment groups in this study.

In the SCATI (Studio sulla Calciparina nell'Angina e nella Trombosi Ventricolare nell'Infarto)[113] randomized trial of 771 patients with acute myocardial infarction, 433 were given the thrombolytic agent streptokinase (1.5 million units over one hour). Half received heparin (12,500 units every 12 hours) and the others no heparin. Of the 235 cases of initial anterior infarction, satisfactory two-dimensional echocardiographic examinations were obtained both early after admission and near the time of discharge in 200. The predischarge echocardiograms showed a significantly lower incidence of left ventricular thrombi in those receiving heparin (18 per cent) than in the control group (37 per cent; $p < 0.01$). The earlier echocardiogram was obtained within 24 hours of admission in 86 per cent of patients, at which time 20 (18 per cent) of those assigned to receive heparin and 13 (14 per cent) of those in the control group showed evidence of thrombi, not a significant difference. Among those free of early echocardiographically manifest thrombi, 6 per cent of those treated with heparin developed thrombi by the time of the predischarge examination, compared with 26 per cent of the controls (relative risk 0.17; 95 per cent confidence interval 0.06 to 0.47; $p < 0.0002$). It is not clear, however, what proportion of these patients were given thrombolytic therapy and whether this intervention affected the rate of development of ventricular thrombi. Stroke occurred in two patients in the control group, and both had echocardiographic evidence of mural thrombi; no strokes were detected in the treated patients. One fatal cerebral hemorrhage occurred in a patient in the heparin group (Fig. 12–4).

Prevention of Embolism with Anticoagu-

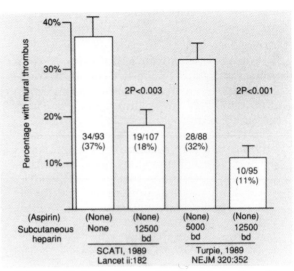

FIGURE 12–4. Incidence of left ventricular thrombi detected by echocardiography in patients with acute myocardial infarction, and effect of therapy with heparin.

lation. Several small and nonrandomized studies[13,72,103,104] explored the impact of anticoagulant therapy to prevent systemic embolism in patients with mural thrombi complicating acute myocardial infarction. Although hampered by limited sample size, and ultimately inconclusive, the outcomes generally favored anticoagulant treatment.

It is clear from these studies that early administration of medium-dose intravenous or high-dose subcutaneous heparin is effective in reducing the incidence of left ventricular thrombus formation, detected echocardiographically, in patients with acute anterior myocardial infarction. It is less clear whether this form of therapy will reduce the occurrence of systemic arterial embolism, since the rate of such events has been too small in these studies to detect any effect of anticoagulant treatment. Administration of heparin is generally begun immediately after the onset of infarction and continues for a period of about ten days. It is not appropriate to await the results of echocardiographic examination before instituting antithrombotic therapy, as treatment is most effective when given as early as possible in the course of acute infarction, and delay may result in reduced efficacy. Furthermore, echocardiography within the first 24 hours after the onset of infarction may fail to detect early thrombus formation,[70] and later studies may detect thrombi too late to avoid embolic complications.

In some patients—those, for example, with ventricular mural thrombi identified by echocardiography or large akinetic regions—heparin therapy may be followed by warfarin. Therapy with warfarin is associated with resolution of echocardiographic features of left ventricular thrombi following myocardial infarction in the majority of cases, and the oral anticoagulant is usually stopped after one to three months unless the risk of thromboembolism remains elevated as a result of heart failure, impaired left ventricular function, or persistent echocardiographic evidence of mural thrombi.

Thrombolytic Therapy and Prevention of Ventricular Thrombi. It is uncertain whether thrombolytic therapy will reduce the likelihood of developing ventricular thrombi. Information from available studies are conflicting, either because of reduced infarct size or concomitant use of anticoagulant medication. Related to this issue is whether short-term anticoagulation designed to prevent

acute coronary reocclusion following thrombolytic therapy is sufficient to maintain prophylaxis against the later development of mural thrombi and cerebral embolism, when the reduction of infarct size is also considered. The impact of thrombolytic therapy was addressed by Natarajan et al.,[114] who described a study of 45 patients with acute myocardial infarction evolving mean serum creatine kinase concentrations of about 1,000 units, half of whom were given streptokinase and half given no antithrombotic therapy. Echocardiography was performed between the seventh and tenth days, finding apical wall-motion abnormalities in all the cases. In 44 per cent of the control group there was evidence of thrombus formation, a surprisingly high prevalence given the modest enzyme levels, but none were found in those given the thrombolytic agent. In the considerably larger Thrombolysis in Myocardial Infarction (TIMI) study,[115] echocardiography was performed 48 to 72 hours after hospitalization in 96 patients with acute myocardial infarction, 43 of whom had received tissue plasminogen activator, 22 streptokinase, and 31 no thrombolytic agents; all were treated with subcutaneous heparin (5,000 units every 12 hours). Infarcts were anterior in about 45 per cent of the cases, and peak serum creatine kinase activity averaged 2,683 units in those given no thrombolytic agents. Left ventricular thrombi were identified in 33 per cent of anterior infarcts as compared with only 4 per cent of inferior infarcts, and rates of thrombus formation were approximately 30 per cent lower in patients who were given lytic therapy than in those who were not. Thrombi were present in 19 per cent of those given tissue plasminogen activator, 5 per cent of patients receiving streptokinase, and 23 per cent of those given no thrombolytic agents; these did not represent statistically significant differences. No emboli were detected in the entire series. Earlier investigators[114] had found decreased left ventricular thrombi with streptokinase, but left ventricular thrombi in that study were detected at a rate of 70 per cent, and ejection fractions were lower. It may turn out, therefore, that left ventricular thrombi relate more to residual systolic myocardial function than to thrombolytic status. Finally, the apparently decreased incidence of ventricular thromboembolism may be mainly a consequence of adjunctive antithrombotic therapy rather than the thrombolytic agents themselves;

however, the recent GISSI 2 study suggests benefit with the lytic agents themselves.[114a]

Platelet Inhibitors for Prevention of Thromboembolism. No trial of sufficient size has yet been reported to establish the role of platelet inhibitor therapy for prevention of left ventricular thrombus formation following acute myocardial infarction. Kouvaris et al.[73] randomly assigned 60 patients to an oral anticoagulant regimen (prothrombin time ratio 1.6 to 2.0), aspirin (650 milligrams/day), or no antithrombotic medication. After 16 months of observation, reduction in size or resolution of echocardiographically manifest thrombi occurred in 15 per cent on patients given the anticoagulant, 13 per cent of those given aspirin, and only 4 per cent of those in the control group ($p < 0.04$). Once again, the size of the population studied was inadequate to produce firm conclusions, but the results support the use of some form of antithrombotic therapy over none at all. In the Second International Study of Infarct Survival (ISIS-2)[116] of 17,187 patients, use of aspirin (160 milligrams/day) reduced brain events. A meta-analysis[117] of individual small studies supports mainly the effectiveness of anticoagulant medication (odds ratios 0.32 with anticoagulant therapy, 0.65 with thrombolytic therapy, and 1.43 with platelet inhibitor therapy compared with respective control groups).

VENTRICULAR DYSFUNCTION FOLLOWING MYOCARDIAL INFARCTION

Quantifying the persistent risk of thromboembolic events in those who survive myocardial infarction with chronic left ventricular dysfunction is one of the most vexing problems facing physicians caring for these patients. For the majority of patients with long-standing ventricular dysfunction related to either dilated cardiomyopathy or coronary disease, there is the need to determine the optimum type and dosage of antithrombotic medication through well-designed prospective clinical trials. The exact roles of echocardiography and other imaging technology as means for selecting patients at high risk of embolic complications for prophylactic treatment are only beginning to unfold.[68,71] Beyond the problem of left ventricular thromboembolism, patients with postinfarctional ventricular dysfunction present a complex situation in which antithrombotic therapy may have implications for prevention of future coronary events. The best approach to prevention of both left ventricular thrombi and complications of underlying coronary atherosclerotic disease are as yet unsettled. As the use of aspirin in patients with acute and chronic forms of ischemic heart disease may increase the risk of bleeding in patients given anticoagulants in conventional doses, physicians face a dilemma: aspirin may be recommended with the intent of preventing coronary complications, but this may not be effective in avoiding cardiogenic embolism.

The Warfarin Reinfarction Study (WARIS)[119] examined the response to warfarin in comparison with placebo among 1,214 survivors of initial myocardial infarction age 75 years or younger followed for a mean of 37 months. In this double-blind, placebo-controlled trial, mortality was reduced 24 per cent ($p = 0.027$) with sustained anticoagulation in the range of 2.8 to 4.8 international normalized ratio (approximate North American prothrombin time ratio 1.5 to 2.0), and the incidence of recurrent infarction was reduced 43 per cent ($p = 0.0001$). The rate of occurrence of stroke was also significantly reduced (61 per cent), from 41 events among patients assigned to placebo to 16 in those assigned to receive warfarin ($p = 0.0001$). Studies were not performed to detect left ventricular mural thrombi; there was no attempt to determine stroke mechanism, and many of these events may have been related to hemorrhage or atherothrombotic phenomena rather than to cardiogenic embolism. Aspirin was not employed in either anticoagulated patients or in those receiving placebo, and the comparative safety and efficacy of platelet inhibitor therapy over the long term following acute myocardial infarction has not yet been evaluated in a trial of sufficient scope. Nevertheless, the value of anticoagulant therapy for prevention of recurrent coronary events, coupled with its effectiveness for prevention of mural thrombosis and probable efficacy for prevention of systemic embolism, would make this form of therapy an appealing option for survivors of acute myocardial infarction were it not for the inconvenience of prothrombin time monitoring. Nevertheless, there is rising interest in the potential use of lower intensity anticoagulant therapy alone or in combination and combinations of an anticoagulant with platelet inhibitory agents such as aspirin. These alternatives as yet remain untested in properly designed clinical trials.

CHRONIC LEFT VENTRICULAR ANEURYSM

In the chronic phase after myocardial infarction, left ventricular mural thrombi may persist or form anew within the cavity of a dyskinetic ventricular aneurysm. In contrast to the prevalence of embolism in acute myocardial infarction, the incidence of embolism in chronic left ventricular aneurysm is significantly lower (0.35 per cent per year).[20] The reason for this difference is probably twofold. First, thrombi formed early after acute infarction are usually mobile, friable, and protrude into the ventricular cavity, whereas thrombi in chronic aneurysms are laminated and more adherent to the endocardium. Second, thrombi located within an aneurysmal sac, which is devoid of contractile fibers, are less prone to propulsion into the ventricular outflow tract. Although some investigators have found a persistent risk of embolism in postinfarction patients,[71] it was not the presence of an aneurysm but rather the mobility and protrusion of thrombus which predicted embolic events. Patients with remote infarction and chronic left ventricular aneurysm therefore appear at lower risk of embolism than patients whose thrombi develop in the setting of acute myocardial infarction. Even within this subset, however, the question of whether anticoagulants should be given to patients with echocardiographic evidence of mobile or protruding thrombi, remains unanswered.

DILATED CARDIOMYOPATHY

Postmortem[120] and echocardiographic[121] studies have found a high prevalence of right and left ventricular mural thrombi in patients with idiopathic dilated cardiomyopathy (over 50 per cent and 36 per cent, respectively). Blood stasis and low shear rate present in a dilated, hypocontractile ventricle lead to activation of coagulation processes. Since the mural thrombus is not mechanically isolated, as occurs in a ventricular aneurysm, embolism of thrombotic material may occur. In one retrospective study, patients treated with anticoagulants had no evidence of systemic embolism, whereas those not anticoagulated had an embolic rate of 3.5 per cent per year.[20] In the absence of a prospective trial of antithrombotic therapy in patients with idiopathic dilated cardiomyopathy, this evidence supports chronic warfarin administration, particularly in those with overt heart failure or atrial fibrillation. As mentioned for cases of chronic dilated cardiomyopathy associated with advanced coronary atherosclerotic heart disease remote from acute myocardial infarction, there are no studies upon which to base a decision regarding the use of anticoagulant medication over a platelet inhibitor such as aspirin, for the purpose of preventing either systemic embolism or mortality related to a recurrent ischemic event.

CONCLUSIONS

Within the cardiac chambers, stasis of blood flow causes coagulation to predominate over platelet activation as the principal mechanism of thrombus formation, and anticoagulant therapy alone seems most appropriate in management of these patients. At highest risk are patients with atrial fibrillation and prior embolism; at somewhat lower but yet substantial risk are those with mitral stenosis or prosthetic heart valves. Patients at medium risk are those immediately following large anterior myocardial infarction and uncompensated dilated cardiomyopathy. For these groups, there is sufficient evidence to indicate chronic anticoagulation. Some patients with nonvalvulopathic atrial fibrillation also benefit from warfarin therapy, but subgroups within this population have not yet been sufficiently defined. At lowest risk are patients under the age of 60 years who have "lone" atrial fibrillation without overt heart disease and those with chronic left ventricular aneurysm, who do not require anticoagulants.

Atrial fibrillation is now recognized as a major risk factor for the development of ischemic stroke, particularly among elderly patients. But the rhythm disturbance represents a marker of associated cardiovascular pathology which may be more directly at the root of many cases of stroke than atrioembolic mechanisms alone. The effectiveness and relative safety of chronic anticoagulant therapy with warfarin has now been validated in three separate clinical trials, supporting a thrombotic mechanism for most of the strokes which occur in patients with nonvalvular atrial fibrillation; the success of therapy with aspirin in younger individuals in one of the studies suggests that administration of this platelet inhibitor may be sufficient for some patients with nonvalvular atrial fibrillation.

Goals for the future include collaborative analysis by investigators involved with ongoing and recently completed trials to further stratify patients in terms of the relative risk of stroke based upon the etiology of the dysrhythmia and associated clinical conditions. Such an effort would greatly enlarge the available data pool, allowing inferences about the optimal therapeutic range for warfarin anticoagulation and selection of some patients for alternative therapy with aspirin. A longer-range view includes the development and testing of even more effective strategies of antithrombotic therapy. For the moment, however, physicians are faced with the challenge of identifying patients with atrial fibrillation who might benefit from antithrombotic therapy and to supervise treatment closely to avoid both the scourges of hemorrhage and stroke.

The best approach to prevention of embolism in patients with acute myocardial infarction cannot yet be defined on the basis of sound data, but it seems reasonable to administer heparin to those with large anterior infarcts during the early phase. Among the many questions left unanswered is whether to regularly perform investigations like echocardiography to detect left ventricular thrombi. Another question is how long to continue prophylactic anticoagulant medication in patients without thrombus formation and when to withdraw anticoagulant medication when thrombus is identified—at the time of the patient's discharge from hospital or after three months. A third issue is whether thrombolytic therapy will reduce the likelihood of developing ventricular thrombi in the first place. Then there is the problem of quantifying the persistent risk of thromboembolic events in those who survive myocardial infarction with chronic left ventricular dysfunction.

In addition to addressing the problem of left ventricular thromboembolism, antithrombotic therapy may have implications for prevention of future coronary events in patients with myocardial infarction. The best approach to prevention of left ventricular thrombi and complications of underlying coronary atherosclerotic disease remains to be defined on the basis of a prospective clinical trial, which might not only compare the safety and efficacy of aspirin and warfarin, but consider as well the potential advantages of a combination of low doses of both forms of antithrombotic medication.

REFERENCES

1. Cerebral Embolism Task Force. Cardiogenic brain embolism. Arch Neurol 1986; 43: 71–84.
2. Cerebral Embolism Task Force. Cardiogenic brain embolism: the second report of the Cerebral Embolism Task Force. Arch Neurol 1989; 46: 727–43.
3. Kannel WB, Abbott RD, Savage DD, McNamara PM. Epidemiologic features of chronic atrial fibrillation: the Framingham Study. N Engl J Med 1982; 306: 1018–22.
4. Wolf PA, Abbott RD, Kannel WB. Atrial fibrillation: a major contributor to stroke in the elderly: the Framingham Study. Arch Intern Med 1987; 147: 1561–4.
5. Halperin JL, Hart RG. Atrial fibrillation and stroke: new ideas, persisting dilemmas (editorial). Stroke 1988; 19: 937–41.
6. Sherman DG, Dyken ML, Fisher M, Harrison MJG, Hart RG. Cerebral embolism. Chest 1986; 89 (suppl): 82S–98S.
7. Fuster V, Halperin JL. Left ventricular thrombi and cerebral embolism: an emerging approach. N Engl J Med 1989; 320: 392–4.
8. Virchow R. Gesammelte abhandlungen zur wissenschaftlichen medtzin. Frankfurt: Meidinger Sohn & Co, 1856: 219–732.
9. Johnson RC, Crissman RS, Didio LJA. Endocardial alterations in myocardial infarction. Lab Invest 1979; 40: 183–93.
10. Hochman JS, Platia EB, Bulkley BH. Endocardial abnormalities in left ventricular aneurysms: a clinicopathologic study. Ann Intern Med 1984; 100: 29–35.
11. Roberts WC, Siegel RJ, McManus BM. Idiopathic dilated cardiomyopathy: analysis of 152 necropsy patients. Am J Cardiol 1987; 60: 1340–55.
12. Mikell FL, Asinger RW, Elsperger KJ, Anderson WR, Hodges M. Regional stasis of blood in the dysfunctional left ventricle: echocardiographic detection and differentiation from early thrombosis. Circulation 1982; 66: 755–63.
13. Asinger RW, Mikell FL, Elsperger J, Hodges M. Incidence of left ventricular thrombosis after acute transmural myocardial infarction: serial evaluation by two-dimensional echocardiography. N Engl J Med 1981; 305: 297–302.
14. Weinrich DJ, Burke JF, Pauletto FJ. Left ventricular mural thrombi complicating acute myocardial infarction: long term follow-up with serial echocardiography. Ann Intern Med 1984; 100: 789–94.
15. Shresta NK, Moreno FL, Narciso FV, Torres L, Calleja HB. Two-dimensional echocardiographic diagnosis of left atrial thrombus in rheumatic heart disease: a clinicopathologic study. Circulation 1983; 67: 341–7.
16. Fulton RM, Duckett K. Plasma-fibrinogen and thromboemboli after myocardial infarction. Lancet 1976; 2: 1161–4.
17. Kumagai K, Fukunami M, Ohmori M, Kitabatake A, Kamada T, Hoki N. Increased intravascular clotting in patients with chronic atrial fibrillation. J Am Coll Cardiol 1990; 16: 377–80.
18. Fuster V, Badimon L, Cohen M, Ambrose JA, Badimon JJ, Chesebro JH. Insights into the pathogenesis of acute ischemic syndromes. Circulation 1988; 77: 1213–20.
19. Cabin HS, Roberts WC. Left ventricular aneurysm, intra-aneurysmal thrombus and systemic embolus in coronary heart disease. Chest 1980; 77: 586–90.
20. Fuster V, Gersh BJ, Giuliani ER, Tajik AJ, Brandenburg RO, Frye RL. The natural history of idiopathic dilated cardiomyopathy. Am J Cardiol 1981; 47: 525–31.
21. Wolf PA, Dawber TR, Thomas HE, Kannel WB. Epidemiologic assessment of chronic atrial fibrillation and risk of stroke: the Framingham Study. Neurology 1978; 28: 973–7.
22. Dunn M, Alexander J, de Silva R, et al. Antithrombotic therapy in atrial fibrillation. Chest 1989; 95(suppl): 118S–127S.

23. Sherman DG, Dyken ML, Fisher M, et al. Antithrombotic therapy for cerebrovascular disorders. Chest 1989; 95(suppl): 140S–155S.

24. Sage JI, Van Uitert RL. Risk of recurrent stroke in patients with atrial fibrillation and nonvalvular heart disease. Stroke 1983; 14: 537–540.

25. Hart RG, Coull BM, Hart PD. Early recurrent embolism associated with nonvalvular atrial fibrillation. Stroke 1983; 14: 688–93.

26. Hurley DM, Hunter AN, Hewett MJ, et al. Atrial fibrillation and arterial embolism in hyperthyroidism. Aust NZ J Med 1981; 11: 391–3.

27. Yuen RWM, Gutteridge DH, Thompson PL, et al. Embolism in thyrotoxic atrial fibrillation. Med J Aust 1979; 1: 630.

28. Staffurth JS, Gibberd MC, Tang Fui SN. Arterial embolism in thyrotoxicosis with atrial fibrillation. Br Med J 1977; 2: 688–90.

29. Bar-Sela S, Ehrenfeld M, Eliakim M. Arterial embolism in thyrotoxicosis with atrial fibrillation. Arch Intern Med 1981; 141: 1191–2.

30. Petersen P, Hansen JM. Stroke in thyrotoxicosis with atrial fibrillation. Stroke 1988; 19: 15–8.

31. Petersen P. Thromboembolic complications in atrial fibrillation. Stroke 1990; 21: 4–13.

32. Brand FN, Abbott RD, Kannel WB, et al. Characteristics and prognosis of lone atrial fibrillation: 30-year follow-up in the Framingham Study. JAMA 1985; 254: 3449–53.

33. Kopecky SL, Gersh BJ, McGoon MD, et al. The natural history of lone atrial fibrillation: a population-based study over three decades. N Engl J Med 1987; 317: 669–74.

34. Wolf PA, Kannel WB, McGee DL, et al. Duration of atrial fibrillation and imminence of stroke: the Framingham Study. Stroke 1983; 14: 664–7.

35. Petersen P, Godtfredsen J. Embolic complications in paroxysmal atrial fibrillation. Stroke 1986; 17: 622–6.

36. Wiener I, Hafner R, Nicolai M, et al. Clinical and echocardiographic correlates of systemic embolism in nonrheumatic atrial fibrillation. Am J Cardiol 1987; 59: 177.

37. Caplan LR, D'Cruz I, Hier DB, et al. Atrial size, atrial fibrillation and stroke. Ann Neurol 1986; 19: 158–61.

38. Tegeler CH, Hart RG. Atrial size, atrial fibrillation and stroke. Ann Neurol 1987; 21: 315–6.

39. Chesebro JH, Fuster V, Halperin JL. Atrial fibrillation—Risk marker for stroke. N Engl J Med 1990; 323: 1556–8.

40. Lapeyre AC, Steele PP, Kazmier FJ, Chesebro JH, Vliestra RE, Fuster V. Systemic embolism in chronic left ventricular aneurysm: incidence and the role of chronic anticoagulation. J Am Coll Cardiol 1985; 6: 534–8.

41. Visser CA, Kan G, Meltzer RS, et al. Embolic potential of left ventricular thrombus after myocardial infarction: a two-dimensional echocardiographic study of 119 patients. J Am Coll Cardiol 1985; 5: 1276–80.

42. Gustafsson C, Blombäck M, Britton M, Hamsten A, Svensson J. Coagulation factors and the increased risk of stroke in nonvalvular atrial fibrillation. Stroke 1990; 21: 47–51.

43. Stein B, Fuster V, Halperin JL, Chesebro JH. Antithrombotic therapy in cardiac disease: an emerging approach based on pathogenesis and risk. Circulation 1989; 80: 1501–13.

44. Tegeler CH. Stroke Prevention in Atrial Fibrillation Study: Carotid Stenosis Study Group: carotid stenosis in atrial fibrillation (abstr). Neurology 1989; 39(suppl): 159.

45. Weinberger J, Rothlauf EB, Materese E, Halperin JL. Noninvasive evaluation of the extracranial carotid arteries in patients with cerebrovascular events and atrial fibrillation. Arch Intern Med 1988; 148: 1785–8.

46. D'Olhaberriague L, Hernandez-Vidal A, Molina L, et al. A prospective study of atrial fibrillation and stroke. Stroke 1989; 20: 1648–52.

47. Bogousslavsky J, van Melle G, Regli F, Kappenberger L. Pathogenesis of anterior circulation stroke in patients with nonvalvular atrial fibrillation: the Lausanne Stroke Registry. Neurology 1990; 40: 1046–50.

48. Feinberg WM, Seeger JF, Carmody RF, Anderson DC, Hart RG, Pearce LA. Epidemiologic features of asymptomatic cerebral infarction in patients with nonvalvular atrial fibrillation. Arch Intern Med 1990; 150: 2340–4.

49. Petersen P, Madsen EB, Brun B, Petersen F, Glydensted

C, Boysen G. Silent cerebral infarction in chronic atrial fibrillation. Stroke 1989; 18: 1098–100.

50. Petersen P, Pedersen F, Johnsen A, et al. Cerebral computed tomography in paroxysmal atrial fibrillation. Acta Neurol Scand 1989; 79: 482–6.

51. Sasaki W, Yanagisawa S, Maki K, Onodera A, Awagi T, Kanazawa T. High incidence of silent small cerebral infarction in patients with atrial fibrillation (abstr). Circulation 1987; 76(suppl IV): 104.

52. Chodosh EH, Foulkes MA, Kase CS, et al. Silent stroke in the NINCDS Stroke Data Bank. Neurology 1988; 38: 1674–9.

53. Kase CS, Wolf PA, Chodosh EH, et al. Prevalence of silent stroke in patients presenting with initial stroke: the Framingham Study. Stroke 1989; 20: 850–2.

54. Coulshed N, Epstein EJ, McKenrick CS, Galloway RW, Walker E. Systemic embolism in mitral valve disease. Br Heart J 1970; 32: 26–34.

55. Burchfiel CM, Hammermeister KE, Krause-Steinrauf H, et al. Left atrial dimension and risk of systemic embolism in patients with a prosthetic heart valve. J Am Coll Cardiol 1990; 15: 32–41.

56. Sherrid MR, Clark RD, Cohn K. Echocardiographic analysis of left atrial size before and after operation in mitral valve disease. Am J Cardiol 1979; 43: 171–8.

57. Moss AJ. Atrial fibrillation and cerebral embolism. Arch Neurol 1984; 41: 707.

58. Presti CF, Asinger RW, Goldman ME. Comparative measurements of the left atrium in patients with constant vs. intermittent nonvalvulopathic atrial fibrillation (abstr). Circulation 1988; 78(suppl II): 600.

59. Ruocco NA, Most AS. Clinical and echocardiographic risk factors for systemic embolization in patients with atrial fibrillation in the absence of mitral stenosis (abstr). J Am Coll Cardiol 1986; 7: 165A.

60. Sanfilippo AJ, Abascal V, Sheehan M, et al. Atrial enlargement as a consequence of atrial fibrillation. Circulation 1990; 82: 792–7.

61. Benjamin EJ, Levy D, Plehn JF, Belanger AJ, D'Agostino RB, Wolf PA. Left atrial size: an independent risk factor for stroke. The Framingham Study (abstr). Circulation 1989; 80(suppl IV): 615.

62. Daniel WG, Angermann C, Engberding, et al. Transesophageal echocardiography in patients with cerebral ischemic events and arterial embolism: a European multicenter study (abstr). Circulation 1989; 80(suppl IV): II–473.

63. Nellessen U, Daniel WG, Matheis G, Oelert H, Depping K, Lichtlen PR. Impending paradoxical embolism from atrial thrombus: correct diagnosis by transesophageal echocardiography and prevention by surgery. J Am Coll Cardiol 1985; 5: 1002–4.

64. Aschenberg W, Schluter M, Kremer P, Schroder E, Siglow V, Bleifeld W. Transesophageal two-dimensional echocardiography for the detection of left atrial appendage thrombus. J Am Coll Cardiol 1986; 7: 163–6.

65. Meltzer RS, Visser CA, Fuster V. Intracardiac thrombi and systemic embolization. Ann Intern Med 1986; 104: 689–98.

66. Visser CA, Kan G, Meltzer RS, Lie KI, Durer D. Long-term follow-up of left ventricular thrombus after acute myocardial infarction: a two-dimensional echocardiographic study in 96 patients. Chest 1984; 86: 532–6.

67. Stratton JR, Lighty GW, Pearlman AS, Ritchie JL. Detection of left ventricular thrombus by two-dimensional echocardiography: sensitivity, specificity and causes of uncertainty. Circulation 1982; 66: 156–66.

68. Stratton JR, Resnick AD. Increased embolic risk in patients with left ventricular thrombi. Circulation 1987; 75: 1004–11.

69. Funke Kupper AJ, Verheugt FWA, Peels CH. Left ventricular thrombus incidence and behavior studied by serial two-dimensional echocardiography in acute anterior myocardial infarction: left ventricular wall motion, systemic embolism and oral anticoagulation. J Am Coll Cardiol 1989; 13: 1514–20.

70. Spirito P, Bellotti P, Chiarella F, et al. Prognostic significance and natural history of left ventricular thrombi in patients with acute anterior myocardial infarction: a two-dimensional echocardiographic study. Circulation 1985; 72: 774–80.

71. Stratton JR, Nemanich JW, Johannessen K-A, Resnick AD. Fate of left ventricular thrombi in patients with remote myocardial infarction or idiopathic cardiomyopathy. Circulation 1988; 78: 1388–93.

72. Tramarin R, Pozzoli M, Febo O, et al. Two-dimensional echocardiographic assessment of anticoagulant therapy in left ventricular thrombosis early after acute myocardial infarction. Eur Heart J 1986; 7: 482–92.

73. Kouvaris G, Chronopoulos G, Soufras G, et al. The effects of long-term antithrombotic treatment on left ventricular thrombi in patients after acute myocardial infarction. Am Heart J 1990; 119: 73–8.

74. Mahoney C, Evans JM, Spain C. Spontaneous contrast and circulating platelet aggregates (abstr). Circulation 1989; 80(suppl IV): 1.

75. de Belder MA, Tourikis L, Leech G, Camm AJ. Spontaneous contrast echos are markers of thromboembolic risk in patients with atrial fibrillation (abstr). Circulation 1989; 80(suppl IV): 1.

76. Maze SS, Kotler MN, Parry WR. Flow characteristics in the dilated left ventricle with thrombus: qualitative and quantitative Doppler analysis. J Am Coll Cardiol 1989; 13: 873–81.

77. Delemarre BJ, Visser CA, Bot H, Dunning AJ. Prediction of apical thrombus formation in acute myocardial infarction based on left ventricular spatial flow pattern. J Am Coll Cardiol 1990; 15: 355–60.

78. Ezekowitz MD, Wilson DA, Smith EO, et al. Comparison of indium-111 platelet scintigraphy and two-dimensional echocardiography in the diagnosis of left ventricular thrombi. N Engl J Med 1982; 306: 1509–13.

79. Penny WJ, Chesebro JH, Heras M, Fuster V. Antithrombotic therapy for patients with cardiac disease. Curr Probl Cardiol 1988; 13: 464–9.

80. Sechtem U, Theissen P, Heindel W, et al. Diagnosis of left ventricular thrombi by magnetic resonance imaging and comparison with angiocardiography, computerized tomography and echocardiography. Am J Cardiol 1989; 64: 1195–9.

81. Roy D, Marchand E, Gagne P, Chabot M, Cartier R. Usefulness of anticoagulant therapy in the prevention of embolic complications of atrial fibrillation. Am Heart J 1986; 112: 1039–43.

82. Petersen P, Boysen G, Godtfredsen J, Andersen ED, Andersen B. Placebo controlled, randomised trial of warfarin and aspirin for prevention of thromboembolic complications in atrial fibrillation: the Copenhagen AFASAK study. Lancet 1989; 1: 175–9.

83. Stroke Prevention in Atrial Fibrillation Study Group Investigators. Preliminary report of the Stroke Prevention in Atrial Fibrillation study. N Engl J Med 1990; 322: 863–8.

84. The Boston Area Anticoagulation Trial for Atrial Fibrillation Investigators. The effect of low-dose warfarin on the risk of stroke in patients with nonrheumatic atrial fibrillation. N Engl J Med 1990; 323: 1505–11.

85. Connolly SJ. Canadian atrial fibrillation anticoagulation (CAFA) study (abstr). Circulation 1990; 82(suppl III): 108.

86. Petersen P, Kastrup J, Helweg-Larsen S, Boysen G, Godtfredsen J. Risk factors for thromboembolic complications in chronic atrial fibrillation: the Copenhagen AFASAK study. Arch Intern Med 1990; 150: 819–21.

87. Stroke Prevention in Atrial Fibrillation Investigators. Design of a multi-center randomized trial for the Stroke Prevention in Atrial Fibrillation Study. Stroke 1990; 21: 538–45.

88. Stein B, Halperin JL, Fuster V. Should patients with atrial fibrillation be anticoagulated prior to and chronically following cardioversion? In: Cheitlin MD, ed. Dilemmas in clinical cardiology. Philadelphia: FA Davis Co, 1990: 231–47.

89. Bjerkelund CJ, Orning OM. An evaluation of DC shock treatment of atrial arrhythmias: immediate results and complications in 437 patients, with long term results in the first 290 of these. Acta Med Scand 1968; 184: 481–491.

90. Bjerkelund CJ, Orning OM. The efficacy of anticoagulant therapy in preventing embolism related to DC electrical conversion of atrial fibrillation. Am J Cardiol 1969; 23: 208–16.

91. Mancini GBJ, Goldberger AL. Cardioversion of atrial fib-

rillation: consideration of embolization, anticoagulation, prophylactic pacemaker, and long-term success. Am Heart J 1982; 104: 617–621.

92. Ikram H, Nixon PGF, Arcan T. Left atrial function after electrical conversion to sinus rhythm. Br Heart J 1968; 30: 80.

93. Rowlands DJ, Logan WFWE, Howitt E, et al. Atrial function after cardioversion. Am Heart J 1967; 74: 149–160.

94. Manning WJ, Leeman DE, Gotch PJ, et al. Pulsed Doppler evaluation of atrial mechanical function after electrical cardioversion of atrial fibrillation. J Am Coll Cardiol 1989; 13: 617–623.

95. Kothari AJ, Paczkowski K, Baker KM, et al. Ventricular thrombi in acute myocardial infarction: incidence, complications and effects of anticoagulation (abstr). J Am Coll Cardiol 1984; 3(suppl): 601.

96. Veterans Administration Cooperative Study Investigators. Anticoagulants in acute myocardial infarction: results of a cooperative clinical trial. JAMA 1973; 225: 724–9.

97. Hilden T, Iversen K, Raaschou F, et al. Anticoagulants in acute myocardial infarction. Lancet 1961; 2: 327–31.

98. Solandt DY, Nassim R, Best CH. Production and prevention of cardiac mural thrombosis in dogs. Lancet 1939; 2: 592–5.

99. Jugdutt BI, Sivaram CA, Wortman C, Trudell C, Penner P. Prospective two-dimensional echocardiographic evaluation of left ventricular thrombus and embolism after acute myocardial infarction. J Am Coll Cardiol 1989; 13: 554–64.

100. Stein B, Halperin JL, Fuster V. Prevention of left ventricular mural thrombosis and arterial embolism during and after acute myocardial infarction. Coron Art Dis 1990; 1: 180–9.

101. Nihoyannopoulos P, Smith GC, Maseri A, Foale RA. The natural history of left ventricular thrombus in myocardial infarction: a rationale in support of masterly inactivity. J Am Coll Cardiol 1989; 14: 903–11.

102. Halperin JL, Fuster V. Left ventricular thrombus and stroke after myocardial infarction toward prevention or perplexity? J Am Coll Cardiol 1989; 14: 912–4.

103. Friedman MJ, Carlson K, Marcus FI, Woolfenden JM. Clinical correlations in patients with acute myocardial infarction and left ventricular thrombus detected by two-dimensional echocardiography. Am J Med 1982; 72: 894–8.

104. Keating EC, Gross SA, Schlamowitz RA, et al. Mural thrombi in myocardial infarction: prospective evaluation by two-dimensional echocardiography. Am J Med 1983; 74: 989–95.

105. Haugland JM, Asinger RW, Mikell FL, Elsperger J, Hodges M. Embolic potential of left ventricular thrombus detected by two-dimensional echocardiography. Circulation 1984; 70: 588–98.

106. Working Party on Anticoagulant Therapy in Coronary Thrombosis. Assessment of short term anticoagulant administration after cardiac infarction: report of the Working Party on Anticoagulant Therapy in Coronary Thrombosis to the Medical Research Council. Br Med J 1969; 1: 335–42.

107. Drapkin A, Merskey C. Anticoagulant therapy after acute myocardial infarction: relation of therapeutic benefit to patient's age, sex and severity of infarction. JAMA 1972; 222: 541–8.

108. Nordrehaug JE, Johannessen K-A, von der Lippe G. Usefulness of high-dose anticoagulants in preventing left ventricular thrombus in acute myocardial infarction. Am J Cardiol 1985; 55: 1491–3.

109. Davis MJE, Ireland MA. Effect of early anticoagulation on the frequency of left ventricular thrombi after anterior wall acute myocardial infarction. Am J Cardiol 1986; 57: 1244–7.

110. Gueret P, Dubourg O, Ferrier E, Farcot JC, Rigaud M, Bourdarias JP. Effects of full-dose heparin anticoagulation on the development of left ventricular thrombosis in acute transmural myocardial infarction. J Am Coll Cardiol 1986; 8: 419–26.

111. Arvan S, Boscha K. Prophylactic anticoagulation for left ventricular thrombi after acute myocardial infarction: a prospective randomized trial. Am Heart J 1987; 113: 688–93.

112. Turpie AGG, Robinson JG, Doyle DJ, et al. Comparison of

high-dose with low-dose subcutaneous heparin in the prevention of left ventricular mural thrombosis in patients with acute transmural anterior myocardial infarction. N Engl J Med 1989; 320: 352–357.

113. SCATI (Studio sulla Calciparina nell'Angina nella Trombosi Ventricolare nell'Infarto) Group. Randomised controlled trial of subcutaneous calcium-heparin in acute myocardial infarction. Lancet 1989; 2: 182–6.

114. Natarajan D, Hotchandani RK, Nigam PD. Reduced incidence of left ventricular thrombi with intravenous streptokinase in acute anterior myocardial infarction: prospective evaluation by cross-sectional echocardiography. Int J Cardiol 1988; 20: 201–7.

114a. Vecchio C, Chiarella F, Lupi G, Bellotti P, Domenicucci S. Left-ventricular thrombus in anterior acute myocardial infarction after thrombolysis: a GISSI-2 connected study. Circulation 1991; 84: 512–519.

115. Held AC, Gore JM, Paraskos J, et al. Impact of thrombolytic therapy on left ventricular mural thrombi in acute myocardial infarction. Am J Cardiol 1988; 62: 310–1.

116. ISIS-2 Collaborative Group. Randomized trial of intravenous streptokinase, oral aspirin, both, or neither among 17,187 cases of suspected acute myocardial infarction. Lancet 1988; 2: 349–60.

117. Eigler N, Maurer G, Shah PK. Effect of early systemic thrombolytic therapy on left ventricular mural thrombus formation in acute anterior myocardial infarction. Am J Cardiol 1984; 54: 261–3.

118. Vaitkus PT, Barnathan ES. Do anticoagulants, thrombolytics or antiplatelet agents reduce the incidence of left ventricular thrombus after anterior myocardial infarction? (abstr.) J Am Coll Cardiol 1991; 17(suppl 2): 146A.

119. Smith P, Arnesen H, Holme I. The effect of warfarin on mortality and reinfarction after myocardial infarction. N Engl J Med 1990; 323: 147–52.

120. Roberts EC, Ferrans VJ. Pathological aspects of certain cardiomyopathies. Circ Res 1974; 34/35(suppl II): 128–44.

121. Gottdiener JS, Gay GA, Van Voorhees L, et al. Frequency and embolic potential of left ventricular thrombus in dilated cardiomyopathy: assessment by two-dimensional echocardiography. Am J Cardiol 1983; 52: 1281–5.

122. Sokolow M, Ball RE. Factors influencing conversion of chronic atrial fibrillation with special reference to serum quinidine concentration. Circulation 1956; 14: 568–583.

123. Goldman MJ. The management of chronic atrial fibrillation: indications for and method of conversion to sinus rhythm. Prog Cardiovasc Dis 1960; 2: 465–479.

124. Lown B, Perlroth MG, Kaidbey S, et al. "Cardioversion" of atrial fibrillation. A report on the treatment of 65 episodes in 50 patients. N Engl J Med 1963; 269: 325–331.

125. Killip T. Synchronized DC precordial shock for arrhythmias: safe new technique to establish normal rhythm may be utilized on an elective or an emergency basis. JAMA 1963; 186: 1–7.

126. Freeman I, Wexler J. Anticoagulants for treatment of atrial fibrillation. JAMA 1963; 184: 1007–10.

127. Rokseth R, Storstein O. Quinidine therapy of chronic auricular fibrillation: the occurrence and mechanism of syncope. Arch Intern Med 1963; 111: 184–9.

128. Morris JJ, Kong Y, North WC, et al. Experience with "cardioversion" of atrial fibrillation and flutter. Am J Cardiol 1964; 14: 94–100.

129. Oram S, Davies JPH. Further experience of electrical conversion of atrial fibrillation to sinus rhythm: analysis of 100 patients. Lancet 1964; 1: 1294–1303.

130. Hurst JW, Paulk EA, Proctor HD, et al. Management of patients with atrial fibrillation. Am J Med 1964; 37: 728–741.

131. Morris JJ, Peter RH, McIntosh HD. Electrical conversion of atrial fibrillation: immediate and long-term results and selection of patients. Ann Intern Med 1966; 65: 216–231.

132. Korsgren M, Leskinen E, Peterhoff V, et al. Conversion of atrial arrhythmias with DC shock: primary results and selection of patients. Acta Med Scand 1965; 431(suppl): 1.

133. Halmos PB. Direct current conversion of atrial fibrillation. Br Heart J 1966; 28: 302–8.

134. Selzer A, Kelly JJ, Johnson RB, et al. Immediate and long-term results of electrical conversion of arrhythmias. Prog Cardiovasc Dis 1966; 9: 90–104.

135. Lown B. Electrical reversion of cardiac arrhythmias. Br Heart J 1967; 29: 469.

136. Resnekov L, McDonald L. Complications in 220 patients with cardiac dysrhythmias treated by phased direct current shock, and indications for electroconversion. Br Heart J 1967; 29: 926–936.

137. Hall JI, Wood DR. Factors affecting cardioversion of atrial arrhythmias with special reference to quinidine. Br Heart J 1968; 30: 84–90.

138. Radford MD, Evans DW. Long-term results of DC reversion of atrial fibrillation. Br Heart J 1968; 30: 91–6.

139. Aberg H, Cullhed I. Direct current countershock complications. Acta Med Scand 1968; 183: 415–21.

140. McCarthy C, Varghese OPJ, Barritt DW. Prognosis of atrial arrhythmias treated by electrical countershock therapy: a three-year follow-up. Br Heart J 1969; 31: 496–500.

141. Henry WL, Morganroth J, Pearlman AS, et al. Relation between echocardiographically determined left atrial size and atrial fibrillation. Circulation 1976; 53: 273–9.

13

UNSTABLE ANGINA—ANTITHROMBOTICS AND THROMBOLYTICS

JOHN A. CAIRNS and MARC COHEN

Unstable angina is a common condition intermediate between stable angina and acute myocardial infarction. Recent understandings about the pathophysiology of coronary atherosclerosis, and the role of thrombosis in its acute complications, have led to numerous clinical trials of antiplatelet, anticoagulant, and thrombolytic drugs for this condition. The results have led to profound changes in the management of patients with unstable angina, and to marked improvements of outcome.

DEFINITION

A spectrum of acute symptomatic manifestations of ischemic heart disease lies between the well-defined diagnosis of stable angina on the one hand, and acute myocardial infarction on the other.[1] Although the predominant manifestation of all syndromes falling within this spectrum is that of ischemic cardiac pain, a variety of terms (for example, acute coronary insufficiency, intermediate coronary syndrome, crescendo angina, preinfarction angina) have been employed, focusing on various aspects of the symptoms. The term unstable angina, in use since 1971[2] is the most simple, inclusive, and descriptive that may be applied to this spectrum and is in general use.

Patients with the following syndromes are generally considered to have unstable angina:

1. Angina of recent onset (previous four weeks).

2. Angina with a progressively severe (crescendo) pattern (previous four weeks).

3. Angina of prolonged duration (more than 15 minutes) at rest (includes patients with variant or Prinzmetal's angina).

4. Angina occurring in the early period (four weeks) after myocardial infarction.

Transient ST and T wave changes may occur, but the development of fixed electrocardiographic (ECG) abnormalities or significant myocardial enzyme elevation indicates that myocardial infarction has occurred. The clinical trials of antithrombotic and thrombolytic therapy have generally been conducted amongst hospitalized patients whose symptoms placed them in category 2 or 3. The requirement for electrocardiographic abnormalities accompanying the pain has varied. A new classification for patients with unstable angina has recently been advocated,[3] which may offer some advantages, but the patient populations in clinical trials done to the present can generally be well described using the above categories.

CLINICAL COURSE AND PREVALENCE

The clinical importance of premonitory chest pain as a sign of impending myocardial infarction was recognized in the late 1930s.[4,5] Larger clinical studies published prior to 1970,[6-9] of patients who received no long-acting nitrates, no anticoagulants, and no beta blocking agents, observed that unstable an-

237

gina was followed by acute myocardial infarction in 21 to 80 per cent of cases, and by death in 1 to 60 per cent. With the recognition of the prognosis of these syndromes, the admission of patients to coronary care units, and the use of varying regimens of long-acting nitrates, beta blockers, and anticoagulation, the rate of acute myocardial infarction had fallen to 7 to 15 per cent, and of early sudden death to 1 to 2 per cent by the 1970s.[10,11] Those patients at highest risk of acute myocardial infarction and sudden death were those with prolonged and recurrent rest pain in hospital, and with ST segment abnormalities accompanying the pain. Although the acute event rates had been sharply curtailed by the 1970s, patients continued to experience a high rate of vascular events over the year following hospitalization for unstable angina. Patients in the placebo groups in two large trials of antiplatelet drug therapy received varying combinations of long-acting nitrates, beta blockers, anticoagulants, and calcium antagonists, and yet the first year mortality was 9.6 per cent in one trial (1974 to 1981)[12] and 8.0 per cent in the other (1979 to 1984).[13] The syndromes of unstable angina are common, accounting for at least 25 per cent of admissions to North American coronary care units.[14]

PATHOPHYSIOLOGY

It has long been recognized that most patients with unstable angina have extensive atherosclerotic coronary artery disease. Although a number of investigators have reported that coronary atherosclerosis is more extensive and severe in patients with unstable angina than in those with stable angina, the biases in such studies diminish their value, and the spectrum of fixed atherosclerotic lesions may be no different in patients with unstable angina.[15,16] However, patients with unstable angina are more likely than those with stable angina to have had recent progression of coronary artery disease.

Moise and co-workers[17] studied the progression of coronary artery disease in 38 patients who had undergone coronary angiography for the evaluation of stable angina, and after a mean of 44 months had developed unstable angina, which was investigated with repeat coronary angiography. When these patients were compared to patients with stable angina who had undergone a second

TABLE 13–1. Comparative Progression of Coronary Artery Lesions Among Patients with Unstable Versus Stable Angina*

	PATIENTS WITH UNSTABLE ANGINA	PATIENTS WITH STABLE ANGINA
Progression	29	12
No progression	9	26
Total†	38	38

* Modified from Moise A, et al. Unstable angina and progression of coronary atherosclerosis. N Engl J Med 1983; 309:685–9, with permission.
† $p < 0.0005$.

angiogram for ongoing stable angina after a mean of 35 months, progression of coronary artery disease was found to be much more marked in those with clinical unstable angina (Table 13–1). It has been noted by other workers that patients with unstable angina may have less collateral formation,[18] and those who fail to respond to medical management may have more extensive and severe atherosclerosis.[19,20] Increasingly, it appears that platelets play a role in the pathogenesis of coronary atherosclerosis and its complications. One of the normal functions of platelets is in hemostasis. Vessel injury results in collagen exposure, which stimulates platelet adhesion and aggregation. Eventually the platelets undergo a "release reaction," with extrusion of active mediators of thrombosis from their cytoplasmic granules, leading to the enzymatic liberation of arachidonic acid, the sequential evolution of prostaglandins, and culminating in the synthesis of thromboxane A_2, an extremely potent vasoconstrictor and platelet aggregant. An irreversible stage of platelet aggregation is reached, which may be followed by the incorporation of fibrin and red blood cells to form a red thrombus.

The atherosclerotic plaque may have its origins in a minimal endothelial injury leading to platelet activation, release of a mitogenic factor that stimulates smooth muscle migration from media to subintima, and subsequent accumulation of lipids[21] (see Chapter 3). The atherosclerotic plaque may become complicated as a result of more marked endothelial injury (particularly atherosclerotic plaque fracture) with the activation of platelets, which release thromboxane A_2 and other mediators, and the sequence may culminate in intraluminal thrombosis.

The observation of Moise,[17] that progression of coronary atherosclerotic stenosis is a common feature of patients with unstable angina, was confirmed by Ambrose.[22] In addition, careful analysis of the morphology of these stenoses indicated that 71 per cent of patients with unstable angina with progression of their coronary lesion to less than complete occlusion, had an eccentric stenosis, and very often the lesion was characterized by "a narrow neck due to one or more overhanging edges or irregular, scalloped borders, or both," the so-called Ambrose type II lesion.[22] It is very likely this is the angiographic appearance of a disrupted atherosclerotic plaque, a partially lysed thrombus, or both. Sherman et al.[23] reported their observations from coronary angioscopy performed during coronary artery bypass surgery in ten patients with unstable angina and ten patients with stable angina. Of the 17 arteries examined in the patients with stable angina, all had partially obstructive atheromas with a smooth surface free of hemorrhage, ulceration, or thrombus. Of the three patients with accelerated angina, all had a complex plaque characterized by ulceration and subendothelial hemorrhage, but no intraluminal thrombus. Of the seven patients with rest angina, all had either a partial or totally occlusive thrombus. The preceding angiography was quite insensitive for the detection of complex plaque and intraluminal thrombosis. A number of reports of the angiographic anatomy of patients with unstable angina have shown considerable variation in the frequency of thrombosis.[24,25] However, the incidence is highest among those patients who undergo angiography within hours of the most recent episode of chest pain, suggesting that spontaneous lysis may have accounted for the relatively low incidence in earlier studies.

In the setting of acute myocardial infarction, the landmark study of DeWood,[26] demonstrating that occlusive coronary thrombosis is an early and important event in more than 80 per cent of transmural infarcts has been confirmed among thousands of patients undergoing angiography in the early hours of acute myocardial infarction. Falk[27] has shown that patients experiencing sudden death preceded by serial episodes of unstable angina, may be shown at autopsy to have an occlusive thrombus composed of layers of platelet thrombi in different stages of organization, corresponding to the clinical episodes of ischemia. Platelet emboli distal to

TABLE 13–2. Presence of Acute Coronary Artery Lesions at Autopsy Among Patients with Cardiac Sudden Death (Test) and Noncardiac Sudden Death (Control)*

	TEST	CONTROL
	Number (%)	Number (%)
Acute lesion	95 (95)	8 (10)
Intraluminal thrombus	74 (74)	0
Intraintimal thrombus with plaque fissure	19 (19)	3 (4)
Intraintimal thrombus only	2 (2)	5 (6)
No acute lesion	5 (5)	70 (90)
Totals	100 (100)	78 (100)

* Modified from Davies MJ, Thomas A. Thrombosis and acute coronary artery lesions in sudden cardiac ischemic death. N Engl J Med 1984; 310:1137–40, with permission.

the site of the occlusive thrombosis have also been observed.[27,28] Davies and Thomas[29] have reported that coronary thrombosis, or plaque injury, or both may be demonstrated in 95 per cent of sudden death victims (Table 13–2). Hence, a pathophysiologic sequence of atherosclerotic plaque disruption, platelet activation, and partial or complete thrombotic coronary occlusion appear to underlie the development of the clinical syndromes of unstable angina and their complications of acute myocardial infarction and sudden death.

Recurrent episodes of pain at rest characterize the symptoms of many patients with unstable angina, and in some instances increased myocardial oxygen demand may underlie such pain patterns.[30] However, as a result of the work of Maseri and colleagues,[15] it is recognized that transient increases in coronary artery tone, usually in the region of an atherosclerotic plaque, likely account for many episodes of angina at rest. In a series of interrelated studies, these investigators showed that in patients with recurrent pain at rest, the initial abnormality observed was myocardial dysfunction, followed by deviation of the ST segment and by chest pain only if the ischemic episode was sufficiently long and extensive. If alterations in blood pressure and heart rate occurred, they followed the development of myocardial dysfunction. Other studies with thallium 201 showed that reversible defects of myocardial perfusion accounted for the change in myocardial function and in the electrocardiogram.[31] Angiography done at the time of chest pain in patients with physiologic evidence of ischemia showed severe coronary artery narrowing in the predicted location, yet when the test was repeated after administration of nitroglycerin and relief of ischemic pain, substantial resolution of the narrowing was observed.[27] A residual atherosclerotic lesion was usually detected in the area of the reversible stenosis. In some instances, the previously reversible spasm became prolonged, and acute myocardial infarction occurred.[33]

An extensive series of investigations make it very likely that platelet activation plays a role in the pathophysiology of recurrent ischemic pain at rest in many patients. In a study of 19 patients with unstable angina at rest, Sobel and colleagues[34] demonstrated that plasma levels of platelet-derived beta-thromboglobulin and platelet factor 4 were significantly elevated in blood samples obtained during or within four hours of an episode of angina. They were unable to observe such a clear association with plasma levels of thromboxane A_2. However, Fitzgerald and colleagues[35] using measurements of 2, 3 dinor-thromboxane B_2, a major urinary enzymatic metabolite of thromboxane A_2, were able to show that among hospitalized patients with unstable angina, 84 per cent of episodes of chest pain were associated with phasic increases of this metabolite. Although platelet activation and thromboxane A_2 release are features of unstable angina, the administration of sufficient aspirin to almost completely suppress the thromboxane A_2 synthesis does not decrease the episodes of recurrent ischemia at rest, indicating that additional factors must play a role in the recurrence of ischemia.[36,37] Folts[38] demonstrated in an experimental model of partial coronary occlusion and endothelial injury in the dog, a cyclic pattern of coronary blood-flow decreases over a few minutes, to be followed by sudden restoration of flow, and repetition of the sequence. Microscopic examination of frozen sections revealed platelet plugging and subsequent dislodgement to underlie the cyclic blood-flow variations. Eventual sustained occlusion often occurs in this model. Administration of aspirin completely abolishes the cyclic flow variation. Ashton and colleagues[39] have extended these observations to demonstrate abolition of the cyclic flow variations by the administration of a thromboxane A_2-prostaglandin H_2 re-

ceptor antagonist, or by a serotonin S_2 receptor antagonist. The effects of epinephrine to produce cyclic flow variations were overcome by the combined administration of antagonists to the thromboxane A_2 receptor and the serotonin receptor. The sequence of platelet accumulation and release, if it occurs in humans, could account for episodic ischemia at rest, and eventual complete occlusion could lead to coronary thrombosis and subsequently myocardial infarction or sudden death. Even in the absence of occlusive thrombosis, platelet embolization, analagous to that which precipitates transient cerebral ischemic attacks in patients with carotid or vertebral atherosclerosis, may cause ischemic complications. Experimental evidence in pigs showed that intracoronary infusion of adenosine diphosphate (ADP) or epinephrine results in platelet plugging and arrhythmic death.[40] Pretreatment with aspirin sharply reduced sudden death.[41] Possibly analogous platelet emboli in the myocardial microcirculation have been noted in studies of human sudden death victims.[27–29,42]

CLINICAL TRIALS OF ANTITHROMBOTIC AND THROMBOLYTIC DRUGS IN UNSTABLE ANGINA

Interest in the possible benefits of these drugs extends back to the 1940s, when the first trials of anticoagulant treatment for the syndromes of unstable angina were initiated. Although the early trials were favorable, increasing skepticism led to diminishing use of anticoagulant therapy. In the 1980s, major trials of aspirin demonstrated startling reductions of coronary events. The delineation of the role of thrombosis in the acute coronary syndromes led to a reevaluation of anticoagulant therapy for unstable angina, and to the conduct of trials of thrombolytic therapy. The management of unstable angina has changed radically in response to the clinical trial results of the past eight years.

Antiplatelet Drugs

Increasing evidence for the role of platelets in the pathogenesis of the complications of coronary artery disease, demonstration of the inhibitory effects of aspirin on platelet function, and the encouraging results from clinical trials in the secondary prevention of acute myocardial infarction and cerebrovascular disease,[43] stimulated the conduct of two major clinical trials of aspirin for the management of unstable angina.[12,13] Somewhat later, these were followed by trials which examined the relative benefits of aspirin alone, heparin alone, and the combination.[44-46]

The Veterans' Administration Cooperative Study[12] of aspirin was conducted in 12 Veterans Administration medical centers between 1974 and 1981 (Table 13–3). A total of 1,338 men entered the study, and after 12 weeks of treatment, there was a marked benefit of aspirin in the reduction of death and nonfatal myocardial infarction.

The target population consisted of patients hospitalized with a clinical diagnosis of unstable angina beginning within one month before and still present within the week before hospital admission. Patients had to have a good clinical history or electrocardiographic evidence of coronary artery disease, and an unstable angina pattern of either crescendo pain or prolonged pain at rest. Acute myocardial infarction was ruled out by electrocardiographic and enzymatic criteria. Of those patients with clinical unstable angina, 27.6 per cent met the study criteria, and 18.3 per cent entered the trial. Subsequently, 72 were found to have developed acute myocardial infarction and were excluded from the primary analysis, leaving 1,266 patients.

Patients entered the study within 51 hours of hospitalization. They were randomly allocated to 324 milligrams of aspirin in an effervescent buffered powder (Alka-Selzer) dissolved in water, or placebo. Coronary angiography was not performed routinely. The principal outcome was death or nonfatal acute myocardial infarction which was reduced from 10.1 to 5.0 per cent (51 per cent reduction, $p = 0.0005$) over the 12-week follow-up period. The other major outcomes and the observed reductions were fatal or nonfatal acute myocardial infarction (55 per cent reduction, $p = 0.001$), nonfatal acute myocardial infarction (51 per cent reduction, $p = 0.005$), and all-cause mortality (51 per cent reduction, $p = 0.054$). An intention-to-treat analysis including all randomized patients indicated reductions in death or nonfatal acute myocardial infarction (41 per cent reduction, $p = 0.004$), and all-cause mortality (34 per cent reduction, $p = 0.17$). Eighty-six per cent of patients were followed-up to one year, with a reduction in mortality of 43 per cent in the aspirin group, from 9.6 to 5.5 per cent ($p = 0.008$).

The Canadian Multicentre Trial[13] of aspirin or sulfinpyrazone, or both, in unstable angina was conducted in seven centers between 1979 and 1984 (Table 13–3). A total of 555 patients (73 per cent men) entered the study, and after a mean follow-up of 18 months, there was a marked benefit from aspirin in the reduction of death and nonfatal

TABLE 13–3. Randomized Trials of Aspirin in Unstable Angina: Study Designs and Outcomes

Study	Year	Patients	Entry Milligram/Day	Window	All Cause Mortality Follow-up	ASA	Placebo	RR	p Value	Cardiac Death or Nonfatal MI ASA	Placebo	RR	p Value
Lewis[12]	1983	1,338	324	51 hours	3 month	1.6	3.3	51	0.054	5.0	10.1	51	0.0005
Cairns[13]	1985	555	1300 (Factorial with 800 milligrams sulfinpyrazone)	8 days	24 month	3.0	11.7	71	0.004	8.6	17.0	51	0.008
Théroux[44]	1988	479	650 (Factorial with heparin infusion)	24 hours	6 day	0	1.7		NS	3.3	12.0	72	0.01
RISC[45]	1990	796	75 (Factorial with heparin every six hours)	72 hours	5 day	0.25	0.25	0	NS	2.5	5.8	57	0.033
					30 day	0.5	2.0	75	NS	4.3	13.4	68	<0.0001
					90 day	1.5	2.5	40	NS	6.5	17.1	62	<0.0001

MI = myocardial infarction; ASA = acetylsalicylic acid (aspirin); RR = risk reduction; NS = not significant.

myocardial infarction. Sulfinpyrazone conferred no benefit.

The target population consisted of patients admitted to a coronary care unit with a clinical (nonangiographic) diagnosis of unstable angina. These patients underwent a detailed interview to delineate good clinical or electrocardiographic evidence of myocardial ischemia, to define an unstable pain pattern, either crescendo pain or prolonged pain at rest, and to rule out myocardial infarction. The study criteria were satisfied by 85 per cent of the 817 patients interviewed after the exclusion process, among whom 159 refused study entry, leaving 555 who entered the trial. Patients were randomly allocated to one of four treatment regimens: aspirin (325 milligrams four times a day) or matching placebo, *plus* sulfinpyrazone (200 milligrams four times a day) or matching placebo, for a total of eight tablets daily to be taken with meals or milk. Coronary angiography was not a prerequisite for study entry.

The primary analysis was one of efficacy, with outcomes to be assessed only among patients who met certain criteria established at the inception of the study, and applied without knowledge of treatment allocated or of clinical outcome. Patients in this analysis had to have been taking at least some study medication within the preceding month. The primary outcome event of cardiac death or

nonfatal myocardial infarction occurred in 36 patients not given aspirin and in 17 taking aspirin, and by two years, the life table rate of these events was 17 per cent versus 8.6 per cent, a risk reduction of 50.8 per cent ($p = 0.008$) (Fig. 13–1). The outcome event of cardiac death alone was reduced from 11.7 to 3 per cent, a risk reduction of 71 per cent ($p = 0.004$) (Fig. 13–2). All deaths were cardiac in this analysis.

In the intention-to-treat analysis, counting all randomized patients and all outcomes, the outcome of cardiac death or nonfatal myocardial infarction was observed in 70 patients, including 17 patients who were excluded from the primary analysis of efficacy. Again, sulfinpyrazone had no significant effect and no interaction with aspirin. The risk reduction with aspirin was 30 per cent ($p = 0.072$). For the outcomes of cardiac death and death from any cause, the corresponding risk reductions with aspirin were 56.3 per cent ($p = 0.009$) and 43.4 per cent ($p = 0.035$), respectively.

Ticlopidine, an antiplatelet drug which appears to act by inhibiting the mobilization of the IIb-IIIa glycoprotein receptor in activated platelets, has been evaluated in several clinical trials among patients with vascular disease. The drug appears to reduce the incidence of subsequent vascular events in patients who have had a previous transient

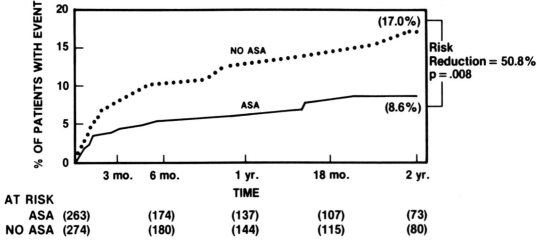

FIGURE 13–1. Occurrence of cardiac death or nonfatal myocardial infarction (MI) in the aspirin (ASA) and no-aspirin group of the Canadian multicenter trial of unstable angina. The graph is a life table depiction of the cumulative risk and time of occurrence of an outcome event, according to aspirin allocation. The numbers of patients at risk are noted below the graph. (From Cairns JA, et al. Aspirin, sulfinpyrazone, or both, in unstable angina. Results of a Canadian multicentre trial. N Engl J Med 1985; 313: 1369–75, with permission.)

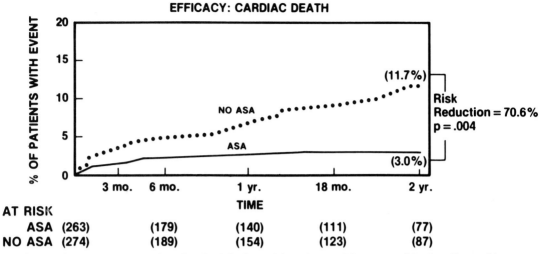

FIGURE 13–2. Occurrence of cardiac death in the aspirin and no-aspirin groups of the Canadian multicenter trial of unstable angina. (From Cairns JA, et al. Aspirin, sulfinpyrazone, or both, in unstable angina. Results of a Canadian multicentre trial. N Engl J Med 1985; 313: 1369–75, with permission.)

cerebral ischemic attack or a stroke,[47,48] to improve symptoms and to reduce vascular events in patients with peripheral vascular disease,[49,50] and to reduce the incidence of aortocoronary venous bypass graft occlusion.[51] Ticlopidine has also been evaluated among patients with unstable angina.

The Studio Della Ticlopidina nell'Angina Instabile Group[52] conducted a randomized, multicenter trial of ticlopidine versus placebo in Italian coronary care units between 1986 and 1987. A total of 652 patients of either sex entered the trial, which demonstrated a statistically significant reduction of the composite outcome of vascular death or nonfatal myocardial infarction.

The target population was patients admitted to the coronary care unit (CCU) during the preceding 48 hours, with a clinical diagnosis of unstable angina of the crescendo or rest pain type. Eligibility required the demonstration of spontaneous or exercise test-induced evidence, while in hospital and before randomization, of transient ischemic ST or T wave abnormalities, without elevation of cardiac enzymes. All patients received intensive conventional therapy, but no aspirin was allowed. Of the 2,438 patients with suspected unstable angina who were screened, a total of 652 (about 26 per cent) were eligible and randomized to ticlopidine 250 milligrams twice a day, plus conventional therapy versus conventional therapy alone, in an open-label manner.

The principal outcome was the composite

of vascular death or nonfatal myocardial infarction, while secondary outcomes were transient ischemic attack, nonfatal stroke, and peripheral vascular accident. During the 24-week follow-up period, an intention-to-treat analysis demonstrated a reduction in the rate of vascular death or nonfatal myocardial infarction from 13.6 to 7.3 per cent by ticlopidine (risk reduction 46.3 per cent, $p = 0.009$) (Fig. 13–3). There were also statistically significant reductions of nonfatal myocardial infarction (46.1 per cent, $p = 0.039$) and the composite of fatal or nonfatal myocardial infarction (53.2 per cent, $p = 0.006$). Analysis of the eligible patients showed still greater risk reductions and levels of significance. Life table analyses of the events were consistent with the simple outcome analyses. During the trial, 17.5 per cent of patients withdrew (19.1 per cent ticlopidine, 16 per cent conventional therapy) for a variety of reasons. Side effects accounted for the withdrawal of 4.8 per cent of the ticlopidine patients, most commonly because of gastrointestinal or skin reactions. Mild bleeding disorders in 1 per cent of patients resolved without stopping ticlopidine, and no clinically important abnormalities of blood cell counts were detected. Coronary revascularization was undertaken in 8.1 per cent of patients.

Anticoagulant Therapy

Heparin and a variety of oral anticoagulants have been used in the therapy of acute

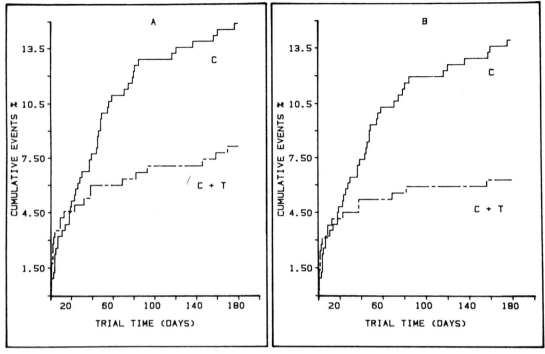

FIGURE 13–3. Occurrence of vascular death or nonfatal myocardial infarction (MI) in the ticlopidine and no-ticlopidine (control) groups of the Italian ticlopidine trial of unstable angina. Graph *A* is a life table depiction of the cumulative risk and time of occurrence of an outcome event, according to ticlopidine allocation, and considering all patients (intention-to-treat). Graph *B* depicts only the eligible patients (efficacy analysis). (From Balsano F, et al. Antiplatelet treatment with ticlopidine in unstable angina. Circulation 1990; 82: 17–26, with permission.)

coronary syndromes since the early 1940s, and indeed the American Heart Association recommended in 1948 that anticoagulation should be employed in the management of most patients with acute myocardial infarction. There were four major trials of the use of anticoagulants in patients with unstable angina reported from 1959 to 1964,[53–56] all of which concluded that such therapy was efficacious, and anticoagulation became standard therapy for unstable angina (Table 13–4). However, none of these trials meets the criteria which are essential for such studies,

calling into question their conclusions of efficacy.[57]

Beamish and Storrie[7] reported the outcome of 100 patients who presented with unstable angina of the crescendo or rest pain type between 1949 and 1957. Eighty-five patients were hospitalized, put at bed rest, and given oral anticoagulants and heparin. The 15 patients who were not hospitalized because of noncompliance or lack of beds were not anticoagulated and were considered to be control subjects. During the six weeks after diagnosis of "acute coronary insuffi-

TABLE 13–4. Early, Nonrandomized Trials of Anticoagulant Therapy of Unstable Angina

		PATIENTS (NUMBER)		FOLLOW-UP	MYOCARDIAL INFARCTION (%)		DEATH (%)	
STUDY	YEAR	*Anticoagulant*	*Control*	*(mo)*	*Anticoagulant*	*Control*	*Anticoagulant*	*Control*
Nichol[53]	1959	318	0	1	6.6		1.5	
Beamish[7]	1960	85	15	1.5	2.4	80	0	60
Wood[8]	1961	100	50	2	3	22	2	16
Vakil[9]	1964	190	156	3	36	49	9.5	24

ciency," two of the 85 anticoagulated patients suffered acute myocardial infarction and none died. Of the 15 untreated patients, 12 had myocardial infarction (all of them outside of hospital), and nine died. The denial of bed rest and hospital nursing care would be expected to have had an adverse effect on the "controls." The authors' conclusion that "prompt administration of anticoagulation appears to influence the outcome favourably" is unjustified, in view of the inadequacies of the study.

Wood[8] studied 150 patients with unstable angina of the rest-pain type from 1947 to 1957. All patients were put at bed rest; 100 received anticoagulants while 50 did not. During the two months after diagnosis, the incidence of myocardial infarction was 3 per cent and of death was 2 per cent among the anticoagulated patients, while the incidences were 22 and 16 per cent, respectively, among the control patients. The allocation was neither randomized nor double-blind, and when there appeared to be an advantage to the first 20 patients who were anticoagulated, there was no further attempt to alternate treated and "control" patients. The last 30 patients to enter the "control" group did so because anticoagulation was deemed to be undesirable for various reasons. Although the therapeutic regimens appeared to differ only with regard to anticoagulation, the unavoidable allocation biases and the small sample size weaken the conclusion that anticoagulation was efficacious.

Vakil[9] conducted a trial of anticoagulant therapy (heparin, oral anticoagulants or both) among 360 patients with angina at rest ("preinfarction syndrome") from 1949 to 1963. All patients were put at bed rest and were sedated. The anticoagulated group (190 patients) and the control group (156 patients) were said to be "well-matched," but the treatment allocation procedure was not specified. Within three months of diagnosis, acute myocardial infarction had occurred in 36.3 per cent of the anticoagulated patients (mortality rate 9.5 per cent) versus in 49.4 per cent of the control patients (mortality rate 23.7 per cent). The conclusion that anticoagulation led to a statistically significant reduction in acute myocardial infarction and particularly in mortality rate must be questioned in view of the study design.

Nichol and associates[53] assembled 318 patients with crescendo or rest angina ("impending myocardial infarction"), all of whom were treated with heparin and oral anticoagulants. At 30 days, the rates of myocardial infarction and death were 6.6 per cent and 1.6 per cent, respectively. The absence of a control group makes interpretation of the results virtually impossible.

Although anticoagulation was widely employed in the treatment of acute myocardial infarction and unstable angina by the mid 1960s, the basis for such therapy began to be widely questioned. The deficiencies in study designs became apparent,[54] the role of coronary thrombosis in the pathogenesis of the acute ischemic syndromes appeared less certain,[55] and outcomes following unstable angina and acute myocardial infarction improved with other advances in medical and surgical therapy. Although eventually three large randomized trials among patients with acute myocardial infarction demonstrated beneficial effects from anticoagulant therapy,[56–58] and a careful overview supported this approach to treatment,[59] anticoagulation was little used in the management of the acute ischemic syndromes.[60]

Interest in the potential value of anticoagulant therapy in unstable angina was rekindled by the results of a clinical trial reported in 1981,[61] and by the increasing evidence for a pathophysiologic role for coronary thrombosis in the acute coronary syndromes. Telford and Wilson[61] conducted a study of heparin and atenolol among patients with unstable angina or subendocardial infarction admitted to a coronary care unit in Northern Ireland between 1977 and 1980. A total of 400 patients were randomized, and there appeared to be a reduction of transmural infarction and death with heparin, but not atenolol.

The target population was patients admitted to the coronary care unit with a clinical diagnosis of unstable angina of the crescendo or rest pain type, or of subendocardial infarction ("cardiac pain associated with ST segment depression and/or T wave inversion with creatinine phosphokinase more than 240 international units/liter or aspartate aminotransferase (AST) more than 60 international units/liter"). Eventually there were 400 patients of either sex who entered the trial, although 186 were later withdrawn "because of incorrect recruitment" (51 did not fill the entry criteria, 84 were incorrectly diagnosed as cardiac pain, 43 had experienced transmural myocardial infarction prior to randomization, and eight were psychologically unstable), leaving 214 patients whose outcomes were analyzable.

Patients were randomly allocated in a double-blind fashion, using a factorial design, to one of four treatment groups: heparin 7,500 to 10,000 international units intravenously every six hours or placebo *plus* atenolol 100 milligrams orally once daily or placebo, during a seven-day treatment period. Patients under age 65 years, who completed the initial course of treatment, were placed on warfarin for the subsequent seven weeks. The principal outcome was transmural myocardial infarction, the incidence of which was no different between atenolol and placebo, but which was reduced from 15 to 3 per cent (80 per cent risk reduction, $p = 0.024$) among the patients receiving heparin. Over the subsequent seven weeks, there were a few additional transmural myocardial infarctions, but the rate was not different between the heparin and no heparin groups. Over the entire eight-week period, there were five deaths (two the first week and three subsequently), all of them among patients not receiving heparin.

A degree of skepticism greeted the results of the Telford trial because of the large number of randomized patients declared ineligible, the borderline statistical significance, and the general lack of enthusiasm for anticoagulant therapy in the acute coronary ischemic syndromes in 1981.

A small study of heparin among 102 patients hospitalized with unstable angina was subsequently reported by Williams et al.[62] The consecutive patients hospitalized with crescendo or rest pain were enrolled from two British hospitals from 1975 to 1978. They were randomly allocated to open-label heparin 10,000 units intravenously every six hours for 48 hours plus warfarin (prothrombin time ratio more than 2) for six months, or control. The composite outcome of recurrent unstable angina, myocardial infarction, or death, was reduced from 34 to 12 per cent in the anticoagulant group ($p < 0.05$).

Neri Serneri et al.[63] evaluated subcutaneous heparin in the long-term management of 30 patients admitted to a coronary care unit in Florence, Italy, demonstrating reduced fibrinopeptide A (FPA) production and fewer episodes of spontaneous angina. The target population was patients hospitalized with rest angina plus evidence of ischemia on Holter monitoring. Over a 20-month period, 30 patients of either sex were

enrolled and 24 completed the study. Patients were randomized, double-blind, to calcium heparin 12,500 international units subcutaneously daily or matching placebo for a six-month period, and then were crossed over to the alternate therapy. They were followed up at two-week intervals for a year with evaluation of clinical symptoms and sampling of blood for fibrinopeptide A. The mean level of fibrinopeptide A was 4.1 ± 3.7 nanograms/milliliter on placebo and 2.3 ± 1.8 nanograms/milliliter on heparin ($p < 0.001$). There was a large and statistically significant decrease in the angina frequency while on heparin. During placebo therapy, the levels of fibrinopeptide A correlated with anginal frequency, whereas on heparin, levels were low and did not correlate with symptoms. Hence, the study indicated that subcutaneous heparin could produce clinical benefit in the long-term management of patients with unstable angina, and suggested that the mechanism was by limiting fibrin formation as reflected by the reduced fibrinopeptide A levels on therapy.

A subsequent study by Neri Serneri and colleagues,[64] comparing heparin, aspirin, and alteplase among hospitalized patients with refractory angina, demonstrated that a continuous infusion of heparin was the most effective therapy for these hospitalized patients.

Aspirin and Anticoagulants

Although the two large trials of aspirin therapy[12,13] demonstrated a marked fall in the incidence of death and nonfatal myocardial infarction over the subsequent 3 to 24 months, neither had shown a reduction in the frequency of recurrent ischemia in hospital. The relatively high incidence of refractoriness to medical therapy in hospital, the increasing probability that acute thrombosis was involved in the pathogenesis, and the evidence of therapeutic benefit from heparin[61,62] led to further trials to examine the potential benefit of heparin alone and in conjunction with aspirin, with a particular focus on short-term outcomes.

Théroux and co-workers[44] conducted a study in two Canadian centers from 1986 to 1988 (Tables 13–3 and 13–5). A total of 479 patients (71 per cent male) entered the study, and after a mean follow-up of six days, there was a marked benefit of heparin for a number

TABLE 13–5. Randomized Trials of Heparin in Unstable Angina: Study Designs and Outcomes

Study	Year	Patient (Number)	Diagnosis	Drug Regimen	Entry Window (hr)	Entry Follow-up	All Cause Mortality (%) Heparin	Placebo	Death or Nonfatal MI (%) Heparin	Placebo	Bleeding
Telford[61]	1981	400	UA or non-Q MI	Random, factorial heparin IV every six hours and/or atenolol	24	1 week	0	1.8	3	15 (MI only)	
						8 week	0	4.4	7	18 (MI only)	
									p = 0.024		
Theroux[44]	1988	497	UA	Random, factorial heparin IV infusion and/or ASA	24	6 day	0	1.7	1.3	7.5	Total 8.3%, 2 × rate on no heparin, most at catheter sites
RISC[45]	1990	796	UA or non-Q MI	Random, factorial heparin IV every six hours and/or ASA	72	5 day			3.4	4.9	1 GI bleed in patient on heparin alone
									p ≤ 0.001		
						30 day			8.1	9.1	
									NS	NS	
						90 day			11.0	12.6	
										NS	

UA = unstable angina; MI = myocardial infarction; GI = gastrointestinal; IV = intravenous; ASA = acetylsalicylic acid (aspirin); NS = not significant.

of outcome events, with somewhat less benefit for the combination, or with aspirin alone. The target population consisted of patients hospitalized with a clinical diagnosis of unstable angina. The diagnosis was based upon a clinical history of accelerating chest pain or chest pain at rest, plus electrocardiographic or clinical evidence of underlying ischemic heart disease. Acute myocardial infarction was ruled out by enzymatic and electrocardiographic criteria, and the patients entered the trial within 24 hours of their most recent episode of pain. Of the patients admitted with unstable angina, 61.6 per cent (479 patients) were randomized to one of four treatment regimens, which were aspirin 650 milligrams orally immediately, followed by 325 milligrams twice daily, or matching placebo, *plus* heparin 5,000 units intravenously, followed by an infusion of 1,000 units/hour, or matching placebo. Infusion rates were varied as necessary by the hospital pharmacist to maintain the partial thromboplastin time (PTT) at 1.5 to 2 times control value, with similar adjustments of placebo infusions also undertaken. Coronary angiography was done a mean of four days after randomization in 91 per cent of patients in accordance with current clinical practice at the participating institutes. The trial therapy was ended when a final management decision was made, usually within 48 hours after coronary angiography.

The three major endpoints were: (a) refractory angina, defined as the presence of recurrent anginal chest pain with ischemic ST-T changes occurring despite full medical therapy, or the need for urgent intervention; (b) myocardial infarction; and (c) death.

Refractory angina occurred in 23 per cent of placebo patients, and was reduced to 8 per cent ($p = 0.002$) by heparin, 11 per cent ($p = 0.011$) by aspirin plus heparin, and 17 per cent ($p = 0.217$) by aspirin alone. Myocardial infarction was reduced from 11.9 per cent on placebo to 0.8 per cent ($p < 0.0001$) by heparin, 1.6 per cent ($p = 0.001$) by heparin plus aspirin, and 3.3 per cent ($p = 0.012$) by aspirin alone. Mortality was 1.7 per cent on placebo, while no deaths occurred on any of the study treatments. Although trends favored heparin and the heparin plus aspirin combination over aspirin alone, there were no statistically significant differences between the treatment groups for any of the major endpoints.

In contrast to the longer-term studies of aspirin,[12,13] which showed no difference in the rate of recurrent ischemia in hospital, the Théroux study,[44] which lasted only six days, found reductions in the rate of refractory angina by heparin or aspirin alone and by the combination, as well as demonstrating reductions of myocardial infarction and mortality during this in-hospital phase.

The principal side effect of concern was bleeding, most often at cardiac catheterization puncture sites. Bleeding occurred in 6.3 per cent of all patients and was twice as common amongst patients receiving heparin. Serious bleeding occurred in 2.1 per cent of patients.

Although gastrointestinal complaints occurred with remarkably similar frequency in the two longer-term trials of aspirin in unstable angina (Lewis 38 per cent,[12] Cairns 39 per cent[13]), a significantly greater frequency of such side effects amongst aspirin-treated patients versus controls was observed only in the Cairns trial ($p = 0.014$)[13] (Table 13–6). In this trial, medication withdrawals were not more common among aspirin groups than nonaspirin groups. Nevertheless, overall withdrawal rate was 28 per cent versus only 1.4 per cent in the Lewis study. This higher withdrawal rate may have arisen in part because the regimen required the ingestion of eight pills per day for two years, rather than only one pill a day for 12 weeks as in the Lewis trial, and the higher dose of aspirin itself may have contributed. In the United Kingdom TIA Aspirin Trial,[65] the only randomized trial in vascular disease to compare two different doses of aspirin (300 milligrams versus 1200 milligrams/day), the smaller dose gave rise to fewer gastrointestinal side effects ($2p < 0.001$) and less gastrointestinal bleeding ($2p < 0.05$), yet was equally efficacious. It is clear therefore that a dose of aspirin of 325 milligrams/day is sufficient for patients with unstable angina. The hope of eliminating gastrointestinal side effects almost completely, possibly limiting inactivation of Prostacyclin (PGI_2) synthesis, and the wish to use aspirin plus anticoagulation has led to trials employing lower-dose aspirin regimens in conjunction with heparin and warfarin.[45,46]

The RISC study group,[45] conducted a study of low-dose aspirin and heparin among 796 men in six Swedish hospitals between 1985 to 1988, (Tables 13–3, 13–5, and 13–6). The rates of myocardial infarction and death were reduced by aspirin. The target population was men hospitalized with un-

TABLE 13–6 Randomized Trials of Aspirin in Unstable Angina: Side Effects, Withdrawals, Revascularization

| Study | Year | Side Effects (%) | | | | Withdrawals (%) | | | | Revascularization (%) | | |
| | | Bleeding | | GI | | "Side Effects" | | Total | | Time (mo) | ASA | Placebo |
		ASA	Placebo	ASA	Placebo	ASA	Placebo	ASA	Placebo			
Lewis[12]	1983	2.6	2.5 (Stool OB)	37.0	39.2	1.4	1.4	4.6	5.6	3	2.6	4.4
Cairns[13]	1985	1.4	1.4 (GI)	43.8	33.6	17	12.1	36.2	32.6	24		31.5
Theroux[44]	1988	2.4	1.7 (Serious)	4.9	5.5	3.7	3.8			3	46.5	50
RISC[45]	1990	"Rare and minor"		6.5	5.5	1.8	1.3	5	5	3	2.5	5.3

GI = gastrointestinal; ASA = acetylsalicylic acid (aspirin).

stable coronary artery disease, defined as the occurrence of non-Q wave infarction or increasing angina taking place within the previous four weeks, and associated with ischemia on a resting electrocardiogram, or at a predischarge exercise test. Eligible patients were randomized double-blind within 72 hours of hospitalization (median 33 hours), to oral aspirin 75 milligram/day or placebo for one year *plus* intermittent intravenous heparin 10,000 units every six hours for 24 hours, followed by 7,500 international units every six hours for four days, or placebo. Of the 945 patients who initially appeared eligible, 149 (16 per cent) were eventually excluded because of the absence of rest or exercise electrocardiographic abnormalities or the presence of Q wave infarction at study entry. The principal outcomes were death and nonfatal myocardial infarction at five, 30, and 90 days. It was intended to follow all patients for one year, but the study was stopped early at the recommendation of the Safety Committee following publication of the ISIS-2 study.

The rates of death or nonfatal myocardial infarction at the five-, 30- and 90-day points were 5.8 per cent, 13.4 per cent, and 17.1 per cent, respectively, and they were reduced by 57 to 61 per cent by aspirin, but not by heparin alone. However, the combination of aspirin and short-term heparin resulted in the lowest rate of events at five days, and slightly lower rates at 30 and 90 days as well (Figs. 13–4 and 13–5). Hemorrhagic side effects were rare, with no fall in mean hemoglobins, and a gastrointestinal bleed in one patient treated with heparin without aspirin. Gastrointestinal symptoms were more frequent with aspirin (5.2 to 6.5 per

cent) than with placebo (0.7 to 1.9 per cent) after three months, but very few patients stopped study therapy.

This study is important because it demonstrated that the marked benefit of aspirin may be achieved at a dose of only 75 milligrams/day. The failure to observe a benefit from heparin alone is inconsistent with the Théroux study[44] and could be explained by the intermittent dose regimen, the later starting time, and the lower acuity of patients in the Swedish study, very few of whom underwent coronary angiography. There is a strong suggestion that the combination of aspirin and heparin for the first five days is preferable to aspirin alone, and there appears to be no increase in bleeding risk.

Cohen et al.[46] conducted a study of aspirin, aspirin plus heparin/warfarin, and heparin/warfarin among 93 patients hospitalized in two New York hospitals with unstable angina or non-Q wave infarction from 1987 to 1989. The results suggest a benefit from aspirin plus heparin/warfarin. The target population was patients hospitalized with non-Q wave infarction or unstable angina with recurrent or rest pain pattern of recent onset, and clinical or electrocardiographic evidence of ischemic heart disease. Within 48 hours of the last pain episode, patients were randomly allocated to open-label therapy with oral aspirin 325 milligrams/day; or intravenous heparin 100 international units/kilogram bolus followed by continuous infusion (partial thromboplastin time 2.0) for three to four days, followed by warfarin (international normalized ratio 3 to 4.5); or aspirin 325 milligram orally stat, followed by 80 milligrams/day *and* heparin/warfarin. The duration of therapy was to be 12 weeks. Ninety-three

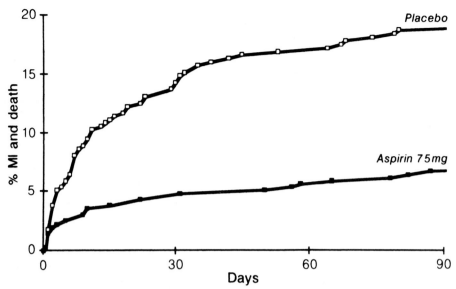

FIGURE 13–4. Occurrence of death or nonfatal myocardial infarction (MI) in the aspirin and no-aspirin (placebo) groups of the RISC Group trial of unstable angina and non-Q wave infarction. The graph is a life table depiction of the cumulative risk and time of occurrence of an outcome event, according to aspirin allocation. (From the RISC Group. Risk of myocardial infarction and death during treatment with low-dose aspirin and intravenous heparin in men with unstable coronary artery disease. Lancet 1990; 336: 827–30, with permission.)

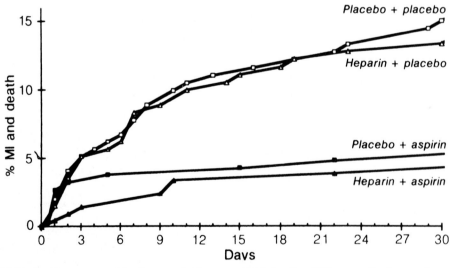

FIGURE 13–5. Occurrence of death or nonfatal myocardial infarction (MI) among the four regimens in the RISC Group trial of unstable angina and non-Q wave infarction. The graph is a life table depiction of the cumulative risk and time of occurrence of an outcome event, according to treatment allocation. (From the RISC Group. Risk of myocardial infarction and death during treatment with low-dose aspirin and intravenous heparin in men with unstable coronary artery disease. Lancet 1990; 336: 827–30, with permission.)

patients (60 per cent male) entered the study and were followed for the principal outcomes of recurrent myocardial ischemia, myocardial infarction, and all-cause mortality.

Meaningful conclusions are difficult because of the small sample size, the high rates of recurrent ischemia (31 per cent overall), and revascularization (50 per cent overall and similar to that in the Théroux study).[44] The rate of infarction and death appeared to be lowest in the group receiving a combination of aspirin and anticoagulation, consistent with observations in the RISC trial, yet there was no spontaneous major bleeding.

Neri Serneri and colleagues[64] conducted a study of heparin, aspirin, and alteplase among 97 patients hospitalized with refractory unstable angina in an Italian coronary care unit. The source population was a group of 302 patients hospitalized with unstable angina of the crescendo or prolonged rest pain type, with clinical or electrocardiographic evidence of myocardial ischemia. These patients were vigorously treated with antianginal therapy, and the target population was those patients who had at least three recurrences of angina or one prolonged episode during the two-day run in period. There were 97 such patients randomized to seven days of treatment with open-label heparin infusion (5,000 international units bolus, 1000 international units/hour, partial thromboplastin time 1.5 to 2), or intermittent heparin (6,000 international units every six hours, partial thromboplastin time less than or equal to 1.5), or buffered aspirin 325 milligrams/day. Eventually the heparin infusion was found to be the most effective treatment, and thereafter patients were randomized to heparin infusion versus alteplase (1.75 milligrams/kilogram over 12 hours).

The heparin infusion reduced the total number of ischemic episodes (symptomatic and silent) by 78 per cent during the first three days of therapy ($p < 0.001$) and was more effective than either of the other regimens. Subsequent comparison of heparin infusion to alteplase showed an 80 per cent reduction of ischemic episodes with heparin, whereas the alteplase produced only a 27 per cent reduction. When heparin infusion was compared to all other treatments, there was a 68 per cent reduction of angina episodes on day zero to three, and a 77 per cent reduction on days four to seven. There was no serious bleeding observed with heparin,

either by continuous infusion or by bolus. The dramatic reduction in episodes of recurrent ischemia is similar to that observed by Théroux,[44] the only other major study to report such an effect as a result of antithrombotic therapy.

Development of monoclonal antibodies to the IIb-IIIa fibrinogen binding site on platelets,[66] and the development of natural and genetically engineered small-molecular inhibitors of thrombin whose action is independent of antithrombin III,[67] is leading to new trials of patients with unstable angina, with the possibility that further reductions of thrombotic outcomes may be possible.

Thrombolytic Therapy

The observations of Moise[17] and Ambrose[22] and others, that angiographic progression of coronary artery stenosis is a common feature in patients with the clinical manifestations of unstable angina, led to a number of studies which attempted to delineate the prevalence of coronary thrombosis in such patients. The apparent incidence of coronary thrombosis has varied considerably, even amongst studies employing rigorous criteria for the angiographic identification of thrombus. In the earlier studies which alerted physicians to the potential role of thrombosis in the etiology of unstable angina, the reported incidence was rather low, ranging from 1 to 12 per cent (Table 13–7)[68–70] However, the mean time from rest pain to angiography was generally rather long (one to three months) in these reports. In more recent studies, in which the time from active symptoms of unstable angina to coronary angiography has generally been two weeks or less, the prevalence of coronary thrombus is considerably higher (Table 13–7).[25,71–78] Endogenous thrombolysis is a potent force in the maintenance of vessel patency, and probably accounts for the lower prevalence of thrombosis when angiography is done following an asymptomatic interval. It is also likely that angiographic criteria that are sufficiently strict to be specific for coronary thrombus are quite insensitive, as observed in an angioscopic study.[23]

Capone et al.[71] carried out the first study in patients with unstable angina to carefully evaluate the prevalence of intracoronary thrombi in relation to the time of angiog-

TABLE 13–7. Prevalence of Intracoronary Thrombus Among Patients with Unstable Angina

STUDY	PATIENTS (NUMBER)	INTRACORONARY THROMBUS PATIENTS (%)	TIME ELAPSED BETWEEN UNSTABLE ANGINA PAIN PATTERN AND ANGIOGRAPHY
Descriptive Studies			
Holmes[68]	1,202	16 (1)	3 months
Zack[69]	83	10 (12)	3 months
Vetrovec[70]	129	8 (6)	1 month
Capone[71]	119	44 (37)	14 days
	44	23 (52)	24 hours
Freeman[25]	24	5 (21)	6.6 days
	54	27 (50)	24 hours
Clinical Trials of Thrombolytic Therapy			
Topol[74]	40	16 (40)	<7 days (pretreatment)
Williams[76]	65	16 (25)	<7 days (pretreatment)
Gold[73]	11	8 (72)	1–3 days (placebo)
Ardissino[77]	20	4 (20)	<48 hours (pretreatment)
Shreiber[75]	11	5 (45)	12–48 hours (aspirin)
deZwaan[79]	41	28 (68)	2–6 hours (median 9 hours)
Gotoh[78]	37	27 (57)	During episode (pretreatment)

raphy following the most recent episode of rest pain. They assembled 119 patients with unstable angina of the rest pain type, confirmed by the presence of angiographic diameter stenosis of 70 per cent or more. Intracoronary thrombus was detected in 52 per cent of 44 patients who had angiography within 24 hours of pain, but in only 28 per cent of patients with pain 1 to 14 days previously. There were no intracoronary thrombi detected among 35 patients with stable angina.

Freeman et al.[25] have also focused on the relationship between the timing of coronary angiography and the most recent episode of rest pain. In a study of hospitalized patients with unstable angina of the rest pain type, they randomized 78 patients to coronary angiography within the first 24 hours (mean 17 ± 6 hours) of hospitalization versus coronary angiography to be performed later (mean 5.7 ± 2.1 days). The overall rate of coronary thrombosis was 42/78 (43 per cent early, 38 per cent delayed, p = not significant). However, one third of the patients randomized to delayed angiography required it urgently because of recurrent ischemia, and the incidence of coronary thrombosis was 75 per cent (mean 3.9 days), whereas in those who could be done in delayed fashion, the incidence of coronary thrombosis was 21 per cent (mean 6.6 days). Hence, of patients who had angiography within 24 hours of rest pain, the prevalence of coronary thrombosis was 50 per cent (27/54) whereas of those who

had late elective angiography, the prevalence of coronary thrombosis was 21 per cent (5/24). The prevalence of complex morphology was no different among the various groups. The presence of coronary thrombus was the strongest independent predictor of in-hospital cardiac events. The presence of ST segment abnormality on the admission electrocardiogram was strongly predictive of coronary thrombus.

Gotoh[78] carried out coronary angiography in 37 patients during an attack of rest angina. Among these patients, 21 (57 per cent) had coronary thrombus present. Each of these patients received an intracoronary infusion of urokinase, and all but one responded with a reduction in the severity of stenosis. Mean stenosis was reduced from 94 per cent to 76 per cent, with no significant further change at the four-week repeat angiography (mean 78 per cent stenosis).

Hence, the clinical data indicate that when coronary angiography is done in close proximity to the most recent episode of rest angina, there is a high prevalence of intracoronary thrombus detected. As the time between rest pain and angiography lengthens, the prevalence of intracoronary thrombus decreases, likely as a result of spontaneous thrombolysis and organization of residual thrombus (Table 13–7).

The increasing evidence for the role of coronary thrombosis in the acute phases of unstable angina, the persisting risk of myocardial infarction and death in spite of conventional medical therapy, and the dramatic evidence of benefit of thrombolytic drugs in acute myocardial infarction, provided a strong rationale for their use in patients with unstable angina. Several uncontrolled case series employing intracoronary streptokinase or urokinase suggested benefit in some patients clinically, but angiographic improvement, although common, was quantitatively rather minor in most series.[72,78-82]

Randomized controlled studies have allowed a more accurate view of the true benefits of thrombolytic therapy for unstable angina (Table 13-8). The first such study, reported by Lawrence in 1980,[83] evaluated 40 hospitalized patients with an unstable pain pattern and clinically "unequivocal evidence of myocardial ischemia." Patients were randomly allocated, single-blind to streptokinase (250,000 international units over one-half hour, 100,000 international units/hour for 24 hours) plus warfarin (prothrombin 5 to 15 per cent of normal), or warfarin alone. Warfarin therapy was sustained over the next six months, by which time there were eight cardiovascular events in the control patients (40 per cent) but only one in the streptokinase group (5 per cent) ($p < 0.02$).

Gold et al.[73] evaluated alteplase in a group of patients hospitalized with chest pain at rest accompanied by 1 millimeter of ST segment elevation or depression within the previous week. Patients were treated with an intensive antianginal regimen for 12 to 28 hours, and were then randomized to intravenous alteplase (0.75 milligrams/kilogram over one hour, 0.5 milligrams/kilogram over four hours, 0.5 milligrams/kilogram over seven hours) versus placebo. Both groups received intravenous heparin by continuous infusion (partial thromboplastin time 1.5 to 2). Patients underwent coronary angiography after one to three days. The efficacy was assessed by comparing the frequency of in-hospital ischemic events over at least four days, the frequency of Holter monitor-detected silent ischemic episodes, and the evidence of intracoronary thrombus. Recurrent ischemic events were fewer in the alteplase group (1/12 versus 6/11, $p < 0.05$), silent ischemia was not seen in either group, and coronary morphology was no different, although subocclusive thrombus was seen only in the placebo group.

Topol et al.[74] evaluated intravenous alteplase in a group of patients hospitalized with rest angina with or without electrocardio-

graphic changes, with more than or equal to 60 per cent stenosis at angiography, and the provocation of ischemia by pacing. A group of 40 patients were randomized to either intravenous alteplase (6 milligrams bolus, total 60 milligrams over one hour, 40 milligrams over two hours, 50 milligrams over five hours, total 150 milligrams) or placebo. All patients received aspirin 325 milligrams orally daily and heparin infusion (partial thromboplastin time 2 to 2.5). Coronary angiography, during which pacing was repeated, was done again after 12 to 24 hours. The principal outcomes were quantitative angiographic stenosis (no difference between groups), pacing threshold (significant increase in alteplase group), and cumulative rates of revascularization procedures (no difference). Complications with percutaneous transluminal coronary angioplasty (PTCA) appeared to be less following alteplase therapy.

Schreiber et al.[75] evaluated urokinase in a group of patients hospitalized with ischemic rest pain associated with electrocardiographic changes who were thought to have unstable angina or non-Q wave infarction in evolution. Within 24 hours of the index pain episode, 25 patients were randomly allocated to open-label intravenous urokinase (3×10^6 units over one-half hour) plus heparin (partial thromboplastin time 1.5 to 2) *or* oral aspirin 325 milligrams, for a seven-day study period. Coronary angiography was performed at 24 to 72 hours after initiation of therapy. The primary endpoint was the occurrence of new ischemic events (myocardial infarction, intractable ischemic pain, or death). Seven of the twenty-five patients proved to have had non-Q wave infarction. New ischemic events were frequent (44 per cent overall), with a trend to fewer events in the urokinase group. The combination of heparin and aspirin was not assessed in this trial, and in view of the clinical efficacy of this combination demonstrated in other trials, the relative roles of the urokinase and heparin in accounting for the positive clinical trend is uncertain. Definite thrombus was detected in 50 per cent of patients, but there was no major difference in angiographic findings between the treatment groups.

Williams et al.[76] evaluated alteplase among a population of hospitalized patients with rest angina associated with ischemic electrocardiographic changes, diagnostic angiography (within seven days after onset of rest angina),

TABLE 13–8. Randomized Clinical Trials of Thrombolytic Therapy in Unstable Angina

Author	Clinical Syndrome	Number of Patients	Therapy	Design	Follow-Up	Benefits of Thrombolytic Therapy	
						Clinical	Angio
Williams[76]	Rest angina ECG ≥80% stenosis	67	High-dose IV alteplase (22) low-dose IV alteplase (23) Placebo alteplase (22) (heparin + ASA in all)	Random, blinded	Angio pre rand. and at 12–48 hours (65/67)	No differences	Minor reduction stenosis severity in all, no differences
Topol[74]	Rest angina ≥60% stenosis Pacing ischemia	40	IV alteplase (20) (150 milligrams over 8 hours) Placebo (20) (heparin + ASA in all)	Random, blinded	Angio pre rand. and at 12–24 hours	Increased pacing threshold ($p = 0.007$), no difference cumulative incidence revascularization	No difference in stenosis severity
Gold[73]	Rest angina ECG	21	IV alteplase (12) (1.75 milligrams/ kilograms over 12 hours) Placebo (11)	Random, blinded	Angio at 24–74 hours	Fewer ischemic events ($p < 0.05$)	No difference coronary morphology, subocclusive thrombus only in placebo
Ardissino[77]	Rest angina ECG Failure of 48-hour intensive therapy	23	IV alteplase (11) (100 milligrams over 5 hours) Placebo (12)	Random, blinded	Angio pre rand. and at 72 hours (20/23)	Fewer Holter ischemic episodes ($p < 0.01$) No difference in persistence of UA >72 hours	No difference in pretreatment and posttreatment quantitative angio
Neri Serneri[64]	Crescendo or rest angina Clinical or ECG Ischemia	39	IV alteplase (20) (1.75 milligrams/ kilograms over 12 hours) Heparin infusion (19)	Random, open	7 days	Less marked decrease of ischemic episodes (alteplase 27%, heparin 80%)	No angio
Shreiber[75]	Rest angina ECG	25	IV UK (12) (3×10^6 international units) plus heparin ASA 325 milligrams/ day (13)	Random, open-label	Angio at 24–72 hours clinical over 7 days	Trend to fewer new ischemic events	No difference

ECG = electrocardiogram; IV = intravenous; ASA = acetylsalicylic acid (aspirin); UK = urokinase; UA = unstable angina;

and a culprit lesion of greater than or equal to 80 per cent diameter stenosis. Within two hours of initial catheterization, 67 patients were randomly allocated to high-dose alteplase (100 milligrams over six hours), low-dose alteplase (0.75 milligram/kilogram over one hour, maximum 60 milligrams, or placebo. All patients received a bolus of heparin at initial catheterization, and a constant infusion to maintain partial thromboplastin time at 1.5 to 2 until follow-up angiography. Daily aspirin 325 milligram was also given and preangiography medications were continued. Repeat angiography was performed at 12 to 48 hours after enrollment. The per cent diameter stenosis of the culprit lesion was less in all three treatment groups at follow-up angiography, with no clear differences amongst the treatment groups. A variety of descriptive classifications for the prevalence of thrombus and the improvement of coronary blood flow also showed improvement at follow-up angiogram for all three treatment groups, with no clear advantage to the alteplase groups. The occurrence of coronary outcomes was not different among the groups. Bleeding was somewhat more common in the alteplase groups, particularly in relation to invasive procedures. The authors were optimistic that alteplase may confer benefit in addition to heparin and aspirin, but acknowledged that it appears modest and that large trials are necessary for a definitive answer.

Ardissino et al.[77] assessed the value of intravenous alteplase in a group of hospitalized patients with recent onset or exacerbation of rest angina, accompanied by ischemic electrocardiographic changes. From a group of 103 such patients, 24 failed to respond to 48 hours of intensive medical therapy and were randomized to intravenous alteplase (10 milligrams bolus, 50 milligrams over one hour, 40 milligrams over four hours, total 100 milligrams), or placebo. Heparin (5,000 units intravenously every six hours, partial thromboplastin time 1.5 to 2) was started in all patients following the five-hour infusion. Angiography was performed in all patients prior to randomization and was repeated after 72 hours. The principal outcomes were recurrent ischemia detected on Holter monitoring, changes from baseline to follow-up coronary angiography, and the persistence of unstable angina after the 72-hour initial follow-up. The alteplase-heparin combination group had no ischemic episodes during the 72-hour early follow-up versus 9/11 heparin-treated patients. Coronary angiographic morphology was unchanged between preinfusion and postinfusion in either group, and unstable angina recurred in most patients over the next several days with no difference in the incidence between the two groups.

In their trial of heparin, aspirin, and alteplase among patients with refractory unstable angina, Neri Serneri et al.[64] randomized 39 patients to heparin infusion (5,000 international units bolus, 1000 international units/hour, partial thromboplastin time 1.5 to 2) or alteplase (1.75 milligrams/kilogram over 12 hours). Over the next three days, there was an 80 per cent reduction in the frequency of ischemic episodes with heparin, but only a 27 per cent reduction with alteplase.

Whereas the benefits of thrombolytic therapy in acute myocardial infarction are unequivocal,[84] there is uncertainty as to its value in unstable angina. Ambrose and Alexoupolos[85] have recently reviewed the controversy. They drew attention to the relatively few available trials, all of which are small, and only a few of which involve randomized comparisons. There is also considerable variability in the patient populations (several of the studies include patients with non-Q wave infarction), the angiographic approaches (none, post-treatment only, pretreatment and post-treatment comparisons, with or without quantitative techniques), the use of aspirin and heparin, thrombolytic protocols (agent, route, dose, duration), and the timing of thrombolytic therapy and follow-up angiography in relation to the most recent pain episode. Although there is a suggestion of more angiographic improvement with thrombolytic therapy, particularly among patients with severe stenosis or clear angiographic evidence of thrombus, the overall benefits are modest and little different from those with heparin. Most controlled studies have shown some reduction in early episodes of ischemia, although generally the rates of later events and the need for revascularization appear to be no different. Failure to achieve the benefits observed among patients with acute myocardial infarction may result from differences in the proportion of the stenosis accounted for by relatively fresh thrombus. It may be that the occlusion of unstable angina develops gradually by recurrent episodes of layered thrombus and that a relatively small proportion of the stenosis is amenable to thrombolysis, by comparison to the sudden formation of a large occlusive thrombus in acute myocardial infarction. Thrombus formation under the atherosclerotic plaque or relatively small amounts of plaque disruption and thrombosis may characterize the pathogenesis of unstable angina in contrast to that of acute myocardial infarction. In any case, with the rather low rates of ischemic events among patients with unstable angina treated with aspirin and heparin, comparison trials with thrombolytic therapy are not justified. Trials evaluating the addition of thrombolytic therapy to heparin and aspirin must include several thousand patients if they are to have any chance of detecting clinically important benefits. The TIMI-3 collaboration is an example of such an undertaking.

SUMMARY AND THERAPEUTIC RECOMMENDATIONS

Unstable angina has long been recognized to carry a much higher risk of acute myocardial infarction and sudden death than does stable angina. Those patients with prolonged episodes of rest pain, accompanied by ST and T wave abnormalities on electrocardiogram, and resistant to antianginal therapy with nitrates, beta blockers, and calcium antagonists, are at particularly high risk. Most patients with unstable angina have relatively severe atherosclerosis. Although unstable angina may result in a few instances from spontaneous increases in myocardial oxygen demand, it is thought that relatively recent changes in myocardial oxygen supply account for most episodes of unstable angina. It is likely that inappropriate increases in coronary tone are an important complement of these reductions in myocardial oxygen supply, and in some patients the excessive tone may be profound (coronary spasm). However, it has been recognized over the past ten years that patients with unstable angina generally have progression of coronary artery stenosis compared to a time when their disease was stable. Careful evaluation of the coronary angiograms, using strict criteria for the presence of intracoronary thrombus, has revealed that the prevalence of such progression is very low among patients with stable angina and high amongst those with unstable angina. The timing of coronary angiography in relation to the most recent episode of rest pain is critical. Studies within

24 hours of pain detect intracoronary thrombus in more than 50 per cent of patients, between one and 14 days in about 30 per cent of patients, and much less commonly beyond one month. It is likely that spontaneous thrombolysis, and the organization of residual thrombus accounts for this temporal phenomenon.

The clinical and angiographic observations are supported by experimental and autopsy studies. There is extensive evidence for the participation of platelets in the process, and the preventative roles of aspirin and of specific blockers of thromboxane A_2 synthase and antagonists of thromboxane A_2 and serotonin receptors. The observation of recurrent formation and disruption of platelet occlusions in the canine coronary stenosis model of Folts, and the effects of various interventions thereon, may closely parallel the situation in human unstable angina. The studies of Falk demonstrating sequential intracoronary thrombosis preceding death in unstable angina, and the studies of Davies and Thomas demonstrating the high prevalence of intramural hemorrhage and/or intraluminal thrombosis among sudden death victims, point to the importance of platelet and fibrin thrombosis in the pathogenesis of unstable angina, acute myocardial infarction, and sudden death. The angiographic studies of DeWood, confirmed in countless clinical studies of coronary thrombolysis, have demonstrated the central role of coronary thrombosis in acute myocardial infarction. Hence, there is a sound pathophysiologic rationale for the use of agents to prevent, limit, and resolve coronary thrombus in the management of patients with unstable angina.

The initial large studies of aspirin[12,13] focused on the reduction of cardiac death and nonfatal infarction over a 3 to 24-month period, reporting dramatic risk reductions of at least 50 per cent. However, there was no reported reduction of recurrent angina or bypass surgery. The Théroux study[44] recruited a higher proportion of very unstable patients early in the hospital course, and observed reductions in cardiac death and nonfatal infarction amongst patients on heparin, aspirin, and the combination by comparison to placebo. However, there were also decreased rates of refractory angina among all active treatment groups, although there was no reduction in the rates of eventual revascularization. The Cohen study[46] found a high rate of recurrent chest pain and ischemia with heparin, aspirin, and the combination, but there was no placebo comparison. Revascularization was required in about 50 per cent of patients by three months, with no differences among the treatment regimens, and similar to that in the Théroux study. In the Neri Serneri study,[64] vigorous heparin therapy by continuous infusion appeared to significantly reduce recurrent ischemic episodes during the early hospital course. Hence there is a large body of evidence indicating that aspirin decreases the incidence of myocardial infarction and cardiac death during the months following the onset of unstable angina. There is considerable evidence that early heparinization is of value in decreasing the early occurrence of myocardial infarction and cardiac death amongst hospitalized patients with unstable angina. The optimal duration of heparin therapy and the need for subsequent warfarin therapy are uncertain. Combination therapy with heparin and aspirin during the period of greater instability in hospital has been evaluated in three studies,[45-46] employing different regimens. In two of these, the combination appeared to offer advantages over either agent alone, yet without significant increased risk of bleeding. The incidence of recurrent ischemia in hospital may be decreased by various heparin and aspirin regimens, although the principal benefit is the reduction in myocardial infarction and cardiac death.

The standard therapy of unstable angina is focused on minimizing the imbalance between myocardial oxygen supply and demand. The patient is placed at bed rest in a coronary care unit, and is sedated. Nitrates, both short and long acting are employed, and either a beta blocker or calcium antagonist is initiated. Patients with recurrent ischemic episodes will be treated with nitrates, a beta blocker, and a calcium antagonist. Antithrombotic therapy has now joined the standard armamentarium of medical therapy, and in selected cases thrombolytic therapy may be effective.

Aspirin therapy is indicated in every patient with unstable angina, unless there are strong contraindications to its use. The definite diagnosis of aspirin allergy is the only absolute contraindication. A history of gastrointestinal hemorrhage is a relative contraindication, but aspirin therapy may still be indicated, particularly in the acute phase of unstable angina. The exact details of the

bleeding history are essential, and if aspirin is to be used, a low-dose enteric-coated preparation and the conjoint use of cytoprotective agents is prudent. Aspirin should be commenced immediately upon the diagnosis of the presence of an acute myocardial ischemic syndrome in the emergency room, as aspirin is of marked benefit both in acute myocardial infarction and unstable angina. The initial dose should be 160 to 325 milligrams (2 to 4 children's aspirins, or ½ to 1 adult aspirin), and should be chewed or dissolved in water and swallowed to achieve the most rapid platelet suppression. The therapy should be maintained at a dose of 160 to 325 milligrams daily of an enteric-coated preparation. Although the longest duration of therapy studied in the trials was two years, the benefits observed in the primary prevention trials suggest that such therapy should be continued indefinitely. Reductions in the incidence of vascular death or nonfatal myocardial infarction in the range of 50 per cent will be observed with this therapeutic regimen. The rate of gastrointestinal side effects will be low, and compliance will be high. There will be a definite increase in the risk of hemorrhage, but most of this is minor, and although the rate of cerebral hemorrhage is probably increased, this is balanced by a lesser incidence of thrombotic stroke, but no overall increase in the incidence of stroke.[86]

The use of heparin appears to be of value in patients hospitalized with unstable angina. In the acute phase of unstable angina, a bolus of heparin, followed by a continuous infusion with maintenance of the partial thromboplastin time in the 1.5 to 2 times normal range may be even more effective than aspirin alone in the prevention of recurrent ischemic episodes and early events. Combination therapy with aspirin and heparin during the early hospital phase may confer additional benefit over either agent used alone. There is likely to be an increase in the risk of bleeding, particularly with the combination, necessitating scrupulous attention to the partial thromboplastin time, and to clinical symptoms and signs of possible hemorrhage. It is recommended that upon the diagnosis of unstable angina, patients receive an initial bolus of 5,000 international units of heparin intravenously, and that the partial thromboplastin time be maintained in the range of 1.5 to 2 times normal (measured at four hours after bolus, and at least at daily intervals) with an initial infusion in the range of 1,000 international units/hour. Aspirin should be initiated immediately, and maintained at a dose of 160 to 325 milligrams/day. A lower daily dose (75 milligrams) may be sufficient, and in conjunction with heparin may be safer, although the evidence in support of such a low dose is relatively small by comparison to that for the higher doses. The heparin should be sustained for at least seven days in sufficient dose intravenously or subcutaneously (SC) to maintain the partial thromboplastin time in the 1.5 to 2 times normal range. The potential value of long-term subcutaneous heparin or of warfarin is uncertain as yet, and such therapies are not recommended except for the most refractory patients where long-term combination therapy with aspirin may be justified.

The value of thrombolytic therapy in patients with unstable angina appears to be modest. Although small controlled studies suggest marginal clinical and angiographic benefits, there is no indication for the routine use of thrombolytic therapy for these patients. The TIMI-3 trial results should permit rational decisions about the role of thrombolytic therapy in unstable angina.

REFERENCES

1. Cairns JA, Fantus IG, Klassen GA. Unstable angina pectoris. Am Heart J 1976; 92: 373–86.
2. Fowler NO. Angina pectoris: clinical diagnosis. Circulation 1972; 46: 1079–7.
3. Braunwald E. Unstable angina: a classification. Circulation 1989; 80: 410–4.
4. Sampson JJ, Eliaser M. The diagnosis of impending acute coronary artery occlusion. Am Heart J 1937; 13: 676–86.
5. Feil H. Preliminary pain in coronary thrombosis. Am J Med Sci 1937; 193: 42–8.
6. Levy H. The natural history of changing patterns of angina pectoris. Ann Intern Med 1956; 44: 1123–35.
7. Beamish RE, Storrie VM. Impending myocardial infarction. Recognition and management. Circulation 1960; 21: 1107–15.
8. Wood P. Acute and subacute coronary insufficiency. Br Med J 1961; 1: 1779–82.
9. Vakil RJ. Preinfarction syndrome-management and follow-up. Am J Cardiol 1964; 14: 55–63.
10. Fulton M, Lutz W, Donald KW, et al. Natural history of unstable angina. Lancet 1972; 1: 860–5.
11. Krauss KR, Hutter AM Jr, Desantis RW. Acute coronary insufficiency course and follow-up. Circulation 1972; 45(suppl I): I-66–71.
12. Lewis HD, Davis JW, Archibald DG, et al. Protective effects of aspirin against acute myocardial infarction and death in men with unstable angina: results of a Veterans' Administration Cooperative Study. N Engl J Med 1983; 309: 396–403.
13. Cairns JA, Gent M, Singer J, et al. Aspirin, sulfinpyrazone, or both, in unstable angina. Results of a Canadian multicentre trial. N Engl J Med 1985; 313: 1369–75.
14. Cairns JA, Singer J, Gent M, et al. Coronary care unit utilization in Hamilton, Ontario, a city of 375,000 people. Can J Cardiol 1988; 4: 25–32.
15. Maseri A, Chierchia S, L'Abbate A. Pathogenetic mechanisms underlying the clinical events associated with ather-

osclerotic heart disease. Circulation 1980; 62(6 pt 2): V3–V13.
16. Rafflenbeul W, Russell RO, Lichtlen PR. Angiographic anatomy of coronary arteries in unstable angina. In: Rafflenbeul W, Lichtlen PR, Balcon R, eds. Unstable Angina Pectoris. Stuttgart: Thieme, 1981:51–7.
17. Moise A, Théroux P, Taeymans Y, et al. Unstable angina and progression of coronary atherosclerosis. N Engl J Med 1983; 309: 685–9.
18. Rafflenbeul W, Smith LR, Rogers WJ, et al. Quantitative coronary arteriography. Coronary anatomy of patients with unstable angina pectoris re-examined 1 year after optimal therapy. Am J Cardiol 1979; 43: 699–707.
19. Bertrand ME. Diagnostic approach to unstable angina with coronary angiography. In: Hugenholtz PG, Goldman BS. eds. Unstable Angina, Current Concepts and Management. Stuttgart: Schattauer, 1985:119–25.
20. Hugenholtz PG, Michels HR, Serruys PW, et al. Nifedipine in the treatment of unstable angina, coronary spasm and myocardial ischemia. Am J Cardiol 1981; 47: 163–73.
21. Ross R. The pathogenesis of atherosclerosis—an update. N Engl J Med 1986; 314: 488–500.
22. Ambrose JA, Winters SL, Arora RR, et al. Angiographic evolution of coronary artery morphology in unstable angina. J Am Coll Cardiol 1986; 7: 472–8.
23. Sherman CT, Litvak F, Grundfest W, et al. Coronary angioscopy in patients with unstable angina pectoris. N Engl J Med 1986; 315: 913–9.
24. Suryapranata H, de Feyter PJ, Serruys PW. Coronary angioplasty in patients with unstable angina pectoris: is there a role for thrombolysis. J Am Coll Cardiol 1988; 12: 69A–77A.
25. Freeman MR, Williams AE, Chisholm RJ, Armstrong PW. Intracoronary thrombus and complex morphology in unstable angina. Relation to timing of angiography and in-hospital cardiac events. Circulation 1989; 80: 17–23.
26. DeWood MA, Spores J, Notske R, et al. Prevalence of total coronary occlusion during the early hours of transmural myocardial infarction. N Engl J Med 1980; 303: 897–902.
27. Falk E. Unstable angina with fatal outcome: dynamic coronary thrombosis leading to infarction and/or sudden death: autopsy evidence of recurrent mural thrombosis with peripheral embolization culminating in total vascular occlusion. Circulation 1985; 71: 699–708.
28. Davies MJ, Thomas AC, Knapman PA, Hangartner JR. Intramyocardial platelet aggregation in patients with unstable angina suffering sudden ischemic cardiac death. Circulation 1986; 73: 418–27.
29. Davies MJ, Thomas A. Thrombosis and acute coronary artery lesions in sudden cardiac ischemic death. N Engl J Med 1984; 310: 1137–40.
30. Cannon DS, Harrison DC, Schroeder JS. Hemodynamic observations in patients with unstable angina pectoris. Am J Cardiol 1974; 33: 17–22.
31. Maseri A, Parodi O, Severi S, et al. Transient transmural reduction of myocardial blood flow demonstrated by thallium-201 scintigraphy, as a cause of varient angina. Circulation 1976; 54: 280–8.
32. Maseri A, L'Abbate A, Pesola A, et al. Coronary vasospasm in angina pectoris. Lancet 1977; 1: 713–7.
33. Maseri A, L'Abbate A, Baroldi G, et al. Coronary vasospasm as a possible cause of myocardial infarction. A conclusion derived from the study of "preinfarction" angina. N Engl J Med 1978; 299: 1271–7.
34. Sobel M, Salzman EW, Davies GC, et al. Circulating platelet products in unstable angina pectoris. Circulation 1981; 63: 300–6.
35. Fitzgerald DJ, Roy L, Catella F, FitzGerald GA. Platelet activation in unstable coronary disease. N Engl J Med 1986; 315: 983–9.
36. Robertson RM, Robertson D, Roberts LF, et al. Thromboxane A_2 in vasotonic angina pectoris: evidence from direct measurements and inhibitor trials. N Engl J Med 1981; 304: 998–1003.
37. Chierchia S, de Caterina R, Crea F, et al. Failure of thromboxane A_2 blockade to prevent attacks of vasospastic angina. Circulation 1982; 66: 702–5.
38. Folts JD, Crowell EB Jr, Rowe GG. Platelet aggregation in

partially obstructed vessels and its elimination with aspirin. Circulation 1976; 54: 365–70.

39. Ashton JH, Golino P, McNatt JM, et al. Serotonin S$_2$ and thromboxane A$_2$-prostaglandin H$_2$ receptor blockade provide protection against epinephrine-induced cyclic flow variations in severely narrowed canine coronary arteries. J Am Coll Cardiol 1989; 13: 755–63.

40. Jorgensen L, Rowsell HC, Hovig T, et al. Adenosine diphosphate-induced platelet aggregation and myocardial infarction in swine. Lab Invest 1967; 17: 616–44.

41. Haft JI, Gershengorn K, Kranz PD, Oestreicher R. Protection against epinephrine-induced myocardial necrosis by drugs that inhibit platelet aggregation. Am J Cardiol 1972; 30: 838–43.

42. Haerem JW. Mural platelet microthrombi and major acute lesions of main epicardial arteries in sudden coronary death. Atherosclerosis 1974; 19: 529–41.

43. Antiplatelet Trialists' Collaboration. Secondary prevention of vascular disease by prolonged antiplatelet treatment. Br Med J 1988; 296: 320–31.

44. Théroux P, Ouimet H, McCans J, et al. Aspirin, heparin, or both to treat acute unstable angina. N Engl J Med 1988; 319: 1105–11.

45. The RISC Group. Risk of myocardial infarction and death during treatment with low-dose aspirin and intravenous heparin in men with unstable coronary artery disease. Lancet 1990; 336: 827–30.

46. Cohen M, Adams PC, Hawkins L, Bach M, Fuster V. Usefulness of antithrombotic therapy in resting angina pectoris or non-Q-wave myocardial infarction in preventing death and myocardial infarction (a pilot study from the Antithrombotic Therapy in Acute Coronary Syndromes Study Group). Am J Cardiol 1990; 66: 1287–92.

47. Gent M, Blakely JA, Easton JD, et al. The Canadian American ticlopidine study (CATS) in thromboembolic stroke. Lancet 1989; 2: 1215–20.

48. Hass WK, Easton JD, Adams HP, et al., for the Ticlopidine Aspirin Stroke Study Group. A randomized trial comparing ticlopidine hydrochloride with aspirin for the prevention of stroke in high-risk patients. N Engl J Med 1989; 321: 501–7.

49. Balsano F, Coccheri S, Libretti A, et al. Ticlopidine in the treatment of intermittent claudication: a 21-month double-blind trial. J Lab Clin Med 1989; 114: 84–91.

50. Boissel JP, Peyrieux JC, Destors JM. Is it possible to reduce the risk of cardiovascular events in subjects suffering from intermittent claudication of the lower limbs? Thromb Haemost 1989; 62: 681–5.

51. Limet R, David JL, Magotteaux P, Larock MP, Rigo P. Prevention of aorta-coronary bypass graft occlusion: beneficial effect of ticlopidine on early and late patency rate of venous coronary bypass grafts: a double-blind study. J Thorac Cardiovasc Surg 1987; 94: 773–83.

52. Balsano F, Rizzon P, Violi F, et al. Antiplatelet treatment with ticlopidine in unstable angina. Circulation 1990; 82: 17–26.

53. Nichol ES, Phillips WC, Casten GG. Virtue of prompt anticoagulant therapy in impending myocardial infarction: experiences with 318 patients during a 10-year period. Am Intern Med 1959; 50: 1158–73.

54. Gifford RH, Feinstein AR. A critique of methodology in studies of anticoagulant therapy for acute myocardial infarction. N Engl J Med 1969; 280: 351–7.

55. Chapman I. The cause-effect relationship between recent coronary artery occlusion and acute myocardial infarction. Am Heart J 1974; 87: 267.

56. Drapkin A, Merskey C. Anticoagulant therapy after acute myocardial infarction: relation of therapeutic benefit to patient's age, sex, and severity of infarction. JAMA 1972; 222: 541–8.

57. Report of the Working Party on Anticoagulation Therapy in Coronary Thrombosis to the Medical Research Council. Assessment of short-term anticoagulant administration after cardiac infarction. Br Med J 1969; 1: 335–42.

58. Anticoagulants in acute myocardial infarction. Results of a cooperative clinical trial. JAMA 1973; 225: 724–9.

59. Chalmers TC, Motta RJ, Smith H Jr, Kunzler A-M. Evidence favouring the use of anticoagulants in the hospital phase of acute myocardial infarction. N Engl J Med 1977; 297: 1091–6.

60. Dalen JE, Goldberg RJ, Gore JM, Struckus J. Therapeutic interventions in acute myocardial infarction. Survey of the ACCP Section on Clinical Cardiology. Chest 1984; 86(2):257–62.

61. Telford AM, Wilson C. Trial of heparin versus atenolol in prevention of myocardial infarction in intermediate coronary syndrome. Lancet 1981; 1: 1225–8.

62. Williams DO, Kirby MG, McPherson K, Phear DN. Anticoagulant treatment in unstable angina. Br J Clin Pract 1896; 40: 114–6.

63. Neri Serneri GG, Abbate R, Prisco D, et al. Decrease in frequency of original episodes by control of thrombin generation with low-dose heparin: a controlled cross-over randomized study. Am Heart J 1988; 115: 60–6.

64. Neri Serneri GG, Gensini GF, Poggesi L, et al. Effect of heparin, aspirin, or alteplase in reduction of myocardial ischaemia in refractory unstable angina. Lancet 1990; 335: 615–8.

65. UK-TIA Study Group, United Kingdom transient ischemic attack (UK-TIA) aspirin Trial: interim results. Br Med J 1988; 296: 316–20.

66. Eisenberg PR. Role of new anticoagulants as adjunctive therapy during thrombolysis. Am J Cardiol 1991; 67: 19A–24A.

67. Gold HK, Coller BS, Yasuda T, et al. Rapid and sustained coronary artery recanalization with combined bolus injection of recombinant tissue-type plasminogen activator and monoclonal antiplatelet GP IIb/IIIa antibody in a canine preparation. Circulation 1988; 77: 670–1.

68. Holmes DR Jr, Hartzler GO, Smith HC, Fuster V. Coronary artery thrombosis in patients with unstable angina. Br Heart J 1981; 45: 411–6.

69. Zack PM, Ischinger T, Aker UT, Dincer B, Kennedy HL. The occurrence of angiographically detected intracoronary thrombus in patients with unstable angina pectoris. Am Heart J 1984; 108: 1408–11.

70. Vetrovec GW, Cowley MJ, Overton BA, Richardson DW. Intracoronary thrombus in syndromes of unstable myocardial ischemia. Am Heart J 1981; 102: 1202–8.

71. Capone G, Wolf NM, Meyer B, Meister SG. Frequency of intracoronary filling defects by angiography in angina pectoris at rest. Am J Cardiol 1985; 56: 403–6.

72. Vetrovec GW, Leinbach RC, Gold HK, Cowley MJ. Intracoronary thrombolysis in syndromes of unstable angina: angiographic and clinical results. Am Heart J 1982; 104: 946–52.

73. Gold HK, Johns JA, Leinbach RC, et al. A randomized, blinded, placebo-controlled trial of recombinant human tissue-type plasminogen activator in patients with unstable angina pectoris. Circulation 1987; 75: 1192–9.

74. Topol EJ, Nicklas JM, Kander NH, et al. Coronary revascularization after intravenous tissue plasminogen activator for unstable angina pectoris: results of a randomized, double-blind, placebo-controlled trial. Am J Cardiol 1988; 62: 368–71.

75. Schreiber TL, Macina G, McNulty A, et al. Urokinase plus heparin versus aspirin in unstable angina and non-Q-wave myocardial infarction. Am J Cardiol 1989; 64: 840–4.

76. Williams DO, Topol EJ, Califf RM, et al. Intravenous recombinant tissue-type plasminogen activator in patients with unstable angina pectoris. Circulation 1990; 82: 376–83.

77. Ardissino D, Barberis P, De Servi S, et al. Recombinant tissue-type plasminogen activator followed by heparin compared with heparin alone for refractory unstable angina pectoris. Am J Cardiol 1990; 66: 910–4.

78. Gotoh K, Minamino T, Katoh O, et al. The role of intracoronary thrombus in unstable angina: angiographic assessment and thrombolytic therapy during ongoing anginal attacks. Circulation 1988; 77: 526–34.

79. de Zwaan C, Bär FW, Janssen JHA, de Swart HB, Vermeer F, Wellens HJJ. Effects of thrombolytic therapy in unstable angina: clinical and angiographic results. J Am Coll Cardiol 1988; 12: 301–9.

80. Rentrop P, Blanke H, Karsch KR, Kaiser H, Kostering H, Leitz K. Selective intracoronary thrombolysis in acute myocardial infarction and unstable angina pectoris. Circulation 1981; 63: 307–17.

81. Mandelkorn JB, Wolf NM, Singh S, et al. Intracoronary thrombus in non-transmural myocardial infarction and in unstable angina pectoris. Am J Cardiol 1983; 52: 1–6.
82. Ambrose JA, Hjemdahl-Monsen C, Borriro S, et al. Quantitative and qualitative effects of intracoronary streptokinase in unstable angina and non-Q-wave infarction. J Am Coll Cardiol 1987; 9: 1156–65.
83. Lawrence JR, Shepherd JT, Bone I, Roger AS, Fulton WFM. Fibrinolytic therapy in unstable angina pectoris. A controlled clinical trial. Thromb Res 1980; 17: 767–77.
84. Cairns JA, Collins R, Fuster V, Passamani ER. Coronary thrombolysis. Chest 1989; 95: 73S–87S.
85. Ambrose JA, Alexopoulos D. Thrombolysis in unstable angina: will the beneficial effects of thrombolytic therapy in myocardial infarction apply to patients with unstable angina? J Am Coll Cardiol 1989; 13: 1666–71.
86. The Steering Committee of the Physician's Health Study Research Group. Final report on the aspirin component of the ongoing Physician's Health Study. N Engl J Med 1989; 321: 129–35.

14

ANTIPLATELET AND ANTICOAGULANT THERAPY IN EVOLVING MYOCARDIAL INFARCTION AND PRIMARY PREVENTION

PATRICIA HEBERT, VALENTIN FUSTER, and
CHARLES H. HENNEKENS

In recent years more reliable data have become available on the benefits of treatment with antiplatelet and anticoagulant drugs for patients with acute evolving myocardial infarction. While the net benefit of antiplatelet therapy is clearly documented, that of anticoagulants is less clear, due at least in part to the higher risks of bleeding. Further, the recently demonstrated benefits and risks of thrombolytic therapy for acute myocardial infarction have raised the question of the added net benefit of adjunctive antithrombotic therapy with either antiplatelet or anticoagulant drugs or both. Finally, recent data have emerged concerning the benefits and risks of antiplatelet therapy in primary prevention of acute myocardial infarction.

ANTIPLATELET AND ANTICOAGULANT THERAPY IN ACUTE MYOCARDIAL INFARCTION

Antiplatelet Therapy

The efficacy of aspirin therapy for evolving myocardial infarction has been demonstrated conclusively in data from a single large-scale trial, the Second International Study of Infarct Survival (ISIS-2).[1] Using a placebo-controlled 2 × 2 factorial design that permitted an evaluation of aspirin alone, as well as streptokinase alone and in combination, the trial randomized 17,187 patients presenting within 24 hours of symptoms, to either a single dose of 162 milligrams of oral aspirin daily for 30 days, 1.5 million units of intravenous streptokinase given over 60 minutes, both, or neither.

The primary endpoint, total vascular mortality, was reduced 23 per cent by aspirin (95 per cent confidence interval: −30 to −15 per cent, $p < 0.00001$) (Table 14–1). The decrease in vascular deaths was similar whether aspirin therapy was initiated 0 to 4 hours (25 per cent), 5 to 12 hours (21 per cent) or 13 to 24 hours (21 per cent) after the onset of clinical symptoms. There were also highly significant reductions for nonfatal reinfarction of 49 per cent and for nonfatal stroke of 46 per cent. For bleeds requiring transfusion, there were no significant differences between the aspirin and placebo groups (0.4 per cent versus 0.4 per cent), although there was a small significant absolute increase of minor bleeds (0.6 per cent, $p < 0.01$) among those allocated to aspirin.

While ISIS-2 provides reliable data about the efficacy of aspirin therapy for acute myocardial infarction, the best dose, frequency of administration, and rate of release for achieving the optimal net benefit on reinfarction, stroke, and vascular death are yet to be determined.

261

TABLE 14–1. Indirect Comparisons of Antiplatelet (Aspirin) and Anticoagulant Therapy in Acute MI: Percent reductions in vascular events observed*

ENDPOINTS	ASPIRIN (ISIS-2)	ANTICOAGULANTS[†]	HEPARIN[‡]
Nonfatal reinfarction	49% ± 9		22% ± 10
Nonfatal stroke	46% ± 17		51% ± 16
Vascular mortality	23% ± 4		
Any vascular event	28% ± 4		21% ± 5
Death		22% ± 7	16% ± 7

* Values are percentage reductions ± standard deviations.
† From overview by Chalmers and others[5–8] of any anticoagulant.
‡ From overview by MacMahon and others[9] of trials of intravenous or subcutaneous heparin.

Basic research is needed to determine the optimal regimen for controlling thromboxane while also sparing prostacyclin and minimizing the occurrence of side effects. The clinical relevance of prostacyclin sparing requires further elucidation. In addition, clinical research is necessary to determine the optimal loading dose during evolving myocardial infarction to achieve the most rapid clinical antithrombotic effect. In this regard, it has been shown that a single dose of aspirin needs to be at least 2 milligrams/kilogram, or about 150 milligrams in a typical male, to produce rapid near-total inhibition of thromboxane metabolites.[2–4] Lower daily doses (for example, 40 to 80 milligrams) take a few days to reach their full antiplatelet effect. These data suggest that to ensure a near-maximal antiplatelet effect of aspirin on the first day, treatment in acute myocardial infarction should be initiated with at least 162 milligrams as in ISIS-2 or even 325 milligrams as in the Gruppo Italiano per lo Studio della Sopravvivenza nell'Infarto Miocardico (GISSI-2).

Anticoagulant Therapy

The efficacy of anticoagulant therapy in evolving myocardial infarction derives primarily from trials of smaller sample size conducted several decades ago. Anticoagulants, in particular heparin, were found to produce a treatment benefit similar in magnitude to that of aspirin.

Thirty-two trials, including approximately 16,000 subjects, were conducted between 1948 and 1973 to assess the efficacy of anticoagulants in the treatment of acute myocardial infarction.[5–7] Twenty-six, all conducted prior to about 1962, used historical controls or nonrandom allocation procedures, mainly alternate allocation schemes. Thus, only six of the 32 trials were strictly randomized. Greater therapeutic benefits were reported in the studies with historical controls or nonrandom allocation procedures than in the randomized trials. The six strictly randomized trials, which included about 3,800 subjects,[5] tested heparin, warfarin (coumadin), and phenindione, either alone or in combination. These data showed statistically significant reductions in overall mortality of 21 per cent ($p < 0.001$) in the initial review, and a 22 per cent reduction (95 per cent confidence interval: −35 to −8 per cent)[8] in a more recent meta-analysis or overview of the same data (Table 14–1).

An overview restricted to heparin alone, given either intravenously or subcutaneously, which included approximately 5,700 subjects showed a 16 per cent reduction in mortality. This effect was similar to the magnitude of the reduction found in a previous overview of all anticoagulant agents (Table 14–1); however, the 95 per cent confidence interval for this reduction is wide, ranging from about zero to about one-third. This overview also suggested that heparin given during the acute phase of myocardial infarction will reduce reinfarction by 22 per cent and stroke by about 51 per cent, but again the 95 per cent confidence intervals are wide.

Comparisons of Antiplatelet and Anticoagulant Therapy in Acute Myocardial Infarction

When comparing the risk reductions in acute myocardial infarction associated with aspirin and anticoagulant therapy, the beneficial effects on mortality appear similar: a 23 per cent reduction in vascular mortality in ISIS-2 versus a 16 to 22 per cent reduction in overall mortality in the overviews of all anticoagulants or, specifically, of heparin, in acute myocardial infarction (Table 14–1).

The risk reductions for aspirin, however, are based on a single large-scale randomized trial of adequate sample size, while those for anticoagulants are based on an overview of numerous smaller trials, most of which were conducted 20 to 30 years ago when methodology was far less rigorous and treatment options in coronary care units far more restricted.

Of greatest importance, however, is the risk of bleeding, which is greater with anticoagulants than with aspirin. However, unlike secondary prevention among survivors where antithrombotic treatment, especially with aspirin, is likely to be given alone, these agents are unlikely to be used as sole treatments in acute myocardial infarction. A major shift in considerations of therapy of acute myocardial infarction has come with the recently established efficacy of thrombolytic agents with and without aspirin and heparin. Since antithrombotic therapy with either or both antiplatelet and anticoagulant drugs may be considered as adjunctive management options, it is important to consider risks and benefits of combined therapy.

ANTIPLATELET OR ANTICOAGULANT THERAPY WITH THROMBOLYSIS

Available data demonstrate conclusively that all three thrombolytic agents in common use—streptokinase (SK), recombinant tissue plasminogen activator (rt-PA), and anisoylated plasminogen streptokinase activator complex (APSAC)—are effective in improving ventricular function and reducing mortality in acute myocardial infarction. Indirect comparisons of the mortality results for patients presenting within six hours of pain onset in the major studies of SK,[1,10,11] of rt-PA,[12] and of APSAC[13,14] indicate a 27 per cent reduction overall with no statistically significant differences among the three drugs.[4] Further, ISIS-3 will provide direct comparisons of the three drugs.[15]

The expanding use of thrombolytics has led to increased interest in the concomitant use of antiplatelet and anticoagulant drugs primarily to reduce the high incidence of reocclusion with these agents (see also Chapter 16). However, a major concern is that more aggressive antithrombotic regimens, particularly when given in combination with thrombolytic agents, may result in an increased incidence of bleeding, especially hemorrhagic strokes.

To date, several published trials have raised the possibility of added net benefits of either or both antiplatelet and anticoagulant drugs. In particular, the use of factorial designs permitted the concomitant evaluation of aspirin or heparin, sometimes alone, or in combination. (See also Chapters 16 and 17.)

Aspirin Added to Thrombolytic Therapy

Conclusive data on the additional net benefit of antiplatelet to thrombolytic therapy comes from ISIS-2.[1] The beneficial effects of aspirin and SK appear to be largely independent of each other, and their combined benefits appear additive. Patients allocated to both agents had a 42 per cent reduction in vascular mortality (95 per cent confidence interval: -50 to -34 per cent, $p < 0.00001$) (Fig. 14–1). Aspirin alone yielded a 23 per cent reduction (95 per cent confidence interval: -30 to -15 per cent) while SK was associated with a 25 per cent reduction (95 per cent confidence interval: -32 to -18 per cent). When treatment with both aspirin and SK was initiated within six hours of the onset of symptoms, the reduction in total vascular mortality was 53 per cent. The combination of aspirin and SK produced significantly fewer reinfarctions than those allocated to SK alone or to no active treatment (1.8 per cent in the combined treatment versus 2.9 per cent in those on no active treatment versus 3.8 per cent in those allocated to SK alone).

The combination of aspirin and SK, like aspirin alone, was associated with a reduction in strokes (0.6 per cent in the combined treatment versus 1.1 per cent in those on no active treatment). Further, there was no significant difference in the frequency of major bleeds; that is, those requiring transfusion, with the addition of aspirin (0.6 per cent in the combined treatment versus 0.5 per cent in the SK, 0.4 per cent in the aspirin, and 0.3 per cent in those on no active treatment).

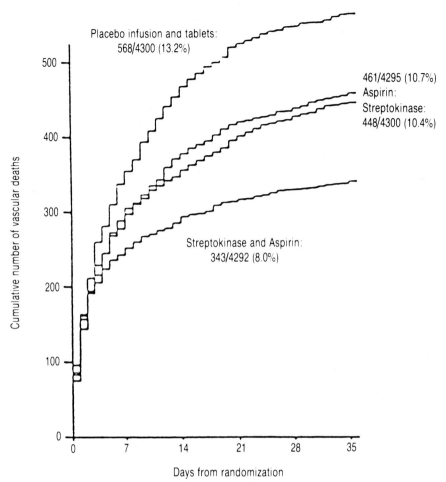

FIGURE 14–1. Cumulative vascular mortality in days 0–35 in patients allocated to streptokinase only, aspirin only, both active treatments, and neither. Data derived from the ISIS-2 (Second International Study of Infarct Survival) Collaborative Group. Randomized trial of intravenous streptokinase, oral aspirin, both, or neither among 17,187 cases of suspected acute myocardial infarction: ISIS-2. Lancet 1988;2: 349–60.

Anticoagulants Added to Thrombolytic Therapy

The two trials of anticoagulants as adjunctive treatment[16,17] have looked at the effect of heparin added to thrombolytic therapy with rt-PA on patency. Heparin was shown to provide no added benefit in one trial[16] assessing early (90-minute) patency, but did appear beneficial in another trial[17] assessing patency at two to three days. In particular, Topol[16] randomized 134 patients within six hours of the onset of symptoms to receive rt-PA alone or rt-PA plus intravenous heparin, 10,000 units bolus administered concurrently with thrombolytic therapy. The

patency rates 90 minutes after initiation of therapy were the same (79 per cent) in the two groups (Table 14–2). Predischarge left ventricular function was also similar in the two groups (50.2 per cent in the rt-PA alone group versus 49.0 per cent in the rt-PA plus heparin group). Bleeding requiring transfusion was not significantly different in the two groups (18 per cent in the rt-PA alone group and 13 per cent in the rt-PA plus heparin group).

However, another trial assessing patency at a later time interval found the possibility of an added benefit of heparin. Bleich et al.[17] randomized 84 patients admitted within six hours of the onset of symptoms to receive

TABLE 14–2. Angiographic Patency Studies:
Intraveous Heparin Added to Thrombolytic Therapy with rt-PA

	PATENCY RATES		P VALUE
	Heparin Plus rt-PA	*rt-PA Alone*	
Topol, et al.[16]			
Angiograph at 90 minutes*	79%	79%	NS
Bleich, et al.[17]			
Angiograph at mean of 57 hours†	71%	43%	0.015

 * Heparin: 10,000 units intravenous bolus administered concurrently with rt-PA.
 † Heparin: 5,000 units intravenous bolus and then 1,000 units per hour titrated to 1.5 to 2.0 times partial thromboplastin time control administered concurrently with rt-PA until angiography.
 Aspirin not given in these two trials.
 NS = not significant.

rt-PA alone or rt-PA plus concurrent intravenous heparin (5,000 units bolus and then 1,000 units/hour titrated to 1.5 to 2 times the partial thromboplastin time control). As shown in Table 14–2, angiography performed at a mean of 57 hours following therapy showed a higher patency rate in the group receiving heparin (71 per cent versus 43 per cent, $p = 0.015$). There was no difference in recurrent ischemia or reocclusion up to seven days after myocardial infarction (11.9 per cent in those treated with rt-PA alone and 7.1 per cent in those with rt-PA plus heparin). Bleeding complications were more common in the group receiving heparin. Moderate or severe bleeding occurred in 2 per cent of the rt-PA alone as compared to 12 per cent in the rt-PA plus heparin group ($p = 0.21$). Since early patency rates do not seem to be surrogates for mortality, comparative trials with this endpoint are needed to provide definitive information on whether there is a net benefit or hazard of adding concurrent intravenous heparin to rt-PA during acute myocardial infarction.

Antiplatelet Therapy Versus Anticoagulants Added to Thrombolytic Therapy

Two patency trials[18,19] directly comparing antiplatelets versus anticoagulants added to thrombolytic therapy have also been conducted. One other study examined infarct size and ventricular function with rt-PA, aspirin, and heparin, as compared to aspirin and heparin alone.

The Heparin-Aspirin Reperfusion Trial (HART)[18] directly compared early intravenous heparin versus low-dose oral aspirin added to thrombolytic therapy with rt-PA. Coronary patency rates were found to be higher with early concomitant treatment with intravenous heparin than with 80 milligrams aspirin, a dose inadequate to achieve a rapid clinical antithrombotic effect. Patients were randomly assigned to receive either immediate (5,000 units bolus) and then continuous intravenous heparin (1,000 units/hour adjusted to maintain partial thromboplastin time at 1.5 to 2 times baseline) (n = 106) or immediate and then daily oral aspirin (80 milligrams) (n = 99) together with rt-PA initiated within six hours of the onset of symptoms. As shown in Table 14–3, patency rates at 7 to 24 hours after beginning therapy were higher in the heparin than in the aspirin group (82 per cent versus 52 per cent, respectively, $p < .0001$). However, at one week when even this low dose of aspirin would have achieved a substantial antithrombotic effect, patency rates in the initially patent vessels were 88 per cent in the heparin group as compared to 95 per cent in the aspirin group ($p = 0.17$). The numbers of bleeds (18 in the heparin and 15 in the aspirin group, $p = 0.72$) were similar. Recurrent ischemic events were more frequent in the heparin group (eight versus two), but this difference did not achieve statistical significance ($p = 0.16$).

In an Australian study,[19] patients enrolled within four hours of symptoms and treated with rt-PA and intravenous heparin for 24 hours were randomly assigned to continue receiving intravenous heparin (n = 99) or to receive aspirin (300 milligrams) plus dipyridamole (300 milligrams) daily (n = 103) for

TABLE 14–3. Angiographic Patency Studies: Direct Comparisons of Antiplatelets Versus Heparin Added to Thrombolytic Therapy with rt-PA

	PATENCY RATES		
	Heparin	*Antiplatelets*	*P* VALUE
Hart Trial[18]			
Angiography at 7 to 24 hours*	82%	52%	<0.0001
Angiography at one week of initially patent vessels	88%	95%	NS
Australian Study[19]†			
Angiography at one week	81.1%	80.2%	NS

* Heparin: Immediate 5,000-unit bolus and then continuous intravenous heparin until second angiography to maintain partial thromboplastin time at 1.5 to 2 times baseline; Aspirin: Immediate and then daily oral aspirin (80 milligrams).

† All patients received intravenous heparin for 24 hours and then were randomly assigned to continue intravenous heparin or to receive aspirin (300 milligrams) plus dipyridamole (300 milligrams) daily.

NS = not significant.

one week. Patency rates at seven to ten days were similar in the groups (81.1 per cent in those on heparin and 80.2 per cent in those on aspirin plus dipyridamole) (Table 14–3). Further, in these patients, the lumen was reduced by 69 ± 2% of normal in the heparin and 67 ± 2% in the aspirin plus dipyridamole group. Mortality and reinfarction rates were both more favorable in the aspirin plus dipyridamole than in the heparin group (two versus five deaths, and two versus five reinfarctions, p = 0.09 for both events). Left ventricular ejection fractions at one month were similar in the two groups (52.4 per cent in the heparin and 51.9 per cent in the aspirin plus dipyridamole group). Thus, this trial suggests that after 24 hours, an antiplatelet regimen is at least as effective as intravenous heparin in maintaining vessel patency, preserving left ventricular function, and preventing reocclusion.

A European Cooperative Study Group (ECSG) trial[20,21] compared the efficacy of treatment with rt-PA, aspirin, and heparin versus aspirin and heparin alone on infarct size and left ventricular function in 721 patients. Treatment was administered within five hours of the onset of symptoms. There were significant reductions in enzymatic infarct size, higher left ventricular ejection fractions, and reductions in diastolic volume and end systolic volume in those treated with rt-PA, aspirin, and heparin. Although deaths were reported, the ECSG trial was not designed to examine mortality, and thus the reported risk reductions are based on small numbers of deaths. There were 47 total deaths, 18 in patients allocated to the three drugs and 29 in those allocated to aspirin

and heparin. At two weeks, the reduction in mortality was 51 per cent (95 per cent confidence interval: −76 to +1 per cent), and at three months it was 36 per cent (95 per cent confidence interval: −63 to +13 per cent) among those receiving rt-PA, aspirin, and heparin as compared to those receiving aspirin and heparin alone. Because of the small number of deaths, the confidence intervals are wide, and at neither individual point in time did the reduction in risk of death achieve conventional levels of statistical significance.

Combined Antiplatelet and Anticoagulant Therapy with Thrombolysis

Because ISIS-2 demonstrated the efficacy of aspirin added to thrombolytic therapy, there has been great interest in determining whether heparin added to a regimen of aspirin and thrombolytic therapy confers an additional net benefit. The European Cooperative Study Group (ECSG-6) trial,[22] a patency study, randomized patients to intravenous rt-PA, aspirin and concomitant intravenous heparin or to rt-PA, aspirin, and heparin placebo. Six hundred fifty-two patients, age 21 to 70 years, were randomized within six hours of the onset of symptoms to rt-PA (100 milligrams) plus aspirin (250 to 300 milligrams followed by 75 to 125 milligrams every other day) plus immediate intravenous heparin (5,000 units bolus followed by 1,000 units/hour) versus the same rt-PA plus aspirin regimen and heparin placebo. Patency rates at 48 to 120 hours (mean 81 hours) were 83.4 per cent in the heparin group as compared to 74.7 per cent in the placebo group ($p = 0.02$). There were no significant differences between the groups in mortality, enzymatic infarct size, recurrent ischemic episodes, or bleeding complications.

The Gruppo Italiano per lo Studio della Sopravvivenza nell'Infarto Miocardico (GISSI-2)[23] and its international extension[24] are the largest mortality trials currently reported in the peer-reviewed literature and provide reliable information about combined antiplatelet and anticoagulant therapy with thrombolysis. These randomized trials directly compared the efficacy of two thrombolytic agents -SK and rt-PA- and also tested whether there are additional net benefits of adding anticoagulation with delayed subcutaneous heparin to low-dose aspirin therapy with thrombolysis. Using a 2 × 2 factorial design, these studies examined the efficacy of rt-PA versus SK and heparin versus no heparin in 20,891 patients randomized to a standard three-hour regimen of rt-PA or a standard 30 to 60 minute regimen of SK. All patients received 300–325 milligrams of aspirin daily, starting at the time of randomization so that it would already have a substantial antithrombotic effect by the time the rt-PA infusion ended. In addition, half of each group were allocated to 12,500 international units subcutaneous heparin twice daily, starting 12 hours after randomization to avoid any undue risk of hemorrhage. There were no clear differences in overall mortality demonstrated between the two thrombolytic agents. There was, however, an apparent nonsignificant ($p = 0.29$) decrease in mortality in those allocated to heparin (8.5 per cent) compared to the nonheparin group

(9.0 per cent). There were no differences in reinfarction and overall stroke in the heparin plus aspirin as compared to the aspirin alone group (Table 14–4) But despite the moderateness of the effects on activated partial thromboplastin time (APTT) and the delayed start of the heparin regimen, the incidence of bleeds requiring transfusion (1.0 per cent versus 0.6 per cent, $p = 0.0002$) was doubled in the heparin group. This randomized comparison is consistent with subgroup data from ISIS-2, which also indicate that heparin increases the risk of bleeding when given in conjunction with thrombolytic therapy. Specifically, for those receiving SK with aspirin, the frequency of bleeds requiring transfusion were lowest among those receiving no heparin, intermediate among those given delayed subcutaneous heparin, and highest among those getting immediate intravenous heparin. Since this subgroup analysis was not a randomized comparison, the finding must be interpreted cautiously.

Using the GISSI-2 data (Table 14–4), it is possible to consider the number of events per 1,000 patients. For mortality, the apparent additional reduction associated with heparin (which was not statistically significant) was 5 deaths per 1,000 (Table 14–5). For major bleeds requiring transfusion, heparin was associated with 4 more events per 1,000 patients. For cerebral bleeds, there was one excess event per 1,000 patients and reinfarction was reduced by heparin by about one per 1,000.

It has been suggested that the delay in heparin treatment until 12 hours after the initiation of thrombolytic treatment as opposed to an immediate intravenous administration may have affected the results and,

TABLE 14–4. Main In-Hospital Results of GISSI-2 and Its International Extension: Subcutaneous Heparin Added to Thrombolytic Therapy Plus Aspirin*

Events in Hospital	Heparin plus Aspirin (n = 10,361)	Aspirin Alone (n = 10,407)	p Value
All Deaths	884 (8.5%)	932 (9.0%)	0.29
Deaths after 12 hours	537 (5.2%)	606 (5.8%)	0.05
Reinfarction	285 (2.8%)	303 (2.9%)	0.51
Stroke	117 (1.1%)	119 (1.1%)	0.98
Transfused bleed	103 (1.0%)	57 (0.6%)	0.0002

* Data Derived from Gruppo Italiano perlo Studio della Sopravvivenza Nell'Infarto Miocardico. GISSI-2. A factorial randomized trial of rt-PA versus streptokinase and heparin versus no heparin among 12,490 patients with acute myocardial infarction. Lancet 1990; 336: 65–71; and The International Study Group. In-hospital mortality and clinical course of 20,891 patients with suspected acute myocardial infarction randomised between rt-PA and streptokinase with or without heparin. Lancet 1990; 336: 71–5, with permission.

TABLE 14–5. Summary of GISSI-2 Results: Absolute Differences per 1,000 Patients Allocated to (Subcutaneous) Heparin Plus Aspirin Versus Aspirin Alone

Deaths	−5
Transfused bleeds	+4
Cerebral bleeds	+1
Reinfarctions	−1

if so, resulted in less favorable mortality reductions with rt-PA relative to SK. The main basis for the objection is the different physiologic action of rt-PA. Unlike SK and APSAC, rt-PA activates plasminogen efficiently only when bound to fibrin, so, although rt-PA dissolves thrombi, it produces less marked depletion of circulating fibrinogen than SK or APSAC. In addition, rt-PA has a shorter life in the circulation; consequently, the possibility has been raised that the most advantageous adjunctive regimen may differ among the different thrombolytic agents. On the other hand, the greater clot lysing ability of rt-PA might also lead to increased hemorrhage, particularly into the brain. In fact, earlier higher doses of rt-PA had to be abandoned because of an unacceptably high risk of cerebral hemorrhage of about 15 per 1,000. The current regimens of rt-PA, SK and APSAC all have demonstrated more acceptable cerebral hemorrhage rates which range from about 5 to 6 per 1,000 treated patients with about a 50% case fatality ratio. At present, it remains unclear whether immediate intravenous administration of heparin offers a net benefit or risk over a delayed regimen, whether intravenous or subcutaneous, until at least after the administration of the thrombolytic agent during evolving myocardial infarction. In order to directly test this hypothesis, a randomized trial is needed with mortality and stroke as endpoints in which aspirin is given to all patients and intravenous heparin administered concurrently with either rt-PA, SK, or APSAC, and compared to delayed administration of heparin.

The Third International Study of Infarct Survival (ISIS-3) is the most recent and largest mortality trial[15] conducted on the combined use of thrombolytic agents, aspirin, and heparin. Final results of this trial have not yet been reported. This randomized trial compared the efficacy of three thrombolytic agents—SK, rt-PA and APSAC—and, in a factorial design, also tested the additional benefit of adding anticoagulation with sub-

cutaneous heparin to low-dose aspirin therapy. All patients in the trial received one month of daily aspirin (162 milligrams). Participants (n = 46,092) with a suspected or definite myocardial infarction were enrolled within 24 hours of the onset of symptoms.

The factorial design also allowed the comparison of the effects of adding heparin (a seven-day fixed-dose course of 12,500 international units administered subcutaneously every 12 hours and begun four hours after randomization) to a one-month daily regimen of aspirin.

Because both GISSI-2 and ISIS-3 examined the benefit of anticoagulation with subcutaneous heparin (after 12 hours or four hours, respectively) added to a regimen of thrombolysis and aspirin therapy, it will be possible to summarize treatment benefits and side effects of therapy across these trials. However, it should be noted that the brand of rt-PA used in ISIS-3 (duteplase) is different from that used in GISSI-2 (alteplase). While duteplase is a predominantly double-chained molecule and the current form of alteplase is single-chained, they have virtually identical 90 minute patency rates (4). Further, based on biologic activity the dosages used were the same. However, based on the gravimetric amounts of material used, the average dose of duteplase was 50 per cent higher than that of alteplase. In the absence of comparative studies between these agents their equivalence for therapeutic purposes (biologic activity in standard clot lysis assays versus their gravimetric amounts) remains unknown.

An overview of the GISSI-2 and ISIS-3 data will provide the most up-to-date and reliable estimates of combined antiplatelet and delayed anticoagulant therapy with thrombolysis. The evaluation of the risks and benefits of immediate versus delayed anticoagulant therapy with antiplatelet therapy and thrombolysis will be determined in a recently begun trial, Global Utilization of SK and rt-PA (GUSTO) for SK but not for rt-PA or APSAC. Further trials will be necessary to resolve the issue of the optimal timing for heparin and whether this differs among the three thrombolytic agents.

ANTIPLATELET THERAPY IN THE PRIMARY PREVENTION OF MYOCARDIAL INFARCTION

Because aspirin had been found to have a significant protective effect in secondary prevention of vascular disease, the possible benefit of aspirin in primary prevention has also been tested. Two randomized trials, the United States Physicians' Health Study[25,26] and the British Doctors' Trial[27] have addressed this question.

The United States Physicians' Health Study[25,26] is a large, double-blind, placebo-controlled trial of 325 milligrams of aspirin taken every other day, conducted among 22,071 United States male physicians, age 40 to 84 years at baseline. At an average of 60.2 months of treatment and follow-up, the randomized aspirin component was terminated early due primarily to the emergence of a statistically extreme 44 per cent reduction in risk of a first myocardial infarction. The number of vascular deaths and total strokes was insufficient upon which to judge whether

there was a possible increase in hemorrhagic strokes. There were, however, 23 hemorrhagic strokes in the aspirin group and 12 in the placebo group ($p = 0.06$).

The British Doctors' Trial,[27] which tested 500 milligrams of aspirin daily among 5,139 male physicians aged 50 to 78 years at baseline, had an open design. Those randomized to the control group were asked to avoid aspirin and aspirin-containing products rather than taking a placebo. At six years of follow-up, there were no significant differences between the treatment groups in the incidence of myocardial infarction, stroke, total cardiovascular mortality, or the combined endpoint of important vascular events (Fig. 14–2). However, when strokes were divided by etiology as well as by the severity of residual disability for nonfatal events, the

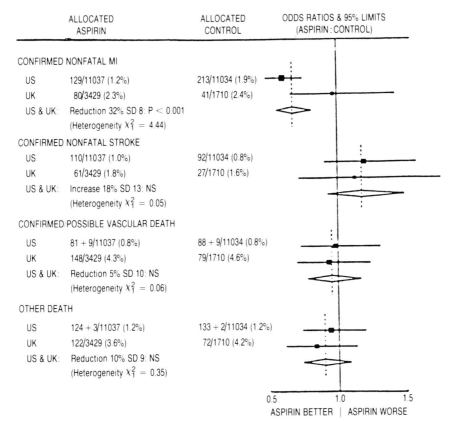

FIGURE 14–2. Overviews of United States[26] and United Kingdom[27] primary prevention trial results for four endpoints: odds ratios (aspirin versus control), overall risk reductions, and heterogeneity tests[30] (sum of four heterogeneity Chi square tests = 4.9, nonsignificant.) For comparability between the two trials, "vascular" deaths include all circulatory causes (9th ICD 390–459), gastric ulcer or hemorrhage (530–535, 578), and sudden or unknown causes (798, 799). For the United States trial, this includes the 94.8 per cent of deaths confirmed as of the final report (81 versus 83). We have also added to the United States trial all reported and unrefuted vascular deaths to date (9 versus 9), including two in the placebo group, which, as fatal lower gastrointestinal hemorrhages, had been classified as nonvascular in the final report (ICD 530–535, 578). Data derived from Hennekens CH, Buring JE, Sandercock P, Collins R, Peto R. Aspirin and other antiplatelet agents in the secondary and primary prevention of cardiovascular disease. Circulation 1989;80:749–56, by permission of the American Heart Association, Inc.

only significant finding was an increased risk of disabling strokes among those assigned to aspirin ($p = 0.05$). This could either reflect more hemorrhagic strokes (which tend to be more severe) among those taking aspirin, or bias resulting from the subjective nature of self-reports of residual impairment in an unblinded trial.

These two primary prevention trials had a number of differences in their designs which may have influenced their results. First, with respect to dose and frequency of administration, the United States trial tested a lower dose of 325 milligrams given every other day, whereas the British trial had a higher dose (500 milligrams) of aspirin administered daily, which could have contributed to the higher level of side effects in the British trial. In addition, the double-blind and placebo-controlled design of the United States trial may have allowed for more unbiased assessments of nonfatal events. On the other hand, the level of compliance appeared similar in the two trials.[28] In the United States trial, 86 per cent of the aspirin group took the drug, and 14 per cent in the placebo group took aspirin at 60.2 months of follow-up, resulting in a difference of 72 per cent in the proportions using aspirin. In the British trial, 70 per cent of those allocated to aspirin reported taking the drug, and 2 per cent of those assigned to aspirin avoidance took aspirin, resulting in a difference of 68 per cent in the proportions using aspirin after 36 months of follow-up.

Probably the most important difference between the two trials, however, is the much larger sample size of the United States trial (22,071 versus 5,139). This resulted in a much greater number of myocardial infarctions in the United States study. However, the number of cardiovascular deaths in the two studies were similar because the rates in the United States trial were so extraordinarily low, and in addition, the British doctors were older. As shown in Figure 14–2, an overview[29] of the results of these two trials demonstrated an overall 33 per cent reduction in nonfatal myocardial infarction that was highly significant ($p < 0.0002$).

Side Effects of Aspirin

In primary prevention, side effects are particularly important, since treatment is administered prophylactically to individuals with no prior history of vascular diseases. For aspirin, the most reliable data concerning side effects derives from the United Kingdom trial of transient ischemic attacks[31] which tested two daily dosages of aspirin versus placebo among 2,345 patients. It was therefore possible to compare directly the frequencies of side effects reported at 300 and 1,200 milligrams/day. As shown in Table 14–6, there was a dose response for each category of side effect including: indigestion, nausea, heartburn, or vomiting; constipation; any gastrointestinal bleeding; and serious gastro-

TABLE 14–6. UK-TIA Trial: Percentage of Patients Ever Reporting Gastrointestinal Side Effects (Mean, Four-Year Follow-Up)

	ALLOCATED TREATMENT			STATISTICAL SIGNIFICANCE OF DIFFERENCE (2 p)	
	Placebo (n = 814)	Aspirin 300 Milligrams/Day (n = 806)	Aspirin 1200 Milligrams/Day (n = 815)	Placebo Versus Both Aspirin	300 Milligrams Versus 1200 Milligrams Aspirin
Indigestion, nausea, heartburn, or vomiting	24.3	29.4	38.8	<0.001	<0.001
Constipation	2.3	5.6	6.0	<0.001	NS
Any gastrointestinal bleed	1.6	2.6	4.7	<0.01	<0.05
Serious gastrointestinal bleed (requiring hospitalization)	0.9	1.5	2.3	<0.05	NS

NS = not significant.
Data derived from the UK-TIA Study Group. United Kingdom transient ischaemic attack (UK-TIA) aspirin trial: interim results. Br Med J 1988;269:316–320.

intestinal bleeding. Indigestion, nausea, heartburn, or vomiting was reported in 24.3 per cent of those receiving placebo, in 29.4 per cent of those on 300 milligrams aspirin daily, and in 38.8 per cent of those receiving 1,200 milligrams/day. The analogous figures for the more serious side effect of any gastrointestinal bleeding were 1.6 per cent, 2.6 per cent, and 4.7 per cent, respectively. For both these categories of symptoms, the difference between the low- and high-dose groups achieved statistical significance. Thus, the side effects of aspirin are clearly dose-related.

CONCLUSIONS

Aspirin as well as heparin have been shown to be of net benefit in the treatment of acute myocardial infarction. The mortality reductions achieved in acute myocardial infarction are similar (about 20 per cent) with the two drugs; however, heparin is associated with more bleeding.

Since therapy for acute myocardial infarction may involve thrombolysis, the adjunctive antithrombotic role of either or both aspirin and heparin assume particular importance. Aspirin in conjunction with streptokinase, and presumably other thrombolytics, is clearly beneficial in acute myocardial infarction. Patients receiving the combination have a greater reduction in vascular mortality than with either agent alone without producing an excess of serious bleeding. The use of aspirin with thrombolysis also protects against the increase in reinfarction that occurs when thrombolytic therapy is given alone.

The tests of heparin added to thrombolysis have been, in general, early patency studies. These lack consistency in their results and are less convincing than mortality studies.

For these reasons, at present the role of heparin remains less well defined than that of antiplatelet treatment with aspirin when given with thrombolytic therapy.

The GISSI-2 mortality study has demonstrated that the addition of heparin to a regimen of aspirin with thrombolytic therapy provides a small added reduction in mortality of about 5 deaths per 1,000 and an excess risk of cerebral hemorrhage of about 1 event per 1,000. Whether or not immediate intravenous heparin will yield a greater benefit or risk in conjunction with rt-PA has not yet been addressed in randomized trials using mortality as an endpoint.

In comparing the net benefits for aspirin, aspirin plus thrombolytic therapy, and heparin added to aspirin and thrombolytics, it is useful to evaluate the ratio of the mortality reduction observed with each treatment regimen to the excess risk of cerebral hemorrhage. For every 1,000 patients who suffer a myocardial infarction, approximately 10 per cent (or 100) will die. Of these, if treated with aspirin, there will be a 23 per cent reduction in mortality (or only 77 of the original 100 would die), and there would be no increase in cerebral hemorrhage (Table 14–7). Thus, this ratio of benefit-to-risk for aspirin alone is infinite. The addition of thrombolytics results in an additional 27 per cent reduction in mortality, resulting in only 50 individuals dying. However, two to three treated patients will suffer a nonfatal cerebral hemorrhage, resulting in a cumulative benefit-to-risk ratio of aspirin and thrombolysis of 19:1. The further addition of subcutaneous heparin results in an additional 5 per cent reduction in mortality (a total of 45 deaths) with an additional excess of one nonfatal cerebral hemorrhage (a cumulative benefit-to-risk ratio of 15:1). Thus it is clear that although there is some additional benefit on

TABLE 14–7. Mortality Reductions and Nonfatal Cerebral Hemorrhage Excesses for Various Therapies of Acute Myocardial Infarction (per 1,000 Patients Treated)

	MORTALITY REDUCTION		CEREBRAL HEMORRHAGE EXCESS		RATIOS	
	Individual	*Cumulative*	*Individual*	*Cumulative*	*Individual*	*Cumulative*
Aspirin	↓ 23	↓ 23	0	0	∞	∞
Thrombolysis	↓ 27	↓ 50	↑ 2.7	↑ 2.7	10:1	19:1
Subcutaneous Heparin	↓ 5	↓ 55	↑ 1.0	↑ 3.7	5:1	15:1

mortality with the addition of heparin to aspirin plus thrombolysis, the benefit-to-risk ratio is reduced. The precise risks and benefits of adding an immediate intravenous or delayed heparin regimen, regardless of whether intravenous or subcutaneous, will require testing in randomized trials.

Finally, for primary prevention, there is conclusive evidence that aspirin reduces the risk of myocardial infarction by about a third. However, the possible effects on cardiovascular death and stroke remain inconclusive owing to an inadequate number of these endpoints in the trials that have been conducted. Further, there are no data from randomized trials of primary prevention in women, and none in men which have tested a very–low-dose aspirin regimen. For all these reasons, any decision to prescribe aspirin to prevent a first myocardial infarction should be based on individual clinical judgement which takes into account the cardiovascular risk profile of the individual as well as side effects of the drug. The prescription of aspirin should be considered only for those men whose risks of a first myocardial infarction are sufficiently high to warrant the adverse effects of long-term administration of the drug.

ACKNOWLEDGEMENTS: We are indebted to Heather Tosteson, Ph.D., for her editorial assistance and to Susan O'Rahilly for her help in preparing the manuscript.

REFERENCES

1. ISIS-2 (Second International Study of Infarct Survival) Collaborative Group. Randomised trial of intravenous streptokinase, oral aspirin, both, or neither among 17187 cases of suspected acute myocardial infarction: ISIS-2. Lancet 1988; 2: 349–60.
2. Patrignani P, Filabozzi P, Patrono C. Selective cumulative inhibition of platelet thromboxane production by low-dose aspirin in healthy subjects. J Clin Invest 1982; 69: 1366–72.
3. Reilly IAG, FitzGerald GA. Inhibition of thromboxane formation in vivo and ex vivo: implications for therapy with platelet inhibitory drugs. Blood 1987; 69: 180–6.
4. ISIS-3 (International Studies of Infarct Survival). Update: scientific background to the ISIS-3 comparisons. Evidence from other studies. Radcliffe Infirmary, Oxford, February 1991.
5. Chalmers TC, Matta RJ, Smith H, Kunzler A-M. Evidence favoring the use of anticoagulants in the hospital phase of acute myocardial infarction. N Engl J Med 1977; 297: 1091–6.
6. Peto R. Clinical trial methodology. Biomed Pharmacother 1978; 28 (special issue): 24–36.
7. Mitchell JRA. Anticoagulants in coronary heart disease—retrospect and prospect. Lancet 1981; 2: 257–62.
8. Yusuf S, Wittes J, Friedman L. Overview of results of randomized clinical trials in heart disease. I. Treatments following myocardial infarction. JAMA 1988; 260: 2088–93.
9. MacMahon S, Collins R, Knight C, Yusuf S, Peto R. Reduction in major morbidity and mortality by heparin in acute myocardial infarction (abstr). Circulation 1988; 78(suppl II): 98.
10. Gruppo Italiano per lo Studio della Streptochinasi nell' Infarto Miocardico (GISSI). Effectiveness of thrombolytic treatment in acute myocardial infarction. Lancet 1986; 1: 397–402.
11. ISAM Study Group. A prospective trial of intravenous streptokinase in acute myocardial infarction (ISAM): mortality, morbidity and infarct size at 21 days. N Engl J Med 1986; 314: 1465–71.
12. ASSET Study Group. Trial of tissue plasminogen activator for mortality reduction in acute myocardial infarction. Lancet 1988; 2: 525–30.
13. AIMS Trial Study Group. Effect of intravenous APSAC on mortality after acute myocardial infarction: preliminary report of a placebo-controlled clinical trial. Lancet 1988; 2: 545–9.
14. AIMS Trial Study Group. Long-term effects of intravenous anistreplase in acute myocardial infarction: final report of the AIMS study. Lancet 1990; 335: 427–31.
15. ISIS-3 (Third International Study of Infarct Survival) Collaborative Group. Preliminary results of the ISIS-3 trial. Presented at the 40th Annual Scientific Session, American College of Cardiology, Atlanta, March 1991.
16. Topol EJ, George BS, Kereiakes DJ, et al., and the TAMI Study Group. A randomized controlled trial of intravenous tissue plasminogen activator and early intravenous heparin in acute myocardial infarction. Circulation 1989; 79: 281–6.
17. Bleich SD, Nichols TC, Schumacher RR, et al. The effect of heparin on coronary arterial patency after thrombolysis with tissue plasminogen activator in acute myocardial infarction. Am J Cardiol 1990; 66: 1412–7.
18. Hsia J, Hamilton WP, Kleiman N, Roberts R, Chaitman BR, Ross AM, for the Heparin-Aspirin Reperfusion Trial (HART) investigators. A comparison between heparin and low-dose aspirin as adjunctive therapy with tissue plasminogen activator for acute myocardial infarction. N Engl J Med 1990; 323: 1433–7.
19. Thompson PL, Aylward PE, Federman J, et al. for the National Heart Foundation of Australia Coronary Thrombolysis Group. A randomized comparison of intravenous heparin with oral aspirin and dipyridamole 24 hours after recombinant tissue-type plasminogen activator for acute myocardial infarction. Circulation 1991;83:1534–42.
20. Van de Werf F, for the Investigators of the European Cooperative Study Group for recombinant tissue-type plasminogen activator. Lessons from the European Cooperative recombinant tissue-type plasminogen activator (rt-PA) versus placebo trial. JACC 1988; 12: 14A–9A.
21. Van de Werf F, Arnold AER, for the European Cooperative Study Group for recombitant tissue-type plasminogen activator. Intravenous tissue plasminogen activator and size of infarct, left ventricular function, and survival in acute myocardial infarction. Br Med J 1988; 297: 1374–9.
22. de Bono DP, Simoons ML, Tijssen J, et al., for the European Cooperative Study Group. Early intravenous heparin enhances coronary patency after alteplase thrombolysis: results of a randomised double blind trial European Cooperative Study Group trial. Br Heart J 1991; in press.
23. Gruppo Italiano per lo Studio della Sopravvivenza Nell'Infarto Miocardico. GISSI-2. A factorial randomized trial of alteplase versus streptokinase and heparin versus no heparin among 12,490 patients with acute myocardial infarction. Lancet 1990; 336: 65–71.
24. The International Study Group. In-hospital mortality and clinical course of 20,891 patients with suspected acute myocardial infarction randomised between alteplase and streptokinase with or without heparin. Lancet 1990; 336: 71–5.
25. The Steering Committee of the Physicians' Health Study Research Group. Preliminary report: findings from the aspirin component of the ongoing Physicians' Health Study. N Engl J Med 1988; 318: 262–4.
26. The Steering Committee of the Physicians' Health Study Re-

search Group. Final report on the aspirin component of the ongoing Physicians' Health Study. N Engl J Med 1989; 321: 129–35.

27. Peto R, Gray R, Collins R, et al. A Randomised Trial of the effects of prophylactic daily aspirin in British male doctors. Br Med J 1988; 296: 313–6.

28. Hennekens CH, Buring JE, Sandercock P, Collins R, Peto R. Aspirin and other antiplatelet agents in the secondary and primary prevention of cardiovascular disease. Circulation 1989; 80: 749–56.

29. Hennekens CH, Peto R, Hutchison GB, Doll R. An overview of the British and American aspirin studies. N Engl J Med 1988; 318: 923–4.

30. Acheson J, Archibald D, Barnett H. et al. Antiplatelet Trialists Collaboration:Secondary prevention of vascular disease by prolonged anti-platelet therapy. Br Med J 1988;296:320–1.

31. UK-TIA Study Group. United Kingdom transient ischaemic attack (UK-TIA) aspirin trial: interim results. Br Med J 1988; 296: 316–20.

15

MYOCARDIAL INFARCTION— THROMBOLYTIC THERAPY IN THE PREHOSPITAL SETTING

W. DOUGLAS WEAVER and J. WARD KENNEDY

THE RATIONALE FOR PREHOSPITAL THROMBOLYTIC THERAPY

Since the initial report from the Gruppo Italiano per lo Studio della Streptochinasi nell' Infarto Miocardico (GISSI-1) placebo-controlled trial of intravenous streptokinase in acute myocardial infarction, which demonstrated a 47 per cent reduction in mortality in the subset of patients treated within the first hour of symptoms, it has become widely recognized and agreed upon that the earlier thrombolytic therapy is initiated, the better the result.[1] Other large and similar trials of intravenous thrombolysis have shown a lesser magnitude of benefit associated with early treatment, but in almost all, there is a consistent attenuation of treatment effect with greater delays from onset of chest pain until initiation of thrombolytic therapy.[2,3] This is evident when stratifying outcome even in the first six hours. Hospital-based trials enroll relatively few patients in the first two hours of symptoms. The other evidence supporting very early treatment is derived from smaller studies of thrombolytic therapy which, because of their small size, are able to detect salvage of myocardium or reduction in mortality only in the subset of patients treated early (Table 15–1).[4,5,37]

It can be argued that the future role of prehospital emergency systems initiating intravenous thrombolytic treatment to patients with acute myocardial infarction is, in many ways, analogous to the situation 20 years ago, when the advent of prehospital management of cardiac arrest dramatically improved the outcome of patients developing out-of-hospital unexpected sudden cardiac death. In earlier years, when prehospital treatment of patients with cardiac arrest consisted of only basic life support (cardiopulmonary resuscitation), and definitive care was delayed until after hospital arrival, survival rates averaged 5 per cent. Since the advent of early paramedic-initiated care, survival rates following unexpected cardiac arrest due to ventricular fibrillation are five to six times higher.[6–11]

Almost every city, small or large, now has an organized system of prehospital emergency medical care. Prehospital assessment, screening, and treatment of patients with chest pain has become routine. Currently, in most communities, this consists of paramedic-initiated cardiac rhythm monitoring, intravenous cannulation, and basic treatment to provide relief of chest pain. If necessary, these personnel are trained to provide cardiac resuscitation and treatment of symptomatic hypotension, pulmonary congestion, and life-threatening arrhythmias, if required.

As there is a consensus that thrombolytic drug therapy should be administered to patients with acute myocardial infarction as rapidly as possible, perhaps the only question to be addressed in the ongoing prehospital studies is whether appropriate patients with chest pain (that is, those with suspected acute coronary thrombosis) can be accurately identified by paramedics working under standing protocols or the guidance of a remote physician in the hospital; and second, whether treatment with thrombolytic therapy can be

TABLE 15–1. Mortality Reduction in Patients with Acute Myocardial Infarction who were Treated Early and Late with Thrombolytic Drugs*

STUDY*	TIME TO TREATMENT (HOURS)	REDUCTION IN MORTALITY	
		Early Treatment (%)	Late Treatment (%)
GISSI-1[1]	<1 versus 2–6	47	15
AIMS[3]	<4 versus 4–6	41	53
ISIS-2[2]	<4 versus 4–12	53	32
Western Washington[5,43]	<3 versus 3–6	54	1
ISAM[4]	<3 versus 3–6	20	12
Average for all		43	22

* Per cent reductions in mortality are shown for each of the trials.

safely begun in that setting. On the other hand, these prehospital studies may be much more important and serve as useful catalysts to widespread implementation of prehospital initiation of thrombolysis if they demonstrate that this treatment strategy is not only feasible, but cost effective in terms of salvaging myocardium and reducing complication rates from acute myocardial infarction over and above results which can be achieved in the hospital setting. These issues have led to several clinical investigations of prehospital-initiated thrombolytic therapy.

IS PREHOSPITAL THERAPY REALLY NECESSARY?

It has been suggested that, analogous to the situation of the severely traumatized victim, there is a "golden hour" in which to screen each patient with chest pain, establish a presumptive diagnosis of acute coronary thrombosis, and initiate thrombolytic drug therapy. The logistics of achieving this goal strongly support prehospital initiation of thrombolytic therapy. Basically, the time delay between onset of chest pain and initiation of therapy has three fundamental components: (a) that associated with patient recognition of the need to seek medical care, (b) the time consumed in transporting the patient to hospital, and (c) the time required for diagnosis and initiation of therapy after hospital arrival.

The Myocardial Infarction, Triage and Intervention (MITI) project is a study which began in Seattle, Washington in 1988 to assess feasibility, safety, and efficacy of prehospital initiation of thrombolytic therapy. It also includes a registry of all patients hospitalized with acute myocardial infarction in the greater Seattle metropolitan area.[12,13] The project has provided the opportunity to accurately assess each of these components of time delay in an unselected case series of patients. The Seattle metropolitan area is typical of many others in the United States, Canada, and Europe. There is an efficient prehospital emergency system staffed primarily by paramedics working under the direction of a remote base station physician. Transport times average 10 to 15 minutes. There are 17 hospitals, including several with tertiary cardiac care capabilities in the Seattle metropolitan area. Because the Seattle emergency medical system was one of the first established, the public served in Seattle may, if anything, be more aware of who to call for help and what to do in case of cardiac emergencies. Transport times may be somewhat shorter than those in either more dense urban or in rural settings. Thus, if anything, the measured delays from chest-pain onset to initiation of treatment in Seattle may conservatively estimate the potential time savings and potential benefit of prehospital-initiated care.

In the early 1990s, patients' failure to recognize the early symptoms of acute infarction and seek emergent care remains the single most significant impediment to very early therapy. Despite the recognized high mortality from cardiac arrest in the first hour of myocardial infarction and the known benefit of rhythm monitoring and rapid defibrillation in patients with suspected acute infarction, only 50 per cent of patients with acute myocardial infarction surveyed in the MITI project sought the care of prehospital emergency medical services (Table 15–2). Also, for those patients who did not seek paramedic

TABLE 15–2. Comparison of Patients with Acute Myocardial Infarction who Call for Paramedic Assistance and Patients who Come to Hospital by Other Means After Symptom Onset*

	EMERGENCY SERVICES	OTHER MEANS	p VALUE
N	2,103 (52%)	1,943 (48%)	
Men	1,359 (65%)	1,792 (67%)	p = NS
Age (yrs ± SD)	67 ± 13	65 ± 13	p <0.001
Pain onset to call/hospital arrival x ± SD (median)	180 ± 508 (60)	628 ± 1,221 (170)	p <0.001
Treated with thrombolytic drugs	649 (31%)	324 (17%)	p <0.0001

* Most of these latter patients arrive by private vehicle, except for 15 per cent who come by private ambulance.
SD = standard deviation; NS = not significant.

services, the delays before coming to hospital were disturbingly long and thereby minimized the opportunity to salvage myocardium. The median delay before seeking care was 60 minutes in patients seeking paramedic services, compared to 2.9 hours in those who came to hospital by other means (p < 0.001). Media-based efforts to increase the proportion of patients seeking prehospital emergency care have thus far yielded disappointing results. In a pilot study carried out in Seattle in which an intensive media campaign was conducted for six weeks, the education effort neither increased the number of people with acute myocardial infarction seeking paramedic services nor shortened the time from chest-pain onset to hospital arrival (2.6 hours before the media education campaign, compared to 2.3 hours after).[14] In a longer, similar effort carried out in Sweden over one year, similar disappointing results were observed.[15] It is apparent that the approach of using mass-media advertising to improve lay public knowledge about heart attack with the hope that they will react sooner to symptoms is inadequate. In addition, such approaches would be even more dismal failures if they disproportionately increased noncardiac emergency department admissions because of anxiety or hysteria.

To determine whether alternative approaches which employ educational methods based on psychological learning theory can yield more effective results, a trial is underway in the Seattle metropolitan area (CALL-FAST) to determine the effectiveness of varied media techniques as well as individual-based layperson education. This trial will determine which, if any, mass-media education technique, including approaches aimed at overcoming denial or which alternatively may cause bystanders to take action and will be effective in reducing the time from symptom onset to arrival at hospital (Fig. 15–1).

Aside from patient recognition of the problem, the prehospital time required for emergency personnel to assess and provide basic treatment including pain relief, monitoring, and intravenous cannulation, added to the hospital transport time and that required in hospital for further clinical assessment and provision of thrombolytic therapy, routinely preclude treatment within the golden hour. Prehospital assessment, initiation of intravenous treatment, and hospital transport routinely consume 30 to 45 minutes. It seems unlikely that these tasks can be accomplished more quickly. Ten to fifteen minutes of this time are required by paramedics to identify the subset of patients with chest pain who have findings suggestive of acute infarction, and another 10 to 15 minutes are used in placing an intravenous cannula to be used for pain relief and to manage cardiac arrest, should it occur and last, and 10 to 15 minutes of transport time is typical.

Hospital delays are also not inconsequential. Sharkey showed that in hospitals participating in the TIMI trial, the hospital time for diagnosis and treatment accounted for 59 per cent of the total delay from chest-pain onset to initiation of treatment.[16] Kereiakes similarly compiled results from six different cities, and also found average delays of 84 ± 55 minutes as well as no time difference for small hospitals versus tertiary cardiac centers.[17] Such delays are being curtailed as awareness of their importance has increased. As shown in Figure 15–2, hospital treatment times recently tabulated in Seattle vary between 27 and 87 minutes with a median of 34 minutes (mean 67 minutes). It is clear from these findings, however, that no matter how quickly hospital staff can initiate thrombolytic therapy, the period for patient recognition, prehospital and hospital care make it impossible to initiate therapy in the hospital

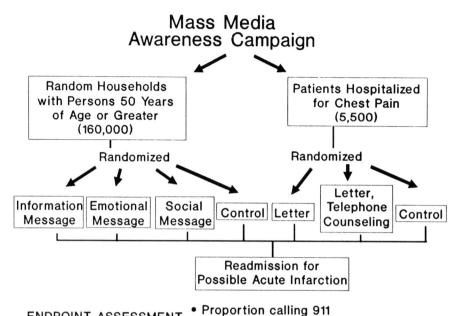

FIGURE 15–1.   CALLFAST Trial. The trial is aimed at assessing the effectiveness of several different media messages, each targeted to a form of reasoning and based on psychosocial learning theories, and to measure the effect of individual counseling in high-risk individuals recently hospitalized because of the suspicion of myocardial ischemia. The trial will determine which, if any, of these approaches increases the proportion of patients with acute infarction seeking emergency medical services care, and determine if any of these methods are effective at reducing the delay from symptom onset to seeking emergent medical care.

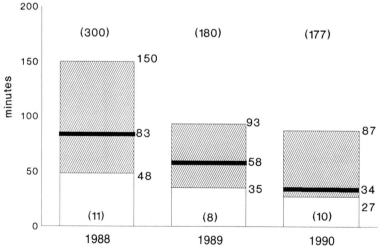

FIGURE 15–2.   Time from hospital arrival to initiation of thrombolytic therapy over a three-year period. The bottom and top of the bars show the 25th and 75th percentiles in minutes for all patients hospitalized with acute myocardial infarction in the Seattle greater metropolitan area. The numbers in parentheses show the fifth and 95th percentiles. The distributions are skewed. The mean times from chest-pain onset to hospital arrival over the three-year period were 101, 75, and 67 minutes, respectively. Hospital treatment times have improved with implementation of the MITI project and increased awareness of the need for rapid treatment. Despite this, the time delay before the patient seeks help, combined with that required for hospital transport added to the above delays, make it logistically improbable to initiate thrombolytic therapy within the first hour of symptoms unless treatment is begun in the prehospital setting.

within the first hour to any significant number of patients. The golden hour ends, on average, about the time paramedics are making the diagnoses.

During the first year or "feasibility phase" of the MITI project, which was primarily aimed at defining optimal patient selection criteria for potential prehospital treatment, the diagnosis of suspected acute coronary thrombosis was made by a remote physician communicating with paramedics, in 59 per cent of patients within the first hour of chest pain.[18] The time required for case identification, including obtaining a 12-lead electrocardiogram was no longer (16 minutes) than it had been in the past, when a nondirected approach was used (18 minutes). Despite the fact that the diagnosis had already been made prior to hospital arrival, *only 3 per cent of these same patients actually received thrombolytic therapy within the first hour after symptom onset.* Thus, even when the diagnosis had been made prior to hospital arrival and staff had done everything to minimize delays after arrival, the logistics simply precluded very early initiation of thrombolytic drug treatment.

CRITERIA TO BE USED FOR ACCURATE PREHOSPITAL PATIENT SELECTION

A successful, effective, and efficient prehospital acute infarction program requires a detailed and exact protocol to be used for evaluating all patients with chest pain, plus an interested physician responsible for providing feedback and to monitor the findings. A single hospital supervisory team (even if responsibility is rotated) would be far superior to a multihospital approach in which responsibility and accountability is unclear. In the MITI Project, a checklist of clinical inclusion and exclusion criteria was developed for use by paramedics to evaluate all patients with presumed cardiac chest pain, the necessary findings of which could be assessed in a five to ten minute brief, directed physical history and examination.[13] The list includes an assessment of the nature of chest pain, duration of symptoms, and a listing of specific illnesses which might place the patient at risk for serious bleeding from thrombolytic therapy. The feedback by paramedics, after using this triage method, indicated that the list provided a far more comprehensive evaluation than the prior, nondirected approach, and that it focused assessment so that diagnosis and treatment decisions occurred much sooner.

Such a checklist approach would likely also be useful if incorporated in the emergency department medical evaluation record. In many cities, emergency departments are overburdened with huge numbers of patients who often have noncritical illnesses and who use the hospital for routine health care needs. This checklist approach, which can be employed by nurses and physicians alike, permits rapid screening of all patients with chest pain for identification of the small but important subset who are potential candidates for reperfusion techniques.

The single most important diagnostic tool to aid in prehospital diagnosis of acute myocardial infarction is the battery powered computer-interpretative 12-lead electrocardiograph. Although in its technological infancy, this devices will likely become a diagnostic tool routinely used by all ambulance systems involved in the triage of chest-pain patients. While at present most such electrocardiographs are single-function devices, they soon will be incorporated with defibrillator-monitors and will probably include quantitative ST segment monitoring, which may prove to be useful for diagnosis as well as to assess the results of treatment.[19] These multipurpose devices will also likely be located in the hospital emergency department, which requires simple and space-efficient technology. The educational program provided to paramedics for familiarization with the checklist criteria and electrocardiograph operation is minimal and, in our case, required only four hours of additional training. The technical quality of the prehospital electrocardiograms has been excellent. No effort was made to teach electrocardiogram interpretation to paramedics, as this would be a time-consuming, inefficient, and expensive.

During the feasibility phase of the MITI project, we compared the accuracy of the remote emergency department physicians to a consensus interpretation of two electrocardiographers and to that of the Marquette Electronics 12-SL (versions 4–6) algorithm (Marquette Electronics, Inc., Milwaukee, Wisconsin). The sensitivity of the electrocardiographers for correctly identifying the subset of patients with acute myocardial infarction and ST segment elevation was 92 per cent, compared to sensitivities of 70 per cent for the emergency physicians, and 70 per cent for the computer-interpretative algorithm, respectively. Of equal or greater importance is the ability to accurately discriminate patients with ST elevation but who do not have acute infarction (for example, early repolarization abnormalities, pericarditis, left ventricular hypertrophy). Although the present computer-interpretative algorithm had lower sensitivity than the electrocardiographer, it was superior at discriminating potentially inappropriate cases.[20] The electrocardiographer and emergency department physicians had false-positive rates of 4 per cent and 7 per cent, respectively—significantly higher than the rate of false-positives for the computer-interpreted electrocardiograph (1 per cent). In most emergency departments, a cardiologist is not immediately available to interpret the electrocardiogram and such consultation would therefore delay treatment and patient transport. Because a combination of full- and part-time physicians often constitute emergency department staff, it is often difficult for emergency department physicians to be experienced with the nuances of changing thrombolysis selection criteria and to be expert electrocardiogram interpreters; thus a reliable means of accurate interpretation is extremely useful. With this in mind, the MITI prehospital trial has utilized the Marquette computer-interpretative algorithm to identify the subset of patients who have diagnostic electrocardiographic abnormalities (ST elevation indicative of epicardial injury) for treatment with thrombolytic therapy, although additional specified criteria are also provided to physicians for including computer-negative electrocardiograms in an attempt to compensate for the present less-than-perfect sensitivity of the algorithm. The digitized electrocardiogram is transmitted by cellular telephone and then printed in the emergency department.[21] It has become clear, during the ongoing trial, that the computer-interpretative electrocardiograph is the only means to consistently provide accurate identification of patients for prehospital thrombolytic treatments. With the use of this approach, the number of false-positive diagnoses is negligible and clearly better than it was without it. Computerized electrocardiography, given the present-day technology, can be used to define a subset of patients with unequivocal evidence of acute coronary thrombosis and who are likely to benefit most from very early initiation of thrombolytic drug therapy while reliably excluding patients with other illness. Patients with complicated medical histories or equivocal electrocardiograms are better managed after further assessment in the hospital. These findings also point out the need for testing any computer algorithm before using it for this purpose. With the electrocardiographic diagnosis being so important for selecting patients for treatment, it becomes imperative that all commercial devices meet acceptable performance levels.

As this and other clinical databases of patients with acute coronary thrombosis expand, the positive predictive accuracy for computer interpretation can be even further improved and may likely become comparable to that of an expert electrocardiographer. In the very near future, computerized electrocardiography should provide almost instantaneous, accurate identification of patients with electrocardiograms consistent with evidence of acute coronary thrombosis.

Is computerized electrocardiography required for prehospital programs? The answer is no, but other approaches will probably result in treating greater numbers of patients with disorders other than acute myocardial infarction. For instance, in the European Myocardial Infarction Project (EMIP) trial of prehospital therapy carried out in Europe, emergency physicians select patients based on their judgment and not using specific electrocardiographic criteria (Boissel J, personal communication). It was recently reported that 10 to 20 per cent of patients enrolled in the trial did not develop evidence of acute myocardial infarction in the hospital, although the vast majority had other coronary ischemic symptoms. An alternative approach obviating the use of telephone transmission of the electrocardiogram to the hospital is that employed by the ambulance system in Sydney, Australia.[22] The prehospital 12-lead electrocardiogram is obtained, computer interpreted, and along with the matrix of ST segment measurements, is printed. A senior cardiologist at a remote hospital then is telephoned and integrates the history, the computer diagnosis, and the ST segment measurements to identify appropriate patients. In screening over 1,300 patients with chest pain, this method has provided an accurate means by which to identify those individuals who are appropriate candidates for initiation of thrombolytic therapy. The method has the advantage in that it does not require specialized electrocardiographic data transmitting or receiving equipment, nor does it incur the cost associated with telephone transmission of the electrocardiogram. Even this will likely become unnecessary when the computer algorithms have been further improved and evaluated, such that transmission is unnecessary for the purposes of "overreading" the electrocardiogram.

A serious impediment to the widespread implementation of prehospital initiation of thrombolytic therapy is the current low-level involvement of cardiologists in the operation of the prehospital emergency medical systems. Yet, patients with chest-pain constitute from 5 to 15 per cent of all medical disorders evaluated and treated by paramedics. *Interested cardiologists need to participate in the teaching and formation of protocols for prehospital management of acute coronary syndromes.* The equipment will soon exist which will allow paramedics to communicate by radio telephone, including sending a 12-lead electrocardiogram within seconds, not only to the emergency department, but to any remote physician.

Prehospital computerized 12-lead electrocardiography benefits all patients with acute infarction, whether or not prehospital thrombolytic therapy is delivered. This technology permits a diagnosis to be made in the subset of patients with ST elevation, allows more appropriate triage of patients with shock or other complications to tertiary cardiac hospitals, and enables a cardiac team to be assembled, even before patient arrival. Last, an electrocardiogram obtained out of hospital shortens the time from hospital arrival to initiation of treatment for patients with acute infarction. Patients in which 12-lead electrocardiograms were obtained by paramedics in the MITI project were treated, on average, 20 minutes sooner than others in whom the electrocardiogram had not been obtained. A randomized trial aimed at assessing the value of prehospital electrocardiography found a similar reduction in the time to treatment.[23] The added time required for the electrocardiogram in both studies was negligible, and yet the hospital delay until treatment was significantly shortened when the diagnosis had been made prior to hospital arrival.

IS THE YIELD WORTH THE EFFORT?

In the first two years of the MITI project, over 4,300 patients with presumed chest pain were evaluated by paramedics. Twelve hundred ninety-three (30 per cent) developed evidence of acute myocardial infarction during hospitalization. Of the patients with evidence of acute myocardial infarction, 464 (36 per cent) received thrombolytic treatment, including 22 per cent who met all of the conservative criteria used for prehospital initiation of therapy. The large number of patients screened for the small number treated should not be surprising. The small proportion of prehospital patients with complaints of chest pain who have both evidence of acute infarction and who are candidates for thrombolytic drug treatment is no different from the situation in the emergency department. That is, several-fold more patients with chest pain are evaluated than those who have evidence of acute myocardial infarction. The proportion of patients who were candidates for thrombolytic therapy is also typical of the in-hospital experience. Currently, either the potential risk of serious bleeding or a nondiagnostic electrocardiogram preclude the majority of patients for consideration for thrombolytic therapy (Fig. 15–3).

On the other hand, the importance of prehospital screening for hastening the initiation of treatment of patients with acute infarction is much greater. In this study, 65 per cent of all patients who were treated with thrombolytic therapy were initially evaluated by paramedics. So the question to be answered is, should the efficiency and yield of prehospital involvement be based on the total number of patients with chest pain (11 per cent), the subset with acute myocardial infarction (47 per cent), or the proportion of patients who are ultimately treated with thrombolytic therapy (65 per cent) (Fig. 15–4)? In order to provide a means for shortening the time to reperfusion following acute coronary thrombosis, prehospital screening and treatment provides a means to speed therapy in more than half of the patients treated, with a time savings of 45 minutes or more.

PREHOSPITAL STUDIES OF THROMBOLYTIC THERAPY

Several studies have been reported of prehospital-initiated thrombolytic therapy (Table 15–3). Most have been designed to evaluate time savings, left ventricular func-

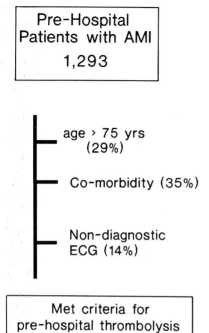

FIGURE 15–3. Twenty-two per cent of all patients with acute infarction who were evaluated initially by paramedics met criteria for prehospital initiation of thrombolytic treatment. The criteria were conservative, specifically excluding elderly patients, and those with a history of uncontrolled hypertension, bleeding, or any prior central nervous system disorder. Of those excluded, almost an equal number were given thrombolytic drug treatment after further hospital evaluation.

tion, infarct size, or mortality differences in those treated in the prehospital setting and those who, instead, are treated after hospital arrival. In a small randomized trial of prehospital- versus hospital-initiated treatment (116 patients) carried out in Israel and aimed at evaluating left ventricular function, there was no difference in resultant left ventricular function, despite a 43-minute time difference between the two treatments. Mortality (a secondary endpoint) was similar for both groups (5.5 and 6.8 per cent, respectively).[24] However, the subset of patients treated within two hours, most of whom were treated in the prehospital setting, had significantly lower mortality than those treated later (Table 15–3).

In another randomized trial of prehospital treatment reported by Shofer, patients with first myocardial infarction associated with significant ST segment elevation were randomized to receive 2 million units of urokinase or placebo in either the prehospital or

hospital setting.[25] As would be expected, patients were treated significantly sooner in the prehospital setting; treatment was begun within two hours in 53 per cent, compared to only 10 per cent when treatment was, instead, initiated after hospital arrival. There were no bleeding complications during transport and overall hospital mortality rates were very low (3.8 per cent). All deaths were due to recurrent myocardial infarction occurring 7 to 14 days later. Randomization was imperfect at balancing the small groups, with prehospital allocated cases having a 47 per cent incidence of anterior infarction compared to only 32 per cent in the control group. The study reported no difference in complications, resulting ejection fraction, or peak creatine kinase levels between the two treatment groups. However, the relatively small sample size (78 patients) and the large standard deviations for each of the endpoints provided little statistical power to measure significant differences. Many other studies have also shown that ejection fraction may be a relatively insensitive indicator of myocardial salvage afforded by very early treatment.

Two larger trials are currently underway to further assess prehospital initiation of thrombolytic therapy. The first is a multicenter study in Europe, the European Myocardial Infarction Project (EMIP) trial. In the most recent available report, 3,800 of an expected 6,000 patients have been enrolled in the study. The time savings of prehospital-initiated therapy has been reported to be 56 minutes.[26–29] The trial is a double-blind, placebo-controlled study of anistreplase administration in the prehospital versus hospital setting. The bolus method of infusion is ideal for the prehospital setting, minimizing difficulties with measured continuous intravenous infusions. The incidence of chest pain at the time of arrival at hospital in patients who received prehospital initiation of anistreplase was significantly lower than in those who received anistreplase after hospital arrival. The overall mortality has been reported to be approximately 10 per cent (Boissel J, personal communication).

This trial is primarily being conducted in Europe, and in most cases, emergency physicians on the ambulance make case selections. Computerized electrocardiography is not used and the physician is given considerable discretion in enrolling patients. Consequently, it has been reported that 10 to 20

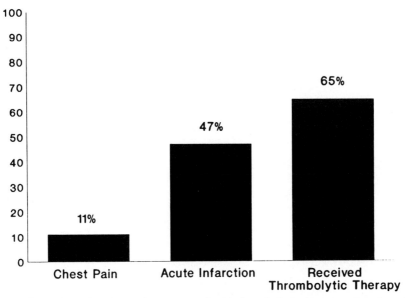

FIGURE 15-4. Proportion of patients who are treated with thrombolytic therapy and evaluated and transported by paramedics. Of all patients with chest pain evaluated by paramedics, 11 per cent are treated with thrombolytic therapy, of which half met the conservative criteria for enrollment in the MITI prehospital trial. On the other hand, of all patients who received thrombolytic therapy, 65 per cent are initially screened by paramedics, pointing out the importance of including prehospital protocols and 12-lead electrocardiography in the emergency medical system in order to provide the best and most rapid care to suitable patients with acute myocardial infarction.

per cent of those enrolled do not develop hospital evidence of acute myocardial infarction. Most patients have other forms of ischemic heart disease and few have noncardiac causes of chest pain. In other large placebo-controlled studies of thrombolytic therapy, there has been no benefit to patient groups other than those with acute infarction. Thus, inclusion of such patients may reduce the statistical power of this prehospital trial; there will have to be at least a 3 per cent or greater difference in mortality to show statistical significance between the two treatment strategies. Thus the major potential problem with the largest of prehospital trials is that it still may not be large enough to detect differences in mortality. There is also the potential for thrombolytic therapy to increase complication rates in the few patients treated with disorders other than acute infarction; for example, aortic dissection, which can at times be confused with acute coronary thrombosis. For example, in the Anglo-Scandinavian Study of Early Thrombosis (ASSET) trial in which strict electrocardiographic criteria were not used, 154 patients (3 per cent) had other disorders and were randomized to either placebo or alteplase. Mortality rates were very high in this group of patients

treated.[30] There is concern about misdiagnosis being an even greater problem in the prehospital setting where prior medical records are not available to help in decision making. Administration of thrombolytic therapy to patients with other disorders is for the most part inconsequential, but on rare occasions, can be catastrophic.[31]

A second large study of thrombolytic therapy is the Seattle MITI prehospital trial. In this trial, unlike the European one, patients with chest pain are screened by *paramedics* using a checklist of clinical inclusion and exclusion criteria. The paramedic then obtains a computer-interpreted electrocardiogram which is transmitted to the emergency department. The decision for enrolling the patient is made by the remote emergency department physician responsible for all paramedic activities. Patients are then randomized to receive aspirin and alteplase in either the prehospital or hospital setting. Heparin is given intravenously upon hospital arrival. The size of the trial was initially dictated by the results of the first Israeli study of prehospital therapy which showed a nine-point improvement in left ventricular ejection fraction in patients who received streptokinase before hospital arrival.[32] The size of the trial

TABLE 15–3. Results of Prehospital Studies of Thrombolytic Therapy*

Study	Type	Drug	Adjunctive Treatment	Number Treated	Findings
Jerusalem[38]	Historical control	750,000 i.u. streptokinase	Intravenous heparin, intravenous aspirin and then 150 milligrams/day	29	54 minute savings; 7-point improvement in ejection fraction
Sydney[34]	Historical control	2 megaunits urokinase	Not stated	51	69–90 minute savings
Rotterdam[33]	Historical control	100 milligrams alteplase	Intravenous heparin for 24 hours	150	47 minute savings
Cincinnati/ Nashville[39]	Historical control	100 milligrams alteplase	Not stated	8	25–60-minute savings
Tel Aviv[24,40]	Randomized	120 milligrams alteplase	250 milligrams aspirin beginning at 24 hours, intravenous heparin for 5 days	87	48-minute savings; no difference in ejection fraction reduction in 60-day and 24-month mortality in group treated within two hours
Hamburg[25]	Randomized	2 megaunits urokinase	Intravenous heparin	78	Patency 61 per cent, 67 per cent, respectively; ejection fraction similar; peak enzymes similar; 52 minute time savings
EMIP[27]	Randomized	30 units anistreplase	Not stated	3,805	56 minute savings; overall mortality 9.8 per cent
Berlin[42]	Randomized	1.5 megaunits streptokinase	Not stated	41	30 minute savings
Antwerp[28]	Concurrent controls	30 units anistreplase	Intravenous heparin after fibrinogen had normalized	13	46 minute savings
Göteburg[41]	Randomized/ placebo	100 milligrams alteplase	Intravenous heparin and then oral anticoagulation for 30 days, 125 milligrams aspirin beta blockers if possible	352	36 minute savings; trial stopped because of reduced mortality in alteplase-treated group

* All studies found that prehospital treatment was feasible and not attenuated by serious arrhythmias or hemmorrhagic complication before hospital arrival.

was thus designed to evaluate resultant left ventricular ejection fraction as well as myocardial infarct size as determined by single photon emission computed tomography three to four weeks after initiation of thrombolytic therapy. In addition, a ranked composite endpoint of worst outcome (mortality) and complications from thrombolytic therapy, and best outcome (small infarct size) is used to monitor outcome between the two treatment groups. Basically, all patients with chest pain of presumed cardiac etiology are initially screened and a prehospital electrocardiogram is acquired from a subset of those who have chest pain for less than six hours, who are under age 75 years, and who have no elevation in systolic blood pressure above 180 mm Hg or other potential illness which would increase the risk of serious bleeding. Only those patients with "positive" computer-interpreted electrocardiograms or those showing marked ST segment elevation (2 millimeters or more in three contiguous leads, or a total of 4 millimeters or more in the inferior limb leads with 2 or more of the leads showing elevation) are considered for enrollment. Verbal consent for participation in the trial is obtained by paramedics.

This trial also has potential shortcomings—again, primarily because of its limited size. Like the larger EMIP trial, it will be a very severe test of thrombolytic therapy, in that the hospital-allocated patients are identified in the prehospital setting and hospital personnel are both notified prior to admission, and are provided the patient's electrocardiogram upon arrival. From a feasibility study, early notification and 12-lead interpreted electrocardiography were of considerable importance in reducing typical hospital treatment delays. Second, the computer algorithm used to identify appropriate patients has a higher sensitivity for inferior (85 per cent) than for anterior (60 per cent) injury and thus could weight case selection toward patients with inferior infarctions—a group in which differences between treatments will be harder to detect.[20] On the other hand, the vast majority of patients treated in the prehospital setting have therapy initiated in the first 60 to 90 minutes, a time period in which few can be treated in the groups receiving treatment after hospital arrival.

In two other cities, paramedic-based systems have set up significant studies of prehospital-initiated thrombolytic therapy. The principal investigators were convinced of the value of early treatment, so these studies were not randomized. In Rotterdam, The Netherlands, 150 patients were treated with prehospital initiation of alteplase. The time saved was estimated to be 47 minutes and the mortality rate was 3 per cent.[33] There were no serious complications.

In Sydney, Australia, over 1,100 patients were screened for prehospital initiation of 2 million units of urokinase. Fifty-two patients were treated. There were no complications and the time savings was estimated to be 60 to 90 minutes.[34]

In summary, the benefit measured by lives saved and reduction in infarct size and complications is yet unclear. However, the studies to date all show that prehospital initiation of therapy is feasible, that it saves time, and that it is the only way to initiate treatment within the first hour of symptoms in any significant proportion of patients.

IMPLEMENTING PROGRAMS

The cost of prehospital programs are relatively inconsequential when compared to the costs of managing patients with acute myocardial infarction in the hospital. However, the cost is considerable when compared to other emergency system costs. The additional training time is modest; three to four hours. The electrocardiographic equipment presently costs $5,000 to $12,000, but it should be recognized that today's equipment is prototypical. Twelve-lead electrocardiography will become part of the standard monitor-defibrillator which is used by all paramedic systems.

Second, the cost for equipment and supplies used in prehospital programs could be borne, at least in part, by the hospitals served. An electrocardiogram acquired from a patient in the prehospital setting during symptoms, or to assess serial changes during transport would be extremely useful in the management of many patients with chest pain. Too often, patients are pain free at the time of the hospital electrocardiogram, and the physician is resigned to admitting them because an electrocardiogram during chest pain is not available. An earlier electrocardiogram might reduce the likelihood of unnecessary hospitalization of many individuals, and the results of serial tracings before and after hospital arrival could greatly aid in making treatment decisions.

It is quite clear that a means needs to be developed that enables the prehospital electrocardiogram to become part of the patient's permanent hospital medical record and be available for serial comparison. Unlike rhythmstrips, the 12-lead electrocardiogram is very useful in serial comparison to make diagnostic and treatment decisions.

COST OF THROMBOLYTIC THERAPY

At the present time, it is not clear that one thrombolytic drug is superior, in terms of mortality reduction, to another. However, the cost for each varies considerably. Thus simple economics would favor the use of streptokinase, but the potential adverse side effect of hypotension might make it less suitable for the prehospital setting, where frequent monitoring of blood pressure during transport is difficult.

Although continuous infusions, which are currently recommended for both alteplase and streptokinase, can be done in the prehospital setting, there is no doubt of the advantage when treatment is given by bolus. On the other hand, if after further hospital assessment it is determined that thrombolysis is not indicated, a continuous infusion can be stopped after a relatively small amount has been given and thus minimize any bleeding risk to the patient. Recently, McKendall et al. evaluated an initial 20-milligram bolus followed 30 minutes later by a continuous infusion, a dosage regimen designed of alteplase for potential use in the prehospital setting.[35] The advantages are that it would be a simple method of administration and that after hospital evaluation 20 to 30 minutes later, the infusion can be continued. In angiographic studies done in a series of 63 patients treated in such a manner, there was a high patency rate—93 per cent with no complications. This may represent the best of regimens—bolus administration, but with a dosage that does not commit the patient inappropriately started on treatment to the risk of full-dose administration, and a drug with no hemodynamic effects.

As some emergency systems are publicly supported and could not afford these drugs, it seems that the most practical way to reimburse for prehospital therapy would be to have each hospital provide replacement drug for each patient brought to that hospital and be, in turn, responsible for billing.

CONSENT FOR THERAPY

Verbal consent in the prehospital setting should include an explanation of the drug, as is the case for all therapies delivered in the prehospital setting.[36] Although thrombolytic therapy can cause serious bleeding including catastrophic intracranial hemorrhage, which is a major concern, other drugs used in the prehospital setting, such as lidocaine, bronchodialators, and epinephrine, can have equally deleterious effects. Written prehospital consent for treatment is impractical in this situation. Most states also provide immunity from civil tort claims for the remote emergency physicians who prescribe emergent prehospital treatment.

SUMMARY

Prehospital initiation of thrombolytic therapy is currently undergoing extensive investigation. It has been shown in several settings, including those in which paramedics screen patients, that accurate identification of patients with acute myocardial infarction is possible. Protocols have been developed which have been helpful in the management of acute myocardial infarction and, in general, speeding treatment in the hospital because of prehospital involvement. It has become quite clear that in the future, prehospital electrocardiography will play a greater role in the management of other ischemic syndromes as well as monitoring changes during transport. Prehospital selection of patients with acute infarction also has the potential to make an accurate diagnosis, so that patients with complicating conditions secondary to acute myocardial infarction can be admitted to tertiary cardiac facilities. The results of several ongoing trials will compare the results of this treatment strategy over rapid hospital-initiated treatment. It is becoming evident that prehospital screening protocols will become part of every program the aim of which is to initiate therapy as rapidly as possible.

REFERENCES

1. Gruppo Italiano per lo Studio della Streptochinasi nell'Infarto Miocadico (GISSI). Effectiveness of intravenous thrombolytic treatment in acute myocardial infarction. Lancet 1986; 1: 397–401.
2. ISIS-2 (Second International Study of Infarct Survival) Collaborative Group. Randomized trial of intravenous streptokinase, oral aspirin, both, or neither among 17,187 cases of suspected acute myocardial infarction: ISIS-2. Lancet 1988; 2: 349–60.
3. AIMS Trial Study Group. Effect of intravenous APSAC on mortality after acute myocardial infarction; preliminary report of a placebo-controlled clinical trial. Lancet 1988; 1: 545–9.
4. The ISAM Study Group. A prospective trial of intravenous streptokinase in acute myocardial infarction. (ISAM) Mortality, morbidity, and infarct size at 21 days. N Engl J Med 1986; 314: 1465–71.
5. Maynard C, Althouse R, Olsufka M, et al. Early versus late hospital arrival for acute myocardial infarction in the western Washington thrombolytic therapy trials. Am J Cardiol 1989; 63: 1296–300.
6. Stults KR, Brown DD, Schug VL, et al. Prehospital defibrillation performed by emergency medical technicians in rural communities N Engl J Med 1984; 310: 219–23.
7. Cobb LA, Werner JA, Trobaugh BG. Sudden cardiac death. 1. A decade's experience with out-of-hospital resuscitation. Mod Concepts Cardiovasc Dis 1980; 49: 31–6.
8. Eisenberg MS, Bergner L, Hallstrom A. Out-of-hospital cardiac arrest: improved survival with paramedic services. Lancet 1980; i: 812–5.
9. Lewis RP, Stang JM, Fulkerson PK, et al. Effectiveness of advanced paramedics in a mobile coronary care system. JAMA 1979; 214: 1902–4.
10. Roth R, Stewart RD, Rogers K, et al. Out-of-hospital cardiac arrest: factors associated with survival. Ann Emerg Med 1984; 13: 237–43.
11. Eisenberg MS, Horwood BT, Cummins RO, Reynolds-Haertle R, Hearne TR. Cardiac arrest and resuscitation: a tale of 29 cities. Ann Emerg Med 1990; 19: 179–86.
12. Kennedy JW, Weaver WD. Potential use of thrombolytic therapy before hospitalization. Am J Cardiol 1987; 64: 8A–11A.
13. Weaver WD. Out of hospital initiation of thrombolytic therapy. In: Jeffery Anderson, ed. Modern management of acute MI in the community hospital. Glenview, IL: Bioliterature, Inc. (in press).
14. Ho MT, Eisenberg MS, Litwin PE, Schaeffer SM, Damon SK. Delay between onset of chest pain and seeking medical care: the effect of public education. Ann Emerg Med 1989; 18: 727–31.
15. Herlitz J, Hartford M, Blohm M, et al. Effect of media campaign on delay times and ambulance use in suspected acute myocardial infarction. Am J Cardiol 1989; 64: 90–3.
16. Sharkey SW, Brunette DD, Ruiz E, et al. An analysis of time delays preceding thrombolysis for acute myocardial infarction. JAMA 1989; 262: 3171–4.
17. Kereiakes DJ, Weaver DW, Anderson JL, et al. Time delays

in the diagnosis and treatment of acute myocardial infarction: a tale of eight cities. Report from the pre-hospital study group and the Cincinnati Heart Project. Am Heart J 1990; 120: 773–80.

18. Weaver WD, Eisenberg MS, Martin JS, et al. Myocardial infarction, triage and intervention project—phase I: patient characteristics and feasibility of pre-hospital initiation of thrombolytic therapy. J Am Coll Cardiol 1990; 15: 925–31.

19. Krucoff MW, Wagner NG, Pope JE, et al. The portable programmable microprocessor driven 12-lead electrocardiographic monitor: preliminary report of a new device for the non-invasive detection of successful reperfusion or silent coronary reocclusion. Am J Cardiol 1990; 65: 143–8.

20. Kudenchuk PJ, Ho MT, Weaver WD, et al., for the MITI Project Investigators. Accuracy of computer-interpreted electrocardiography in selecting patients for thrombolytic therapy. J Am Coll Cardiol 1991; 17: 1486–91.

21. Grim P, Feldman T, Martin M, Donovan R, Nevins V, Childers RW. Cellular telephone transmission of 12-lead electrocardiograms from ambulance to hospital. Am J Cardiol 1987; 60: 715–20.

22. O'Rourke M, Cook A, Gallagher D, Caroroll G, Hall J. Electrocardiographic diagnosis of evolving myocardial infarction without telemetry for paramedic-initiated pre-hospital thrombolysis (abstr). J Am Coll Cardiol 1991; 17(suppl): 331A.

23. Karagounis L, Ipsen SK, Jessop MR, et al. Impact of field-transmitted electrocardiography on time to in-hospital thrombolytic therapy in acute myocardial infarction. Am J Cardiol 1990; 66: 786–91.

24. Roth A, Barbash GI, Hod H, et al. Should thrombolytic therapy be administered in the mobile intensive care unit in patients with evolving myocardial infarction? A pilot study. J Am Coll Cardiol 1990; 15(5): 932–6.

25. Schofer J, Buttner J, Geng G, et al. Prehospital thrombolysis in acute myocardial infarction. Am J Cardiol 1990; 66: 1429–33.

26. Castaigne AD, Duval AM, Dubois-Rande JL, Herve C, Jan F, Louvard Y. Prehospital administration of anisoylated plasminogen streptokinase activator complex in acute myocardial infarction. Drugs 1987; 33(suppl 3): 231–4.

27. Report of the European Myocardial Infarction Project (EMIP) Subcommittee. Potential time savings with pre-hospital intervention in acute myocardial infarction. Eur Heart J 1988; 9: 118–24.

28. Bossaert LL, Demey HE, Colemont LJ, et al. Prehospital thrombolytic treatment of acute myocardial infarction with anisoylated plasminogen streptokinase activator complex. Crit Care Med 1988; 16(9): 823–30.

29. Villemant D, Barriot P, Riou B, et al. Achievement of thrombolysis at home in cases of acute myocardial infarction. Lancet 1987; 1: 228–9.

30. Wilcox RG, von der Lippe G, Olsson CG, Jensen G, Skene AM, Hampton JR (for the ASSET Study Group). Trial of tissue plasminogen activator for mortality reduction in acute myocardial infarction. Anglo-Scandinavian Study of Early Thrombolysis (ASSET). Lancet 1988; 2: 525–30.

31. Blankenship X, Almquist AK. Cardiovascular complications of thrombolytic therapy in patients with a mistaken diagnosis of acute myocardial infarction. J Am Coll Cardiol 1989; 14: 1579–82.

32. Koren G, Weiss AT, Hasin Y, et al. Prevention of myocardial damage in acute myocardial ischemia by early treatment with intravenous streptokinase. N Engl J Med 1985; 313: 1384–9.

33. Bouten MJM, Simoons ML, Hartman JAM, van Miltenburg AJM, van de Poese, Pool J. Snellere behandeling van het acute myocardinfarct door toediening van alteplase (rtPA) voor opname. Ned Tijdsckd 1990; 50: 2434–8.

34. O'Rourke M, Gallagher D, Healey J, et al. Paramedic-initiated pre-hospital thrombolysis using urokinase in acute coronary occlusion (TICO2) (abstr). J Am Coll Cardiol 1991; 17(suppl): 246A.

35. McKendall G, Woolard R, McDonald MJ, Williams DO. Feasibility of pre-hospital acute myocardial infarction diagnosis: results of pre-hospital administration of t-PA (PATS) study (abstr). Circulation 1990; 82(4): III667.

36. Grim PS, Singer PA, Gramelspacher GP, et al. Informed consent in emergency research. Prehospital thrombolytic therapy for acute myocardial infarction. JAMA 1989; 262(2): 252–5.

37. Ritchie JL, Cerqueira M, Davis K, Maynard C, Kennedy JW. Western Washington intravenous streptokinase in myocardial infarction trial: radionuclide ventricular function and infarct size. J Am Coll Cardiol 1988; 11: 689–97.

38. Weiss AT, Fine DG, Applebaum D, et al. Prehospital coronary thrombolysis. A new strategy in acute myocardial infarction. Chest 1987; 92: 124–8.

39. Gibler WB, Kereiakes DJ, Dean EN, et al., and the investigators of the Cincinnati Heart Project and the Nashville Prehospital TPA Trial. Prehospital diagnosis and treatment of acute myocardial infarction: a north-south perspective. Am Heart J 1991; 121: 1–11.

40. Barbash GI, Roth A, Hod H, et al. Improved survival but not left ventricular function with early and prehospital treatment with plasminogen activator in acute myocardial infarction. Am J Cardiol 1990; 66: 261–6.

41. The Thrombolysis Early in Acute Heart Attack Trial Study Group. Very early thrombolytic therapy in suspected acute myocardial infarction. Am J Cardiol 1990; 65(7): 401–7.

42. Bippus PH, Haux R, Schroder R. Prehospital intravenous streptokinase in evolving myocardial infarction: a randomised study about feasibility, safety, and time-gain (abstr). Eur Heart J 1987; 8(suppl): 103.

43. Kennedy JW, Martin GV, Davis KB, et al. Western Washington intravenous streptokinase in acute myocardial infarction trial. Circulation 1988; 77(2): 345–52.

16

THROMBOLYSIS IN THE TREATMENT OF ACUTE MYOCARDIAL INFARCTION

BURTON E. SOBEL

Several recent reviews have emphasized specific aspects of thrombolysis in the treatment of acute myocardial infarction.[1-7] This chapter synthesizes and reconciles diverse views whenever possible, identifies seminal contributions, and focuses on rapidly evolving areas. Its overall objective is to provide the information needed for thoughtful and appropriate judgments required in the use of thrombolytic agents for the treatment of patients with acute myocardial infarction without purveying an algorithmic "cookbook" formula that would be simplistic and could be constructed to supplant the need for clinical decision-making predicated on knowledge. General principles are emphasized. Specific recommendations are included only as guidelines rather than all-encompassing "recipes."

EARLY EVOLUTION OF CORONARY THROMBOLYSIS

Many clinicians labor under the misapprehension that coronary thrombolysis is a novel approach in the treatment of acute myocardial infarction. In fact, its history is rich and extensive.[8] It had been shown as early as 1903 that chloroform treatment of serum gave rise to a proteolytic enzyme that could dissolve clots,[9] and as early as 1933 that filtrates of cultures of streptococci contain a component capable of inducing lysis of clots formed in plasma.[10] An important observation in 1941 by Millstone demonstrated that the streptococcal product (what is now called

streptokinase [SK]) was not active in the absence of plasma or an euglobulin fraction and hence that it required an intermediate target (what is now called plasminogen) for induction of clot lysis.[11] Millstone's observation led to the conclusion that lysis of fibrin clots formed from fibrinogen by thrombin occurred only when the fibrinolytic streptococcal product activated a component of plasma that in turn elicited lysis.

This component, plasminogen, was identified in 1945 by Christensen, who recognized that it was a circulating zymogen; that is, a precursor of an active proteolytic enzyme, and that the zymogen was converted to active enzyme (plasmin) by streptokinase.[12] Within a short time, the modern view of the fibrinolytic system emerged based in part on the observation that plasminogen binds to clots (albeit quite weakly), that activators such as streptokinase convert plasminogen to plasmin, and that clot-associated plasmin is the critical component generated by the activation of the fibrinolytic system that is responsible for clot lysis.[13]

We now know that proteolysis of fibrin by plasmin is not specific and that it depends physiologically to a large extent on the localization of plasminogen to the fibrin domain mediated by the weak interaction of lysine binding sites in plasminogen. Pharmacologic inhibitors of fibrinolysis such as epsilon-aminocaproic acid (EACA), a lysine analog, compete with plasminogen for binding to clots. Physiologic inhibition of plasmin activity in the circulation is mediated by several circulating inhibitors, the most important of which is alpha$_2$-antiplasmin, which forms complexes in a 1:1 M ratio with a lysine binding site (rapid interaction) and the active catalytic site (somewhat slower interaction) of plasmin. Other inhibitors such as alpha$_2$-macroglobulin can modulate overall plasmin activity in plasma when alpha$_2$-antiplasmin has been consumed. Because of the presence of circulating inhibitors, under physiologic conditions even maximal activation of the fibrinolytic system does not result in plasminemia.[14] However, when pharmacologic activators of the fibrinolytic system are used, particularly first-generation agents such as streptokinase, urokinase, and anisoylated plasminogen streptokinase activator complex (APSAC: generic name, anistreplase; Eminase) that do not discriminate between circulating and fibrin-associated plasminogen, concentrations of free alpha$_2$-antiplasmin decline rapidly. Under these conditions plasminemia inevitably ensues, with consequent degradation of numerous circulating proteins including coagulation factors, fibrinogen, and plasminogen, among many others. Such phenomena, in aggregate, are referred to as a systemic lytic state and may predispose to or potentiate bleeding.[15,16]

Early Treatment of Acute Myocardial Infarction

Predicated on rapidly accelerating advances in the understanding of the fibrinolytic system at the time, attempts were made to treat acute myocardial infarction with fibrinolytic agents as early as 1958.[17] The feasibility of administering streptokinase intravenously for treatment of evolving myocardial infarction was demonstrated initially in 24 patients even though the importance of coronary thrombosis as the proximate cause of acute myocardial infarction was at that time still hotly debated. Endpoints for clinical investigation of potential benefits of thrombolysis in patients with acute myocardial infarction were unfortunately quite primitive, however, and the practical utility of the approach was not widely accepted. Some investigators demonstrated that jeopardized, ischemic myocardium could apparently be protected by induction of reperfusion in animals subjected to coronary thrombosis, but even this compelling observation did not shift the pendulum toward clinical acceptance.[18]

Following the initial feasibility studies in 1958,[17] several large-scale investigations were performed with streptokinase and occasionally other activators of the fibrinolytic system given intravenously. Angiographic evaluations were generally not available, and accordingly, mortality was the primary endpoint. Many patients were not treated for as long as 72 hours after the onset of infarction; thus, it is not surprising that results of these ambitious but somewhat ill-conceived (judging from the current perspective) clinical trials were ambiguous. One study demonstrated a 50 per cent reduction of mortality six months after treatment with streptokinase within 12 hours of the onset of infarction,[19,20] but in concert, the numerous cooperative trials of the era, despite their large size and extensive acquisition of data, did not lead to changes in practice.

During the 1970s, much of the research focusing on ischemic heart disease was dominated by the concept that preservation of jeopardized, ischemic myocardium could be best achieved by reduction of myocardial oxygen requirements.[21] A link between prognosis and the extent of infarction had been established,[22,23] and results of studies in experimental animals had demonstrated that timely reduction of myocardial oxygen requirements could indeed delay necrosis or preserve myocardium indefinitely. However, clinical application of these principles led to the ultimate realization that the impact on myocardial preservation of reduction of myocardial oxygen requirements was modest, at best.[24] Thus, the stage was set for a paradigm shift. Induction of salvage of myocardium by early recanalization of occluded coronary arteries was demonstrated in experimental animals,[25] and investigators and clinicians were becoming increasingly certain that survival after acute myocardial infarction was inversely proportional to the extent of myocardium undergoing irreversible injury and that optimal treatment of incipient or evolving infarction should be designed to preserve jeopardized, ischemic myocardium by restoring its nutritive perfusion.

Several factors accounted for an explosive evolution of coronary thrombolysis at this time. A long-standing debate regarding the role of coronary thrombosis as the proximate cause of acute myocardial infarction was resolved by a pivotal angiographic study by DeWood and co-workers,[26] who demonstrated that intracoronary thrombi were present in a preponderant majority of patients who could be studied immediately after the onset of acute myocardial infarction. Although these results did not unequivocally prove that thrombosis precedes infarction, they strongly supported the hypothesis, particularly because the incidence of apparent thrombosis declined rapidly with prolongation of the interval between the apparent onset of infarction and the performance of angiography. A second clinical observation of seminal importance was the angiographic documentation of clot lysis after administration of intracoronary fibrinolytic agents.[27,28] The impact of this observation was augmented by frequent, concomitant reduction of chest pain experienced by patients given intracoronary thrombolytic agents, accelerated regression of electrocardiographic abnormalities indicative of acute infarction and accelerated evolution of Q waves, and the increasing confidence of many angiographers in evaluating critically ill patients with evolving myocardial infarction based on reassuring experience in previous angiographic studies of acutely ill patients with coronary spasm.[29]

Nevertheless, much skepticism surrounded coronary thrombolysis in the early 1980s. Recognition of potential risks (primarily hemorrhage) was widespread.[30] The possibility that coronary vasospasm, calcium overload accompanying suffusion of jeopardized myocardium with blood from recanalized vessels, and the "no reflow" phenomenon (microvascular compromise secondary to platelet and leukocyte plugging, endothelial swelling, or vasoconstriction) might compromise benefit otherwise conferred to jeopardized myocardium was seriously entertained. The myth of reperfusion injury was rampant.[31] The success of early reperfusion in reducing virtually all signs of irreversible injury[32] in hearts of animals, the striking benefits of very early reperfusion on salvage of myocardium in patients,[33] the difficulty of determining whether reperfusion injury (manifest by contraction band necrosis and myocytolysis) extends or simply substitutes for coagulative necrosis indicative of ischemic injury in the region at risk, and the relatively modest or absent benefit of attenuation of putative mediators of reperfusion injury such as oxygen-centered free radicals in enhancing salvage of myocardium accompanying reperfusion underlie the predominant current view that reperfusion injury[34] is not a critical factor in the pathogenesis of myocardial infarction treated with thrombolytic drugs. Many were fearful that arrhythmogenicity in surviving islands of myocardium would augment the incidence of sudden cardiac death among patients in whom recanalization was successful.[34] Differentiation between regional wall-motion abnormalities reflecting irreversible injury from those associated with myocardial stunning was difficult, rendering assessment of functional benefit of recanalization difficult.

At about this time, progress was being made in a related area—namely, the development of second-generation activators of the fibrinolytic system.[15,35-40] Such agents preferentially induce activation of fibrin-associated compared with circulating plasminogen and accordingly exhibit relative clot selectivity. They were developed based on the premise that clot selectivity would be associated with increased safety and efficacy by virtue of likelihood that pharmacologically effective doses could be administered without inducing a systemic lytic state or compromising hemostasis. Tissue-type plasminogen activator (t-PA) was the first example. The recombinant deoxyribonucleic acid (DNA)-produced, predominantly single-chain form of human tissue-type plasminogen activator, alteplase, is the only second-generation plasminogen activator approved for clinical use today. It was initially isolated in pharmacologic quantities from Bowes melanoma cell conditioned media by Rijken and Collen.[41] The clinically approved form, alteplase, was produced subsequently by recombinant deoxyribunucleic acid technology. In 1983, melanoma cell human tissue-type plasminogen activator was administered intravenously to dogs and shown to lyse experimentally induced coronary thrombi within a few minutes without inducing a systemic lytic state.[35] Positron-emission tompography demonstrated recovery of previously jeopardized ischemic myocardium. Based on these observations, a pilot study was performed in seven patients with total thrombotic coronary occlusions in whom parenterally administered tissue-type plasminogen activator restored perfusion in 19 to 57 minutes (in six of the seven patients) without appreciable fibrinogenolysis or induction of bleeding.[38] Subsequent, analogous studies were soon undertaken with a predominantly two-chain form of human tissue-type plasminogen activator produced by recombinant deoxyribonucleic acid technology and harvested from Chinese hamster ovary cells cultured in roller bottles, first in dogs in which coronary thrombolysis was induced without eliciting a systemic lytic state,[36] and subsequently in patients in which intravenously administered tissue-type plasminogen activator recanalized 75 to 80 per cent of occluded coronary arteries within 60 to 90 minutes in doses well below those presently used clinically.[40]

The promise of second-generation fibrinolytic drugs intensified interest in the clinical value of coronary thrombolysis for primary treatment of acute myocardial infarction in the early 1980s. Results of studies in experimental animals defined a temporal window of efficacy[42] by demonstrating that optimal salvage of jeopardized myocardium required rapid induction of clot lysis and that the amount of myocardium preserved was inversely proportional to the interval between the onset of ischemia and the induction of recanalization. Results of clinical studies demonstrated that the extent of recovery of regional wall motion was governed by the same principle and that reliance on assessment of global indexes such as ejection fraction for defining functional benefits of recanalization was hazardous.[43] The Gruppo Italiano per lo Studio della Streptochinasi nell'Infarto Miocardio (GISSI-1) results[44] demonstrated that reduction of mortality was attainable with intravenously administered streptokinase, and furthermore, that the magnitude of reduction of mortality was greatest when the interval between the onset of infarction and administration of the fibrinolytic agent was brief. Another large, placebo-controlled trial with intravenous streptokinase, the Second International Study of Infarct Survival (ISIS-2), confirmed these results.[45]

By the mid 1980s, a consensus had emerged regarding the preferable route of administration of thrombolytic drugs.[3] Although intracoronary administration of fibrinolytic agents had been required in several pivotal studies designed to assess efficacy of clot lysis, it was recognized that intravenous administration was more universally applicable and the more desirable general approach. Despite the fact that spontaneous recanalization occurs in many patients victimized by acute myocardial infarction, it was appreciated that induction of recanalization rapidly, with fibrinolytic agents, resulted in substantial salvage of jeopardized ischemic myocardium, improvement of ventricular function, and enhancement of survival. Anx-

iety regarding induction of potentially catastrophic intracerebral hemorrhage had abated because of persuasive analysis based on evaluation of approximately 40,000 patients who had been studied in diverse clinical trials with first- and second-generation fibrinolytic agents that demonstrated that the overall risk of stroke is virtually identical in appropriately selected patients managed with fibrinolytic agents and in those managed with anticoagulation alone.[46] Although it had been feared that initially successful pharmacologically induced coronary thrombolysis would require cardiac catheterization in massive numbers of patients to identify those requiring early angioplasty, results of several trials, including the Thrombolysis and Angioplasty in Myocardial Infarction study (TAMI-3),[47] the European Cooperative Study Group trial (ECSG-4),[48] and the Thrombolysis and Myocardial Infarction trial (TIMI II)[49] were concordant and compelling in demonstrating that a conservative strategy was superior. Accordingly, it was shown that catheterization and angioplasty, if indicated, could be delayed until and unless signs or symptoms of spontaneous or provoked ischemia became evident, and the epigrammatic guideline that "deferred is preferred" for angioplasty after successful coronary thrombolysis gained credence.

Despite the efficacy of coronary thrombolysis as primary therapy for acute myocardial infarction attributable to coronary thrombosis, only approximately 140,000 of the 700,000 patients hospitalized with acute myocardial infarction are presently being treated with thrombolytic agents.[50] Persistent uncertainty regarding principles underlying the use of thrombolytic agents, the setting in which they should be administered, indications and contraindications, and benefits and risks of concomitant use of adjunctive and conjunctive agents have inhibited optimal utilization of coronary thrombolysis in clinical practice. Information pertinent to resolving each of these areas of uncertainty is now extensive.

PRINCIPLES UNDERLYING THE TREATMENT OF ACUTE MYOCARDIAL INFARCTION WITH THROMBOLYTIC DRUGS

The only established mechanism by which coronary thrombolysis confers benefit in patients with acute myocardial infarction is through recanalizing infarct-related arteries. Clarity regarding this unifying principle has been obscured by misconceptions in interpreting the "open-artery hypothesis," which holds that some benefit can be conferred by coronary thrombolysis even when it must be delayed so long that salvage of jeopardized, ischemic myocardium cannot be anticipated. As discussed later in consideration of the open-artery hypothesis, even late recanalization may reduce late arrhythmogenicity, reduce late potentials that may be harbingers of anatomic substrates of lethal arrhythmias detectable by high-resolution electrocardiography, improve ventricular remodeling, augment development of collaterals because of the presence of the recanalized infarct-related artery as a conduit, diminish development of ventricular aneurysms or their arrhythmogenicity, and improve healing in the peri-infarct zone. Although benefits of early recanalization in salvaging jeopardized, ischemic myocardium, preserving ventricular function, and enhancing survival have been established firmly, proof that late recanalization in the absence of early patency (sic) confers independent benefit is not yet available. However, the open-artery hypothesis and the concept that maximal benefit accompanies very early reperfusion are not antithetical. They are, in fact, complementary ideas. Each recanalization must be accompanied by sustained patency if benefits are to be optimal. Late recanalization alone may be better than no recanalization. Regardless, however, all of the benefits attributable to an open infarct-related artery at the time of hospital discharge depend on recanalization of the infarct-related artery rather than some numinous attribute of thrombolytic drugs.

It has been thought by some that the benefits of coronary thrombolysis may be related in part to mechanisms independent of recanalization of the infarct-related artery,[51,52] including diminution of plasma viscosity with drugs that induce a systemic lytic state and consequent facilitation of maintenance of a higher cardiac output than would be the case otherwise, induction of hypotension (usually inadvertent and unwelcome consequences of the use of drugs such as streptokinase or anistreplase, which contains primarily streptokinase, in which the manifestation may reflect immune-mediated vasodilation or activation of the kinin system), which has been proposed as a means of diminishing myocar-

dial oxygen requirements, or other nonspecific actions. A powerful argument against the importance of such mechanisms is the equivalent or even superior benefit of first-generation thrombolytic agents in salvaging myocardium and improving ventricular performance when they are administered directly into the coronary circulation at much lower doses than those required systemically. Under these conditions, the nonspecific effects (with a fall in fibrinogen of 70 per cent or more in 88 per cent of patients[53] given the conventional intracoronary doses of streptokinase and a decline to 88 ± 70 milligrams/deciliter six hours after intracoronary administration of 240,000 units of streptokinase[54]) are reduced but not eliminated. Despite the less intense lytic state, recanalization is not attenuated. The same observation lays to rest the claim[55] that induction of a systemic lytic state is necessary for rapid clot lysis or prevention of reocclusion. In fact, the frequency and rapidity[56–59] (Figs. 16–1 and 16–2) of recanalization seen with clot-selective fibrinolytic drugs that induce a moderate systemic lytic state exceed those with first-generation, non–clot-selective drugs that induce a more intense one.

The Dynamic Nature of Infarction

When coronary care units were first developed in the early 1960s, acute myocardial infarction was conceptualized as a discrete event from which a patient either survived or succumbed. Such units were justified on the basis of their being able to respond to malignant ventricular arrhythmias with alacrity, reversing the otherwise lethal effects of primary or secondary ventricular fibrillation early in the hospital course. As is now widely recognized, they reduced the death rate from acute myocardial infarction in hospitalized patients from approximately 30 per cent to approximately 15 per cent. It soon became apparent, however, that many patients who survived infarction with or without the need for electrical defibrillation ultimately succumbed because of refractory cardiogenic shock, or survived for a brief interval only to be disabled by refractory congestive heart failure.

The concept that myocardial infarction is a dynamic process, evolving over hours rather than only a few minutes, and that its net effect is attributable to a large extent to the

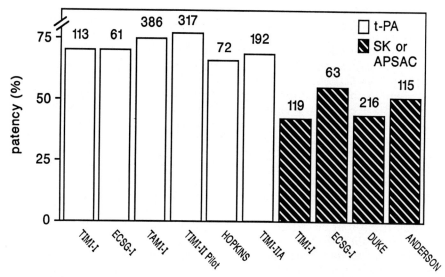

FIGURE 16–1. Angiographic patency of infarct-related arteries 90 minutes after treatment with intravenous streptokinase, tissue-type plasminogen activator (alteplase), or anistreplase, as reported in ten major trials (for review of trials see references 47, 48, 56, 88, 91, 124, 165–168).

amount of myocardium undergoing irreversible injury emerged as a result of numerous observations in experimental animals and in patients in studies testing the hypothesis that infarct size could be reduced by interventions that reduce myocardial oxygen requirements, augment myocardial oxygen supply, or both. This dynamic property of acute myocardial infarction—its evolution over minutes to hours even though it is often initiated by a

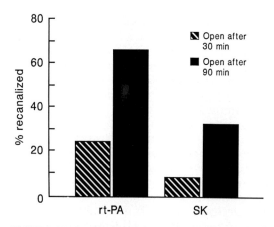

FIGURE 16–2. Percentages of patients in the TIMI I trial in whom recanalization was documented by arteriography 30 and 90 minutes after the onset of the infusion of streptokinase or recombinant tissue-type plasminogen activator (alteplase). (Data from Chesebro SH, et al. Thrombolysis in Myocardial Infarction (TIMI) trial, Phase I. A comparison between intravenous tissue plasminogen activator and intravenous streptokinase. Circulation 1987; 76: 142–54, with permission.)

discrete insult interrupting blood flow through an infarct-related artery—constitutes an important principle in the conceptual framework of coronary thrombolysis. It portends a temporal window of as much as several hours during which reperfusion of jeopardized myocardium can be anticipated to salvage at least some of the ischemic tissue at risk. The enhancement of survival of myocardium in proportion to the brevity of the antecedent interval of ischemia preceding reperfusion is readily demonstrable in studies of experimental animals. Furthermore, results of such studies have indicated that some tissue can be salvaged when reperfusion is initiated as late as three hours after the interruption of blood flow to a region of myocardium at risk.

In patients, the temporal window may be wider than it is in laboratory animals for several reasons. Occlusion of the infarct-related artery may be intermittent rather than sustained because of activation of the endogenous fibrinolytic system, contributions of vasospasm and its relief to cyclic changes in perfusion through the infarct-related artery, and the dynamic nature of thrombosis, hemorrhage, and fissuring of atherosclerotic plaques underlying many thrombotic coronary occlusions. Thus, infarction may be stuttering, and the use of fibrinolytic drugs may diminish the incidence or severity of subsequent thrombotic events that would have exacerbated infarction in their absence. Accordingly, even though improved left ventricular function and survival are most marked when thrombolytic agents can be administered within one hour after the onset of symptoms, benefit attributable to salvage of jeopardized ischemic myocardium has been seen in some cases with treatment initiated as late as four to six hours after the onset of symptoms. Additional factors that may broaden the temporal window of therapeutic opportunity in patients are the influence of collaterals and the difficulty of timing, with certitude, the onset of infarction in patients as opposed to the case in experimental animals in which a discrete insult is induced at a defined time. Many patients experience intermittent chest pain that cannot be differentiated from the pain of infarction (unstable angina) without proceeding to develop a frank infarction. Conversely, some infarctions are, of course, clinically silent. The time of onset of elevation of enzymes in plasma indicative of infarction after chest pain is perceived as variable even though the corresponding interval in experiments in animals subjected to coronary ligation is remarkably constant. Electrocardiographic criteria of the time of onset of infarction are imprecise because those that are most sensitive (such as ST segment elevation) are not specific for tissue necrosis (in contrast to criteria such as the later evolution of Q waves). Accordingly, in clinical practice, the treating physician is often unable to define the time of onset of infarction precisely even when the time of onset of symptoms of the index infarction in question is known accurately (which is often not the case). Thus, one is faced with the need to err on the side of prolongation of the temporal window of opportunity for treatment with thrombolytic drugs.[60] As noted previously, late recanalization in the established absence of early patency is hypothesized, although not proven, to confer benefit that does not depend on salvage of initially jeopardized ischemic myocardium (benefit implied by the open-artery hypothesis). If such benefit is shown to occur when early patency is indeed absent, initiation of treatment with thrombolytic drugs would be justified for patients whose infarcts may have occurred more than four to six hours earlier.

Despite these considerations, the treating physician ought not be cavalier. An overwhelming body of information supports the view that the extent of salvage of myocardium is remarkably dependent on the brevity of the interval of ischemia before recanalization and that salutary influences of thrombolysis on ventricular performance and survival are largely dependent on the amount of myocardium that can be salvaged.[42,44,61] (See Chapter 15.) Thus, as has been said epigrammatically "time is muscle" (Sarnoff J, personal communication). In fact, many believe that induction of recanalization of an infarct-related artery an average of 15 minutes after the onset of occlusion will exert strikingly more favorable effects on prognosis than induction of recanalization an average of 30 or 45 minutes after the onset of occlusion in otherwise similar patients.

The Timing of Recanalization

Recanalization should be induced as quickly as possible after the onset of myocardial infarction attributable to coronary thrombosis.[44,45,61-68] Thus, once the diagnosis is strongly suspected and possible contraindications to the use of thrombolytic drugs have been appropriately considered and excluded, treatment should be initiated with the agent deemed to be most effective as soon as possible. Some investigators advocate primary angioplasty as treatment for acute myocardial infarction, a strategy that will be discussed briefly below, but such an approach is not applicable to the vast majority of patients who can be treated with thrombolytic drugs administered intravenously virtually immediately in settings that would not permit immediate catheterization. Successful therapy with thrombolytic agents is predicated on induction of rapid recanalization, assurance of persistence of recanalization, and judicious and aggressive use of adjunctive and conjunctive measures to ensure sustained patency. The unfortunate reliance by some on acquisition of laboratory results such as elevated activities of plasma enzymes to definitively establish the diagnosis of acute myocardial infarction before implementing treatment with thrombolytic drugs is inappropriate. Plasma enzyme activities may not exceed the upper limits of normal ranges for several hours after the onset of unequivocal transmural infarction, and delay in implementing recanalization is not justified simply so that the treating physician can be unequivocally certain that an infarction is indeed established. Coronary thrombolysis is well worth the risk in appropriately selected patients when treatment can be initiated within three hours after the apparent onset of infarction. It is likely to be most effective when it can be initiated even earlier, and optimally, it should be initiated as soon as possible after the onset of ischemia. Most investigators agree that benefits attributable to salvage of ischemic myocardium can be anticipated even when its implementation must be delayed for three to six hours after the onset of apparent infarction, and many contend that even later implementation of coronary thrombolysis is justified in some patients because of considerations implicit in the open-artery hypothesis and the potential value of coronary thrombolysis in interrupting stuttering infarction. (See also Chapter 15.)

The Simultaneity of Thrombosis and Thrombolysis

Because benefits of coronary thrombolysis depend primarily or exclusively on recanalization, much attention has been devoted to the determinants of restoration of patency of an occluded infarct-related artery. Generally, occlusive thrombi form on a nidus of an active, complex, rupturing or fissuring atherosclerotic plaque as a result of local activation of platelets and the coagulation system.[69] Exposure of circulating blood to thrombogenic substances in the vessel wall including collagen (which activates platelets), von Willebrand factor (which binds platelets through the surface receptor glycoprotein Ib-alpha under conditions of high sheer stress),[70] and tissue factor (which, when complexed with activated factor VII, activates the extrinsic pathway of coagulation) may initiate or potentiate thrombosis.[71] Generation of thrombin through activation of the extrinsic pathway of coagulation, the intrinsic pathway, or both (with the tissue/activated factor VII complex potentially activating factor IX as well as factor X), can accelerate clotting directly and exert positive feedback on the intrinsic pathway of coagulation by activating factor V and factor VIII.[72] Furthermore, as clots undergo pharmacologically induced lysis, they elaborate and release components such as thrombin that may potentiate the simultaneously occurring local thrombosis. In addition, nonspecific and potentially undesirable effects of free plasmin (unbound to fibrin) can induce procoagulant effects that

may attenuate the rate or extent of recanalization.[73-75] Thus, the time course, frequency, and completeness of recanalization depend on the extent to which the pharmacologically induced thrombolysis exceeds the countervailing, contemporaneous, locally and systemically stimulated ongoing thrombosis.

Recognition of these phenomena has led to a rapidly growing appreciation of the essentiality of measures that have been called conjunctive.[4,76] Such measures are designed to potentiate thrombolysis by inhibiting the simultaneously ongoing thrombosis, not only to prevent early thrombotic reocclusion, but also to accelerate recanalization. Awareness of these phenomena has led also to a more critical appraisal of results of clinical studies performed to assess the efficacy of coronary thrombolysis and more critical assessments of their design and of study endpoints.

Types of Clinical Trials

Three major types of clinical studies have been performed to define the therapeutic efficacy of coronary thrombolysis. Recanalization trials are the most informative.[3] They require angiographic documentation of the presence of an occlusive thrombus before treatment is initiated as well as angiographic documentation of clot lysis and resultant recanalization of the infarct-related artery. Results of such trials are the most definitive with respect to comparison of efficacy of diverse thrombolytic agents, diverse therapeutic regimens with conjunctive or adjunctive agents, and the rapidity of induction of recanalization with specific agents. Unfortunately, however, such studies require coronary angiography before treatment and thereby entail at least some delay. The impact of results of recanalization studies on the development of coronary thrombolysis has been profound, but the frequency with which they can be performed presently is limited because of ethical considerations mandating against delay before the onset of treatment.

Patency trials utilize angiography in a different fashion. They define the presence of a patent infarct-related artery at a given interval after the apparent onset of infarction and usually employ angiography only after treatment has been implemented. Results of such studies have been used to document efficacy but are not as conclusive as those obtained in recanalization trials because some patients are included as "successes" in whom complete occlusion had never been present; others are included as failures in whom the thrombolytic agent had recanalized the infarct-related artery transiently but in which reocclusion occurred before angiography was performed; and some are included as successes in whom the drug failed to open the infarct-related artery but in whom spontaneous recanalization occurred subsequently before angiography. The ambiguity has led to much unnecessary confusion. It is well appreciated that infarct-related arteries recanalize spontaneously (over many hours to days) in at least a majority of patients with transmural myocardial infarction. Results of a patency trial in which angiography is performed only several days after the onset of infarction will therefore often fail to show differences between any regimens being compared because of the overriding impact of spontaneous restoration of patency at a time when salvage of myocardium is unlikely (the so-called "catch-up" phenomenon), obscuring marked differences that had been present with respect to early recanalization. Accordingly, the coupling between the discerned incidence of late patency and salvage of myocardium is extraordinarily loose and potentially markedly misleading. Even though some observers[77] have ascribed similarities to different thrombolytic drugs on the basis of similarities in late patency, such conclusions do not appear to be justified.

The third type of clinical evaluation of efficacy of thrombolytic agents relies on nonangiographic endpoints to define indirectly the apparent incidence of restoration of patency of infarct-related arteries by measuring endpoints such as persistent regional wall-motion abnormalities, impaired global left ventricular function, or mortality. Because the endpoints are only loosely coupled to the absolute rate, incidence, and persistence of recanalization; because the statistical variance of each of these endpoints is wide in any given sample; and because some of the endpoints such as mortality occur with low frequency in populations studied, such studies require large numbers of patients, often in excess of 10,000, to detect statistically and clinically significant differences attributable to differences in the rate and incidence of recanalization.

Interpretation of results of such studies is confounded by additional difficulties, one of which is exemplified by consideration of ef-

fects of coronary thrombolysis on left ventricular function. This endpoint, relied upon by many, might be anticipated at first blush to reflect the benefits of recanalization in a direct fashion. However, interpretation must be circumspect. In general, ventricular function has been assessed with global indexes such as ejection fraction. Global indexes are limited to an accuracy of only ± 5 per cent, a range within which induced changes may fall and often fail to reflect the functional status of the left ventricle and its improvement as a result of thrombolysis because of concomitant changes in preload and afterload that detract from their sensitivity. In addition, improvement in regional wall motion in the risk region may be offset by diminished compensatory hyperfunction in nonjeopardized myocardium with no net change in the global index.[78] Accordingly, characterization of regional function is likely to be more specific and less ambiguous.

Unfortunately, however, even endpoints defining regional function do not entirely circumvent difficulties that obscure interpretation. As pointed out by Van der Werf,[79] reperfusion may improve regional function in jeopardized ischemic myocardium in individual patients but fail to improve it in groups of treated compared with control patients because of unappreciated and confounding effects on survival. If treatment increases survival, and particularly if it increases survival among patients with markedly depressed ventricular function, regional wall motion in the entire group of treated patients who survive may be no better (and perhaps worse) than that in the surviving group of control patients from which mortality has already claimed those with the most depressed ventricular function. This dichotomy, which has been called the ventricular function/mortality paradox, appears to account for the inverse relationship between overall improvement in survival and overall improvement in ventricular function evident from careful analysis of results in survivors in many clinical trials of thrombolytic agents.

Effects of Thrombolysis on Ventricular Function

Despite these caveats, coronary thrombolysis unequivocally improves ventricular function as judged from results before and after treatment of patients given thrombolytic agents in recanalization and patency trials. Left ventricular ejection fraction increased significantly in patients treated with intracoronary streptokinase[80] when thrombolysis was successful but did not change when it failed. Improvement has been seen also in treated patients in randomized trials with intracoronary streptokinase[5] in comparison with results in controls. In other studies, improved regional wall motion without improvement in global ejection fraction was evident at the time of hospital discharge in patients in whom recanalization was successful with intracoronary streptokinase,[78] with no change evident in patients in whom persistent recanalization had not been induced. Analogous results have been reported with intravenous streptokinase.[81-84]

Preservation of global ventricular function has been demonstrated in randomized trials of other thrombolytic agents as well, such as tissue-type plasminogen activator given to patients within four hours of the apparent onset of infarction[68] who were compared with those given a placebo. Analogous results were obtained in the double-blind, randomized, multicenter Thrombolysis in Acute Coronary Occlusion (TICO) trial[67] in which treated patients had a global ejection fraction of 62 per cent compared with 54 per cent in controls given placebo. A similar difference was seen when ejection fraction was measured one week after the onset of infarction.[68] In general, as judged from results of diverse trials, the earlier the administration of thrombolytic agents, the greater the preservation of regional left ventricular function.[61,82-88]

Favorable effects on ventricular performance appear to be more prominent among patients with anterior as opposed to inferior infarction.[65] Nevertheless, improvement has been seen in some patients with inferior infarction[89] as well. Thus, even though many studies have failed to show improvements in left ventricular function assessed with global or even regional indexes in comparisons of

TABLE 16–1. Ejection Fraction Three Weeks After Myocardial Infarction*

		EJECTION FRACTION	
	NUMBER	Streptokinase or Urokinase	Tissue-Type Plasminogen Activator
Studies comparing thrombolytic agents			
White	270	58 ± 12	58 ± 12
PAIMS	171	53 ± 10	55 ± 11
GAUS	246	52 ± 14	53 ± 12
Thrombolysis with or without coronary angioplasty		+PTCA	−PTCA
TAMI 1	386	53	56
ECSG	367	49	49
TIMI IIa	389	50	49
TIMI IIb	3262	50	50.4†
SWIFT	800	51.7 ± 15	50.7 ± 15
Adjunctive agents		Treatment	Placebo
Captopril	38	52.4 ± 11.5	48.9 ± 13.8
Superoxide dismutase	120	52.4 ± 13.7	55.6 ± 12.6
Prostacyclin	50	48.0 ± 9.4	50.4 ± 9.8‡
Beta blockers	1390	50.5	50
Nifedipine	149	54.0 ± 11	56.0 ± 15

* Reprinted with permission, from Califf RM, et al. Left ventricular ejection fraction may not be useful as an end point of thrombolytic therapy comparative trials. Circulation 1990; 82: 1847–53.
† By gated blood pool scintigraphy.
‡ Not randomized.
PAIMS = Plasminogen Activator Italian Multicenter Study; GAUS = German Activator Urokinase Study; (+) (−) PTCA = (with) (without) percutaneous transluminal coronary artery angioplasty; TAMI = Thrombolysis and Angioplasty in Myocardial Infarction; ECSG = European Cooperative Study Group; TIMI = Thrombolysis in Myocardial Infarction; SWIFT = Should We Intervene Following Thrombolysis?

treated and untreated groups, perhaps because of the ventricular function/mortality paradox, and despite the insensitivity of indexes of global function for comparison of diverse regimens[90] (Table 16–1), analysis of regional wall motion in studies employing serial observations have been remarkably concordant in demonstrating a significant but modest benefit conferred by coronary thrombolysis. A corollary of these observations is that the conclusion[77] that similarity of global ventricular function in survivors after treatment with disparate thrombolytic drugs implies equivalence of agents is not justified.

Effects on Mortality

Because early mortality associated with acute myocardial infarction is relatively low (on the order of 12 to 20 per cent during the past ten years with perhaps an even lower overall mortality rate accompanying recent improvements in management), and because many patients treated with a specific regimen in comparative trials will require interventions during the hospital course and early convalescent interval that may make independent contributions to outcome, it has been difficult to definitively assess the impact of coronary thrombolysis on survival. The large GISSI-1 trial of more than 12,000 patients demonstrated an overall reduction in 21-day mortality from 13.0 to 10.7 per cent attributable to treatment with intravenous streptokinase, and perhaps even more important, documented a 47 per cent reduction of mortality in patients who could be treated within the first hour after the onset of symptoms.[44] Analysis of pooled data from four trials that compared a first-generation thrombolytic drug (streptokinase) with a second-generation agent (tissue-type plasminogen activator)[3,56,87,91,92] indicated an 8 per cent 21- to 30-day absolute mortality rate for patients treated with streptokinase and a 4 per cent mortality among those treated with tissue-type plasminogen activator.[3] Accordingly, it was surprising to many that the results of the recently completed GISSI-2 and t-PA/SK International trials, which directly compared tissue-type plasminogen activator with streptokinase in 20,891[93] patients, failed to demonstrate a significant difference in mortality with the two drugs and reported an overall early mortality of 8.7 per cent. These results are at variance with the recently summarized[4]

(Fig. 16–3) overall early mortality in several studies of second-generation, clot-selective drugs of 5.6 per cent in 8,501 patients from 19 trials, a rate substantially lower than the 9.4 per cent rate among 16,824 patients treated with first-generation fibrinolytic agents including streptokinase, urokinase, and anistreplase studied in the same and similar trials during the same interval. A summary of the early mortality in studies with thrombolytic drugs preceding the GISSI-2, t-PA/SK International, and ISIS-3 trials is shown in Table 16–2.

The overall high mortality rate in the GISSI-2 and t-PA/SK International trials appears to be attributable at least in part to the lack of adequate concomitant anticoagulation, as discussed later under conjunctive treatment. Because of the potentially protective anticoagulant effects of elevated concentrations of fibrinogen degradation products induced by plasminemia many hours after thrombolysis, the lack of adequacy of anticoagulation in these trials would be expected to detract more from the efficacy of treatment with tissue-type plasminogen activator, the second-generation fibrinolytic agent used (alteplase), than from that of the first-generation drug (streptokinase). Accordingly the lack of difference between early mortality with streptokinase and alteplase in these trials may be a manifestation of the same fundamental deficiency in design—namely lack of adequate anticoagulation—as is, in part, the overall high mortality seen with both drugs.

A recent analysis of the effect of adequate anticoagulation on the success of coronary thrombolysis (vigorous treatment with intravenously administered heparin) points toward the importance of anticoagulation (Table 16–3). In those trials in which intravenous heparin was not used concomitantly, mortality in the treatment group averaged 9.3 per cent. In those in which intravenous heparin was used concomitantly, mortality averaged 5.5 per cent. The data from which these averages were computed are summarized in Table 16–4 (studies without concomitant intravenous heparin) and Table 16–5 (studies with concomitant intravenous heparin). Judging from the pooled data acquired in studies employing principles of practice that more closely resemble conventional procedures in the United States than do the procedures mandated by the protocols used in the GISSI-2 and ISIS-3 trials, one can conclude that thrombolytic agents without

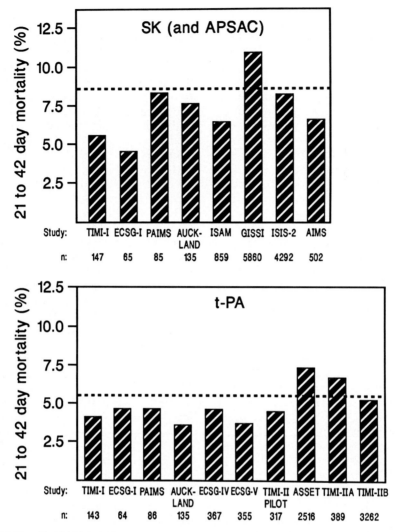

FIGURE 16–3. Absolute mortality reported at 21 to 30 days in eight major trials of streptokinase and anistreplase (*top*) (for review of trials, see references 44, 45, 56, 63, 82, 87, 91, 92), and eight major trials of tissue-type plasminogen activator (alteplase) (*bottom*) (for review of trials, see references 48, 56, 61, 64, 87, 91, 92, 167). Dashed line indicates mortality for all patients in each panel. In placebo-controlled studies, "n" refers to the number of patients receiving active drug. ISIS-2 data (*top*) are reported for patients given streptokinase plus aspirin (mortality was 10.4 per cent in 4,300 patients given streptokinase alone).

concomitantly administered intravenous heparin reduce early mortality by 29 per cent, and that with concomitantly administered intravenous heparin they reduce it much more, by 39 per cent, regardless of which thrombolytic agent is used.

The favorable effects of coronary thrombolysis on mortality extend well beyond the interval early after infarction. They are sustained for at least one year as judged from results in the AIMS trial (with anistreplase)[94] and in the GISSI-1 trial (with streptokinase) in which only a very small fraction of patients underwent angioplasty or coronary bypass

grafting during the year after infarction. They are sustained for at least a comparable interval as judged from the low initial mortality (4.9 per cent) in the more than 3,000 patients treated with intravenous tissue-type plasminogen activator in the TIMI-II trial, only 50 per cent of whom were randomized to the "early angioplasty if indicated and feasible" arm.[49]

The favorable effects of coronary thrombolysis on mortality appear to depend directly on recanalization of the infarct-related artery. Thus, the more marked reductions in mortality seen in most studies of second-genera-

TABLE 16–2. Early Mortality in Trials with Thrombolytic Drugs Preceding GISSI-2 and the t-PA/SK International Trial*

	PLACEBO GROUP		FIRST-GENERATION DRUGS		SECOND-GENERATION DRUGS	
TRIAL	Number	% Mortality (Number)	Number	% Mortality (Number)	Number	% Mortality (Number)
AIMS	502	12.2 (62)	502(APSAC)	6.4 (32)		
GAUS			121(UK)	4.1 (5)	124(t-PA)	4.8 (6)
ISAM	463	7.1 (33)	477(SK)	6.3 (30)		
PAIMS			85(SK)	8.2 (7)	86(t-PA)	4.7 (4)
PRIMI			203(SK)	4.9 (10)	198(scu-PA)	3.5 (7)
TIMI I			147(SK)	8.2 (12)	143(t-PA)	4.9 (7)
TICO (Sydney/Auckland)	71	5.6 (4)			74(t-PA)	5.4 (4)
ECSG (1979)	106	30.6 (32)	125(SK)	15.6 (20)		
ECSG-1 (1985)			65(SK)	4.6 (3)	64(t-PA)	4.7 (3)
ECSG-2 (1985)	65	6.2 (4)			64(t-PA)	1.6 (1)
ECSG-3 (1987)					123(t-PA)	4.9 (6)
ECSG-4 (1988)					184(t-PA)	3.0 (6)
					183(t-PA + 2 hour PTCA)	7.0 (13)
ECSG-5 (1988)	366	5.7 (21)			355(t-PA)	2.8 (18)
GISSI-1†	5852	13.0 (761)	5860(SK)	10.7 (627)		
New Zealand-1	93	12.9 (12)	79(SK)	2.5 (2)		
New Zealand-2			135(SK)	7.4 (10)	135(t-PA)	3.7 (5)
ISIS-2†‡	8595	12.0 (1031)	8592(SK)	9.2 (790)		
HART					106(t-PA)	2.0 (2)
HART†					99(t-PA)	3.0 (3)
SCATI			218(SK + intravenous followed by subcutaneous heparin)	4.5 (10)		
			215(SK w/o subcutaneous heparin)	8.8 (19)		
ASSET	2495	9.8 (245)			2516(t-PA)	7.9 (181)
NHF Australia	71	2.8 (2)			73(t-PA)	9.6 (7)
TIMI II pilot					317(t-PA)	4.4 (14)
TIMI IIa					195(t-PA + 2 hour PTCA)	5.2 (11)
					200(t-PA + 24 hour PTCA)	7.4 (15)
TIMI IIb					3262(t-PA)	4.9 (160)
Total	18,679	11.8 (2204)	16,824	9.4 (1577)	8501	5.6 (476)

* Reprinted with permission, from Tiefenbrunn AJ, Sobel BE. Thrombolysis and Myocardial Infarction. Fibrinolysis 1991;5: 1–15.
† Intravenous heparin was not included in the protocol.
‡ Intention to treat with intravenous heparin in a minority of treated patients.
AIMS = APSAC (anisoylated plasminogen streptokinase activator complex) Intervention Mortality Study; GAUS = German Activator Urokinase Study; ISAM = Intravenous Streptokinase in Acute Myocardial Infarction Study; PAIMS = Plasminogen Activator Italian Multicenter Study; PRIMI = Prourokinase in Myocardial Infarction Study; TICO = Thrombolysis in Acute Coronary Occlusion; ECSG = European Cooperative Study Group; GISSI = Gruppo Italiano per lo Studio della Streptochinasi nell'Infarto Miocardio; ISIS = International Study of Infarct Survival; HART = Heparin-Aspirin Reperfusion Trial; SCATI = Studio sulla Calciparini nell'Angina nella Trombosi Ventriculare nell' Infarto; ASSET = Anglo-Scandinavian Study of Early Thrombolysis; NHF = National Heart Foundation; TIMI = Thrombolysis in Myocardial Infarction. SK = streptokinase; t-PA = tissue-type plasminogen activator; UK = urokinase; scu-PA = single-chain urokinase plasminogen inhibitors.

TABLE 16–3. Pooled Data on Early Mortality (≤42 Days) in Trials of Intravenous Streptokinase or Tissue-Type Plasminogen Activator (alteplase) With and Without Heparin*

	PLACEBO GROUP		TREATMENT GROUP		% REDUCTION IN MORTALITY (TREATMENT VERSUS PLACEBO)
	Number	*% Mortality (Number)*	*Number*	*% Mortality (Number)*	
With intravenous heparin	3090	9.2 (284)	9,298	5.5 (514)	39
Without intravenous heparin	16,331	13.1 (2,144)	34,581	9.3 (3,226)	29

* Reprinted with permission, from Tiefenbrunn AJ, Sobel BE. Thrombolysis and myocardial infarction. Fibrinolysis 1991; 5: 1–15.

tion compared with first-generation agents parallel consistent differences in the incidence of recanalization induced with the two types of drugs. Patency 90 minutes after treatment with intravenous streptokinase is evident in approximately 50 per cent of patients studied angiographically. Patency estimated at the same interval after the onset of treatment with tissue-type plasminogen activator (alteplase) in otherwise similar studies averages approximately 75 per cent (Figure 16–1). Analogous results have been obtained in those studies in which recanalization was measured directly[40,95] or estimated based on patency early after treatment[91] when streptokinase and tissue-type plasminogen activator were compared directly in the same trial. The observed difference in the incidence of early recanalization (approximately 75 per cent with tissue-type plasminogen activator

compared with 50 per cent with streptokinase) would be expected to translate into a 33 per cent difference in early mortality, a value entirely in keeping with the difference in mortality that has been observed in studies with second-generation as opposed to first-generation agents (Table 16–2).

Such differences in sustained patency may have been absent in the GISSI-2, the t-PA/SK International, and ISIS-3 trials because of the lack of utilization of concomitantly administered intravenous heparin. As shown in the recently published Heparin or Aspirin Reocclusion Trial (HART)[96] study in which the primary endpoint was angiographically documented patency one day after induction of coronary thrombolysis, patency in patients given heparin with tissue-type plasminogen activator was 82 per cent. In contrast, it was significantly less (only 52 per cent) among

TABLE 16–4. Early Mortality (≤42 Days) in Trials of Intravenous Thrombolytic Drugs Without Heparin*

TRIAL	PLACEBO GROUP		TREATMENT GROUP	
	Number	*% Mortality (Number)*	*Number*	*% Mortality (Number)*
GISSI-1				
Times to treatment				
≤12 hours	5,852	13.0 (761)	5,860	10.7 (627)
≤1 hour	642	15.4 (99)	635	8.2 (52)
≤3 hour	3,078	12.0 (369)	3,016	9.2 (277)
3–6 hour	1,800	14.1 (254)	1,849	11.7 (216)
6–9 hour	659	14.1 (93)	693	12.6 (87)
GISSI-2/Int'l t-PA/SK		N/A	10,364(t-PA)	8.9 (922)
			10,385(SK)	8.5 (883)
ISIS-2	4300	13.2 (568)	1,463	9.6 (140)
			(SK + ASA)	
HART		N/A	99	3.0 (3)
SCATI		N/A	217	8.8 (19)
Total	16,331	13.1 (2,144)	34,581	9.3 (3,226)

* Reprinted with permission, from Tiefenbrunn AJ, Sobel BE. Thrombolysis and myocardial infarction. Fibrinolysis 1991; 5:1–15. Abbreviations are as in Table 16–2. ASA = aspirin; N/A = not applicable.

TABLE 16–5. Early Mortality (≤42 Days) in Trials of Intravenous Thrombolytic Drugs With Heparin*

	Placebo Group		Treatment Group	
Trial	Number	% Mortality (Number)	Number	% Mortality (Number)
ASSET	2,495	9.8 (245)	2,516	7.2 (181)
ECSG-1		N/A	64(t-PA)	4.7 (3)
			65(SK)	4.6 (3)
ECSG-2	65	6.2 (4)	64(t-PA)	1.6 (1)
ECSG-3			123(t-PA)	4.9 (6)
ECSG-4		N/A	367	5.0 (18)
ECSG-5	366	5.7 (21)	355	2.8 (10)
HART			106	2.0 (2)
			1,024 (SK +	6.4 (66)
ISIS-2 ("intention to treat" with intravenous heparin)			ASA)	
NHF Australia	71	2.8 (2)	73	9.6 (7)
New Zealand-1	93	12.9 (12)	79	2.5 (2)
New Zealand-2		N/A	135(t-PA)	3.7 (5)
			135(SK)	7.4 (10)
SCATI		N/A	218	4.5 (10)
TIMI II pilot		N/A	317	4.4 (14)
TIMI IIa			195(t-PA + 2 hour PTCA)	5.2 (11)
			200(t-PA + 24 hour PTCA)	7.4 (15)
TIMI IIb		N/A	3,262	4.9 (160)
Total	3,090	9.2 (284)	9,298	5.5 (514)

* Reprinted with permission, from Tiefenbrunn AJ, Sobel BE. Thrombolysis and myocardial infarction. Fibrinolysis 1991; 5: 1–15. Abbreviations are as in Table 16–2. ASA = aspirin; N/A = not applicable.

patients who were not given heparin concomitantly with the tissue-type plasminogen activator. Similar results were reported by Bleich and co-workers,[97] who observed patency in 71 per cent of patients approximately 2.5 days after treatment with tissue-type plasminogen activator plus conjunctive heparin compared with only 44 per cent in those to whom intravenous heparin was not administered. A third comparison in which patency was assessed even later, at a mean of 81 hours (48 to 120 hours)[98] found a directionally similar (83.4 per cent versus 74.7 per cent) and statistically significant difference, but one smaller than that seen in the HART and Bleich studies, perhaps because patency was assessed so late that "catch-up" attributable to the well-recognized contributions of late spontaneous recanalization had occurred. In a prospective double-blind trial, patients with acute myocardial infarction were treated with saruplase (80 milligrams over 60 minutes) and randomly assigned to receive 5,000 units heparin or placebo at the start of treatment with the thrombolytic drug. At the end of the saruplase infusion, patency in patients treated with saruplase plus heparin was 80.8 per cent compared with only 60.4 per cent

in patients treated with saruplase without heparin (p = 0.03).[99] Results of these four studies (Table 16–6) indicate that anticoagulation is particularly important in sustaining patency induced with thrombolytic agents (particularly second-generation, clot-selective drugs that give rise to lower concentrations of fibrinogen degradation products with their consequent anticoagulant effects than do first-generation agents). Even though the incidence of induction of patency in 90 minutes after tissue-type plasminogen activator appears to be comparable whether or not heparin is given concomitantly,[100] results of these four recent angiographic studies indicate that the incidence of reocclusion and consequent compromise of benefit of initially successful thrombolysis will be greater when anticoagulation is not sufficiently vigorous and intravenously administered heparin is not employed concomitantly. Because reduction of early mortality depends not only on induction of recanalization but also on its persistence, results of the GISSI-2 and ISIS-3 trials should not be expected to reflect the apparent differences in the incidence of early recanalization and it persistence seen with second-generation compared with first-generation

TABLE 16–6. Coronary Patency in Patients Treated With Alteplase or Saruplase With or Without Conjunctive, Intravenous Heparin (See also Chapter 17)

STUDY	NUMBER	TIME OF ANGIOGRAPHY AFTER TREATMENT (HOURS)		PATENCY OF THE INFARCT-RELATED ARTERY		DRUG
		Mean	*Range*	*With Heparin*	*Without Heparin*	
HART	205	18	(7–24)	82% (−ASA)*	48% (+ASA)	Alteplase
Bleich et al.	83	57	(48–72)	71% (−ASA)	44% (−ASA)	Alteplase
ECSG-6	609	81	(48–120)	84% (+ASA)	75% (+ASA)	Alteplase
Tebbe	118	8	(6–12)	81%	60%	Saruplase

* ASA refers to the use (+) or lack (−) of protocol-mandated aspirin.

thrombolytic agents administered with appropriately vigorous, concomitant anticoagulation.

Risks Associated with Coronary Thrombolysis

The major risk accompanying the use of thrombolytic drugs is hemorrhage.[101] Concern was heightened by experience reported from early recanalization trials in which the incidence of bleeding was reported meticulously and patients were subjected to repetitive vascular access. In clinical practice, the overall incidence of bleeding is substantially less than it is in such trials. However, any plasminogen activator can induce catastrophic hemorrhage if a protective clot is present (such as one forming during the early stages of healing of a peptic ulcer or preventing bleeding in a previously ruptured Berry aneurysm). None available presently (or perhaps ever) can discriminate between such protective clots and the therapeutic targets of fibrinolysis in coronary arteries. Such catastrophic episodes can, however, be generally avoided by appropriate selection of patients, exclusion of those with specific contraindications discussed in detail below, and possibly weight-adjusted dose regimens.

Patients with acute myocardial infarction are, of course, subject to other manifestations of atherosclerosis as well, in view of the generalized nature of the disorder, and to complications of infarction that may be manifest by hemorrhage exacerbated by fibrinolytic drugs (such as embolization from a ventricular mural thrombus to the brain with conversion of an embolic to a hemorrhagic cerebrovascular accident). Some patients may be compromised by the use of oral anticoagulant agents before an index infarction, which could exacerbate bleeding induced by any fibrinolytic drug. A small minority of patients may be at increased risk of bleeding because of pregnancy, a postpartum state, or active menstruation—all of which are relative contraindications to the use of fibrinolytic agents. Nevertheless, with increasing experience, the remarkable safety of judiciously implemented coronary thrombolysis has been demonstrated amply.[3,4,43]

The most serious risk associated with fibrinolytic drugs, intracranial hemorrhage, appears to be increased only minimally when fibrinolytic agents are administered to appropriately selected patients. In the Anglo-Scandinavian Study of Early Thrombolysis (ASSET) trial, patients treated with tissue-type plasminogen activator exhibited an incidence of stroke of 1.1 per cent—virtually identical to the 1.0 per cent incidence in placebo-treated controls.[64] Among the first 3,000 patients treated with conventional doses of tissue-type plasminogen activator in studies in the United States, the overall incidence of cerebrovascular accident was less than 0.5 per cent.[3] Results of early studies with intravenous streptokinase indicated that patients over the age of 75 were at greater risk for major hemorrhagic complications, including intracranial hemorrhage[102] than younger patients, and anecdotal information in the dose-finding portion of the TIMI II study[103] in which 5 of 326 patients (1.5 per cent) treated with 150 milligrams of tissue-type plasminogen activator manifested intracranial bleeding compared with 0.6 per cent in the remainder after the dose had been reduced to 100 milligrams over three hours indicates that suprapharmacologic doses of thrombolytic agents may predispose to this devastating complication. However, in an analysis of five large, placebo-controlled clinical trials with a variety of thrombolytic agents involving approximately 40,000 patients, the overall incidence of stroke (thromboembolic and hemorrhagic) in patients treated with a thrombolytic agent was found to be 0.9 per cent, a value virtually identical to that in patients given placebo in the same trials.

Second-generation agents appear to be somewhat safer than first-generation agents judging from the lower transfusion requirements and the lower incidence of spontaneous, major bleeding encountered with their use.[3,43,87,101] However, with judicious selection of patients, use of all available thrombolytic agents is remarkably safe and well worth the risk in treatment of patients with acute myocardial infarction.

Consolidation of Benefits

Because benefits of coronary thrombolysis depend primarily on rapidly induced and sustained recanalization, and because the rate of restoration of patency of a thrombotically occluded infarct-related artery is a reflection of the predominance of thrombolysis over ongoing concomitant thrombosis, vigorous, concomitant anticoagulation is necessary. It is necessary also to prevent early thrombotic reocclusion that may compromise benefit otherwise conferred by initially successful thrombolysis.

Several factors that can potentiate local thrombosis may retard recanalization or predispose to early thrombotic reocclusion. Exposure of blood to thrombogenic factors including von Willebrand factor and tissue factor within the arterial wall and to complex atherosclerotic plaques may initiate the deposition of platelets and their activation and may activate the coagulation cascade directly.[69,70] Thrombin is a potent activator of platelets, and recent information is compatible with the view that a major determinant of platelet activation in the vicinity of thrombi undergoing lysis is thrombin elaborated from the dissolving clot or generated locally as a result of activation of the coagulation system.[72] Diminished release of prostacyclin and heparin-like proteoglycans from dysfunctional or damaged endothelium or walls of vessels with denuded endothelium can contribute. Surprisingly, the fibrinolytic agents themselves may paradoxically accelerate thrombosis, which is of course generally

masked by their predominant, clot-lysing effects.[73-75] In patients given thrombolytic agents, increases occur in the concentration of fibrinopeptide A in plasma, a marker of continuing thrombin activity. Concentrations of metabolites of thromboxane increase in urine in patients treated with thrombolytic agents as well, reflecting platelet activation in vivo accompanying fibrinolysis[104] even though neither plasminogen activators themselves (such as tissue-type plasminogen activator) nor plasmin exert direct effects on washed platelets maintained in solutions with physiologic concentrations of calcium.[105] Procoagulant effects of plasminogen activators are demonstrable in vitro and are reflected by paradoxical acceleration of clotting in recalcified citrated plasma supplemented with products of incubation of plasma with tissue-type plasminogen activator. These effects can be simulated by plasmin and inhibited by antiplasmins, suggesting that the procoagulant effects of plasminogen activators in vivo reflect plasminemia and consequent nonspecific proteolytic effects of plasmin on procoagulant proteins (Eisenberg PR, personal communication). Such procoagulant effects of plasminogen activators appears to be more prominent with first- as opposed to second-generation fibrinolytic drugs, in keeping with their more intense elaboration of plasmin in the fluid phase of blood because of lack of clot selectivity.[74] This may explain, in part, the more rapid recanalization seen with second- compared with first-generation fibrinolytic agents. However, procoagulant effects can be seen with high concentrations of drugs of both types. In view of these considerations, it is not surprising that concomitant inhibition of coagulation, diminution of activation of platelets, or both appear to accelerate and sustain recanalization induced with fibrinolytic agents after coronary thrombolysis in experimental animals and in patients.

Adjunctive and Conjunctive Agents

It is useful to consider two categories of pharmacologic agents used in association with fibrinolytic drugs for treatment of coronary thrombosis.[3,76] Adjunctive agents have been defined as drugs designed to attenuate irreversible myocardial injury secondary to ischemia or reperfusion by diminishing myocardial oxygen requirements (such as vasodilators used to diminish ventricular preload and afterload), inhibiting deleterious effects of noxious metabolites accumulating in ischemic or reperfused myocardium (such as oxygen-centered free radicals), and diminishing calcium overload among other mechanisms. Along with other interventions, including the administration of oxygen, adjunctive agents are, in a sense, anti-injury agents. Conjunctive agents have been defined as agents designed to potentiate thrombolysis per se, that is, to accelerate recanalization, to sustain it, or both. Examples include anticoagulants and antiplatelet agents as well as interventions under investigation[106] targeted against induction of prothrombotic effects of plasminogen activators. Adjunctive and conjunctive agents of diverse types, many of which are investigational, are listed in Table 16–7. Those often used concomitantly with fibrinolytic agents in patients with myocardial infarction and the dose of each are indicated in Table 16–8.

Examples of conjunctive agents with particular promise are those that inhibit the major receptor mediated platelet aggregation in vivo (the surface glycoprotein receptor, glycoprotein IIb-IIIa, which interacts with fibrinogen among other adhesive proteins). Both monoclonal antibodies to the glycoprotein IIb-IIIa receptor[107] and synthetic, low molecular weight competitive antagonists (fibrinogenomimetics) have been effective[108] in studies in experimental animals. Retardation of thrombotic reocclusion has been demonstrated with heparin in animals as well,[109] but the effect is modest for reasons delineated below. More powerful, direct-acting antithrombins such as hirudin are more effective in both accelerating recanalization and retarding or preventing early thrombotic reocclusion in animals treated with fibrinolytic agents after induction of thrombosis secondary to injury to the vessel wall. It appears that antithrombins such as intravenously administered heparin can prevent both activation of the coagulation cascade and platelet deposition to a considerable extent in such preparations, suggesting that the proximate cause of thrombosis complicating fibrinolysis is activation of the coagulation system and generation of thrombin.[71,109] Inhibition of the extrinsic pathway of coagulation with lipoprotein-associated coagulation inhibitor (LACI) is effective as well, consistent with this hypothesis.[106]

Clinical experience is consistent with these

TABLE 16–7. Adjunctive and Conjunctive Agents Under Investigation*

CONJUNCTIVE AGENTS
Platelet antagonists
  Thromboxane A₂ inhibitors
    Cylooxygenase inhibitor (aspirin)
    Thromboxane A₂ receptor inhibitor
  Serotonin receptor inhibitor
  Eicosanoids (prostacyclin and prostaglandin E₁)
  Glycoprotein IIb-IIIa receptor blockers
    Murine monoclonal antibody
    Disintegrins
      Synthetic arginine-glycine-aspartate (RGD) peptides
      Snake venom peptides
  Anti-von Willebrand factor, antiglycoprotein Ib-IX
  Ticlopidine
  Eicosapentanoic acid
  Combined fibrinolytic drugs to augment fibrinogen degradation products
Thrombin inhibitors
Antithrombin III dependent (indirect)
Heparin
  Heparin fragments
  Antithrombin III independent (direct)
    Hirudin
    Synthetic hirudin analogs (hirugen, hirulog, hirullin)
    Arginine analogs (argatroban)
    D-phenylalanyl-L-prolol-L-arginyl choloromethylketone (PPACK)
Other anticoagulants
  Activated protein C, thrombomodulin-like peptides, lipoprotein-associated coagulation factor (LACI)
  Fibrinogen depletors (batroxibin, ancrod)
  Plasminogen activator inhibitor type-1 antagonists
  Factor Xa inhibitor (tick anticoagulant peptide)
  Factor XIII inhibitors
ADJUNCTIVE AGENTS
Beta blockers
Angiotensin-converting enzyme inhibitors
Calcium-channel blockers
Oxygen free radical scavengers
  Superoxide dismutase
  Dimethylthiourea
  Deferoxamine
  Mercaptopropionyl
  N-acetylcysteine
Neutrophil inhibitors
  Adenosine
  Ibuprofen
  Perfluorochemicals
  Prostacyclin
  Leukocyte surface protein antibody

* Reprinted with permission, from Popma JJ, Topol EJ: Adjuncts to thrombolysis for myocardial infarction. Ann Intern Med 1991; 115: 34–44.

observations. In the International Study of Infarct Survival (ISIS-2) trial,[45] one-month mortality among patients treated with streptokinase was 8.3 per cent among patients in whom the intention to treat with intravenous

TABLE 16–8. **Conjunctive and Adjunctive Agents in General Use**

DRUG	ROUTE OF ADMINISTRATION	DOSE AND DURATION	OPTIMAL CANDIDATES	MECHANISM OF BENEFIT
Conjunctive Agents				
Aspirin	Oral	160–325 milligrams/day, first dose as soon as possible	All patients	↓ Reinfarction, recurrent ischemia
Heparin	Intravenous	5000-unit bolus at time of therapy, 1000 units/hour to titrate activated partial thromboplastin time to twice baseline value for ≤48 hours	All patients	↓ Reinfarction, recurrent ischemia
Adjunctive Agents				
Beta blockers			Patients without specific contraindications, e.g., hypotension, bradycardia, reactive airway disease	↓ Reinfarction, recurrent ischemia ↓ Cardiac rupture ↓ Intracerebral hemorrhage
Atenolol	Intravenous	5 milligrams twice, then 50 milligrams orally daily		
Metoprolol	Intravenous	Three doses of 5 milligrams, then 50 milligrams orally twice a day		
Nitrates	Intravenous	Titrate systolic blood pressure to 10 per cent decrease	Patients with persistent chest pain, ischemia, elevated blood pressure	↓ Preload

heparin applied compared with 10.1 per cent in those in whom it did not. However, these data must be interpreted cautiously because definitive information regarding how much heparin was actually administered and when it was given is not available. Favorable effects of heparin were demonstrated also in the Studio sulla Calciparina nell'Angina e nella Trombosi Ventricolare nell'Infarto (SCATI) trial in which addition of heparin to a strep-tokinase regimen reduced in-hospital mortality from 8.8 per cent to 4.5 per cent.[110] Several trials have demonstrated that conjunctive treatment with *intravenous* heparin results in a higher incidence of patency from one to several days after the onset of treatment with tissue-type plasminogen activator, consistent with the view that effective anti-coagulation diminishes the likelihood of early thrombotic reocclusion, especially since early patency (assessed angiographically at 90 minutes) appears to occur with the same frequency whether or not heparin is administered concomitantly with tissue-type plasminogen activator as judged from the results of the TAMI-3 trial.[100] As noted previously, the lack of concomitantly administered intravenous heparin may explain the relatively high early mortality in the GISSI-

2, the t-PA/SK International, and the ISIS-3 trials, and may have obscured differences in the efficacy of the fibrinolytic drugs tested in GISSI-2. (See also Chapters 16 and 17.)

Anticoagulation with Heparin. Unfortunately, heparin is a suboptimal anticoagulant for several reasons.[72] Its antithrombin activity depends on the presence of adequate concentrations of circulating antithrombin III, which may be compromised in some patients. Because of steric effects, the heparin–antithrombin III complex cannot penetrate thrombi, and accordingly, heparin is not effective in antagonizing the activity of clot-bound thrombin. Similar considerations explain its relative inefficacy against thrombin associated with fibrin, fibrin fragments, or fibrinogen degradation products. Thus, heparin is only partially effective against thrombin that may initiate coagulation in the setting of thrombolysis.[111]

Another more serious difficulty relates to the pharmacokinetics and pharmacodynamics of heparin.[112] Clearance of heparin proceeds by two independent mechanisms. The first involves binding to endothelial cell constituents that must be saturated before appreciable concentrations of heparin appear in plasma. Once concentrations of heparin in plasma begin to rise, clearance is determined primarily by a nonsaturable renal mechanism. Thus, initial clearance of heparin is rapid and subsequent clearance slow. Accordingly, the half-life of heparin increases with progressively higher plasma concentrations.

Regardless of the route of administration, anticoagulant effects of modest doses of heparin are delayed because of the predominance over early events of the saturable mechanism of clearance. In normal volunteers, administration of intravenous heparin as a continuous infusion over 24 hours in a total dose of 10,000 units elicits no obvious effects of heparin in plasma. Only when the dose is increased to 30,000 units over 24 hours does binding-site saturation occur sufficiently to give rise to therapeutic levels of heparin in plasma. When heparin is administered subcutaneously, it enters the circulation slowly. Accordingly, the saturation mechanism is not exceeded because previously occupied endothelial binding sites rapidly become available with a consequent lack of elevation of concentration of heparin in plasma. A single subcutaneous dose of at least 20,000 units is required to elicit heparin blood levels within the therapeutic range for the prevention of arterial thrombosis. Lower doses, even if repeated at intervals such as 12 hours, will not elicit therapeutic levels for at least 24 to 48 hours, if at all.

The delay in onset of therapeutic concentrations of heparin in plasma and anticoagulant effects accompanying them can be diminished by initiating treatment with an intravenous bolus dose of approximately 5,000 units to saturate the endothelial cell binding sites. When continuous intravenous infusion follows, therapeutic levels can be initiated promptly and sustained. However, as shown by Turpie and co-workers, the regimen of 12,500 units of heparin administered subcutaneously twice daily, favored by many European investigators, fails to elicit therapeutic concentrations of heparin in plasma throughout the entire period of treatment in as many as 50 per cent of patients.[113] This regimen, used in the GISSI-2 and t-PA/SK International trials, certainly does not elicit adequate anticoagulation within the first 12 to 24 hours after the onset of treatment with fibrinolytic agents, and accordingly, can be anticipated to be associated with a high incidence of reocclusion of initially recanalized vessels.

Despite its limitations, anticoagulation with heparin is the most practical approach presently available for concomitant treatment of patients given fibrinolytic drugs. Administration of an intravenous bolus injection of 5,000 units followed by an infusion of 1,000 units/hour for three to five days is appropriate. Such a regimen should generally double the activated partial thromboplastin time. Although not used in routine clinical management, demonstrable suppression of elevations of fibrinopeptide A is a theoretically attractive criterion of adequacy of dose. Judging from the favorable results already available from studies in experimental animals and the probable advantages of direct-acting, low molecular weight antithrombins, it appears likely that agents such as hirudin, hirulog, and argatroban will undergo vigorous clinical evaluation and may become part of the therapeutic armamentarium in the near future. Other anticoagulants such as the tic anticoagulant protein, which inhibits activated coagulation factor X, accelerate thrombolysis and retard reocclusion in experimental animals[114] and may enhance anticoagulation clinically as well. (See also Chapters 6 and 7.)

Antiplatelet Agents. Another approach to prevention of reocclusion has entailed the use of antiplatelet agents. Indirect criteria of platelet activation associated with administration of fibrinolytic agents to animals were acquired by Fitzgerald and co-workers, who detected increased concentrations of metabolites of thromboxane in urine indicative of activation of platelets in vivo.[115] Subsequently, the same workers extended their observations to patients given activators of the fibrinolytic system.[104] Although plasminogen activators and/or plasmin generated by them have been alleged to exert direct effects on platelets, thereby potentially accounting for activation of platelets in vivo, when washed platelets are maintained in solution with physiologic concentration of calcium, neither tissue-type plasminogen activator nor plasmin induces activation.[105] Furthermore, it appears that activation of the coagulation system by plasminogen activators precedes activation of platelets in vitro and in vivo and that preclusion of activation of the coagulation system with the use of thrombin inhibitors prevents the associated activation of platelets that would be seen otherwise.[116] The remarkably protective effects of powerful, direct-acting antithrombin agents such as hirudin on reocclusion after thrombolysis in vessels with deep arterial wall injury[116] or electrically induced intimal damage,[109] insults likely to predispose to formation of platelet-rich thrombi, suggest that the activation of platelets in vivo is largely dependent on thrombin even in these settings that simulate thrombosis associated with atherosclerotic plaque rupture. Accordingly, it appears likely that platelet activation does contribute to reocclusion after pharmacologically induced thrombolysis, that antiplatelet agents such as aspirin (which inhibits thromboxane-but not thrombin-induced platelet aggregation) may therefore diminish the incidence or retard the occurrence of reocclusion, but that the primary culprit in platelet activation is thrombin generated by activation of the coagulation system or thrombin and perhaps other procoagulants leading to elaboration of thrombin released locally. In view of these considerations, the most effective means to prevent activation of platelets in the setting of coronary thrombolysis may be intense anticoagulation with effective antithrombin agents.

Platelets can be activated through at least four pathways (a thrombin-, collagen-, or epinephrine-stimulated pathway; an adenosine diphosphate- or serotonin-stimulated pathway initiated by moieties released from platelet-dense granules; a thromboxane-mediated pathway; and a platelet-activating factor-mediated pathway). Only the thromboxane-stimulated pathway of platelet activation is sensitive to inhibition with aspirin, and accordingly, despite the favorable results seen with aspirin in trials such as ISIS-2 on survival after treatment with fibrinolytic agents, it appears likely that more powerful inhibitors of platelets or inhibitors of factors activating them such as thrombin will be needed to induce optimal inhibition of their contribution to reocclusion. This rationale underlies the evolution of monoclonal antibodies to platelet glycoprotein receptors such as the glycoprotein IIb-IIIa receptor, competitive antagonists of such receptors, inhibitors of platelet-activating factor,[117] and other antiplatelet drugs (Table 16–7). However, the advent of novel, powerful, and direct-acting antithrombins as well as other effective inhibitors of the coagulation system may obviate the need for antiplatelet drugs in the setting of coronary thrombolysis, if, in fact, platelet activation is largely or exclusively mediated by thrombin under such circumstances.

In current clinical practice, the most effective anticoagulant (heparin) exhibits some unavoidable limitations including inefficacy with respect to thrombin bound to fibrin and thrombin associated with fibrin and fibrinogen degradation products as well as dependence for activity on antithrombin III. Accordingly, concomitant use of antiplatelet drugs, generally aspirin, is presently recommended as conjunctive therapy (Table 16–8). (See also Chapters 16 and 17.)

Maintenance of Recanalization with Early Angioplasty

The potential utility of angioplasty for preventing reocclusion has been examined and its other potential applications in the setting of acute myocardial infarction have been explored vigorously. Angioplasty is designed to attack the stenosis and atherosclerotic plaque underlying coronary thrombosis, as suggested when combined thrombolysis and angioplasty were employed in 1982.[118,119] Several strategies have been addressed,[120] including primary or direct angiography, in which angioplasty is used to initiate reperfusion; immediate angioplasty intended to augment the coronary blood flow early after successful thrombolysis; rescue angioplasty in which balloon dilation is performed only if thrombolytic therapy has failed to induce recanalization of the infarct-related artery; routine or prophylactic angioplasty, in which all patients with suitable coronary vascular anatomy (residual high-grade lesions in the infarct vessel amenable to angioplasty) are treated; and selective angioplasty performed only to treat either spontaneously symptomatic or exercise-induced ischemia after thrombolysis. Each has been evaluated clinically and in randomized trials.

Primary angioplasty was first reported by Hartzler and colleagues in 1983.[121] The first 500 patients they studied consecutively have been reported.[122] Together with results from several other studies,[120] the results demonstrate that primary angioplasty induces reperfusion in more than 90 per cent of patients treated. The incidence of recanalization compares favorably with that seen with intravenous administration of thrombolytic drugs, but several practical limitations must be considered. First, primary angioplasty requires rapid transfer to an interventional cardiac catheterization laboratory, immediate availability of operators at all times, inherent time delays associated with performance of the procedure, and cost. Second, mechanical trauma to the affected arterial segment may be deleterious. In most cases, the infarct-related vessel already exhibits plaque fissuring or rupture, with attendant platelet aggregation and fibrin accretion. This may contribute to an early reocclusion rate of approximately 15 per cent.[120] Third, sudden, intense reperfusion may elicit serious arrhythmias, conceivably a marker of reperfusion injury.[122] Fourth, a procedure for prompt surgical backup must be in place at all times.

Primary angioplasty can be advocated in patients for whom thrombolysis is contraindicated, such as those with recent stroke or major surgery. It may be particularly worthwhile when it can be implemented very promptly, as is the case when a patient's myocardial infarct occurs in or in the immediate vicinity of a catheterization laboratory.

Immediate coronary angioplasty after initially successful thrombolysis was an attractive approach a priori, but this strategy was found wanting in three randomized trials. In the TAMI-1, ECSG-4, and TIMI IIA studies,[47,48,123,124] immediate compared with deferred angioplasty (or conservative management) led to no apparent benefit in terms of global or regional left ventricular function but was associated with increased risk of reocclusion, abrupt vessel closure (during the procedure), the need for emergency bypass surgery, and bleeding. In aggregate, the data from these three trials argue cogently for a "deferred is preferred" approach to angioplasty in this setting.[47,48,120,124]

Indications for rescue angioplasty remain unclear. Balloon-mediated restoration of patency of the infarct-related vessel after failure of pharmacologic thrombolysis can be accomplished in more than 85 per cent of patients,[120,125] but the extent of actual clinical benefit conferred has not yet been established. Initial efforts were plagued by very high reocclusion rates, approaching 30 per cent.[47] Conversely, as was clear from sequential angiographic studies performed 90 minute and 24 hours after thrombolysis, delayed restoration of patency of the infarct-related vessel can and does occur even without rescue angioplasty.[126] As summarized in Table 16–9, results with rescue angioplasty depend in part on the specific thrombolytic agent used.[125] In patients given a non–clot-selective activator such as streptokinase or urokinase or those given a combination of a clot-selective agent plus a nonselective agent, reocclusion occurs less frequently and technical success of rescue angioplasty is enhanced[125] (Table 16–9).

The right coronary artery appears to be

TABLE 16–9. Meta-Analysis of Results of Coronary Angioplasty*

Author	Number of Patients	Thrombolytic Agent(s)	Patients in Whom Therapy was Successful (%)	Patients With Reocclusion (%)	Change in Ventricular EF (Baseline to Day 7)	Mortality (%)
Fung et al.[127]	13	SK	92	16	+10	7.6
Holmes et al.[128]	34	SK	71	NR	NR	3.0
Grines et al.[129]	8	t-PA + SK	92	12	+5	NR
Grines et al.[130]	12	t-PA + SK	100	8	NR	NR
Topol et al.[57]	27 (22)†	t-PA + UK	86	3	NR	5.4
Califf et al.[58]	15	t-PA	87	15	+1	NR
	25	UK	84	12	+1	NR
	12	t-PA + UK	92	0	+2	NR
O'Connor et al.[131]	90	SK	89	14	−1	17.0
Baim et al.[132]	37	t-PA	NR	26	NR	5.4
Topol et al.[47]	96 (86)†	t-PA	73	29	−1	10.4
	216	Pooled SK, UK, or combination	186/216 (86%)‡	20/182 (10.9%)§		
	138	Pooled t-PA only	76/101 (75%)‡	37/138 (26.8%)§		

* Reprinted with permission, from Topol EJ, Holmes D, Rogers W. Coronary angiography after thrombolysis for acute myocardial infarction. Ann Intern Med 1991; 114: 877–885.
† Number of patients in whom rescue angioplasty was actually attempted.
‡ $p = 0.026$.
§ $p = 0.0004$.
EF = ejection fraction; NR = not reported; t-PA = tissue-type plasminogen activator; UK = urokinase; SK = streptokinase.

especially prone to complications with rescue angioplasty.[123] This may be attributable to embolization of a more extensive clot burden in the right compared with the left coronary artery, an exaggerated Bezold-Jarisch reflex eliciting hypotension, or more extensive reperfusion injury because of increased flow (lower diastolic, tissue pressure) in the right compared with the left ventricle or in the right compared with the left coronary bed after restoration of patency.

Rescue angioplasty after failure of pharmacologic thrombolysis should be considered for patients with cardiogenic shock or extensive exterior wall myocardial infarction. Its value should be clarified when results from ongoing randomized trials become available.[125]

Presently, it is difficult to identify definitively those patients in whom thrombolysis elicits recanalization in the absence of angiography.[134] However, continuous, digital 12-lead electrocardiography may help. Recent advances in the development of biochemical markers of reperfusion are particularly promising. Sudden washout into the circulation of myoglobin or the tissue subform (isoform) of the MM or MB isoenzyme of creatine kinase (CK) that has been released into extracellular fluid from myocytes undergoing necrosis accompanies recanalization and provides a sensitive and specific index of reperfusion that can be observed rapidly by measuring plasma myoglobin and plasma MM or MB creatine kinase isoforms.[135-137] More universal use of macromolecular markers of recanalization may permit more effective selection of patients who require rescue angioplasty because thrombolysis has failed and prompt and accurate recognition of patients in whom reperfusion has been initially successful without the need for routine angiography.[120,125]

Two trials have assessed the value of routine compared with selective use of angioplasty after thrombolysis. In the TIMI II trial,[49] more than 3,000 patients were given tissue-type plasminogen activator and randomly assigned to either cardiac catheterization in 18 to 48 hours with angioplasty of the infarct-related vessel if its anatomy was appropriate (invasive strategy) or to no cardiac catheterization or angioplasty unless mandated by spontaneously or symptomatic predischarge exercise-induced recurrent ischemia (conservative strategy). The two approaches led to no differences in mortality, reinfarction, or cardiac function. Thus, it appears that angioplasty should be performed only as necessary to ameliorate recurrent ischemia rather than prophylactically or routinely.[49] Similar conclusions were reached in the Should We Intervene Following Thrombolysis? (SWIFT) trial in which the two approaches were evaluated after treatment with anistreplase in 800 patients.[133] Routine angioplasty was not only without benefit but also deleterious in that it was associated with a higher rate of reinfarction.[138] Thus, angioplasty need be performed only in patients who manifest signs of recurrent ischemia after initially successful thrombolysis.

Properties of Plasminogen Activators Used in the Treatment of Acute Myocardial Infarction

The fundamental distinction between thrombolytic agents and one that is of primary clinical import is based on relative fibrin specificity and hence clot selectivity. First-generation agents activate plasminogen similarly whether it is encountered in the fluid phase of circulating blood or in association with fibrin in clots. Agents of this type available for clinical use include streptokinase, anisoylated plasminogen streptokinase activator complex (Eminase; generic name, anistreplase), and urokinase. Second-generation agents activate plasminogen in the fibrin domain preferentially. The only one presently available for clinical use is a tissue-type plasminogen activator that has the same primary structure as the native, human tissue-type plasminogen activator and is available as a primarily single-chain preparation (Activase, Actilyse; generic name, alteplase). A recombinant, single-chain, unglycosylated urinary-type plasminogen activator (scu-PA; generic name, saruplase) is still investigational. Second-generation agents are stimulated when they are associated with fibrin, which also binds their physiologic substrate, plasminogen, thereby juxtaposing the activator and its substrate. Fibrin-associated plasminogen is activated as much as 1,000-fold more intensely by tissue-type plasminogen activator compared with plasminogen in plasma.[1] Despite initial expectations, anistreplase exhibits no fibrin specificity in human subjects. Accordingly, it is not a second-generation agent in this classification scheme because it is not clot selective.[43]

Clot selectivity is a relative phenomenon. First-generation agents do not exhibit any clot selectivity regardless of what route of administration is used (including the intracoronary as well as the intravenous route). Consequently, they elicit plasminemia in all doses that are therapeutically effective. As a result, a systemic lytic state is induced reflected by diminution in the concentrations in plasma of numerous circulating proteins, including plasminogen, fibrinogen, alpha$_2$-antiplasmin, and coagulation factors V and VIII. The action of plasmin in fibrinogen gives rise to increased concentrations in the circulation of B-beta1-42, a fibrinogen degradation product that reflects the presence of a systemic lytic state.

Second-generation agents elicit much less plasminemia in therapeutically effective doses. Suprapharmacologic doses can, of course, elicit plasminemia with all its consequences. No currently available agent is entirely clot selective. Nevertheless, with therapeutic doses of tissue-type plasminogen activator (alteplase), the concentrations of plasminogen, fibrinogen, alpha$_2$-antiplasmin, and other targets of proteolytic activity in plasma decline much less markedly than is the case with streptokinase, anistreplase, or urokinase; the augmentation of concentrations in plasma of B-beta1-42 is of much less magnitude or entirely absent; and potentially deleterious consequences of plasminemia can be avoided.

One disadvantage of plasminemia is a predisposition to bleeding that, although manageable and acceptable clinically, leads to a greater transfusion requirement with first- than with second-generation agents. Another is "plasminogen steal," a phenomenon reflecting conversion of plasminogen in blood to plasmin with consequent leeching of fibrin-associated plasminogen from the clot into the circulating blood as a result of mass action.[139] The diminution of fibrin-associated plasminogen reduces the efficacy of any plasminogen activator exposed to the thrombus, and accordingly, reduces the intensity of fibrinolysis. This phenomenon may contribute to the slower rates of recanalization and decreased frequency of recanalization seen with first-generation agents such as streptokinase compared with second-generation agents such as tissue-type plasminogen activator because of the more marked conversion of circulating plasminogen to plasmin that they induce. In studies in vitro, impairment of fibrinolysis attributable to plasminogen steal can be overcome by supplementation of blood with exogenous plasminogen sufficient to maintain the concentration of plasminogen in the physiologic range. However, this approach is impractical in vivo because of the prodigious quantities of plasminogen that would be required.

A third disadvantage of plasminemia is procoagulation that can be induced by all plasminogen activators.[73–75] Increased concentrations of fibrinopeptide A, the initial cleavage product of thrombin's action on fibrin, are seen when blood is exposed to plasminogen activators in vitro and in vivo and are indicative of activation of the coagulation system. Such increases are much more marked with first- than with second-generation plasminogen activators and can be inhibited by antiplasmins in vitro. Plasmin can activate coagulation factor V directly[140] and can elicit the formation of thrombin from prothrombin. It may act also at other points in the coagulation cascade involved in both the intrinsic and extrinsic systems (Eisenberg PR, personal communication). Induction of procoagulation by plasminogen activators, particularly first-generation agents, may retard recanalization (because of diminution of the predominance of thrombolysis compared with thrombosis early in the course of treatment) and predispose to early thrombotic reocclusion. Such effects may account, in part, for the lower incidence of early patency seen with first-generation agents compared with tissue-type plasminogen activator as judged from comparison of results from angiographic trials (Figure 16–1).

Second-generation agents were developed initially based on the premise that they would provide increased safety as a result of their relative clot selectivity. They do appear to induce less spontaneous bleeding than first-generation agents, and their use has been associated with somewhat lower transfusion requirements. However, when used judiciously in appropriately selected patients, both first- and second-generation agents are remarkably safe. Second-generation agents appear, however, to be more powerful fibrinolytic agents in that they induce recanalization more rapidly and more often than first-generation agents, probably in part because of the factors noted in consideration of the consequences of clot selectivity.

Induction of a systemic lytic state with first-generation agents such as streptokinase has been claimed to offer potential advantages. The marked elevations seen of fibrinogen degradation products, known to exhibit anticoagulant and antiplatelet effects, may in fact diminish the likelihood of early, thrombotic reocclusion in inadequately anticoagulated patients. However, the retardation of the coagulation process induced by fibrinogen degradation products cannot be assumed to reflect conditions that are as protective as those induced by heparin because of differential mechanisms involved in the two instances. The potentially protective effects of fibrinogen degradation products (with respect to reocclusion 90 minutes or more after treatment) probably appear later than the deleterious prothrombotic effects accompanying plasminemia and reflected by elevated fibrinopeptide A in plasma (which may retard recanalization or potentiate very early reocclusion) because of gradual accumulation of fibrinogen degradation products secondary to their long circulating half-life.

Clinically available activators of the fibrinolytic system can be differentiated with respect to several other properties that may be important in individual patients. Antibodies to streptokinase are present in virtually all patients and may increase markedly in concentration after exposure to streptokinase or anistreplase (which contains approximately 1.25 million units of streptokinase in the conventionally used dose of 30 units or milligrams). Accordingly, allergic reactions with these agents are common, as is hypotension that may be potentiated by decreased plasma viscosity accompanying fibrinogenolysis and activation of the kinin system as a result of plasminemia.[43] In the ISIS-3 trial, allergic reactions causing persistent shock occurred in 0.3 per cent of streptokinase-treated patient and in 0.6 per cent of anistreplase-treated patients; the corresponding figures for profound hypotension requiring drugs were 6.8 per cent and 7.2 per cent (data presented by the ISIS-3 investigators at the 1991 National Meeting of the American College of Cardiology). Such reactions can complicate the care of patients with already precarious hemodynamics as a result of evolving myocardial infarction. Retreatment, when necessary because of threatened or overt thrombotic reocclusion, is feasible with tissue-type plasminogen activator and urokinase, but not advisable with streptokinase or anis-

treplase because of the likelihood of antibody-mediated resistance to plasminogen activation and allergic reactions.[141]

The half-life of tissue-type plasminogen activator is on the order of only a few minutes, in contrast to the much more prolonged half-lives in the circulation of streptokinase, anistreplase, and urokinase. This may be an advantage in patients likely to require aggressive, invasive interventions including surgery early after the onset of treatment with thrombolytic drugs, because thrombolytic activity in plasma declines very rapidly after termination of intravenous infusions of tissue-type plasminogen activator in contrast to streptokinase, anistreplase, and urokinase. Sustained fibrinolytic activity in the circulation can be induced, if necessary under special circumstances, with continuing low-dose infusions of tissue-type plasminogen activator as judged from results in experimental animals[142] and patients.[143]

The prolonged persistence of intravenously administered tissue-type plasminogen activator in the interstices of clot present during the infusion leads to persistent action on targeted thrombi long after the concentration of tissue-type plasminogen activator in the blood has declined to baseline.[144] This may explain the efficacy of front-loaded regimens of tissue-type plasminogen activator,[145] including even regimens employing a bolus, intravenous dose only.[146]

A comparison of salient clinical features, including dose of plasminogen activators available for clinical use (saruplase is still investigational), is shown in Table 16–10.

Use of Different Fibrinolytic Agents in Combination

Some investigators[58,147,148] have sought to take advantage of the more rapid and frequent induction of recanalization possible with tissue-type plasminogen activator and the retardation of reocclusion attributed to elevated concentrations of fibrinogen degradation products in plasma accompanying induction of a systemic lytic state with streptokinase or urokinase by administering a combination of tissue-type plasminogen activator (sometimes in reduced or half conventional dosage) with streptokinase[147] or urokinase. Combination regimens have been advocated as being potentially beneficial in reducing costs of treatment, reducing the

TABLE 16–10. Thrombolytic Agents Used Clinically

DRUG	COMMON NAME	DOSE	ADVANTAGES/DISADVANTAGES
Alteplase	t-PA	100 milligrams over 1.5–3 hour	Clot selective; nonimmunogenic; most rapid restoration of patency; expensive
Duteplase*	t-PA		
Streptokinase	SK	1.5 million units over 1 hour	Immunogenic; inferior frequency of early patency but low incidence of reocclusion (≤12%); inexpensive
Anistreplase	APSAC	30 milligrams over 2–5 minutes	Convenient, bolus administration; contains only SK as the plasminogen activator; expensive
Urokinase	UK	1.5 million unit bolus + 1.5 million units over 1 hour	Patency profile similar to SK with low incidence of reocclusion (<10%); expensive
Saruplase	scu-PA	20 milligram bolus + 60 milligrams over 1 hour	Exhibits clot selectivity; investigational in the United States

* Duteplase is not likely to be made commercially available, and therefore information about dose and advantages and disadvantages of its use are not enumerated.

incidence of reocclusion, or both. However, they entail potential disadvantages as well: they may elicit varying concentrations of fibrinogen degradation products that may exert varying anticoagulant effects at unanticipated intervals, exacerbate prothrombotic effects because of the plasminemia induced, induce a variable intensity of fibrinolysis because of rapidly changing net concentrations of plasminogen activator in the circulation, and potentially exacerbate bleeding risk because of plasminemia. As judged from the remarkable progress being made in studies of direct-acting antithrombins in animals, the increasing evidence of limitations of heparin as an anticoagulant in patients given thrombolytic drugs, advantages of clot-selective fibrinolytic agents used singly with respect to avoidance of plasminemia and the rapidity and frequency of recanalization, and the likelihood that optimal prevention of reocclusion will depend on optimal anticoagulation and inhibition of platelet activation likely to be readily achievable by appropriately targeted drugs, a strong argument can be made for use of second-generation fibrinolytic agents with the best available regimens for anticoagulation as the treatment of choice. The contention[55] that effective thrombolysis and prevention of reocclusion require induction of a systemic lytic state cannot be supported in view of the high incidence of prompt and sustained recanalization induced by tissue-type plasminogen activator when the agent has been administered with appropriate, concomitant anticoagulation.

Results with Individual Fibrinolytic Agents

Based on the monumental amount of information that has been acquired during the past decade, much of which has been reviewed recently,[3,43] several aspects of coronary thrombolysis have been established unequivocally (Table 16–11). As shown in early angiographic studies, intracoronary strepto-

TABLE 16–11. Thrombolysis and Acute Myocardial Infarction—Established Tenets*

Importance of thrombosis in pathophysiology of acute myocardial infarction
Induction of thrombolysis pharmacologically
Favorable impact of thrombolysis on morbidity and mortality of patients with acute myocardial infarction
Importance of early reperfusion
Superiority of second-generation agents in eliciting early reperfusion
Lack of need for universal emergency percutaneous transluminal coronary angioplasty after thrombolysis
Value of adjunctive pharmacologic therapy in laboratory animals subjected to coronary thrombolysis
Importance of conjunctive antithrombin agents
Importance of conjunctive antiplatelet agents
Lack of need for universal elective percutaneous transluminal coronary angioplasty after thrombolysis
Value of adjunctive beta blockade in patients undergoing thrombolysis
Potential for increased rate and/or rapidity of successful thrombolysis with novel drug regimens
Safety justifying broadening of criteria for use of thrombolytic agents

* Reprinted with permission, from Tiefenbrunn AJ, Sobel BE. Thrombolysis and myocardial infarction. Fibrinolysis 1991; 5: 1–15.

kinase recanalizes approximately 70 per cent of infarct-related arteries. In contrast, intravenous streptokinase induces early patency in only approximately 50 per cent when strict recanalization criteria are applied to the analysis of data.[149] The frequency of early recanalization and patency assessed approximately 90 minutes after the onset of treatment is remarkably constant when all first-generation drugs are considered (streptokinase, anistreplase, and urokinase), as shown in Figure 16–1, which covers results that were available through 1988.

Second-generation fibrinolytic drugs such as tissue-type plasminogen activator induce recanalization more rapidly and more often than first-generation agents.[38,40,91,95]

The GISSI-I trial[44] established the efficacy of streptokinase in reducing mortality. As shown in Table 16–2, which compiles information from studies of more than 42,000 patients, early mortality is consistently lower in studies with second- as opposed to first-generation agents, in keeping with their apparently more effective induction of prompt recanalization. Early mortality was, however, virtually identical with a first-generation (streptokinase) and a second-generation (tissue-type plasminogen activator) drug in the GISSI-2 and t-PA (alteplase)/SK International trials and in ISIS-3 (duteplase), and was substantially greater in both treatment groups compared with early mortality in many other trials of either first- or second-generation agents (Table 16–2). As noted previously, intravenous heparin was not used in the combined GISSI-2 and t-PA/SK International trial and ISIS-3. These studies employed only subcutaneously administered heparin beginning four hours (ISIS-3) or 12 hours (GISSI-2) after the onset of treatment with a fibrinolytic agent. Two-week mortality was 8.7 per cent for the GISSI-2 trial as a whole. Results with tissue-type plasminogen activator and streptokinase were not significantly different.

Several investigators have suggested that these anomalous results reflect the lack of adequate anticoagulation in both treatment groups in view of the omission of any heparin in 50 per cent of the patients studied and the relative inefficacy of subcutaneous heparin in the low and frequent dosing used (given to 50 per cent of the patients treated with each fibrinolytic agent) as a conjunctive agent.

Inadequate anticoagulation is likely to have affected results with alteplase and duteplase even more adversely than those with streptokinase because of the marked elevation in fibrinogen degradation products induced by streptokinase, which may partially protect against reocclusion in the first day after treatment. Thus, differences in the rates and frequency of initial recanalization and their clinical consequences including survival may have been obscured by an inordinately high incidence of early reocclusion among a larger fraction of patients given alteplase or duteplase in whom initial recanalization may have been induced more often. Because of the lack of adequate anticoagulation, neither the GISSI-2 and t-PA/SK International trials nor the ISIS-3 investigation can provide definitive information permitting objective comparison of the benefits of a second-compared with a first-generation fibrinolytic agent.

Regardless of the thrombolytic agent used, early treatment of acute myocardial infarction attributable to coronary thrombosis is clearly beneficial. In patients treated within a few hours after the onset of infarction, improvement in regional wall motion in the jeopardized zone can be anticipated, reflecting salvage of myocardium; the extent of infarction delineated electrocardiographically and enzymatically can be reduced; and early mortality can be diminished by as much as 50 per cent.[3,4,43] Even when treatment is initiated later, some benefits attributable to salvage of myocardium may accrue. Treatment that cannot be initiated until more than six hours after the onset of apparent infarction is unlikely to salvage clinically significant amounts of myocardium, but preliminary observations indicate that at least in some patients, benefits may be anticipated including reduction of arrhythmogenicity, augmentation of collateral perfusion, improved ventricular remodeling,[60] improved healing in the peri-infarct zone, and reduction of formation of ventricular aneurysms and their associated arrhythmogenicity. Ancillary benefits may include reduction of the incidence, severity, or complications of ventricular mural thrombi. Despite the apparent resistance to recanalization of the right coronary artery compared with other vessels[56,150,151] and the higher incidence of reocclusion in the right compared with the left coronary artery,[152] benefits can be obtained in patients with right as well as left coronary artery occlusions, inferior as well as anterior infarction, and involvement of the right ventricle. The apparent lack of reduction in mortality in some studies of patients with inferior infarction may reflect the relatively low mortality among all patients in this group, the lack of sufficiently prompt induction of treatment after the onset of infarction, or the relatively greater collateralization of obstructed right compared with left coronary arteries.[153]

Unfortunately, the full therapeutic potential of coronary thrombolysis has not been realized because only a small fraction (approximately 20 per cent)[50] of patients with acute myocardial infarction admitted to hospitals in the United States are being treated with these agents. Even with appropriate exclusion of patients who are not suitable candidates according to the criteria presented below, it is clear that many patients who should be benefiting from fibrinolytic drugs are not being treated.

Principles Underlying Dosing with Fibrinolytic Drugs

Again regardless of what fibrinolytic agent is used, the fundamental principle underlying its use is the urgency of initiation of treatment as soon as possible after the onset of infarction. Appropriate patient selection is essential (see below for criteria), and can generally be accomplished within only a few minutes. As stated above, there is no justification for delaying the onset of treatment until results of laboratory tests such as plasma enzyme determinations are available because salvage of myocardium is so dependent on the brevity of ischemia preceding recanalization and because results of such tests may not become positive for several hours after the onset of infarction.

Conventional doses of clinically available thrombolytic agents are shown in Table 16–10. A few specific considerations merit attention.

Dosing with streptokinase has to be arbitrary because the impact of circulating antibody varies from patient to patient and cannot be readily anticipated or titrated. Although anistreplase elaborates fibrinolytic activity only slowly as it undergoes deacylation in vivo, its primary component is streptokinase (1.25 million units of streptokinase in the 30-unit conventional dose of anistreplase). Accordingly, arbitrary doses (fixed doses or units/kilogram body weight) are used because interactions between the streptokinase component and antibody are just as difficult to define prospectively or by titration as they are with streptokinase.

Tissue-type plasminogen activator has been given in both fixed-dose and body-weight-adjusted dose regimens (the latter particularly attractive for use in diminutive patients, especially if elderly) developed with reference to fibrinolytic activity induced in plasma and limitation of induction of a systemic lytic state. Most early large-scale trials used fixed-dose regimens, but efficacy and safety may be enhanced with weight-adjusted regimens and front-loaded dosing in which a large fraction of the total dose is administered over a compressed interval. The Neuhaus regimen,[145] for example, consists of a 15-milligram bolus followed by 50 milligrams given intravenously over 30 minutes and a subsequent 35 milligrams over the next hour with a total of 100 milligrams being administered over 90 minutes. With this regimen, early patency (within 90 minutes) has been reported to be 91 per cent consistent with persistence of activation of clot-associated plasminogen even when plasma concentrations of tissue-type plasminogen activator have declined markedly.[144] Alternative, front-loaded regimens include the extreme case, namely administration of a single bolus injection of tissue-type plasminogen activator (1 milligram/kilogram body weight) intravenously. Patency with this regimen is remarkably high (80 per cent) despite only minimal reduction of the concentration of circulating fibrinogen.[146]

Persistent infusion of subthrombolytic doses of tissue-type plasminogen activator may prevent early reocclusion.[142,143] However, vigorous anticoagulation coupled with the use of antiplatelet drugs is probably a better approach because prolonged persistence in the circulation of any activator of plasminogen can lead to consumption of $alpha_2$-antiplasmin, plasminemia, and induction of a systemic lytic state that may be deleterious.

Risks of Treatment with Fibrinolytic Agents

The emergence of coronary thrombolysis as primary treatment for acute myocardial infarction was retarded by considerable early apprehension. Because of the marked depletion of fibrinogen seen with the first-generation agents that had been used to treat other conditions such as pulmonary embolic disease, the recognized 0.8 to 1.3 per cent incidence of stroke even among patients with infarction who are not treated with fibrinolytic agents or anticoagulants,[43] and the obvious theoretical risk of inducing devastating intracranial bleeding or converting a thromboembolic stroke into a lethal hemorrhagic one, many clinicians and investigators were reluctant to use plasminogen activators in the treatment of acute myocardial infarction. Initial experience in carefully controlled, multicenter, large-scale clinical trials paradoxically intensified anxiety because the most widely publicized randomized, multicenter studies utilized protocols involving repetitive vascular access. They reported higher overall incidences of bleeding, including that from catheterization and vascular access sites as well as spontaneous bleeding.

Early experience demonstrated that the risk of intracranial hemorrhage with fibrinolytic agents is greater in patients with a history of cerebrovascular events or refractory, severe hypertension,[43] age greater than 75 years, and possibly with suprapharmacologic doses of fibrinolytic drugs such as the 150-milligram dose of tissue-type plasminogen activator used in a portion of the TIMI II study. However, as shown by analysis of data from almost 40,000 patients studied, the overall incidence of stroke among patients treated with fibrinolytic agents is 0.9 per cent, identical to the incidence in patients treated with placebo in the same trials. Although a modest increase in the proportion of strokes that are hemorrhagic can be anticipated with thrombolytic drugs, the overall, beneficial impact of coronary thrombolysis on survival far outweighs the negative impact of conversion of a small number of thromboembolic to hemorrhagic strokes.[46]

Unfortunately, there is no simple relationship between an easily measurable laboratory value and the risk of bleeding. Gimple, Gold, and their colleagues[154] have suggested that prolongation of bleeding time may correlate with an increased risk of spontaneous bleeding, but routine determination of bleeding time is neither required nor definitive. A general but loose concordance between bleeding risk and the presence of a lytic state is evident. Among patients who develop spontaneous hemorrhage after treatment with fibrinolytic agents, the intensity of the lytic state is often although not always striking. Conversely, however, many patients with an intense, lytic state develop no spontaneous bleeding. Clot-selective agents confer some benefit with respect to spontaneous bleeding as shown by the ECSG trial,[91] by analysis of data from head-to-head comparisons between first- and second-generation thrombolytic agents in relatively small trials[3] (Fig. 16–4), and by results of large-scale multicen-

FIGURE 16–4. Average incidence of major spontaneous bleeding from four recent studies (for review of trials, see references 56, 87, 91, 168) directly comparing the incidence in patients treated with streptokinase and those treated with tissue-type plasminogen activator (alteplase). (Reprinted with permission, from Tiefenbrunn AJ, Sobel BE. Thrombolysis and myocardial infarction. Fibrinolysis 1989; 3: 1–15.)

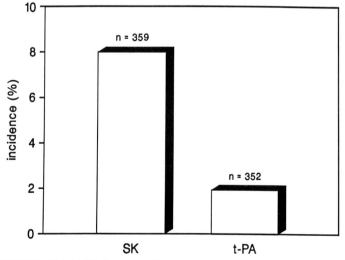

*TIMI-I, ECSG-I, PAIMS, Dorent et al.
For reference: Fibrinogen decrease in 3 hr averaged 57% (SK) and 26% (t-PA) with bleeding correlating with FDP elevations (Rao et al.) in TIMI-I

ter trials comparing the two.[93] Although the difference in bleeding incidence may be as much as twofold, the absolute incidence of bleeding induced by any fibrinolytic agent in judiciously selected patients treated with conventional dose regimens is modest. For patients who may require emergency surgery, avoidance of induction of a systemic lytic state may be particularly desirable as may use of a thrombolytic agent with a short half-life in the circulating blood.

Selection of Patients

Although the clinical value of coronary thrombolysis is no longer in dispute, its provision to all patients with infarction who can benefit has been elusive. It is no longer tenable to confine the use of thrombolytic agents to tertiary facilities equipped for cardiac catheterization, angioplasty, or surgery.[50] Administration of thrombolytic agents by paramedical personnel will undoubtedly emerge just as electrical defibrillation, initially the province solely of physicians, exerted its most beneficial effects when nurses and other nonphysician personnel were empowered to use it. Progress in achieving more universal implementation of coronary thrombolysis will depend, however, on optimal selection of patients. Several principles apply in interpreting studies addressing patient selection and in formulating clinical judgments regarding individual patients. Unfortunately, a decision to treat or not to treat with thrombolytic drugs can be made only rarely in absolute terms by relying on the presence or absence of absolute contraindications.

Much confusion regarding patient selection has occurred because of the difference between protocol requirements in multicenter, large-scale clinical trials and characteristics of patients encountered in clinical practice. For example, a trial may elect to define an exclusion criterion of advanced age as 60, 70, or any other arbitrary number of years. Accordingly, its results will pertain only to populations that exclude patients exceeding the arbitrary age limit. Unfortunately, however, many argue by implications that the use of agents tested in such a trial is contraindicated in patients exceeding the arbitrary age limit even though no patients exceeding this limit were actually exposed to the drug, and hence no data are available regarding the

risk-to-benefit ratio pertinent to them. The clinician is, of course, faced daily with the need to extrapolate from knowledge of mechanisms of action of thrombolytic agents, individual characteristics of patients who are candidates for treatment, results of pilot and large-scale trials, and numerous other factors that constitute the underpinnings of "clinical judgment" used in making therapeutic decisions. It cannot be assumed that any simplistic algorithm will suffice.

Criteria for patient selection differ markedly from one clinical investigation to another. Early mortality in victims of acute myocardial infarction has been declining substantially because of numerous advances including earlier and more accurate diagnosis, electrical defibrillation, treatment with antiarrhythmics such as lidocaine, use of beta-adrenergic blockers and vasodilators, circulatory support, emergency revascularization, and pharmacologic thrombolysis, to note but a few. Accordingly, risk-to-benefit ratios suggested by results of well-done large trials in the past may not be directly pertinent to patients encountered today or tomorrow.

All agree that thrombolysis should be implemented as soon as possible after the time of onset of infarction and that the relative benefits that can be anticipated diminish as the interval between the onset of infarction and the onset of treatment increases. However, even here, one is faced with a difficult dilemma. For example, even if we assume that treatment eight hours or more after the onset of infarction is not likely to salvage any myocardium and may therefore be considered to entail excessive risk in an elderly patient with an inferior myocardial infarction, we often cannot define with acceptable accuracy that time of onset of infarction when a specific decision has to be made. Chest pain, elecrocardiographic ST segment and T wave changes, arrhythmias, and other clinical criteria are notoriously unreliable for this purpose. The clinician is not justified in waiting to make a decision until laboratory results such as plasma enzyme values are available. Even when such results are known, they simply define the presence or absence of infarction one to two hours earlier (because of the lag time between the onset of infarction and elevation of plasma enzyme activity), but not its time of onset.

Because of the possibility of stuttering infarction, the implications of the open-artery hypothesis, and imprecision in identifying the time of onset of infarction, it may be desirable to implement therapy with thrombolytic agents relatively long after the onset of chest pain or other clinical manifestations of an incipient or evolving infarction in some instances. An initial infarction may have implications quite different from those of a subsequent infarction in a given patient in whom no additional loss of ventricular myocardium may be tolerated. Conversely, less overall benefit may be attainable in a patient with a subsequent infarction because of the extensive loss of functional myocardium already present. An analogous paradox requiring clinical judgment for resolution exists in considering whether to treat an elderly subject in whom the risk of induction of bleeding is clearly increased but the benefit of thrombolysis may be substantial because of the extraordinarily high risk of nonattenuated infarction—as has been shown to be the case with invasive interventions in elderly patients by Rahimtoola.[155] Such judgments must take into account the locus of infarction (with greater benefit of treatment anticipated with anterior as opposed to inferior infarction), its nature (with Q wave infarction with acute ST segment elevation having been more definitively demonstrated to be responsive but suspected infarction encountered before Q waves could have evolved potentially providing even greater opportunity for salvage of myocardium by prevention of ischemic injury), and the apparent extent of infarction (as judged from the electrocardiographically discerned risk region, with large incipient infarctions presaging high mortality and offering the best opportunity for a favorable therapeutic response).

Perhaps of most importance, patient selection must be based on knowledge of relative and absolute contraindications to the use of thrombolytic agents.[156] A recent compilation of commonly accepted contraindications to the use of thrombolytic agents is shown in Table 16–12. Those pertaining to central nervous system lesions, recent trauma or surgery, and active bleeding or a predisposition to bleeding have the most force in clinical decision making. Another compilation of contraindications divided into absolute and relative contraindications was presented in the recent published ACC/AHA Guidelines for the Early Management of Patients with Acute Myocardial Infarction[157] (Table 16–13).

TABLE 16–12. Contraindications to Thrombolysis*

Past cerebrovascular event or known intracranial aneurysm, arteriovenous malformation, or neoplasm
Recent trauma, including prolonged cardiopulmonary resuscitation within the past two weeks
Major surgery within the last two months, especially intracranial or spinal surgery
Gastrointestinal or genitourinary bleeding presently or within the preceding four weeks
Known bleeding disorders, including those secondary to severe hepatic or renal disease
Oral anticoagulant therapy
Pregnancy
Diabetes with proliferative retinopathy
Previous coronary artery bypass graft surgery
Previous myocardial infarction in the same site (because of impairment of electrophysiologic diagnosis of infarction)
Left bundle branch block (because of impairment of electrophysiologic diagnosis of infarction)
Cardiogenic shock (although some have reported striking improvement with thrombolytics)
Likelihood of left atrial or left ventricular thrombus, including mitral valve disease and chronic atrial fibrillation
Advanced age, often considered as greater than 75 years

* Reprinted with permission, from Muller DWM, Topol EJ. Selection of patients with acute myocardial infarction for thrombolytic therapy. Ann Intern Med 1990; 113: 949–60.

Management of Patients after Coronary Thrombolysis

Once thrombolysis agents have been administered, several steps are essential. Conjunctive treatment, generally aspirin and intravenous heparin, is necessary unless constrained by specific contraindications to prevent reocclusion, recurrent ischemia, and reinfarction. Despite use of such therapy, "breakthrough episodes" (early thrombotic reocclusions) may occur.[152] Accordingly, vigorous surveillance is required to detect episodes of myocardial ischemia. Approximately 80 per cent of recurrent ischemic events occur within the first 48 hours.[152] Thus, continuous electrocardiographic monitoring is essential during this interval. Serial 12-lead electrocardiograms and serial plasma enzyme determinations are useful to enhance interpretation of clinical sequelae that may be indicative of recurrent ischemia as well. Customary supportive care is essential, including analgesics for relief of chest pain, administration of oxygen if hypoxia supervenes, and treatment of congestive heart failure and arrhythmias with vasodilators, diuretics, and cardiotonic and antiarrhythmic drugs.

TABLE 16–13. Contraindications to Thrombolysis*

ABSOLUTE

Active internal bleeding
Aortic dissection
Prolonged or traumatic cardiopulmonary resuscitation
Recent head trauma or known intracranial neoplasm
Diabetic hemorrhagic retinopathy or other hemorrhagic ophthalmic condition
Pregnancy
Previous allergic reaction to the thrombotic agent (streptokinase or anistreplase)
Recorded blood pressure >200/120 mm Hg
History of cerebrovascular accident known to be hemorrhagic

RELATIVE

Recent trauma or surgery >two weeks; trauma or surgery more recent than two weeks, which could be a source of rebleeding, is an absolute contraindication
History of chronic severe hypertension with or without drug therapy
Active peptic ulcer
History of cerebrovascular accident
Known bleeding diathesis or current use of anticoagulants
Significant liver dysfunction
Prior exposure to streptokinase or anistreplase (this contraindication is particularly important in the initial six- to nine-month period after administration of streptokinase or anistreplase and applies to reuse of any streptokinase-containing agent, but does not apply to tissue-type plasminogen activator or urokinase)

* Extracted with permission, from ACC/AHA Guidelines for the Early Management of Patients with Acute Myocardial Infarction. A Report of the American College of Cardiology/ American Heart Association Task Force on Assessment of Diagnostic and Therapeutic Cardiovascular Procedures (subcommittee to develop guidelines for the early management of patients with acute myocardial infarction). Circulation 1990; 82: 664–707.

Unnecessary venous and arterial access should be avoided. Neurologic status should be assessed frequently for immediate detection of any finding that might be indicative of intracranial hemorrhage. Measurements of fibrinogen, activated partial thromboplastin time, and platelet count may be useful in facilitating detection of undue risk of bleeding, adjusting doses of anticoagulants, and timing the withdrawal of previously inserted vascular sheaths. In some circumstances, assessment of thrombin activity in vivo by measurement of fibrinopeptide A may be helpful in ensuring adequacy of anticoagulation as well.

For patients who have not manifested signs or symptoms of recurrent ischemia leading to angiographic evaluation, assessment of cardiac perfusion in response to physiologic stress is appropriate before discharge. Such functional testing provides a measure of functional capacity that may enhance confidence as the patient returns home. It also identifies patients with provoked ischemia who may benefit from revascularization by angioplasty or coronary artery bypass surgery and who are therefore candidates for angiographic evaluation.

Functional testing has serious limitations. As shown in the five-year follow-up of the Dutch Inter-University Reperfusion Trial,[158] a negative functional test after coronary thrombolysis is not a powerful descriptor of low risk for subsequent infarction or ischemia. The explanation may lie in the overwhelming importance of the infarct-related artery itself, which may manifest repeat plaque fissuring or rupture precipitating reinfarction that cannot be recognized or presaged by functional testing.

Several functional tests are employed. No one is clearly superior. Exercise thallium testing, symptom-limited treadmill exercise with electrocardiography only, thallium scintigraphy with dipyridamole or adenosine, stress echocardiography with exercise or dobutamine, or gated blood pool imaging may suffice.[125] For patients who cannot exercise, testing may be deferred or performed in a fashion avoiding the need for exercise (for example, thallium with dipyridamole or adenosine). For patients with either spontaneously manifest or provoked ischemia, cardiac catheterization is indicated before discharge, with evaluation for potential revascularization.[125]

Anticipated Developments

The following can be anticipated as use of coronary thrombolysis for primary treatment of acute myocardial infarction becomes more universally applicable.

Earlier Administration of Fibrinolytic Agents. Aggressive public education as well as heightened awareness by physicians and paramedical personnel should lead to more prompt access of patients with incipient or evolving myocardial infarction to the health care system, more prompt implementation of coronary thrombolysis after onset of infarction in appropriate candidates, and consequently even greater salvage of myocardium, preservation of ventricular function, and enhancement of survival than that already attainable. It is likely that thrombolytic agents will be administered not only by emergency room personnel but also by paramedical personnel in ambulances who would be guided by immediate, telephonic transmission of electrocardiograms to support or refute the diagnosis of suspected myocardial infarction, instantaneous communication with cardiologists when the need arises, and experience in rapid determination of the suitability of candidates for treatment with thrombolytic drugs. The feasibility of intramuscular administration of fibrinolytic agents such as tissue-type plasminogen activator with appropriate enhancers of absorption has been demonstrated in studies in animals in which coronary thrombolysis has been elicited promptly without local or systemic adverse effects.[159-161] Telephonic electrocardiographic surveillance such as that used routinely for patients at high risk of lethal arrhythmia and recipients of pacemakers who may require immediate diagnosis from a distance is likely to be a necessary component of self-administration of fibrinolytic agents, which would be undertaken only after the diagnosis of acute myocardial infarction had been confirmed electrocardiographically and potentially confounding diagnoses excluded by direct, telephonic communication with a member of the medical care team.

Evolution of Novel Agents. Several guiding principles have emerged that will condition developments in pharmacology ultimately leading to even more effective, novel fibrinolytic agents. Targets include modification of half-life in the circulation for use of novel agents in specific settings[162] (for example, those with a longer half-life being suitable for treatment of conditions such as acute pulmonary embolism with intermittent administration rather than a continuous infusion or for administration of fibrinolytic agents intramuscularly); functional "invisibility" to inhibitors such as plasminogen activator inhibitor-1, which may attenuate exogenous or endogenous fibrinolysis because of augmented synthesis from endothelial cells, the liver, or both;[163,164] and increased clot selectivity with avoidance of procoagulant effects and plasminogen steal with consequently more rapid and sustained recanalization.

Development of Promising Conjunctive Agents. More effective acceleration of recanalization and retardation or prevention of reocclusion will undoubtedly accompany the development of powerful regimens designed to prevent prothrombotic effects of fibrinolytic drugs, inhibit activation of platelets that may, of course, depend in part or wholly upon such effects, or both. Direct-acting antithrombins such as hirudin (synthesized by recombinant deoxyribonucleic acid technology), its lower molecular weight cogeners, and synthetic antithrombin inhibitors such as argatroban are particularly promising because they can inhibit thrombin without having to interact with antithrombin III as heparin does, and accordingly, can inhibit thrombin associated with clots or fibrinogen degradation products as well as free thrombin, in contrast to heparin. Inhibition of the extrinsic pathway of coagulation with lipoprotein-associated coagulation inhibitor, which complexes with tissue factor, factor VII, and activated factor X, and inhibition of activated coagulation factor X, a key component in both the extrinsic and intrinsic pathways, provide additional, promising targets for conjunctive agents that will enhance fibrinolysis. To whatever extent platelet activation persists and attenuates the net benefit of fibrinolysis despite optimal anticoagulation, antiplatelet agents such as inhibitors of the glycoprotein IIb-IIIa surface glycoprotein receptor for fibrinogen, including analogs of the domains binding to the integrin and antibodies to the receptor, may be useful as well. Development of all such conjunctive agents will require rigorous preclusion of the absence of serious side effects that could predispose to thrombocytopenia or frank hemorrhage.

Further Elucidation of Pathophysiology and Enhancement of the Efficacy of Coronary Thrombolysis. The contributions of molecular biology, cell biology, and pharmacology to the development of novel fibrinolytic and conjunctive agents will not be confined to therapeutics. Agents evaluated will be of considerable value in determining the extent to which specific pathophysiologic mechanisms influence the course of coronary thrombolysis and accordingly will help to identify the most promising targets for safely accelerating and sustaining recanalization. Modification of the genetic expression of specific components of the endogenous coagulation and fibrinolytic systems with orally active agents may be possible and beneficial. In view of the potential importance of altered concentrations of specific components of the fibrinolytic system such as plasminogen activator inhibitor-1 as markers and perhaps determinants of risk of accelerated vascular disease, modification of their expression with exogenous agents or gene therapy may evolve as part of the therapeutic armamentarium as well. Coronary thrombolysis has already reduced the toll from acute myocardial infarction dramatically. Its impact on attenuation of infarction, salvage of jeopardized myocardium, preservation of ventricular function, and enhancement of survival will undoubtedly continue to grow as its exciting evolution proceeds.

ACKNOWLEDGMENTS: Substantial information was provided for several sections of this chapter, particularly those concerning angioplasty and management of patients after treatment with thrombolytic drugs, by Dr. Eric J. Topol to whom the author and editors are deeply indebted. The editorial and secretarial assistance of Beth Engeszer and Lori Dales is appreciated.

REFERENCES

1. Collen D, Lijnen HR, Verstraete M, eds. Thrombolysis: biological and therapeutic properties of new thrombolytic agents. Edinburgh: Churchill Linginstone, 1985.
2. Sobel BE, ed. Cardiology Clinics: thrombolysis and the heart. Philadelphia: WB Saunders Co., 1987.
3. Tiefenbrunn AJ, Sobel BE. The impact of coronary thrombolysis on myocardial infarction. Fibrinolysis 1989; 3: 1–15.
4. Tiefenbrunn AJ, Sobel BE. Thrombolysis and myocardial infarction. Fibrinolysis 1991; 5: 1–15.
5. Vermeer F, ed. Thrombolysis in acute myocardial infarction. Assen/Maastricht: Van Gorcum, 1987.
6. Goa KL, Henwood JM, Stolz JF, Langley MS, Clissold SP. Intravenous streptokinase: a reappraisal of its therapeutic use in acute myocardial infarction. Drugs 1990; 39: 693–719,.
7. Anderson JL. Summary of U.S. clinical trials program for evaluation of anistreplase. Clin Cardiol 1990; 13(suppl V): 33–8.
8. Sherry S. The fibrinolytic system and its pharmacologic activation for thrombolysis. In: Sobel BE, ed. Cardiology clinics: thrombolysis and the heart. Philadelphia: WB Saunders Co., 1987: 1–11.
9. Delezenne C, Pozerski E. Action du sérum sanguin sur la gélatine en présesnce du chloroforme. C R Soc Biol (Paris) 1903; 55: 327–9.
10. Tillett WS, Garner RL. The fibrinolytic activity of hemolytic streptococci. J Exp Med 1933; 58: 485–502.
11. Milstone H. A factor in normal human blood which participates in streptococcal fibrinolysis. J Immunol 1941; 42: 109–16.
12. Christensen LR. Streptococcal fibrinolysis: a proteolytic reaction due to a serum enzyme activated by streptococcal fibrinolysis. J Gen Physiol 1945; 28: 363–83.
13. Sherry S, Fletcher AP, Alkjaersig N. Fibrinolysis and fibrinolytic activity in man. Physiol Rev 1959; 39: 343–82.
14. Tiefenbrunn AJ, Graor RA, Robison AK, Lucas FV, Sobel BE. Pharmacodynamics of tissue-type plasminogen activator (t-PA) characterized by computer-assisted simulation. Circulation 1986; 73: 1291–9.
15. Collen D, Stassen JM, Verstraete M. Thrombolysis with human extrinsic (tissue-type) plasminogen activator in rab-

bits with experimental jugular vein thrombosis. Effect of molecular form and dose of activator, age of the thrombus, and route of administration. J Clin Invest 1983; 71: 368–76.
16. Collen D, Lijnen HR. The fibrinolytic system in man: an overview. In: Collen D, Lijnen HR, Verstraete M, eds. Thrombolysis: biological and therapeutic properties of new thrombolytic agents. Edinburgh: Churchill Livingstone, 1985: 1–14.
17. Fletcher AP, Sherry S, Alkjaersig N, Smyrniotis FE, Jick S. The maintenance of a sustained thrombolytic state in man. II. Clinical observations on patients with myocardial infarction and other thromboembolic disorders. J Clin Invest 1959; 38: 1111–9.
18. Sherry S, Fletcher AP, Alkjaersig N. The fibrinolysin system: some physiological considerations. In: Page I, ed. Connective tissues, thrombosis and atherosclerosis. New York: Academic Press, 1959: 241–58.
19. European Cooperative Study Group for Streptokinase Treatment in Acute Myocardial Infarction. Streptokinase in acute myocardial infarction. N Engl J Med 1979; 301: 797–802.
20. Verstraete M, van de Loo J, Jesdinsky HL, eds. Streptokinase in acute myocardial infarction. Acta Med Scand 1981; 648 (suppl): 1–117.
21. Maroko PR, Kjekshus JK, Sobel BE, et al. Factors influencing infarct size following experimental coronary artery occlusions. Circulation 1971; 43: 67–82.
22. Sobel BE, Bresnahan GF, Shell WE, Yoder RD. Estimation of infarct size in man and its relation to prognosis. Circulation 1972; 46: 640–8.
23. Geltman EM, Ehsani AA, Campbell MK, et al. The influence of location and extent of myocardial infarction on long-term ventricular dysrhythmia and mortality. Circulation 1979; 60: 805–14.
24. Roberts R, Croft C, Gold HK, et al. Effect of propranolol on myocardial infarct size in a randomized, blinded, multicenter trial. N Engl J Med 1984; 311: 218–25.
25. Ginks WR, Sybers HD, Maroko PR, et al. Coronary artery reperfusion. II. Reduction of myocardial infarct size at one week after the coronary occlusion. J Clin Invest 1972; 51: 2717–23.
26. DaWood MA, Spores J, Notska RN, et al. Prevalence of total coronary occlusion during the early hours of transmural myocardial infarction. N Engl J Med 1980; 303: 897–903.
27. Chazov EL, Matteeva LS, Mazaev AV, et al. Intracoronary administration of fibrinolysis in acute myocardial infarction. Ter Arkh 1976; 48: 8–19.
28. Rentrop P, Blanka H, Karsch KR, et al. Acute myocardial infarction: Intracoronary application of nitroglycerin and streptokinase in combination with transluminal recanalization. Am J Cardiol 1979; 2: 354–63.
29. Maseri A, L'Abbate A, Baroldi G, et al. Coronary vasospasm as a possible cause of myocardial infarction. N Engl J Med 1978; 299: 1271–7.
30. Bresnahan GF, Roberts R, Shell WE, Ross J Jr, Sobel BE. Deleterious effects due to hemorrhage after myocardial reperfusion. Am J Cardiol 1974; 33: 82–6.
31. Fox KAA, Saffitz JE, Corr PB. Pathophysiology of myocardial reperfusion. In: Sobel BE, ed. Cardiology clinics: thrombolysis and the heart. Philadelphia: WB Saunders Company, 1987: 31–48.
32. Maroko PR, Libby P, Ginks WR, Shell WE, Ross J Jr. Coronary artery reperfusion. I. Early effects on myocardial contractility and myocardial necrosis. J Clin Invest 1972; 51: 2710–6.
33. Rentrop P, Blanke H, Karsch KR, Kaiser H, Kostering H, Leitz K. Selective intracoronary thrombolysis in acute myocardial infarction and unstable angina pectoris. Circulation 1981; 63: 307–17.
34. Fox KAA, Bermann SR, Sobel BE. Pathophysiology of myocardial reperfusion. In: Creger WP, ed. Annual review of medicine. Palo Alto: Annual Reviews Inc., 1985: 125–44.
35. Bergmann SR, Fox KAA, Ter-Pogossian MM, Sobel BE, Collen D. Clot-selective coronary thrombolysis with tissue-type plasminogen activator. Science 1983; 220: 1181–3.
36. Van de Werf F, Bergmann SR, Fox KAA, et al. Coronary

thrombolysis with intravenously administered human tissue-type plasminogen activator produced by recombinant DNA technology. Circulation 1984; 69: 605–10.

37. Sobel BE, Bergmann SR. The impact of coronary thrombolysis and tissue-type plasminogen activator (t-PA) on acute myocardial infarction. In: Collen D, Verstraete M, eds., Thrombolysis. Edinburgh: Churchill Livingstone, 1985: 61–84.

38. Van de Werf F, Ludbrook PA, Bergmann SR, et al. Coronary thrombolysis with tissue-type plasminogen activator in patients with evolving myocardial infarction. N Engl J Med 1984; 310: 609–13.

39. Sobel BE, Geltman EM, Tiefenbrunn AJ, et al. Improvement of regional myocardial metabolism after coronary thrombolysis induced with tissue-type plasminogen activator or streptokinase. Circulation 1984; 69: 983–90.

40. Collen D, Topol EJ, Tiefenbrunn AJ, et al. Coronary thrombolysis with recombinant human tissue-type plasminogen activator: a prospective, randomized, placebo-controlled trial. Circulation 1984; 70: 1012–7.

41. Rijken DC, Collen D. Purification and characterization of the plasminogen activator secreted by human melanoma cells in culture. J Biol Chem 1981; 256: 7035–41.

42. Bergmann SR, Lerch RA, Fox KAA, et al. Temporal dependence of beneficial effects of coronary thrombolysis characterized by positron tomography. Am J Med 1982; 73: 573–81.

43. Fry ETA, Sobel BE. Coronary thrombolysis. In: Zipes DP, Rowlands DJ, eds. Progress in cardiology Vol. 3/1. Philadelphia: Lea & Febiger, 1990: 199–239.

44. Gruppo Italiano per lo studio della streptochinasi nell'infarto miocardio (GISSI). Effectiveness of intravenous thrombolytic treatment in acute myocardial infarction. Lancet 1986; 1: 397–401.

45. ISIS-2 (Second International Study of Infarct Survival) Collaborative Group: randomised trial of intravenous streptokinase, oral aspirin, both or neither among 17,187 cases of suspected acute myocardial infarction: ISIS-2. Lancet 1988; 2: 349–60.

46. Tiefenbrunn AJ, Ludbrook PA. Coronary thrombolysis— it's worth the risk. JAMA 1989; 261: 2107–8.

47. Topol EJ, Califf RM, George BS, et al. A multicenter randomized trial of intravenous recombinant tissue plasminogen activator and immediate angioplasty in acute myocardial infarction. N Engl J Med 1987; 317: 581–8.

48 Simoons ML, Arnold AER, Betriu A, et al. Thrombolysis with tissue plasminogen activator in acute myocardial infarction: no additional benefit from immediate percutaneous coronary angioplasty. Lancet 1988; 1: 197–202.

49. The TIMI Study Group. Comparison of invasive and conservative strategies after treatment with intravenous tissue plasminogen activator in acute myocardial infarction. Results of the Thrombolysis in Myocardial Infarction (TIMI) Phase II Trial. N Engl J Med 1989; 320: 618–27.

50. Braunwald E. Optimizing thrombolytic therapy of acute myocardial infarction. Circulation 1990; 82: 1510–3.

51. Marder VJ, Sherry S. Thrombolytic therapy: current status (1). N Engl J Med 1988; 318: 1512–20.

52. Marder VJ, Sherry S. Thrombolytic therapy: current status (2). N Engl J Med 1988; 318: 1585–95.

53. Cowley MJ, Hastillo A, Vetrovec GW, Fisher LM, Garrett R, Hess ML. Fibrinolytic effects of intracoronary streptokinase administration in patients with acute myocardial infarction and coronary insufficiency. Circulation 1983; 67: 1031–8.

54. Rogers WJ, Mantle JA, Hood WP Jr, et al. Prospective randomized trial of intravenous and intracoronary streptokinase in acute myocardial infarction. Circulation 1983; 68: 1051–61.

55. Rapaport E. Systemic lytic state called reocclusion key. Medical World News 1990; November: 12.

56. Chesebro JH, Knatterud G, Roberts R, et al. Thrombolysis in Myocardial Infarction (TIMI) trial, phase I: a comparison between intravenous tissue plasminogen activator and intravenous streptokinase. Circulation 1987; 76: 142–54.

57. Topol EJ, Califf RM, George BS, et al. Coronary arterial thrombolysis with combined infusion of recombinant tissue-type plasminogen activator and urokinase in patients with acute myocardial infarction. Circulation 1988; 77: 1100–7.

58. Califf RM, Topol EJ, Stack RS, et al. Evaluation of combination thrombolytic therapy and timing of cardiac catheterization in acute myocardial infarction. Results of Thrombolysis and Angioplasty in Myocardial Infarction— Phase 5 randomized trial. Circulation, 1991; 83: 1543–56.

59. von Essen R, et al. TAPS: t-PA vs APSAC: patency study in acute myocardial infarction. Presented at the George Washington University Sixth International Symposium and preceding the 1990 National Meeting of the American Heart Association.

60. Braunwald E. Myocardial reperfusion, limitation of infarct size, reduction of left ventricular dysfunction, and improved survival. Should the paradigm be expanded? Circulation 1989; 79: 441–4.

61. Van de Werf F, Arnold AER, for the European Cooperative Study Group for Recombinant Tissue-type Plasminogen Activator. Intravenous tissue plasminogen activator and size of infarct, left ventricular function, and survival in acute myocardial infarction. Br Med J 1988; 297: 1374–9.

62. Dalen JE, Gore JM, Braunwald E, et al. Six- and twelve-month follow-up of the phase I Thrombolysis in Myocardial Infarction (TIMI) Trial. Am J Cardiol 1988; 62: 179–85.

63. AIMS Trial Study Group. Effect of intravenous APSAC on mortality after acute myocardial infarction: preliminary report of a placebo-controlled clinical trial. Lancet 1988; 2: 545–9.

64. Wilcox RG, von der Lippe G, Olsson CG, Jensen G, Shene AM, Hampton JR, for the ASSET Study Group. Trial of tissue plasminogen activator for mortality reduction in acute myocardial infarction: Anglo-Scandinavian Study of Early Thrombolysis (ASSET). Lancet 1988; 2: 525–30.

65. Ritchie JL, Cerqueria M, Maynard C, Davis K, Kennedy W. Ventricular function and infarction size: the Western Washington Intravenous Streptokinase in Myocardial Infarction Trial. J Am Coll Cardiol 1988; 11: 689–97.

66. White HD, Norris RM, Brown MA, et al. Effect of intravenous streptokinase on left ventricular function and early survival after acute myocardial infarction. N Engl J Med 1987; 317: 850–5.

67. O'Rourke M, Baron D, Keogh A, et al. Limitation of myocardial infarction by early infusion of recombinant tissue-type plasminogen activator. Circulation 1988; 77: 1311–5.

68. National Heart Foundation of Australia Coronary Thrombolysis Group. Coronary thrombolysis and myocardial salvage by tissue plasminogen activator given up to 4 hours after onset of myocardial infarction. Lancet 1988; 1: 203–8.

69. Stein B, Fuster V, Halperin J, Chesebro JH. Antithrombotic therapy in cardiac disease: an emerging approach based on pathogenesis and risk. Circulation 1989; 80: 1501–15.

70. Roth GJ. Developing relationships: arterial platelet adhesion, glycoprotein Ib, and leucine-rich glycoproteins. Blood 1991; 77: 5–19.

71. Webster MWI, Chesebro JH, Mruk JS. Antithrombotic therapy during and after thrombolysis for acute myocardial infarction. Coronary Artery Dis 1990; 1: 190–8.

72. Eisenberg PR. Mechanism of action of heparin and anticoagulation therapy: implications for the prevention of arterial thrombosis and the treatment of mural thrombosis. Coronary Artery Dis 1990; 1: 159–65.

73. Eisenberg PR, Sherman L, Rich M, et al. Importance of continued activation of thrombin reflected by fibrinopeptide A to the efficacy of thrombolysis. J Am Coll Cardiol 1986; 7: 1255–62.

74. Eisenberg PR, Miletich JE, Sobel BE, Jaffe AS. Differential effects of activation of prothrombin by streptokinase compared with urokinase and tissue-type plasminogen activator (t-PA). Thromb Res 1988; 50: 707–17.

75. Rapold HJ, Kuemmerli H, Weiss M, Baur H, Haeberli A. Monitoring of fibrin generation during thrombolytic therapy of acute myocardial infarction with recombinant tissue-type plasminogen activator. Circulation 1989; 79: 980–9.

76. Sobel BE. Coronary thrombolysis. Coronary Artery Dis 1990; 1: 3–7.

77. Rapaport E. Thrombolytic agents in acute myocardial infarction. N Engl J Med 1989; 320: 861–4.

78. Stack RS, Phillips HR III, Grierson DS, et al. Functional improvement of jeopardized myocardium following intracoronary streptokinase infusion in acute myocardial infarction. J Clin Invest 1983; 72: 84–95.

79. Van de Werf F. Discrepancies between the effects of coronary reperfusion on survival and left ventricular function. Lancet 1989; 1: 1367–8.

80. Reduto LA, Smalling RW, Freund GC, et al. Intracoronary infusion of streptokinase in patients with acute myocardial infarction: effects of reperfusion on left ventricular performance. Am J Cardiol 1981; 48: 403–9.

81. Schröder R, Biamino GV, Leitner E-R, et al. Intravenous short-term infusion of streptokinase in acute myocardial infarction. Circulation 1983; 67: 536–48.

82. The ISAM Study Group. A prospective trial of intravenous streptokinase in acute myocardial infarction (ISAM): mortality and infarct size at 21 days. N Engl J Med 1986; 314: 1465–71.

83. Koren G, Weiss AT, Hasin Y, et al. Prevention of myocardial damage in acute myocardial ischemia by early treatment with intravenous streptokinase. N Engl J Med 1985; 313: 1384–9.

84. Sheenan FH, Braunwald E, Canner P, et al. The effect of intravenous thrombolytic therapy on left ventricular function: a report on tissue-type plasminogen activator and streptokinase from the Thrombolysis in Myocardial Infarction (TIMI Phase I) trial. Circulation 1987; 75: 817–29.

85. Durand P, Asseman P, Pruvost P, et al. Effectiveness of intravenous streptokinase on infarct size and left ventricular function in acute myocardial infarction: prospective and randomized study. Clin Cardiol 1987; 10: 383–92.

86. Topol EJ, Weiss JL, Brinker JA, et al. Regional wall motion improvement after coronary thrombolysis with recombinant tissue plasminogen activator: importance of coronary angioplasty. J Am Coll Cardiol 1985; 6: 426–33.

87. Magnani B, for the PAIMS Investigators. Plasminogen Activator Italian Multicenter Study (PAIMS): comparison of intravenous recombinant single-chain human tissue-type plasminogen activator (rt-PA) with intravenous streptokinase in acute myocardial infarction. J Am Coll Cardiol 1989; 13: 19–26.

88. Guerci AS, Gerstenblith G, Brinker JA, et al. A randomized trial of intravenous tissue plasminogen activator for acute myocardial infarction with subsequent randomization to elective coronary angioplasty. N Engl J Med 1987; 317: 1613–8.

89. Bates ER, Topol EJ, Kline EM, et al. Early reperfusion therapy improves left ventricular function after acute inferior myocardial infarction associated with right coronary artery disease. Am Heart J 1987; 114: 261–7.

90. Califf RM, Harrelson-Woodlief L, Topol EJ. Left ventricular ejection fraction may not be useful as an end point of thrombolytic therapy comparative trials. Circulation 1990; 82: 1847–53.

91. Verstraete M, Bernard R, Bory M, et al. Randomised trial of intravenous recombinant tissue-type plasminogen activator versus intravenous streptokinase in acute myocardial infarction. Lancet 1985; 1: 842–7.

92. White HD, Rivers JT, Norris RM, et al. Is rt-PA or streptokinase superior for preservation of left ventricular function after myocardial infarction? (abstr). Circulation 1988; 78(suppl II): II-303.

93. Gruppo Italiano per lo Studio della Sopravvivenza nell'Infarto Miocardio (GISSI-2). A fraction randomised trial of alteplase versus streptokinase and heparin versus no heparin among 12,490 patients with acute myocardial infarction. Lancet 1990; 336: 65–71.

94. AIMS Trial Study Group. Long-term effects of intravenous anistreplase in acute myocardial infarction: final report of the AIMS study. Lancet 1990; 335: 427–31.

95. TIMI Study Group. Special report: the thrombolysis in myocardial infarction (TIMI) trial. N Engl J Med 1985; 312: 932–6.

96. Hsia J, Hamilton WP, Kleiman N, et al. A comparison between heparin and low-dose aspirin as adjunctive therapy with tissue plasminogen activator for acute myocardial infarction. N Engl J Med 1990; 323: 1433–7.

97. Bleich SD, Nichols T, Schumacher R, et al. The role of heparin following coronary thrombolysis with tissue plasminogen activator (t-PA) (abstr). Circulation 1989; 80(suppl II): II-113.

98. de Bono DP, Simoons ML, Tijssen J, et al. The effect of early intravenous heparin on coronary patency, infarct size and bleeding complication after alteplase thrombolysis: results of a randomised, double-blind European Cooperative Study Group Trial. Br Heart J, in press.

99. Vermeer F, Massberg I, Meyer J, et al. Saruplase, a new fibrin specific thrombolytic agent: efficacy and safety in the first 1000 patients (abstr). J Am Coll Cardiol 1991; 17(suppl): 152A.

100. Topol EJ, George BS, Kereiakes DJ, et al. A randomized controlled trial of intravenous tissue plasminogen activator and early intravenous heparin in acute myocardial infarction. Circulation 1989; 79: 281–6.

101. Sobel BE. Safety and efficacy of tissue-type plasminogen activator produced by recombinant DNA technology (rt-PA). J Am Coll Cardiol 1987; 10: 40B–4B.

102. Lew AS, Hod H, Cercek B, Shah PK, Ganz W. Mortality and morbidity rates of patients older and younger than 75 years with acute myocardial infarction treated with intravenous streptokinase. Am J Cardiol 1987; 59: 1–5.

103. Braunwald E, Knatterud GL, Passamani E, Robertson TL, Solomon R. Update form the Thrombolysis in Myocardial Infarction Trial (letter). J Am Coll Cardiol 1987; 10: 970.

104. Fitzgerald DJ, FitzGerald GA. Antiplatelet and anticoagulant therapy during coronary thrombolysis. TCM 1991; January/February: 29–39.

105. Torr SR, Winters KJ, Santoro SA, Sobel BE. The nature of interactions between tissue-type plasminogen activator and platelets. Thromb Res 1990; 59: 279–93.

106. Haskel EJ, Torr SR, Day KC, et al. Prevention of arterial reocclusion after thrombolysis with recombinant lipoprotein-associated coagulation inhibitor (LACI). Circulation, in press.

107. Yasuda T, Gold HK, Leinbach RC, et al. Lysis of plasminogen activator-resistant platelet-rich coronary artery thrombus with combined bolus injection of recombinant tissue-type plasminogen activator and antiplatelet GPIIb/IIIa antibody. J Am Coll Cardiol 1990; 16: 1728–35.

108. Haskel EJ, Adams SP, Feigen LP, et al. Prevention of reoccluding platelet-rich thrombi in canine femoral arteries with a novel peptide antagonist of platelet glycoprotein IIb/IIIa receptors. Circulation 1989; 80: 1775–82.

109. Haskel EJ, Prager NA, Adams SP, Feigen LP, Sobel BE, Abendschein DR. The relative efficacy of antithrombin compared with antiplatelet agents in accelerating coronary thrombolysis and preventing early reocclusion. Circulation 1991; 83: 1048–56.

110. The SCATI (Studio sulla Calciparini nell'Angina nella Thrombosi Ventriculare nell'Infarto) Group. Randomised controlled trial of subcutaneous calcium-heparin in acute myocardial infarction. Lancet 1989; 2: 182–6.

111. Weitz JI, Huboda M, Massel D, Maraganore D, Hirsh J. Clot-bound thrombin is protected from inhibition by heparin-antithrombin III but is susceptible to inactivation by antithrombin III independent inhibitors. J Clin Invest 1990; 86: 385–91.

112. Hirsh J. Heparin. N Engl J Med, 1991; 324: 1565–74.

113. Turpie AGG, Robinson JH, Doule DJ, et al. Comparison of high-dose with low-dose subcutaneous heparin to prevent left ventricular mural thrombosis in patients with acute transmural anterior myocardial infarction. N Engl J Med 1989; 320: 352–7.

114. Vlasuk G, Sitko G, Shebuski R. Specific factor Xa inhibition enhances thrombolytic reperfusion and prevents acute reocclusion in the canine copper coil model of arterial thrombosis (abstr). Circulation 1990; 82(suppl III): III-603.

115. Fitzgerald DJ, Wright F, FitzGerald GA. Increased thromboxane biosynthesis during coronary thrombolysis. Evidence that platelet activation and thromboxane A_2 modulate the response to tissue-type plasminogen activator in vivo. Circ Res 1989; 65: 83–94.

116. Chesebro JH. Antithrombotic therapy in coronary artery disease. Review in depth. Coronary Artery Dis 1990; 2: 147–90.

117. Nohara R, Bergmann SR. Reduction of stenosis-induced

cyclic flow variations by inhibition of platelet-activating factor in dogs. Coronary Artery Dis 1990; 1: 347–54.

118. Meyer J, Merx W, Schmitz H, et al. Percutaneous transluminal coronary angioplasty immediately after intracoronary streptolysis of transmural myocardial infarction. Circulation 1982; 66: 905–13.

119. Swan HJC. Thrombolysis in acute myocardial infarction: treatment of the underlying coronary artery disease. Circulation 1982; 66: 914–6.

120. Topol EJ. Coronary angioplasty for acute myocardial infarction. Ann Intern Med 1988; 109: 970–80.

121. Hartzler GO, Rutherford BD, McConahay DR. Percutaneous transluminal coronary angioplasty: application for acute myocardial infarction. Am J Cardiol 1984; 53: 117C–21C.

122. O'Keefe JH, Rutherford BD, McConahay DR, et al. Early and late results of coronary angioplasty without antecedent thrombolytic therapy for acute myocardial infarction. Am J Cardiol 1989; 64: 1221–30.

123. Ramos RG, Patel C, Gangadharan V, Gordon S, Timmis GC. Outcome of coronary angioplasty (PTCA) following thrombolytic therapy in acute myocardial infarction (abstr). Circulation 1986; 74(suppl II): II–124.

124. TIMI Research Group. Immediate vs delayed catheterization and angioplasty following thrombolytic therapy for acute myocardial infarction. JAMA 1988; 260: 2849–58.

125. Topol EJ, Holmes DR, Rogers WJ. Coronary angiography for acute myocardial infarction: a critical appraisal. Ann Intern Med, 1991; 114: 877–85.

126. PRIMI Trial Study Group. Randomised double-blind trial of recombinant pro-urokinase against streptokinase in acute myocardial infarction. Lancet 1989; 1: 863–7.

127. Fung AY, Lai P, Topol EJ. Value of percutaneous transluminal coronary angioplasty after unsuccessful intravenous streptokinase therapy in acute myocardial infarction. Am J Cardiol 1986; 58: 686–91.

128. Holmes DR Jr, Gersh BJ, Bailey KR et al. Rescue percutaneous transluminal coronary angioplasty after failed trombolytic therapy 4 year follow-up. J Am Cardiol 1989; 13(2): 193a.

129. Grines CL, Nissen SE, Booth DC et al. A new thrombolytic regimen for acute myocardial infarction using combination half dose tissue-type plasminogen activator with full dose streptokinase: a pilot study. J Am Coll Cardiol 1989; 14: 573–80.

130. Grines CL, Nissen, Booth DC et al. A prospective randomized trial comparing combination half dose TPA with streptokinase to full dose TPA in acute myocardial infarction preliminary report. J Am Coll Cardiol 1990; 15(2): 4a.

131. O'Connor CM, Mark DB, Hinohara T, et al. Rescue coronary angioplasty after failure of intravenous streptokinase in acute myocardial infarction: in-hospital and long-term outcomes. J Inv Cardiol 1989; 1: 85–95.

132. Baim DS, Diver DJ, Knatterud GL. PTCA salvage for thrombolytic failures implications from TIMI II-A. Circulation 1988; 78: 112.

133. Gacioch GM, Topol EJ. Sudden paradoxic clinical deterioration during angioplasty of the occluded right coronary artery in acute myocardial infarction. J Am Coll Cardiol 1989; 14: 1202–9.

134. Califf RM, O'Neill W, Stack RS, et al. Failure of simple clinical measurements to predict perfusion status after intravenous thrombolysis. Ann Intern Med 1988; 109: 658–62.

135. Hashimoto H, Abendschein DR, Sobel BE. Early detection of myocardial infarction in conscious dogs by analysis of plasma MM creatine kinase isoforms. Circulation 1985; 71: 363–9.

136. Nohara R, Myears DW, Sobel BE, Abendschein DR. Optimal criteria for rapid detection of myocardial reperfusion by creatine kinase MM isoforms in the presence of residual high-grade stenosis. J Am Coll Cardiol 1989; 14: 1067–73.

137. Abendschein DR, Ellis AK, Eisenberg PR, Klocke FJ, Sobel BE, Jaffe AS. Prompt detection of coronary recanalization by analysis of rates of change of concentrations of macromolecular markers in plasma. Coronary Artery Dis 1991; 2: 201–12.

138. SWIFT (Should We Intervene Following Thrombolysis?) Trial Study Group. SWIFT trial of delayed elective intervention v conservative treatment after thrombolysis with anistreplase in acute myocardial infarction. Br Med J 1991; 302: 555–60.

139. Sobel BE, Nachowiak DA, Fry ETA, Bergmann SR, Torr SR. Paradoxical attenuation of fibrinolysis attributable to "plasminogen steal" and its implications for coronary thrombolysis. Coronary Artery Dis 1990; 1: 111–9.

140. Lee CD, Mann KG. The activation of human coagulation factor V by plasmin (abstr). Blood 1987; 70: 389A.

141. Barbash GI, Hod H, Roth A, et al. Repeat infusions of recombinant tissue-type plasminogen activator in patients with acute myocardial infarction and early recurrent myocardial ischemia. J Am Coll Cardiol 1990; 16: 779–83.

142. Fox KAA, Robison AK, Knabb RM, Rosamond TL, Sobel BE, Bergmann SR. Prevention of coronary thrombosis with subthrombolytic doses of tissue-type plasminogen activator. Circulation 1985; 72: 1346–54.

143. Gold KH, Leinbach RC, Garabedian HD, et al. Acute coronary reocclusion after thrombolysis with recombinant human tissue-type plasminogen activator: prevention by a maintenance infusion. Circulation 1986; 73: 347–52.

144. Eisenberg PR, Sherman LA, Tiefenbrunn AJ, Ludbrook PA, Sobel BE, Jaffe AS. Sustained fibrinolysis after administration of t-PA despite its short half life in the circulation. Thromb Haemost 1987; 57: 35–40.

145. Neuhaus K-L, Feuerer W, Jeep-Tebbe S, Niederer W, Vogt A, Tebbe U. Improved thrombolysis with a modified dose regimen of recombinant tissue-type plasminogen activator. J Am Coll Cardiol 1989; 14: 1566–9.

146. Tranchesi B, Verstraete M, Vanhove P, et al. Intravenous bolus administration of recombinant tissue plasminogen activator to patients with acute myocardial infarction. Coronary Artery Dis 1990; 1: 83–8.

147. Grines CL, Nissen SE, Booth DC, et al. A prospective, randomized trial comparing combination half dose t-PA with streptokinase to full dose t-PA in acute myocardial infarction: preliminary report (abstr). J Am Coll Cardiol 1990; 15(suppl): 4A.

148. The Urokinase and Alteplase in Myocardial Infarction Collaborative Group. Combination urokinase and alteplase in the treatment of myocardial infarction. Coronary Artery Dis 1991; 2: 225–35.

149. Rentrop KP. Thrombolytic therapy in patients with acute myocardial infarction. Circulation 1985; 71: 627–31.

150. Califf RM, Topol EJ, George BS, et al. Characteristics and outcome of patients in whom reperfusion with intravenous tissue-type plasminogen activator fails: results of the Thrombolysis and Angioplasty in Myocardial Infarction (TAMI) I trial. Circulation 1988; 77: 1090–9.

151. Tendera MP, Campbell WB, Tennant SN, Ray WA. Factors influencing probability of reperfusion with intracoronary ostial infusion of thrombolytic agent in patients with acute myocardial infarction. Circulation 1985; 71: 124–8.

152. Ohman EM, Califf RM, Topol EJ, et al. Consequences of reocclusion after successful reperfusion therapy in acute myocardial infarction. Circulation 1990; 82: 781–91.

153. Stadius ML, Maynard C, Fritz JK, et al. Coronary anatomy and left ventricular function in the first 12 hours of acute myocardial infarction: the Western Washington Randomized Intracoronary Streptokinase Trial. Circulation 1985; 72: 292–301.

154. Gimple LW, Gold KH, Leinbach RC, et al. Correlation between template bleeding times and spontaneous bleeding during treatment of acute myocardial infarction with recombinant tissue-type plasminogen activator. Circulation 1989; 80: 581–8.

155. Rahimtoola SH, Grunkemeier GL, Starr A. Ten year survival after coronary artery bypass surgery for angina in patients aged 65 years and older. Circulation 1986; 74: 509–17.

156. Muller DWM, Topol EJ. Selection of patients with acute myocardial infarction for thrombolytic therapy. Ann Intern Med 1990; 113: 949–60.

157. Gunnar RM, Bourdillon PDV, Dixon DW, et al. ACC/AHA Guidelines for the early management of patients with acute myocardial infarction. Circulation 1990; 82: 664–707.

158. Simoons ML, Vos J, Tijssen JGP, et al. Long-term benefit

of early thrombolytic therapy in patients with acute myo-cardial infarction: 5 year follow-up of a trial conducted by the Interuniversity Cardiology Institute in The Netherlands. J Am Coll Cardiol 1989; 14: 1609–15.

159. Sobel BE, Fields LE, Robison AK, Fox KAA, Sarnoff SJ. Coronary thrombolysis with facilitated absorption of intra-muscularly injected tissue-type plasminogen activator. Proc Natl Acad Sci USA 1985; 82: 4258–62.

160. Sobel BE, Saffitz JE, Fields LE, et al. Intramuscular ad-ministration of tissue-type plasminogen activator in rabbits and dogs and its implications for coronary thrombolysis. Circulation 1987; 75: 1261–72.

161. Sobel BE, Sarnoff SJ, Nachowiak DA. Augmented and sus-tained plasma concentrations after intramuscular injections of molecular variants and deglycosylated forms of tissue-type plasminogen activators. Circulation 1990; 81: 1362–73.

162. Lucore CL, Fry ETA, Nachowiak DA, Sobel BE. Bio-chemical determinants of clearance of t-PA from the cir-culation. Circulation 1988; 77: 906–14.

163. Sobel BE. Coronary thrombolysis and the new biology. J Am Coll Cardiol 1989; 14: 850–60.

164. Fujii S, Hopkins WE, Sobel BE. Mechanisms contributing to increased synthesis of plasminogen activator inhibitor type-2 in endothelial cells by constituents of platelets and their implications for thrombolysis. Circulation 1991; 83: 645–51.

165. Stack RS, O'Connor CM, Mark DB, et al. Coronary per-fusion during acute myocardial infarction with a combined therapy of coronary angioplasty and high-dose intravenous streptokinase. Circulation 1988; 77: 151–61.

166. Anderson JL, Rothbard RL, Hackworthy RA, et al. Mul-ticenter reperfusion trial of intravenous anisoylated plas-minogen streptokinase activator complex (APSAC) in acute myocardial infarction: controlled comparison with intra-coronary streptokinase. J Am Coll Cardiol 1988; 11: 1153–63.

167. Passamani E, Hodges M, Herman M, et al. The Throm-bolysis in Myocardial Infarction (TIMI) phase II pilot study: Tissue plasminogen activator followed by percutaneous transluminal coronary angioplasty. J Am Coll Cardiol 1987; 10: 51B–64B.

168. Dorent R, Vahanian A, Michel P, Verdy E, Conard J. Bleed-ing complications of thrombolytic therapy in patients with acute myocardial infarction (M.I.) receiving I.V. infusion of SK or 1 chain rt-PA (abstr). Finbrinolysis 1988; 2(suppl I): 85.

17

MYOCARDIAL INFARCTION: ADJUNCTIVE ANTITHROMBOTIC THERAPY TO THROMBOLYSIS

ALLAN M. ROSS

There has been intense interest of late regarding post-thrombolytic anticoagulation as a strategy to prevent early reocclusion of reperfused coronary arteries following initial treatment for acute myocardial infarction. Several important new studies have been completed, but by no means have they quieted the controversy that exists regarding appropriate therapeutic approaches. Further, the issues surrounding debate over adjunctive anticoagulation, heparin in particular, figure prominently in the larger arena in which disputes over the relative merits of the specific fibrinolytic activators themselves are conducted.

An analysis of these issues must begin with an understanding of the pathophysiologic milieu at the site of the acute coronary thrombosis that initiates myocardial infarction. While discussed in considerable detail in Chapters 2 and 3 of this volume, it is to be recalled that thrombus formation is not a random event but rather is initiated by an intense stimulus, usually severe endothelial (or deeper) injury of the arterial wall owing to rupture of the fibrous cap which lies over an atherosclerotic plaque; hence, the equilibrium normally present between procoagulant and anticoagulant components of blood plasma are skewed in favor of thrombosis when the passing blood elements encounter the thrombogenic components of the plaque interstices.

Additionally, the augmented perturbation of the flow pattern at the site of this intraluminal deformity contributes further impetus for platelet deposition and aggregation compounding the prothrombotic environment.

The therapeutic administration of a potent plasminogen activator leading to dissolution of the clot in no way removes the original cause of clot formation. Thus, the environment exists for another bout of thrombosis. In point of fact, lysis itself, predominantly owing to thrombin release is yet another procoagulant component. Owen et al.[1] demonstrated an increase in thrombin activity in myocardial infarction patients treated with streptokinase, while Gulba and associates[2] have demonstrated increased thrombosis activity following urokinase or alteplase administration. The dissolving clot serves as a reservoir of continuously released thrombin free to catalyze a new round of fibrinogen to fibrin conversion and free to stimulate further platelet activation. The plasminogen activators themselves have either no (i.e., alteplase) or only weak (i.e., streptokinase) anticoagulant properties (deriving chiefly from fibrinogen depletion and the release of fibrin and fibrinogen degradation products). Deducing from these observations one would almost expect all episodes of thrombolysis to be followed by rethrombosis unless intense adjunctive anticoagulation was coadministered with the plasminogen activator.

Actually, in a sense, rethrombosis may be

the common early postlytic scenario. Angiographic and angioscopic observations of thrombus behavior, when influenced by plasminogen activators, demonstrate the process of lysis to be a stuttering one.[3] Open channels for antegrade arterial flow occur and close again in the early stages of lysis.

The thrombus proceeds from a dense and occlusive plug, through a "swiss-cheese"–like stage with transient full and partial perforations until in successful cases, the lytic forces seem to win out and increasing flow occurs (Fig. 17–1). Similar stuttering cycles of thrombosis to reperfusion to thrombosis have been carefully documented in animal models of coronary occlusion.

When the procoagulant forces predominate, there is either no demonstrable reperfusion or there is temporary patency followed by rethrombosis and reocclusion. The actual frequency of reocclusions in plasminogen activator-treated patients is not known precisely, and as will be shown, is in part a function of the anticoagulant regimen administered, as well as (perhaps, in part) a function of the thrombolytic drug selected and the dosing regimen employed.

Precise quantification of rethrombosis is virtually impossible in the clinical setting. One would need, for each and every treatment regimen of interest, to perform pretreatment angiography, since the reocclusion risk for spontaneously reperfused arteries is much different (that is, much lower than for those pharmacologically achieved). Pretreatment angiography is now generally deemed inappropriate due to the delay it imposes in starting effective therapy. Furthermore, to accurately measure reocclusion, patients would need to undergo numerous coronary angiograms per day, at least over the first few days. This would be necessitated because: (a) clinical suspicion of reocclusion is unreliable; (b) reinfarction is an inadequate surrogate since it is often unidentifiable in the earliest hours of the index myocardial infarction, or may be absent despite documented reocclusion; and (c) reocclusion need not be "permanent," that is, thrombolysis may be successful on the day of infarction; reocclusion might occur on day two or three but be followed by spontaneous reperfusion on day four. The notion that one pair of angiograms (the first at 90 minutes after the start of therapy, and the second seven days later) defines the entire issue, is scientifically naive (Figs. 17–2 and 17–3). No investigator is, therefore, likely to ever perform a perfect reocclusion study given these caveats. However, we do have general knowledge about the broad range of the phenomenon in clinical practice.

The earliest literature on this subject derives from the era of direct intracoronary infusion of streptokinase (Table 17–1). As can be appreciated, the range is enormous, from 0 per cent to nearly 50 per cent. More recent estimates of reocclusion with diverse intravenously administered activators, dosing schemes, and anticoagulant regimens place the approximate reocclusion incidence for the period from 90 minutes after treatment to about a week in the 10 to 15 per cent range with all thrombolytic agents. There has been a suspicion that the shorter acting and more fibrin-specific plasminogen activators,

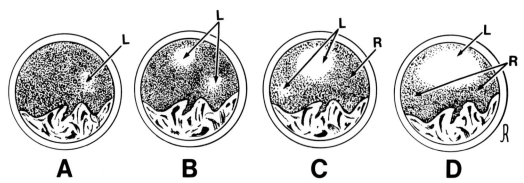

A   **B**   **C**   **D**

FIGURE 17–1. Schematic representation of the competing lytic and thrombotic forces acting upon a dissolving thrombus. Some areas of initial lysis (L) are closed again quickly by rethrombosis (R). In this example, lysis predominates overall, resulting in effective reperfusion. In the first postreperfusion hours and days, however, substantial clot persists with the attendant risk of further thrombin induced clotting. (Drawing by Jed Ross)

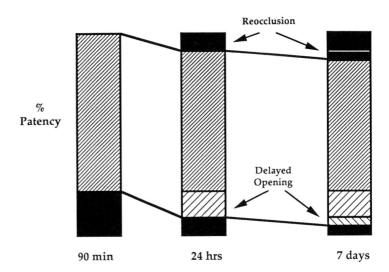

FIGURE 17–2. Reperfusion and reocclusion profile following alteplase-induced thrombolysis. Early (90-minute) patency is approximately 80 per cent. Subsequently, some open arteries reocclude, while others, initially occluded, show late patency. Angiography at any single point in time incompletely characterizes the dynamic events. Solid black portions of bars represent the percentage with a totally occluded artery at each point in time.

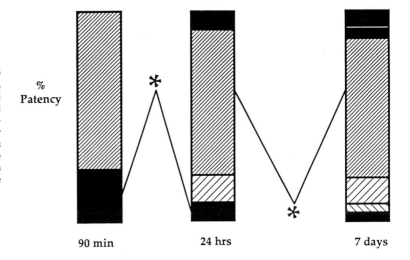

FIGURE 17–3. Even multiple angiograms in a single patient, that is, 90 minutes, 24 hours, and a week after lytic therapy would fail to identify vessels that underwent transient reperfusion or reocclusion between the studies (indicated by asterisks). Yet the clinical outcome in such patients might be influenced by these transient events.

TABLE 17–1. The Range of Angiographically Proven Reocclusion After Reperfusion with Intracoronary Streptokinase. Reocclusion in the TIMI-1 Trial with Intravenous Alteplase or Streptokinase are Included as a Reference

STUDY	DRUG/ROUTE	REOCCLUSION	%
Merx[4]	Streptokinase/intracoronary	29/88	33
Serruys[5]	Streptokinase/intracoronary	7/41	17
Urban[6]	Streptokinase/intracoronary	9/59	15
Ferguson[7]	Streptokinase/intracoronary	7/34	21
Anderson[8]	Streptokinase/intracoronary	0/16	0
Leiboff[9]	Streptokinase/intracoronary	5/11	45
		57/249	23
TIMI-1[10]	Streptokinase/Intravenous	4/29	14
TIMI-1[10]	Alteplase/Intravenous	15/62	24

particularly if used without intense antico-agulation (as will be detailed later), may be associated with more reocclusion than seen with nonspecific or "systemic" lytic agents.

New information on the timing of reocclu-sion and its clinical impact is particularly relevant and revealing. Ohman et al.,[11] by compiling the angiographic and clinical re-sults from the highly instructive series of Thrombosis in Acute Myocardial Infarction (TAMI) trials reported on the follow-up of 810 acute myocardial infarction patients with coronary angiography 90 minutes after the start of thrombolytic therapy. A very respect-able 88 per cent of these patients had one or more follow-up angiograms.

The overall reocclusion rate was 12 per cent; importantly, only half of these events were clinically recognizable. The highest fre-quency of acute reclosure occurred within 12 hours of reperfusion, and 50 per cent of all identified reocclusions were within the first 24 hours. After the first post-treatment day, the rate of this untoward event declined substantially to about 1 per cent per day for the remainder of the first week.

Perhaps the most important observation made in this report was the impact of reclo-sure on mortality during the hospital course. Persistent patency was associated with a 4.5 per cent mortality rate, whereas reocclusion led to an 11 per cent fatality rate. The message appears to be that reclosure occurs early (consistent with the pathophysiologic notion that early after the start of lysis the stimulus for rethrombosis is greatest) and with a severe clinical outcome penalty. Thus the heightened interest in post-thrombolysis antithrombotic therapy.

ANTITHROMBOTIC APPROACHES TO PREVENT REOCCLUSION

Role of Aspirin

The antithrombotic agents, those presently available and newer agents under develop-ment, have been discussed in Chapters 5 and 6. Substantial angiographically based throm-bolytic clinical trial experience with such agents exists for heparin only.

There is also an extensive literature on the use of aspirin, given for its antiplatelet effects, as primary or secondary prevention of ath-erosclerotic sequelae. Used in the acute set-ting, however, information has been mostly limited to studies of unstable angina and in the case of acute myocardial infarction; solely, the important Second International Study of Infarct Survival (ISIS-2) study.[12]

The precise relevance of unstable angina studies extrapolated to suggest the impact of an agent like aspirin in the acute infarction patient is speculative at best. Nonetheless, important parallels exist in the two condi-tions; chiefly, the presence of an unstable atherosclerotic plaque, and usually some components of intracoronary thrombus.[13]

These features of unstable angina have led to trials of antiplatelet, anticoagulant, and combination therapies in the condition. Two large trials of aspirin showed benefit in re-duction of death and myocardial infarc-tion.[14,15] Subsequent investigations have compared aspirin, heparin, and a combina-tion of both.

In a report by Theroux et al.[16] utilizing combined endpoints of refractory angina, myocardial infarction, and death over a six-day period, continuous intravenous heparin produced the lowest event rate (9.3 per cent). Heparin plus daily oral aspirin led to an 11.5 per cent rate, and oral aspirin alone led to a 16.5 per cent rate. Endpoints occurred in 26 per cent of patients receiving placebo only.

A heparin-to-aspirin comparison was also performed by Neri Serneri et al.[17] comparing the effects of intravenous heparin or oral aspirin on recurrent ischemia. In this trial, heparin was highly effective, whereas aspirin was not. Thus, the older literature (on un-stable angina) would seem to indicate that if used as monotherapy, the antithrombin ef-fect of heparin produced superior clinical outcome than the antiplatelet effect of aspi-rin. It was the ISIS-2 trial, however, that produced the most impressive results with the use of 160 milligrams of oral aspirin daily, in acute ischemia/infarction patients.[12] Details of this prestigious study have been widely disseminated. Certain features, how-ever, deserve remention here in an effort to fully dissect the impact of aspirin, alone or in conjunction with streptokinase, on five-week mortality. Unlike most other large in-farct studies in the current era, ISIS-2 pur-posely widened entry criteria by accepting patients late after pain onset (up to 24 hours), and even those without electrocardiographic criteria specific for acute infarction.

By so doing, the investigators were able to shed light on some continuously perplexing issues regarding patient selection. The cost of this strategy, however, is a cohort less well defined and to some degree (presumably) diluted by individuals with syndromes other than acute myocardial infarction (including unstable angina).

The information derived (and still forthcoming) from ISIS-2 has been tremendously enlightening, but of all its results, the mortality reduction of more than 20 per cent afforded by aspirin alone was in many ways the most dramatic. One hundred sixty milligrams of aspirin reduced mortality as much as full-dose streptokinase given alone, and the two active agents were additive, reducing death rate to 8 per cent (from 13.2 per cent for double placebo).

A still unanswered challenge is to understand the mechanisms by which aspirin exerted so powerful an effect. The causes of death after myocardial infarction are only a few: major pump failure, cardiac rupture, stroke, and arrhythmia. What effects of aspirin impacted which of these mechanisms? Aspirin's suppression of platelet aggregation is its principally recognized cardiovascular effect, but this aspect presumably comes into play primarily by preventing reocclusion-reinfarction after initial coronary artery reperfusion. This seems to be confirmed in ISIS-2, as the highest rate of reinfarction seen was in the active streptokinase no-aspirin group.

The statistics, however, would not support this antireocclusion mechanism as fully explanatory of the aspirin (used alone) mortality reduction, particularly since in the group receiving no active streptokinase, early reperfusion can be assumed to have been infrequent. Reocclusion cannot be directly interrogated in this nonangiographic trial, but the ISIS-2 study does contain specific reinfarction data. The reinfarction rate reported for the double-placebo group was low, 3 per cent (in the very large trials like ISIS-2 with abbreviated case report forms and no requirement for continuous enzyme sampling, reported reinfarction rates tend to be half of that as reported from more closely controlled studies). Aspirin reduced reported reinfarction by 1.2 patients per 100 treated. Were reinfarction universally fatal (which it is not), the mechanism for aspirin's favorable mortality effect as monotherapy would still remain elusive. Small reductions for aspirin-treated patients in the other potentially fatal events recorded in the study (cardiac rupture, arrhythmia, and stroke) do not account for

the "gap." In any event, with or without a full explanation, the excellent empirically observed results with aspirin in ISIS-2 raised questions about the need for systemic heparin in conjunction with plasminogen activators: might oral aspirin be an adequate and less toxic surrogate? Indirectly, this possibility was seminal in stimulating some of the heparin trials discussed below. (See also Chapters 14 and 16.)

HEPARIN

The antithrombin effects of heparin have been utilized for decades in acute myocardial infarction, but formerly as much for demonstrated benefits in reducing late complications (deep vein thrombosis, left ventricular mural thrombosis formation, and pulmonary embolism) as for its potential adjunctive role in treating the proximate cause of the myocardial infarction, thrombotic coronary occlusion.

Over the past decade, however, in the era of reperfusion, heparin has been extensively used and debated for its role in promoting thrombolysis initiated with a plasminogen activator, and for its utility in preventing postlytic recurrent coronary thrombosis. The majority of large-scale thrombolytic trials (ISAM,[18] AIMS,[19] the TAMI,[20] and European Cooperative Study Group [ECSG] trials[21]) all began with the empiric use of systemic heparinization carried forward from earlier experiences demonstrating the need for an effective strategy to prevent reocclusion after direct intracoronary lytic agent reperfusion. Notable exceptions to incorporation of intravenous heparin into recent clinical trials are the important most recent studies performed by the ISIS and GISSI collaborators, (GISSI-2[22] and ISIS-3[23]) which will be discussed later. (See also Chapters 14 and 16.)

HEPARIN-THROMBOLYTIC "SYNERGISM"

There has been an incompletely resolved uncertainty regarding the possible synergistic combination of plasminogen activators and heparin. In an animal arterial thrombus model, Cercek et al.[24] demonstrated very significantly enhanced reduction in thrombus weight 15 minutes after alteplase and heparin treatment, compared with alteplase alone. They made similar observations utilizing streptokinase or urokinase as the activator.[25] Their interpretation of this data, however, is that the usual competing processes of clot lysis and new clot formation is influenced in favor of the lytic process by the presence of an antithrombin drug. From a semantic point of view, this would not be considered true "synergism."

In the only clinical study of this issue, Topol et al.[26] randomized alteplase-treated infarct patients to immediate or 90-minute delayed intravenous heparin. At the 90-minute angiogram, both groups showed an infarct-related coronary artery patency rate of 79 per cent. A smaller cohort within this study had their initial angiogram in the 30- to 75-minute postinfusion onset time window. Their patency with immediate intravenous heparin was 88 per cent; when heparin was delayed, 81 per cent (Califf R., personal communication). This small number of patients cannot lead to a firm conclusion regarding heparin's role in promoting lysis, though some impact is possible.

HEPARIN TO PREVENT RETHROMBOSIS

As mentioned previously, heparin had been utilized empirically and extensively in clinical practice to prevent reocclusion, but the outstanding benefit seen with aspirin in ISIS-2 raised questions about the possible substitution of aspirin for heparin, possibly with a savings in hemorrhagic complications. There had also been conflicting data on the efficiency of heparin to sufficiently inhibit rethrombosis. Johns et al.[27] reported a small randomized trial (52 patients) of postlytic strategies. After a 90-minute alteplase infusion, patients received either continuous intravenous heparin alone or four hours of additional intravenous alteplase at a dosage of 0.8 milligrams/kilogram, plus heparin. Acute reocclusion occurred in 19 per cent of those in the heparin-only arm, and in none of those given additional alteplase. Additionally, a broad range of measures including rate of thrombus dissolution and late recurrent ischemic events all favored the group receiving prolonged lytic infusion. The strong inference was that intravenous heparin was inadequate to prevent rethrombosis, and was certainly inferior to prolonged acti-

vator infusion. In dramatic contrast to the report from Johns was that of Verstraete et al. (ECSG-3).[28] Utilizing a similar trial design, 81 infarct patients with alteplase-induced infarct artery patency 90 minutes after the start of treatment were managed on continuous intravenous heparin alone (plus an alteplase placebo), or heparin plus an additional 30 milligrams of alteplase over a subsequent six-hour period.

Angiography 6 to 24 hours later revealed very low reocclusion frequency; 6 per cent for heparin alone, 5 per cent for heparin plus prolonged alteplase. There was a suggestion of faster residual clot dissolution with prolonged alteplase use, but the investigators reached just the opposite of the opinion of Johns and concluded that when utilizing intravenous heparin, additional prolonged plasminogen activator infusion was not necessary to inhibit rethrombosis.

RECENT ALTEPLASE-HEPARIN TRIALS

The similarities and differences of the studies herein described is displayed in Figure 17–4. The Heparin-Aspirin-Reperfusion Trial (HART),[29] was designed to further study the interaction of antiplatelet or anticoagulant drugs with alteplase. The hypothesis was that oral aspirin would inhibit reocclusion as effectively as intravenous heparin. Two hundred five acute infarction patients received a 100-milligram infusion of alteplase and were randomized to concomitant oral aspirin (80 milligrams chewed and swallowed, plus 80 milligrams/day for a week), or to immediate and continuous intravenous heparin (5,000-unit bolus, then 1,000 units/hour to maintain partial thromboplastin time 1.5 to 2 times control). The primary endpoint was angiographic patency at 7 to 24 hours and was actually performed at a mean of 18 hours post-treatment (Fig. 17–5).

This time period was selected to encompass the period of highest reocclusion risk. In fact, HART was not strictly a reocclusion study, since no pretreatment angiogram was required. Rather, it was assumed, based upon previous studies, that the patient selection and alteplase infusion regimen (identical to that used in TIMI-2)[30] would produce 90-minute patency approximately 80 per cent (documented in TIMI-2, TAMI). At a mean of 18 hours after treatment onset, patency

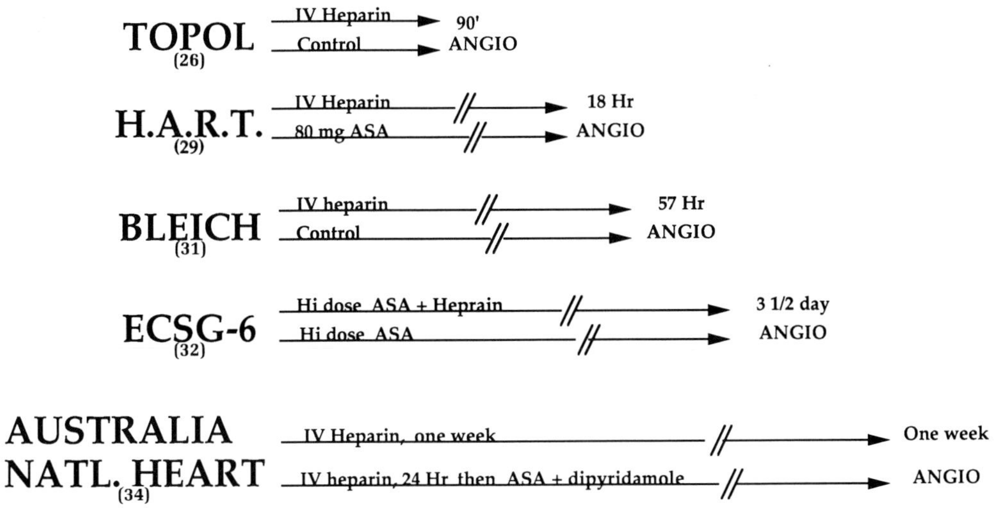

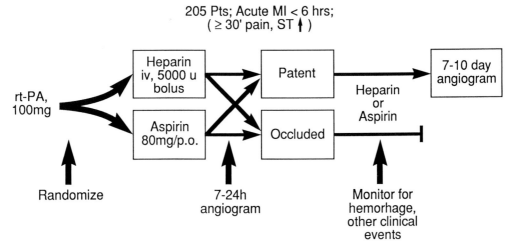

$$
\begin{aligned}
&\text{TOPOL}_{(26)} &&\underset{\text{Control}}{\overset{\text{IV Heparin}}{\longrightarrow}} &&\overset{90'}{\longrightarrow}\text{ANGIO}
\end{aligned}
$$

TOPOL (26)
  IV Heparin → 90'
  Control → ANGIO

H.A.R.T. (29)
  IV Heparin —//— 18 Hr
  80 mg ASA —//— ANGIO

BLEICH (31)
  IV heparin —//— 57 Hr
  Control —//— ANGIO

ECSG-6 (32)
  Hi dose ASA + Heprain —//— 3 1/2 day
  Hi dose ASA —//— ANGIO

AUSTRALIA NATL. HEART (34)
  IV Heparin, one week —//— One week
  IV heparin, 24 Hr then ASA + dipyridamole —//— ANGIO

FIGURE 17–4. Differences in protocol design of five clinical trials which examined the alteplase/heparin interaction. Arrow length represents time to patency-determining angiogram. See text for details.

for alteplase plus heparin was 82 per cent. Somewhat surprising, and in contrast, there was only a 52 per cent patency seen in the group receiving alteplase and oral aspirin in place of heparin. This difference was highly significant ($p < 0.0001$).

There has since been much question and some criticism of the study for having selected the TIMI[30] dose of aspirin (that is, 80 milligrams) as the alternative to heparin. The TIMI investigators had chosen this dose since it had been shown more than sufficient to interdict platelet cyclooxygenase activity and hence platelet aggregation. But the possibility that a higher initial dose of aspirin might accomplish this goal in a shorter time period

has not been fully evaluated. The ISIS-2 dose of aspirin, it is to be recalled, was 160 milligrams. The potential for an additional "baby" aspirin to have substantially altered the outcome in the HART study remains speculative.

Other predeclared endpoints in this study showed little difference comparing the two adjunctive strategies. "Late" reocclusion was determined comparing patency at a five- to seven-day angiogram in patients whose arteries were open on the first study.

For the heparin and aspirin groups, sustained patency was documented in 88 and 95 per cent, respectively (p = not significant). No different in bleeding was observed (low in both groups, 1.7 per cent heparin, 3.0 per

FIGURE 17–5. The protocol design of the Heparin Aspirin Reperfusion Trial (HART).

cent aspirin). In the heparin group there were two deaths and one instance of intracerebral bleeding.

A similar though smaller study, with similar results, was done by Bleich et al.[31] In this trial of 84 acute myocardial infarction patients, randomization was to alteplase plus intravenous heparin versus alteplase with no adjunctive therapy. Aspirin was not used in either treatment group. The patency determining coronary angiogram was performed a mean 57 hours after treatment had begun. Similar to the HART trial results, there was a nearly 30 per cent patency advantage for the group treated with concomitant intravenous heparin compared with those not immediately anticoagulated (71 per cent versus 43 per cent, $p < 0.02$). It should be appreciated that no aspirin was given to the "controls."

The most recent and largest investigation of the need for early intravenous heparin in alteplase-treated infarct patients was the sixth from the European Cooperative Study Group (ECSG-6).[32] Six hundred eighty-seven patients were included in this double-blind, randomized multicenter trial with two distinctive features: whereas only one treatment arm was randomized to early intravenous heparin (the other arm receiving a placebo infusion), both groups got early high-dose aspirin; also, the patency-determining angiogram was relatively late, three to five days after the infarct. A statistically significant patency advantage of 8 per cent for the heparin group was observed (83 per cent versus 75 per cent), $p < 0.01$).

In this ECSG study, whereas the patency rate for intravenous heparin-treated patients is in line with previously cited studies, the 75 per cent patency for the no-heparin group is somewhat high. There are at least two possible explanations—the time of angiography and the aspirin regimen.

Regarding angiography time, it has been well appreciated that the majority of infarct coronary arteries are recanalized eventually, whether or not a thrombolytic drug is given. At about a week after a myocardial infarction, 50 to 70 per cent of infarct-related arteries are patent (although most presumably became open too late to result in appreciable myocardial salvage). Hence, a dilemma for investigators: study a reperfusion strategy quite early and risk "missing" the peak frequency of reocclusion; or do the angiogram relatively late and risk diluting the effect of

the treatment strategy by some late recanalization events that may be unrelated to the treatment under investigation. In the ECSG-6 the angiogram was performed quite late in the hospital course.

The high-dose aspirin regimen in ECSG-6 represents the other possible explanation for higher patency seen in the no-heparin arm of this trial, compared with those previously cited, and is another argument for using a dose greater than 80 milligrams in the infarct setting. The initial dose of aspirin was either 250 milligrams intravenously or 300 milligrams orally. The degree to which these factors contributed to the ECSG-6 outcome is presently unknowable.

Further data analysis of the ECSG-6 patient cohort uncovered strong additional evidence to link heparin anticoagulation and preserved postalteplase patency (Verstraete M., personal communication). In 159 patients, partial thromboplastin time levels during the study period were available and could be divided into those with persistent prolongation and those whose heparin dosing proved subtherapeutic (the heparin instructions in this study were to begin with an intravenous bolus of 5,000 units and then maintain a 1,000 units/hour infusion rate; although partial thromboplastin times were often obtained and recorded, heparin dose was not adjusted on the basis of the laboratory value).

For the cohort with therapeutic range anticoagulation, the three- to five-day patency was 93 per cent; with partial thromboplastin times below the usual target range, patency was significantly less frequent, only 77 per cent. The outcome of these alteplase-heparin trials displayed in juxtaposition is shown in Figure 17–6.

The need-for-intravenous-heparin issue has also recently been examined in patients receiving the plasminogen activator saruplase (or single chain urokinase plasminogen activator [SCUPA], or pro-urokinase). This agent has many similarities to alteplase including human protein origin, fibrin specificity, short half-life, and very rapid induction of coronary thrombus lysis. Tebbe et al.[33] performed a randomized trial in 118 infarct patients given saruplase with and without early intravenous heparin. The time from treatment onset to patency-determining angiogram was 6 to 12 hours. Eighty-one per cent of those receiving intravenous heparin had a patent infarct-related artery, compared with only 60 per cent in those in whom heparin was omit-

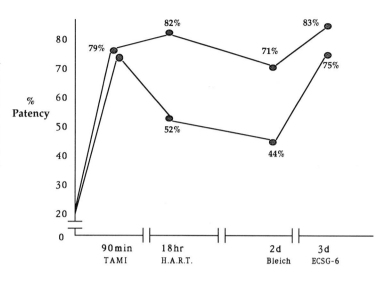

FIGURE 17–6. The magnitude of heparin-induced patency advantage after alteplase treatment shown to be (in part) a function of the time frame in which coronary angiography is performed. The upper curve represents patients treated with early intravenous heparin; the lower, heparin omitted: for details see text.

ted ($p < 0.02$), recapitulating the previously described alteplase trials.

The apparent conclusion from these multiple confirmatory studies is that the short-acting, relatively fibrin-specific human origin plasminogen activators (alteplase, saruplase) should be administered with adjunctive ("conjunctive"?) early and adequately dosed (intravenous) heparin anticoagulation sufficient to achieve and sustain therapeutic prolongations of the partial thromboplastin time.

DURATION OF HEPARIN ANTICOAGULATION

The desirable duration of heparin therapy after thrombolysis is yet another issue incompletely characterized. To study this question, the Australian National Heart Foundation trial[34] treated 202 patients with alteplase and 24 hours of intravenous heparin. Subsequently, patients were randomized to an additional six days of intravenous heparin or oral aspirin and dipyridamole instead. Angiography to quantitate sustained patency was done at the end of a week and demonstrated the same rate (80 per cent) for both groups.

This apparently most critical period of the first 24 hours during which intravenous heparin may have its major impact is compatible with previously cited evidence that later in the recovery phase the risk of reocclusion diminishes markedly. Confirmatory studies would, however, be desirable before hepar-

inization for as brief a period as only one day could be comfortably endorsed.

SUBCUTANEOUS HEPARIN

This route of administration has the advantage of simplicity and has been used in a variety of settings, particularly as prophylaxis for such events as deep vein thrombosis, pulmonary embolism, and left ventricular mural thrombosis following infarction. In the study of subcutaneous heparin efficacy for these indications, much has been learned about the pharmacodynamics of this route of administration. Heparin is given to increase the affinity of antithrombin III for thrombin which occurs when the heparin-antithrombin III complex is formed. Other nonspecific binding sites for heparin exist, however, and compete with antithrombin III for the heparin. Chiefly, these competitive binding sites are on vascular endothelial cells, and heparin molecules trapped in this fashion are cleared rapidly with no anticoagulant effect. The endothelial sites become free again to combine with new heparin molecules. While this clearance route is easily saturated by bolus intravenous heparin injections or high-dose constant intravenous infusions (leaving most of the heparin available to effect its anticoagulant properties), the slow release following subcutaneous administration has quite a different profile. Turpie et al.[35] have shown that following a 5,000-unit subcutaneous regimen of heparin every 12 hours, no effective anticoagulation occurs, presumably due to the fact that most or all of the agent is cleared by the mechanism cited above. With very–high-dose subcutaneous heparin, clearance binding sites can eventually be saturated, leading to the desired antithrombin effect, but quite variably so among patients, and only after a considerable time delay. Hull et al.[36] found that a majority of patients managed with subcutaneous heparin do not achieve therapeutic levels of anticoagulation.

Another problem associated with subcutaneous heparin observed by Turpie, is the substantial delay from the beginning of the treatment to the achievement of significant partial thromboplastin time prolongations. As opposed to intravenous heparin, which rapidly anticoagulates, high-dose subcutaneous heparin usually takes hours—up to one and a half days—to achieve the desired effect.

SUBCUTANEOUS HEPARIN AND ALTEPLASE

Despite the previous discussion regarding the timing of reocclusion, its apparent partial prevention by the use of early intravenous heparin, and the marginal pharmacodynamics of subcutaneous heparin for this purpose, the possible substitution of delayed subcutaneous heparin in conjunction with alteplase was investigated in the GISSI-2/International alteplase-Streptokinase Study (Table 17–2).[22,37] No clinical benefit, specifically, no reduction in deaths or reinfarctions, was achieved by adding delayed (12 hours after alteplase) subcutaneous heparin at a dose of 12,500 units every 12 hours. In contrast, for patients in this trial given streptokinase, additional late subcutaneous heparin seemed to be of benefit as will be detailed below.

DIFFERING ANTICOAGULANT NEEDS WITH DIFFERENT PLASMINOGEN ACTIVATORS?

The chief difference between agents like alteplase and agents like streptokinase or anistreplase are the origin of the protein (that is, human versus bacterial), and the relative binding specificity of the molecule or complex. In clinical medicine, the differences are that following alteplase administration, plasmin formation and proteolysis occurs mainly at the site of fibrin or thrombus, whereas the circulating streptokinase-plasmin activator molecule is a more indiscriminate proteolytic catalyst. The differences in measurable laboratory perturbation are considerable, particularly the effects on two key coagulation parameters: fibrinogen levels and fibrin (and fibrinogen) degradation product (FDPs). With exceptions, fibrinogen depletion associated with alteplase administration is modest, and fibrinogen degradation product release is minor.

Since these effects act concordantly (that is, low fibrinogen and high fibrinogen degradation products diminish the likelihood of new clot formation), alteplase-treated patients exhibit minimal inhibition of rethrombosis risk. In contrast, typical intravenous streptokinase does effect profound reduction in fibrinogen levels and marked elevations of fibrinogen degradation product levels. Moreover, the effects of clinical doses of alteplase are short lived, whereas those following streptokinase or anistreplase use are prolonged.[38,39] Despite a two- to fivefold increase in the derangement of coagulation factors and the duration of these changes, it is evident that streptokinase administration by no means provides sufficient protection against recurrent thrombosis when given as monotherapy (Table 17–1). One might theorize, however, that the temporal urgency and required magnitude of poststreptokinase anticoagulation to prevent reinfarction might be less than following alteplase, but the theory has not been adequately tested.

HEPARIN AND SYSTEMIC PLASMINOGEN ACTIVATORS

In comparison to the extensively studied issue of patency and reocclusion with the relatively fibrin-specific plasminogen activators given with or without intravenous heparin, such information is not available for agents like streptokinase or anistreplase. This, despite the fact that empiric use of early concomitant high-dose intravenous heparin originated in that era a decade or so ago, when direct intracoronary infusion of streptokinase was en vogue as a reperfusion strategy. Reocclusion was recognized to be a frequent phenomenon and anticoagulation assumed to be a necessity.

In an early report from the intravenous streptokinase literature, Kaplan et al.[40] recognized a strong correlation between heparin (and the degree of partial thromboplastin time prolongation it induced) and the likelihood of recurrent (postlytic) episodes of ischemia. In their report, early recurrent events were two to four times more likely in the face of subtherapeutic partial thromboplastin time levels, and were particularly common shortly after heparin was also continued. In the absence of specific angiographically based heparin-streptokinase reocclusion studies, inferences may be made from trials in which heparin's impact on reinfarction or mortality has been compiled.

In the SCATI study (Studio sulla Calciparina nell' Angina E Nella Trombosi Ventricolare nell infarto),[41] 711 infarct patients were randomly assigned to a heparin or no-heparin group, along with streptokinase if within six hours of symptom onset, without streptokinase if later into the infarction. Heparin was administered as an intravenous bolus of 2,000 units followed nine hours later by the first of 12-hourly doses of 12,500 units given subcutaneously until hospital discharge or beyond.

Impact of heparin in the late-treated group (which did not receive lytic therapy) on the major endpoints of recurrent ischemia, recurrent infarction, and death, was minimal. In the early group (less than six hours), however, heparin substantially improved the outcome following streptokinase treatment, particularly in the hospital fatality rate (4.5 per cent with heparin, 8.8 per cent without, $p < 0.05$). The reduction in recurrent ischemia (28 per cent less frequent) and reinfarction (15 per cent fewer) did not reach a statistically significant level in this sample size.

The ISIS-2 study has been previously described in some detail. Although the primary factorial randomization concerned streptokinase and oral aspirin, the reporting form did request information regarding plans for use of heparin, which was left to the individual clinician's discretion. With caution, analysis of outcome (mortality) can be performed on the basis of heparin-related subgroups. For patients receiving intravenous heparin, the mortality rate was lowest, 6.7 per cent at five weeks postmyocardial infarction. Patients in the subcutaneous heparin group had an intermediate mortality rate of 7.4 per cent (not statistically different from the intravenous group) and patients in whom there were no plans to administer heparin had the highest mortality rate (8.5 per cent, $p < 0.01$) compared with both heparin subgroups.

The GISSI-2/International Study more directly interrogated the heparin issue. Primary randomization was to streptokinase or alteplase in this investigation, but a second randomization assigned patients to either no heparin (only oral aspirin) or subcutaneous heparin plus aspirin. The heparin group had the drug's administration delayed for 12 hours after the plasminogen activator was given, a strategy selected partly on the basis of a desire to minimize bleeding complications that might be augmented by heparinizing patients still in a "lytic state." For patients assigned to late heparin treatment, the drug was given as 12,500 unit subcutaneous injections twice daily. Results from the entire patient cohort show no mortality benefit for alteplase-treated patients derived from adjunctive subcutaneous heparin versus none (9.2 per cent versus 8.7 per cent, $p =$ not significant). In streptokinase-treated patients, however, mortality was lower with heparin (7.9 per cent) compared with the no-heparin group (9.2 per cent).

In view of the fact that heparin treatment was delayed for 12 hours, and that, as discussed, the onset of action following this route of administration is further delayed, it was of interest to inspect the mortality impact amongst patients who survived the first 12 hours in order to be eligible for anticoagulation. Among 10,074 such patients who had received streptokinase, adjunctive heparin led to a 5.0 per cent mortality rate compared to 6.2 per cent if given no heparin ($p < 0.01$).

A similar subgroup analysis for survivors (at least to 12 hours) amongst alteplase recipients shows no such late subcutaneous heparin benefit, and a 5.9 per cent subsequent mortality rate was seen with or without the anticoagulant (subgroup analysis presented but not yet published from the large ISIS-3 trial also showed a trend toward lower mortality rate for streptokinase patients who additionally received delayed subcutaneous heparin, further discussed below).

It might be surmised from these agent-specific differences in late heparin's impact on mortality rate that the longer and more profound disturbance of coagulation factors following streptokinase use does in fact reduce the requirements, in time and magnitude, for achieving heparinization compared with the need following alteplase for prevention of reocclusion and its negative clinical sequelae. Also, it could be argued that an earlier and more effective heparin regimen in the streptokinase- and alteplase-treated patients in the trial might have led to even better outcome as observed in the aforementioned SCATI study. The arbiter of this issue, a large trial in which streptokinase plus early intravenous heparin is compared with streptokinase and delayed subcutaneous heparin, has not yet been performed.

THE RISKS OF ANTIPLATELET/ ANTICOAGULANT ADJUNCTS TO THROMBOLYTIC THERAPY

Thrombolytic agents, anticoagulants, and antiplatelet agents (in descending order) share hemorrhagic complications as their major risks. Predictably, combinations of these classes of drugs will augment such risks. Hence, it is important to determine that the net benefit of the various strategies outweighs the adverse effects.

The multiple combinations and permutations resultant from differing plasminogen activators (and doses), differing heparin regimens, and even differing aspirin doses presents a formidable array for attempted analysis of risks. Additionally, definitions and reporting requirements have not been uniform in published studies. Finally, protocols requiring angiography and attendant vascular punctures in patients at risk cannot be directly compared with trials not involving vessel trauma. Nonetheless, some tabulation of drug-related hemorrhagic complications is available for inspection.

The specific augmented risk of an immediate dose of 160 milligrams of aspirin at the time of streptokinase infusion (and continued daily thereafter) can be partially deduced from tabular data in the ISIS-2 report by subtracting the event rates for the combination arm (streptokinase plus aspirin) from those in the column for streptokinase (with or without aspirin).

Such an exercise indicates an aspirin-related increase in major bleeding (requiring transfusion) of approximately 4 patients per 1,000. There were five confirmed cases of intracerebral bleeding in the four thousand patient combination group and two in the equal-sized streptokinase/no aspirin cohort: but total cerebral vascular accidents (intracerebral bleeding plus thromboembolic stroke) were lower by 3 events per 1,000 with the use of aspirin. Hence, this salicylate dose cannot be considered an important source of

risk when combined with the plasminogen activator.

A larger body of information exists regarding the excess bleeding risks associated with the use of heparin. The combination of streptokinase or alteplase with heparin has been studied in large and small trials, with the anticoagulant given intravenously, subcutaneously, or both. In the SCATI study,[41] with myocardial infarction patients randomized to a heparin or control group, serious bleeding was seen almost exclusively in patients who received streptokinase and the early intravenous plus delayed subcutaneous heparin. The frequency of retroperitoneal and intracerebral bleeds amongst 360 heparinized patients was one patient each; gastrointestinal bleeding was observed in two, cutaneous hematoma in three, and other "minor" bleeds in nine patients. Thus, the overall bleeding rate was 16/360 or 4.4 per cent; however, it should be noted that 142 of these 360 did not receive streptokinase, hence the real denominator is lower and the bleeding rate, therefore, somewhat higher. In nonheparinized patients, the total bleeding rate was two patients (0.6 per cent), both gastrointestinal in origin.

In the HART trial,[29] there were 14/106 patients who had bleeding episodes in the alteplase plus heparin intravenous treated cohort, and 10/99 in the alteplase plus aspirin group. There was only one episode of intracerebral bleeding in the trial (a no-heparin patient), suggesting a very modest hemorrhagic risk.

In contrast, a higher frequency was cited in the study by Bleich et al.[31] which listed hemorrhagic complications by category; "minor," "major," and "severe." The rates amongst those receiving intravenous heparin with alteplase were 52 per cent, 10 per cent, and 2 per cent, respectively, whereas those randomized to no heparin suffered minor bleeds in 36 per cent and major events in 2 per cent.

The two recent largest trials, GISSI-2[22] and ISIS-3,[23] provide the most information on the subject, despite rather brief reporting requirements. These studies, however, only shed light on the adverse effects of the delayed subcutaneous use of heparin.

The GISSI trial was reported separately for the Italian component and the international extension, both delaying by 12 hours the use of heparin (12,500 subcutaneous twice daily). The Italian report does not

TABLE 17–2. Incidence of Strokes by Type, Major Hemorrhage, and Pulmonary or Systemic Embolism in the GISSI-2 Trial

Event	Heparin (%)	No Heparin (%)
Any cerebrovascular accident	1.0	1.0
Intracranial bleeding	0.3	0.3
Ischemic	0.4	0.4
Undefined	0.3	0.3
Major bleeds	1.0	0.6
All thromboembolism	0.5	0.9

separate heparin and no-heparin patients according to their assigned plasminogen activator. There were no differences, based upon the heparin/no-heparin randomization in hemorrhagic nor total strokes. Major hemorrhage was 1 per cent with heparin, 0.6 per cent without, while minor bleeds were seen in 9.6 per cent and 5.3 per cent, respectively.

The report from the international collaborators[42] gives complications for the entire combined cohort of nearly 21,000 patients, stratified by activator. Concerning strokes, hemorrhagic or otherwise, the four subgroups (streptokinase with and without heparin and alteplase with or without heparin) were all clustered within a narrow range with variation never exceeding 3 events per 1,000. Other major bleeding was 0.8 per cent for alteplase with heparin, 0.5 per cent without; for streptokinase it was 1.2 per cent with heparin and 0.6 per cent without.

The most controversy over the adverse effects of heparin added to a plasminogen activator was generated at the March 1991, American College of Cardiology Annual Scientific Sessions where the preliminary results of ISIS-3 were presented.[23] This study of more than 40,000 patients contained six major subgroups: treatment with streptokinase, anistreplase, or duteplase (a tissue type plasminogen activator) each with and without subcutaneous heparin delayed four hours from the start of lytic therapy and given as 12,500 units twice daily. The precise numbers cannot be considered final at this time, but major bleeding requiring transfusion was increased from 0.8 per cent to 1.1 per cent by the addition of heparin, and "probable" cerebral bleeding increased from 0.4 per cent to 0.6 per cent.

Acting in the other direction, heparin decreased recurrent infarction from 3.6 per cent to 3.3 per cent and decreased all-cause in-hospital mortality from 7.5 per cent to 7.0 per cent ($p < 0.03$). Hence, on balance, the largest studies, which used delayed subcutaneous heparin, appear to show a small favorable net effect for anticoagulation.

Overall, one can deduce that aggressive thrombolytic plus heparin strategies used in protocols requiring arterial puncture increase minor bleeding substantially but that major bleeding is augmented on the order of 1 or 2 per cent. Delayed subcutaneous heparin does produce fewer such episodes. Perhaps most importantly, the most severe bleeding complication (that is, intracerebral bleeds) seems augmented by heparin use only by a magnitude of 1 to 3 patients per 1,000 and is fully offset by an overall mortality reduction of equal or greater magnitude.

CONCLUSIONS

The expected clinical course after thrombolytic therapy for acute myocardial infarction is influenced by a variety of recognized factors including patient age, gender, infarct location, and time from symptom onset; but failure to achieve patency or recurrence of thrombotic occlusion figure prominently amongst (negative) outcome predictors. The local prothrombotic factors within the culprit artery are not substantially impacted by the plasminogen activators themselves, hence adjunctive or conjunctive pharmacological measures assume major importance. Early suppression of platelet function can be in part achieved by aspirin and with minimal augmented hemorrhagic risk, and hence should be routinely employed at a starting dose of at least 160 milligrams. This agent probably should be continued indefinitely in the postmyocardial infarction patients.

Heparin appears to exert a more powerful salutary effect, certainly on the angiographic endpoint of reocclusion, and particularly when given intravenously in concert with relatively fibrin-specific plasminogen activators. More controversial is the suitability of subcutaneous heparin as an alternative to the intravenous route and particularly if the start of such therapy is delayed resulting in the absence of measurable anticoagulation during the first 12 to 24 hours of the infarction when reocclusion risk is highest. Adverse

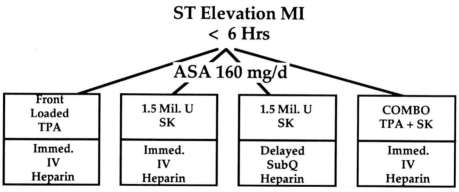

FIGURE 17–7. The treatment strategies are under investigation in the ongoing GUSTO trial.

(hemorrhagic) complications ascribable to heparin are modest and appear to be outweighed by clinical benefit. Evidence exists to support controlling heparin dose by partial thromboplastin time measured to achieve full anticoagulation. Some data also exists to suggest that this need substantially decreases after the first post-treatment day.

The possibility that the non–fibrin-specific activators (that is, streptokinase) exhibit a lessened requirement for aggressive anticoagulation has been hypothesized but not proven. This question, amongst others, is a subject of the latest and ongoing "mega" clinical trial in reperfusion therapy, the "GUSTO" study (Global Utilization of Streptokinase and TPA for Coronary Occlusion). In two of the four randomly assigned treatment areas of this protocol (Fig. 17–7) infarct patients will receive streptokinase; one arm with immediate and continued intravenous heparin, the other with delayed subcutaneous heparin as in the ISIS-3 protocol (also, all patients will receive aspirin).

The underlying hypothesis to be tested in GUSTO would be: "regimens that promote earlier and sustained infarct artery patency will lead to superior clinical benefits." The two treatment arms predicted to provide earliest patency are a front-loaded alteplase regimen and a combination arm, alteplase plus streptokinase for possible further reocclusion suppression. These latter groups will receive early intravenous heparin in doses sufficient to accomplish full anticoagulation. This trial will also include an extensive angiographic substudy in order to document the temporal course of patency achieval and the reocclusion rate with the various therapies.

It would be anticipated that information heretofore generated and currently being collected regarding today's antiplatelet and antithrombin agents used in the thrombolytic setting will guide therapeutic decisions as the next generation of activators and adjuncts reach the clinical arena.

REFERENCES

1. Owen J, Friedman KD, Grossman BA, Wilkins C, Berke AD, Powers ER. Thrombolytic therapy with tissue plasminogen activator or streptokinase induces transient thrombin activity. Blood 1988; 72(2): 616–20.
2. Gulba DC, Barthels M, Westhoff-Bleck M, et al. Increased thrombin levels during thrombolytic therapy in acute myocardial infarction. Circulation 1991; 83: 937.
3. Hackett D, Davies G, Chierchia S, Maseri A. Intermittent coronary occlusion in acute myocardial infarction. Value of combined thrombolytic and vasodilator therapy. N Engl J Med 1987; 317: 1055.
4. Merx W, Dorr R, Rentrop P, et al. Evaluation of the effectiveness of intracoronary streptokinase infusion in myocardial infarction: postprocedure management and hospital course in 204 patients. Am Heart J 1981; 102: 1181.
5. Serruys PW, Wijns W, van den Brand M, et al. Is transluminal coronary angioplasty mandatory after successful thrombolysis? Br Heart J 1983; 50: 257.
6. Urban PL, Cowley M, Goldberg S, et al. Intracoronary thrombolysis in acute myocardial infarction: clinical course following successful myocardial reperfusion. Am Heart J 1984; 108: 873.
7. Ferguson DW, White CW, Schwartz JL, et al. Influence of baseline ejection fraction and success of thrombolysis on mortality and ventricular function after acute myocardial infarction. Am J Cardiol 1984; 54: 705.
8. Anderson JL, Marshall HW, Bray BE, et al. A randomized trial of intracoronary streptokinase in the treatment of acute myocardial infarction. N Engl J Med 1983; 308: 1305.
9. Leiboff RH, Katz RJ, Wasserman AG, et al. A randomized, angiographically controlled trial of intracoronary streptokinase in acute myocardial infarction. Am J Cardiol 1984; 53: 404.
10. Chesebro JH, Knatterud G, Roberts R, et al. Thrombolysis in Myocardial Infarction (TIMI) trial, Phase I: a comparison between intravenous tissue plasminogen activator and intravenous streptokinase. Circulation 1987; 76: 142.
11. Ohman EM, Califf RM, Topol EJ, et al. Consequences of reocclusion after successful reperfusion therapy in acute myocardial infarction. Circulation 1990; 82: 781.

12. ISIS-2 (Second International Study of Infarct Survival) Collaborative Group. Randomised trial of intravenous streptokinase, oral aspirin, both, or neither among 17,187 cases of suspected acute myocardial infarction: ISIS-2. Lancet 1988; 2: 349.

13. Sherman CT, Litvak F, Grundfest W, et al. Coronary angioscopy in patients with unstable angina. N Engl J Med 1986; 315: 913.

14. Lewis HD Jr, Davis JW, Archibald DG, et al. Protective effects of aspirin against acute myocardial infarction and death in men with unstable angina: results of a Veterans Administration Cooperative Study. N Engl J Med 1983; 309: 396.

15. Cairns JA, Gent M, Singer J, et al. Aspirin, sulfinpyrazone, or both in unstable angina: results of a Canadian multicenter trial. N Engl J Med 1985; 313: 1369.

16. Theroux P, Ouimet H, McCans J, et al. Aspirin, heparin, or both to treat acute unstable angina. N Engl J Med 1988; 319: 1105.

17. Neri Serneri GG, Gensini GF, Poggesi L, et al. Effect of heparin, aspirin or alteplase in reduction of myocardial ischaemia in refractory unstable angina. Lancet 1990; 335: 615.

18. The I.S.A.M. Study Group. A prospective trial of intravenous streptokinase in acute myocardial infarction (I.S.A.M.). N Engl J Med 1986; 314: 1465.

19. AIMS Trial Study Group. Effect of intravenous APSAC on mortality after acute myocardial infarction: preliminary report of a placebo-controlled clinical trial. Lancet 1988; 1: 545.

20. Topol EJ, Califf RM, George BS, et al. A randomized trial of immediate versus delayed elective angioplasty after intravenous tissue plasminogen activator in acute myocardial infarction. N Engl J Med 1987; 317: 581.

21. Verstraete M, Bernard R, Bory M, et al. Randomised trial of intravenous recombinant tissue-type plasminogen activator versus intravenous streptokinase in acute myocardial infarction. Lancet 1985; 1: 842.

22. Gruppo Italiano Per Lo Studio Della Sopravvivenza Nell-Infarto Miocardico. GISSI-2: a factorial randomised trial of alteplase versus streptokinase and heparin versus no heparin among 12,490 patients with acute myocardial infarction. Lancet 1990; 336: 65.

23. Sleight P. Preliminary outcome data, ISIS-3 presented at the American College of Cardiology Annual Scientific Meeting, March 1991, Atlanta, GA.

24. Cercek B, Lew AS, Hod H, et al. Enhancement of thrombolysis with tissue-type plasminogen activator by pretreatment with heparin. Circulation 1986; 74: 583.

25. Cercek B, Lew AS, Satoh Y, et al. Heparin enhances experimental thrombolysis by preventing new fibrin deposition. Circulation 1985; 72(suppl III): 111.

26. Topol EJ, George BS, Kereiakes DJ, et al. A randomized controlled trial of intravenous tissue plasminogen activator and early intravenous heparin in acute myocardial infarction. Circulation 1989; 79: 281.

27. Johns JA, Gold HK, Leinbach RC, et al. Prevention of coronary artery reocclusion and reduction in late coronary artery stenosis after thrombolytic therapy in patients with acute myocardial infarction. Circulation 1988; 78: 546.

28. Verstraete M, Arnold AER, Brower RW, et al. Acute coronary thrombolysis with recombinant human tissue-type plasminogen activator: initial patency and influence of maintained infusion on reocclusion rate. Am J Cardiol 1987; 60: 231.

29. Hsia J, Hamilton WP, Kleiman N, et al. A comparison between heparin and low-dose aspirin as adjunctive therapy with tissue plasminogen activator for acute myocardial infarction. N Engl J Med 1990; 323: 1433.

30. The TIMI Research Group, Baltimore. Immediate vs Delayed Catheterization and Angioplasty Following Thrombolytic Therapy for Acute Myocardial Infarction, TIMI II Results. JAMA 1988; 260: 2849.

31. Bleich SD, Nichols TC, Schumacher RR, et al. Effect of heparin on coronary arterial patency after thrombolysis with tissue plasminogen activator in acute myocardial infarction. Am J Cardiol 1990; 66: 1412.

32. European Cooperative Study Group. A randomized trial of heparin versus placebo after rt-PA. Presented at the 12th Congress of European Cardiologists. Stockholm, Sweden, September 1990.

33. Tebbe U. A randomized trial of heparin versus placebo after pro-urokinase induced thrombolysis. Presented at the George Washington University 6th International Workshop on Thrombolysis and Interventional Therapy in Acute Myocardial Infarction, Dallas, TX., Nov. 1990.

34. National Heart Foundation of Australia Coronary Thrombolysis Group. A randomized comparison of oral aspirin/dipyridamole versus intravenous heparin after rTPA for acute myocardial infarction. Circulation 1989; 80(suppl II): II-114.

35. Turpie AGG, Robinson JG, Doyle DJ, et al. Comparison of high-dose with low-dose subcutaneous heparin to prevent left ventricular mural thrombosis in patients with acute transmural anterior myocardial infarction. N Engl J Med 1989; 320: 352.

36. Hull RD, Raskob GE, Rosenbloom D. Heparin for 5 days as compared with 10 days in the initial treatment of proximal venous thrombosis. N Engl J Med 1990; 322: 1260.

37. The International Study Group. In-hospital mortality and clinical course of 20,891 patients with suspected acute myocardial infarction randomised between alteplase and streptokinase with or without heparin. Lancet 1990; 336: 71.

38. Rao AK, Pratt C, Berke A. Thrombolysis in myocardial infarction trial (TIMI)—phase I: hemorrhagic manifestations, complications, and changes in plasma fibrinogen and fibrinolytic system in patients treated with recombinant tissue plasminogen activator and streptokinase. J Am Coll Cardiol 1988; 11: 1.

39. Magnani B, for the PAIMS Investigators. Plasminogen Activator Italian Multicenter Study (PAIMS): comparison of intravenous recombinant single-chain human tissue-type plasminogen activator (rt-PA) with intravenous streptokinase in acute myocardial infarction. J Am Coll Cardiol 1989; 13: 19.

40. Kaplan K, Davison R, Parker M. Role of heparin after intravenous thrombolytic therapy for acute myocardial infarction. Am J Cardiol 1987; 59: 241.

41. The SCATI (Studio Sulla Calciparina Nell'Angina E Nella Trombosi Ventricolare Nell'Infarto) Group. Randomised controlled trial of subcutaneous calcium-heparin in acute myocardial infarction. Lancet 1989; 2: 182.

42. The International Study Group. In house mortality and clinical course of 20891 patients with suspected acute myocardial infarction randomized between alteplase and streptokinase with or without heparin. Lancet 1990; 336: 71–75.

18

ANTITHROMBOTIC THERAPY IN THE CHRONIC PHASE OF MYOCARDIAL INFARCTION

Pål Smith

Patients with nonfatal myocardial infarction face a high risk of a recurrence, and the risk of succumbing to cardiovascular disease in the next two to three years amounts to 15 to 20 per cent.[1] Even if the mortality rate eventually decreases, the stabilized annual mortality rate after six months is about four to eight times that faced by a comparable noncoronary population.[2]

Two different approaches may be applied to prolong life and avoid nonfatal complications in postinfarction patients. First, intervention that aims at reducing known risk factors for myocardial infarction including cigarette smoking, hypertension, diabetes, and hypercholesterolemia. The second strategy is therapy that may reduce the risk, regardless of known risk for a recurrent event. There is now strong evidence that thrombosis plays a major role in ischemic heart disease. Thus, an antithrombotic regimen may be beneficial in preventing further cardiovascular attacks. This chapter deals with the rationale for antithrombotic therapy in the secondary prevention of myocardial infarction and the experiences from a number of clinical trials. Finally, an attempt has been made to evaluate the efficacy of different antithrombotic drugs in this setting.

THE RATIONALE FOR ANTITHROMBOTIC PROPHYLAXIS IN THE SECONDARY PREVENTION OF MYOCARDIAL INFARCTION

Pathology

Deterioration of stable ischemic heart disease may follow progression of atherosclerosis, formation of platelet aggregates, coronary thrombosis, and coronary artery spasm. The association of thrombosis and atherosclerosis has long been recognized,[3] and presence of fibrin and other components of the clotting system in human atherosclerotic plaques has been documented,[4] suggesting that development and progression of atherosclerotic lesions may be accelerated and amplified by activation of the clotting cascade. To what extent antithrombotic therapy may retard the progression of stenosing atherosclerotic lesions is currently not known.

Occlusive thrombi in the offending artery, preponderantly at the site of a cracked atherosclerotic lesion, is a common finding in evolving myocardial infarction[5,6] (see Chapters 2 and 3). Disordered platelet function may contribute to the occlusive vascular lesions by aggregation, or by inducing vasospasm and coagulation, which in turn encourages fibrin deposition and formation of a fibrin-rich thrombus.[7] Repeated deposition of thrombotic material causes a gradual narrowing of the vessel lumen. Microinfarction due to fragmentation and embolization downstream is a frequent finding.[6]

The "Thrombotic Burden" in Cardiovascular Disease

Epidemiologic studies have convincingly shown an association of risk for cardiovascular disease and increased levels of fibrinogen and clotting factor VII (see Chapter 4).

343

In 1980, Meade and colleagues reported an association of coagulation factors with cardiovascular death. In their prospective study on apparently healthy subjects, high levels of fibrinogen and clotting factor VII at entry were found to be associated with increased risk of subsequent coronary mortality and morbidity.[8] Other prospective studies have confirmed these observations.[9-12] Coronary artery disease has been associated with an impaired fibrinolytic capacity,[13] and elevated levels of the rapid inhibitor of tissue plasminogen activator (PAI-1) has been shown to be a risk factor for recurrent myocardial infarction.[14] These findings support the idea that an imbalance in procoagulant, anticoagulant, or the fibrinolytic activities may facilitate thrombus formation in coronary artery disease.

Goals of Antithrombotic Therapy

The aims of antithrombotic therapy after myocardial infarction are to reduce or prevent: (a) early infarct extension, (b) cardiac chamber thrombus formation, and (c) recurrence of myocardial infarction and death. The idea that antithrombotic therapy may retard progressive atherothrombosis is interesting, but not yet confirmed. Thrombotic mechanisms may be modified pharmacologically by continuous suppression of platelet activity, by sustained inhibition of the clotting cascade, by inhibition of activated thrombin, and by stimulation of the fibrinolytic system. The superior way to obtain reliable information on the efficacy of various drugs to achieve these goals, is the controlled clinical trial. So far, platelet inhibitors and anticoagulants were tested in large-scale trials after myocardial infarction. Albeit the fibrinolytic capacity may be chronically stimulated by anabolic steroids, no trial on such treatment has been reported on the prevention of arterial thrombosis.

A simplistic model of risk reduction by antithrombotic intervention after nonfatal myocardial infarction is depicted in Figure 18-1. Effective prevention of coronary and cardiac chamber thrombosis reduces the risk for myocardial reinfarction and cardiogenic stroke. Noncardiogenic stroke, resulting from the common underlying atherosclerotic disease, may be prevented as well. Prevention of further damage to the myocardium reduces the risk of heart failure, and prevention of stroke prevents the disability often associated with cerebrovascular accidents. As myocardial infarction is a common disorder in all westernized countries, effective prophylaxis may produce a substantial benefit in terms of saved lives and averted morbidity.

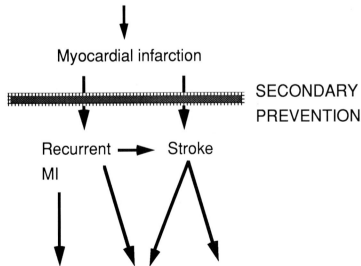

FIGURE 18–1. A model of action of secondary prophylaxis after acute myocardial infarction.

CLINICAL TRIAL EVALUATION

Single Trials

*We should not just accept the results
of separate clinical trials, but scrutinize
the premises for the conclusions that are drawn*

The randomized controlled trial is widely recognized as a valuable tool for evaluating the efficacy of drug therapy. However, the validity of a trial is contingent upon adequate design, randomization, proper control, and a sufficient sample size. Even so, the trial may not provide relevant information if the study does not reflect the clinical condition to which the study regimen will be referred. Figure 18–2 lists essential information that should be looked for in trials claiming benefit from a specific treatment. Outcome measures in postmyocardial infarction studies are generally expressed on the broad categories failure or success. Most antithrombotic trials have evaluated the effect on mortality and reinfarction, and some have also investigated the influence of therapy on cerebrovascular endpoints. Whether all-cause mortality or cardiovascular mortality is the most appropriate endpoint may be debatable. On one hand, death is not necessarily a measure of thrombus formation. Sudden cardiac death is thought to be due principally to arrhythmias, even though some data suggest an association of sudden death with thrombosis.[15] On the other hand, the results of the large clofibrate trial[16] showed that even though the incidence of myocardial infarction was reduced on clofibrate, mortality from all causes was significantly higher in the actively treated group. Thus, to cover also the possibility of a harmful effect of the drug, all-cause mortality should always be considered, especially in trials involving long-term

Design of trial
No of included patients
Delay before treatment is commenced
Time of observation
Drug dose
Concomitant drugs
Withdrawals
Outcome measures
Intention-to-treat analysis?
Efficacy in terms of averted events
Generalizability

FIGURE 18–2. Keypoints of design and results of clinical trials.

drug administration. The assessment of a trial should also take into account the delay before treatment is commenced, and the duration of therapy. The impact of therapy may not be the same if begun immediately or some time after the event. Moreover, a short-term effect does not automatically imply that the effect will be maintained over time. Optimal drug dose needs to be assessed, and it should be kept in mind that the study results apply to that dose only. Another important issue is the impact of concomitant drugs; for instance, an unequivocal effect on mortality has been demonstrated by beta-blockade after myocardial infarction.[1,17] Several studies have suggested, albeit weak, an antiplatelet action of unselective beta-antagonists.[18,19] The practical implications of this finding is uncertain, but there is a reasonable chance that weak platelet inhibitors might not add benefit to that brought about by a beta-blocker.

Basically, results of clinical trials may be analyzed two ways. The most conservative approach is the intention-to-treat analysis, which takes into consideration all results from all randomized patients. The explanatory approach, which is more likely to express the true drug effect in the specific trial, includes results only from those patients with valid entry criteria who complied with the protocol. The on-treatment analysis may provide the most useful information on the actual benefit that may be derived. An issue that seldom is raised is whether the results are generalizable, which implies that patients not entered have the same susceptibility for the clinical outcome measure as participants. If not so, extrapolating from the study population may not be justified. Selection bias may have occurred in trials entering only fractions of the screened population.

In some trials, analyses were performed in order to identify subgroups with varying degree of benefit from treatment. Subgroup analyses do involve a number of problems (for example, loss of power, statistical multiplicity, uneven distribution of risk factors across the various subgroups). Also, investigated subgroups should be prespecified in the study protocol. Thus, results of subgroup analyses should be considered with caution.

Numerous clinical trials on antithrombotic therapy in and after acute myocardial infarction have been published. During the past two decades, clinical trial methodology has improved considerably. Even so, most if not all trials have their limitations. Thus, we should not just accept the results of separate clinical trials, but should scrutinize the premises for the conclusions that are drawn. In this chapter, emphasis has been put on the large, well-designed, and long-term secondary prevention studies. Trials implementing short-term therapy, or therapeutic interventions in the acute phase of myocardial infarction are discussed in Chapter 11.

Meta-Analysis

If available, the discussion of the separate antithrombotic agents includes the results of at least one meta-analysis. Put briefly, meta-analysis is the use of formal statistical techniques to sum up a body of separate (but similar) experiments.[20] The rationale of a meta-analysis of data from different trials is that, despite the advances made in clinical trial methodology, one may often be faced with the challenge of interpreting results from trials too small to have achieved a statistically significant result, or to have ruled out a medically important result. There are some limitations in the interpretation of a meta-analysis, even when performed according to strict rules, not the least because of the great variation in design and performance between individual trials.

ANTITHROMBOTIC DRUGS

Platelet Inhibitors

SULFINPYRAZONE

Two studies have evaluated the prophylactic effect of platelet inhibition by sulfinpyra-

zone after myocardial infarction[21,22] (Table 18–1). The daily dose was 800 milligrams in both. The Anturane Reinfarction Trial[21] randomized 1,629 patients of either sex who had survived acute myocardial infarction by 25 to 35 days to sulfinpyrazone or matching placebo. Follow-up averaged 16 months, and total withdrawal rate during the study was 26.6 per cent. At end of study (Table 18–1), a 29 per cent reduction in mortality was noted. The most remarkable result was a 74 per cent reduction in risk of sudden death at seven months, and a reduction by 43 per cent at end of study. However, deaths occurring within the first seven days of therapy, deaths more than seven days after dropout, deaths in noncompliers, and deaths in association with surgical procedures were considered nonanalyzable in this study. Because of design and analysis, the study was heavily attacked. The United States Food and Drug Administration (FDA) published a formal critique of the study,[23] and refused to approve a claim that the drug reduced the risk for sudden death during the first six months after acute myocardial infarction. Another trial on sulfinpyrazone was reported by the Anturan Reinfarction Italian Study Group.[22] In this trial, 727 patients were randomized to either active treatment or placebo. After averaged 19 months follow-up, mortality was similar in the two groups, while the rate of combined fatal and nonfatal myocardial reinfarction was 56 per cent lower in the actively treated group. The rate of sudden death was similar in the two groups (3 per cent versus 2.5 per cent in treated and placebo groups), strikingly in contrast to the results of the Anturane Reinfarction Trial.[21]

TABLE 18–1. Distribution of Endpoints in the Different Antiplatelet Trials According to Treatment Groups

Study (Year)	Drug	Treatment Time (Months)	Treatment Type Control	Treatment Type Treatment	Mortality (%) Control	Mortality (%) Treatment	Nonfatal Myocardial Infarction (%) Control	Nonfatal Myocardial Infarction (%) Treatment	Nonfatal Cerebrovascular Attacks (%) Control	Nonfatal Cerebrovascular Attacks (%) Treatment	Averted Event
ART (1980)[21]	Sulfinpyrazone	16	783	775	6.3	4.1	3.5	1.3	—	—	4.3
ARIS (1982)[22]	Sulfinpyrazone	19	362	365	5.5	5.2	7.7	3.2	1.6	0.2	6.2
STAI (1990)[37]	Ticlopidine	6	338	314	4.7	2.5	8.9	4.8	—	—	6.3
Elwood (1974)[28]	Aspirin/dipyridamole	12	624	615	9.7	7.6	—	—	—	—	2.1
CDPA (1976)[29]	Aspirin/dipyridamole	22	771	758	8.3	5.8	4.1	3.6	1.0	1.1	2.9
Elwood (1979)[30]	Aspirin/dipyridamole	12	850	832	14.8	12.3	7.4	3.7	—	—	6.2
GAMIS (1980)[31]	Aspirin/dipyridamole	24	309	317	10.3	8.5	5.1	3.4	—	—	3.5
AMIS (1980)[32]	Aspirin/dipyridamole	36	2,257	2,267	9.7	10.7	9.4	7.7	2.0	1.1	1.6
PARIS I (1980)[33]	Aspirin/dipyridamole	41	406	1,620‡	12.8	10.6	9.9	7.4	2.0	1.1	5.6
PARIS II (1986)[34]	Aspirin/dipyridamole	23	1,565	1,563	7.2	7.1	4.5	2.1	2.1	1.3	3.5

* Total death, nonfatal myocardial reinfarction and nonfatal stroke averted per 100 patients treated for 0.5 to 3.5 years.
† On treatment analysis.
‡ Combined active treatment arms, for details see text.

No subgroup analyses were performed in any of the two studies, and no separate meta-analysis has been published. For this purpose, data from these trials have been assessed together with data from trials on other platelet inhibitors.[24] Theoretically, the effective range may be increased if the antiplatelet substance also has antiarrhythmic properties. *Sulfinpyrazone* offer such theoretical possibilities,[21] but due to the controversy following the conflicting findings of the two studies that have been performed, and due to some side effects of the drug, sulfinpyrazone has not come into common use in the secondary prophylaxis after myocardial infarction.

DIPYRIDAMOLE

Dipyridamole inhibits the enzyme phosphodiesterase. Its precise mechanism of action is not yet fully understood, but it seems that dipyridamole inhibits platelet adhesion to subendothelial vessel structures.[25] It also inhibits platelet aggregation in vivo. The drug has been widely tested in a variety of clinical settings, but experience with the agent as monotherapy after myocardial infarction relates to a single study only. In that study, no benefit was found of dipyridamole 400 milligrams/day compared with placebo, either in terms of prevention of thromboembolic complications, or myocardial reinfarction and death.[26] However, the study groups were small, and follow-up lasted only one month.

ASPIRIN

Aspirin irreversibly acetylates the enzyme cyclooxygenase, which is necessary for the conversion of platelet arachidonic acid to thromboxane A_2. The latter is a powerful platelet aggregating agent and vasoconstrictor. Cyclooxygenase also converts endothelial arachidonic acid to prostacyclin, which is a powerful inhibitor of platelet aggregation and a potent vasodilator. Prostacyclin may therefore help keep the vessel wall "clean." The effect of aspirin is measurable within a few hours after ingestion. The ideal dose of aspirin would be the one that inhibited the production of thromboxane A_2, but at the same time did not interfere with the formation of prostacyclin. In secondary prophylactic trials after myocardial infarction, daily doses have varied from 300 to 1,500 milligrams. These doses are known to inhibit cyclooxygenase both in vessel wall and platelets.[27]

Clinical Trials on Aspirin. Current literature includes a number of reports on the effect of aspirin in cardiovascular disease. Seven randomized studies,[28-34] involving 620 to 4,524 patients, have evaluated the prophylactic effect of aspirin after myocardial infarction (Table 18–1, Fig. 18–3). The time between the index infarction and onset of treatment varied considerably across these studies—from one study which included most of the patients within one week, to that which included the majority of the participants after more than five years. The most early trial administered a comparatively low dose of aspirin (300 milligrams/day), while larger doses (900–1,500 milligrams/day) were given in subsequent trials.

In 1974, Elwood and his group randomized 1,239 men to receive either aspirin 300 milligrams/day or placebo on the average ten weeks after acute myocardial infarction.[28] Average length of follow-up was 12 months. Ten per cent of those entered were withdrawn during the study. Numerically, more deaths were observed in the placebo group than in the aspirin group. However, the difference did not attain statistical significance. No other endpoints were studied.

In the Coronary Drug Project aspirin study of 1,529 men, mortality in the aspirin group was 5.8 per cent as compared with 8.3 per cent in the placebo group over 22 months.[29] No important benefit was found pertaining to reinfarction or stroke in this study. The mortality rate in the control group was low, probably owing to the fact that more than five years had elapsed since the index infarction in the majority of patients. Furthermore, all patients in this trial had received either dextrothyroxine or varying doses of estrogen as part of another study, the Coronary Drug Project, for some time between the index infarction and recruitment. Even though the hormone medication was discontinued 6 to 25 months prior to enrollment into the aspirin study, the possibility of an impact of this treatment causes some uncertainty as for the generalizability of the findings.

A follow-up study by Elwood and colleagues in 1979 was conducted in 1,682 patients of either sex.[30] One fourth of the patients were entered within three days, and the majority of patients were included within one week after the qualifying infarction. Dropouts during the trial numbered 228 in each group. A reduction of 17.3 per cent in risk of death by aspirin was found, but again this reduction was not statistically significant.

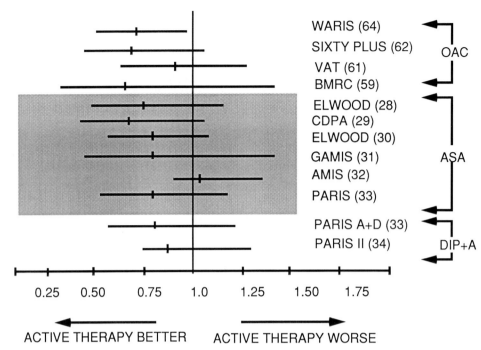

0.25 0.50 0.75 1.0 1.25 1.50 1.75

ACTIVE THERAPY BETTER   ACTIVE THERAPY WORSE

FIGURE 18–3. Results of long-term antithrombotic trials on mortality. Reductions are given as odds ratios and the horizontal lines represent 95 per cent confidence intervals. Results are based on the intention-to-treat principle apart from reference 28, where such data are not available. Numbers in brackets represent reference number. OAC-oral anticoagulants, ASA (A)-aspirin, DIP(D)-dipyridamole.

Data on reinfarctions were limited and uncertain according to the authors. These data are included in the summary in Table 18–1, but omitted in graphic presentation of the various trials in Figure 18–4.

The German-Austrian trial[31] investigated three test arms: aspirin 1,500 milligrams/day or matching placebo, and an open group receiving oral anticoagulants (reviewed later in this chapter). Survivors of myocardial infarction of either sex were entered into this trial five to six weeks after the event. Of the patients, 317 took aspirin and 309 took placebo. Mean follow-up averaged two years. More than 30 per cent dropped out for reasons other than a documented endpoint. Total mortality was 8.5 per cent in the aspirin group and 10.3 per cent in the placebo group, a reduction by aspirin of 17 per cent. Neither this difference nor the difference in reinfarction or stroke was statistically conclusive.

The largest study on aspirin after myocardial infarction ever performed was the Aspirin Myocardial Infarction Study.[32] This National Heart, Lung and Blood Institute-sponsored randomized double-blind study involved 4,524 men and women, recruited eight weeks to five years after an acute myocardial infarction. The test medication consisted of aspirin 1,000 milligrams/day or matching placebo. Mortality from any cause after averaged 36 months follow-up was 10.8 per cent in the aspirin group and 9.7 per cent in the placebo group. The difference was statistically not significant. When fatal endpoints other than total mortality were analyzed, there again was no evidence of a benefit by aspirin. Both the incidence of recurrent nonfatal myocardial infarction and stroke was lower among those taking aspirin (Table 18–1), but owing to a large number of significant tests performed during and after follow-up, the authors correctly stated that ". . . exact statements of statistical significance are impossible to make in this situation" (from AMIS Research Group).

Dipyridamole was added to aspirin in two studies. The Persantine-Aspirin Reinfarction Study[33] had three therapy arms consisting of one group receiving dipyridamole plus aspirin, one group receiving aspirin alone, and one placebo group (Table 18–1). The 1,759 men and 267 women were entered into the trial two months to five years after the qualifying infarction, and allocated to treatment with 972 milligrams aspirin daily (n = 810),

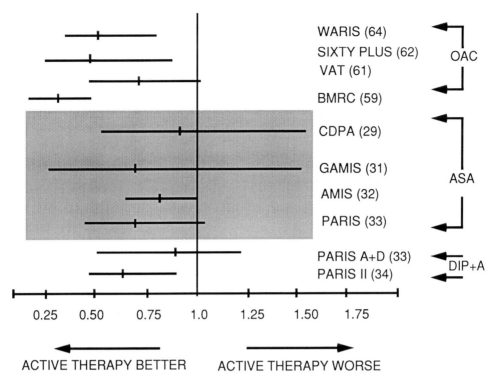

FIGURE 18–4. Effect of long-term antithrombotic trials on myocardial reinfarction. Reductions are given as odds ratios and the horizontal lines represent 95 per cent confidence intervals. Results are based on the intention-to-treat principle apart from reference 28, where such data were not available. Reliable data on reinfarction not available for references 25 and 27, which have been omitted. Numbers in brackets represent reference number. OAC = oral anticoagulants, ASA (A) = aspirin, DIP(D) = dipyridamole.

972 milligrams aspirin plus dipyridamole 225 milligrams daily (n = 810), or placebo matching the aspirin group (n = 406). Mean follow-up was 41 months, and mortality in the placebo group during that time was 12.8 per cent. Total mortality was 10.5 per cent in the group assigned to aspirin alone, and 10.7 per cent in the group taking the combination of dipyridamole and aspirin. As for reinfarction and stroke rates, only small and unimpressive reductions by aspirin or the combined treatment were found (Table 18–1). A follow-up study with a two-group design was published in 1986.[34] In that study, 3,128 patients were entered earlier, with an entry window of four weeks to four months after myocardial infarction. The test medication was aspirin 330 milligrams plus dipyridamole 75 milligrams three times daily or matching placebo medication. Mean observation time was 23 months. There was no difference in total mortality or stroke, while a significant reduction in non-fatal myocardial infarction from 7.1 per cent in the control group to 4.5 per cent in the actively treated group was observed.

Subgroup Analyses. Subgroup analyses were performed in some of the trials in order to pursue the idea that treatment would have a different (that is, better) effect in some categories. Hence, attempts were made in some of the studies to see if outcome was affected by sex, age, having had a previous myocardial infarction, varying intervals between infarction and beginning of treatment, or concomitant drugs.[28,31,33,34] No effect was found for women (regarding mortality) in one study,[31] but the benefit for men was still not large enough to attain statistical significance. No age effect was observed in the only study addressing that issue.[28] It is difficult to envisage a clear time effect, but the difference between the treatment and control groups appeared to be greater among those entered "early" as compared to those included "late" in one study.[33] Larger differences between treatment and placebo groups in "coronary incidence" was observed in one study for patients whose qualifying myocardial infarction was their first.[34] A notable result of the Persantin-Aspirin Reinfarction (PARIS II)

Study[34] was a larger effect of dipyridamole and aspirin among patients using beta-receptor blocking agents than in the subgroup not using these agents. In conclusion, the evidence for differing treatment effects in subgroups is conflicting. No subgroup has yet been identified that is more likely than another to benefit from treatment with aspirin.

TICLOPIDINE

A metabolite of this pyridine derivative has broad antiplatelet activity. It irreversibly inhibits, in a concentration-dependent manner, platelet aggregation induced by adenosine diphosphate, and indirectly, the aggregation induced by low concentrations of collagen, epinephrine, platelet-activating factor, and thrombin. The bleeding time is prolonged, with a maximum effect after five to six days of repeated oral administration with a lag time of three to five days. Ticlopidine inhibits ex vivo fibrinogen binding to the glycoprotein IIb-IIIa complex, the fibrinogen receptor found on the platelet membrane, but does not prevent the formation of thromboxane A_2, prostacyclin, or cyclic adenosine monophosphate phosphodiesterase.[35] Ticlopidine also reduces plasma fibrinogen and increases red cell deformability.[36]

In a strict sense, no large-scale trial in ticlopidine has been reported in the post-myocardial infarction setting. Recently, however, a study including patients with unstable angina was reported[37] (Table 18–1). Because the patients were followed-up for six months, it appears justified to evaluate the results of this study. Altogether, 652 patients (25 per cent of those screened) were randomized either to conventional therapy (beta-blocker, calcium channel blocker, or nitrates [n = 338]), or to conventional therapy plus ticlopidine 250 milligrams twice daily (n = 314).

The risk of vascular death and fatal myocardial infarction was reduced (16 events among the control group versus 8 in the ticlopidine group), but the reduction was statistically not significant. However, total events (including also nonfatal reinfarction) was 13.6 per cent in the conventionally treated group as compared with 7.3 per cent in the ticlopidine group, a reduction of 46 per cent ($p = 0.009$). Three nonfatal strokes occurred in the control group as compared with none in the ticlopidine group.

The distribution of primary endpoints was assessed by the authors in relation to sex and prior myocardial infarction. While no relation of sex to efficacy of ticlopidine was apparent, reduction of events seemed to be greater for patients with previous myocardial infarction in the ticlopidine group. No multivariate analysis was performed, hence confounding was not controlled for.

Side Effects of Platelet Inhibitors. Treatment with aspirin and the combination of aspirin with dipyridamole resulted in a raised frequency of side effects. Dipyridamole, either alone or combined with aspirin was associated with increased incidences of headache. The rate of gastrointestinal symptoms was almost doubled in studies using a daily dose of 1,000 milligrams aspirin or more.[32-34] Bleeding complications occurred chiefly in the gastrointestinal tract and presented as hematemesis, bloody stool, and black tarry stool. Table 18–2 summarizes frequency and severity of side effects as reported by the various study groups. The incidence of adverse side effects causing withdrawal of treatment for any reason other than death, cardiovascular events, or cancer, was approximately doubled in patients receiving ticlopidine compared with placebo.[36] In a placebo-controlled trial evaluating 1,053 patients over a three-year period, ticlopidine

TABLE 18–2. Distribution of Fatal and Serious Nonfatal Bleedings as Reported in Platelet Inhibitor Studies

Study	Aspirin Milligram/Day	Dipyridamole Milligram/day	Fatal (%) Control	Fatal (%) Treatment	Nonfatal (%) Control	Nonfatal (%) Treatment	Combined (%) Control	Combined (%) Treatm
Elwood I[28]	300	—	—	—	—	—	—	—
CDPA[29]	972	—	—	—	4.6	6.2	4.6	6.2
Elwood II[30]	900	—	—	—	0.4	0.9	0.4	0.9
GAMIS[31]	1,500	—	—	—	0.0	2.9	0.0	2.9
AMIS[32]	1,000	—	—	—	49	8.2	4.9	8.2
PARIS I[33]	972	225	—	—	1.7	3.4	1.7	3.4
PARIS II[34]	972	225	—	—	0.9	1.5	0.9	1.5

was associated with adverse effects in 54 per cent of patients and in 34 per cent of those receiving placebo. Of these adverse symptoms, 8 per cent were considered severe in the ticlopidine group (versus 3 per cent in the placebo group), and treatment was withdrawn in 12 versus 3 per cent of patients. The most commonly reported adverse effects are gastrointestinal (nausea, diarrhea), rash, and bleeding, but the most feared are neutropenia and agranulocytosis. The latter hematological disorders appear early in treatment (first 12 weeks), but are reversible on discontinuation of treatment[36] Few, and only minor adverse reactions were observed in the trial on ticlopidine. Those observed were mild gastrointestinal disorders and rash. No bleeding disorders were reported.

Trials have tended to use progressively lower doses of aspirin as these still inhibit platelet aggregation and have less effect on synthesis of prostacyclin. However, the dose of aspirin required to inhibit platelet aggregation in response to differing stimuli varies, and presently we do not know which stimuli are relevant in arterial thrombosis in man.[38] Doses as low as 75 milligrams/day still can cause gastric mucosal bleeding, but at a low incidence.[24]

Meta-Analysis. The Antiplatelet Trialists' Collaboration Group concluded in 1988 that the results from pooling all platelet inhibitor trials on postmyocardial infarction treatment together favors aspirin over placebo, with a reduction in cardiovascular mortality of 13 per cent, a reduction in recurrent nonfatal reinfarction by 31 per cent, and a reduction in nonfatal strokes of 42 per cent.[24]

Conclusions Pertaining to Platelet Inhibitors. Seven trials on aspirin or the combination of aspirin with dipyridamole have been evaluated, one of which has been conducted recently. The results are fairly consistent, demonstrating a statistically nonsignificant reduction in the risk of death, and a more pronounced reduction in the incidences of reinfarction and stroke. No single trial has produced evidence in terms of a statistically significant reduction in total mortality in favor of aspirin over placebo. In contrast, reduction in the risk of recurrent myocardial infarction has been more promising. The impact on stroke by platelet inhibitors has, in turn, been less impressive. A meta-analysis suggests a reduction in cardiovascular mortality by platelet inhibitors of 13 per cent, a reduction in nonfatal reinfarction of 31 per

cent, and a reduction in the incidence of nonfatal stroke of 42 per cent.[24] However, even small absolute reductions may suggest a major relative reduction if the incidence rate in the control group is low. Hence, avoided events per 100 patients treated may be a more informative way to assess the benefit of treatment. The reductions in event rates achieved in the different trials (Table 18–1) consistently suggest that long-term treatment with platelet inhibitors avoids two to six major events per 100 treated patients, when treatment is given for from 1 to 3.5 years. The associated risk for serious bleeding varies considerably across the studies, probably owing to different criteria. Apparently, gastrointestinal bleeding has not been separated from gastrointestinal symptoms in many studies, and only one study explicitly reports that no bleedings were fatal.[31] This may of course be due to absence of such events, but fatal cerebral and gastrointestinal bleeding may also have been categorized as stroke and death caused by "nonatherosclerotic cardiovascular disease." Table 18–2 contains data on bleeding as provided in the different study reports. An attempt has been made to include in this summary only those bleeding episodes reported by the authors as being clinically important. It appears that aspirin doubles the risk of significant bleeding. All aspirin trials in this review used doses varying from 300 to 1,500 milligrams/day. Low-dose aspirin caused less gastrointestinal upset and less occult blood loss (Table 18–2). It is not clear if enteric-coated preparations of aspirin carry any additional advantage in reducing gastrointestinal blood loss. Data indicate that even lower doses (80 to 150 milligrams/day) may have an antithrombotic effect in man.[40] At present the optimum dose of aspirin for secondary prevention after acute myocardial infarction is not firmly established.

Most aspirin trials had a wide entry window. Thus, caution is warranted when applying the findings of these trials to the immediate postmyocardial infarction situation. On the other hand, given the decline in complication rate over time, the late entry may possibly have led to an underestimation of the potential benefit of the drug.

The following consensus statement on the use of aspirin in coronary heart disease was issued in 1989 by the Australian National Heart Foundation:

1. Aspirin reduces the risk of clot formation (thrombosis) within blood vessels of the heart. This is the likely basis of its action in reducing the risk of heart attack.

2. The benefits of aspirin in heart disease can be achieved with doses as low as 100 to 300 milligrams/day.

3. Carefully conducted research has established a role for aspirin in patients with acute heart attack or unstable angina and after recovery from heart attack or coronary artery bypass surgery.

4. Asymptomatic patients at high risk of suffering a heart attack may reduce this risk by taking aspirin. However, a decision to take aspirin in an attempt to reduce the risk of heart attack should be made by a general practitioner or specialist after detailed consideration of all the medical risks versus the benefits.

5. Unwanted effects of aspirin include minor bleeding from the stomach, activation of peptic ulcers, an increased tendency to bruising, hypersensitivity reactions, and a slightly increased risk of significant bleeding.

6. While aspirin may significantly reduce the risk of stroke due to clot formation in the blood vessels in the brain, this benefit is offset by a slight increase in the risk of stroke due to brain hemorrhage.

7. If aspirin is used to prevent a heart attack, this should only be in association with an overall program of coronary prevention including diet, cessation of cigarette smoking, control of blood pressure, and regular exercise.

Anticoagulant Drugs

HEPARIN

The anticoagulant action of heparin is due to binding to antithrombin III, which thereby accelerates the latter's rate of inhibition of the major coagulation enzymes: thrombin, factor IX, X, XI, and XII.[41] A stimulating effect on fibrinolysis has been reported in one report.[42] Conflicting evidence exists for an antiplatelet effect in vitro.[43,44]

Clinical Trials on Heparin. The long-term effect of heparin after myocardial infarction has been investigated in one trial.[45] In this study, 3,859 patients were screened and 728 eventually were entered. The patients were recruited 6 to 18 months after myocardial infarction and randomly assigned

to a daily subcutaneous injection of 12,500 international units unfractionated heparin daily during an average of 23 months, or no heparin. Age ranged from 50 to 75 years. About 15 per cent of the patients were taking beta-blockers. Moreover, more than 30 per cent of those assigned to heparin and more than 40 per cent of those allocated to the control group took antiplatelet agents concurrently. There were few dropouts (7.7 per cent in the heparin group versus 6.3 per cent among controls). Heparin treatment reduced the cumulative mortality rate by 34 per cent on intention-to-treat basis (not significant), and by 48 per cent on on-treatment basis ($p < 0.05$). The accumulated reinfarction rate was significantly lower in the heparin group (63 per cent), whatever was employed in the analysis. Stroke was not reported as an endpoint. There were only minor side effects.

This study provides evidence of a benefit of heparin therapy after myocardial infarction. However, the impact of concurrent antiplatelet medication may have been substantial. Despite the appeal of a fixed-dose regimen of subcutaneous heparin, with no need for laboratory control, the parenteral route is probably less feasible than orally administered drugs in a long-term setting.

ORAL ANTICOAGULANTS

Oral anticoagulants (coumarins, indanediones) inhibit the carboxylation of glutamic acid to gamma-carboxyglutamic acid residues on some proteins involved in blood coagulation, the four coagulation factors (II, VII, IX, and X), and the two physiologic inhibitors (protein C and protein S). After a latent period, peculiar to each type of oral anticoagulant (18 to 72 hours), the production of vitamin K-dependent proteins is reduced, and the speed with which their concentration in the blood decreases is in proportion to their individual half-life. After a few days, a new equilibrium is established between the rates of synthesis and degradation (metabolism) of the vitamin K-dependent proteins.[46] Even if all oral anticoagulants are thought to have the same mode of action, varying pharmacokinetic properties may contribute to differing efficacy and risk profile.

Clinical Trials. Few topics have engendered as much controversy in cardiological practice as oral anticoagulant therapy in the long-term management of patients after myocardial infarction, the purpose of which would be to prevent recurrent coronary thrombosis, cardiogenic emboli, and perhaps atherothrombotic progression. The main reason for the controversy is because conclusive evidence of a benefit of such therapy has long been lacking.[47]

The first studies with heparin and oral anticoagulants administered in the acute phase of a myocardial infarction revealed a clear reduction in cerebral and peripheral arterial emboli, deep venous thrombosis, pulmonary emboli, and mortality. The latter finding is questionable in view of more recent studies, and many cardiologists limit the use of oral anticoagulants during the acute phase of myocardial infarction to those patients with a large infarction, extensive wall-motion defects, intracavitary thrombi, and a clearly increased risk of deep vein thrombosis. After a report on the efficacy of anticoagulation during the first six weeks after myocardial infarction by Wright et al. in 1948,[48] anticoagulation was officially endorsed by the American Heart Association. In following trials, the investigators were probably so convinced of the benefit of such treatment that the need for appropriate control groups was neglected. A critical review of the previous anticoagulant trials was published by Gifford and Feinstein in 1969.[49] They showed that only 2 out of 32 clinical studies[50,51] satisfied criteria for what would be adequate trial design, and that methodological shortcomings had been especially serious in those studies claiming benefit from anticoagulation. That set the stage for the end of the recommendation to use anticoagulants in the acute phase of myocardial infarction.

A subsequent report of the International Anticoagulant Review Group analyzed 2,487 cases from long-term trials carried out between 1950 and 1965.[52] However, neither the 20 per cent reduction of mortality in patients given anticoagulants reported in this review nor the publication of more optimistic reports[53,54] could reverse a steady decline in the popularity of anticoagulant therapy. Uncertainties about optimal intensity of treatment[55] were probably also contributing factors to the dwindling enthusiasm, as were changing views as to the pathogenesis of myocardial infarction that led to increased use of antiplatelet agents.[56,57] The introduction of beta-adrenoceptor blocking drugs and studies focusing on the ability of these agents to reduce postinfarction mortality probably also played a role.[1,17,58]

Of the 19 randomized clinical trials on long-term oral anticoagulants after myocardial infarction up to 1990, only four were of sufficient size and design to permit appropriate interpretation (Table18–3, Figs. 18–3 and 18–4). The British Medical Research Council Trial (BMRC),[59] was a double-blind comparison of a high dose (anticoagulant group) with an inert dose (low dose) of phenindione. The size of the background population is unknown. Patients were randomized within four to six weeks of infarction and followed-up for at least two years. Of the 383 persons entered into this trial, 11 were lost for follow-up. Although both mortality (7.7 per cent in the high-dose group versus 11.7 per cent among the control group) and nonfatal reinfarction (13.3 per cent in the high-dose group against 36.7 per cent in the control group) was reduced by anticoagulation, only the difference for myocardial reinfarction attained statistical significance. The incidence of thromboembolic morbidity, including pulmonary embolism and stroke, was low and did not permit separate assessment. Recently, low-dose anticoagulant therapy proved effective in reducing the incidence of venous thromboembolic complications following major gynecological surgery.[60] To what extent, if any, an effect of the low-dose

TABLE 18–3. Distribution of Endpoints in the Different Anticoagulant Trials

STUDY (YEAR)	DRUG	TREATMENT TIME (MONTHS)	TREATMENT TYPE		MORTALITY (%)		NONFATAL MYOCARDIAL INFARCTION (%)		NONFATAL CEREBROVASCULAR ATTACKS (%)		AVERTED EVENTS*
			Control	Treatment	Control	Treatment	Control	Treatment	Control	Treatment	
IHS (1987)[15]	Heparin	23	365	363	6.3	4.1	3.5	1.3†	—	—	4.3
BMRC 1964[59]	Oral anticoagulants	>24	188	195	11.1	7.6	36.7	13.3	—	—	26.9
VAT (1969)[61]	Oral anticoagulants	24–60	350	385	32.6	31.2	20.8	15.5	—	—	6.7
Sixty Plus (1980)[62]	Oral anticoagulants	24	439	439	15.7	11.6	8.4	4.1	3.4	1.3	10..5
WARIS (1990)[64]	Oral anticoagulants	37	607	607	20.2	15.4	12.3	6.2	7.2	3.2	14.9

* Total deaths, nonfatal myocardial reinfarction and nonfatal stroke averted per 100 patients treated for 2 to 5 years.
† On treatment data.

regimen may have reduced relatively the benefit observed in the high-dose group remains uncertain.

The Veterans Administration Trial entered 747 patients into the study within 21 days of the acute event.[61] Twelve of those admitted were excluded from the final data analysis. Patients allocated to anticoagulation received bishydroxycoumarin. The anticoagulated group suffered less deaths and reinfarctions than the placebo group during the three years of follow-up ($p < 0.01$), but the difference was less impressive at five years. Patients in the anticoagulant group were less frequently readmitted to hospital for recurrent myocardial infarction than those taking placebo (66 versus 92 events). A reduction in other thromboembolic events also was seen (17 in the anticoagulant group and 39 among those assigned to placebo). Notably, the achieved level of anticoagulation was not satisfactory according to the intensity recommended today.

The design of the Sixty Plus Trial was different from that of the others.[62] This study entered patients older than 60 years who had already been treated with oral anticoagulants (acenocoumarin or phenprocoumon) for at least six months, median six years. The patients received either continued anticoagulation or matching placebo. When patients who deviated from the protocol were included in the analysis, the difference in total mortality (51 deaths in the anticoagulant group versus 69 in the control group) attained borderline statistical significance ($p = 0.07$). Those who continued anticoagulation fared considerably better with respect to total reinfarction (29 in the actively treated as compared with 64 in the placebo group), a difference yielding statistical significance ($p = 0.0005$). Notably, the number of intracranial events due to any cause, was impressively reduced by anticoagulation (12 in the anticoagulant group versus 20 in the control group). Moreover, even if there were more deaths attributable to intracranial bleeding, total number of deaths owing to intracranial events was higher in the placebo group than in the anticoagulant group.

The design of this trial did cause some concern, and most critics argued that it had demonstrated the risk of stopping anticoagulant therapy at 60 years of age in subjects that apparently had benefited from such therapy over years. Moreover, as all subjects enrolled were over 60 years, the generalizability of the results to younger patients is uncertain. Hence, even though the results were encouraging and, indeed, stimulated the debate, the need for a study with a more appropriate design was explicitly formulated.[47,63]

The Warfarin Reinfarction Study (WARIS). The WARIS trial was planned and designed as a response to the debate on long-term oral anticoagulation following the Sixty Plus study. It was a prospective, double-blind, and placebo-controlled study, and evidence of success or failure was based primarily on the total death rate.[64] Other endpoints were recurrent myocardial infarction and cerebrovascular accidents. A large number of previous studies made it possible to estimate a reduction in risk by active treatment with reasonable certainty, which in tern enabled the calculation of a realistic number of patients. Treatment allocation was stratified for chronic beta-blockade to ensure even distribution of subjects on such drugs in the two study groups.

Patients of either sex aged 75 or less were eligible at discharge from hospital after a documented myocardial infarction if they exhibited no indication for or specific contraindication against treatment with oral anticoagulants, lived in the study area, had anticipated acceptable compliance, and gave their informed consent. Physicians at the hospital providing the initial care decided whether an indication for oral anticoagulants was present. Chronic atrial fibrillation, left ventricular mural thrombi, or a high risk for thromboembolic disease other than myocardial infarction were generally considered as indications for long-term anticoagulation.

During the accrual period from January 10, 1983 through March 24, 1986, 1,918 eligible patients were identified of whom 1,214 (63 per cent) were entered into the study. Overall duration on test medication averaged 37 months. Endpoints were taken to have occurred on treatment if occurring within 28 days after stopping test medication. For the intention-to-treat analysis, all events after randomization were counted. The target range of anticoagulation was an international normalized ratio of 2.8 to 4.8 which is equivalent to a prolongation of 1.5 to 2 times control using a typical North-American thromboplastin reagent. An international normalized ratio between 2.5 and 4.8 has been proposed for prevention of arterial thrombosis.[55] Blood was drawn from all patients at the follow-up visits which, after initial stabilization of the prothrombin time, were scheduled every four to six weeks. In the placebo group, the dosage was changed according to preset criteria.

Total mortality was reduced significantly by anticoagulation from 20.2 per cent in the control group to 15.4 per cent in the warfarin group, and so was total reinfarction rate (20.4 per cent versus 13.5 per cent). Nonfatal reinfarction on treatment occurred in 12.3 per cent of the patients in the placebo group compared with 6.2 per cent of those in the warfarin group, a reduction by 49 per cent. An appreciable reduction of 55 per cent in the number of strokes was noted in the warfarin group as compared with the placebo group (7.2 versus 3.2 per cent, $p = 0.0015$). Four fatal intracerebral hemorrhages (one of which occurred more than one year after termination of test medication) occurred in warfarin-treated patients, while no thromboembolic strokes were observed. By contrast, no fatal hemorrhagic strokes and ten fatal thromboembolic strokes were seen in patients taking placebo.

Adequacy of Anticoagulant Control. The importance of adequately applied anticoagulation has been emphasized in a number of reports demonstrating protection against cerebral and systemic thromboembolism in patients with rheumatic heart disease and patients with prosthetic heart valves.[65,66] In a review of al prospective randomized trials to assess the effect of long-term anticoagulation in patients with coronary artery disease, Loeliger convincingly demonstrated a correlation between level and stability of anticoagulation with degree of benefit. The more intensive regimens apparently achieved the better results.[67] Notably, the intensity of treatment achieved in the WARIS trial[64] was more in keeping with recent recommendations for intensity of anticoagulant therapy[55] than that in the Veterans Administration Study,[61] whereas it was comparable with that of the BMRC and Sixty Plus studies.[59,62]

Subgroup Analyses. Subgroup analyses were performed in some trials, but only subgroup data from the WARIS trial were subjected to multivariate analyses, in order to control for confounding factors (unpublished data). Even so, it is prudent to view these data with caution.

One of the striking results of the BMRC trial[59] was the apparently larger reduction in the risk of death and reinfarction among patients under the age of 55 as compared with those who were older. This difference was not observed in the Veterans Administration study, which instead claimed an increased benefit among subjects with a myocardial infarction prior to the qualifying event.[59] Treatment with warfarin, age, diabetes mellitus, and concurrent beta-blockade all explained important differences in the incidence of death in the WARIS trial. Hence, treatment with warfarin and age were recognized as independent prognostic factors for relapsing myocardial infarction. Compared with the overall effects, reduction in mortality was more pronounced in patients having sustained their first infarction than when all patients were analyzed together. Similarly, the reinfarction rate was further reduced by warfarin when considering patients in whom the qualifying infarction was their first, and in nondiabetic subjects. There was a trend favoring younger subjects over elderly in terms of drug efficacy, but the difference did not attain statistical significance. Data from both the BMRC and the Veterans Administration studies suggest that the benefit from oral anticoagulation disappears over time. These findings are contradicted, however, by the results of the Sixty Plus Study (more than six years after the qualifying event and yet the advantage of continuing therapy) and the results of the WARIS study (Fig. 18–5). Figure 18–5 demonstrates that the cumulative reinfarction rates for the two WARIS study groups do not converge during two to five years of follow-up, hence confirming an effect over time. Thus, neither of the two largest and best documented trials support the contention of a decline of benefit after two to three years.

Meta-Analysis. In 1977, Chalmers et al. pooled the data from all randomized trials on oral anticoagulants in the acute phase of myocardial infarction and concluded that treatment with anticoagulants did reduce mortality by about 21 per cent.[68] Reanalysis, using more rigorous statistical methods, supports Chalmers and coworkers' conclusion.[69] In an analysis of seven anticoagulant trials after myocardial infarction, Leizorovicz and Boissel conclude that oral anticoagulation reduces mortality by a statistically significant 28 per cent and relapsing myocardial infarction by 45 per cent.[70] Their analysis included only trials meeting certain criteria, hence an extensive meta-analysis on the efficacy of oral

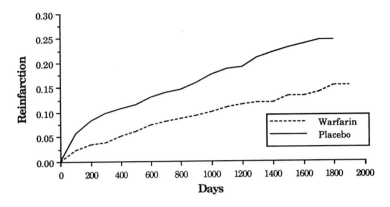

FIGURE 18–5. Cumulative total reinfarction rates (on treatment) in warfarin and control group in the WARIS study.

anticoagulants after myocardial infarction is still pending.

Side Effects. One of the main concerns about oral anticoagulation is the associated risk of bleeding. This risk is clearly related to the intensity of anticoagulation.[71] Table 18–4 contains data on reported bleeding complications in the anticoagulant trials. Similar to the evaluation of side effects pertaining to platelet inhibitory drugs (Table 18–2), this table is also limited to major bleedings. In the BMRC study, major bleeding occurred more frequently in the anticoagulant group (3 versus 0), and one case was fatal.[59] Serious bleedings were also more frequent in the anticoagulated group in the Veterans Administration Study, which noted four fatal events versus none in the control.[61] In the Sixty Plus Study,[62] four deaths were associated with hemorrhage. In the WARIS trial,[63] five patients in the warfarin group suffered an intracranial hemorrhage while on treatment, three of which were fatal (0.16 fatal events per 100 patients per year). Major extracranial bleeding associated with warfarin therapy occurred in eight patients. Minor bleeding, requiring dose adjustment, was observed in 69 patients, 25 of whom were in the placebo group. In seven of the patients with major extracranial bleeding, this was

associated with peptic ulcer, cancer, or forbidden intake of antiplatelet drugs. The low risk of bleeding in the WARIS trial, amounting to a combined incidence of serious bleeding of 0.6 per 100 years at risk, may be due to at least two important factors. First, the prothrombin time reagent used for all controls in the WARIS trial, is extremely sensitive at the therapeutic level. By contrast, a number of North-American thromboplastin reagents have shown less sensitivity to the reduction of vitamin K-dependent clotting factors.[72] Relatively insensitive reagents may lead to overtreatment, and hence increase the risk of bleeding.[73] A second point is that, compared with the Sixty Plus Study, considerably less patients in the WARIS trial exhibited international normalized ratio values exceeding the upper therapeutic limit during follow-up.

Conclusions Pertaining to Oral Anticoagulants. Five anticoagulant studies have been reviewed; one on heparin, and four on oral anticoagulants. For most practical purposes, the orally administered drugs are the most interesting. The two most recently published studies on oral anticoagulation, the Sixty Plus Study and the WARIS trial, fulfill both methodological requirements for modern clinical trials: large sample size, double-

TABLE 18–4. Distribution of Fatal and Serious Nonfatal Bleedings Reported in Studies on Oral Anticoagulants

STUDY	FATAL (%)		NONFATAL (%)		COMBINED (%)	
	Control	Treatment	Control	Treatment	Control	Treatment
BMRC[59]	0	0.5	0.0	8.2	0.0	8.7
VAT[61]	0	1.0	2.8	15.0	2.8	16.0
Sixty Plus[62]	0	1.1	1.1	5.0	1.1	6.1
WARIS[64]	0	0.4	0.0	1.3	0.0	1.7

blind and placebo-controlled design, and analysis according to the intention-to-treat principle. As for yet, the WARIS trial is the only study on any antithrombotic regimen proving efficacy by reduction of total death. However, all studies revealed a statistically significant reduction in relapsing myocardial infarction. The findings of the WARIS trial are supported not only by trends in other anticoagulant trials.[59,61,62] but are also substantiated by analyses on aggregated data.[68–70] Moreover, the effect of anticoagulation was demonstrable even though a vast proportion of the patients received concurrent beta-blockade in both the Sixty Plus Study and the WARIS trial. As seen in Table 18–3, anticoagulant therapy averts 4 to 26 events per 100 patients treated for two to three years. Given the results from the two trials applying the most adequate control,[62,64] avoidance of 10 to 14 events seems to be a realistic gain. With reasonable conduction of the anticoagulant therapy, especially with the use of suitable control methods, the incidence of bleeding may be kept at a low level.

A more frequent use of oral anticoagulants implies questions related to inconvenience and health care resources. The risk of hemorrhage with anticoagulant therapy has resulted in the usual practice of monitoring the level of anticoagulation at monthly intervals. However, available data provide no conclusive evidence that this arbitrarily chosen interval is appropriate for all patients, and longer control intervals have been proposed for suitable patients.[74] Self-monitoring may be a way to reduce costs and inconvenience, and perhaps also to improve patient compliance. To this end, devices for measuring the anticoagulant effect that are affordable, accurate, reliable, and easy to use, are essential. Such instruments are being made and have been successfully tested on a smaller scale in a clinical setting,[75] and even in a randomized clinical trial.[76]

Aspirin versus Anticoagulants

Until now, two studies were a head-to-head comparison of acetylsalicylic acid and oral anticoagulants. Both were designed in an unblinded fashion. In the German-Austrian Myocardial Infarction Study (GAMIS), patients were randomized to treatment with phenprocoumon (n = 320), aspirin (n = 317), or placebo (n = 309).[31] This study was basically a study on aspirin with a matching placebo group, but an open anticoagulant group was also included. Seven centers participated in the study, and patients were enrolled within five to six weeks after the index infarction and allocated to aspirin or matching placebo or a dicoumarin derivative aiming at a prolongation of the prothrombin time from 2.1 to 4.8 in terms of international normalized ratio. No statistically significant difference was detectable between the groups, either for the endpoint mortality, or for reinfarction. However, about 10 per cent in each treatment group were lost for follow-up. The accomplished level of anticoagulation showed that the patients in the anticoagulant group were within the target range for less than 60 per cent of the time. The test medication was withdrawn in 9 patients on aspirin and in 12 on anticoagulants because of bleeding, none of which were fatal. One stroke occurred in each of the actively treated groups.

In the EPSIM Study,[77] which was a multicenter open trial, patients were entered on average 11 days after myocardial infarction, and allocated at random to anticoagulant therapy (n = 651) or aspirin (n = 652). Patients assigned to aspirin received 500 milligrams/day, while those in the anticoagulant group received a dosage of oral anticoagulants aiming for a prothrombin time range from 25 to 35 per cent of normal. Mean follow-up was 29 months. More patients in the aspirin group than in the anticoagulant group were withdrawn during the study (139 versus 82). There were 67 deaths in the anticoagulant group and 72 in those taking aspirin. The rate of reinfarction was higher (n = 32) in the aspirin group than in the anticoagulant group (n = 20), but neither difference was statistically significant. The accomplished level of anticoagulation was not of an intensity compatible with what is now regarded to be optimal.[55] Deaths attributable solely to bleeding occurred in one subject in each study group. There was no apparent difference in the frequency of cerebrovascular diseases, but there were more gastrointestinal events in the aspirin group. A statement by the authors is rather confusing: ". . . the cohort of patients enrolled in the trial was not a representative subset of patients with recent infarction" (adapted from the EPSIM Research Group).

For obvious reasons it is difficult to compare the pharmacotherapeutic potential and safety of drugs as observed in different trials. Even though populations at different risk have been studied, the present data suggest a superiority of anticoagulants compared with antiplatelet drugs, with more deaths and morbidity averted by anticoagulants (Tables 18–1 and 18–3). The presentations based on odds ratios provide no information on the amount of avoided events. Nevertheless, three out of four anticoagulant trials exhibit greater reductions in mortality and reinfarction than all antiplatelet studies (Figs. 18–3 and 18–4). Notably, the 95 per cent confidence interval for the WARIS trial is the only one not to also include the possibility of an adverse effect in terms of mortality. As for the endpoint, myocardial reinfarction, the anticoagulant studies yield confidence intervals that are narrower (and which to a larger extent indicate a benefit) than do the antiplatelet studies. This superiority is plausibly explained by evidence indicating that thrombin is probably the most potent platelet aggregating agent in vivo.[78] As outlined in Tables 18–2 and 18–4, the risk of hemorrhage resulting from antiocoagulant therapy appears to be only slightly increased as compared with the risk of bleeding induced by aspirin.

AGENTS WITH MINOR ANTITHROMBOTIC PROPERTIES

Beta-blockers and Calcium Channel Blockers

The beneficial and protective effects of beta-adrenergic blockers in ischemic heart disease is well documented. Studies have shown that both propranolol and timolol possess platelet antiaggregatory properties.[18,19] Calcium antagonists inhibit platelet aggregation and adenosine triphosphate release, but evidence of a positive benefit has been contradictory. The Danish Verapamil Infarction Trial II[79] recently reported some promising results, but neither the reduction in mortality rate, nor the reduction in risk of reinfarction by verapamil attained statistical significance at a conventional level. Presently, it is not known whether the anti-ischemic effects of beta-blockers and calcium channel blockers are related to platelet inhibitory actions.

Polyunsaturated Fatty acids

Greenland eskimos have an age-adjusted mortality from myocardial infarction that is approximately one tenth that among Danes or North Americans. This difference has been linked to a high daily intake of the long-chain n-3 polyunsaturated fatty acids eicosapentaenoic acid and docosahexaenoic acid that have been found to exhibit antithrombotic and antiatherogenic properties. Both eicosapentaenoic acid and docosahexaenoic acid compete with arachidonic acid in several ways: by inhibition of the synthesis of arachidonic acid and by substituting arachidonic acid as a substrate for the cyclooxygenase, thus limiting the production of thromboxane A_2 by platelets.[80] The net result is a shift toward a more vasodilatory state and toward platelets less prone to aggregate. Recently, a randomized trial on the effect of dietary intervention in the secondary prevention of myocardial infarction reported a significant reduction in death in patients who followed advice to increase fish intake.[81] A disturbing point was that the two-year incidence of reinfarction plus death from ischemic heart disease was not significantly altered by the fish-rich diet, thus contradicting the idea of an antithrombotic action.

FUTURE DIRECTIONS

In consideration of the results of the WARIS trial, aspirin (or another platelet inhibitor) and oral anticoagulants should now be directly compared to establish if there really is a difference in efficacy. For this purpose, a specifically designated trial is urgently needed. Such a trial may also evaluate the risk of bleeding associated with each of the two types of drugs. On the basis of the present limited knowledge, the following questions need to be examined in greater detail:

1. Does long-term anticoagulation retard atherosclerosis?
2. Does anticoagulation aiming at a lower level of intensity suffice in preventing cardiovascular events in the secondary prevention of myocardial infarction?
3. How does aspirin, or other platelet inhibitors, perform against oral anticoagulants in a head-to-head comparison?
4. Does low-dose aspirin (for instance,

150 milligrams/day) combined with oral anticoagulants at a lower level of anticoagulation (for example, an international normalized ratio of 2.0 to 2.5) offer any advantage over either therapy alone in prevention of myocardial infarction, but not at the cost of safety?

CLINICAL IMPLICATIONS AND CONCLUSION

To close this chapter, some remarks on differences between the various types of antithrombotic drugs after myocardial infarction deserve renewed attention. The abrupt conversion from stable ischemic heart disease to unstable angina and the subsequent progression to acute myocardial infarction may result from platelet aggregation, coronary artery spasm, and activation of the clotting cascade at the site of a stenotic coronary lesion. The relative importance of platelets compared with the clotting system in terms of formation of a significant thrombus remain uncertain. Though imperfect, the controlled clinical trial is our most effective tool to evaluate clinical therapy in this setting. The scrutiny of the trials has been made in the perspective of a practicing cardiologist. Thus, not only the type and magnitude of event reduction, but also the problems related to side effects and generalization of the results have been highlighted.

The benefit derived both from platelet inhibitors and anticoagulant drugs is in accord with the theory that there are at least two mechanisms involved in arterial thromboembolism, one of which has a significant coagulation component; the other is largely dependent on platelets. However, little is known of the relative importance of the various thrombogenic mechanisms in coronary thrombosis.

Each patient should, as always in good clinical practice, have an individually tailored therapy after myocardial infarction. Antithrombotic therapy is an adjunct, not an alternative to reduction of conventional risk factors and beta-blockers. Aspirin and oral anticoagulants are presently the options for the majority of cases requiring antithrombotic therapy. Because a conclusive trial comparing aspirin and anticoagulants has not yet been conducted, we do not know if the apparent superiority of anticoagulants is real.

REFERENCES

1. The Norwegian Multicenter Study Group. Timolol-induced reduction in mortality and reinfarction in patients surviving acute myocardial infarction. N Engl J Med 1981; 304: 801–7.
2. Furberg CD. Secondary prevention trials after acute myocardial infarction. Am J Cardiol 1987; 60: 28A–32A.
3. Smith EB, Staples EM, Dietz HS. Role of endothelium in sequestration of lipoprotein and fibrinogen in aortic lesions, thrombi, and graft pseudo-intimas. Lancet 1979; 2: 812–6.
4. Smith EB, Staples EM. Haemostatic factors in human aortic intima. Lancet 1981; 1: 1171–4.
5. DeWood M, Spores J, Notske R, et al. Prevalence of coronary occlusion during the early hours of transmural myocardial infarction. N Engl J Med 1980; 303:897–902.
6. Falk E. Unstable angina with fatal outcome: dynamic coronary thrombosis leading to infarction and/or sudden death. Circulation 1985; 71: 699–708.
7. Fuster V, Badimon L, Cohen M. Ambrose JA, Badimon JJ, Chesebro J. Insights into the pathogenesis of acute isochemic syndromes. Circulation 1988; 77:1213–20.
8. Meade TW, Chakrabarti R, Haines AP, et al. Haemostatic function and cardiovascular death: early results of a prospective study. Lancet 1980; 1: 1050–4.
9. Wilhelmsen L, Svärdsudd K, Korsan-Bengtsen K, Larsson B, Welin L, Tibblin G. Fibrinogen as a risk factor for stroke and myocardial infarction. N Engl J Med 1984; 311: 501–5.
10. Kruskal JB, Commerford PJ, Franks JJ, Kirsch RE. Fibrin and fibrinogen-related antigens in patients with stable and unstable coronary artery disease. N Engl J Med 1987; 317: 1361–5.
11. Stone MC, Thorp JM. Plasma fibrinogen—a major coronary risk factor. J R Coll Gen Pract 1985; 35: 565–9.
12. Kannel WB, Wolf PA, Castelli WP, D'Agostino RB. Fibrinogen and risk of cardiovascular disease. JAMA 1987; 258: 1183–6.
13. Francis RB, Kawanishi D, Baruch T, Mahrer P, Rahimtoola S, Feinstein DL. Impaired fibrinolysis in coronary artery disease. Am Heart J 1988; 115: 776–80.
14. Hamsten A, Walldius G, Szamosi A, et al. Plasminogen activator inhibitor in plasma: risk factor for recurrent myocardial infarction. Lancet 1987; 2: 3–9.
15. Davies MJ, Thomas A. Thrombosis and acute coronary artery lesions in sudden cardiac ischemic death. N Engl J Med 1984; 310: 1137–40.
16. Committee of Principal Investigators. WHO cooperative trial on primary prevention of ischaemic heart disease using clofibrate to lower serum cholesterol: mortality follow-up. Lancet 1980; 2: 379–85.
17. Betablocker Heart Attack Trial Research Group. A randomized trial of propranolol in patients with acute myocardial infarction. JAMA 1982; 247: 1707–14.
18. Weksler BB, Gillick M, Pink J. Effect of propranolol on platelet function. Blood 1977; 49: 185–96.
19. Thaulow E, Kjekshus J, Erikssen J. Effect of timolol on platelet aggregation in coronary heart disease. Acta Med Scand 1982; 651 (suppl): 101–9.
20. Sacks HS, Berrier J, Reitman D, Ancona-Berk VA, Chalmers TC. Meta-analyses of randomized controlled trials. N Engl J Med 1987; 316: 450–5.
21. The Anturane Reinfarction Trial Research Group. Sulfinpyrazone in the prevention of sudden death after myocardial infarction. N Engl J Med 1980; 302: 250–6.
22. Anturan Reinfarction Italian Study. Sulphinpyrazone in post-myocardial infarction. Lancet 1982; 1: 237–42.
23. Temple R, Pledger GW. The FDA's critique of the Anturane Reinfarction Trial. N Engl J Med 1980; 303: 1488–92.
24. Antiplatelet Trialists' Collaboration. Secondary prevention of vascular disease by prolonged antiplatelet treatment. Br Med J 1988; 296: 320–31.
25. Harker LA, Kadatz RA. Mechanism of action of dipyridamole. Thromb Res 1983; suppl IV: 39–46.
26. Gent AE, Brook CGD, Foley TH, Miller TN. Dipyridamole: a controlled trial of its effect in acute myocardial infarction. Br Med J 1968; 4: 366–8.
27. Preston FE, Whipps S, Jackson CA, French AJ, Wyld PJ, Stoddard CJ. Inhibition of prostacyclin and platelet throm-

boxane A$_2$ after low-dose aspirin. N Engl J Med 1981; 304: 76–9.

28. Elwood PC, Cochrane AL, Burr ML, et al. A randomized controlled trial of acetyl salicylic acid in the secondary prevention of mortality from myocardial infarction. Br Med J 1974; 1: 436–40.

29. The Coronary Drug Project Research Group. Aspirin in coronary heart disease. J Chron Dis 1976; 29: 625–42.

30. Elwood PC, Sweetnam PM. Aspirin and secondary mortality after myocardial infarction. Lancet 1979; 2: 1313–5.

31. Breddin K, Loew D, Lechner K, Überla K, Walter E. Secondary prevention of myocardial reinfarction: a comparison of acetylsalicylic acid, placebo and phenprocoumon. Haemostasis 1980; 9: 325–44.

32. Aspirin Myocardial Infarction Study Research Group. A randomized, controlled trial of aspirin in persons recovered from myocardial infarction. JAMA 1980; 243: 661–9.

33. The Persantine-Aspirin Reinfarction Study Research Group. Persantine and aspirin in coronary heart disease. Circulation 1980; 62: 449–61.

34. Klimt CR, Knatterud GL, Stamler J, Meier P. Persantine-aspirin reinfarction study. Part II. Secondary prevention with persantine and aspirin. J Am Coll Cardiol 1986; 7: 251–69.

35. Saltiel E, Ward A. Ticlopidine: a review of its pharmacodynamic and pharmacokinetic properties, and therapeutic efficacy in platelet dependent disease states. Drugs 1987; 34: 222–62.

36. McTavish D, Faulds D, Goa KL. Ticlopidine. An updated review of its pharmacology and therapeutic use in platelet-dependent disorders. Drugs 1990; 40: 238–59.

37. Balsano F, Rizzon P, Violi F, et al. Antiplatelet treatment with ticlopidine in unstable angina. Circulation 1990; 82: 17–26.

38. Herd CM, Rodgers SE, Lloyd JV, Bochner F, Duncan EM, Tunbridge LJ. A dose-ranging study of the antiplatelet effect of enteric coated aspirin in man. Aust NZ J Med 1987; 17: 195–200.

39. Prichard PJ, Kitchingman GK, Walt RP, Daneshmend T, Hawkey CJ. Human gastric mucosal bleeding induced by low dose aspirin, but not warfarin. Br Med J 1989; 298: 493–6.

40. Burch JW, Stanford N, Majerus PW. Inhibition of platelet prostaglandin synthetase by oral aspirin. J Clin Invest 1978; 61: 314–9.

41. Björk I, Lindahl U. Mechanism of the anticoagulant action of heparin. Mol Cell Biochem 1982; 48: 161–82.

42. Arnesen H, Engebretsen LF, Ugland OM, Seljeflot I, Kierulf P. Increased fibrinolytic activity after surgery induced by low dose heparin. Thromb Res 1987; 45: 553–9.

43. O'Brien JR, Shoobridge SM, Finch WJ. Comparison of the effect of heparin and citrate on platelet aggregation. J Clin Pathol 1969; 22: 28–31.

44. Thomson C, Forbes CD, Prentice CRM. The potentiation of platelet aggregation and adhesion by heparin in vitro and in vivo. Clin Sci Mol Med 1973; 45: 485–94.

45. Serneri GGN, Gensini GF, Carnovali M, Rovelli F, Pirelli S, Fortini A. Effectiveness of low-dose heparin in prevention of myocardial reinfarction. Lancet 1987; 1: 937–42.

46. Kelly JG, O'Malley K. Clinical pharmacokinetics of oral anticoagulants. Clin Pharmacokinet 1979; 4: 1–15.

47. Mitchell JRA. Anticoagulants in coronary heart disease—retrospect and prospect. Lancet 1981; I: 257–62.

48. Wright IS, Marple CD, Beck DF. Anticoagulant therapy of coronary thrombosis with myocardial infarction. JAMA 1948; 138: 1074–9.

49. Gifford RH, Feinstein AR. A critique of methodology in studies of anticoagulation for acute myocardial infarction. N Engl J Med 1969; 280: 351–7.

50. Carleton RA, Sanders CA, Burack WR. Heparin administration after acute myocardial infarction. N Engl J Med 1960; 263: 1002–5.

51. Wasserman AJ, Gutterman LA, Yoe KB, Kemp VE, Richardson RW. Anticoagulants in acute myocardial infarction: the failure of anticoagulants to alter mortality in randomized series. Am Heart J 1966; 71: 43–9.

52. International Anticoagulant Review Group. Collaborative analysis of long-term anticoagulant administration after acute myocardial infarction. Lancet 1970; 1: 203–9.

53. Loeliger EA, Hensen A, Kroes F, et al. A double-blind trial

54. Meuwissen OJAT, Vervoorn AC, Cohen O, Jordan FLJ, Nelemans FA. Double blind trial of long-term anticoagulant treatment after myocardial infarction. Acta Med Scand 1969; 186: 361–8.

55. Loeliger EA. The optimal therapeutic range in oral anticoagulation. History and proposal. Thromb Haemost 1979; 42: 1141–52.

56. Weiss HJ, Tschopp TB. Impaired interaction (adhesion-aggregation) of platelets with the subendothelium in storage-pool disease and after aspirin ingestion. N Engl J Med 1975; 293: 619–23.

57. Baumgartner HR, Muggli R, Tschopp TB, Turito VT. Platelet adhesion, release and aggregation in flowing blood: effects of surface properties and platelet function. Thromb Haemost 1976; 35: 124–38.

58. Multicentre International Study. Reduction in mortality after myocardial infarction with long-term betaadrenoceptor blockade. Br Med J 1977; 2: 412–21.

59. British Medical Research Council. An assessment of long-term anticoagulant administration after cardiac infarction. Br Med J 1964; 2: 837–43.

60. Douglas AS, McNicol GP. Anticoagulants after myocardial infarction (letter). Lancet 1981; 1: 717.

61. Ebert RV, Borden CW, Hipp HR, et al. Long-term anticoagulant therapy after myocardial infarction. JAMA 1969; 207: 2263–7.

62. The Sixty Plus Reinfarction Study Research Group. A double-blind trial to assess long-term oral anticoagulant therapy in elderly patients after myocardial infarction. Lancet 1980; 2: 989–93.

63. Poller L, McKernan A, Thomson JM, Elstein M, Hirsch PJ, Jones JB. Fixed minidose warfarin: a new approach to prophylaxis against venous thrombosis after major surgery. Br Med J 1988; 295: 1309–12.

64. Smith P, Arnesen H, Holme I. The effect of warfarin on mortality and reinfarction after myocardial infarction. N Engl J Med 1990; 323: 147–52.

65. Friedli B, Aerichide N, Grondin P, Campeau L. Thromboembolic complication of heart valve prostheses. Am Heart J 1971; 81: 702–8.

66. Björk VO, Henze A. Encapsulation of the Björk-Shiley aortic disc valve prosthesis caused by the lack of anticoagulant treatment. J Thorac Cardiovasc Surg 1973; 7: 17–20.

67. Loeliger EA. Oral anticoagulation in patients surviving myocardial infarction. A new approach to old data. Eur J Clin Pharmacol 1984; 26: 137–9.

68. Chalmers TC, Matta RJ, Smith H, Kunzler A-M. Evidence favoring the use of anticoagulants in the hospital phase of acute myocardial infarction. N Engl J Med 1977; 297: 1091–6.

69. Peto R. Clinical trial methodology. Biomed Pharmacother 1978; 28 (special issue): 24–36.

70. Leizorovicz A, Boissel JP. Oral anticoagulant in patients surviving myocardial infarction. Eur J Clin Pharmacol 1983; 24: 333–6.

71. Landefeld CS, Goldman L. Major bleeding in outpatients treated with warfarin: incidence and prediction by factors known at the start of outpatient therapy. Am J Med 1989; 87: 144–52.

72. Zucker S, Cathey MH, Sox PJ, Hallec EC. Standardization of laboratory tests for controlling anticoagulant therapy. Am J Clin Pathol 1970; 53: 348–54.

73. Hirsh J. Mechanism of action and monitoring of anticoagulants. Semin Thromb Hemost 1986; 12: 1–11.

74. Rospond RM, Quandt CM, Clark GM, Bussey HI. Evaluation of factors associated with stability of anticoagulation therapy. Pharmacotherapy 1989; 9: 207–13.

75. Ansell J, Holden A, Knapic RN. Patient self-management of oral anticoagulation guided by capillary (fingerstick) whole blood prothrombin times. Arch Intern Med 1989; 149: 2509–11.

76. White RH, McCurdy SA, von Marensdorff H, Woodruff DE, Leftgoff L. Home prothrombin time monitoring after the initiation of warfarin therapy. Ann Intern Med 1989; 111: 780–7.

77. The E.P.S.I.M. Research Group. A controlled comparison

of aspirin and oral anticoagulants in prevention of death after myocardial infarction. N Engl J Med 1982; 307: 701–8.

78. Mustard JF, Packham MA. Factors influencing platelet function: adhesion, release and aggregation. Pharmacol Rev 1970; 22: 97–187.

79. The Danish Study Group on Verapamil in Myocardial Infarction. Effect of verapamil on mortality and major events after acute myocardial infarction (DAVIT II). Am J Cardiol 1990; 66: 779–85.

80. Goodnight SH, Harris WS, Connor WE, Illingworth DR. Polyunsaturated fatty acids, hyperlipidemia, and thrombosis. Arteriosclerosis 1982; 2: 87–113.

81. Burr ML, Fehily AM, Gilbert JF, et al. Effects of changes in fat, fish, and fibre intakes on death and myocardial reinfarction: Diet And Reinfarction Trial (DART). Lancet 1989; 2: 757–61.

19

CHRONIC CORONARY DISEASE

JAN J. C. JONKER and JAMES H. CHESEBRO

Sluggish circulation and changes in the quality of blood may produce thrombosis as postulated by Virchow nearly 150 years ago.[1] Zahn described as early as in 1874 the development of thrombosis after injuring a blood vessel wall.[2] Thrombosis and atherosclerosis are closely related in the pathogenesis of coronary artery disease (see Chapter 3).

Coronary thrombi cause acute ischemic events in coronary heart disease and intimately participate in the long-term progression of atherosclerosis and chronic ischemia. Thrombi have a strong tendency to form on atherosclerotic plaques at sites of stenosis, rupture, or hemorrhage, and may lead to acute or chronic narrowing of the lumen and subsequent ischemia. By organization and incorporation of thrombi into the arterial wall, they contribute to the growth of plaques and perpetuation of ischemia. Even small, nonocclusive mural thrombi contribute to stenosis and progression of ischemia by incorporating into the arterial wall. The larger thrombi or thromboemboli may completely obstruct the arterial lumen and produce acute ischemia or subsequent infarction. The pathogenesis of thrombosis (see Chapter 2) and atherosclerosis and thrombosis (see Chapter 3) were discussed in depth and will only be briefly reviewed in this chapter in the context of therapy.

Chronic coronary disease is broadly defined as a state with previous or current clinical manifestations of stable angina pectoris, or angiographically documented coronary disease of at least one coronary artery (more than 20 per cent stenosis) with or without associated symptoms, or the chronic state weeks or months remote from myocardial infarction. It is probably six months after myocardial infarction before the risk of thrombosis with recurrent ischemia or myocardial infarction is decreased to the chronic medium risk of two to five per cent per year or with the stress of noncardiac surgery.[3-5] However, there is a decreasing risk over the first six months after myocardial infarction (especially the second three-month period compared with the first). It is practical to include trials which started in the first few months after myocardial infarction as patients are entering this chronic stage.

STATUS OF CORONARY ARTERIES

There is a wide spectrum of atherosclerosis in patients with chronic coronary disease. Based on patients who present with the acute coronary syndromes of unstable angina or acute myocardial infarction or have worsening symptoms of ischemia and undergo coronary angiography, one third to one half of patients have single-vessel coronary artery disease (50 per cent or more stenosis) and the remainder approximately equally divided between two- or three-vessel disease; 5 to 8 per cent have left main coronary disease.[6-8]

Nearly all patients have dysfunctional (but anatomically intact, type I injury) endothelium with small focal spots of mildly injured (type II or subendothelial injury) endothelium.[9-13] This allows focal platelet or white cell deposition as documented by scanning electron microscopy.[13,14] Variable degrees of lipid incorporation are present in the arterial wall at extracellular (often bound to glycosaminoglycans) or intracellular (foam cells derived from macrophages or smooth muscle cells) locations. The most critical lipid accumulations related to thrombotic risk are focal pools of lipid covered by a fibrous cap which contains monocytes (see Chapter 3).[15] There appears to be enzymatic degradation of collagen in the fibrous cap to a thin and weakened latticework which may eventually rupture.

Plaque rupture leads to mural thrombosis or arterial occlusion and the conversion of chronic coronary disease to the acute coronary syndromes of unstable angina, myocardial infarction, or sudden death (see Chapter 2).[13-19] Only about one quarter of acute ischemic events appear to be associated with mild injury and a focal hour-glass stenosis with a platelet aggregate which is usually in a distal or branch coronary artery.[15] Three quarters of acute ischemic events appear to be associated with plaque rupture and a firmly anchored mural thrombus.

Arterial substrates increase thrombogenicity of this deep injury and make it difficult to treat. These substrates include tissue thromboplastin, collagen types I and III, glycosylated collagen in diabetes, lipids, lack of prostacyclin and endothelium-derived relaxing factor (both potent platelet-inhibitors), and increased thrombin content with binding to arterial wall matrix.[19-23] Experimental studies show that aspirin reduces the incidence of mural thrombosis by approximately 50 per cent and heparin will do the same at high doses.[24,25] Arterial thrombosis after deep injury is highly thrombin dependent, since specific thrombin inhibition totally prevents mural thrombosis in vivo and limits platelet deposition to a single layer.[25,26] In addition, it takes five times higher dose of thrombin inhibition to prevent platelet thrombi than fibrin thrombi in the absence of arterial injury in the rat.[27]

The rheology of blood flow (see Chapter 2) is also altered by coronary disease with both diffuse narrowing, discrete stenoses, or dilation (uncommon in coronary arteries). With narrowing, increased shear forces (related directly to velocity of blood flow and inversely to the third power of the diameter) cause red cells to force platelets to the periphery, increase platelet deposition, and increase cellular surface adenosine diphosphate. Aneurysmal dilation of arteries reduces shear force, leads to stasis of blood flow, more fibrin than platelet deposition,

and is best treated with anticoagulation. Platelet deposition is greatest in the minimal lumen diameter of the stenosis where there is often a "whitish" thrombus. Distal to this there is stasis and thus often a "reddish," fibrin-rich thrombus.

These experimental observations are consistent with clinical observations of coronary thrombosis made in the first half of this century.[28-32] There is a chronic risk of acute myocardial infarction of 2 to 5 per cent per year and a gradation of risk depending on the number and severity of risk factors.[3] The clinical risk factors for coronary artery disease are also consistent with the arterial substrates and systemic factors which increase the risk of arterial thrombosis (see Chapter 2).[5,20,21] Risk of clinical thrombotic events may be decreased by reducing these risk factors (such as decreasing low-density lipoprotein cholesterol and increasing high-density lipoprotein cholesterol to prevent plaque rupture and the conversion of chronic mild disease to plaque rupture and acute coronary events.[33-36]

MODIFICATION AND INHIBITION OF THROMBUS FORMATION

During platelet activation and fibrin formation, four endogenous mechanisms may limit thrombosis (see also Chapter 1). The *first* mechanism is prostacyclin, the potent inhibitor of platelet aggregation, formed in the vascular wall and present on the endothelial surface. It is formed either from prostaglandin G_2 or arachidonic acid by the action of prostacyclin synthetase. The release of prostacyclin into the vascular lumen depends primarily on the integrity of the endothelium.[37] Prostacyclin synthesis is increased by pulsatility of flow, increased shear stress, hypoxia, vasoactive mediators such as bradykinin, angiotensin and histamine, and high-density lipoproteins. Conversely, increased lipid peroxidases, low-density lipoprotein, and atherosclerotic lesions are associated with a decreased production of prostacyclin by vascular tissue. In addition, both nicotine and cigarette smoking itself inhibit prostacyclin production and augment platelet reactivity. Prostacyclin stimulates adenyl cyclase which increases cyclic adenosine monophosphate and thus inhibits both platelet secretion and aggregation.[38] Its concentration depends on the activity of adenyl cyclase and phosphodiesterase. Thromboxane A_2 has opposite biologic effects.

The *second* mechanism is the action of antithrombin III. A proteolytic enzyme inhibitor was described in 1895.[39] Brinkhous described antithrombin III in 1939,[40] and in 1973 it was purified and further characterized by Rosenberg and co-workers.[41] Antithrombin III prevents the escape of thrombin into the circulation by forming thrombin–antithrombin III complexes (on the endothelium and in circulating blood) and also inhibits activated factors, IX, X, XI, and XII.[42] Its action is markedly enhanced by heparin, which complexes with antithrombin III.[43] Although antithrombin III binds tightly, it acts slowly, accesses activated factors within thrombus or bound to membranes, and is limited by natural inhibitors such as fibrin II monomer and platelet factor 4.

The *third* mechanism is protein C, a vitamin K-dependent protease. It is activated by the binding of thrombin with thrombomodulin on the endothelial cell.[44] The activated form together with its cofactor protein S is a powerful inhibitor of activated factor V and factor VIII, and thus a potent endogenous anticoagulant.[45] Activated protein C is not inhibited by heparin and antithrombin III. It is an experimental stimulator of fibrinolysis by activating plasminogen and neutralizing a circulating inhibitor of tissue plasminogen activator.[46]

The *fourth* mechanism is the fibrinolytic system, which activates plasminogen to plasmin and hydrolyzes fibrin into soluble fragments.[47] It also degrades fibrinogen, and factors V, VIII, and II. The proteolytic activity of plasmin occurs at the fibrin and endothelial surfaces and may spill out into the plasma as alpha$_2$-antiplasmin is depleted. When fibrin degradation is almost completed, plasmin itself is rapidly inactivated by alpha$_2$-plasmin inhibitor. A specific plasminogen activator inhibitor (PAI-I) has been identified in human platelets and in the extracellular matrix of cultured endothelial cells,[48] has been characterized,[49] and probably is critical in the resistance to lysis of compared to venous thrombi.[50]

HEMODYNAMIC FACTORS IN CORONARY THROMBOSIS

In the coronary circulation, unique conditions exist that may predispose to thrombosis, when compared with other arterial systems. During systole there is minimal flow in the coronary arteries. The pulsating heart may interrupt flow at every cycle and alter flow by angulation of the arteries. The proximal left anterior descending coronary artery is the "artery of death" or the site where thrombotic occlusion occurs most frequently.[51] A raised plaque may cause local flow disturbances, increasing the shear stress at the site of the luminal obstruction. The high shear stress at the plaque external surface, decreased tensile strength of the fibrous cap, and the sudden decrease in pressure distal to a stenosis may cause collapse and possibly disruption of a soft plaque.[15-19] The fibrous cap is often very thin and heavily infiltrated with foam cells, indicating erosion of the cap from within. A thin cap is very fragile and may rupture even with normal hemodynamic stress such as bending and twisting of the arteries, which occurs during every heartbeat. In addition, changes in distending pressure (for example, pulsating variations of blood flow) and changes in vascular tone can cause disruption of the fragile plaque.[15-18] Rupture of the plaque may be considered a random event in the evolution and growth of the atherosclerotic lesions, and may occur when the cap is so attenuated that even normal hemodynamic stress disrupts it.

There is a marked circadian variation in the frequency of the onset of acute coronary events, with the largest number of events beginning between 6 AM and noon.[52-54] A possible explanation is that a hypercoagulable state occurs after arising from sleep and interacts with an arterial atherosclerotic plaque to produce arterial thrombosis. There is an enhanced platelet aggregability in the early morning[55] and a circadian rhythm in fibrinolytic activity (low in the morning and high in the afternoon).[56,57] An increase in the activity of the sympathetic nervous system in the presence of atherosclerotic plaques may also contribute to the circadian rhythm of intracoronary thrombosis and platelet aggregation. The activity of the sympathetic nervous system is increased after arising. Heart rate, mean arterial pressure, and norepinephrine levels are all at a minimum at approximately 6 AM and rise sharply to maximum levels at 9 AM. In addition, the low level of plasma norepinephrine that occurs during sleep is associated with upregulation of beta-adrenergic receptors. Thus, on awakening, the upward surge of catecholamine levels may combine with a transient period of increased responsiveness of receptors.

First, increased activity of the sympathetic nervous system may increase platelet aggregability[53] and combine with a hypercoagulable state to lead to arterial thrombosis. Second, the rapidly rising blood pressure and heart rate in the morning may produce disruption of plaques with arterial thrombosis. Third, an increase in tone of the coronary arteries in the morning has been demonstrated.[58] In the presence of coronary atherosclerosis, such an increase in tone may decrease flow with subsequent promotion of arterial thrombosis. It is likely that interaction of all three processes occurs. In addition, disturbances of coronary vasomotion frequently occur at sites of atherosclerotic stenosis.[59]

A large number of arterial dilators, including muscarinic cholinergic agonists such as acetylcholine, relax blood vessels indirectly by stimulating the release of an endothelium-derived relaxing factor.[12,60] It has been shown that when the endothelium is removed, the release of the endothelium-derived relaxing factor is lost and the normal vasodilator response to acetylcholine is instead replaced by a paradoxical vasoconstriction resulting from the direct effects of acetylcholine on vascular smooth muscle cells. Progressive narrowing of all prestenotic, stenotic, and poststenotic coronary segments was observed in response to stepwise infusions of acetylcholine in vessels with advanced stenosis, leading to transient complete vessel occlusion in the majority of the patients.[10] Without preexistent stenosis there is usually no significant thrombosis in the absence of plaque rupture or deep injury.[61] Approximately 80 per cent of coronary thrombi have a layered structure indicating an episodic growth by repeated mural deposits.[19] A ruptured plaque is found underneath in more than 80 per cent of coronary thrombi.[15,17-19] During the evolution of a coronary thrombus, episodic growth appears to alternate with thrombus disintegration and peripheral embolization as seen by the frequent finding of small fragments of thrombus material impacted in intramyocardial arteries downstream to evolving coronary thrombi, often associated with microinfarcts.[17-19] It is likely that platelet aggregates or the freely floating thrombus that forms poststenotically has a high potential to embolize. Therefore, arterial thrombus during formation within and distal to a ruptured plaque may be in dynamic change in which the thrombus waxes and wanes in size

over hours and even days.[62,63] The difference between stable and unstable angina pectoris seems to be qualitative with intact versus disrupted plaque surface. The severity of stenosis seems to be a powerful predictor for the natural progression to thrombotic occlusion. However, progression to total occlusion is more often asymptomatic than a clinical event and results in myocardial infarction in less than one in five patients.[34,64]

CORONARY THROMBOSIS AND CARDIAC ISCHEMIA

The concept that coronary thrombosis is the primary cause of obstruction, with subsequent myocardial ischemia or infarction, is now widely accepted. Blood flowing through a vessel is not only suddenly accelerated as it passes through an area of stenosis, but it is also immediately decelerated distal to the stenosis. This acceleration of blood flow induces flow separations and recirculation zones (vortices) downstream from the stenosis. The combination of a higher shear rate area at the stenosis activating predominantly platelets and the low shear rate area beyond the stenosis (recirculation zones) leading to deposition of fibrin, contributes to the "head" of the fixed thrombus being composed mainly of platelets and the "tail" containing larger amounts of fibrin in a meshwork, which traps a large number of red cells (see Chapter 2).

Patients with coronary artery disease may have an increased whole blood viscosity,[65] increased plasma viscosity,[66] and elevated fibrinogen levels.[67] Fibrinogen is the major plasma determinant of blood viscosity and of red cell aggregation. The mechanism responsible for the elevation of fibrinogen in patients with coronary artery disease remains uncertain. Increased biosynthesis and turnover of this protein have been implicated.[68] Fibrinogen and factor VII are recognized as major independent risk factors for coronary disease.[67,69,70] The convective transport of relevant solutes is influenced by the rheology of blood flow. Increased aggregation of red cells and increased blood viscosity reduce the rate of convective movement. Areas of low oxygen tension or concentrated procoagulants would also have increased blood viscosity, particularly in regions of low or disturbed flow distal to a stenosis. A more recent study demonstrated that the presence of fibrinogen, fibrin, and their degradation products may be present in advanced atherosclerotic lesions with stenosis.[71] Thus recurrent episodes of plaque disruption and thrombosis may lead to progressive stenosis of coronary arteries. Acute ischemic episodes may be the consequence of larger plaque fissures, larger thrombi, or thrombotic processes out of control.

The degree, suddenness, and duration of progression of the thrombotic process, the surface area of deep injury, substrates in the arterial wall, and the size of the involved vessel determine the presence and nature of the clinical event. The prevalence of these processes are unknown. They have important clinical significance for prevention of thrombotic episodes and progression of atherosclerosis by reducing modifiable risk factors and designing new therapy.

MYOCARDIAL INFARCTION AND PROGRESSION OF DISEASE

The risk of a myocardial infarction is not related to the severity of the underlying coronary disease. In a five-year prospective angiographic study of patients with known coronary disease followed for five years, asymptomatic total occlusions of coronary arteries usually involved more severely stenosed arteries (56 per cent of patients who developed silent total occlusions had a stenosis more than 75 per cent). Of all the patients who developed a total occlusion of a coronary artery, only 17 per cent developed a myocardial infarction, probably because of preexisting collateral flow associated with the high-grade baseline lesion. However, in patients who developed myocardial infarction, 85 per cent had a preexisting lesion with less than 75 per cent stenosis, and more than half had a stenosis less than 50 per cent.[34] This is consistent with retrospective angiographic studies that also showed that more than half of patients who developed myocardial infarction had a preexisting lesion of the infarct-related artery with less than 50 per cent stenosis.[35,36] Thus with so many minor lesions antedating plaque rupture and myocardial infarction, exercise testing will not necessarily predict patients prone to myocardial infarction. These clinical observations are consistent with the underlying pathophysiology of plaque rupture and thrombosis (see Chapters 2 and 3).[15-19]

The major mechanism of coronary disease progression appears to be repeat rupture of coronary artery plaques.[15] Thus reduction of risk factors which lead to plaque rupture are capable of reducing both coronary event rates and progression of coronary artery disease.[33]

Based on the high thrombogenicity of the local arterial substrates, systemic factors favoring thrombosis, and the rheology of blood flow, prophylactic treatment of thrombosis after plaque rupture may reduce acute coronary events such as myocardial infarction, but will probably not be able to prevent asymptomatic mural thrombosis and the slower growth of lesions by smaller rupture of plaques.

ANTITHROMBOTIC THERAPY IN CHRONIC CORONARY ARTERY DISEASE

Our attention is focused on patients with low to medium risk for experiencing acute thrombotic phases that lead to acute clinical events. It has been advocated that therapy for a patient with coronary artery disease is not satisfactory if the physician attempts to treat only anginal episodes, but that the goal should be the total eradication of all ischemic episodes instead and therefore the elimination of the total ischemic burden. Although this goal may be conceivably valid, its pursuit may result in more harm than good. The first concern is that if medical therapy is pursued beyond the point of eliminating symptomatic episodes of ischemia, the medications required may lead to adverse side effects that may have a deleterious impact on the quality of life and perhaps even on survival. Thus, attention should focus on the risk-to-benefit ratio of therapeutic strategies.

It should also be emphasized that in chronic coronary artery disease with stable angina pectoris, the role of platelet activation and thrombin generation is usually not detectable with conventional laboratory examinations.[72-75] Even pacing and exercise-induced ischemia could not significantly activate the coagulation system.[73,74] However, after induction of coronary spasm by injected acetylcholine, fibrinopeptide A is released in the circulation while beta-thromboglobulin levels remained unchanged, indicating no detectable activation of platelets, but rather an activation of the coagulation system.[76] The important contributions of modifying risk factors and their effects on the progression of atherosclerosis are beyond the scope of this chapter. The incidence of coronary heart disease and mortality can be favorably reduced by lowering cholesterol.[77] Greater reduction of risk and even regression of coronary atherosclerosis are possible by also raising high-density lipoprotein cholesterol.[33]

If the platelet–vessel wall interaction plays a dominant role in atherogenesis, then inhibition of platelet adhesion may be beneficial in preventing or inhibiting progression of atherosclerosis. Unfortunately, no drug with this property is currently available. Even if platelet adhesion could be completely prevented, the ultimate risk of bleeding would prohibit its long-term use.

Secondary Prevention after Myocardial Infarction

During the first year after myocardial infarction, approximately 10 per cent of patients die. Factors contributing to this mortality include recurrent ischemia, rethrombosis, ventricular arrhythmias, and left ventricular dysfunction. The incidence of death and recurrent myocardial infarction is lower six months to one year after myocardial infarction. Thereafter the early incidence of myocardial infarction is approximately 2 to 5 per cent per year. The incidence of death is mainly dependent upon left ventricular function. Following thrombolysis, mortality may be very low, in part due to selection of patients with good left ventricular function, but there do appear to be advantages of maintaining patency of the infarct-related artery.[3–5,78–80] There have been nine trials of platelet inhibitor therapy after myocardial infarction; seven using aspirin with or without dipyridamole, and two using sulfinpyrazone. These are summarized in Table 19–1.

In the first Medical Research Council (MRC-I) Trial, 1,239 men were randomized to aspirin (300 milligrams/day) or placebo by Elwood et al.[81] Although patients treated with aspirin had a lower mortality by 24 per cent, this was not statistically significant. In patients entered within six weeks of infarction, mortality was reduced by 41 per cent.

In the Coronary Drug Project Aspirin Study (CDP), 1,529 male patients were randomized five years or more after infarction to aspirin 325 milligrams three times per day

or placebo.[82] There was a 30 per cent reduction in mortality (not statistically significant) after 22 months of follow-up.

In the German-Austrian Reinfarction Study (GARS), 946 patients were randomized slightly more than a month after infarction to aspirin 500 milligrams three times daily, oral anticoagulation, or placebo.[83] Although patients treated with aspirin had a 40 per cent lower incidence of cardiac death and coronary events (not statistically significant), there was no difference in total mortality between the three groups.

In the second Medical Research Council Trial (MRC-II), 1,682 patients were randomized a mean of one week after infarction to aspirin 300 milligrams three times daily or placebo.[84] The primary endpoint was total mortality. Although the aspirin group had a 17 per cent reduction in total mortality at one year, this was not significantly different. In the aspirin group, there was a 28 per cent reduction in cardiac death plus nonfatal reinfarction ($p < 0.05$).

In the Aspirin After Myocardial Infarction Study (AMIS), the largest individual study, 4,525 patients were randomized to aspirin 500 milligrams twice daily or placebo a mean of 25 months after infarction and followed-up for three years.[85] The endpoints were total and coronary mortality, myocardial infarction, and stroke; these were not significantly different between groups. Although reinfarction was slightly lower, and total and coronary mortality slightly higher in the aspirin group, patients in the aspirin group had a greater number of cardiac risk factors which may have accounted for these trends.

In the first Persantine-Aspirin Reinfarction Study (PARIS-I), 2,206 patients were randomized to aspirin 325 milligrams three times per day, aspirin plus dipyridamole (75 milligrams three times daily), or placebo a mean of 20 months after infarction. The endpoints were total and coronary mortality and coronary incidence which was 20 to 25 per cent lower in the treated groups at 41 months of follow-up, but this was not statistically significant. Aspirin alone was as effective as aspirin plus dipyridamole. Patients entered within six months of infarction derived the greatest benefit from therapy with a 50 per cent reduction in event rate.[86]

In the second Persantin-Aspirin Reinfarction Study (PARIS-II), 3,128 patients were randomized within four months of infarction to aspirin plus dipyridamole (325 milligrams

TABLE 19–1. Randomized Trials of Platelet Inhibitors for Secondary Prevention of Myocardial Infarction

			REDUCTION IN EVENT RATE WITH THERAPY (%)		
TRIAL	PATIENTS	DRUG (MILLIGRAMS/DAY)	Total Mortality	Cardiac Mortality	Coronary Events
MRC-I[81]	1,239	Aspirin (300)	24	NA	NA
CDP[82]	1,529	Aspirin (972)	30	28	22
GARS[83]	626	Aspirin (1,500)	18	42	37
MRC-II[84]	1,682	Aspirin (900)	17	22	28*
AMIS[85]	4,524	Aspirin (1,000)	(−10)	(−8)	5
PARIS-I[86]	2,206	Aspirin (972)	18	21	24
		Aspirin (972) + dipyridamole (225)	16	24	25
PARIS-II[86]	3,128	Aspirin (990) + dipyridamole (225)	3	6	24*
ART[88,89]	1,558	Sulfinpyrazone (800)	28†	24†	NA
ARIS[90]	727	Sulfinpyrazone (800)	5	5	56‡

* $p < 0.05$.
† Lower total and cardiac mortality are due to a marked reduction in early sudden death.
‡ $p < 0.01$.
AMIS = Aspirin Myocardial Infarction Study; ARIS = Anturane Reinfarction Italian Study; ART = Anturane Reinfarction Trial; CDP = Coronary Drug Project; GARS = German-Austrian Reinfarction Study; MRC-1 = Medical Research Council (1974); MRC-II = Medical Research Council (1979); NA = not available; PARIS-I = Persantine-Aspirin Reinfarction Study (1980); PARIS-II = Persantine-Aspirin Reinfarction Study (1986).

and 75 milligrams, three times per day, respectively) or placebo and followed for 23 months.[87] Although cardiac mortality was 20 per cent lower in treated patients at one year, there was only a 6 per cent reduction at the end of the study at a mean of 23 months. However, coronary incidence (death plus nonfatal reinfarction) and nonfatal reinfarction alone were significantly reduced by 24 and 36 per cent, respectively ($p < 0.05$). The greatest benefit appeared in patients with a non-Q wave infarction where aspirin plus dipyridamole reduced the coronary incidence by 51 per cent. Thus, patients with the highest risk of recurrent ischemia derived the greatest benefit.

In the Anturane Reinfarction Trial (ART), 1,558 patients were randomized a mean of one month after infarction to sulfinpyrazone 200 milligrams four times per day or placebo.[88] After reanalysis because of initial incomplete analysis of fatalities, a revised report showed 24 per cent fewer cardiac deaths in the treated group, but this was not statistically significant.[89] In those who had sudden cardiac death, this modus was reduced by 57 per cent in the treated group ($p = 0.02$).

In the Anturane Reinfarction Italian Study (ARIS), 727 patients were randomized a mean of two weeks after infarction to sulfinpyrazone 400 milligrams two times daily or placebo and followed for a mean of 19 months.[90] Although there was a significant reduction in reinfarction by 56 per cent ($p < 0.01$), there was no difference in cardiac mortality or sudden death. We find that sulfinpyrazone (as opposed to aspirin) does not significantly reduce quantitative platelet deposition or mural thrombosis after acute arterial injury by balloon dilatation (biologic tissue as substrate).[91] Nor does it reduce reinfarction or mortality in patients with unstable angina (another arterial thrombotic problem).[92] Thus sulfinpyrazone is not a consistently effective antithrombotic agent in arterial disease and injury.

Because of limited size and length of follow-up, no single study provided clear direction for therapy. Thus pooling data from properly executed randomized trials may provide better guidance. Meta-analysis of randomized trials in cardiovascular and cerebrovascular disease has been reported and included more than 18,000 patients treated with platelet inhibitor therapy after myocardial infarction.[93] With platelet inhibitor therapy there was a reduction in nonfatal reinfarction by 31 per cent, cardiovascular mortality by 13 per cent, nonfatal stroke by 42 per cent, and vascular events (infarction, stroke, and death) by 25 per cent. All aspirin-containing therapies with or without dipyridamole were effective.

There are five large randomized controlled trials using anticoagulants after myocardial infarction. Four trials entered patients soon after myocardial infarction and followed them for several years.[94–98] Only one trial showed a significant reduction in mortality.[98] In the Medical Research Council Study, anticoagulant therapy reduced reinfarction by 60 per cent. The Sixty Plus Reinfarction Study[96] has a unique design. Patients over age 60 who had been on anticoagulant therapy for a median of six years after infarction were randomized to continuation of this therapy or placebo. After two years of follow-up, those continuing anticoagulation had a 26 per cent lower death rate ($p = 0.07$) and a large reduction of 55 per cent in the incidence of reinfarction ($p = 0.0005$). The applicability of this trial to the general population of general coronary artery disease has been questioned because of the selection of patients from a group who may have been dependent on chronic anticoagulation.

In the EPSIM (Enquepe de Prevention Secondaire de l'Infarctus du Myocarde) Trial,[97] anticoagulant therapy was compared with aspirin without any control group in patients after myocardial infarction. After follow-up for 29 months there was no significant difference in the incidence of reinfarction or total and cardiac mortality.

In the recently reported Warfarin Re-Infarction Study (WARIS) Study,[92] 1,214 patients age 75 or less were randomized four weeks after myocardial infarction to warfarin (international normalized ratio 2.8 to 4.8) or placebo and followed for a mean of 37 months. Total mortality was significantly reduced by 24 per cent from 20 per cent in the placebo to 15 per cent in the warfarin group (95 per cent confidence interval 4 to 44 per cent, $p = 0.027$). Recurrent myocardial infarction (either fatal or nonfatal) was significantly reduced by 34 per cent from 20 per cent in the placebo to 14 per cent in the warfarin group (95 per cent confidence interval 19 to 54 per cent, $p = 0.0007$). Cerebrovascular accidents (hemorrhagic and nonhemorrhagic were also significantly reduced by 55 per cent, from 7.2 per cent in the placebo to 3.3 per cent in the warfarin group ($p = 0.0015$). Serious bleeding occurred in 0.6 per cent warfarin treated patients per year. (See also Chapter 19.)

Stable Angina

Disruption of minor atherosclerotic plaques in coronary arteries with variable mural thrombosis, with or without clinical symptoms, appears to be the major mechanism of progression of coronary artery disease.[99]

Antiplatelet therapy with oral aspirin and dipyridamole in pigs fed a 2 per cent cholesterol diet for six months significantly reduced the proportion of pigs with more than 10 per cent atherosclerotic plaque in the aorta from 8/11 (73 per cent) of pigs in the control group to 1/7 (14 per cent) of pigs taking aspirin (15 milligrams/kilogram/day) and dipyridamole (6 milligrams/kilogram/day). Likewise, the mean surface area of plaque in the aorta was reduced from 18 per cent of the aortic surface in the control group to 8 per cent ($p < 0.05$) in the platelet inhibitor group. Later we found that pigs do not absorb oral dipyridamole and therefore that all of the effects were due to aspirin. Pigs with von Willebrand's disease had even less plaque (1/7 or 14 per cent of pigs had significant aortic plaque, and plaque involved only 3 per cent of the aortic surface, $p < 0.01$).[100]

Thus the effect of aspirin (975 milligrams/day) plus dipyridamole (225 milligrams/day) on angiographic coronary disease progression and cardiovascular endpoints was assessed in a five-year, prospective, randomized, double-blind, placebo trial with 373 patients with low-risk (mean ejection fraction 59 per cent), medically treated coronary artery disease.[101] The groups were well matched for baseline criteria. Two angiograms were performed in 296 patients (80 per cent), 4.6 ± 0.1 years apart, and reviewed blindly by two panels of two angiographers with discrepancies resolved by third panel.

There were fewer myocardial infarcts in treated (4 per cent) compared with placebo patients (12 per cent, $p = 0.007$). New coronary lesions (mean stenosis 45 per cent) were reduced to involve 21 per cent of treated patients compared with 30 per cent of placebo patients ($p = 0.06$). Using Brensike criteria, there was no treatment effect on definite lesion progression (41 per cent of treated versus 39 per cent of placebo patients), probable progression (11 per cent of treated versus 13 per cent of placebo patients), mixed progression/regression (21 per cent of treated versus 28 per cent of placebo patients), no change (16 per cent of treated versus 19 per cent of placebo patients), probable regression (5 per cent of treated versus 0 per cent of placebo patients, or a definite regression (4 per cent of treated versus 2 per cent of placebo patients). There was no difference in total mortality (6 per cent in each group) or cardiac death (4 per cent in each group). Stroke or transient cerebral ischemia was significantly reduced from 4 per cent in the placebo to 0 per cent in the treated ($p = 0.007$).

Thus platelet inhibitor therapy reduced myocardial infarction and stroke or transient ischemic attack and appears to lessen new lesion formation but does not prevent progression of coronary artery disease in patients with preexisting coronary lesions.[101]

Approximately two thirds of patients have angiographic progression of coronary disease over five years. Plasma total cholesterol correlated poorly with angiographic disease progression. The strongest negative predictor of progression of coronary disease was apolipoprotein A_1/total cholesterol, followed by high-density lipoprotein/total cholesterol ratio.[101,102]

Dipyridamole alone does not significantly reduce platelet deposition or mural thrombosis in pigs after acute arterial injury. Similarly, low-dose aspirin alone (1 milligram/kilogram/day) is as effective as aspirin plus dipyridamole in pigs.[91] Aspirin alone is as effective as combined aspirin plus dipyridamole in preventing aortocoronary vein graft occlusion (see Chapter 20) and in reducing recurrent infarction after the initial myocardial infarction as previously discussed. Thus the addition of dipyridamole to aspirin therapy does not appear to be necessary.

The current recommendation for therapy is aspirin at 80 to 325 milligrams/day for patients with stable coronary artery disease and after myocardial infarction. Warfarin appears to be at least equally effective after myocardial infarction (see Chapter 18). However, a trial of combined warfarin plus low-dose aspirin compared with either therapy alone is needed. Improved strategies for preventing progression of preexisting coronary lesions are needed and may center on therapies for lowering low-density lipoprotein cholesterol plus raising high-density lipoprotein cholesterol,[33] longer-term specific thrombin inhibition,[25,26,99] or both.

REFERENCES

1. Virchow R. Gesammelte Abhandlungen zur wissenschaftlichen medium, IV. Thrombose und Embolie, Veränderungen des Thrombosis. Frankfurt a.M., 1855: 323.

2. Zahn FW. Untersuchungen über Thrombose. Virchows Arch F Path Anat 1874; 62: 82.

3. Kannel WB, Wolf PA, Garrison RJ. Survival following initial cardiovascular events. Framingham Study, Section 35. U.S. Department of Health and Human Services, National Institutes of Health. U.S. Department of Commerce. National Technical Information Center. Publication No. PB 88-204029, 1988.

4. Steen TA, Tinker JH, Tarhan S. Myocardial reinfarction after anesthesia and surgery. JAMA 1978; 239: 2366–70.

5. Caselli WP, Garrison RJ, Wilson PWF, Abbott RD, Kalousdian S, Cannel WB. Incidence of coronary heart disease and lipoprotein cholesterol levels: Framingham Study. JAMA 1986; 256: 2835–8.

6. Fuster V, Frye RL, Connolly DC, Danielson MA, Elveback LR, Kurland LT. Arteriographic patterns early in the onset of coronary syndromes. Br Heart J 1975; 37: 1250–5.

7. Chesebro JH, Knatterud G, Roberts R, et al. Thrombolysis in Myocardial Infarction (TIMI) Trial, Phase I: a comparison between intravenous tissue plasminogen activator and intravenous streptokinase: clinical finding through hospital discharge. Circulation 1987; 76: 142–54.

8. TIMI Study Group. Comparison of invasive and conservative strategies after treatment with intravenous tissue plasminogen activator in acute myocardial infarction. N Engl J Med 1989; 320: 618–27.

9. Ip JH, Fuster V, Badimon L, Badimon J, Taubman MB, Chesebro JH. Syndromes of accelerated atherosclerosis: Role of vascular injury and smooth muscle cell proliferation. J Am Coll Cardiol 1990; 15: 1667–87.

10. Ludmer PL, Selwijn AP, Shook TL, et al. Paradoxical vasoconstriction induced by acetylcholine in atherosclerotic coronary arteries. N Engl J Med 1986; 315: 1046–51.

11. Zeiher AM, Drexler H, Wollschlaeger H, Saurbier B, Just H. Coronary vasomotion in response to sympathetic stimulation in humans: importance of the functional integrity of the endothelium. J Am Coll Cardiol 1989; 14: 1181–90.

12. Furchgott RF, Zawadski JV. The obligatory role of endothelial cells in the relaxation of arterial smooth muscle by acetylcholine. Nature 1980; 288: 373–6.

13. Davies MJ, Woolf N, Rowles PM, Peper J. Morphology of the endothelium over atherosclerotic plaques in human coronary arteries. Br Heart J 1988; 60: 459–64.

14. Ross R. The pathogenesis of atherosclerosis—an update. N Engl J Med 1986; 314(8): 488–500.

15. Davies MJ. A macro and micro view of coronary vascular insult in ischemic heart disease. Circulation 1990; 82(suppl II): II-38–46.

16. Fuster V, Stein B, Ambrose JA, Badimon L, Badimon JJ, Chesebro JH. Atherosclerotic plaque rupture and thrombosis: evolving concepts. Circulation 1990; 82(suppl II): II-47–59.

17. Davies NJ, Thomas AC. Plaque fissuring—the cause of myocardial infarction, sudden ischaemic death, and cresendo angina. Br Heart J 1985; 53: 363–73.

18. Falk E. Morphologic feature of unstable atherothrombotic plaques underlying acute coronary syndromes. Am J Cardiol 1989; 63: 114E–20E.

19. Falk E. Unstable angina with fatal outcome: dynamic coronary thrombosis leading to infarct and/or sudden death. Autopsy evidence of recurrent mural thrombosis with peripheral embolization culminating in total vascular occlusion. Circulation 1985; 71: 699–708.

20. Chesebro JH, Zoldhelyi P, Fuster V. Pathogenesis of thrombosis in unstable angina. Am J Cardiol 1991, (in press).

21. Fuster V, Badimon L, Cohen M, Ambrose JA, Badimon JJ, Chesebro JH. Insights into the pathogenesis of acute ischemic syndromes. Circulation 1988; 77: 1213–20.

22. Crowley JG, Pierce RA. The affinity of platelets for subendothelium. Am J Surg 1981; 47: 529–32.

23. Bar-Shavit R, Eldora A, Vlodavsky Y. Binding of thrombin to subendothelial extracellular matrix: protection and expression of functional properties. J Clin Invest 1989; 84: 1096–104.

24. Lam JYT, Chesebro JH, Steele PM, Badimon L, Fuster V. Is vasospasm related to platelet deposition? Relationship in a porcine preparation of arterial injury in vivo. Circulation 1987; 75: 243–8.

25. Heras M, Chesebro JH, Penny WJ, Bailey KR, Badimon L, Fuster V. Effects of thrombin inhibition on the development of acute platelet-thrombus deposition during angioplasty in pigs: heparin versus recombinant hirudin, a specific thrombin inhibitor. Circulation 1989; 79: 657–65.

26. Heras M, Chesebro JH, Webster MWI, et al. Hirudin, heparin, and placebo during deep arterial injury in the pig. The in vivo role of thrombin in platelet-mediated thrombosis. Circulation 1990; 82: 1476–84.

27. Markwardt F, Kaiser B, Novak G. Studies on antithrombotic effects of recombinant hirudin. Thromb Res 1989; 54: 377–88.

28. Herrick JB. Clinical features of sudden obstruction of the coronary arteries. JAMA 1912; 59: 2015–20.

29. Hamman L. The symptoms of coronary occlusion. Bull Johns Hopkins Hosp 1926; 38: 273–319.

30. Parkinson J, Bedford DE. Cardiac infarction and coronary thrombosis. Lancet 1928; 1: 4–11.

31. Levine SA, Brown CL. Coronary thrombosis: its various clinical features. Medicine 1929; 8: 245–418.

32. Benson RL, Hunter WC, Manlove CH. Spontaneous rupture of the heart. Report of 40 cases in Portland, Oregon. Am J Pathol 1933; 9: 295–328.

33. Brown G, Albers JJ, Fisher LD, et al. Regression of coronary artery disease as a result of intensive lipid lowering therapy in men with high levels of apolipoprotein B. N Engl J Med 1990; 232: 1337–9.

34. Webster MWI, Chesebro JH, Smith HC, et al. Myocardial infarction and coronary artery occlusion: a prospective 5-year angiographic study (abstr). J Am Coll Cardiol 1990; 15(suppl): 218A.

35. Ambrose JA, Tannenbaum MA, Alexopoulos D, et al. Angiographic progression of coronary artery disease and the development of myocardial infarction. J Am Coll Cardiol 1988; 12: 56–62.

36. Little WC, Constantinescu M, Applegate RJ, et al. Can coronary angiography predict the site of a subsequent myocardial infarction in patients with mild-to-moderate coronary artery disease? Circulation 1988; 78: 1157–66.

37. Weksler BB. Prostaglandins and vascular function. Circulation 1984; 70(suppl III): III-63–61.

38. Haslam RJ, Davidson MML, Fox JEB, Lynham JA. Cyclic nucleotides in platelet function. Thromb Haemost 1978; 40: 232–40.

39. Contejean C. Recherches sur les injections intraveineuses de peptone et leur influence sur la coagulabilite du sang chez le chien. Arch Physiol Norm Pathol 1895; 7: 45.

40. Brinkhous KM, Smith HP, Warner EP, Seegers WH. Inhibition of blood clotting: unidentified substance which acts in conjunction with heparin to prevent conversion of prothrombin into thrombin. Am J Physiol 1939; 125: 683–7.

41. Rosenberg RD, Damus PS. The purification and mechanism of action of human antithrombin-heparin cofactor. J Biol Chem 1973; 248: 6490.

42. McNeely TB, Griffith MJ. The anticoagulant mechanism of action of heparin in contact-activated plasma; inhibition of factor X activation. Blood 1985; 65: 1226–31.

43. Rosenberg RD. Heparin-antithrombin system. In: Colman RW, Hirsh J, Marder VJ, Salzman EW, eds. Hemostasis and Thrombosis. Philadelphia: JB Lippincott, 1987: 962–85.

44. Esmon CT, Owen WG. Identification of an endothelial cell cofactor for thrombin-catalyzed activation of protein C. Proc Natl Acad Sci USA 1981; 78: 2249–52.

45. Stenflo J. A new vitamin K-dependent protein. Purification from bovine plasma and preliminary characterization. J Biol Chem 1976; 251: 355.

46. Van Hinsbergh VWM, Bertina RM, van Wijngaarden A, et al. Activated protein C decreases plasminogen activator inhibitor activity in endothelial cell conditioned medium. Blood 1985; 65: 444–51.

47. Robbins KC. The plasminogen-plasmin enzyme system. In: Colman RW, Hirsh J, Marder VJ, Salzman EW, eds. Hemostasis and Thrombosis. Philadelphia: JB Lippincott, 1987: 623–39.

48. Mimuro J, Schleef RR, Loskutoff DJ. Extracellular matrix of cultured bovine aortic endothelial cells contains functionally active type 1 plasminogen activator inhibitor. Blood 1987; 70: 721–8.

49. Fay WP, Owen WG. Platelet plasminogen activator inhibitor: purification and characterization of interaction with plasminogen activators and activated protein C inhibitor. Biochemistry 1989; 28: 5773–8.

50. Jang IK, Gold H, Ziskind AA, et al. Differential sensitivity of erythrocyte-rich and platelet-rich arterial thrombi to lysis with recombinant tissue-type plasminogen activator: a possible explanation for resistance to coronary thrombolysis. Circulation 1989; 79: 920–8.

51. Schwartz CJ, Mitchell JRA. The relation between myocardial lesions and coronary artery disease. I. An unselected necropsy study. Br Heart J 1962; 24: 761–861.

52. Muller JE, Tofler GH, Willich SN, Stone PH. Circadian variation of cardiovascular disease and sympathetic activity. J Cardiovasc Pharmacol 1987; 10(suppl 2): S104–9.

53. Muller JE, Ludmer PL, Willich SN, et al. Circadian variation in the frequency of sudden death. Circulation 1987; 75: 131–8.

54. Ridker PM, Manson JE, Buring JE, Muller JE, Hennekens CH. Circadian variation of acute myocardial infarction and the effect of low-dose aspirin in a randomized trial of positions. Circulation 1990; 82: 897–902.

55. Tofler GH, Czeisler CA, Rutherford J, Williams GH, Muller JE. Increased platelet aggregability after arising from sleep. J Am Coll Cardiol 1986; 7: 116A.

56. Kluft C, Kie FH, Rijken DC, Verheyen JH. Daytime fluctuations in blood of tissue type plasminogen activator (t-PA) and its fast-acting inhibitor (PAI-1). Thromb Haemost 1988; 59: 329–32.

57. Urano T, Sumiyoshi K, Nakamura M, Mori T, Takada Y, Takada A. Fluctuation of TPA and PAI-1 antigen levels in plasma: difference of their fluctuation patterns between male and female. Thromb Res 1990; 60: 55–62.

58. Yasue H. Circadian variation in response to exercise: an important variable in interpretation of the exercise stress test. Pract Cardiol 1983; 9: 43–5.

59. Roberts WC, Curry RC Jr, Isner JM, et al. Sudden death in Prinzmetal's angina with coronary spasm documented by angiography: analysis of three necropsy patients. Am J Cardiol 1982; 50: 203–10.

60. Ganz P, Davies PF, Leopold JA, Gimbrone MA Jr, Alexander RW. Short and long-term interactions of endothelium and vascular smooth muscle in coculture: effects on cyclic GMP production. Proc Natl Acad Sci USA 1986; 83: 3552–6.

61. Badimon L, Badimon JJ, Galvez A, Chesebro JH, Fuster V. Influence of arterial damage and wall shear rate on platelet deposition. Ex vivo study in a swine model. Arteriosclerosis 1986; 6: 312–20.

62. Lowe GDO. Blood rheology in arterial disease. Clin Sci 1986; 71: 137–46.

63. Dintenfass L. The rheology of blood in vascular disease. J R Coll Physicians Lond 1971; 5: 231–40.

64. Ellis S, Aldeman E, Coin K, Fisher L, Sanders W, Bourassa M, the CASS investigators. Prediction of risk of anterior myocardial infarction by lesion severity and measuring method of stenosis in the left anterior descending coronary distribution: a CASS Registry Study. J Am Coll Cardiol 1988; 11: 908–16.

65. Rainer C, Kawanishi DT, Chandraratna PAN, et al. Changes in blood rheology in patients with stable angina pectoris as a result of coronary artery disease. Circulation 1987; 76: 15–20.

66. Fuchs J, Weinberger I, Rotenberg Z, et al. Plasma viscosity in ischaemic heart disease. Am Heart J 1984; 108: 435.

67. Meade TW, Mellows S, Brozovic M, et al. Haemostatic function and ischaemic heart disease: principal results of the Northwick Park Heart Study. Lancet 1986; 2: 533–7.

68. Pilgeram LO. Hemostatic factors and coronary heart disease. Biomedicine 1982; 36: 187.

69. Stone MC, Thorpe JM. Plasma fibrinogen—a major coronary risk factor. J R Coll Gen Pract 1985; 35: 565–9.

70. Kannel WB, Castelli WP, Meeks SL. Fibrinogen and cardiovascular disease. J Am Coll Cardiol 1985; 5: 517.

71. Bini A, Fenoglio JJ, Mesa-Tejada R, Kudryk B, Kaplan KL. Identification and distribution of fibrinogen, fibrin, and fibrin(ogen) degradation products in atherosclerosis: use of monoclonal antibodies. Arteriosclerosis 1989; 9: 109–21.

72. Verheugh FW, Seeruys PW, van Vliet H, Spijkers A, Hugenholz PG. Intracoronary platelet release in patient with and without coronary artery disease. Thromb Haemost 1983; 49: 28–31.

73. Nicols AB, Gold KD, Marcella JJ, Canon PJ, Owen J. Effect of pacing-induced myocardial ischemia on platelet activation of fibrin formation in the coronary circulation. J Am Coll Cardiol 1987; 10: 40–5.

74. McGill D, McGuiness J, Lloyd J, Ardlie N. Platelet function and exercise induced myocardial ischaemia in coronary heart disease patients. Thromb Res 1989; 56: 147–58.

75. Kruskal JB, Commerford PJ, Franks JJ, Kirsch RE. Fibrin and fibrinogen-related antigens in patients with stable and unstable coronary artery disease. New Engl J Med 1987; 317: 1361–5.

76. Oshima S, Yasue H, Ogawa H, Okumura K, Matsuyama K. Fibrinopeptide A is released into the coronary circulation after coronary spasm. Circulation 1990; 82: 2222–5.

77. Holme I. An analysis of randomized trials evaluating the effect of cholesterol reduction on total mortality and coronary heart disease incidence. Circulation 1990; 82: 1916–24.

78. Gersh BJ. Benefits of the open artery: beyond myocardial salvage. J Myocardial Ischemia 1990; 2: 15–37.

79. Califf RM, Topol EJ, Gersh BJ. From myocardial salvage to patient salvage in acute myocardial infarction: the role of reperfusion therapy. J Am Coll Cardiol 1989; 14: 1382–8.

80. Dalen JE, Gore JM, Braunwald E, et al. Six- and Twelve-month follow-up of the phase I thrombolysis in myocardial infarction (TIMI Trial). Am J Cardiol 1988; 62: 179–85.

81. Elwood PC, Cochrane AL, Burr ML, et al. A randomized controlled trial of acetylsalicylic acid in the secondary prevention of mortality from myocardial infarction. Br Med J 1974; 1: 436–40.

82. Coronary Drug Project Group. Aspirin in coronary heart disease. J Chronic Dis 1976; 29: 625–42.

83. Breddin K, Loew D, Lechner K, Oberla K, Walter E. The German-Austrian Aspirin Trial: a comparison of acetylsalicylic acid, placebo and phenprocoumon in secondary prevention of myocardial infarction. Circulation 1980; 62(suppl V):V-63–72.

84. Elwood PC, Sweetman PM. Aspirin and secondary mortality after myocardial infarction. Lancet 1979; 2: 1313–5.

85. Aspirin Myocardial Infarction Study Research Group. A randomized controlled trial of aspirin in persons recovered from myocardial infarction. JAMA 1980; 243: 661–9.

86. The Persantine-Aspirin Reinfarction Study Group. Persantine and aspirin in coronary heart disease. Circulation 1980; 62: 449–61.

87. Klimt CR, Knatterud GL, Stamler J, Meier P, and the Persantine Aspirin Reinfarction Study Research Group. Part II. Secondary coronary prevention with persantine and aspirin. J Am Coll Cardiol 1986; 7: 251–69.

88. The Anturane Reinfarction Trial Research Group. Sulfinpyrazone prevention of suden death after myocardial infarction. N Engl J Med 1980; 302: 250–6.

89. The Anturane Reinfarction Trial. Re-evaluation of outcome. N Engl J Med 1982; 306: 1005–8.

90. Report from the Anturane Reinfarction Italian Study. Sulfinpyrazone in post-myocardial infarction. Lancet 1982; 1: 237–42.

91. Lam JYT, Chesebro JH, Steele PM, et al. Antithrombotic therapy for arterial injury by angioplasty: efficacy of common platelet-inhibitors versus thrombin inhibition in pigs. Circulation 1991 (in Press).

92. Cairns JA, Gent M, Singer J, et al. Aspirin, sulfinpyrazone, or both in unstable angina. N Engl J Med 1985; 213: 1369–75.

93. Antiplatelet Trialists' Collaboration. Secondary prevention of vascular disease by prolonged antiplatlet treatment. Br Med J 1988; 296: 320–31.

94. Second Report of the Working Party on Anticoagulant Therapy in Coronary Thrombosis to the Medical Research Council. An assessment of long-term anticoagulant administration after cardiac infarction. Br Med J 1964; 2: 837–43.

95. Ebert RV, Borden CW, Hipp HR, et al. Long-term anticoagulant therapy after myocardial infarction: final report of the Veterans Administration Cooperative Study. JAMA 1969; 207: 2263–7.

96. Report of the Sixty-Plus Reinfarction Study Research Group. A double-blind trial to assess long-term oral anticoagulant therapy in elderly patients after myocardial infarction. Lancet 1980; 2: 989–93.

97. The E.P.S.I.M. Research Group. A controlled comparison of aspirin and oral anticoagulants in prevention of death after myocardial infarction. N Engl J Med 1982; 307: 701–8.

98. Smith P, Arnesen H, Holme I. The effect of warfarin on mortality and reinfarction after myocardial infarction. N Engl J Med 1990; 323: 147–52.

99. Fuster V, Badimon L, Chesebro JH. Coronary artery disease progression and acute coronary syndromes. New Engl J Med 1991, In Press.

100. Fuster V, Bowie EJW, Chesebro JH. Inhibition of early atherosclerotic lesions in pigs with von Willebrands disease or treatment with platelet inhibitors. Thromb Haemost 1979; 42: 270.

101. Chesebro JH, Webster MWI, Smith HC, et al. Antiplatelet therapy in coronary disease progression: reduced infarction and new lesion formation. Circulation 1989; 80(suppl II): II-266.

102. Webster MWI, Chesebro JH, Kottke BA, et al. Apoplipoprotein AI and coronary disease progression: A 5-year angiographic study. J Am Coll Cardiol 1990; 15: 114A.

20

CORONARY ARTERY BYPASS SURGERY:
Antithrombotic Therapy

JAMES H. CHESEBRO, and STEVEN GOLDMAN

PATHOGENESIS OF OCCLUSION

The pathogenesis of acute and chronic occlusion of aortocoronary vein grafts is depicted in Figure 20–1.[1] Acute intraoperative angioscopy of vein grafts showed that only intraluminal examination may reveal technical faults in suturing at the distal anastomosis; this may occur in up to 20 per cent of grafts and may cause low flow and increased risk for early occlusion.[2] Disease of vein grafts is a form of accelerated atherosclerosis which begins with acute vascular injury, mural thrombosis, and smooth muscle cell proliferation.[1] Injury to the vein graft, which begins with the endothelium, results from procurement of vein from the leg, surgical handling, delays before insertion in the aortocoronary position, the type of preservation solution, and the increased shear forces of the pulsatile arterial system.[3,4] As soon as blood flows through the vein graft, immediate platelet deposition occurs with formation of mural thrombus which is evident histologically in three quarters of vein grafts in animals or patients who succumb within 24 hours of operation.[3–6] The internal mammary artery (IMA) is more protected (technically, genetically, or both) from generalized injury and platelet deposition because of less extensive surgical handling, previous adaptation to arterial shear forces, and partially intact vasa vasorum.

With vascular injury there is platelet deposition and secretion of growth and chemotactic factors for smooth muscle cells and white cells. Cellular injury may also induce growth factor secretion (such as basic fibroblast growth factor) and expression and rapid changes in gene expression during the first 48 hours.[7,8] Type II injury (endothelial denudation) occurs throughout the vein graft and type III, deep injury, at the anastomotic sites. Vein graft distension to high pressures is no longer carried out because of the added injury from this stretch response and recent evidence that this stimulates marked medial smooth muscle cell proliferation within 48 hours.[9,10]

Thrombosis

Platelet deposition within vein grafts begins during the operation as soon as blood flows through the graft. This information led to the approach that maximal antithrombotic protection should be started perioperatively to protect high-risk vein grafts in which blood flow is low (especially less than 40 milliliters/minute) or the distal coronary artery is small (less than 1.5 millimeters).[3,5,11] Occlusion within the first month after operation is related to thrombosis, which is in part due to technical problems, injury, and associated coronary atherosclerosis.[2,4,12] The extent of asymptomatic mural thrombus within vein grafts is likely considerable and probably underestimated at angiography unless it is quite extensive (Fig. 20–2).

Smooth Muscle Cell Proliferation

Smooth muscle cell proliferation is evident histologically about a month after operation

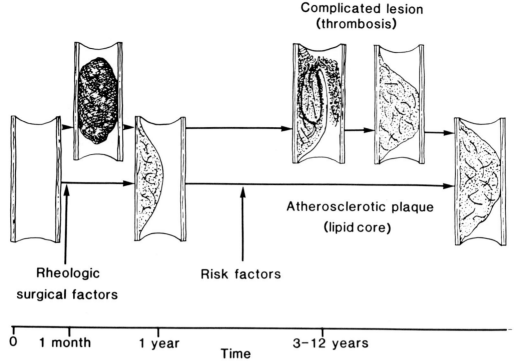

FIGURE 20–1. Stages of atherosclerotic vein graft disease are depicted (see text). Stage I involves acute injury and thrombosis within the first month after operation and appears related to surgical and rheologic factors. Stage II occurs mainly between 1 and 12 months and involves accelerated smooth muscle cell proliferation and matrix synthesis. Stage III involves lipid incorporation into the vein graft wall and atherosclerotic plaque formation with rupture of the complicated lesion and subsequent thrombosis. (Modified from Fuster V, Chesebro JH, Role of platelets and platelets inhibitors in aortocoronary artery vein-graft disease. Circulation 1986; 73: 227–32, with permission.)

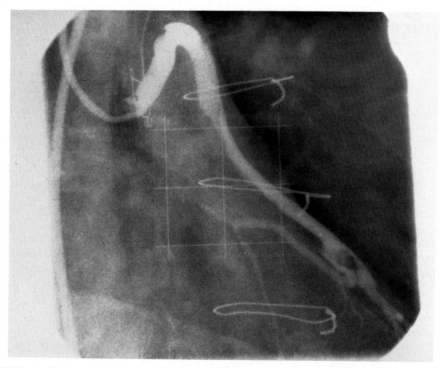

FIGURE 20–2. Vein graft to left anterior descending coronary artery in the asymptomatic patient eight days after operation. Note diffuse narrowing of mid and distal vein graft and filling defect adjacent to distal anastomosis, all of which is consistant with mural thrombus.

and is the main cause of occlusion between 1 and 12 months after operation.[12–14] Experimentally, smooth muscle cell proliferation can be divided into three phases. In phase I, there is medial smooth muscle cell hyperplasia which peaks at 48 hours, appears to be due to vascular stretching and injury, appears closely related to basic fibroblast growth factor (bFGF), is probably not related to platelets, but may be enhanced by thrombin.[8–10,15–18] During phase II (4 to 14 days), or the intermediate phase, smooth muscle cells migrate from media to intima and proliferate within the intima.[7,15] Migration and intimal proliferation are separable phenomena. Both may depend upon platelets and platelet-derived growth factor (PDGF); however more growth factors (including bFGF which is not platelet-derived) also cause proliferation.[7,17] In phase III (more than 14 days), or late smooth muscle cell proliferation, there is intimal hypertrophy and production of extracellular matrix.[15,19] Porcine studies in our laboratory suggest that deep arterial injury with mural thrombus leads to greater smooth muscle cell proliferation than mild injury with a single layer of platelets.[20] Likewise, therapy which reduces mural thrombus in canine vein grafts reduces intimal thickening.[4,13] Regrowth of endothelium appears to inhibit continued proliferation, but endothelium is known to regulate proliferation via synthesis of inhibitors or facilitators of growth. The process of accelerated atherosclerosis and smooth muscle cell proliferation has been recently reviewed.[1]

The stages of accelerated atherosclerosis in vein grafts are depicted in Figure 20–1. In stage I there is thrombosis, which usually occurs during the first few weeks. The stage of rapid proliferation begins within a month, is probably greatest within the early months, but appears to mature over the first year. Few changes occur during the second and third year. Beyond the third year, lipid incorporation becomes evident with formation of complex atherosclerotic lesions which contain a lipid core. Mechanisms contributing to this are outlined in Figure 20–3 and have been reviewed.[21,22] Lipid entry into the vessel wall attracts monocytes with conversion to macrophages which engulf lipid and evolve into foam cells. Foam cells may also develop from lipid incorporation by smooth muscle cells. The lipid core attracts more monocytes, which also invade the fibrous cap covering the lipid pool. It appears that the fibrous cap becomes thinner with dissolution of the collagen matrix. This results in rupture of the fibrous plaque and acute thrombus formation.[21,22] The presence of coronary risk factors increases the likelihood of complex lesion formation, plaque rupture, and associated thrombosis. These risk factors include lipids (increased low-density lipoprotein cholesterol, triglycerides, and lipoprotein (a), decreased high-density lipoprotein cholesterol), cigarette smoking, diabetes, and hypertension.[23,30] Continued smoking is particularly associated with thrombus in vein grafts.[27,28] Thrombus in vein grafts is most frequently observed between five and ten years after operation.[29] Thrombus is present in one half to three quarters of vein grafts from patients who undergo reoperation or come to autopsy.[6,14,27] Thrombus is associated with a ruptured plaque or an aneurysmal dilatation. By five to ten years after operation, clinical problems are related equally to atherosclerosis in vein grafts and progression of the underlying coronary artery disease.[23,24]

Prevalence of Vein Graft Occlusion

In the first few weeks after operation, as many as 10 to 15 per cent of grafts may be occluded, and 20 to 30 per cent of patients may have one or more vein graft occlusions. This may be reduced by 50 to 70 per cent with appropriately administered antithrombotic therapy.[31–33] At one year, approximately 25 per cent of grafts may be occluded. This may be reduced by 30 to 56 per cent with antithrombotic therapy. These occlusions may involve 40 to 50 per cent of patients, and antithrombotic therapy may reduce this to 21 to 53 per cent of patients with one or more occlusions. Variability in rates of occlusion with therapy may in part be related to patient compliance, arterial rheology (flow and lumen diameter), and arterial substrates exposed with the operation.[34,35] Beyond one year, the occlusion rate is 2 to 4 per cent per year over the first five years, when 35 per cent of vein grafts may be occluded. By ten years after operation, approximately 50 per cent of vein grafts are occluded.[24,25] By contrast, occlusion of the internal mammary artery graft is considerably lower at approximately 10 per cent, seven to ten years after operation.[36–41] The marked decrease in occlusion of the internal mammary artery graft probably relates in

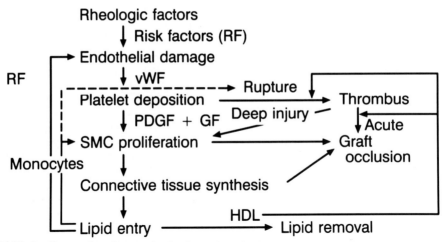

FIGURE 20–3. Proposed pathogenesis of vein graft occlusion and chronic disease (see text). Acute endothelial damage is due to surgical factors. Late endothelial dysfunction or injury is associated with risk factors. Platelet deposition early is more prominent in regions of deeper injury, especially at the distal anastomotic site where shear forces are higher as the vein joins a smaller coronary artery lumen. Thrombus formation late is related to a ruptured atherosclerotic plaque. Because vein grafts have no branches, thrombus often propagates proximally to fill the whole graft proximal to the site of thrombosis. Accelerated smooth muscle cell (SMC) proliferation occurs early in stage II and appears significantly related to platelet-derived growth factor (PDGF) and probably also other growth factors (GF). Slower and more chronic proliferation may also occur, especially in the presence of abnormal risk factors. Increased connective tissue matrix occurs in the later phases of SMC proliferation. Lipid entry into the vein graft wall marks the beginning of stage III with the formation of a complex lesion which may rupture and lead to spontaneous deep injury and acute thrombosis. High-density lipoprotein cholesterol may remove lipid from the wall and carries an important inhibitor of coagulation, lipoprotein associated coagulation inhibitor (LACI) which inhibits the interaction between tissue factor and activated factor VII early in the coagulation cascade. Thus particular attention to maintaining high levels of high-density lipoprotein cholesterol appears important. Elevated low-density lipoprotein and triglycerides may attract monocytes with more foam cell development and increase risk for complex atherosclerotic lesions with plaque rupture.

part to decreased injury at the time of operation with partial preservation of the vasa vasorum and the inherent decreased risk of atherosclerotic involvement of this artery.[42]

RATIONALE FOR OPTIMAL ANTITHROMBOTIC THERAPY

Because platelet deposition starts as soon as blood flows through the vein graft, perioperative antithrombotic therapy is critical for its reduction. This was shown experimentally[4,5] prior to designing large trials for the prevention of aortocoronary vein graft occlusion.[31,32] Reduction of acute thrombus with perioperative antiplatelet therapy also significantly reduced subsequent intimal proliferation two to three months after operation in the canine model (Figs. 20–4A, 20–4B, and 20–4C).[13] This may be more easily accomplished in the canine model where the

stimulus for thrombosis is less, runoff is better, and platelets are probably more sensitive to antiplatelet therapy. Thus antithrombotic therapy can intervene in stage I of vein graft disease (Fig. 20–1). This has been confirmed in several clinical trials.[31–35] Success is not achieved when therapy is started too late, as shown by an earlier trial which started therapy three to four days after operation.[43] The effect of timing of antiplatelet therapy is summarized in Figure 20–5. Note that the best early patency (triangles) was achieved when therapy was started either before or within the first day after operation.

Dipyridamole by itself does not significantly reduce platelet deposition or mural thrombus formation on the deeply injured artery, but it does reduce platelet deposition on artificial surfaces.[53] Experimentally, dipyridamole decreased platelet activation and maintained the platelet count during cardiopulmonary bypass when given as an infusion during the operation.[54,56] In humans, when

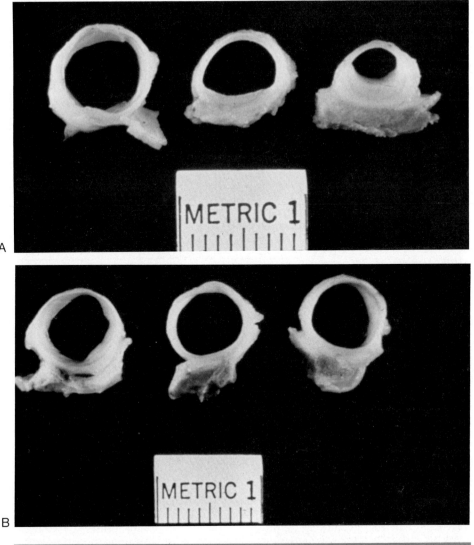

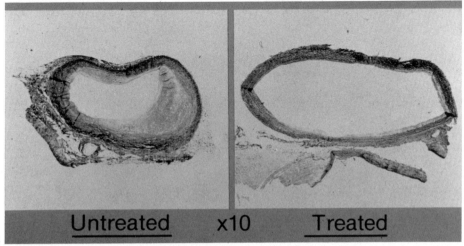

FIGURE 20–4A.   Cross sections (proximal, mid, and distal from left to right) of canine vein graft in control group at three months after aortocoronary bypass operation. Note extensive distal narrowing of vein graft. *B.*   Canine vein graft cross section (proximal, mid, and distal left to right) at three months after coronary bypass operation in groups treated with dipyridamole and aspirin starting perioperatively. Note the absence of distal narrowing. *C.*   Representative histologic cross-sections for distal vein grafts at three months after operation in a control group on the left (shows eccentric intimal proliferation) and from animal treated with antiplatelet therapy on the right (shows minimal eccentric proliferation).

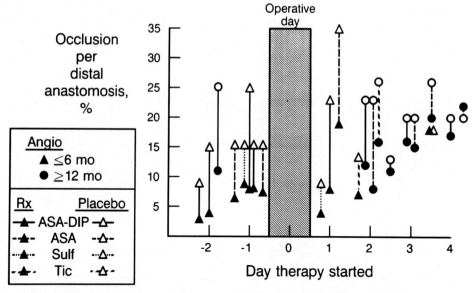

FIGURE 20–5. Relationship of vein graft occlusion to the day of starting platelet inhibitor therapy (Rx) before (day −2 or −1) or after (day 1, 2, 3, or 4) operation. Studies in which therapy was started before or soon after operation were the most successful in preventing subsequent vein graft occlusion. The time of angiography (Angio) is shown by the shape of the symbol, the drugs administered by the type of lines between symbols, and open symbols depict placebo and closed symbols treatment as shown in the key. ASA = acetylsalicylic acid (aspirin); DIP = dipyridamole; SULF = sulfinpyrazone. This figure shows studies from references 29, 30, 32, 33, 40, 41, 43–52. (Modified from Chesebro JH, et al. J Am Coll Cardiol 1986; 8: 56B–66B, with permission.)

administered preoperatively at 100 milligrams four times a day and during the operation at 0.24 milligrams/kilogram/hour, dipyridamole maintained platelet counts above 150 times 10⁹/liter in 71 per cent of patients compared with only 28 per cent of patients in the control group; in addition, dipyridamole reduced total blood loss from 1,550 milliliters in the control to 850 milliliters in the treated, and packed red blood cell transfusions from 3.3 liters in the control group to 1.9 liters in the treated group.[55] Thus oral plus intravenous dipyridamole may be a positive approach for reducing bleeding and platelet consumption in vein grafts. Thus more clinical studies are needed in humans with intravenous perioperative dipyridamole to more fully evaluate the effect on bleeding and reduction of blood transfusion.

The use of compounds during or soon after operation which block fibrinolysis or increase coagulation factors such as aprotinin or desmopressin (desamino-8-arginine vasopressin, DDAVP), may enhance mural thrombosis in vein grafts; although these compounds may not increase early overt

occlusion, they may increase the risk of late vein graft disease. This danger is very real, since thrombosis enhances intimal proliferation,[3,4,13,20] and thrombosis and thrombolysis are simultaneous and dynamic processes which start as soon as the vein graft is placed. More preclinical animal studies are required with aprotinin or infusion of factor VIII and von Willebrand factor (to mimic desmopressin which does not have an effect in animals) to quantitatively determine if platelet deposition and mural thrombus are increased in vein grafts with this type of therapy.

The current role of perioperative dipyridamole for therapy in patients is uncertain. A recent study showed that preoperative oral dipyridamole and intraoperative intravenous dipyridamole significantly increased vein graft blood flow but did not significantly reduce vein graft occlusion one year later (23 per cent occluded in dipyridamole group versus 28 per cent occlusion in the placebo group, $p = 0.08$).[57] Unfortunately, early postoperative vein graft occlusion rates were not assessed, since this would have the greatest chance of showing a difference, if it does exist.

Platelet Inhibitor Dosages

Dosages of platelet inhibitor therapy were originally chosen on the basis of prolongation of a shortened platelet survival in humans and their ability to significantly reduce quantitative indium-111-labeled platelet deposition in animals.[4,5,58–61] This led to the dosages employed in the two major platelet inhibitor trials in coronary bypass operations.[31,32,34,35] The conduct of these trials was also based upon the principles learned from animal studies and discussed above. Therapies employed in the Mayo Clinic Study and the Veterans Administration Cooperative Study are summarized in Tables 20–1 and 20–2, respectively. In these trials, angiography was performed both early (one week) and late (one year) after operation.

In the Mayo Clinic Study, angiography was performed in 88 per cent of patients early after operation (median, eight days) and the results are summarized in Figure 20–6. The 70 per cent reduction in vein graft occlusion was present in more than 50 subgroups including patients at higher and lower risk for occlusion as determined by vein graft blood flow, coronary artery lumen diameter, or presence or absence of endarterectomy.[31] In the Veterans Administration Cooperative Study, early catheterization was done a mean of nine days after operation and within 60

TABLE 20–1.   The Mayo Clinic Study. Platelet-Inhibitor Therapy for Patients Undergoing Aortocoronary Bypass Graft Operation*

Two days before operation
  Dipyridamole (Persantin), 100 milligrams, orally four times daily
On day of operation
  2 hours before operation: dipyridamole, 100 milligrams, orally
  1 hour after operation: dipyridamole, 100 milligrams, via nasogastric tube (clamp, 1.5 hours)
  7 hours after operation: dipyridamole, 75 milligrams, and aspirin, 325 milligrams via nasogastric tube (clamp, 1.5 hours)
On day after operation and daily thereafter
  Dipyridamole, 75 milligrams, and aspirin, 325 milligrams orally three times daily

* No other aspirin or prostaglandin-inhibiting drugs, especially nonsteroidal anti-inflammatory agents (sulindac [Clinoril] would least interfere), inhibitors of gastric acid secretions (for example, cimetidine or ranitidine) or simultaneous antacid should be given. For patients with only internal mammary artery bypass grafts and no vein grafts, empiric therapy is advised for three months to allow healing at anastomotic sites.

TABLE 20–2.   Veterans Administration Cooperative Study. Platelet-Inhibitor Therapy for Patients Undergoing Aortocoronary Bypass Graft Operation*

All drugs started before operation:
  Aspirin 325 milligrams daily
  Aspirin 325 milligrams three times daily
  Aspirin 325 milligrams and dipyridamole 75 milligrams, both three times daily
  Sulfinpyrazone 267 milligrams three times daily

* All therapy was started 48 hours before operation except aspirin which was administered as a single dose 12 hours before operation. The first dose of therapy was administered six hours after operation by a nasogastric tube which was then clamped for 1.5 hours. Therapy was continued every eight hours down the nasogastric tube until regular oral dosing could be substituted.

days in 72 per cent of patients. These results are summarized in Figures 20–7. There was no significant difference in early vein graft occlusion in any of the aspirin-containing drug regimens. Sulfinpyrazone was of borderline benefit and resulted in transient renal insufficiency in 5.3 per cent of patients.[32]

In the Mayo Clinic Study, new occlusion of vein grafts beyond the first month after operation and up to one year after operation in patients with all types of grafts (proven to be patent by angiography at early study) is shown in the middle panel of Figure 20–8 (occlusion of distal anastomoses on the left and by patients with one or more occlusions on the right). There was a significant reduction in new occlusions from 27 per cent of patients in the placebo group to 16 per cent in the treated group. Overall, one year after operation, 25 per cent of grafts were occluded in the placebo group compared to 11 per cent in the treated; this involved 47 per cent of patients with one or more occlusions in the placebo compared with 22 per cent in the treated group. Eighty-four per cent of patients were restudied late after operation.[34] In the Veterans Administration Cooperative Study, new occlusions from nine days after operation to one year later occurred in just under 10 per cent of grafts, this was not significantly different in treated or control groups. A possible explanation for this difference from the Mayo Clinic Study may be the extent to which risk factors were modified or patient compliance in taking therapy. The overall rates of occlusion of vein grafts at one year after operation in the Veterans Admin-

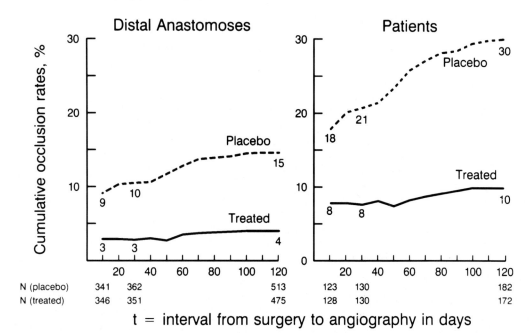

FIGURE 20–6. (*Left*) Occlusion rate of vein graft-coronary artery distal anastomoses totally occluded on angiography at *t* days after operation. (*Right*) Occlusion rate of patients with one or more distal anastomoses occluded on angiography at *t* days after operation (for group difference, *p* value and 95 per cent confidence limits were as follows: at $t = 10$, $p = 0.003$, 5 to 22 per cent; at $t = 30$, $p = 0.0004$, 7 to 23 per cent; at $t = 120$, $p < 10^{-6}$, 14 to 30 per cent). The range of *t* was 7 to 180 days. The occlusion rates did not change from 120 to 180 days after operation, when only six more patients underwent angiography. N = total number of distal anastomoses or patients in treated and placebo groups at 10, 30, and 120 days after operation. (Reprinted with permission from Chesebro JH, et al. A platelet-inhibitor-drug trial in coronary-artery bypass operations: benefit of perioperative dipyridamole and aspirin therapy on early postoperative vein-graft patency. N Engl J Med 1982; 307: 73–8.)

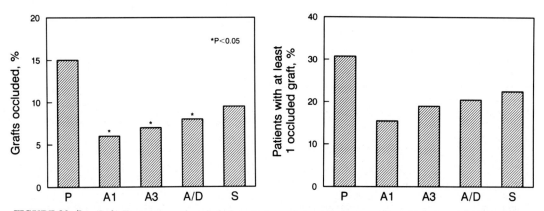

FIGURE 20–7. (*Left*) Percentage of occluded grafts in each treatment group from Veterans Administration Trial. P = placebo; A1 = aspirin once daily; A3 = aspirin three times daily; A/D = aspirin/dipyridamole; S = sulfinpyrazone. *$p < 0.05$ refers to comparison between each treatment group and placebo by cluster analysis. The 95 percent confidence intervals of the differences are: A1 versus P, difference 8.4 per cent (1.7, 15.0 confidence intervals); A3 versus P, difference 7.2 per cent (0.5, 13.8 confidence intervals; A/D versus P, difference 6.8 per cent (0.1, 13.4 confidence intervals); S versus P, difference 5.1 per cent (−1.6, 11.8 confidence intervals). (*Right*) Percentage of patients with at least one occluded graft. P = placebo; A1 = aspirin once daily; A3 = aspirin three times daily; A/D = aspirin/dipyridamole; S = sulfinpyrazone. The 95% confidence intervals of the differences are: A1 vs P, difference 13.4% (−0.2, 27.1 CI); A3 vs P, difference 11.2% (−2.5, 24.9 CI); A/D vs P, difference 9.2% (−4.5, 22.9 CI); S vs P, difference 8.1% (−5.5, 21.9 CI). (Reproduced from Goldman S, et al. Improvement in early saphenous vein graft patency after coronary artery bypass surgery with antiplatelet therapy: results of a Veterans Administration Cooperative Study. Circulation 1988; 77: 1324–32, with permission.)

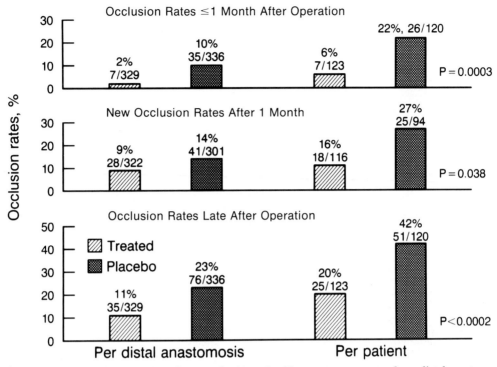

Occlusion rates, %

Occlusion Rates ≤1 Month After Operation

30
20   2%   10%   6%   22%, 26/120
10   7/329   35/336   7/123
0   P = 0.0003

New Occlusion Rates After 1 Month

30   27%
20   9%   14%   16%   25/94
10   28/322   41/301   18/116
0   P = 0.038

Occlusion Rates Late After Operation

50   42%
40   ▨ Treated   51/120
30   ▧ Placebo   23%   20%
20   76/336   25/123
     11%
10   35/329   P<0.0002
0
     Per distal anastomosis   **Per patient**

FIGURE 20–8. Occlusion rates for all types of vein grafts. The rates are expressed per distal anastomosis and per patient (proportion with at least one occlusion). Occlusion is shown as events occurring within one month (95 per cent confidence limits for the per patient difference, 8 to 24 per cent), as new events occurring beyond one month (in distal anastomoses and patients without occlusion within one month of operation) from angiography performed one year later (per patient, $p = 0.048$; 95 per cent confidence limits for the difference, 0 to 22 per cent) and as events at a median of one year after operation (95 per cent confidence limits for the per patient difference, 11 to 34 per cent). These subsets include only patients who had angiography within one month of operation and again one year later. Below each percentage is shown the ratio of distal anastomoses or patients with occlusion to total distal anastomoses or patients. (Reprinted with permission from Chesebro JH, et al. Effect of dipyridamole and aspirin on late vein-graft patency artery coronary bypass operations. N Engl J Med 1984; 310: 209–14.)

istration Cooperative Study are summarized in Figure 20–9. The proportion of patients with one or more occlusions one year after operation was 44 per cent in the placebo group compared with 35 per cent in the treated group ($p = 0.10$). Angiography was performed late after operation in 65 per cent of the patients.[35] Thus there do not appear to be significant differences between aspirin-containing regimens for treatment of patients with aortocoronary bypass graft operation.

Perioperative Bleeding

In the Mayo Clinic Study, dipyridamole was started before operation, but aspirin was started seven hours after operation. There was no difference in chest-tube blood loss, transfusion requirements for red cells, platelets or fresh frozen plasma, or reoperation

for bleeding (4 to 5 per cent of patients in each group).[31] In the Veterans Administration Cooperative Study, preoperative aspirin was associated with a significant increase in chest-tube blood loss to slightly over 1,100 milliliters in the worst of three aspirin groups compared with slightly over 800 milliliters in the placebo group. In addition, 6.1 per cent of patients underwent reoperation for bleeding in the preoperative aspirin group compared with 1.9 per cent of patients in the placebo and sulfinpyrazone groups.[32]

The Veterans Administration Cooperative Study Group has recently compared preoperative versus postoperative administration of aspirin (325 milligrams versus placebo the night before).[62] All patients received aspirin 325 milligrams six hours after operation and daily thereafter. Angiography was performed in 72 per cent of patients an average of eight days after operation. Vein graft occlusion was

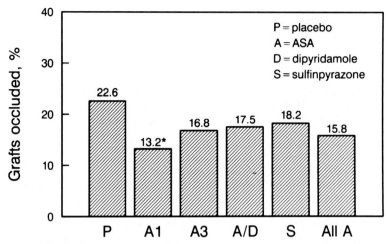

FIGURE 20–9. Bar graph of percentage of occluded graphs in each treatment group and overall for aspirin from the Veterans Administration Cooperative Study one year after operation. P = placebo; A1 = aspirin once daily; A3 = aspirin three times daily; A/D = aspirin/dipyridamole; S = sulfinpyrazone; A1 versus P, 9.4 per cent difference (95 per cent confidence intervals: 0.0, 18.7); A3 versus P, 5.8 per cent difference (95 per cent confidence intervals: −3.6, 15.2); A/D versus P, 5.1 per cent difference (95 per cent confidence intervals: −4.2, 14.5); S versus P, 4.6 per cent difference (95 per cent confidence intervals: −4.9, 13.8); all versus P, 6.8 per cent difference ($p = 0.029$). (Reproduced with permission from Goldman S, et al. Saphenous vein graft patency 1 year after coronary artery bypass surgery and effects of antiplatelet therapy: results of a Veterans Administration Cooperative Study. Circulation 1989; 80: 1190–7.)

similar in both groups (7.4 per cent with preoperative aspirin versus 7.8 per cent without). In the group taking preoperative aspirin, none of 22 distal anastomoses in Y-grafts were occluded compared with 7 per cent of 43 distal anastomoses in the nonaspirin group; in addition, in the preoperative aspirin group, none of 131 internal mammary artery grafts were occluded compared with 2.4 per cent in 125 internal mammary artery grafts in the nonaspirin group. These results in internal mammary artery grafts were of borderline significance and were retrospective observations which warrant a further prospective study. The median blood loss 35 hours after operation was 1,150 milliliters in the preoperative aspirin group compared with 1,045 milliliters in the nonaspirin group, red cell transfusion 900 milliliters versus 725 milliliters and reoperation for bleeding 6.3 per cent versus 2.4 per cent in the preoperative aspirin versus nonaspirin groups, respectively.[62]

Aspirin 325 milligrams/day has been administered as early as one hour after operation down the nasogastric tube and compared to placebo.[63] Vein graft angiography performed in 97 per cent of patients a median of seven days after operation showed occlusion in 1.6 per cent of distal anastomoses in the aspirin group and 6.2 per cent in the

placebo group with no difference in chest-tube blood loss or blood transfusion requirements between groups. The reoperation rate for bleeding was 4.8 per cent in the aspirin group and 1 per cent in the placebo group.

Other Antithrombotic Inhibitor Therapies

In a study of 173 patients, ticlopidine 250 milligrams twice daily or placebo was administered starting two days after operation. Over 90 per cent of patients were restudied by digital angiography at 10, 180, and 360 days after operation. The proportion of distal anastomoses occluded was reduced at ten days from 13.4 per cent in the placebo group to 7.1 per cent in the treated ($p < 0.05$), at 180 days from 24.0 per cent to 15 per cent ($p < 0.02$), and at 360 days from 26.1 per cent to 15.9 per cent ($p < 0.01$), in the placebo and treated groups, respectively.[52] This single study needs confirmation. Ticlopidine has a delayed onset of action of one to two days and reaches a maximal effect at three to five days.

In other studies, aspirin dosage has been reduced to 100 to 150 milligrams/day with significant reductions in vein graft occlusion in both studies.[41,64] Oral anticoagulation has also successfully reduced aortocoronary vein graft occlusion when heparin and dipyridamole were administered three times daily for seven days prior to starting oral anticoagulation versus no further therapy.[33] Eight weeks after operation there was a significant reduction in occlusion of distal anastomoses (from 15 per cent in the placebo group to 10 per cent in the oral anticoagulation group) and proportion of patients with one or more occlusions (33 per cent of patients in the placebo group compared with 19 per cent of patients in the oral anticoagulation group).

In a well-executed study comparing aspirin 50 milligrams (started the night before operation) plus dipyridamole 400 milligrams (started two days before operation) in two divided doses per day compared with oral anticoagulation (international normalized ratio 2.5 to 5.0) started on the first day after operation, graft angiography was obtained in 99 per cent of patients two weeks after operation and 95 per cent of patients one year after operation.[65] Early graft occlusion occurred in 7 per cent of both groups (16 per cent and 19 per cent of patients, respectively) and late graft occlusion in 16 per cent of distal anastomoses when therapy was continued for one year and in 23 per cent of distal anastomses if patients were switched to placebo at three months after operation. This confirms the efficacy of oral anticoagulation and the need for therapy for at least one year after operation.

CURRENT RECOMMENDATIONS

Aspirin reduces infarction and death in patients with unstable angina (see Chapter 13). In addition, more than half of patients presenting to hospital with acute coronary syndromes are on aspirin, which probably reduced the severity of their syndrome from myocardial infarction to unstable angina. These benefits of reduced arterial thrombosis in these patients appear to outweigh the risks of a slightly greater need for reoperation for bleeding after bypass operation. Early withdrawal of antithrombotic therapy in patients with unstable angina increases the risk of recurrent ischemia and myocardial infarction (see Chapter 13).

Thus in patients presenting with unstable angina who are awaiting aortocoronary bypass graft operation, aspirin may be continued daily up to the time of operation. In patients with rest angina, a heparin infusion to maintain the activated partial thromboplastin time at approximately twice control is also advisable before operation. When used with heparin, aspirin should be reduced to 80 milligrams/day. Aspirin 160-milligrams loading dose will acutely minimize thromboxane A_2 production, and 80 milligrams/day will maintain this effect with the lowest risk of side effects.[66] A new, slow-release formulation of low-dose aspirin preserves vascular prostacyclin production, inhibits thromboxane A_2, and needs clinical testing.

As noted above, preoperative dipyridamole therapy is of uncertain antithrombotic value, and does not need to be used routinely. However, it may be beneficial in decreasing intraoperative platelet consumption and in contributing to reduced blood loss (see above). If patients have not been on aspirin before operation, aspirin should be started one hour after operation down the nasogastric tube at a minimum dose of 160 milligrams/day for loading, and thereafter may be administered at 80 to 325 milligrams/day and continued indefinitely. Patients who are at high risk (see Chapter 23) with low vein graft blood flow (less than 40 milligrams/minute) or a small coronary artery lumen at the point of vein graft insertion (smaller than 1.5 millimeters), or with associated endarterectomy of the bypassed coronary artery, may be considered for combination therapy with oral anticoagulation (started on the first postoperative day) plus low-dose aspirin at 80 milligrams/day. In these high-risk patients, heparin may be administered at a relatively low dose initially to maintain the activated partial thromboplastin time at just above the upper normal value in the recovery room. The dosage may be increased to prolong the activated partial thromboplastin time to 1.5 times control after the chest tubes are removed. This may then be switched to oral anticoagulation maintaining the prothrombin time at 1.5 to 1.8 times control (international normalized ratio 3.0 to 4.5).

It is also critical to reduce all coronary risk factors including cessation of smoking, treatment of hypertension and diabetes, and correction of lipid abnormalities. Progression of both aortocoronary vein graft disease and native coronary artery disease has been shown to be significantly reduced in patients with reduced low-density lipoprotein cholesterol and increased high-density lipoprotein cholesterol.[67,70] The only studies which have shown a significant regression in vein graft or coronary artery disease have been those where the high-density lipoprotein cholesterol has been increased with specific therapy, such as with niacin.[69,70] Unless impossible from an anatomic or technical standpoint, at least one internal mammary bypass graft should be included, and this is usually to the largest and most significant vessel for myocardial supply, the left anterior descending coronary artery. Use of the internal mammary artery graft appears responsible for reducing graft occlusion in retrospective and a prospective study[36–42,66] and improving survival in retrospective studies.[36–41]

Prevention of Late Vein Graft Disease and Occlusion

No currently available therapy prevents the accelerated atherosclerotic process which leads to late occlusion in vein grafts. The Veterans Administration Cooperative Study Group is currently collecting data on the effects of aspirin 325 milligrams/day on vein graft patency at three years after operation; this is the time when late vein graft disease begins to appear. Control of risk factors such as cessation of smoking, reduction of low-density lipoprotein cholesterol, and increase of high-density lipoprotein cholesterol, appear very promising since this may reduce the atherosclerotic process and the incidence of plaque rupture. This is suggested by the reduction in number of coronary events by this therapy.[69,70] In patients with incomplete correction of risk factors, consideration might be given to long-term anticoagulant therapy along with low-dose aspirin at 80 milligrams/day in order to prevent the disastrous consequences of plaque rupture in a vein graft. This leads not only to local occlusion, but also to occlusion of the entire graft proximal to the ruptured lesion, since vein grafts have no branches and thus are prone to long segments of occlusion. Thus large amounts of thrombus accumulate in vein grafts, which makes them very risky for performing balloon angioplasty or atherectomy.

Prolonged selective urokinase infusion combined with heparin plus aspirin therapy may be beneficial for clearing thrombus and preparing the patient for subsequent angioplasty.[71]

Thrombosis of Late Vein Graft Occlusion

In vein grafts with late occlusion after zero to six months (penetrable with a guide wire) local infusion of urokinase 50,000 to 100,000 international units per hour for 17 to 70 hours (mean 24 hours) has been used with successful recanalization in 79 per cent (Hartmann J, personal communication, 1991). An alternative may be direct and serial injection into the thrombus 1 to 2 centimeters at a time with a 5 French Sones catheter using urokinase 20,000 international units/centimeters of thrombus (Schneider E, personal communication, 1991). Simultaneous heparin 5,000-unit bolus and activated partial thromboplastin time 2.0 to 2.5 times control may reduce simultaneous rethrombosis and may be followed by percutaneous transluminal coronary angioplasty if necessary after all thrombus is cleared. Long-term therapy starting at hospital dismissal based on pathogenesis and risk (see Chapter 23) would be oral anticoagulation (international normalized ratio 3.0 to 4.5, or prothrombin time 1.5 to 1.8 times control) plus aspirin 80 milligrams/day.

The timing, duration, and intensity of antithrombotic therapy, as well as the duration of lytic therapy needs further study. In addition, the role of chronic oral anticoagulation in preventing the massive accumulation of thrombus which often accompanies plaque rupture in vein grafts, also needs study.

REFERENCES

1. Ip JH, Fuster V, Badimon L, Badimon J, Taubman MB, Chesebro JH. Syndromes of accelerated atherosclerosis: role of vascular injury in smooth muscle cell proliferation. J Am Coll Cardiol 1990; 15: 1667–87.
2. Grundfest WS, Litvack F, Sherman T, et al. Delineation of peripheral and coronary detail by intraoperative angioscopy. Ann Surg 1985; 202: 394–400.
3. Fuster V, Chesebro JH. Role of platelets and platelet inhibitors in aortocoronary artery vein-graft disease. Circulation 1986; 73: 227–32.
4. Josa M, Lie JT, Bianco RL, Kaye MP. Reduction of thrombosis in canine coronary bypass vein grafts with dipyridamole and aspirin. Am J Cardiol 1981; 47: 1248–54.
5. Fuster V, Dewanjee MK, Kaye MP, Josa M, Metke MP, Chesebro JH. Noninvasive radioisotopic technique for detection of platelet deposition in coronary artery bypass grafts in dogs and its reduction with platelet inhibitors. Circulation 1979; 60: 1508–12.
6. Bulkley BH, Hutchins GM. Pathology of coronary artery bypass graft surgery. Arch Pathol Lab Med 1978; 102: 273–80.
7. Majesky MW, Reidy MA, Bowen-Pope DF, Hart CE, Wilcox JN, Schwartz SM. PDGF ligand and receptor gene expres-

sion during repair of arterial injury. J Cell Biol 1990; 111: 2149–58.

8. Lindner V, Lappi DA, Baird A, Majack RA, Reidy MA. Role of basic fibroblast growth factor in lesion formation. Circ Res 1991; 68: 106–13.

9. Webster MWI, Chesebro JH, Heras M, Mruk JS, Grill DE, Fuster V. Effect of balloon inflation on smooth muscle cell proliferation in the porcine carotid artery. J Am Coll Cardiol 1990; 15: 165A.

10. Capron L, Bruneval P. Influence of applied stress on mitotic response of arteries to injury with a balloon catheter: quantitative study in rat thoracic aorta. Cardiovasc Res 1989; 23: 941–48.

11. Chesebro JH, Fuster V. Platelets and platelet-inhibitor drugs in aortocoronary vein bypass operations. Int J Cardiol 1983; 2: 511–6.

12. Uni KK, Kottke BA, Titus JL, Frye RL, Wallace RB, Brown AL. Pathologic changes in aortocoronary saphenous vein grafts. Am J Cardiol 1974; 34: 526–32.

13. Metke MP, Lie JT, Fuster V, Josa M, Kaye MP. Reduction of intimal thickening in canine coronary bypass vein grafts with dipyridamole and aspirin. Am J Cardiol 1979; 43:1144–8.

14. Lie LT, Lawrie GM, Morris GC. Aortocoronary bypass saphenous vein graft atherosclerosis. Am J Cardiol 1977; 40: 906–14.

15. Clowes AW, Reidy MA, Clowes MM. Kinetics of cellular proliferation after arterial injury. I. Smooth muscle growth in the absence of endothelium. Lab Invest 1983; 49: 327–33.

16. Fingerle J, Johnson R, Clowes AW, Majesky MW, Reidy MA. Role of platelets in smooth muscle cell proliferation and migration after vascular injury in rat carotid artery. Proc Natl Acad Sci USA 1989; 86: 8412–6.

17. Fingerle J, Au WPT, Clowes AW, Reidy MA. Intimal lesion formation in rat carotid arteries after endothelial denudation in absence of medial injury. Arteriosclerosis 1990; 10:1082–7.

18. Berk BC, Taubman MB, Gragoe EJ, Fenton FW, Griendling KK. Thrombin signal transduction mechanisms in rat vascular smooth muscle cells. Calcium and protein kinase C-dependent and -independent pathways. J Biol Chem 1990; 265: 17334–40.

19. Snow AD, Bolender RP, Wright TN, Clowes AW. Heparin modulates the composition of the extracellular matrix domain surrounding arterial smooth muscle cells. Am J Pathol 1990; 137: 313–30.

20. Webster MWI, Chesebro JH, Grill DE, Badimon JJ, Badimon L. Influence of deep and mild arterial injury on smooth muscle cell proliferation after angioplasty (abstr). Circulation 1991; 84 (Suppl IV), in press.

21. Fuster V, Stein B, Ambrose JA, Badimon L, Badimon JJ, Chesebro JH. Atherosclerotic plaque rupture and thrombosis: evolving concepts. Circulation 1990; 82(suppl II): II-47–59.

22. Davies MJ. A macro and micro view of coronary vascular insult in ischemic heart disease (abstr). Circulation 1990; 82(suppl II): II-38–46.

23. Bourassa MG, Campeau L, Lesperance J, Grondin CM. Changes in grafts and coronary arteries after saphenous vein aortocoronary bypass surgery: results at repeat angiography. Circulation 1982; 65(suppl II): II-90–7.

24. Campeau L, Enjalbert M, Lesperance J, Vaislic C, Grondin CM, Bourassa MG. Atherosclerosis and late closure of aortocoronary saphenous vein grafts: sequential angiographic studies at 2 weeks, 1 year, 5 to 7 years, and 10 to 12 years after surgery. Circulation 1983; 68(suppl II): II-1–7.

25. Fuster V, Chesebro JH. Current concepts of thrombogenesis: role of platelets. Mayo Clin Proc 1981; 56: 102–12.

26. Palac RT, Meadows WR, Hwang MH, Loeb HS, Pifarre R, Gunnar RM. Risk factors related to progressive narrowing in aortocoronary vein grafts studied 1 and 5 years after surgery. Circulation 1982; 66(suppl I): I-40–4.

27. Neitzel GF, Barboriak JJ, Pintar K, Qureshi I. Atherosclerosis in aortocoronary bypass grafts: morphologic study and risk factor analysis 6 to 12 years after surgery. Arteriosclerosis 1986; 6: 594–600.

28. Solymoss BC, Nadeau P, Millette D, Campeau L. Late

29. Walts AE, Fishbein MC, Matloff JM. Thrombosed, ruptured atheromatous plaques in saphenous vein coronary artery bypass grafts: 10 years' experience. Am Heart J 1987; 114: 718–23.

30. Hoff HF, Beck GJ, Skibinski CI, et al. Serum Lp(a) level as a predictor of vein graft stenosis after coronary artery bypass surgery in patients. Circulation 1988; 77: 1238–44.

31. Chesebro JH, Clements I, Fuster V, et al. A platelet-inhibitor-drug trial in coronary-artery bypass operations: benefit of perioperative dipyridamole and aspirin therapy on early postoperative vein-graft patency. N Engl J Med 1982; 307: 73–8.

32. Goldman S, Copeland J, Moritz T, et al. Improvement in early saphenous vein graft patency after coronary artery bypass surgery with antiplatelet therapy: results of a Veterans Administration Cooperative Study. Circulation 1988; 77:1324–32.

33. Gohlke H, Gohlke-Barwolf C, Sturzenhofecker P, et al. Improved graft patency with anticoagulant therapy after aortocoronary bypass surgery: a prospective randomized study. Circulation 1981; 64(suppl II): II-22–7.

34. Chesebro JH, Fuster V, Elveback LR, et al. Effect of dipyridamole and aspirin on late vein-graft patency after coronary bypass operations. N Engl J Med 1984; 310: 209–14.

35. Goldman S, Copeland J, Moritz T, et al. Saphenous vein graft patency 1 year after coronary artery bypass surgery and effects of antiplatelet therapy: results of a Veterans Administration Cooperative Study. Circulation 1989; 80: 1190–7.

36. Loop FD, Lytle BW, Cosgrove DM, et al. Influence of the internal-mammary-artery graft on 10-year survival and other cardiac events. N Engl J Med 1986; 314: 1–6.

37. Spencer FC. The internal mammary artery: the ideal coronary bypass graft? N Engl J Med 1986; 314: 50–1.

38. Lytle BW, Loop FD, Cosgrove DM, Ratliff NB, Easley K, Taylor PC. Long-term (5–12 years) serial studies of internal mammary artery and saphenous coronary bypass grafts. J Thorac Cardiovasc Surg 1985; 89: 248–58.

39. Barner HB, Swartz MT, Mudd JG, Tyras DH. Late patency of the internal mammary artery as a coronary bypass conduit. Ann Thorac Surg 1982; 34: 408–12.

40. Techtor AJ, Schmahl TM, Janson B, Kallies JR, Johnson D. The internal mammary artery graft: its longevity after coronary bypass. JAMA 1981; 246: 2181–3.

41. Grondin CM, Campaeau L, Lesperance J, Engalbert M, Bourassa MG. Comparison of late changes in internal mammary artery and saphenous vein grafts in 2 consecutive series of patients 10 years after operation. Circulation 1984; 70(suppl I): I-208–12.

42. Sims FH. A comparison of coronary and internal mammary arteries and implications of the results in etiology of arteriosclerosis. Am Heart J 1983; 105: 560–6.

43. Pantely GA, Goodnight SH Jr, Rahimtoola SH, et al. Failure of antiplatelet and anticoagulant therapy to improve patency of grafts after coronary-artery bypass. N Engl J Med 1979; 301: 962–6.

44. Rajah SM, Salter MCP, Donaldson DR, et al. Acetylsalicylic acid and dipyridamole improve the early patency of aorta-coronary bypass grafts: a double-blind, placebo-controlled, randomized trial. J Thorac Cardiovasc Surg 1985; 89: 373–7.

45. Baur HR, VanTassel RA, Pierach CA, Gobel FL. Effects of sulfinpyrazone on early graft closure after myocardial revascularization. Am J Cardiol 1982; 49: 420–4.

46. Mayer JE, Lindsay WG, Castaneda W, Nicoloff DM. Influence of aspirin and dipyridamole on patency of coronary artery bypass grafts. Ann Thorac Surg 1981; 31: 204–10.

47. Lorenz RL, Weber M, Kotzur J, et al. Improved aortocoronary bypass patency by low-dose aspirin (100 mg daily). Lancet 1984; i: 1261–4.

48. Brown BG, Cukingnan RA, DeRouen T, et al. Improved graft patency in patients treated with platelet-inhibiting therapy after coronary bypass surgery. Circulation 1985; 72: 138–46.

49. Brooks N, Wright J, Sturridge M, et al. Randomized placebo controlled trial of aspirin and dipyridamole in the prevention of coronary vein graft occlusion. Br Heart J 1985; 53: 201–7.

50. McEnany MT, Salzman EW, Mundth ED, et al. The effect of antithrombotic therapy on patency rate of saphenous vein coronary artery bypass grafts. J Thorac Cardiovasc Surg 1982; 83: 81–9.

51. Sharma GVRK, Khuri SF, Josa M, Folland ED, Parisi AF. The effect of antiplatelet therapy on saphenous vein coronary artery bypass graft patency. Circulation 1983; 68(suppl II): II-218–21.

52. Limet R, David JL, Magotteaux P, Larock MP, Riego P. Prevention of aorto-coronary bypass graft occlusion: beneficial effect of ticlopidine on early and late patency rates of venous coronary bypass grafts: double-blind study. J Thorac Cardiovasc Surg 1987; 94: 773–83.

53. Pumphrey CW, Fuster V, Dewanjee MK, Chesebro JH, Vlietstra RE, Kaye MP. Comparison of the antithrombotic action of calcium antagonist drugs with dipyridamole in dogs. Am J Cardiol 1983; 51: 591–5.

54. Nuutinen LS, Pihlajaniemi R, Saarela E, Karkola P, Hollmen A. The effect of dipyridamole on the thrombocyte count and bleeding tendency in open-heart surgery. J Thorac Cardiovasc Surg 1977; 74: 295–8.

55. Toteoh KH, Christakis GT, Weisel RD, et al. Dipyridamole preserved platelets and reduced blood loss after cardiopulmonary bypass. J Thorac Cardiovasc Surg 1988; 96: 332–41.

56. Becker RM, Smith MR, Dobell ARC. Effect of platelet inhibition on platelet phenomenon in cardiopulmonary bypass in pigs. Ann Surg 1974; 179: 52–7.

57. Ekeström SA, Gunnes S, Brodin UB. Effect of dipyridamole (persantin) on blood flow and patency of aortocoronary vein bypass grafts. Scand J Thorac Cardiovasc Surg 1990; 24: 191–6.

58. Fuster V, Chesebro JH. Current concepts of thrombogenesis: role of platelets. Mayo Clin Proc 1981; 56: 102–12.

59. Harker LA, Ross R, Slichter SJ, Scott CR. Homocystine-induced arteriosclerosis: the role of endothelial cell injury and platelet response in its genesis. J Clin Invest 1976; 58: 731–41.

60. Steele P, Rainwater J, Vogel R. Platelet suppressant therapy in patients with prosthetic cardiac valves: relationship of clinical effectiveness to alteration of platelet survival time. Circulation 1979; 60: 910–3.

61. Donadio JV, Anderson CF, Mitchell JC, et al. Membrano-proliferative glomerulonephritis: a prospective clinical trial of platelet-inhibitor therapy. N Engl J Med 1984; 310: 1421–6.

62. Goldman S, Copeland J, Moritz T, et al. Starting aspirin before operation: effects on early graft patency. Circulation 1991; 84 (2): 520–526.

63. Gavaghan TP, Gebski V, Baron DW. Immediate postoperative aspirin improves vein graft patency early and late after coronary artery bypass graft surgery. Circulation 1991; 83: 1526–33.

64. Sanz G, Pajaron A, Alegria E, et al. Prevention of early aortocoronary bypass occlusion by low-dose aspirin and dipyridamole. Circulation 1990; 82: 765–73.

65. Pfisterer M, Jockers G, Regenass, et al. Trial of low-dose aspirin plus dipyridamole versus anticoagulants for prevention of aortocoronary vein graft occlusion. Lancet 1989; 2(8653): 1–7.

66. Clarke RJ, Mayo G, Price P, FitzGerald GA. Preservation of systemic prostacyclin biosynthesis by controlled release aspirin: biochemical selectivity for thromboxane A_2. N Engl J Med 1991 (in press).

67. Brensike FJ, Levy PR, Kelsey SF, Passamani ER, et al. Effects of therapy with cholestyramine on progression of coronary arteriosclerosis: results of the NHLBI Type II Coronary Intervention Study. Circulation 1984; 69: 313–24.

68. Arntzenius AC, Kromhout D, Barth JD, et al. Diet, lipoproteins, and the progression of coronary atherosclerosis. The Leiden Intervention Trial. N Engl J Med 1985; 312: 805–11.

69. Blankenhorn DH, Nessim SA, Johnson RL, Sanmarco ME, Azen SP, Cashin-Hemphil L. Beneficial effects of combined colestipol-niacin therapy on coronary atherosclerosis and coronary venous bypass graft. JAMA 1987; 257: 3233–40.

70. Brown G, Albers JJ, Fisher LD, et al. Regression of coronary artery disease as a result of intensive lipid-lowering therapy in men with high levels of apolipoprotein B. N Engl J Med 1990; 323: 1289–98.

71. Sharaf BL, Bier JD, Ledley GS, Williams DO. Prolonged selective urokinase infusion versus PTCA from totally occluded coronary saphenous vein bypass grafts (abstr). J Am Coll Cardiol 1991; 17: 337A.

21

PERCUTANEOUS TRANSLUMINAL CORONARY ANGIOPLASTY:
Prevention of Occlusion and Restenosis

ROBERT M. CALIFF and JAMES T. WILLERSON

Percutaneous interventional techniques have become a common part of the practice of cardiovascular medicine. The reported number of angioplasty procedures performed in the coronary arteries has increased from 100,000 in 1985 to over 250,000 in 1989.[1] With recent data suggesting an advantage for angioplasty over medical therapy in symptomatic single-vessel disease,[2] the number of angioplasty procedures is likely to continue to grow in the foreseeable future. Furthermore, multiple new technologies have now been introduced to reduce obstructive lesions using shaving, pulverizing, and vaporizing techniques, thereby expanding percutaneous techniques to more complex and challenging coronary lesions.[3]

Percutaneous techniques for intervening to reduce the degree of coronary stenosis are limited primarily by three factors: physical inaccessibility of the lesion, abrupt closure after initial success, and restenosis. Although thrombosis cannot be implicated as a major factor with regard to physical access, abrupt closure and restenosis have both been closely linked to the response of the thrombotic system to mechanically-induced arterial injury. This chapter will review the clinical profile and pathophysiology of each problem. A summary of past, current, and future clinical trials will then follow with a unifying theme of examining the possible impact of

the thrombotic response to the injury induced in the process of failure of intravascular intervention, within the context of what is known about the mechanisms and clinical outcomes associated with the procedure.

PATHOPHYSIOLOGY

Routine Angioplasty

The mechanism of successful percutaneous intervention with current techniques always involves deep injury to the arterial wall. Whether the device is routine angioplasty, atherectomy, or laser, the process of widening the arterial lumen involves producing thermal or mechanical injury to the atherosclerotic plaque and its immediate vicinity. A recent report described a normal appearance of the post PTCA region by angiography in 64 per cent of patients undergoing angioplasty, although angioscopy, which gives a more precise visual image, demonstrated intimal trauma in every case,[4] a finding that confirms previous pathological studies.[5] The short-term and long-term response to the process of inducing injury is the basis for a successful or a failed procedure.

Routine balloon angioplasty has been the most carefully studied procedure in a variety of situations. The technique of balloon angioplasty involves fracturing the atherosclerotic plaque with remodeling of the arterial wall including stretching of the normal component of the arterial wall. Waller and colleagues[6,7] have described four basic mechanical responses to the trauma (Fig. 21–1). In some cases only superficial intimal cracks are produced, and the predominant mechanism of producing a wider lumen comes from stretching of the more normal part of the arterial wall when the lesion is eccentric or from concentric stretching of the vessel wall when a concentric lesion is present. These types of responses were associated with a "smooth" appearance on coronary angiography. Lesions with a "hazy" appearance on angiography tended to have deep intimal-medial cracks with associated fibrin–platelet thrombi. When an angiographic appearance of "intimal splitting" was observed on angiography, the pathology demonstrated a deep intimal-medial crack with dissection through the media, creating an intimal-medial flap. Finally, when the angiographic description was labeled as a dissection, a true lumen and

a false lumen created by the balloon trauma was usually identifiable. Each of these different traumatic lesions forming the spectrum of mechanisms can result in "successful" angioplasty with symptomatic improvement owing to an increase in the lumen available for coronary blood flow. Both the exact geometry of the vessel after the traumatic violation and the degree to which thrombosis is stimulated must have some role in determining the final outcome for the patient.

Abrupt Closure

The clinical definition of abrupt closure has been somewhat variable from study to study. In most series, abrupt closure has been defined as angiographically documented complete occlusion of the vessel at any time after the lesion has been approached with a mechanical instrument. One obvious exception, of course, would be a vessel with total occlusion prior to the procedure when that lesion is never crossed. Some series have also

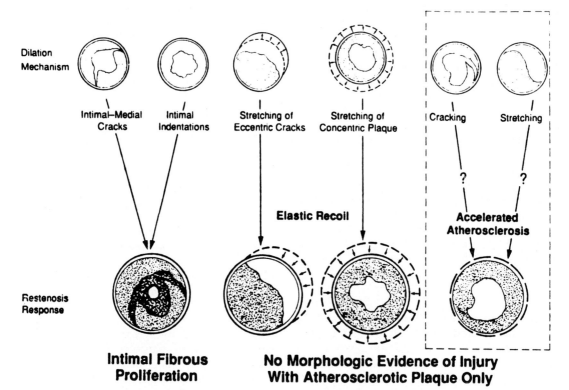

FIGURE 21–1. Proposed mechanisms of luminal widening with balloon angioplasty (cracking and stretching) and the two major subgroups of restenosis lesions: intimal fibrous proliferation and elastic recoil. (Reproduced with permission from Waller BF. Pathology of transluminal balloon angioplasty used in the treatment of coronary heart disease. Hum Pathol 1987; 18: 476–84.)

included patients with a widely patent artery on angiography, but with a marked reduction in flow leading to ischemia. This phenomenon has also been called the "no reflow" phenomenon by clinicians, and may result from microvascular plugging or vasospasm downstream from the angioplasty site. When abrupt closure occurs after the patient has already left the angiographic suite, sometimes flow is restored before repeat angiography is obtained, or angiography cannot be repeated owing to other complications or death. Thus all clinical series of abrupt closure must be regarded as imprecise because of different detection rates.

As described in detail in Chapters 2 and 3, a tremendous stimulus to thrombosis is created by exposure of the circulating blood to tissue factor and other components of the undersurface of the plaque. The demonstration by Waller and colleagues that the extent of arterial injury can range from a fissure or crack to a large intimal dissection with a creation of a flap in the artery provides a rationale for the hypothesis that variable stimulation of the clotting system may occur in the setting of percutaneous intervention.[8] When the procedure is successful, the assumption is made that the propensity for thrombosis is overcome by the intrinsic antithrombotic and fibrinolytic system and reinforced by the influence of potent antithrombin and antiplatelet agents administered therapeutically. Abrupt closure may be due predominantly to a mechanical process in which the intimal flap falls against the opposite wall of the artery, or to an exuberant clotting process. In Waller's review, a "folded, curled up" large intimal flap was found in the majority of cases of abrupt closure coming to autopsy. Of course, most cases of abrupt closure involve at least some component of each process, since a larger dissection should be expected to produce a greater stimulus to clotting. Why some abrupt closures occur in the absence of a large mechanical tear in the vessel remains unclear.

Restenosis

The exact definition of restenosis continues to be debated, but all observers agree that the loss of lumen initially gained with the interventional procedure is a major problem of all presently available percutaneous interventional techniques.[9–12] The difference between the lumen at the site of intervention immediately after the procedure and at a follow-up time thus defines the degree to which restenosis has occurred. Binary classification rules have been sought for convenience. The most commonly used definition when a visual assessment is made is recurrence of more than 50 per cent luminal diameter stenosis after initial reduction of the lesion by at least 20 per cent, and to less than 50 per cent stenosis by visual or caliper assessment, or loss of more than 0.72 millimeter in luminal diameter from immediately postprocedure to follow-up by quantitative angiography. Neither definition is ideal. The diameter stenosis definition fails to take into account the degree of initial lumen enlargement (an increase in stenosis from 45 per cent to 55 per cent would be counted as restenosis), or the fact that a recurrent stenosis greater than 50 per cent in a large vessel may not be flow limiting. Requirement of an encroachment of greater than 0.72 millimeter by quantitative angiography leads to a systematic overestimation of restenosis rates in large vessels, and a systematic underestimation in small vessels. These differences in definition can obviously lead to large fluctuations in reported restenosis rates.

The process of restenosis is complex and multifactorial. Three major classes of factors can be invoked in the process (Fig. 21–2). First, since the process of angioplasty itself is critically dependent on mechanical trauma to the abnormal vessel wall and stretching of the normal vessel wall, the natural tendency of the tissue to recoil is a major factor to be considered. In one study, Rensing and coworkers[13] describe loss of 50 per cent of the theoretical initial maximal gain almost immediately after angioplasty. Similarly, Nobuyoshi and colleagues demonstrated that 16 per cent of angioplasty patients had a loss of more than 0.5 millimeter in luminal diameter in the first 24 hours after the procedure.[14]

The second important process is the formation of thrombus on the surface and inside of the disrupted plaque. Waller and others have demonstrated that in many cases dissection into the plaque then leads to hemorrhage which can serve to displace the plaque into the lumen or cause the plaque mass to grow. A similar process is thought to account for some of the growth of atherosclerotic plaques after plaque rupture in de novo atherosclerotic pathophysiology.[15,16] The intensity of thrombus formation could serve to reduce

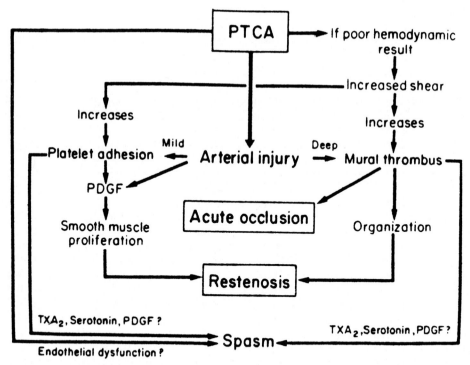

FIGURE 21–2. Proposed mechanisms underlying abrupt closure and chronic restenosis after percutaneous intervention. PTCA = percutaneous intervention; PDGF = platelet-derived growth factor; TXA2 = thromboxane A_2. (Courtesy of Dr. V. Fuster.)

the initial gain in lumen both by adding to the plaque mass and by elaborating more growth factors.

The final process which has led to the most intense interest has been the impact of mitogenic factors released by platelets, monocytes, and by components of the intact parts of the vascular wall. Even endothelium, although generally protective, can produce growth factors[17,18]; smooth muscle cells produce growth factors and respond to growth factors by proliferating.[19,20] Monocytes, which are attracted to the area of injury by chemotactic factors, including the growth factors themselves, also produce potent growth factors.

Endothelial injury at sites of coronary artery stenosis causes recurrent platelet attachment and dislodgement. The frequency and severity of this process of cyclical coronary blood flow alteration is directly related to the subsequent severity of neointimal proliferation in experimental canine models. Furthermore, the administration of a combined thromboxane A_2 synthesis inhibitor and receptor antagonist and serotonin receptor antagonist for 14 days after experimental injury prevents cyclical coronary blood flow altera-

tions.[21,22] Follow-up studies in the canine model demonstrate marked attenuation of neointimal proliferation.

Forrester and colleagues[23] have recently synthesized information about the intimal proliferative component of restenosis into an attractive hypothesis that restenosis simply represents an exaggerated form of the normal healing process (Fig. 21–3). They conceptualized a temporal sequence of events, all triggered by the denudation of endothelium and stretching of the entire vessel wall, including the normal portion of the vessel. The accumulation of platelets produces a variety of substances including growth factors and an endoglycosidase, which removes heparin from the injured cell,[24] thus making the cell more receptive to growth factors.[25] During the second to fourth days after vessel-wall trauma, smooth muscle cells change to the synthetic phenotype and migrate to the area of injury, while endothelial cells migrate to the lateral borders of the plaque fracture. Between the fifth and tenth days, extracellular matrix is formed by the transformed smooth muscle cells. In this paradigm of normal healing, intimal hyperplasia would reach a peak in 4 to 12 weeks after the

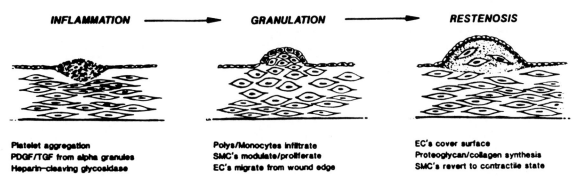

INFLAMMATION ⟶ GRANULATION ⟶ RESTENOSIS

Platelet aggregation
PDGF/TGF from alpha granules
Heparin-cleaving glycosidase

Polys/Monocytes infiltrate
SMC's modulate/proliferate
EC's migrate from wound edge

EC's cover surface
Proteoglycan/collagen synthesis
SMC's revert to contractile state

FIGURE 21–3. Hypothetical mechanisms for the process of restenosis after mechanical intervention. PDGF = platelet-derived growth factor; Polys = polymorphonuclear cells; SMC = smooth muscle cells; TGF = transforming growth factor. (Reproduced with permission from Forrester JS, et al. A paradigm for restenosis based on cell biology: clues for the development of new preventive therapies. J Am Coll Cardiol 1991; 17: 758–69.)

injury,[26] after which the smooth muscle cells would revert to the contractile phenotype. By 120 to 180 days the vessel-wall dynamics would have reverted to normal unless the endothelium remained denuded.

Therefore, the time course of arterial luminal renarrowing is a complex process that begins at the time of initial balloon dilation. If the process leads to sudden complete occlusion, it is termed abrupt closure. If the acute process leads to incomplete occlusion, the patient may not be identified as having a procedural failure until enough narrowing occurs to produce symptoms, at which time the process will be termed restenosis. The proportion of overall renarrowing events owing to each of the three major identified pathophysiologic phenomena—architecture, thrombosis, and intimal proliferation—remains uncertain. In fact, in many cases, the pathophysiology is very much interrelated, since larger intimal-medial tears may lead to creation of an occlusive intimal flap and to more intense thrombosis, which in turn may lead to a greater amount of intimal proliferation.

CLINICAL EPIDEMIOLOGY

Incidence of Abrupt Closure

The frequency of abrupt closure has been inconsistent among reports for the reasons mentioned above (Table 21–1), but the overall reported frequency with standard balloon angioplasty has varied from 1.5 per cent to 10 per cent in the catheterization laboratory and from 1 per cent to 4 per cent after leaving the laboratory. In general, approxi-

mately 70 per cent of episodes of abrupt closure occur in the angioplasty suite, while 30 per cent occur at a later time. Over 95 per cent of episodes of complete abrupt closure occur within the first 24 hours. The differences among studies could also result from underreporting in less rigorous studies, since events in the interventional catheterization laboratory are difficult to capture.

Most pathological studies in humans and animals demonstrated platelet-rich thrombi on the surface of the plaque within 12 hours of the procedure, whereas several angioscopic studies have verified that the plaque tearing or intimal denudation with subsequent clot formation is a common occurrence, even in successful angioplasty.[4,27] In one study evaluating angiograms, 44 per cent of abrupt closure cases had visible thrombus, while 80 per cent had visible dissections.[28] This finding that over half of abrupt closures appear to be mostly mechanical has been a consistent finding since the era of pretreatment with aspirin and the aggressive use of heparin.

Risk Factors for Abrupt Closure

Risk factors for abrupt closure can be considered in three broad categories: patient-related (systemic), lesion-related, and procedure-related. Patient-related risk factors refer to characteristics describing the overall clinical state of the patient. Lesion-related factors are the specific characteristics of each lesion that might be approached with percutaneous techniques. Current methods of characterizing lesions rely on angiography, although in the future angioscopy and intra-

TABLE 21–1. Rates of Abrupt Closures During and After Angioplasty

SOURCE	YEARS	TOTAL NUMBER PATIENTS	REPORTED RATE (%)
Simpfendorfer[109]*	1983–1985	1,500	2.0
Gablinani[47]*	1983–1987	1,238	1.8
Marquis[110]	1982–1983	164	11
Sinclair[27]	1981–1986	1,160	4.7
Shin[111]		240	8.6
Ellis[30]	1982–1986	4,772	4.4
Hollman[112]	1980–1982	935	2.1
Burkhard[113]	1984–1988	750	6.9
Steffino[114]	1983–1986	500	6.8
Mahin[115]	1979–1983	223	8.0
Stolz[116]		240	10.4
Gaul[117]	1980–1986	3,548	3.1
Meyerovitz[118]	1984–1986	516	8.5
NHLBI I[33]	1978–1981	1,155	4.5
NHLVI II[52]	1985–1986	3,548	6.8
deFeyter[34]	1986–1988	1,423	7.3

* In laboratory reocclusions only.

vascular ultrasound[29] may provide more precise characterization of the lesions. Procedure-related characteristics can be loosely interpreted to include the level of expertise and choice of equipment, as well as the clinical strategy, including pharmacologic manipulation.

Numerous studies have evaluated patient-related factors, but most have lacked adequate statistical power to reliably detect significant relationships.[1] A common thread through these studies, however, has been the identification of unstable angina, particularly refractory angina up to the time of angioplasty, as a risk factor. Patients with recent myocardial infarction and acute myocardial infarction have similarly been found to be at high risk of abrupt closure. The only other consistent findings have been an increased risk in women and diabetics in most studies.[1]

Lesion-related characteristics have been found to be significantly associated with abrupt closure. In an early study, Ellis and colleagues[30] have found the following characteristics to be associated with abrupt closure in 140 cases of abrupt closure drawn from 4,772 patients at Emory University: degree of stenosis prior to angioplasty, lesion length greater than two luminal diameters, bend point greater than 45 per cent, branch point, appearance of thrombus, multiple stenoses in the same vessel, and multivessel disease.

A more detailed follow-up study involving a multicenter collaboration of centers with a higher volume of multivessel angioplasty found that many specific morphologic characteristics of the lesions were significantly predictive of abrupt closure.[31] The American Heart Association/American College of Cardiology classification scheme was developed to classify lesions according to the likelihood of success or acute complication.[32] The classification scheme was initially devised based on "clinical wisdom" without an empirical base for the hierarchy (Table 21–2). When Ellis and colleagues evaluated the system, the classification was found to stratify risk, as the ACC/AHA class was the most powerful predictor of acute complications of multivessel angioplasty. Even after including the score in a regression model, however, the presence of high-grade stenosis, bend stenosis 60 per cent or more, chronic total occlusion, or "excessive" tortuosity, defined as a stenosis distal to three or more bends in the artery, were independently associated with complications. When the risk of a complication per lesion was assessed, type A lesions were associated with a 2.8 per cent risk. Lesions with one type B characteristic had a 4.4 per cent risk of a complication, while lesions with two or more type B characteristics had a 9.7 per cent risk of complication. Finally, those with at least one type C characteristic had a 20 per cent risk of a complication.

In a larger but less detailed experience of the National Heart, Lung and Blood Institute Percutaneous Transluminal Coronary Angioplasty Registry (NHLBI), 6.8 per cent of patients had an abrupt closure (4.9 per cent in the laboratory and 1.9 per cent outside the laboratory).[33] Lesion characteristics as-

TABLE 21–2. American Heart Association/American College of Cardiology Classification

Type A lesions
  Discrete (<10 millimeters length)
  Concentric
  Readily accessible
  Nonangulated segment, <45°
  Smooth contour
  Little or no calcification
  Less than totally occlusive
  Not ostial
  No major branch involvement
  Absence of thrombus
Type B lesions
  Tubular (10–20 millimeters length)
  Eccentric
  Moderate tortuosity
  Moderate angulated segment (>45°, <90°)
  Irregular contour
  Moderate to heavy calcifications
  Total occlusion <3 months old
  Ostial focation
  Bifurcation lesions
  Thrombus present
Type C lesions
  Diffuse (>2 centimeters length)
  Excessive tortuosity of proximal segment
  Extremely angulated segments >90°
  Total occlusion >3 months
  Inability to protect major sidebranch
  Degenerated vein graft

sociated with increased risk of abrupt closure included severe stenosis before the procedure, diffuse or multiple discrete morphology, thrombus, and collateral flow from the lesion. The odds ratios for each of these factors exceeded 1.5, indicating a substantial increase in risk. Unfortunately, the data col-

lection for the registry did not allow for collection of the entire AHA/ACC classification.

Preventive Treatment of Abrupt Closure

Evaluations of outcomes when abrupt closure occurs have consistently shown a disappointing (less than 60 per cent) reopening rate. In the NHLBI Registry only 49 per cent of arteries of patients with abrupt closure could be reopened after abrupt closure occurred.[33] Surprisingly, similar results have been found in two more recent series. Lincoff and colleagues[11] reported that successful reversal of abrupt closure occurred in only 43 per cent of patients despite a variety of maneuvers including coronary stents and thrombolytic therapy. Importantly, use of the stent was an independent predictor of successful reopening. Ten of sixty-three patients who could not be successfully reopened died in hospital. De Feyter and co-workers reported similar findings from the Dutch Thorax Center.[34] These findings make it clear that the first choice of therapy should be preventive, but that potent interventions are needed when abrupt closure occurs.

The prevention of abrupt closure has focused on three approaches: platelet inhibition, thrombin antagonism, and mechanical improvement in the lumen. Each of these therapies has produced evidence of benefit from observational studies, but only platelet

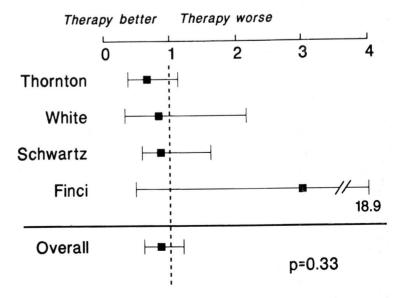

FIGURE 21–4. Overview of trials evaluating the effect of aspirin on restenosis rates. Results are displayed as odds ratios with 95 per cent confidence intervals. (Reproduced with permission from Califf RM, et al. Restenosis after coronary angioplasty: an overview. J Am Coll Cardiol 1991; 17: 2B–13B.)

inhibition has been studied in randomized trials (Table 21–3). Nevertheless, a rational approach to patient management and a sound basis for future development of more potent therapies has evolved.

Many early observational studies indicated that antiplatelet agents were associated with a reduction in the risk of abrupt closure at the time of angioplasty.[35–37] A randomized trial conducted by the Montreal Heart Institute demonstrated this point definitively.[38] In this trial, patients were randomized to either one 330-milligram aspirin tablet and 75-milligram dipyridamole tablets daily or to placebo. The treated patients had a 1.6 per cent rate of Q wave myocardial infarction compared with 6.9 per cent in the placebo group. The second study compared three therapies: ticlopidine 250 milligrams three times daily, aspirin 325 milligrams twice daily and dipyridamole 75 milligrams three times daily, and placebo.[39] Ischemic complications occurred in 1.8 per cent of ticlopidine-treated patients, 5.4 per cent of aspirin-treated patients, and 13.6 per cent of placebo-treated patients. These observational studies and randomized trials demonstrate beyond any doubt that antiplatelet therapy is a prerequisite for percutaneous intervention.

The dose of aspirin needed for maximum benefit and minimum risk remains a topic of controversy in this area as in most other areas of aspirin use. Several randomized trials at Emory University have evaluated this issue.[40] In one trial, patients were randomized to 80 milligrams or 1,500 milligrams of aspirin starting the day before the procedure. No difference in acute ischemic complications was reported. A second study evaluated the benefit of adding dipyridamole 75 milligrams three times daily to a twice daily dose of 325 milligrams of aspirin.[41] Again, no difference in acute ischemic complications was found. These studies in aggregate point to a generally accepted recommendation of once daily dosing of 160 to 325 milligrams of aspirin, starting at least 24 hours before the procedure if possible. This protocol makes the preangioplasty dose equivalent to the recommended dose for acute myocardial infarction, unstable angina, and coronary bypass graft patency.

The data regarding heparin administration are much less well controlled, but the nature of the observations are so powerful as to mandate antithrombotic therapy at the time of angioplasty. In several animal models, heparin has been found to be highly effective in preventing platelet and thrombus deposition in the experimental angioplasty setting. The most convincing experimental evidence comes from a porcine model investigated by Heras and co-workers.[42] In arterial segments with deep injury in this model, the degree of thrombus formation was inversely proportional to the logarithm of the number of heparin units given per unit of body weight. Observational evaluations in humans have shown a marked reduction in abrupt closure in patients treated with heparin for several days prior to angioplasty in the setting of unstable angina[43–45] or angiographically vis-

TABLE 21–3. Trials of Antiplatelet Agents in the Prevention of Abrupt Closure*

TRIAL	NUMBER OF PATIENTS	TREATMENT	COMPLICATION RATE (%)
† White[39]	333	Aspirin & Dipyridamole	5.0
		Ticlopidine	2.0
		Placebo	14.0
† Schwartz[38]	376	Aspirin	1.6
		Placebo	6.9
† Chesebro[119]	207	Aspirin & Dipyridamole	11.0
		Placebo	20.0
‡ Barnathon[35]	220	Aspirin	1.8
		Aspirin & Dipyridamole	0
		None	
‡ Kent[36]	500	Aspirin	1.3
		None	6.5

* Adapted with permission from Stein et al. Platelet inhibitor agents in cardiovascular disease: an update. J Am Coll Cardiol 1989; 14: 813–36.
† Randomized trial.
‡ Observational studies.

ible thrombus in the vessel.[46] Another study has documented a clustering of reocclusive events at the time of discontinuation of heparin therapy.[47]

Although the use of heparin is now accepted as standard and necessary therapy at the time of angioplasty, considerable controversy remains concerning the duration, dose, and proper monitoring of heparin therapy. From the experimental models, high-dose, prolonged, intravenous heparin infusions would seem to be advantageous. One randomized trial has been conducted comparing 18 to 24 hours of intravenous heparin therapy to heparin use only during the immediate procedure.[48] This study randomized only 208 patients in each group and excluded patients with a substantial intimal tear or dissection. There was a statistically insignificant trend (1.8 per cent with heparin compared with 2.4 per cent without heparin) toward a lower risk of abrupt closure in the heparin-treated group. Clearly, the sample size would have needed to be much larger in order to demonstrate the statistical significance of such a trend. The exclusion of patients with complicated procedures or angiographic evidence of filling defects at the completion of the procedure further limited the power of the study.

Ample evidence is now available to demonstrate that a "standard" dose of heparin (5,000-unit bolus and an intravenous infusion of 1,000 units/hour) is inadequate for many patients undergoing angioplasty. Monitoring of the activated partial thromboplastin time or of the activated clotting time (ACT) in the angioplasty laboratory has since become standard practice in the conduct of angioplasty. Several centers have now reported that patients with only a modest elevation of the activated partial thromboplastin time or activated clotting time despite "standard" heparin therapy have an increased risk of abrupt closure. In the largest series, Dougherty and co-workers[49] demonstrated that patients with an activated clotting time above 300 seconds had a significantly reduced risk of ischemic events and no increased risk of bleeding, while 79 per cent of the patients with a procedural complication had an activated clotting time below 250 seconds. In one small study of 94 patients, no relationship was found between the procedural response of the activated clotting time to heparin and the subsequent risk of restenosis.[50] Similar findings with regard to the activated partial thromboplastin time and abrupt closure have been reported by McGarry and colleagues.[51] In patients with an activated partial thromboplastin time three times control or higher the mortality rate was 0.4 per cent and the myocardial infarction rate was 2.6 per cent, while in patients with activated partial thromboplastin time values below three times control, the death rate was 1.5 per cent and the myocardial infarction rate was 10.7 per cent. These findings have led to a strategy in which large doses of intravenous heparin are commonly used in the setting of angioplasty with constant surveillance with bedside monitoring of the activated partial thromboplastin time or activated clotting time.

Treatment of Abrupt Closure

The initial treatment of abrupt closure involves immediate redilation whenever possible, generally using standard balloon technology. This approach fails in over 40 per cent of cases.[11,34,52] No clinical trials have been completed to guide the physician once the standard approach has been found to be unsuccessful. A variety of mechanical approaches have been advocated in addition to the use of thrombolytic therapy.

The major problem with clinical management once abrupt closure has occurred is that prolonged efforts to reestablish stable patency of the artery can lead to disaster if significant myocardial damage occurs and the patient goes to surgery in an unstable hemodynamic state. Furthermore, the use of potent anticoagulants, thrombolytic agents, or devices that can lead to arterial perforation or extended mechanical dissection make the operation much more complex and add to the risk of prolonged cardiopulmonary bypass and bleeding. Thus, the acute percutaneous or pharmacologic management of abrupt closure is a "double-edged sword" that holds the promise of averting the need for emergency bypass or preventing myocardial necrosis when the percutaneous method is successful, but the risk of delaying surgical revascularization when the percutaneous approach fails.

In general, a detailed angiographic assessment is made. If the occlusion appears to be predominantly thrombotic, thrombolytic therapy may be used after rapid testing with the activated clotting time or the activated partial thromboplastin time to ensure that adequate heparin anticoagulation has been achieved. If no evidence of thrombus is apparent, most operators proceed directly to mechanical salvage procedures, including prolonged balloon inflation, "hot" balloon technology, atherectomy, or stenting.

The results with thrombolytic therapy have been less favorable than expected. In a recent series,[34] intracoronary streptokinase at a mean dose of 750,000 international units was given to 34 patients with abrupt closure. Clinical success occurred in only 53 per cent of patients, while a major complication occurred in the remainder, including death, nonfatal infarction, and emergency coronary bypass surgery. At the University of Michigan[11] 43 of 110 patients with abrupt closure were treated with thrombolytic therapy. The majority of patients received urokinase; despite this therapy six patients required bypass surgery and two required coronary stenting. In a multivariate analysis, thrombolytic therapy was not found to be associated with a better outcome.

The increasingly preferred method of dealing with abrupt closure has been the employment of more sophisticated mechanical technology. Perfusion balloon devices were initially developed as "bail-out" devices to seat across a lesion that had previously occluded and could not be reopened while efforts were made to proceed with bypass grafting.[53,54] Observational studies have indicated that maintenance of perfusion while going to the operating room substantially reduces morbidity associated with emergency surgery. These devices evolved into perfusion balloon catheters, which have the capability of maintaining distal perfusion while a standard or prolonged angioplasty procedure is carried out.[55] Recent studies have demonstrated a substantial salvage rate using perfusion balloon catheters to "tack-up" large dissections causing abrupt closure.[56]

Substantial salvage rates in the setting of abrupt closure have recently been described with heated laser. The neodymium-yttrium-aluminum-garnet laser investigated by Jenkins and Spears[57] has been shown to produce a better appearance of the artery and to prevent the need for emergency bypass surgery in 84 per cent of patients. Further work with other methods, including the combination of a radiofrequency heated perfusion balloon catheter that would allow gradual heating to "weld" the artery are currently under investigation. An animal investigation indicated that a smoother lumen with a less thrombogenic environment could be produced, theoretically by sealing planes of dissection as they are formed.[58]

Atherectomy is a procedure in which a part of the plaque mass is excised and extracted from the artery. A small experience has now been generated with the use of atherectomy to salvage a patent vessel after abrupt closure with routine angioplasty. In a series of 30 patients with failed angioplasty, Vetter and colleagues[59] found that directional atherectomy succeeded in achieving a 50 per cent or less stenosis in 26 patients (87 per cent). Recently, however, a report of a coronary perforation in this setting has been published.[59] More experience will be needed, especially since the primary use of directional atherectomy is associated with a 4.2 per cent risk of abrupt closure.[10]

Much recent effort has been expended on the use of coronary stents in the setting of abrupt closure. Several different stent designs have now been used in observational clinical studies.[60–62] In the largest study with clinical follow-up to date, Serruys and colleagues[63] reported that with the Wallstent, a self-expanding stainless steel stent, complete occlusion occurred in follow-up in 25 of 105 patients treated with stents. The vast majority of these occlusions occurred in the first two weeks after implantation, mostly from an obvious episode of thrombosis. Another four patients did not have assessment of the status of the stent because they had died, while four patients refused restudy and two patients had technically inadequate studies.

A major issue with the current generation of stents is that the stent material is quite thrombogenic. The current antithrombotic regimen for stent implantation is extensive compared with previous anticoagulation regimens. The regimen for the Palmaz-Schatz stent includes the following: aspirin 325 milligrams daily and dipyridamole 75 milligrams three times daily for 48 hours before procedure and for three months after the procedure; low molecular weight dextran 40 (100 milliliters/hour intravenously to a total dose of 1 liter); heparin 10,000-unit bolus and then 2,500 units/hour during the procedure; then a heparin infusion to maintain the activated partial thromboplastin time at 1.5 to 2.5 times baseline; intracoronary urokinase (up to 500,000 units) if thrombus is visible;

and warfarin started on the day of the procedure and maintained for three months.

INCIDENCE OF RESTENOSIS

Clinical studies of the epidemiology of restenosis continue to be plagued by substantial difficulties with definition and experimental design. A large number of definitions for restenosis have been used, although in general when visual criteria have been used, a satisfactory initial result has been defined as both a 20 per cent improvement in luminal diameter and a reduction of the stenosis to less than 50 per cent of the luminal diameter. Restenosis has been defined as a recurrence of more than 50 per cent stenosis after an initially successful procedure. Reiber and colleagues have suggested that since the degree of intimal proliferation or encroachment on the lumen of the vessel is the main issue, restenosis should be defined as an absolute change in vessel lumen beyond the variability seen over time in lesions not treated with angioplasty. In a study done at the Dutch Thorax Center, these investigators determined that an encroachment of more than 0.72 millimeter exceeded two standard deviations from the mean change in lumen size over time.[64,65] While this definition is an improvement over previous standards, it does not take into account the overall size of the vessel, and may lead to underestimation of the clinically important restenosis rates in small vessels in which an increase of only 0.5 millimeter could lead to a physiologically significant stenosis.[9]

Given these limitations, the best estimates of restenosis rates come from studies with high degrees of angiographic and clinical follow-up. These studies have consistently shown a restenosis rate of more than 35 per cent when visual criteria have been used and when the occurrence of at least one restenotic lesion, regardless of the number of lesions initially dilated, includes the patient in the group with restenosis.[18] Interestingly, the restenosis rate in symptomatic patients ranges from 44 to 92 per cent, and in asymptomatic patients the restenosis rate ranges from 2 to 32 per cent.[1] Therefore, clinical studies of restenosis may make numerous classification errors unless angiographic data are available.

The timing of the restenotic process has been defined by several detailed angiographic studies. In a carefully designed follow-up study, Serruys and co-workers[65] demonstrated that the average luminal diameter initially increased from 2.06 millimeters at baseline to 2.11 millimeters at 30 days, and then gradually diminished to 1.93 millimeters at 60 days, 1.77 millimeters at 90 days, and 1.69 millimeters at 120 days. Using the quantitative definition of loss of lumen more than 0.72 millimeter, only 3 per cent of patients were classified as having restenosis between three and four months. Noboyushi and co-workers[14] extended these observations by finding no further restenosis between three months, six months, and one year when the average luminal diameter was evaluated in a large series of patients.

The clinical incidence of restenosis is a pivotal issue in the choice of revascularization therapies, and the potential impact of an effective treatment for restenosis on the use of percutaneous intervention is obvious when these rates are considered. Fortunately, the risk of restenosis in each individual lesion is not completely independent. Since the risk in a single lesion is 35 to 40 per cent, the risk to the patient of at least one restenosis event (assuming independence of risk) can be calculated as in Table 21–4. Multiple studies have now shown that the risk of restenosis in multiple lesions is, in fact, *interdependent.*[1] Therefore, the risk of at least one lesion developing restenosis is lower than predicted in multivessel disease, although the risk of at least one lesion having restenosis does increase to some extent as a function of the number of lesions dilated.[66]

Only a few studies have directly addressed the financial implications of restenosis. In an early study from the Mayo Clinic,[67] the first year follow-up charges were $10,641 in patients with restenosis, while the follow-up charges for patients without restenosis were $2,123. The follow-up charges for patients treated with coronary artery bypass grafting instead of angioplasty were $1,422 during

TABLE 21–4.

Number of Lesions Treated	Expected Restenosis Rate	Actual Restenosis Rate
1	0.40	0.40
2	0.64	0.51
3	0.78	0.58
4	0.87	0.72

the first year of follow-up. Making a few simple assumptions, it has been estimated that reducing the restenosis rate from 33 per cent to 25 per cent would reduce long-term procedural costs from $15,424 per patient to $13,734.[1] Not counting the gained revenue from time lost from work, this modest reduction in restenosis rates would save over $300 million annually to the United States economy alone.

Despite a multitude of observational studies in thousands of patients, few patient-related factors have been found to be consistently associated with the risk of restenosis. Perhaps the most consistent finding has been that instability of angina as measured by a number of definitions has been associated with an odds ratio for restenosis of 1.03 to 2.04.[1,9] The replication of this finding in multiple studies leads to a great degree of confidence in its importance. In our own series at Duke University, patients continuing to have unstable symptoms at the time of angioplasty despite maximal medical therapy have the highest rate of restenosis (above 50 per cent).[68] The only other patient-related factor that has been consistently related to restenosis is the presence of diabetes.[1,69,70] The odds ratio for restenosis in studies of diabetic patients has ranged from 1.60 to 2.91.

The other traditional risk factors including hypertension, family history, elevated cholesterol, gender, and cigarette smoking have not been found to be major factors in the majority of studies. In the largest series to date, neither past nor current cigarette smoking was found to have any relationship with restenosis.[9] Similarly, total cholesterol in the major subfractions of cholesterol were not found to be related to restenosis, although a modest trend toward a reduction in restenosis was observed in patients with a high-density lipoprotein cholesterol value above 40 milligrams/deciliter.[71] Although male gender was initially identified as a risk factor for restenosis, more recent large studies have not consistently confirmed this finding. This observation has led to speculation that newer technology may have produced better initial improvement in luminal diameter in men with large vessels, thus explaining the apparent loss of importance of gender as a risk factor for restenosis.

Recent studies have begun to evaluate the potential role of the hemostatic and fibrinolytic system in restenosis. In one small study,

elevation of plasminogen activator inhibitor-1 (PAI-1) levels was found to be a predictor of restenosis.[72] Another small study showed elevation of multiple procoagulant factors (plasminogen activator inhibitor-1, tissue plasminogen activator antigen, fibrinogen, factors VII and VIII) and depression of inducible fibrinolytic response in patients with restenosis at follow-up.[73] A prospective study at Duke University demonstrated a significant relationship between baseline fibrinogen levels and subsequent restenosis.[1]

The relationship between lesion-related characteristics and restenosis has not been addressed by many studies with adequate angiographic follow-up rates. Available data have indicated an increased propensity for restenosis in lesions located in the proximal left anterior descending artery.[74,75] In the Duke series of over 3,000 patients, we found no difference in restenosis rates according to lesion location.[66] One possible explanation is that in studies with low rates of angiographic follow-up, functional testing for ischemia is more likely to be definitive with a proximal left interior descending lesion, leading to a greater chance of detection of recurrent stenosis. The presence of a lesion in a saphenous vein bypass graft has been a consistent indicator of high risk of restenosis.[76,77] Finally, the risk of restenosis as defined by recurrence of stenosis above 50 per cent has been directly related to the severity of stenosis prior to dilation.[1] This finding has been particularly striking for chronically occluded vessels, which have a restenosis risk exceeding 50 per cent in most series.[78]

Unfortunately, little data currently exist relating detailed morphological lesion characteristics to risk of restenosis. The M-HEART study[18] which was predominantly designed to evaluate the impact of intravenous steroid therapy on the risk of restenosis, found that only stenosis length, preprocedure per cent stenosis, and adjacent artery diameter were related to the subsequent probability of restenosis. A smaller study by Halon and co-workers[79] found that in patients with unstable angina the risk of restenosis was related to location in the proximal left anterior descending artery, but also to the presence of irregularities in the contour of the lesion, angiographic appearance of thrombus, and to a collateral perfusion greater than perfusion in the vessel dilated. This information leads to the conclusion that the risk of restenosis is increased in lesions with complex morphologic characteristics.

Procedure-related factors and restenosis have been difficult to evaluate because of the complex interaction between the patient and lesion-related characteristics and the procedure itself. The degree of stenosis at the end of the procedure has consistently been found as a critical predictor of restenosis, regardless of whether standard balloon angioplasty or other percutaneous interventional techniques are used. This factor serves as an excellent example of the difficulty in sorting out the role of the procedure relative to other factors. Common sense would dictate that patients with a 49 per cent residual stenosis at the end of the procedure would be more likely to develop a more than 50 per cent stenosis at follow-up than patients with an initial 25 per cent stenosis. However, the conclusion does not necessarily follow that persisting in an effort to achieve the widest lumen possible will lead to a better clinical result, since the reason for more substantial residual stenosis may be the plaque architecture rather than the methods used in the interventional procedure. Complex preprocedure patient and lesion characteristics may limit the ability to achieve a wide lumen independently of the technique.

Various reports have found a higher restenosis rate with lower balloon inflation pressures,[80] lower balloon-to-artery ratios,[81] and fewer balloon inflations.[82] Follow-up trials evaluating each of these phenomena have failed to find a consistent effect.[81] Generally, an "oversized" balloon will lead to a higher abrupt closure rate, and higher pressures and multiple inflations probably reflect the difficulty of dilating the lesion.

An interesting procedure-related factor has been the creation of an angiographically visible dissection. Several studies have reported a low risk of restenosis in patients with a dissection.[83,84] Both studies found, however, that when the dissection resulted in a significant pressure gradient across the stenosis, the risk of restenosis was higher. These findings have led to speculation that production of greater injury may actually accelerate the healing process.

Prolonged, slow inflation of the balloon has been advocated as a method of producing remodeling of the vessel to improve the luminal widening with a decrease in the amount of trauma to the vessel wall.[55] Animal studies[85] have supported this concept, while preliminary human data are also suggestive.[55,86] A large, randomized clinical trial is presently underway comparing a standard one-minute inflation with a 15-minute inflation with a perfusion balloon catheter, which allows gradual, prolonged balloon inflation. This type of inflation is made possible because of continuous perfusion of the distal vessel through a central core in the balloon.

Percutaneous atherectomy was developed as a method of removing the plaque from the artery by a combination of cutting and physical extraction, thereby creating a wider lumen at the end of the procedure. The creation of a smooth lumen theoretically should also have the advantage of producing less turbulent flow in the area of the intervention. Restenosis rates of approximately 40 per cent have been reported with both the Simpson Atherocath,[87] which has been approved by the Food and Drug Administration, and with the Transluminal Extraction Endarterectomy Catheter (TEC),[88] which is still investigational. Coronary stents with several different designs have now been deployed in a substantial number of patients outside of the previously discussed setting of abrupt closure. In animal models a proliferative response is elicited by stent implantation with currently available materials. However, the creation of an initially widened lumen by preventing elastic recoil may allow for intimal proliferation without substantial compromise of the lumen. Early angiographic follow-up has not been as encouraging as initially hoped for, however.[61,63]

At this point, most clinical studies investigating laser therapy for coronary stenosis have evaluated lasers that do not truly ablate atheroma, but use thermal energy, which leads to a marked proliferative response. As expected, initial reports have found a similar restenosis rate to standard angioplasty. A recent report[89] documented a substantial proliferative response in a patient who came to autopsy several months after an excimer laser procedure, although the authors felt that the degree of the response was less than frequently seen with standard balloon angioplasty.

Treatment of Restenosis

A number of approaches to the prevention of restenosis with pharmacologic therapy have been considered (Table 21–5). These

TABLE 21–5. Approaches to Restenosis

APPROACH	STATUS OF TRIALS
Platelet inhibition	
Aspirin	2
Thromboxane receptor blockade	3
GP IIb-IIIa antagonists	4
Fish oil	2
Ketanserin	4
Thrombin inhibition	
Heparin	2
Hirudin	4
Hirulog	4
Smooth muscle cell proliferation inhibition	
Low molecular weight heparin	3
Angiotensive converting enzyme inhibitors	3
Lipid reduction	3
Direct growth factor inhibitor	
Angiopeptin	3
Mechanical	
Stent	2
Laser	2
Heater balloon	2
Atherectomy	3

1 = evidence substantially negative; 2 = evidence equivocal; 3 = trials substantially underway, no results yet; 4 = trials in planning phase.

approaches can be conveniently divided into categories according to the major pathophysiologic target. The first area to attack has been the activation of platelets, either by inhibitory steps in the multiple pathways of platelet activation or by blocking platelet-specific receptors. Other pharmacologic strategies have focused on prevention of the formation of thrombin at the site of angioplasty. General approaches to inhibit smooth muscle cell proliferation have been tested. More specific approaches to blocking the effects of growth factors are now becoming available. Finally, enhanced mechanical approaches, combined with local delivery of potent pharmacological therapy have become the topic of intense research efforts.

A variety of antiplatelet agents have been shown to reduce both platelet deposition and intimal proliferation after experimental vascular injury in animal models. The impact of aspirin on the risk of restenosis has been evaluated in seven randomized trials including over 1,500 patients[1] (Fig. 21–4). Although no significant difference has been found in any individual study, when the results of all available trials were combined in a meta-analysis, a trend toward a reduction in restenosis rates was found with doses of aspirin

at 325 milligrams or less per day (Fig. 21–5). Overall, in the seven studies a statistically insignificant 11 per cent reduction in the risk of restenosis was observed.

Other agents affecting platelet function or the balance of thromboxane and prostacyclin have also been evaluated.[90] In several studies with ticlopidine, an insignificant trend toward a lower restenosis rate has been observed as with aspirin, although the most recent study showed a trend in the opposite direction.[91] Two small trials with prostacyclin analogs have also shown a trend toward benefit, although the most substantial reduction was in clinical events rather than angiographic restenosis rates. All of these individual studies were plagued by a sample size too small to reliably detect less than a 50 per cent reduction in the rate of restenosis.

The specific effects of anticoagulant drugs have been studied in only two completed clinical trials to date. In a comparison of coumadin and aspirin, the Emory group found a 25 per cent lower restenosis rate with aspirin, although the study was limited by several methodologic difficulties.[92] Only 248 patients were randomized, thus severely restricting the power of the study. Furthermore, general compliance with the coumadin arm was only 74 per cent, and only 35 per cent of patients had a "therapeutic" prothrombin time.

The study by Ellis and colleagues[48] found no advantage to more prolonged (18 to 24 hour) heparin administration compared with heparin during the procedure only. The study did not address the issue of high-dose heparin, however. In the porcine model, high-dose heparin has been found to reduce the deposition of platelets and to impede subsequent intimal proliferation after vascular injury.[42] Another interesting aspect of heparin is the finding that the nonanticoagulant heparin fragments decrease intimal hyperplasia, but only when given in the first three days after arterial injury.[93–95] Two randomized trials are underway comparing enoxaparin, a low molecular weight heparin fragment, with placebo in the treatment of restenosis. Giving standard heparin in high doses has the potential to combine the anticoagulant effects of standard heparin with antiproliferative effects of both standard heparin and the low molecular weight fragments.

Some of the most interesting results of clinical trials to date have come from evaluation of omega-3 fatty acids and restenosis.[96]

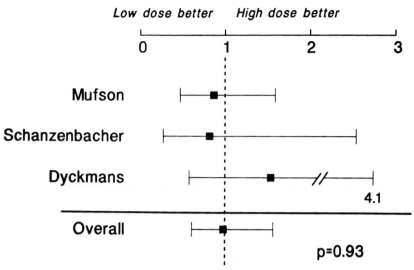

FIGURE 21–5. Overview of trials evaluating the effect of high-dose (1,000 to 1,500 mg/day) and low-dose (80 to 320 mg/day) aspirin in restenosis. Results are shown as odds ratios with 95 per cent confidence intervals. (Reproduced with permission from Califf RM, et al. Restenosis after coronary angioplasty: an overview. J Am Coll Cardiol 1991; 17:2B–13B.)

Large numbers of studies have now demonstrated that high doses of omega-3 fatty acids have a variety of physiologic effects that may improve the environment for performing angioplasty.[96] Effects on platelet function include an increased bleeding time, reduced platelet aggregation to standard stimuli such as collagen and adenosine diphosphate, and prolonged time to occlusion of prosthetic grafts. Platelet counts are also reduced by omega-3 fatty acids, although the degree of reduction is not major. Evidence is accumulating for a favorable effect on platelet–vessel wall interactions as evidenced by reduction in intimal hyperplasia after arterial wall injury. Furthermore, omega-3 fatty acids appear to have a generally favorable influence on endothelial-dependent vascular responses, as evidenced by a diminished tendency for spasm and response to various stimuli in arteries with both preserved and damaged endothelium. Other potentially favorable effects of omega-3 fatty acids include a decrease in whole blood viscosity owing to increased deformibility of red blood cells, enhanced endothelial-derived relaxing factor release, and a more salutary balance between endogenous tissue plasminogen activator and its inhibitors.

To date, five randomized trials evaluating omega-3 fatty acids in the prevention of restenosis have been completed (Fig. 21–6). Unfortunately, these studies all had relatively small sample sizes (less than 150 patients)

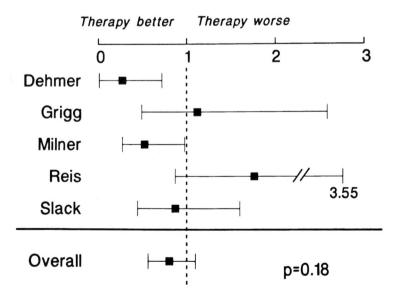

FIGURE 21–6. Overview of trials evaluating the effect of omega-3 fatty acids on restenosis rates. Results are displayed as odds ratios with 95 per cent confidence intervals. (Reproduced with permission from Califf RM, et al. Restenosis after coronary angioplasty: an overview. J Am Coll Cardiol 1991; 17: 2B–13B.)

and vary considerably in the dose and timing of drug administration, in addition to the completeness of angiographic follow-up. The most promising study by Dehmer and co-workers had the advantage of starting the omega-3 fatty acid one week before the angioplasty procedure and having complete angiographic follow-up with quantitative angiography.[97] Despite the hazards of meta-analysis when trials of different methodology are combined, an overview demonstrates a substantial trend ($p = 0.18$) toward a reduction in restenosis rates.

Several small trials have evaluated the role of coronary vasodilators in the prevention of restenosis. These drugs might be beneficial by providing an environment with greater blood flow and therefore less of a tendency for clot formation. The two studies with calcium channel blockers were both negative, although neither study had enough patients to reliably detect a restenosis reduction of less than 50 per cent.[98,99] The only substantial effort to directly inhibit proliferation of smooth muscle cells has recently been reported. The M-HEART Study Group randomized 915 patients to either placebo or to a 1-gram bolus of methylprednisolone prior to angioplasty.[18] The restenosis rate was 39 per cent in treated patients and 40 per cent in the control group. A further evaluation of the data suggested that a lower restenosis rate occurred in patients with low-risk morphologic characteristics. Since this finding was not a prespecified analysis in the protocol, it must be replicated before adoption in the clinical practice.

Future Trials

At least 11 placebo control trials of restenosis are currently underway (as shown in Table 21–5). As compared with the generation of trials with insufficient statistical power previously discussed, these trials in general have the statistical power to detect a 33 per cent reduction in the rate of restenosis. Unfortunately, the lack of a reliably predictive animal model has limited the enthusiasm for any of the current approaches, although all have been shown to inhibit intimal proliferation after experimental vascular injury.

A pair of randomized trials with GR32191, a specific thromboxane A_2 receptor antagonist, have recently completed enrollment, although final angiographic and clinical follow-

up results are not available. These studies will also provide an interesting comparison with aspirin during the acute phase of the angioplasty procedure. Solutroban, another specific thromboxane receptor antagonist, is also being evaluated in a randomized trial. Whether blocking platelet function by another pathway (perhaps more intensely, also) than the one inhibited by the aspirin effect will have a more profound impact on intimal proliferation hopefully will be known when present trials with over 2,000 patients are reported.

Another interesting approach to the modulation of the platelet effect in the setting of angioplasty is to inhibit the effects of serotonin. A series of studies have now identified serotonin as a potent mediator in platelet aggregation and coronary vasoconstriction.[100,101] Detailed human studies have found that serotonin concentrations are increased in the setting of unstable angina and complex plaque morphology.[102] Furthermore, serotonin has been shown to lead to increased deoxyribonucleic acid synthesis and proliferation of vascular smooth muscle cells.[103] Ketanserin, a serotonin S_2-receptor antagonist, blocks the effects of serotonin on platelet aggregation and mitogenesis. A large trial evaluating ketanserin is presently underway.

Pilot studies in the setting of angioplasty are now underway with 7E3.[104] These early studies have demonstrated a dramatic effect on platelet function with an intravenous bolus or infusion of this antibody which blocks the glycoprotein IIb-IIIa receptor. Over 75 patients have now undergone angioplasty after pretreatment with this agent with good results to date. A large randomized clinical trial with a combined endpoint of abrupt closure and restenosis is planned for 1991 to 1992.

Finally, several studies are underway evaluating particular growth factor antagonists. In models involving injury to arterial walls, cilazapril, an angiotensin-converting enzyme inhibitor has been shown to dramatically inhibit myointimal hyperplasia.[105] Demonstration of angiotensin receptors and converting enzyme activity in arterial walls[106] has provided further rationale for a role of angiotensin-converting enzyme inhibitors in restenosis. Angiopeptin, which appears to be a nonspecific antagonist of multiple growth factors, including insulin-like growth factor I and epidermal growth factor, has also been shown to inhibit myointimal proliferation in both rabbit and primate models.[107,108] A large trial is currently underway evaluating this agent.

CURRENT CLINICAL RECOMMENDATIONS

Based on current clinical knowledge, therapeutic recommendations for standard balloon angioplasty related to the thrombotic system are fairly simple. First, whenever possible, patients with unstable ischemic syndromes should be "cooled off" with antianginal, antiplatelet, and antithrombin therapy because of the apparent higher risk of abrupt closure and restenosis in these patients. If the patient cannot be stabilized, intensive antithrombotic therapy during and after the procedure is needed. Second, pretreatment with aspirin 165 to 325 milligrams/day and heparin to achieve a high level of anticoagulation is necessary to reduce the risk of abrupt closure. Third, careful monitoring of anticoagulation during the procedure and in the immediate postprocedure period is mandatory. Unfortunately, since no therapy has been shown to reduce restenosis rates in patients with a successful initial procedure, the only current antithrombotic recommendation in postpercutaneous transluminal coronary angioplasty patients is one aspirin per day as in all patients with advanced coronary artery disease. As previously described, recommendations for intracoronary device use or implantation are more complex and subject to change at this time.

THE FUTURE

The process by which percutaneous interventions result in a successful or failed procedure are complex, involving the interaction of mechanical factors, the thrombotic system, and growth factors. More sophisticated devices will almost certainly provide an improved outlook in terms of treating abrupt closure and producing a wider lumen with successful procedures. Whether pharmacologic approaches that attack only one component of the complex pathophysiology can have a major impact by interrupting a causal chain remains unclear. An alternative approach would be to inhibit multiple pathways simultaneously, hoping to achieve additive or synergistic effects. This approach has been effective in the treatment of acute myocardial infarction with thrombolytic and antiplatelet therapy.

Finally, for high-risk lesions, the combination of a mechanical device such as a stent and a pharmacologic approach may be most effective. In particular, the development of biodegradable polymers may allow for a less thrombogenic substrate in which intensive pharmacologic therapy can be delivered locally at the site of the mechanical intervention. Regardless of the approach used, a more directed approach to modification of thrombosis will make the margin of safety and efficacy much greater for percutaneous intervention.

REFERENCES

1. Califf RM, Ohman EM, Frid DJ, et al. Restenosis: the clinical issues. In: Topol EJ, ed. Textbook of intervention cardiology. Philadelphia: WB Saunders Co., 1990: 363–94.
2. Parisi AF, Hartigan P, Folland ED, VA ACME. Initial clinical results of the randomized VA acme trial of angioplasty vs. medicine for single vessel disease. JACC 1991; 2: 30A.
3. Waller BF. "Crackers, breakers, stretchers, drillers, scrapers, shavers, burners, welders and melters"—the future treatment of atherosclerotic coronary artery disease? A clinical-morphologic assessment. J Am Coll Cardiol 1989; 13: 969–87.
4. Uchida Y, Hasegawa K, Kawamura K, Shibuya I. Angioscopic observation of the coronary luminal changes induced by coronary angioplasty. Am Heart J 1989; 117: 769–76.
5. Potkin BN, Roberts WC. Effects of coronary angioplasty on atherosclerotic plaques and relation of plaque composition and arterial size to outcome. Am J Cardiol 1988; 62: 41–50.
6. Waller BF. Pathology of transluminal balloon angioplasty used in the treatment of coronary heart disease. Hum Pathol 1987; 18: 476–84.
7. Waller BF. Morphologic correlates of coronary angiographic patterns at the site of percutaneous transluminal coronary angioplasty. Clin Cardiol 1983; 11: 817–23.
8. Waller BF. Early and late morphologic changes in human coronary arteries after percutaneous transluminal coronary angioplasty. Clin Cardiol 1983; 6: 363–72.
9. Califf RM, Fortin DF, Frid DJ, et al. Restenosis after coronary angioplasty: an overview. J Am Coll Cardiol 1991; 17: 2B–13B.
10. Popma JJ, Topol EJ, Pinkerton CA, Whitlow PL, Hartzler GO, Selmon MR. Abrupt closure following directional coronary atherectomy: clinical, angiographic and procedural outcome. JACC 1991; 2: 23.
11. Lincoff MA, Popma JJ, Ellis SG, Hacker JA, Topol EJ. Abrupt vessel closure complicating coronary angioplasty: clinical, angiographic, and therapeutic profile. Submitted 1991; CIRC, in press.
12. Popma JJ, Califf RM, Topol EJ. Clinical trials of restenosis following coronary angioplasty: will the ends be justified by the means? Submitted 1991; CIRC, in press.
13. Rensing BJ, Serruys PW, Beatt KJ, Suryapranata H, Laarman GJ, deFeyter PJ. Densitometrically observed differences in elastic recoil of the 3 main coronary arteries after percutaneous transluminal coronary angioplasty. J Am Coll Cardiol 1990; 15: 43.
14. Nobuyoshi M, Takeshi K, Nosaka H, et al. Restenosis after successful percutaneous transluminal coronary angioplasty: serial angiographic follow-up of 229 patients. J Am Coll Cardiol 1988; 12: 616–23.
15. Davies MJ, Thomas AC. Plaque fissuring: the cause of acute

myocardial infarction, sudden ischemic death, and crescendo angina. Br Heart J 1985; 53: 363–73.

16. Falk E. Unstable angina with fatal outcome, dynamic coronary thrombosis leading to infarction and/or sudden death: autopsy evidence of recurrent mural thrombosis with peripheral embolization culminating in total vascular occlusion. Circulation 1985; 71: 699–708.

17. DiCorleto PE, Chisolm GM. Participation of the endothelium in the development of the atherosclerotic plaque. Prog Lipid Res 1986; 25: 365–74.

18. Pepine CJ, Hirshfeld JW, MacDonald RG, et al. A controlled trial of corticosteroids to prevent restenosis after coronary angioplasty. Circulation 1990; 81: 1753–61.

19. Haudenschild CC, Grunwald J. Proliferative heterogeneity of vascular smooth muscle cells and its alteration by injury. Exp Cell Res 1985; 157: 364–70.

20. Grunwald J, Haudenschild CC. Intimal injury in vivo activates vascular smooth muscle cell migration and explant outgrowth in vitro. Arteriosclerosis 1984; 4: 183–8.

21. Willerson JT, Yao SK, McNatt J, et al. Frequency and severity of cyclic flow alterations and platelet aggregation predict the severity of neointimal proliferation following experimental coronary stenosis and endothelial injury. Proc Natl Acad Sci USA 1991; AAP (Presentation).

22. Willerson JT, Eidt JF, McNatt J, et al. Role of thromboxane and serotonin as mediators in the development of spontaneous alterations in coronary blood flow and neointimal proliferation in canine models with chronic coronary artery stenosis and endothelial injury. J Am Coll Cardiol 1991; 17: 101B–10B.

23. Forrester JS, Fishbein M, Helfant R, Fagin J. A paradigm for restenosis based on cell biology: clues for the development of new preventive therapies. JACC 1991; 17: 758–69.

24. Castellot JJ, Wong K, Hoover HB, et al. Binding and internalization of heparin by vascular smooth muscle cells. J Cell Physiol 1985; 124: 13–20.

25. Campbell GR, Campbell JH, Manderson JA, Horrigan S, Rennick RE. Arterial smooth muscle: a multifunction mesenchymal cell. Pathol Lab Med 1988; 112: 977–86.

26. Mizuno Y, Miyamotot A, Shibuya T, et al. Changes of angioscopic macromorphology following coronary angioplasty. Circulation 1988; 78: 289.

27. Sinclair IN, McCabe CH, Sipperly ME, Baim DS. Predictors, therapeutic options, and long-term outcome of abrupt reclosure. Am J Cardiol 1988; 61: 61G–6G.

28. Pryor DB, Harrell FE Jr, Rankin JS, et al. The changing survival benefits of coronary revascularization over time. Circulation 1987; 76(suppl V): V13–20.

29. Yock PG, Linker DT. Catheter-based two dimensional ultrasound imaging. In: Topol EJ, ed. Textbook of interventional cardiology. Philadelphia: WB Saunders Co., 1990: 42–3.

30. Ellis SG, Roubin GS, King SB. Angiographic and clinical predictors of acute closure after native vessel coronary angioplasty. Circulation 1988; 77: 372–9.

31. Ellis SG, Vandormael MG, Cowley MJ, et al. Coronary morphologic and clinical determinants of procedural outcome with angioplasty for multivessel coronary disease: implications for patient selection. Circulation 1990; 82: 1193–202.

32. Ryan TJ, Faxon DP, Gunnar RM, et al. Guidelines for percutaneous transluminal coronary angioplasty: a report of the American College of Cardiology/American Heart Association Task Force on Assessment of Diagnostic and Therapeutic Cardiovascular Procedures (subcommittee on percutaneous transluminal coronary angioplasty). J Am Coll Cardiol 1988; 12: 529–45.

33. Detre K, Holmes DM, Holubkov R, et al. Incidence and consequences of perioprocedural occlusion. The 1985–1986 National Heart, Lung, and Blood Institute Percutaneous Transluminal Coronary Angioplasty Registry. Circulation 1990; 82: 739–50.

34. deFeyter PJ, van den Brand M, Jaarman G, vanDomburg R, Serruys PW, Suryapranata H. Acute coronary artery occlusion during and after percutaneous transluminal coronary angioplasty. Circulation 1911; 83: 927–36.

35. Barnathan ES, Schwartz JS, Taylor L, et al. Aspirin and dipyridamole in prevention of acute coronary thrombosis complicating coronary angioplasty. Circulation 1987; 76: 125–34.

36. Kent KM. Restenosis after percutaneous transluminal coronary angioplasty. Am J Cardiol 1988; 6: 67G–70G.

37. Cunningham DA, Kumar B, Siegal BA, Gillula LA, Totty WG, Welch MJ. Aspirin inhibition of platelet deposition at angioplasty sites: demonstration by platelet scintigraphy. Radiology 1984; 151: 487–90.

38. Schwartz L, Bourassa MG, Lesperance J, et al. Aspirin and dipyridamole in the prevention of restenosis after percutaneous transluminal coronary angioplasty. N Engl J Med 1988; 318: 1714–9.

39. White CW, Chaitman B, Lassar TA, Ticlopidine Study Group. Antiplatelet agents are effective in reducing the immediate complications of PTCA: results from the ticlopidine multicenter trial. Circulation 1987; IV: 400.

40. Mufson L, Black A, Roubin G, et al. A ramdomized trial of aspirin in PTCA: effect of high vs. low dose aspirin on major complications and restenosis (abstr). J Am Coll Cardiol 1988; 11: 236A.

41. Lembo NJ, Black AJ, Roubin GS, et al. Does the addition of dipyridamole to aspirin decrease acute coronary angioplasty complications? The results of a prospective randomized clinical trial (abstr). J Am Coll Cardiol 1988; 11: 237A.

42. Heras M, Chesebro JH, Penny WJ, et al. Importance of adequate heparin dosage in arterial angioplasty in a porcine model. Circulation 1988; 78: 654–60.

43. Lukas MA, Deutsch E, Lakey WF. Beneficial effect of heparin therapy on PTCA outcome in unstable angina (abstr). J Am Coll Cardiol 1988; 11: 132A.

44. Ogilby JD, Koeplman HA, Klein LW, Agarwal JB. Adequate heparinization during PTCA: assessment using activated clotting time (abstr). J Am Coll Cardiol 1988; 11: 237A.

45. Hettleman BD, Aplin RL, Sullivan PR, Lemla H, O'Connor GT. Three days of heparin pretreatment reduces major complications of coronary angioplasty in patients with unstable angina. J Am Coll Cardiol 1990; 15: 154A.

46. Sugrue DD, Holmes DR, Smith HC, et al. Coronary artery thrombus as a risk factor for acute vessel occlusion during percutaneous transluminal coronary angioplasty: improving results. Br Heart J 1986; 53: 363–73.

47. Gabliani G, Deligonul U, Kern M, Vandormael M. Acute coronary occlusion occurring after successful transluminal angioplasty: temporal relationship to discontinuation of anticoagulation. Am Heart J 1988; 116: 696–700.

48. Ellis SG, Roubi GS, Wilentz J, Douglas JS, King SB. Effect of 18–24 hour heparin administration for prevention of restenosis after uncomplicated coronary angioplasty. Am Heart J 1989; 117: 777–82.

49. Dougherty KG, Marsh KC, Edelman SK, Gaos CM, Ferguson JJ, Leachman R. Relationship between procedural activated clotting time and in-hospital post PTCA outcome. Abstracts of the 63rd Scientific Sessions 1991; III–189.

50. Perin EC, Turner SA, Ferguson JJ. Relationship between the response to heparin and restenosis following PTCA. Circulation 1990; 173: III–189.

51. McGarry T, Gottlieb R, Zelenkofske S, et al. Relationship of anticoagulation level and complications after successful percutaneous transluminal coronary angioplasty (PTCA). Abstracts of the 63rd Scientific Sessions 1991; III–189.

52. Detre KM, Holmes DR, Holubkov R, et al. Incidence and consequences of perioprocedural occlusion. Circulation 1990; 82: 739–50.

53. Sundram P, Harvey JR, Johnson RG, Schwartz MJ, Baim DS. Benefit of the perfusion catheter for emergency coronary artery grafting after failed percutaneous transluminal coronary angioplasty. Am J Cardiol 1989; 282: 285.

54. Ferguson TB, Hinohara T, Simpson J, Stack RS, Wechsler AS. Catheter reperfusion to allow optimal coronary bypass grafting following failed transluminal coronary angioplasty. Ann Thorac Surg 1986; 42: 399–405.

55. Stack RS, Quigley PJ, Collins G, Phillips HR. Perfusion balloon catheter. Am J Cardiol 1988; 61: 77G–80G.

56. Smith JE, Quigley PJ, Tcheng JE, Bauman RP, Thomas J, Stack RS. Can prolonged perfusion balloon inflations sal-

vage vessel patency after failed angioplasty? (abstr). Circulation 1989; 80: 11–373.

57. Jenkins RD, Spears JR. Laser balloon angioplasty. A new approach to abrupt coronary occlusion and chronic restenosis. Circulation 1990; 81: IV-101–8.

58. Buller CE, Skethc MH, Phillips HR, Stack RS. Thermal perfusion balloon angioplasty. J Am Coll Cardiol 1911; 2: 123A.

59. Topol EJ. Emergency strategies for failed percutaneous transluminal coronary angioplasties. Am J Cardiol 1989; 63: 249–50.

60. Sigwart U, Urban P, Svein G, et al. Emergency stenting for acute occlusion after coronary balloon angioplasty. Circulation 1988; 78: 1121–7.

61. Schatz RA, Baim DS, Leon M, et al. Clinical experience with the Palmaz-Schatz coronary stent: Initial results of a multicenter study. Circulation 1991; 83: 148–61.

62. Roubin GS, Douglas LS, Lembo NJ, Black AJ, King SB. Intracoronary stenting for acute closure following percutaneous transluminal coronary angioplasty (PTCA). Circulation 1988; 78: II-407.

63. Serruys PW, Strauss BH, Beatt KJ, et al. Angiographic follow-up after placement of a self-expanding coronary artery stent. N Engl J Med 1991; 324: 13–7.

64. Reiber JHC, Serruys PW, Kooijman CJ, et al. Assessment of short, medium, and long term variations in arterial dimensions from computer-assisted quantitation of coronary cincangiograms. Circulation 1985; 71: 280–8.

65. Serruys PW, Luijten HE, Beatt KJ, Incidence of restenosis after successful coronary angioplasty: a time-related phenomenon: a quantitative angiographic study in 342 consecutive patients are 1, 2, 3, and 4 months. Circulation 1988; 77: 361–71.

66. Tcheng JE, Frid DJ, Fortin DF, Nelson CL, Stack RK, Peter RH, Stack RS, Califf RM. Restenosis: angiographic predictors, clinical outcomes. JACC 1991; 17: 345A.

67. Reeder GS, Krishan I, Nobrega FT, et al. Is percutaneous coronary angioplasty less expensive than bypass surgery? N Engl J Med 1984; 311: 1157–62.

68. Frid DJ, Fortin DF, Lam LC, et al. Effects of unstable symptoms on restenosis. Circulation 1990; 82: III-427.

69. Frid DJ, Fortin DF, Gardner LW, et al. The effect of diabetes on restenosis. JACC 1991; 17: 268A.

70. Margolis JR, Chen C, Glemser E. Restenosis after PTCA is increased in diabetic patients. Eur Heart J 1989; 10: III-5.

71. Harlan WR, Fortin DF, Frid DJ, et al. Are serum lipoprotein levels important in predicting restenosis after coronary angioplasty? Abstracts of the 63rd Scientific Sessions 1991; III-427.

72. Huber K, Jorg M, Resch I, et al. Association of a significant increase of plasminogen activator inhibitor-1 with the development of a coronary restenosis in patients after PTCA. J Am Coll Cardiol 1990; 15: 209.

73. Kirschstein W, Simianer S, Dempfle CE, et al. Impaired fibrinolytic capacity and tissue plasminogen activator release in patients with restenosis after PTCA. Thromb Haemost 1989; 62: 772–5.

74. Leimgruber PP, Roubin GS, Hollman J, et al. Restenosis after successful coronary angioplasty in patients with single vessel disease. Circulation 1986; 73: 710–7.

75. Mata LA, Bosch X, David PR, Rapold HJ, Corcos T, Bourassa MG. Clinical and angiographic assessment 6 months after double vessel percutaneous coronary angioplasty. J Am Coll Cardiol 1985; 6: 1239–44.

76. Cote G, Myler RK, Stertzer SH, et al. Percutaneous transluminal angioplasty of stenotic coronary artery bypass grafts: 5 years experience. J Am Coll Cardiol 1987; 9: 8–17.

77. Douglas JS, Gruentzig AR, King SB, et al. PTCA in patients with prior coronary bypass surgery. J Am Coll Cardiol 1983; 2: 745–54.

78. Serruys PW, Umans V, Heyndrickx GR, van den Brand M, deFeyter PJ, Wijns W, Jaski B, Hugenholtz PG. Elective PTCA of totally occluded coronary arteries not associated with acute myocardial infarction: short-term and long-term results. Eur Heart J 1985; 6: 2–12.

79. Halon DA, Merdler A, Shefer A, Flugelman MY, Lewis BS.

Identifying patients at high risk for restenosis after PTCA for unstable angina pectoris. Am J Cardiol 1989; 64: 289–93.

80. Meier B, Gruentzig AR, King SB, et al. Higher balloon dilatation pressure in coronary angioplasty. Am Heart J 1984; 107: 213–9.

81. Roubin GS, Douglas JS, King SB, et al. Influence of balloon size on initial success, acute complications, and restenosis after percutaneous transluminal coronary angioplasty: A prospective randomized study. Circulation 1988; 78: 557–65.

82. Uebis R, Schmitz E, VomDahl J, Blome R, vonEssen R, Hanrath P. Single versus multiple balloon inflations in coronary angioplasty: late angiographic results and recurrence. J Am Coll Cardiol 1989; 13: 58.

83. Leimgruber PP, Roubin GS, Anderson HV, et al. Influence of intimal dissection on restenosis after successful angioplasty. Circulation 1985; 72: 530–5.

84. Matthews BJ, Ewels CJ, Kent KM. Coronary dissection: a predictor of restenosis? Am Heart J 1988; 115: 547–54.

85. Perez JA, Mikat EM, Ramirez NM, Collins GJ, Phillips HR, Stack RS. Effect of prolonged balloon inflation on arterial hyperplasia in rabbits. Circulation 1987; 76: 184.

86. Quigley PJ, Kereiakes DJ, Abbottsmith CW, et al. Prolonged autoperfusion angioplasty: immediate clinical outcome and angiographic follow-up. J Am Coll Cardiol 1989; 13: 155.

87. Hinohara T, Rowe M, Sipperly ME, et al. Restenosis following directional coronary atherectomy after native coronary arteries. J Am Coll Cardiol 1990; 15: 196.

88. Stack RS, Phillips HR, Quigley PJ, et al. Multicenter registry of coronary atherectomy using the transluminal extraction-endarterectomy catheter. J Am Coll Cardiol 1990; 15: 196.

89. Karsch KR, Haase KK, Wehrmann M, Hassenstein S, Hanke H. Smooth muscle cell proliferation and restenosis after stand alone coronary excimer laser angioplasty. JACC 1991; 4: 29.

90. Turner BM, Beratis NG, Hirschhorn K. Cell-specific differences in membrane beta-glucosidase from normal and Gaucher cells. Biochim Biophys Acta 1977; 480: 442–9.

91. Bertrand ME, Allain H, Lablanche JM. Results of a randomized trial of ticlopidine versus placebo for prevention of acute closure and restenosis after coronary angioplasty (PTCA). Circulation 1990; 82: III-190.

92. Thornton MA, Gruentzig AR, Hollman J, King SB, Douglas JS. Coumadin and aspirin in prevention of recurrence after transluminal coronary angioplasty: a randomized study. Circulation 1984; 69: 721–7.

93. Guyton JR, Rosenberg RD, Clowes AW, Karnovsky MJ. Inhibition of rat arterial smooth muscle cell proliferation by heparin. In vivo studies with anticoagulation and nonanticoagulant heparin. Thromb Res 1980; 46: 625–34.

94. Gordon JB, Berk BC, Bettman MA, Selwyn AP, Rennke H, Alexander RW. Vascular smooth muscle cell proliferation following balloon injury is synergistically inhibited by low molecular weight heparin and hydrocortisone. Circulation 1987; 76: 213.

95. Clowes AW, Karnowsky MJ. Suppression by heparin of smooth muscle cell proliferation in injured arteries. Nature 1977; 265: 625–6.

96. Dehmer GJ. Omega-3 Fatty acids. In: Topol EJ, ed. Textbook of interventional cardiology. Philadelphia: WB Saunders Co., 1990: 121–52.

97. Dehmer GJ, Popma JJ, vandenBerg EK, et al. Reduction in the rate of early restenosis after coronary angioplasty by a diet supplemented with n-3 fatty acids. N Engl J Med 1988; 319: 733–40.

98. Korcos T, David PR, Val PG, et al. Failure of diltiazem to prevent restenosis after PTCA. Am Heart J 1985; 109: 926–31.

99. Whitworth HB, Roubin GS, Hollman J, et al. Effect of nifedipine on recurrent stenosis after percutaneous transluminal coronary angioplasty. J Am Coll Cardiol 1986; 8: 1271–6.

100. Golino P, Ashton JH, Buja LM, et al. Local platelet activation causes vasoconstriction of large epicardial canine

coronary arteries in vivo. Thromboxane A2 and serotonin are possible mediators. Circulation 1989; 79: 154–66.

101. Benedict CR, Matheur B, Cartwright J, Sordahl LA. Correlation of plasma serotonin changes with platelet aggregation an in vivo dog model of spontaneous occlusive coronary thrombus formation. Circulation 1986; 58: 58.

102. vandenBerg EK, Schmitz JM, Benedict CR, Malloy CR, Willerson JT, Dehmer GH. Transcardiac serotonin concentration is increased in selected patients with limiting angina and complex lesion morphology. Circulation 1989; 79: 116–24.

103. Nemecek GM, Coughlin SR, Handley DA, Moskowitz MA. Stimulation of aortic smooth muscle cell mitogenesis by serotonin. Proc Natl Acad Sci USA 1986; 83: 674–8.

104. Ellis SG, Bates ER, Schaible T, Weisman HF, Pitt B, Topol EJ. Prospects for the use of antagonists to the platelet glycoprotein IIb/IIIa receptor to prevent postangioplasty restenosis and thrombosis. J Am Coll Cardiol 1991; 17: 89B–95B.

105. Powell JS, Muller RK, Bumgartner HR. Suppression of the vascular response to injury: the role of angiotensin-converting enzyme inhibitors. JACC 1991; 17: 137B–42B.

106. Ehlers MRW, Riordan JF. Angiotensin converting enzyme: new concepts concerning its biological role. Biochemistry 1989; 28: 5311–8.

107. Conte JV, Foegh ML, Calcagno D, Wallace RB, Ramell PW. Peptide inhibition of myointimal proliferation following angioplasty in rabbits. Transplan Proc 1989; 4: 3695–6.

108. Lundergan C, Foegh ML, Ramwell P. Peptide inhibition of myointestinal proliferation hyangiopeptin, a somafostatin analogue. JACC 1991; 17: 132B–6B.

109. Simpendorfer C, Belardi J, Bellamy G, Gallan K, Frankco I, Hollman J. Frequency, management, and follow-up of patients with acute coronary occlusions after percutaneous

110. Marquis JF, Schwartz L, Aldridge H, Majid P, Henderson M, Matushinsky E. Acute coronary artery occlusion during percutaneous transluminal coronary angioplasty treated by redilation of the occluded segment. J Am Coll Cardiol 1984; 4: 1268–71.

111. Shiu MF, Silverton NP, Oakley D, Cumberland D. Acute coronary occlusion during percutaneous transluminal coronary angioplasty. Br Heart J 1985; 54: 129–33.

112. Hollman J, Gruentzig AR, Douglas JS, King SB, Ischinger T, Meier B. Acute occlusion after percutaneous transluminal coronary angioplasty: a new approach. Circulation 1983; 68: 725–32.

113. Burkhard-Meier C, Vonarnim TH, Stablein A, Werdan K, Hofling B. Major complications of PTCA: analysis of 500 patients. Eur Heart J 1988; 9: 218.

114. Steffenion G, Meier B, Finci L, et al. Acute complications of elective coronary angioplasty: a review of 500 consecutive procedures. Br Heart J 1988; 59: 151–8.

115. Mabin TA, Holmes DR, Smith HC, et al. Intracoronary thrombus: role in coronary occlusion complicating percutaneous transluminal coronary angioplasty. J Am Coll Cardiol 1985; 5: 198–202.

116. Stolz RI, Varricchione TR, Kellett MA, Christelis EM, Ryan TJ, Faxon DP. Abrupt reocclusion in PTCA: angiographic characteristics ad clinical consequences. J Am Coll Cardiol 1987; 9: 181.

117. Gaul C, Hollman J, Simpendorfer C, Franco I. Acute occlusion in multiple lesion coronary angioplasty: frequency and management. J Am Coll Cardiol 1989; 13: 283–8.

118. Meyerovitz MF, Friedman PL, Ganz P, Selwyn AP, Levin DC. Acute occlusion developing during or immediately after percutaneous transluminal coronary angioplasty: non-surgical treatment. Radiology 1988; 169: 491–4.

22

STROKE AND TRANSIENT ISCHEMIC ATTACK:
Thromboembolism and Antithrombotic Therapy

DAVID G. SHERMAN and ROBERT G. HART

Incidence and Prevalence of Stroke

Stroke is the third most common cause of death in the United States and the leading cause of neurologic disability in adults. Each year 500,000 new strokes occur, with 150,000 of these dying as a result of their stroke. Two million individuals are alive with various degrees of neurologic sequelae following a previous stroke.[1] Seventy per cent have some impaired vocational capacity, and 30 per cent require assistance in their activities of daily living. Twenty per cent need help with walking, and 15 per cent are institutionalized. There has been a steady decline in the mortality from stroke over the past 15 years. Because of the increasing mean age of the population in most Western nations, the absolute number of strokes continues to increase.

Economic Impact of Stroke

The annual cost of stroke in the United States is about $13 billion. One third of the 2 million persons surviving a stroke are potential wage earners younger than age 65.

Classification of Cerebrovascular Disorders

The term "stroke" is used to describe a number of brain disorders with the common feature of an abnormality of the brain's vasculature. Strokes are classified according to whether they are ischemic or hemorrhagic; they are described by the vascular territory involved, their temporal profile, and by their etiology.

ISCHEMIC AND HEMORRHAGIC STROKES

Arterial occlusion with brain ischemia and infarction accounts for most strokes. These occlusions arise by a number of mechanisms and account for about 85 per cent of all strokes. When progressive arterial stenosis occurs, blood flow declines to the area of brain supplied by the artery. As blood flow drops below a critical level, the deprived brain ceases to function. If blood flow is maintained through collateral circulation or a residual lumen at a minimal level (about 15 milliliters/100 grams/minute) the neurons maintain their integrity while remaining electrically and functionally silent. If blood flow can be restored promptly, these cells recover. If this minimal level of flow is persistent or decreases further, cells are no longer able to maintain their biochemical and structural integrity. The brain region involved in whole or part passes from reversible ischemia to irreversible infarction. The goal of restoring blood flow to ischemic brain is further complicated by the potential for reperfusion injury to ischemic brain as a result of the formation of free radicals and other poten-

409

tially deleterious substances. These principles form the theoretical basis for therapies of acute ischemic stroke. The aim is to rescue brain with reversible ischemia through means directed at improving flow or preserving viable ischemic neurons and thereby minimizing the amount of brain infarction and neurological disability. The clinical corollary of reversible neuronal ischemia is the transient ischemic attack (TIA). Here, regional ischemia produces a focal neurologic deficit that resolves completely because of restoration of normal flow and metabolism prior to the development of irreversible ischemia and infarction.

Hemorrhagic strokes occur when blood leaks out of a brain vessel. Subarachnoid hemorrhage occurs when a vessel, usually an arterial aneurysm, ruptures with bleeding into the subarachnoid space. Intracerebral hemorrhages occur with bleeding from a small artery within the brain parenchyma. A patient may have both subarachnoid and intracerebral bleeding, depending on the location of the ruptured vessel. As with ischemic stroke, a number of vascular pathologies may produce a hemorrhagic stroke. Hemorrhagic strokes account for about 15 per cent of all strokes. An important distinction is between a primary intracerebral hemorrhage wherein the initial event is rupture of an artery within the brain, and a secondarily hemorrhagic infarction wherein initially a vascular occlusion produces brain ischemia with subsequent reperfusion allowing leakage of blood from damaged vascular elements into the ischemic brain. As a general rule, hemorrhagic stroke carries a worse prognosis, with a mortality rate of about 40 per cent, compared to a 15 to 20 per cent mortality in ischemic stroke. Computerized tomography (CT) and magnetic resonance imaging (MRI) scanning have allowed the detection of intracerebral bleeding that was previously clinically occult.

TEMPORAL PROFILE OF BRAIN ISCHEMIA

All ischemic brain episodes are described based on the temporal profile of their neurologic deficit. A transient ischemic attack is a focal ischemic neurologic event that has completely resolved clinically within 24 hours. This time interval is arbitrary, and in fact most transient ischemic attack last less than 30 minutes. One type of transient ischemic attack is amaurosis fugax or transient monocular blindness (TMB). In this case there is transient ischemia to the retinal circulation. A focal ischemic episode that persists for greater than 24 hours and is not clearly worsening or improving at that point is called a "completed stroke." A stroke that undergoes resolution of the neurologic deficit within three weeks is sometimes referred to as a "reversible ischemic neurologic deficit (RIND)." The term "progressing stroke" or "stroke in evolution" is used to denote the situation where over minutes or hours there is worsening of the stroke deficit because of expansion of the area of ischemia. These terms do not imply an etiology for a patient's focal ischemic symptoms. The temporal profile is but one of the clinical, radiologic, and laboratory features of an ischemic event that point to a probable etiology.

VASCULAR TERRITORY

Strokes are also classified based on the vessel involved in causing the stroke symptoms. The patient's symptoms, signs, and brain imaging studies allow inference about the vessel responsible for the stroke. Strokes are thus said to be in the right or left carotid artery distribution, in the vertebrobasilar artery territory, involving one of the major intracranial arteries (middle, anterior, or posterior cerebral) or involving small named and unnamed arteries. As with the temporal profile, the vascular territory has little etiologic implication independent of other features of the stroke or transient ischemic attack.

PATHOPHYSIOLOGY OF CEREBROVASCULAR DISORDERS

There are multiple potential causes for stroke. Disease (especially atherosclerosis) of the large and small arteries accounts for the majority of ischemic strokes. Other disorders of the arterial wall, disorders of coagulation, and cardiac sources of emboli may act alone or in combination to produce vascular thrombosis.

Carotid and Intracranial Artery Pathology

What is the nature of carotid artery disease in the population of patients with cerebral ischemia? Harrison et al. examined the angiographic appearance of the carotid arteries in 215 patients with transient ischemic attacks, reversible ischemic neurologic deficits, or completed strokes.[2] They found that 20 per cent of patients had normal carotid arteries. An equal fraction had carotid artery occlusion and the remaining 60 per cent had a spectrum of carotid atherosclerotic plaques and stenotic changes. When Bogousslavsky examined 380 patients with a cortical middle cerebral artery territory stroke, he found that 17 per cent had internal carotid artery occlusion, 32 per cent had a normal internal carotid artery, and the remainder had varying degrees of carotid artery stenosis.[3] Of the 230 patients undergoing cerebral angiography, 112 showed occlusion of a branch of the middle cerebral artery. In 50 cases, carotid artery atherosclerosis with distal embolization was felt to be the cause, whereas in 44 cases (40 per cent), cardiogenic embolism was the suspected mechanism. Thus, an embolus arising from an atherosclerotic carotid artery plaque was a common mechanism for the genesis of stroke symptoms in the middle cerebral artery territory.

In another prospective study of 80 patients with focal ischemic symptoms undergoing angiography within six hours, a complete arterial occlusion was present in 76 per cent. Two thirds of these were intracranial occlusions. Seventy per cent of the occlusions that were assessed in one week showed recanalization. Potential embolic sources for the intracranial occlusions were the carotid artery (30 of 80), the heart (17 of 80), either the heart or the carotid arteries (20 of 80), or no cardiac or arterial source apparent in 13 of 80.[4]

RISK FACTORS FOR CEREBROVASCULAR DISEASE

The major risk factors for stroke can be viewed as either untreatable or potentially treatable. Untreatable risk factors include age, sex, family history, and ethnic origin. The major potentially treatable risk factors include hypertension, cardiac disease, cerebrovascular disease, transient ischemic attack, cigarette smoking, and diabetes mellitus.

Age, Gender, and Race

The incidence of stroke is strongly related to age, and more than doubles in each successive decade. The incidence is generally 25 per cent higher in men than in women.[5]

Hypertension

The presence of hypertension increases the risk of stroke by six to seven times in both men and women.[6] In borderline hypertension the adjusted relative risk of stroke is about double.[7]

Smoking

Cigarette smoking has been shown to be a risk factor for stroke, particularly in men under age 65 and women over the age of 65.[8] Smoking increases the risk of subarachnoid hemorrhage by fivefold with the risk related to the amount of smoking and gender. Heavy smokers, more than 20 cigarettes daily, have an odds ratio of 19.8 for subarachnoid hemorrhage. Women have an odds ratio of 7.4 compared to men with a ratio of 2.9.[9] Recently, tobacco use has been linked to extracranial carotid artery atherosclerosis.[10,11]

Cholesterol and Lipids

The relationship of serum cholesterol to stroke is somewhat paradoxical. The risk of stroke is increased with either low or high serum cholesterol.[12] Men with cholesterol levels of under 4.14 millimoles/liter (160 milligrams/deciliter) had a three-times-higher risk of death from intracranial hemorrhage than did men with higher cholesterols. Conversely, the risk of nonhemorrhagic stroke increased progressively in patients with elevated serum cholesterol levels.[13]

Atherosclerotic Vascular Disease

Atherosclerosis affects arteries throughout the body. Atherosclerosis in one vascular territory is a marker for disease in other susceptible arteries. Patients with coronary or peripheral vascular disease have a higher risk for cerebral atherosclerosis.

There are a number of ways in which one can detect carotid artery disease. A carotid bruit can be heard in a little over 4 per cent of the general population over the age of 45.

By age 65, some 6 to 7 per cent of asymptomatic individuals will be found to have a carotid bruit.[14-16] The presence of a bruit, while useful as a marker of atherosclerotic disease and increased risk for stroke, is not highly predictive of carotid stenosis. In one study of 500 patients with asymptomatic neck bruits, almost one half (n = 230) had less than 30 per cent carotid artery stenosis by noninvasive studies. Only 113 (23 per cent) had the minimum degree of stenosis considered sufficient to impede flow.[17]

The carotid ultrasound has been most widely used to attempt to define individuals at increased risk for stroke.[17,18] When carotid stenosis progresses to occupy 75 per cent or greater of the luminal diameter, there is a sharp increase in the risk for the development of ischemic symptoms. The majority of time the initial symptoms take the form of tran-sient ischemic attacks which may later culminate in a stroke. Some patients in this group experience stroke unheralded by transient ischemic attack. In addition to the degree of stenosis as a predictor of subsequent symptoms, it has also been observed that heterogeneous and low-density plaques more likely become symptomatic (Figs. 22–1 and 22–2). These low-density areas may represent regions of intraplaque hemorrhage which may disrupt the surface of the plaque or may account for a sudden progression of the stenosis.[19,20] Chambers and Norris found that 18 per cent of their patients with a 75 per cent or greater carotid artery stenosis experienced transient ischemic attack or stroke within one year, with 5 per cent of patients experiencing a completed stroke and 3 per cent experiencing a stroke without a preceding ischemic attack.[17] Langsfield fol-

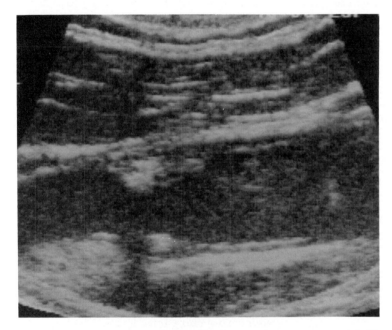

FIGURE 22–1. The high echogenicity area seen at the bifurcation represents a hard plaque with calcification. This causes acoustic shadowing of the region below near the external carotid artery (not visualized in this frame).

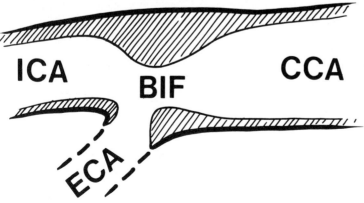

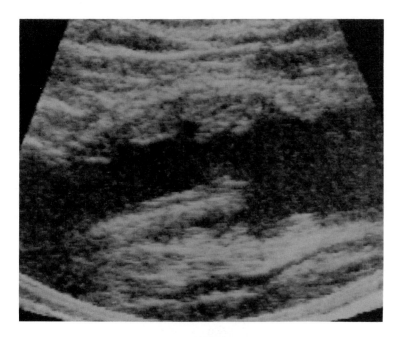

FIGURE 22-2. Soft plaque with ulceration seen in the internal carotid artery (ICA). The external carotid artery (ECA) is not seen in this frame because its course is not in the same plane as the other vessels. ICA = internal carotid artery; BIF = bifurcation; ECA = external carotid artery; CCA = common carotid artery.

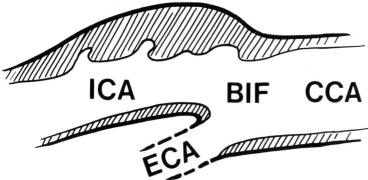

lowed the carotid artery contralateral to an endarterectomy in 289 patients and the carotid arteries in 130 asymptomatic patients referred for evaluation of bruits. Over a 15-month period of observation, about half of the carotid arteries did not change appreciably. About one fourth increased in the degree of stenosis or in the degree of echolucency of the plaque. Similarly, about one fourth were noted to have a reduction in the degree of stenosis or became more echodense. Ten of the two hundred eighty-nine patients (3.5 per cent) suffered a stroke on the side contralateral to the endarterectomy. Two patients (1.5 per cent) in the asymptomatic group experienced a stroke. The patients most likely to develop cerebrovascular symptoms were those with complex, echolucent plaques and those with stenosis of greater than 75 per cent.[21] Moore et al. noted

the importance of compound ulcerations in asymptomatic carotid arteries as predictors of subsequent stroke.[22] Others have failed to show such a strong relationship between the presence of plaque ulceration and the subsequent development of symptoms in the carotid artery.[23]

Cardiac Disorders

About 15 per cent of all ischemic strokes are due to a cardiogenic embolism. The most common underlying conditions are nonrheumatic atrial fibrillation, rheumatic heart disease, acute myocardial infarction, left ventricular thrombi remote from a myocardial infarction, and prosthetic cardiac valves.[24,25] Small embolic fragments, only 3 to 4 millimeters in diameter, can occlude the middle cerebral artery and cause devastating stroke. The cardiac disorders are reviewed in other chapters.

Nonrheumatic atrial fibrillation carries a risk of stroke of about 5 per cent per year. The risk of stroke in this population is more than five times that of a comparable population without atrial fibrillation. Myocardial infarcts occur in approximately 500,000 people per year. About 3 per cent (15,000) of patients with an acute myocardial infarction suffer a stroke while still in the hospital.

Coagulation and Hematologic Disorders

A variety of disorders of the blood elements and coagulation factors may cause or contribute to stroke.[26,27] Some 5 per cent of young adults with stroke have a hematologic disorder as the primary mechanism for their stroke. There may be uncertainty as to whether a hematologic finding is causally related to a given patient's stroke. At times the relationship may be indisputable, while at other times the etiologic association is uncertain. Inherited deficiencies of coagulation inhibitors have been associated with thrombosis of cerebral arteries and veins. These include antithrombin III, protein C, and protein S deficiencies. Hereditary abnormalities of fibrinolysis associated with ischemic stroke include dysfibrinogenemia and deficiency of plasminogen, plasminogen activator, factor XII, and prekallikrein. Elevation of factors VIII and V have been observed in patients with ischemic stroke and suggested as contributing to thrombosis. Erythrocyte disorders associated with stroke include polycythemia vera, sickle cell disease and trait, sickle-C disease, beta-thalassemia, paroxysmal nocturnal hemoglobinuria, and secondary polycythemia. Platelet disorders promoting stroke include essential thrombocythemia, secondary thrombocytosis, and acquired hyperaggregable ("sticky") platelets. Autoantibodies may develop in some patients and promote thrombosis. The lupus anticoagulant and antiphospholipid antibodies have been associated with increased risk of stroke and stroke recurrence.

Increased blood viscosity may contribute to diminished brain blood flow and ischemia. Blood and plasma viscosity are increased in patients with stroke and transient ischemic attack and also in patients with risk factors for cerebrovascular disease compared to controls.[28] The major contributors to increased blood viscosity are increased fibrinogen, decreased albumin, and elevated hematocrit.

NATURAL HISTORY OF TRANSIENT ISCHEMIC ATTACK AND STROKE

Diagnosis of Transient Ischemic Attack and Stroke

AMBIGUITY IN DIAGNOSIS

The first objective in managing a patient with transient ischemic attack or stroke is to determine the cause for their brain ischemia. This task is complicated by the lack of specificity of the patient's symptoms and signs and by the frequent coexistence of several potential causes for the brain ischemia. Even in the hands of stroke specialists, some 10 to 30 per cent of patients with a focal cerebral ischemic event will not have a specific cause for their transient ischemic attack or stroke determined. In at least another one third, coexistent disease of the arterial wall, the heart, and blood elements make precise definition of the cause difficult, if not impossible.

There is frequently uncertainty about whether carotid atherosclerotic disease demonstrated in an individual is, in fact, the cause for their ischemic stroke. Many of these patients have coexistent small-vessel disease involving the intracranial circulation, and many also have cardiac disorders capable of producing cardiogenic emboli to the brain. About 30 per cent of patients with carotid system ischemic stroke have a potential cardiac source of embolus, and 30 per cent of these have carotid atherosclerosis or occlusion, making definite determination of the cause difficult.[29] One fifth of patients with carotid system transient ischemic attack have both carotid atherosclerosis and a possible cardiac source of embolus.[30] There is a tendency to overestimate rather than underestimate carotid atherosclerosis as a cause of ischemic stroke. Carotid atherosclerosis is common in the general population and can be demonstrated reliably by carotid ultrasound or angiography. On the other hand, small-vessel intracranial disease is difficult to confirm and generally is inferred from the overall clinical picture. Likewise, many cardiac sources of emboli are relatively hidden from the eyes and ears of the echocardiogram and stethoscope. Acquired and hereditary prothrombotic conditions may lead to brain ischemia alone or in concert with structural disorders of the heart or cerebral vessels.

The symptoms and signs produced with a transient ischemic attack or a stroke are rarely helpful in sorting out one potential cause from others. Amaurosis fugax and its variant, transient monocular visual loss with exposure to bright light, are perhaps most specific in suggesting carotid artery occlusion or stenosis, although other mechanisms such as mitral valve prolapse and migraine may also cause temporary retinal ischemia. A rare form of "limb-shaking transient ischemic attack" is also indicative of carotid occlusion or high-grade stenosis with impaired hemispheric perfusion. A history of repeated stereotyped transient ischemic attacks is more commonly seen with carotid atherosclerotic disease than it is with cardiogenic embolism. Atherothrombotic strokes are more likely to have their onset while the patient is sleeping, and are apparent on awakening, with a stuttering course. Cardiogenic emboli more often produce the sudden onset of a maximal neurologic deficit while the patient is awake and active.

Much of the cerebral white matter, basal ganglia, thalamus, and brainstem is supplied by tiny penetrating arteries which originate from the medium-sized cerebral arteries (for example, middle cerebral artery, anterior cerebral artery). These thread-like vessels are beyond the resolution of arteriography and are named in groups: lenticulostriates, thalamogeniculates, for example. Since the mid 1960s, distinct clinical syndromes have been recognized when these arteries are occluded, leading to small subcortical "lacunar" (from *lacuna,* meaning "hole") strokes. The majority of these small subcortical strokes are due to intrinsic intracranial cerebrovascular disease, although a small fraction can be attributed to emboli from the heart or cervical carotid arteries. If lesions are multiple and bilateral, primary intracranial artery disease is almost certainly the cause. While acute mortality of lacunar infarction is low (1 per cent in 30 days), the rate of recurrence is particularly high (15 per cent in the first year).[31,32] These small subcortical lacunar infarcts, accounting for some 20 per cent of carotid territory strokes are commonly attributed to disease of the small penetrating arteries originating from the middle and posterior cerebral arteries. One cannot, however, exclude other stroke mechanisms, because the clinical, computed tomographic, or magnetic resonance imaging findings suggest a "lacunae." Emboli from the carotid artery or the heart may occlude these small penetrating vessels, emphasizing the need to consider the spectrum of stroke mechanisms as a cause for small infarcts of the basal ganglia and internal capsule.

The abrupt onset of maximal neurologic deficit in an individual less than 55 years of age is particularly suggestive of cardiogenic embolism, especially if there is a history of cardiac disease. All patients should be questioned regarding symptoms of coronary ischemia, congestive heart failure, cardiac arrhythmias, and rheumatic fever. If the history, physical examination, chest x-ray, and electrocardiogram fail to suggest cardiac disease, and the patient is over the age of 55, an extensive cardiac work-up should not be undertaken until other vascular causes for stroke or transient ischemic attack have been eliminated. Even patients with suspected cardiogenic embolus and a known cardiac source of embolus, and those patients with clinical and radiologic features characteristic of lacunar stroke should generally have noninvasive studies of the carotid arteries considered in their diagnostic work-up. The absence of major carotid atherosclerotic disease supports these other stroke mechanisms and helps define that group of patients with unsuspected carotid artery disease as the cause for their transient ischemic attack or stroke. The majority of the remaining patients are those with risk factors for atherosclerotic disease, absent or minimal cardiac disease, and a clinical profile that is atypical for a lacunae. In these patients, if the patient is considered a potential candidate for carotid endarterectomy, it is advisable to proceed either directly to cerebral angiography or, in some cases, to first obtain noninvasive studies of the carotid arteries, and if the potentially operative lesion is suggested by noninvasive studies, to proceed with cerebral angiography.

NATURAL HISTORY

What is the natural history of transient ischemic attack or minor stroke untreated? The risk of subsequent stroke is generally estimated at about 5 per cent per year for the first three years and 3 per cent annually thereafter. The risk is somewhat greater in the first month following a transient ischemic attack. One half of the patients with transient ischemic attack will suffer a myocardial infarction within the next five to seven years, emphasizing the importance of a transient ischemic attack as a marker for atherosclerosis in other circulations. The predictive value of the number of transient ischemic attacks is somewhat controversial. A study of patients seen at the Mayo Clinic found that the probability of stroke within 30 days of one, two to four, or five or more transient ischemic attacks was 6, 7, and 20 per cent.[33]

ANTIPLATELET AGENTS AND CEREBROVASCULAR DISORDERS

Aspirin for Transient Ischemic Attack and Stroke

Aspirin is the antiplatelet agent most widely used for stroke prevention in patients at risk. There have been some ten randomized clinical trials of in excess of 4,500 patients with transient ischemic attack examining the benefits of aspirin. Overall, aspirin use has reduced the occurrence of primary stroke by 21 per cent.[34] Eight trials looked at the value of aspirin following prior stroke and found a 26 per cent reduction in stroke recurrence in these patients.

Aspirin and Secondary Stroke Prevention

The United Kingdom-Transient Ischemic Attack Study was a multicenter trial of 2,435 patients with transient ischemic attack or minor stroke. Patients were randomized to placebo or aspirin 300 or 1,200 milligrams/day and were followed for a mean of four years. There was an 18 per cent reduction in the risk of myocardial infarction, recurrent stroke, or death in the aspirin-treated patients. There was a 7 per cent reduction in the risk of disabling stroke or vascular death.[35]

The European Stroke Prevention Study was a multicenter trial of 2,500 patients with transient ischemic attack (33 per cent), reversible ischemic neurologic deficit (7 per cent), or stroke (60 per cent). Patients were randomized to placebo or aspirin 975 milligrams and dipyridamole 225 milligrams/day and followed for two years. There was a 33.5 per cent reduction in the risk of recurrent stroke or death and a 38 per cent reduction in the risk of stroke only.[36,37]

The Dutch TIA Trial compared two doses of aspirin in patients with transient ischemic attack or minor stroke.[38] In this study, 3,150 patients with transient ischemic attack or minor stroke were randomized in a double-blind fashion to aspirin 30 milligrams or 360 milligrams/day. Patients were followed for an average of 2.6 years. The primary endpoints were vascular death, stroke, and myocardial infarction. Primary endpoints occurred in 6 per cent of the patients, with no significant difference in the two doses of aspirin. The investigators conclude that there is no difference in the efficacy of these two doses of aspirin. The event rate was low, suggesting possibly a low-risk population and raising the issue of comparability of the population studied to other studies. The relative value of higher doses of aspirin, 900 to 1,300 milligrams/day, compared to these lower doses was not addressed in this study.

Aspirin and Primary Stroke Prevention

The United States and British physicians' studies of aspirin in the prevention of cardiovascular disease have raised questions regarding the use of aspirin by individuals free of cardiac and cerebrovascular disease. The U.S.A. Physicians' Health Study compared alternate-day aspirin (325 milligrams) and placebo in 22,071 male physicians aged 40 to 84 during a mean follow-up of 4.8 years.[39] Of 293 myocardial infarctions (MIs), only 23 (7.8 per cent) were fatal. Nonfatal myocardial infarction was reduced by 43 per cent, but the absolute magnitude of reduction was only 0.14 per cent/year owing to the low prevalence of myocardial infarctions in this population. Death from all cardiovascular causes was identical in the two groups and extraordinarily low (only 0.08 per cent/year). Strokes were about half as common as myocardial infarctions, only 5 per cent were fatal. Disabling and fatal strokes increased by 64 per cent in the aspirin arm. Disabling and fatal hemorrhagic strokes were increased fivefold (10 versus 2), with an absolute risk increase of 0.02 per cent/year. In this population of 22,000 male physicians, there were 13 fewer fatal myocardial infarctions and 9 more disabling or fatal strokes in the aspirin-treated patients. While there has been concern expressed over the routine use of aspirin in light of a potential increased risk for hemorrhagic stroke, the absolute risk is small: over 5,000 individuals would be required to take aspirin for a year before one would suffer a disabling stroke.

The British Physicians' Study randomized 5,139 male physicians to take 300 to 500 milligrams of aspirin daily or to avoid aspirin (unblinded, no placebo administration).[40] Mean follow-up was 5.5 years. The rate of death in the British study was 10.3 times that of the U.S.A. Physicians' trial. There were no significant differences between treatment arms in the rates of fatal or nonfatal myocardial infarction. While transient ischemic attacks were significantly reduced (0.28 per cent/year vs. 0.16 per cent/year), the rates of disabling or fatal stroke were 75 per cent higher (0.20 per cent/year versus 0.35 per cent/year). Overall, the outcome in the aspirin-treated patients was worse owing to the increased rate of disabling and fatal strokes. While the number of enrolled physicians was smaller than in the United States trial, the vascular event rates were five to ten times higher and were more serious events.

These two large studies lead to the conclusion that the routine use of aspirin in healthy men may not be justified when the risks of a disabling or fatal stroke are compared to the benefits in reducing nonfatal myocardial infarction. (See also Chapter 14.)

Ticlopidine for Transient Ischemic Attack and Stroke

MECHANISM OF ACTION

Ticlopidine is a platelet antiaggregating agent whose mechanism of action is incompletely understood. Ticlopidine has a time- and dose-dependent inhibition of platelet aggregation which persists for more than 72 hours after discontinuation of treatment with a return to baseline values after four to ten days. One effect of ticlopidine is to interfere with platelet membrane function by inhibiting adenosine diphosphate-induced platelet-fibrinogen binding. It differs from aspirin and other antiplatelet agents in that it is not a cyclooxygenase (aspirin effect) or phosphodiesterase (dipyridamole effect) inhibitor: its action is not dependent on prostaglandin formation effects. Platelet aggregation inhibition is detected within two days of initiation of therapy. Maximum platelet inhibition is achieved within five to eight days. Bleeding

times are prolonged with ticlopidine, with maximal effect seen after five to six days. Clopidogrel is an analogue of ticlopidine, which is 50 to 100 times more potent in animal models.

CLINICAL TRIALS

The Ticlopidine Aspirin Stroke Study (TASS) compared the efficacy of ticlopidine (250 milligrams twice daily) and aspirin (650 milligrams twice daily) in patients with a recent transient ischemic attack or minor stroke for the reduction of stroke and death.[41] This multicenter trial enrolled 3,069 patients and followed them for a mean of 3.3 years. Stroke occurred in 13.8 per cent (212 of 1,540) patients on aspirin and in 11.2 per cent (172 of 1,529) patients receiving ticlopidine (Table 22–1). This represents a 21 per cent reduction in stroke risk. Death occurred in 12.7 per cent of the aspirin-treated patients and in 11.4 per cent of those on ticlopidine. The period of greatest risk reduction was in the first year, when the risk of stroke or death combined was reduced by 41 per cent from 7.9 per cent to 4.6 per cent.

The Canadian American Ticlopidine Study (CATS) was a multicenter trial comparing ticlopidine (250 milligrams twice daily) and placebo in 1,053 patients with completed stroke followed for a mean of 1.1 years.[42] The combined endpoint of stroke, myocardial infarction, or vascular death occurred in 22.3 per cent (118 of 528) patients receiving placebo (Table 22–2). The patients treated with ticlopidine had a combined event rate of 14.1 per cent (74 or 525). This difference represents a 30 per cent reduction in the ticlopidine-treated patients.

TABLE 22–1. Ticlopidine Aspirin Stroke Study (TASS)

	TICLOPIDINE	ASPIRIN
Number	1,529	1,540
Deaths	175	196
	(11.4%)	(12.7%)
Stroke	172	212
	(11.2%)	(13.8%)
Intracranial hemorrhage	7	7
Diarrhea plus gastrointestinal symptoms	20%	10%
White blood cell count less than 450	13	0
Cholesterol	+9%	+2%

TABLE 22–2. Canadian America Ticlopidine Study (CATS)

	TICLOPIDINE	PLACEBO
Number	531	541
Stroke/myocardial infarction/ vascular death	74 (14.1%)	118 (21.8%)
Intracranial hemorrhage	2	0
Diarrhea	2.3%	0.7%
Neutropenia	0.8%	0.2%

Ticlopidine was effective in reducing stroke in both men and women.

RISKS OF THERAPY

The limiting side effects of ticlopidine are diarrhea and neutropenia. Diarrhea was reported in about 13 per cent of patients on ticlopidine, with half of these being withdrawn from therapy because of the diarrhea. Neutropenia of some degree developed in 2.4 per cent of patients receiving ticlopidine. This neutropenia was severe (less than 450 absolute neutrophil count) in 0.8 per cent of patients. The neutropenia occurs within three months of initiating ticlopidine therapy and is reversible when the drug is discontinued.

Dipyridamole in Cerebrovascular Disorders

Dipyridamole has almost always been used in combination with aspirin for the prevention of stroke following transient ischemic attack or minor stroke. When dipyridamole alone was compared to aspirin, there appeared to be no benefit in stroke prevention.[43–45] The European Stroke Prevention Study compared aspirin and dipyridamole in combination to placebo in 2,500 patients with prior transient ischemic attack or minor stroke.[37] Over a two-year period of follow-up, there was a 33 per cent reduction in the primary endpoints of stroke and death. Thus the combination of aspirin and dipyridamole in this large study showed a greater benefit than previous studies of aspirin alone had shown. Nevertheless, when dipyridamole alone has been directly compared to aspirin in combination with dipyridamole in the same trial, the latter drug did not add significant benefit.

ANTICOAGULANTS AND CEREBROVASCULAR DISORDERS

Heparin in Acute Ischemic Stroke

RATIONALE

The use of heparin in acute ischemic stroke is based on the assumption that anticoagulants will prevent worsening of ischemia by preventing propagation of thrombus or reembolization of thrombotic material. About 20 per cent of ischemic strokes will progress during the few days from onset. These patients with stroke-in-evolution or progressive stroke have increased morbidity and mortality. Small randomized studies conducted in the 1960s looked at the use of heparin in patients developing a progressive stroke. These studies suggested a benefit in reduced mortality with anticoagulants, at the price of an increased frequency of bleeding complications. The mortality rate in untreated patients was 40 to 60 per cent. It is possible that some of the patients actually had hemorrhagic strokes prior to treatment because these studies were conducted prior to the use of computed tomography or magnetic resonance imaging. Based on these small studies and clinicians' concern about the high morbidity and mortality in these patients, the standard of practice in most areas is still to anticoagulate any patient with an ischemic stroke who is felt to be "progressing."

RECENT CLINICAL TRIALS

In addition to using heparin in patients with progressing stroke, some physicians began to anticoagulate patients with transient ischemic attack or mild to moderate neurologic deficits from ischemia in hopes of preventing the development of a progressive stroke. Reports of series of nonrandomized patients suggested a benefit in the prevention of stroke progression and recurrence.[46,47] Other studies failed to show a reduction in stroke occurrence in patients treated with heparin.[48] A randomized, double-blind trial of 225 patients with completed stroke treated an average of 27 hours from onset showed no statistically significant difference in rates of progression of 17 per cent in the heparin-treated and 19.5 per cent in the placebo-treated groups.[49] A randomized clinical trial is currently underway examining low molecular weight heparin for the prevention of stroke progression and recurrence.

RISKS OF HEPARIN ANTICOAGULATION

Heparin anticoagulation in the setting of acute stroke or transient ischemic attack is accompanied by a bleeding risk of 1 to 4 per cent.[50] Symptomatic brain hemorrhage is the most feared complication. The patients at greatest risk for brain hemorrhage are those with large brain infarct, those with embolic stroke mechanism, and those who are anticoagulated at the time of their stroke. The risk of heparin-induced thrombocytopenia in patients treated for transient ischemic attack or stroke is about 2 per cent.[51,52]

Warfarin in Cerebrovascular Disorders

PRIMARY PREVENTION

The Warfarin Reinfarction Study randomly assigned 1,214 patients to warfarin or placebo a mean of 27 days following myocardial infarction. After an average of 37 months follow-up there was a significant reduction in death (minus 24 per cent), recurrent myocardial infarction (minus 34 per cent), and in stroke (minus 55 per cent).[53] The other randomized trials studying warfarin for primary stroke prevention have involved patients with atrial fibrillation. All have shown a reduction of stroke of from 50 to 85 per cent with the use of warfarin anticoagulation.

SECONDARY PREVENTION

There are no randomized clinical trials of sufficient size to judge the merits of warfarin for the prevention of stroke following transient ischemic attack or stroke. Small randomized trials comparing warfarin and aspirin found no superiority with anticoagulation.[54,55]

Ancrod in Cerebrovascular Disorders

Ancrod is the purified proteolytic fraction of the venom of the Malayan pit viper. Its mechanism of action is to cleave the A-fibrinopeptides but not B-fibrinopeptides from fibrinogen. Following intravenous or subcutaneous administration, there is a rapid reduction in plasma fibrinogen concentration, a corresponding rise in fibrinogen degradation products, and a reduction in plasma plasminogen.[56] Blood viscosity declines along with the decrease in fibrinogen levels. The rationale for the use of ancrod in the treatment of acute ischemic stroke is that (a) it produces improved flow by reducing blood viscosity; (b) thrombolysis occurs as a result of the release of plasminogen activator; and (c) further thrombosis is inhibited via ancrod's anticoagulant properties.

Small clinical trials of ancrod in ischemic stroke have been done. A randomized, single-blind study evaluated subcutaneous ancrod in patients with acute ischemic stroke.[57] Fifteen patients treated with ancrod were compared to 15 controls. Fibrinogen levels declined to 100 to 130 milligrams/deciliter. There was a trend in favor of the ancrod-treated patients toward improved neurologic scores and reduced mortality. A second study was a double-blind, randomized, placebo-controlled trial comparing ten patients treated with ancrod to ten receiving placebo.[58] Mean plasma fibrinogen level was reduced from 385 milligrams/deciliter at baseline to 116 milligrams/deciliter at six hours and to 52 milligrams/deciliter at 24 hours after initiation of therapy. No significant bleeding or toxic effects of the ancrod were noted. The ancrod-treated patients showed improved outcome in their neurologic scores at three months following stroke. A double-blind, randomized, placebo-controlled trial of ancrod treatment begun within six hours of ischemic stroke onset is currently in progress.

THROMBOLYSIS AND CEREBROVASCULAR DISORDERS

Experimental Studies

Thrombolytic agents have been looked at in animal stroke models to address the issue of clot lysis and brain hemorrhage. An embolic stroke model in rabbits showed rates of clot lysis by angiogram from 70 to 100 per cent using tissue-type plasminogen activator (t-PA) and from 40 to 90 per cent with streptokinase. Hemorrhagic infarction has been noted in 30 to 35 per cent of animals receiving tissue-type plasminogen activator as opposed to 70 to 90 per cent of those receiving streptokinase and in 20 to 25 per cent of control animals. Thus, this and other animal models have shown that tissue-type plasminogen activator and other thrombolytic agents can open embolically occluded cerebral arteries and that secondary hemorrhagic infarction tends to be mild and not associated with large hematoma formation and neurologic worsening.[59]

Human Studies

The first experiences with thrombolytic agents for the treatment of acute stroke resulted in an excessively high rate of bleeding complications and death. In these studies, thrombolytic agents were administered many hours or days after stroke onset. Thereafter, thrombolytic agents were abandoned as potential therapies for acute stroke until recent studies in coronary occlusion rekindled interest. In addition to concerns about bleeding into the ischemic brain, there are also concerns about distal migration of clot. Reperfusion of ischemic brain might worsen brain edema and potentiate the adverse effects of calcium, potassium, excitatory neurotransmitters, and free radicals. Experimental and clinical experience with tissue-type plasminogen activator more recently has suggested the possibility of recanalization and benefit with acceptably low complication rates.[60–68]

Recently, tissue-type plasminogen activator was administered in one study to patients with angiographically documented arterial occlusions. Seventy-one patients were treated within eight hours of stroke onset. Repeat angiography showed recanalization in 41 per cent of the patients following tissue-type plasminogen activator. Six of the seventy-one patients (8.4 per cent) developed an intracerebral hemorrhage; four of these worsened, with three deaths. The frequency of intracerebral hemorrhage or hemorrhagic infarction was less (20 per cent) in the patients treated within six hours compared to those treated between six and eight hours, where the rate was 58 per cent.[69] Clinical improvement was more likely in those patients with recanalization. In this study, the risk of bleeding did not appear to be related to the dose of tissue-type plasminogen activator. In another study, tissue-type plasminogen activator was studied in an open-label, dose-escalation design for ischemic stroke treated within 90 minutes of onset.[70] Seventy-four patients received tissue-type plasminogen activator in doses from 10 to 87 milligrams. Intracerebral hematoma occurred within the presumed region of infarction in two patients

and outside the region of infarction in one patient. Neurologic improvement within six hours occurred in 29 patients. A larger study of similar design is currently in progress which enrolls patients within either 90 or 180 minutes of ischemic stroke onset.

SUMMARY

Stroke is a major cause of death and disability in adults. Stroke occurs with increasing frequency with advancing age, suggesting that it will assume greater rather than lesser importance as our population ages. The risk factors for stroke parallel those for arterial thrombosis in noncerebral circulations. The causes of stroke are multiple and obscure often enough that at least in a third of the cases no clear stroke etiology can be identified. There are at present no proven therapies for ischemic stroke despite vigorous searches in the form of randomized clinical trials and experimental investigations. This fact underscores the importance of preventive therapy. Risk factors must be identified and treated. Antithrombotic therapy is of proven benefit in a number of situations where patients at risk for stroke can be identified. Nevertheless, many strokes continue to occur in individuals not known to be at risk and in too large a number of those having their risk factors addressed. Despite gains and promising new discoveries, much remains to be done.

REFERENCES

1. 1989 Stroke facts. American Heart Association publication.
2. Harrison MJG, Marshall J. Prognostic significance of severity of carotid atheroma in early manifestations of cerebrovascular disease. Stroke 1982; 13: 567–9.
3. Bogousslavsky J, Van Melle G, Regli F. Middle cerebral artery pial territory infarcts: a study of the Lausanne stroke registry. Ann Neurol 1989; 25: 555–60.
4. Fieschi C, Argentino C, Lenzi GL, Sacchetti ML, Toni D, Bozzao L. Clinical and instrumental evaluation of patients with ischemic stroke within the first six hours. J Neurol Sci 1989; 91: 311–22.
5. Dyken ML, Wolf PA, Barnett HJM, et al. Risk factors in stroke: a statement for physicians by the subcommittee on risk factor and stroke of the stroke council. Stroke 1984; 15: 1105–11.
6. Castelli WP, Anderson K. A population at risk. Prevalence of high cholesterol levels in hypertensive patients in the Framingham Study. Am J Med 1986; 80: 23–32.
7. Wolf PA, Kannel WB, McGee DL. Prevention of ischemic stroke: risk factors. In: Barnett HMJ, et al., eds. Stroke: pathophysiology, diagnosis and management. Vol 2. New York: Churchill Livingstone, 1986: 967–88.
8. Gill JS, et al. Cigarette smoking: a risk factor for hemorrhagic

and nonhemorrhagic stroke. Arch Intern Med 1989; 149: 2053–7.

9. Longstreth WT, Nelson L, Koepsell TD, van Belle G. Risk factors for subarachnoid hemorrhage (abstr). Stroke 1991; 22: 149.

10. Whisnant JP, Homer D, Ingall TJ, Baker HL, O'Fallon M, Weibers DO. Duration of cigarette smoking is the strongest predictor of severe extracranial carotid artery atherosclerosis. Stroke 1990; 21: 707–14.

11. Tell GS, Howard G, McKinney WM, Toole JF. Cigarette smoking cessation and extracranial carotid atherosclerosis. JAMA 1989; 261: 1178–80.

12. Wolf PA, D'Agostino RD, Belanger AJ, Kelly-Hayes M, Kase CS, Kannel WB. Are blood lipids risk factors for stroke (abstr). Stroke 1991; 22: 150.

13. Iso H, Jacobs DR, Wentworth D, Neaton JD, Cohen JD, for the MRFIT Research Group. Serum cholesterol levels and six-year mortality from stroke in 350,977 men screened for the multiple risk factor intervention trial. N Engl J Med 1989; 320: 904–10.

14. Heyman A, Wilkinson WE, Heyden S, et al. Risk of stroke in asymptomatic persons with cervical arterial bruits. A population study in Evans County, Georgia. N Engl J Med 1980; 302: 838–41.

15. Wolf PA, Kannel WM, Sorlie P, McNamara P. Asymptomatic carotid bruit and risk of stroke. The Framingham Study. JAMA 1981; 245: 1442–5.

16. Sandok BA, Whisnant JP, Furlan AJ, Mickell JL. Carotid artery bruits: prevalence survey and differential diagnosis. Mayo Clin Proc 1982; 52: 227–30.

17. Chambers BR, Norris JW. Outcome in patients with asymptomatic neck bruits. N Engl J Med 1986; 315: 860–5.

18. Autret A, Pourcelot L, Sardear D, Marchal C, Bertrand PH, deBoisvilliers S. Stroke risk in patients with carotid stenosis. Lancet 1987; 1: 888–90.

19. Johnson JM. Natural history of asymptomatic carotid plaque. Arch Surg 1985; 120: 1010–2.

20. Hunter WM, Sterpetti AV, Shultz R, Feldhuas J. Carotid plaque ulceration: its significance in cerebral ischemia (abstr). Stroke 1989; 20: 158.

21. Langsfeld M, Gray-Weale AC, Lusby RJ. The role of plaque morphology and diameter reduction in the development of new symptoms in asymptomatic carotid arteries. J Vasc Surg 1989; 9: 548–57.

22. Moore WS, Boren C, Malone JM, et al. Natural history of nonstenotic, asymptomatic ulcerative lesions of the carotid artery. Arch Surg 1978; 113: 1352–9.

23. Kroener J, Dorn PL, Shoor PM, et al. Prognosis of asymptomatic ulcerating carotid lesions. Arch Surg 1980; 115: 1387–92.

24. Cerebral Embolism Task Force. Cardiogenic brain embolism: the second report of the Cerebral Embolism Task Force. Arch Neurol 1989; 46: 727–43.

25. Cerebral Embolism Task Force. Cardiogenic brain embolism. Arch Neurol 1986; 43: 71–84.

26. Hart RG, Kanter MC. Hematologic disorders and ischemic stroke. Stroke 1990; 21: 1111–21.

27. Schafer AI. The hypercoaguable states. Ann Intern Med 1985; 102: 814–28.

28. Coull BM, Beamer N, deGarmo P, et al. Chronic blood hyperviscosity in subjects with acute stroke, transient ischemic attack, and risk factors for stroke. Stroke 1991; 22: 162–8.

29. Olsen TS, Skriver EB, Herning M. Cause of cerebral infarction in the carotid territory. Its relation to the size and the location of the infarct and to the underlying vascular lesion. Stroke 1985; 16: 459–66.

30. Bogousslavsky J, et al. Cardiac and arterial lesions in carotid transient ischemic attacks. Arch Neurol 1986; 43: 223–8.

31. Miller V. Lacunar stroke, a reassessment. Arch Neurol 1983; 40: 129–34.

32. Bamford JM, Sandercock P, Jones L, Warlow C. The natural history of lacunar infarction: the Oxfordshire Community Stroke Project. Stroke 1987; 18: 545–51.

33. Keith DS, Phillips SJ, Whisnant JP, Nishimaru K, O'Fallon WM. Heparin therapy for recent transient focal cerebral ischemia. Mayo Clin Proc 1987; 62: 1101–6.

34. Antiplatelet Trialists' Collaboration. Secondary prevention

of vascular disease by prolonged antiplatelet treatment. Br Med J 1988; 26: 320–31.

35. UK-TIA Study Group. The UK-TIA aspirin trial. The interim results. Br Med J 1988; 296: 316–20.

36. ESPS Study Group. The European Stroke Prevention Study (ESPS): principal endpoints. Lancet 1987; 2: 1351–4.

37. ESPS Group. European Stroke Prevention Study. Stroke 1990; 21: 1122–30.

38. Van Gijn J. Results of the Dutch Aspirin Trial. In Press.

39. The Steering Committee of the Physicians' Health Study Research Group. Preliminary report; findings from the aspirin component of the ongoing physicians' health study. N Engl J Med 1988; 318: 262–4.

40. Peto R, Gray R, Collins R, Wheatley K, et al. Randomized trial of prophylactic daily aspirin in British male doctors. Br Med J 1988; 296: 313–6.

41. Hass WK, Easton JD, Adams HP, et al., for the Ticlopidine Aspirin Stroke Study Group. A randomized trial comparing ticlopidine hydrochloride with aspirin for the prevention of stroke in high-risk patients. N Engl J Med 1989; 321: 501–7.

42. Gent M, Blakely JA, Easton JD, et al. The Canadian American Ticlopidine Study (CATS) in thromboembolic stroke. Lancet 1989; 1: 1215–20.

43. Bousser MG, Eschwege E, Haguenau M, et al. "AICLA" controlled trial of aspirin and dipyridamole in the secondary prevention of atherothrombotic cerebral ischaemia. Stroke 1983; 13: 5–14.

44. Guiraud-Chaumeil B, Rascol A, David J, Boneu B, Clanet M, Bierme R. Prevention des recidives des accidents vascularires cerebraux ischemiques par les anti-aggregants plaquettaires. Rev Neurol (Paris) 1982; 138: 367–85.

45. The American-Canadian Co-Operative Study Group. Persantin aspirin trial in cerebral ischemia, part II: endpoint results. Stroke 1985; 16: 406–15.

46. Putman SF, Adams HP Jr. Usefulness of heparin in initial management of patients with recent transient ischemic attacks. Arch Neurol 1985; 42: 960–2.

47. Ramirez-Lassepas M, Quinones MR, Nino HH. Treatment of acute ischemic stroke open trial with continuous intravenous heparinization. Arch Neurol 1986; 42: 386–90.

48. Haley EC Jr, Kassell NF, Torner JC. Failure of heparin to prevent progression in progressing ischemic infarction. Stroke 1988; 19: 10–4.

49. Duke RJ, Bloch RF, Trupie AGG, Trebilcock R, Bayer N. Intravenous heparin for the prevention of stroke progression in acute partial stable stroke: a randomized controlled trial. Ann Intern Med 1986; 105: 825–8.

50. Keith DS, Phillips SJ, Whisnant JP, Nishimaura K, O'Fallon WM. Heparin therapy for recent transient focal cerebral ischemia. Mayo Clin Proc 1987; 62: 1101–6.

51. Ramirez-Lassepas M, Quinones MR. Heparin therapy for stroke: hemorrhagic complications and risk factors for intracerebral hemorrhage. Neurology 1984; 34: 114–7.

52. Rao AK, White GC, Sherman L, Colman R, Lan G, Ball AP. Low incidence of thrombocytopenia with porcine mucosal heparin. Arch Int Med 1089; 149: 1285–8.

53. Smith P, Arneses H, Holme I. The effect of warfarin on mortality and reinfarction after myocardial infarction. N Engl J Med 1990; 323: 147–52.

54. Buren A, Ygge J. Treatment program and comparison between anticoagulants and platelet aggregation inhibitors after transient ischemic attack. Stroke 1981; 12: 578–80.

55. Garde A, Samuelsson K, Fahlgran H, Hedberg E, Hjerne LG, Ostman J. Treatment after transient ischemic attacks: a comparison between anticoagulant drug and inhibition of platelet aggregation. Stroke 1983; 14: 677–81.

56. Bell WR. Defibrinogenating enzymes. In: Colman RW, Hirsh J, Marder V, Salzman E, eds. Hemostasis and thrombosis: basic principles and clinical practice. Philadelphia: JB Lippincott Co., 1987; 886–900.

57. Hossman V, Heiss WD, Bewermeyer H, Wiedemann G. Controlled trial of ancrod in ischemic stroke. Arch Neurol 1983; 40: 803–8.

58. Olinger CP, Brott TG, Barsan WG. Use of ancrod in acute or progressing ischemic cerebral inaction. Ann Emerg Med 1988; 17: 1208–9.

59. Lyden PD, Zivin JA, Clark WA, et al. Tissue plasminogen activator-mediated thrombolysis of cerebral emboli and its

effect on hemorrhagic infarction in rabbits. Neurology 1989; 39: 703–8.

60. Hacke W, Zeumer H, Ferbert A, Bruckmann H, Del Zoppo GJ. Intra-arterial thrombolytic therapy improves outcome in patients with acute vertebrobasilar occlusive disease. Stroke 1988; 19: 1216–22.

61. Del Zoppo GJ, Ferbert A, Otis S, et al. Local intra-arterial fibrinolytic therapy in acute carotid territory stroke. A pilot study. Stroke 1988; 19: 307–13.

62. Bruckmann H, Ferbert A, del Zoppo GJ, Hacke W, Zeumer H. Acute vertebral basilar thrombosis: angiologic-clinical comparison and therapeutic implications. Acta Radiol 1987; 369: 38–42.

63. Zeumer H, Hundgen R, Ferbert A, Ringelstein EB. Local intraarterial fibrinolytic therapy in inaccessible internal carotid occlusion. Neuroradiology 1984; 26: 315–7.

64. Wildemann B, Hutschenreuter M, Krieger D, Hacke W, von Kummer R. Infusion of recombinant tissue plasminogen activator for treatment of basilar artery occlusion. Stroke 1990; 21: 1513–4.

65. Zivin JA, Lyden PD, DeGirolami U, et al. Tissue plasminogen activator: reduction of neurologic damage after experimental embolic stroke. Arch Neurol 1988; 45: 387–91.

66. Zivin JA, Fisher M, DeGirolami U, et al. Tissue plasminogen activator reduces neurological damage after cerebral embolism. Science 1985; 230: 1289–92.

67. Kissel P, Chehrazi B, Seibert JA, Wagner FC Jr. Digital angiographic quantification of blood flow dynamics in embolic stroke treated with tissue-type plasminogen activator. J Neurosurg 1987; 67: 399–405.

68. Papadopoulos SM, Chandler WF, Salamat MS, Topol EJ, Sackellares JC. Recombinant human tissue-type plasminogen activator therapy in acute thromboembolic stroke. J Neurosurg 1987; 67: 394–8.

69. The t-PA/Acute Stroke Study Group. An open safety/efficacy trial of rt-PA in acute thromboembolic stroke: final report (abstr). Stroke 1991; 22: 153.

70. Brott T, Haley C, Levy D, et al. Safety and potential efficacy of tissue plasminogen activator (tPA) for stroke (abstr). Stroke 1990; 21: 181.

23

PERIPHERAL ARTERIAL OCCLUSION:

Thromboembolism and Antithrombotic Therapy

RAYMOND VERHAEGHE and HENRI BOUNAMEAUX

The most common cause of obstructive arterial disease in the lower limbs is slowly progressive atherosclerosis, often complicated by thromboembolic events. Other types of degenerative or inflammatory arteriopathy (Table 23–1) which also result in narrowing of the lumen and obstruction of blood flow are rare in comparison with atherosclerosis. In this chapter, we will mainly deal with the atherosclerotic type of peripheral arterial occlusive disease and particularly focus on antithrombotic and thrombolytic therapy. Other therapeutic principles and general management are discussed in the context of thrombosis, embolism, and their prevention.

ATHEROSCLEROSIS AND THROMBOSIS IN PERIPHERAL ARTERIAL DISEASE—PRIMARY PREVENTION

Atherosclerosis is a multiorgan disorder characterized by localized plaque formation in selected sites of the arterial tree. Coronary arteries and the carotid bifurcation are particularly prone to plaque deposition, as are the leg arteries, which are more often affected than arteries of similar size in the arms. This difference may be partly due to a different hydrostatic pressure, but also to more marked exercise-related variations of blood flow in the lower extremities.

Clinical manifestations of atherosclerosis in the legs include acute, thrombotic or embolic, occlusion of a leg artery and chronic arterial insufficiency resulting in intermittent claudication or rest pain and gangrene. The management of these two clinical conditions will be discussed in specific sections at the end of this chapter. In fact, the risk of a leg amputation is relatively low (5 per cent or less), but the patients suffering from intermittent claudication have a life expectancy which is reduced by about ten years as compared with the general population. Their overall mortality at 5, 10, and 15 years is

TABLE 23–1. Etiology of Peripheral Arterial Occlusive Disease in the Legs

Degenerative arterial disease
  Atherosclerosis
  Mönckeberg's medial sclerosis
  Medial cystic degeneration
  Fibromuscular dysplasia
Inflammatory arterial disease
  Thromboangiitis obliterans (Buerger's disease)
  Systemic giant cell arteritis (Horton)
  Takayasu's disease
  Arteritis associated with connective tissue disease
Arterial thrombosis
  Idiopathic
  Associated with protein C or protein S deficiency
  Immunologic (for example, associated with lupus-like anticoagulant or heparin induced)
Miscellaneous
  Peripheral arterial embolism
  Arterial trauma
  Arterial spasm (drug-induced or spontaneous)

about 30, 50, and 70 per cent, respectively, owing to cardiovascular causes (myocardial infarction, stroke) in two thirds of the cases and to noncardiovascular causes (for example, lung cancer) for the remaining third.[1] Thus, the therapeutic approach of these patients should achieve two complementary goals: first, it should aim at reducing the symptoms in the leg; and second, it should slow down the progression of the atherosclerotic disease, particularly the incidence of its thrombotic complications (secondary prevention).

The pathogenesis of atherosclerosis and thrombosis is discussed in detail in Chapter 3. Briefly, no single etiologic factor of atherosclerosis is known and our knowledge is mostly based on the epidemiologic characteristics of patients with the disease as well as on observations of pathologists. Atherosclerotic disease of the lower extremities is strongly related to cigarette smoking, hypercholesterolemia (particularly low-density lipoprotein and very–low-density lipoprotein-hypercholesterolemia), diabetes mellitus, and hypertension. Almost all patients in whom claudication starts before the age of 70 have a long history of cigarette smoking. In a recent update of the Framingham Study, Kannel and McGee[2] show that cigarette smoking doubles the incidence of intermittent claudication both in men and women, whereas hypertension increases the risk 2.5- and 4-fold, in men and women, respectively. Direct information is lacking on how these risk factors are related to the cellular interactions which determine the development and progression of atherosclerosis, but according to the response-to-injury hypothesis, hypercholesterolemia may stimulate plaque formation by growth-factor release from monocytes and platelets (platelet-derived growth factor [PDGF]), whilst cigarette smoking, hypertension, and diabetes would act directly on the endothelium to release mitogens that can induce smooth muscle cell migration and proliferation.

Primary prevention of peripheral arterial occlusive disease is basically a battle against risk factors of atherosclerosis. As long as the genetic basis that underlies the increased susceptibility of some persons to this disease and the relative resistance of others has not been elucidated, emphasis should be put on cessation of cigarette smoking, and on lowering of blood pressure and serum cholesterol level. The campaigns against smoking

were reinforced by several reports which show that even ambient smoke is hazardous to the health. For example, in the Multiple Risk Factor Intervention Trial (MRFIT), the relative risk of dying was increased by 79 per cent ($p < 0.01$) in nonsmoking males whose wives smoked when comparing with nonsmokers whose wives did not.[3] These data lent impetus to the antitobacco movement in many Western countries. Campaigns to convince people that smoking is no longer socially acceptable resulted in a clear-cut progressive reduction of tobacco use. In the United States, the prevalence of cigarette smoking in men decreased from 52 per cent in 1965 to 33 per cent in 1985, the corresponding figures in women being 34 and 28 per cent, respectively. At the same time, improved detection and treatment of hypertension (for example, with thiazide diuretics or beta blockers), reduction of blood cholesterol owing to changes in dietary habits, and an improved level of fitness in the population may have contributed to the decline of mortality from coronary heart disease in the United States over the past 20 years. As far as leg arterial disease is concerned, most data are on secondary prevention. Cessation of smoking was associated with an improvement of 86 per cent of the maximum treadmill walking distance compared to only 24 per cent in the subjects who continued smoking.[4] Lowering of plasma cholesterol was able to slow down the arteriographic progression of femoral atherosclerosis[5] and a similar effect has been obtained with antiplatelet drugs in a placebo-controlled trial.[6] However, the question whether these drugs should be used as a primary prevention of leg arterial disease in an unselected population or at least in high-risk subgroups (for example, smokers, familial hypercholesterolemia) has never been addressed.

THERAPEUTIC PRINCIPLES TO RELIEVE ARTERIAL OCCLUSION

Vascular Surgery

When surgical repair is considered for arterial disease of the legs, several important factors have to be evaluated: the severity of the patient's symptoms, the level of the main obstructive lesion, the physical condition and general prognosis of the patient, and the expected result of the surgical procedure.

Surgeons continue to debate on the opportunity of a vascular reconstruction in a patient with intermittent claudication as chief complaint. Many feel that surgical intervention should be reserved for patients with critical leg ischemia, a term which refers to ischemia that endangers the limb (see Treatment of Critical Limb Ischemia) (so-called limb salvage surgery), but others may propose surgery to patients with disabling claudication as well. Since the success of surgery depends on the level of the obstruction, the localization of the lesions has to be evaluated in conjunction with the severity of the symptoms. Patients with a limited walking distance owing to aortoiliac disease are better surgical candidates than their counterparts with femoropopliteal disease, certainly if the obstructive lesions extend beyond the tibiofibular bifurcation. Physical examination of the patient is instructive: mild claudication in the presence of normal arterial pulses in the groin suggests femoropopliteal disease, which does not require immediate surgery so that the need for invasive testing may be questioned. On the other hand, a systolic bruit in the groin may reveal an osteal stenosis of the deep femoral artery, a lesion which is easily corrected with a limited surgical procedure (profundaplasty). Patients with critical ischemia deserve full investigation of their lesions to determine their operability. If no vessels are seen in the lower leg, one should not too hurriedly conclude to inoperability, because low flow may prevent visualization of distal vessels.

The age, life expectancy, and physical condition of the patient are equally important determinants to select patients for vascular surgery. In addition, these factors help to determine the choice of the surgical procedure. Some vascular reconstructions impose less burden on elderly patients than a major amputation, but at increasing age, claudication is an insufficient justification for arterial surgery. If the patient is unfit for major abdominal surgery, alternative techniques may be considered, such as a retroperitoneal approach to the aorta or an extra-anatomical reconstruction (for example, an axillofemoral or femorofemoral crossover graft).

The long-term results of arterial reconstruction depend on the distal run-off and of the material used for grafting. The flow through the reconstruction decreases if the circulation in the distal bed is impaired, and long-term patency will be much lower. Surgery under these conditions will be reserved for true limb salvage. The choice of the graft material is particularly important for infrainguinal reconstructions. Although there is a clear preference for the autologous saphenous vein, an increasing proportion of elderly patients have no adequate vein available and require a prosthetic graft.

Two basic techniques of revascularization are used: thromboendarterectomy and bypass grafting of the obstructive lesions (Fig. 23-1). Thromboendarterectomy has limited applications: localized aortoiliac disease without heavy calcification or aneurysmal dilatation and stenotic lesions at the femoral bifurcation. Thromboendarterectomy of the proximal part of the deep femoral artery (profundaplasty) is a well-tolerated operation to improve the collateral blood supply to the limb when the superficial femoral artery is occluded. Infrainguinal thromboendarterectomy has poor late patency rates and therefore this technique is largely abandoned in the femoropopliteal region. The implantation of an aortofemoral Dacron graft is a simpler procedure than aortoiliac endarterectomy. The graft usually starts with a terminoterminal anastomosis on the aorta and ends on the femoral artery. A proximal terminolateral anastomosis saves the normal pelvic circulation and decreases the risk of postoperative impairment of erection. For femoropopliteal reconstruction, the saphenous vein bypass graft remains the preferred material. The saphenous vein is totally removed, reversed because of its valves, and sewn proximally on the common femoral and distally on the popliteal or tibial artery. In most patients, the distal anastomosis descends below the knee joint. A prosthetic graft is a second choice at this level with poorer results. An elegant but delicate technique for long reconstructions is the venous bypass in situ. The proximal saphenous vein is slightly moved and anastomosed on the femoral artery in the groin, while the smaller distal end is mobilized and fixed on the popliteal or tibial artery. Side branches are ligated and the valves are destroyed with a suitable instrument.

Many patients who undergo vascular surgery have multisegmental arterial occlusive disease. This is almost certainly the case if they have critical ischemia. The proximal lesion is repaired first either by aortoiliac endarterectomy or, more commonly, by aortofemoral bypass grafting. The operative mortality of aortoiliac surgery is low (1 to 2

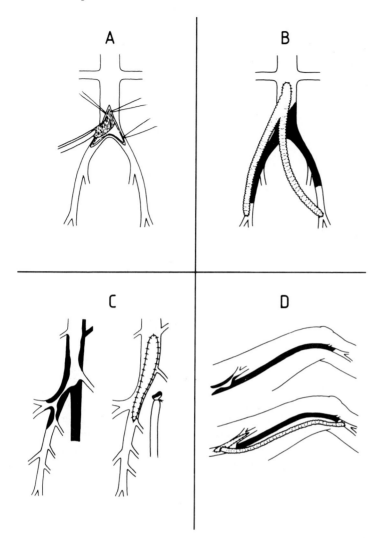

FIGURE 23–1. Schematic presentation of common surgical procedures. (*A*) Open thromboendarterectomy. (*B*) Aortofemoral bypass graft. (*C*) Profundaplasty with ligation of occluded superficial femoral artery. (*D*) Femoropopliteal bypass graft.

per cent), but it increases in patients with critical ischemia (4 to 5 per cent). The long-term patency rate is fairly high (90 per cent at 10 years and 85 per cent at 15 years in patients with severe claudication) (Fig. 23–2), but a considerable number of reinterventions is needed over the years to achieve this result.[7]

Surgical repair of a femoropopliteal occlusion is normally restricted to patients with critical ischemia and to selected patients with multilevel disease who receive an aortofemoral graft simultaneously. The long-term results of infrainguinal bypass surgery depend largely on the particular selection of the patients considered. Factors that affect late outcome are, for example, the site of the terminal anastomosis and the graft material used. In general, autologous vein grafts carry

better patency rates than prosthetic grafts and the difference is magnified with more distal terminal anastomosis.[8] Approximate one-year patency rates for infrainguinal reconstructive procedures vary as much as from 25 per cent for prosthetic distal tibial grafts to 85 per cent for autologous vein bypasses with above-knee terminal anastomosis.[9]

Percutaneous Revascularization Procedures

Introduced by Dotter and Judkins in 1964, the transluminal treatment of atherosclerotic obstructive lesions of the leg arteries became popular only after the development by Grüntzig of a double-lumen polyvinyl balloon catheter in 1974. Later, percutaneous translu-

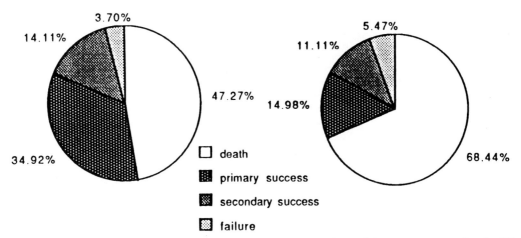

FIGURE 23–2. Outcome 10 (*left*) and 15 years (*right*) after aortofemoral Dacron reconstruction in **371** patients with severe claudication. Primary and secondary success denotes normal graft function without and with secondary intervention, respectively. (Courtesy of Dr. A. Nevelsteen).

minal angioplasty (PTA) was also used to treat arterial obstruction in other regions and particularly in the coronary arteries. We will focus here on the use of percutaneous transluminal angioplasty in the leg arteries and briefly comment on recent developments of the transluminal technique.

PERCUTANEOUS TRANSLUMINAL ANGIOPLASTY OF THE LEG ARTERIES

Procedure. The percutaneous transluminal angioplasty procedure can be described in three phases: (a) an artery is punctured using the classical Seldinger technique, (b) a guide wire is advanced beyond the arterial lesion, and (c) the balloon catheter is passed over the guide wire and inflated under fluoroscopic monitoring until adequate enlargement of the arterial lumen is obtained (Fig. 23–3). Percutaneous transluminal angioplasty was shown to produce longitudinal fissures in the atherosclerotic plaque which is detached from the intima. In the healing phase, the intimal tear retracts and the arterial lumen is enlarged. The femoral artery in the groin is commonly used as puncture site; it has the advantage of being well compressible. The ankle pressure is measured before the procedure and again after the procedure to test the hemodynamic result of the percutaneous transluminal angioplasty.

Clinical Application. The clinical indications for percutaneous transluminal angioplasty are listed in Table 23–2. As for surgery, the procedure is only justified if symptoms are disabling the patient or endanger the limb. Percutaneous procedures have a theo-

retical advantage for young patients in whom they can postpone vascular surgery for a number of years. They would be even more useful in poor-risk elderly patients, but widespread arterial disease frequently prevents their application in this population.

The initial technical result as demonstrated on a control angiography at the end of the procedure determines the primary success rate. Patency rate is defined as the percentage of patients in whom the artery is still open for a given period of observation after initial technical success of the procedure and is calculated by means of the life-table method. The cure rate is obtained by multiplying the patency rate by the primary success rate. In a prospective series of 984 percutaneous transluminal angioplasties, Johnston et al.[10] identified several factors that are important for the long-term prognosis. The following variables, when considered individually, were significantly ($p < 0.05$) associated with success of percutaneous transluminal angioplasty by means of the Cox proportional hazards regression model: (a) clinical stage (claudication versus limb salvage), (b) site (common iliac artery versus other), (c) severity of the lesion (stenosis versus occlusion), (d) distal run-off (good versus poor). Thus an analysis of the results of percutaneous transluminal angioplasty has to take into account the type and localization of the lesion as well as the clinical stage.

Primary success rates of 90 per cent and more have been reported after percutaneous transluminal angioplasty at iliac level with patency rates and cure rates at three years of

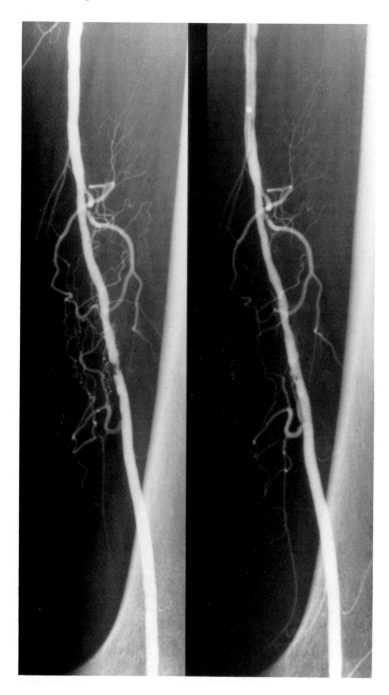

FIGURE 23–3. Percutaneous transluminal angioplasty of the superficial femoral artery. (*Left*) Before percutaneous transluminal angioplasty, 90 per cent stenosis of the artery resulting in a ankle-arm systolic pressure gradient of 40 mm Hg and pain-free walking distance of 100 meters. (*Right*) After the procedure, restoration of a normal arterial lumen with simultaneous diminution of the ankle-arm systolic pressure gradient to 10 mm Hg and doubling of the walking distance. (Courtesy of Dr. PA Schneider.)

about 85 and 80 per cent, respectively (Table 23–3). Lower success rates in other series may be due to a higher proportion of patients with critical ischemia. In the femoropopliteal region, primary success rates are some 10 per cent lower than at the iliac level, with patency rates and cure rates at three years of about 65 and 60 per cent, respectively (Table 23–4). Very few data exist on the use of percutaneous transluminal angioplasty in infrapopliteal vessels. Technical advances and increased experience in treating lesions below the knee in the last years yielded results which are comparable to the results of distal bypass surgery.[11] Bakal et al.[12] performed 57 procedures in 53 patients, all but one being performed for limb salvage. Primary success was reached in 72 per cent with limb salvage

TABLE 23–2. Indications for Percutaneous Transluminal Angioplasty

Optimal lesions
  Short stenosis of the common or external iliac artery
  Isolated stenosis of the superficial femoral or popliteal artery
  Isolated short obstruction (less than 3 centimeters) of the superficial femoral artery
  Stenosis at surgical anastomosis
Possibly treatable
  Isolated, proximal stenosis of the internal iliac artery
  Multiple stenoses of the superficial femoral artery
  Longer obstruction (3 to 10 centimeters) of the superficial femoral artery
  Short obstruction of distal popliteal artery
  Stenosis of the proximal deep femoral artery
  Stenosis of the abdominal aorta
For limb salvage only
  Longer obstruction (>10 centimeters) of the femoropopliteal axis (?)
  Stenosis of the calf arteries

in 58 per cent. When flow to the foot through the main arteries was restored (29 procedures), prompt clinical improvement was the rule.

The complications of percutaneous transluminal angioplasty are listed in Table 23–5. According to Mahler's recent overview,[13] they occur with an overall frequency of 5 per cent, the mortality of the procedure being 0.07 per cent, and the need for surgery 0.8 per cent.

NEW DEVELOPMENTS IN PERCUTANEOUS REVASCULARIZATION

Since percutaneous transluminal angioplasty with Grüntzig's double-balloon catheter was accepted as an effective method of treatment, modifications in design of the catheters were proposed, and several new concepts of transluminal treatment using different devices were developed. All of them, however, are auxiliary methods to complement classical balloon percutaneous transluminal angioplasty rather than to replace it. Local thrombolysis is discussed separately later (see Thrombolytic Therapy).

Simpson Atherectomy. The peripheral Simpson atherectomy catheter is designed for percutaneous removal of plaque material from peripheral vessels.[27] Residual plaques are thought to contribute to restenosis after percutaneous transluminal angioplasty. Thus, their removal might reduce the restenosis rate, which is about 5 per cent per year. The essential feature of the catheter is a cylindrical metal housing with a longitudinal window over one third of its circumference, and an integrated, externally controllable, rotating cutter. The catheter is positioned so that the stenotic plaque protrudes into the window of the housing. A low-pressure balloon opposite the window is then inflated to compress the housing onto the atheroma. The motor-driven rotating cutter is slowly advanced so that 1-millimeter slices of the plaque up to 15 millimeters long are excised and trapped within the distal housing cap (Fig. 23–4).

The ideal lesion to remove with the Simpson catheter is a short eccentric stenosis. The reported primary success rate exceeds 90 per cent in several series, but long-term follow-up is still scarce. The technique was also found to be useful for removal of obstructive intimal flaps in patients following classical percutaneous transluminal angioplasty.[28] A definitive place for percutaneous atherectomy remains to be established.

TABLE 23–3. Immediate and Long-Term Results After Iliac Percutaneous Transluminal Angioplasty

AUTHORS (YEAR)	NUMBER	PRIMARY SUCCESS (%)	FOLLOW-UP (YEARS)	PATENCY RATE (%)	CURE RATE (%)
Grüntzig[14] (1980)	54	92	3	83	76
Spence et al.[15] (1981)	148	92	3	79	73
Freiman et al.[16] (1981)	120	90	2	83	75
Kumpe and Jones[17] (1982)	71	82	3	96	79
Schneider et al.[18] (1982)	200	93	5	85	79
Colapinto[19] (1983)	195	94	3	82	77
Dotter et al.[20] (1983)	1082	90	3	81	73
Kadir et al.[21] (1983)	141	96	3	89	85
Gallino et al.[22] (1984)	131	95	5	87	83
van Andel et al.[23] (1985)	185	96	7	90	86
Kammerlander[24] (1989)	85	75	3	82	62

TABLE 23–4. Immediate and Long-Term Results After Femoropopliteal Percutaneous Transluminal Angioplasty

AUTHORS (YEAR)	NUMBER	PRIMARY SUCCESS (%)	FOLLOW-UP (YEARS)	PATENCY RATE (%)	CURE RATE (%)
Grüntzig[14] (1980)	236	83	3	70	58
Spence et al.[15] (1981)	96	84	3	70	59
Freiman et al.[16] (1981)	88	93	2	67	62
Kumpe and Jones[17] (1982)	50	86	3	56	48
Colapinto[19] (1983)	108	93	3	59	55
Dotter et al.[20] (1983)	2104	90	3	67	60
Schneider et al.[18] (1982)	682	88	5	68	60
Gallino et al.[22] (1984)	280	84	5	67	56
Krepel et al.[25] (1985)	138	84	5	70	59
Hewes et al.[26] (1986)	91	83	3	65	54
Kammerlander[24] (1989)	54	85	3	84	71

Rotational Angioplasty. The Kensey catheter[29] is a new mechanical rotational device that is claimed to produce extremely small particles that pass through the capillary bed. This so-called micropulverization is obtained by a self-centering, high-speed, rotating cam which is theoretically not able to damage viscoelastic material such as normal arterial wall. However, a pathological study performed on fresh amputated legs[30] suggests that larger debris is produced as well, and dissection and perforation of the wall occur. These observations clearly call for well-controlled, prudent clinical investigation.

The Rotablator is a very flexible, high-speed, rotating, abrasive burr coated with diamond clips designed to preferentially grind harder surfaces such as plaque material while minimizing damage to the vessel wall. Seventy-five per cent of the particles produced are smaller than 10 to 15 microns, and less than 5 per cent are from 200 to 250 microns. Preliminary clinical experience shows a high primary success rate of rotary ablation of segmental stenoses, but the restenosis rate within the first year may be considerable. Several other rotational devices are being tested clinically.

Laser-Assisted Angioplasty. The ability of lasers to cut channels through even the toughest materials led to the consideration of their use to recanalize blood vessels occluded by atherosclerosis. Several lasers are available of which the argon laser, the neodymium:yttrium-aluminium-garnet (Nd:YAG) laser, and the excimer laser have been used in a number of clinical studies. Reported primary success rates to recanalize femoral and iliac vessels vary from 70 to 95 per cent. Restenosis or reocclusion within the first year occurs in up to 40 per cent of the patients. Lateral damage to the arterial wall with perforations is observed in up to 10 per cent of the patients. The costs of the procedure have to be weighed in view of the advantages and potential hazards. Laser-assisted angioplasty still has to be considered as an experimental procedure.[31]

Ultrasonic Angioplasty. Ultrasound energy applied through a catheter delivery system can be used to open completely obstructed atherosclerotic vessels. A first report describes reopening of three out of four occluded vessels and a reduction of four stenoses. All lesions were further treated with balloon angioplasty. There were no major complications. The limitations of the system appear to be the lack of ease of steering and flexibility.[32]

Stents. In an attempt to improve the apparent limitations of conventional balloon percutaneous transluminal angioplasty (restenosis), balloon-expandable, intraluminal stents were permanently implanted in areas of atherosclerotic stenoses following percutaneous transluminal angioplasty. A preliminary report of a multicenter study performed on 15 patients was published by the end of 1988.[33] Smooth and regular lumens

TABLE 23–5. Complications of Percutaneous Transluminal Angioplasty

Hematoma at the puncture site	0.8%
Peripheral embolization	2%
Dissection of the arterial wall	Extremely rare
Arterial wall rupture	1%
Formation of a false aneurysma	0.3%

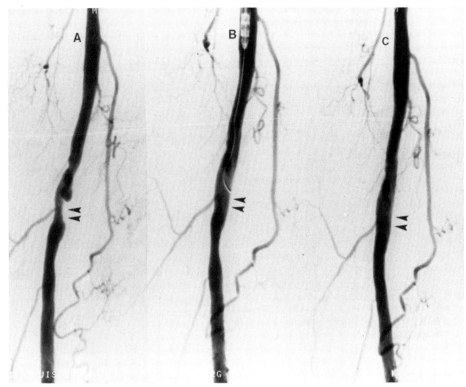

FIGURE 23–4. Percutaneous atherectomy of eccentric atheromatous plaque on the superficial femoral artery (arrowheads). Angiographic view before (A) and at the end of the procedure (B and C). The Simpson catheter is visible in the proximal part of the artery (B). (Courtesy of Dr. G. Wilms.)

were obtained with the stent, which should prevent the development of luminal irregularities after percutaneous transluminal angioplasty. Stent thrombosis occurred in one patient, which could be lysed with local urokinase. In all cases, an improved clinical and hemodynamic status has been maintained during the 6 to 12 months of follow-up. Limitations of the procedure include the reduced capability of negotiating the tortuous iliac vessels because of the relative rigidity of the stent material, and potential triggering of thrombus formation and of intimal hyperplasia. More experience will be necessary in order to establish the exact indications of this new supportive method.

Thrombolytic Therapy

Systemic thrombolytic therapy has been used for almost three decades in the treatment of acute and chronic arterial occlusions in the limbs. Intravenous administration of relatively high doses of streptokinase (SK) was shown to restore patency in almost two thirds of recently occluded arteries. In chronic obstruction the success rate was lower and almost no lysis was obtained in thrombi older than three months in the iliac or femoral artery. This therapeutic effect was obtained at the expense of a serious bleeding tendency. The incidence of major hemorrhagic complications was considerable, and fatal bleeding occurred in 1 to 3 per cent of the patients. With the exception of a few well-experienced European centers, which tend to use ultrahigh doses of streptokinase, the systemic infusion of thrombolytic enzymes for peripheral disease has therefore been gradually abandoned and largely replaced by surgical procedures with a lower risk to the patient.

Following initial reports in the early 1970s that demonstrated lysis of thrombi in peripheral arteries with a low dose of locally delivered streptokinase, this intra-arterial infusion technique has gained wide acceptance over the past decade for a variety of clinical conditions in various vascular beds. The objective is to achieve optimal thrombolysis at the

TABLE 23–6. Agents and Therapeutic Schemes in Local Thrombolysis for Peripheral Arterial Disease

Streptokinase
  1,000–3,000 international units every 5–15 minutes
  5,000 international units/hour continuously; eventually
    initial bolus: 20,000 international units
    initial rapid infusion: 2,000 international units/minute (20 minutes)
Urokinase
  75,000 international units initial dose and 37,500 international units/hour maintenance dose
  20,000 or 25,000 international units/hour continuously
  440 international units/kilogram/hour continuously
  1,000 international units/kilogram/hour (+ lys-plasminogen) continuously
  4,000 international units/minute until initial recanalization; thereafter 1,000–2,000 international units/minute
Alteplase
  0.025 to 0.1 milligrams/kilogram/hour continuously
  0.25 to 10 milligrams/hour continuously

occlusion site and at the same time minimize the bleeding risks associated with the systemic fibrinolytic effect by reducing the dose of the thrombolytic enzyme.

PROCEDURE

As in percutaneous transluminal angioplasty, a suitable catheter is introduced into the occluded vessel for local delivery of the thrombolytic agent (Table 23–6). Ideally, the catheter is inserted into the proximal part of the occluding thrombus. An easily compressible puncture site is chosen. Streptokinase has been the most widely used agent. Several therapeutic regimens have been tried, but they basically fit into one of the two following schemes. The first consists of repeated intrathrombotic injections: 1,000 to 3,000 international units/hour streptokinase are delivered into the clot every 5 to 15 minutes. Between two infiltrations, the catheter is advanced step by step with or without a guide wire. The procedure is continued until the thrombus is completely infiltrated and the open distal lumen is reached. The mechanical effect of catheter movement may add to the thrombolytic effect. The second and more popular scheme is a continuous infusion of 5,000 international units/hour administered with the aid of an arterial infusion pump. Apparently, this dose was arbitrarily determined as 1/20th of the systemically used

maintenance dose of 100,000 international units/hour.

The experience with locally administered urokinase (UK) is more limited, but the number of reports is rising. With this agent, the proposed dose varies from 5,000 to 100,000 international units/hour and even higher. A popular high-dosage scheme in the United States is to administer 240,000 international units/hour until initial recanalization has occurred, followed by 60,000 to 120,000 international units/hour until complete lysis occurs. Over the last five years, a few reports have been published with alteplase (recombinant tissue-type plasminogen activator [rt-PA]). The doses used varied from 0.025 to 0.1 milligrams/kilograms/hour and from 0.25 to 10 milligrams/hour. The duration of treatment is determined by the individual patient's response. For a short thrombus, an infusion of limited duration (one to a few hours) may suffice to obtain complete lysis, but an extended occlusion occasionally requires several days to clear. Apart from clinical evaluation and noninvasive testing, progression of clot lysis is followed by fluoroscopy or angiography via the catheter every 12 to 24 hours or earlier if rapid clearance is anticipated. As soon as evidence for partial clot lysis is obtained, the catheter can be advanced into the proximal edge of the remaining clot and the infusion is continued. Thrombolytic treatment is considered to have failed, and normally stopped, if after 24 to 48 hours no lysis is observed.

There is no unanimity as to the concomitant use of antithrombotic drugs to prevent the development of catheter-related thromboembolism. Some discontinue all anticoagulants at the initiation of the procedure, whereas others advocate the simultaneous use of heparin, either intra-arterially (250 to 800 international units/hour), intravenously, or even subcutaneously. After a successful procedure, most patients receive antithrombotic prophylaxis with aspirin or a similar drug. Others prefer systemic heparin followed by coumarinic drugs (see Antithrombotic Therapy in Percutaneous Revascularization Procedures).

CLINICAL APPLICATION

Clinical experience with local thrombolysis in *acute* limb ischemia is still limited (Fig. 23–5). Reported series are small and contain a mixed population of patients with arterial

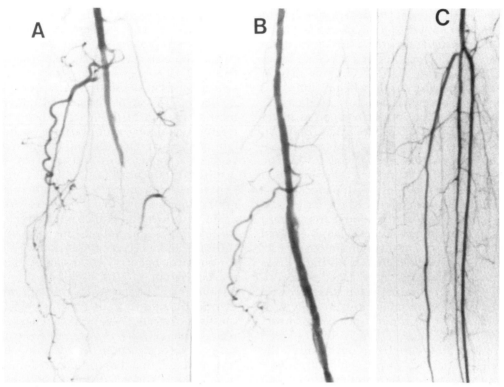

FIGURE 23–5. Acute occlusion of the superficial femoral artery in a 56-year-old woman (*A*). Local thrombolysis with alteplase (50 milligrams over five hours) restored patency in the femoral artery (*B*) and in the distal arteries (*C*).

occlusions of different origin, location, extent, and with a variable degree of ischemia. The therapeutic success rate thus largely differs (25 to 50 per cent). Arteriographic evidence of complete or partial lysis normally leads to immediate clinical improvement, but limb salvage can ultimately not be achieved in all of them either because of absent runoff vessels or due to irreversible ischemia, if the circulation was restored too late. Recurrent thrombosis is one of the main reasons for ultimate failure in those series. Most investigators stress the need to look carefully for a causative lesion on the postlytic angiography, and to complement the lytic therapy with either transluminal angioplasty or a surgical procedure in order to improve the circulation to the limb further and to prevent early rethrombosis. Others use local infusion of thrombolytic agents as an adjunct to balloon-catheter embolectomy or thrombectomy in limb-threatening ischemia, if, after removal of all thrombus material accessible to the balloon-catheter, the operative arteriography shows residual thrombus distal to the popliteal artery and if the viability of the involved extremity is still questionable (intraoperative thrombolysis).[34]

A particular situation arises when thrombosis occurs during angiography or percutaneous angioplasty. Here, it appears almost natural to exchange the catheter for an infusion catheter and to start thrombolytic therapy immediately.

In *chronic* arterial obstruction intra-arterial thrombolysis has become an attractive alternative to surgery and angioplasty in recent years, but the question as to which patients it should be applied as the treatment of choice remains to be answered. Some investigators reported lysis of an occluded iliac artery in a small number of patients. However, well-established surgical techniques are available to treat aortoiliac occlusions with an acceptable risk to most patients. To demonstrate that local thrombolytic therapy might be superior to current surgical practice in restoring and maintaining patency in the aortoiliac segment would be a formidable if not impossible task. Whether selected subgroups of patients with chronic iliac occlusion might benefit from local thrombolysis appears to be a more realistic approach. The contralateral access to an iliac occlusion carries an additional risk: pericatheter thrombosis may in this case jeopardize a nonischemic limb.

A more substantial amount of data has been published on local thrombolysis in femoropopliteal occlusion. Reported results on a large number of patients with an arterial occlusion are summarized in Table 23–7. The cited studies differ from each other in several respects. A few used step-by-step intrathrombotic injections in patients who refused vascular surgery or were unsuitable for surgical procedures, but most investigators infused the thrombolytic enzyme continuously. Factors with a presumed impact on the success rate were differently appreciated, too. Primary recanalization correlated inversely with the age of the thrombus and the length of the occluding clot in most series; the impact of the clinical stage (II to IV of Fontaine) was rarely considered. In our center, the overall lysis rate was 77 per cent, but patients who present with a short femoral occlusion (less than 10 centimeters) and claudication only have a 90 per cent chance of complete lysis.[68] It may be argued that short femoral occlusions can be recanalized with balloon angioplasty without preceding thrombolysis. However, with angioplasty, the primary success rate declines rapidly to roughly one third if the length of the occlusion exceeds 3 centimeters. On the other hand, angioplasty is used as an aid to intra-arterial thrombolysis when an offending stenotic lesion is unmasked by the clot lysis. Information on the long-term patency after primary recanalization is still scarce: cumulative patency after five years approaches 60 per cent. Early rethrombosis occurs in 5 to 15 per cent of the patients and is followed by a yearly reocclusion rate of 5 to 8 per cent.[51] Differences between individual centers may reflect the particular patient selection in each center.

Numerous reports describe successful treatment of *occluded bypass grafts* with local low-dose streptokinase, urokinase, and alteplase. The primary recanalization rate varies from 20 to 80 per cent. As for the native arteries, this wide scatter can probably be ascribed to the small numbers of patients in most series and to the heterogeneity of the treated population with grafts of various origin and anatomic location. Some reports suggest a higher lysis rate in vein grafts compared with prosthetic grafts. Preliminary experience with alteplase in occluded bypass grafts suggests a higher lysis rate with this agent, but the number of patients treated up to now imposes a cautious interpretation of the data, and a direct comparison with other thrombolytic agents is not available. Thrombolytic therapy in graft occlusion offers two advantages. The postlytic arteriogram can identify all sites of graft stenosis, which can mostly be treated by percutaneous angioplasty, but occasionally requires secondary surgical reconstruction. In addition, thrombus material that has propagated into the distal vessels can be dissolved at the same time. Nevertheless, the long-term patency after a successful lysis is not brilliant. Rethrombosis occurs within three months in one third and within the first year in two thirds; these poor late results are still better than what can be achieved with surgical thrombectomy.[70] Patients with a recently thrombosed hemodialysis access fistula can also benefit from local thrombolytic treatment, with a high chance of recanalization.

COMPLICATIONS

If the basic philosophy of intra-arterial thrombolysis with low-dose thrombolytic agents holds true, the incidence of hemorrhagic complications should be substantially lower than with systemic therapy. Local bleeding from the arterial puncture site occurs in 10 to 30 per cent of the patients, but is usually minor and can be controlled with

TABLE 23–7. Local Thrombolysis in Arterial Occlusion

	STREPTOKINASE	UROKINASE	ALTEPLASE
Number of reports*[35–69]	22	11	8
Number of patients	1130	411	271
Complete lysis (angiography)			
Number	760	291	239
Per cent	67	71	88

prolonged local compression. Major hematoma or retroperitoneal hemorrhage occasionally requires blood transfusion. Remote bleeding is observed in 3 to 5 per cent of the treated patients, although it is absent in some series. Severe gastrointestinal or intracranial hemorrhage was reported in a number of patients, and a few fatal bleedings occurred. In fact, evidence for systemic fibrinolytic effects of the locally infused enzyme can be obtained with sensitive tests in almost all patients as the time of infusion increases.

Episodes of distal embolization by fragments of the lysing clot (or rarely from other sites, such as cardiac mural thrombi or aneurysm contents) are observed in up to 10 per cent of the patients. Small emboli in tiny arteries are usually lysed during the course of continued thrombolysis. They cause transient pain sometimes accompanied by visible signs of localized ischemia. Emboli that occlude larger distal arteries are potentially more harmful. Although some subsequently dissolve by additional fibrinolytic agent or even lyse spontaneously in the first hours after therapy, prompt surgical intervention may be required if profound leg ischemia develops.

Catheter manipulation in the arterial lumen entails a definite risk of thrombosis, wall dissection, or vessel spasm. Pericatheter thrombosis was reported in up to one fourth of the patients with intra-arterial infusions of streptokinase in an early study. This figure is much higher than during diagnostic angiography, probably because of the low flow rate with ensuing hypercoagulability proximal to the occlusion. In general, the risk of pericatheter thrombosis increases with the duration of the procedure. Whereas many of these newly formed clots would lyse with further infusion of the thrombolytic agent, some may cause severe ischemia and require urgent surgery. Several measures have been proposed to obviate this local thrombotic tendency: to use thin catheters or catheters with side holes, to increase the fibrinolytic dose rate, or to add heparin to the fibrinolytic drugs. Others, though, believe that the simultaneous administration of thrombolytic agents and heparin leads to a marked increase of the bleeding tendency, which outweighs the additional antithrombotic benefit.

Intra-arterial infusion of thrombolytic agents has renewed interest in thrombolysis of arterial obstructions in the limb and is now recognized as a newly established therapeutic tool to restore vascular patency by nonoperative means. The main issue at this moment is determining in which patient local thrombolysis is the treatment of choice in comparison with other, better established therapeutic modalities. Therefore, data on larger and more homogeneous groups of patients are needed than are presently available. In addition, patients should be followed more extensively to gain better insight into the long-term results. Although serious bleeding still remains a potential hazard, the original idea of reducing the risk of severe hemorrhage seems to have materialized to such an extent that local thrombolysis is realized in conditions in which systemic thrombolysis would be inconceivable. A direct comparison between the main thrombolytic agents would be welcome to determine which agent is the most efficacious and the safest.

ANTITHROMBOTIC THERAPY IN SECONDARY PREVENTION

Antithrombotic Therapy and Natural History of Peripheral Arterial Disease

The natural history of atherosclerotic disease of the leg arteries is characterized by a relatively benign local evolution. It can be estimated that in general, three out of four men presenting with intermittent claudication will never have a very serious problem necessitating vascular reconstruction, and no more than 5 per cent are ever likely to require a major amputation.[1] However, whereas the functional prognosis is rather favorable with stabilization or even improvement of the symptoms in most patients, the underlying atherosclerotic disease progresses with time. In half of the legs with a normal circulation at the first presentation, the arteries become obliterated at follow-up. Thus, initially unilateral disease frequently ends bilaterally. This local evolution is well illustrated in the recently published Prevention of Atherosclerotic Complications with Ketanserin (PACK) trial.[71] In this large double-blind study, 3,899 patients with intermittent claudication of varying severity were randomized to receive either ketanserin, a serotonin-2-antagonist, or placebo, and were followed over at least one year. The 1,869 placebo patients provide valuable information on the short-term prognosis of claudication patients. At one year, the mean pain-free walking distance increased by 25 per cent, but the systolic ankle pressure index did not improve, and 5 per cent of the patients had progression of their symptoms to the extent that surgical intervention was required.[72]

Although the natural history of atherosclerotic disease of the leg arteries is characterized by a relatively benign local evolution, the general prognosis of patients with peripheral arterial obstructive disease is rather grim. They have high prevalences of coronary disease and cerebrovascular disease, but the exact percentages depend on the way patients are selected for screening and on which methods are used for their evaluation. Clinical screening combined with electrocardiography detects 40 to 60 per cent of patients with coronary artery disease among claudication patients, whereas systematic preoperative coronary angiography detects 90 per cent. Similarly, few patients with leg arterial disease have a history of cerebrovascular disease, but when noninvasive tests are applied to preoperative patients, almost 30 per cent appear to have significant extracranial arterial disease. The annual incidence of nonfatal coronary and cerebrovascular events in patients with intermittent claudication is uncertain; in the PACK trial, it was 1 per cent under placebo.[71] There is ample evidence that patients presenting with intermittent claudication have a mortality which is two to three times more than expected.[1] In the PACK trial, 4 per cent mortality was observed within one year; in this study the systolic pressure gradient between arm and ankle, an index of the severity of leg arterial disease, correlated positively with mortality. Overall, vascular mortality is responsible for almost two thirds of the total mortality.

Since thrombosis of atherosclerotic arteries is only the final step of a long evolution, long-term oral anticoagulation is rather unlikely to represent a serious advance in the pharmacological prevention of progression of peripheral arterial occlusive disease. A few early trials have shown a favorable trend with oral anticoagulants, but their design and size do not allow a definite conclusion. There are two prospective studies on the value of oral anticoagulants in patients suffering from intermittent claudication. In the first, all of the included patients initially received oral anticoagulant therapy for at least six months and were then randomly assigned to switch to placebo or to continue oral anticoagulation.

TABLE 23–8. Effect of Antithrombotic Therapy on Natural History

Anticoagulants
  Decrease fatal myocardial infarction[73]
  Lower incidence of vascular events[74]
  Retard progression of leg arterial disease[74]
  Decrease mortality in surgical patients[75]
Antiplatelet drugs
  Improve general prognosis (vascular death, myocardial infarction, stroke)[76–78]
  Decrease thrombotic occlusion of stenotic artery[79]
  Retard angiographic progression of disease[6,80]

This trial was interrupted prematurely because of a significant surplus of deaths from myocardial infarction in the placebo group.[73] In the second and still unpublished trial, no benefit of anticoagulants on total mortality was found, although there was a lower incidence of vascular events (peripheral, cerebrovascular, cardiovascular). In addition, the progression of the leg arterial disease appeared delayed as evidenced by a slower deterioration of the ankle pressure index in patients treated with anticoagulants.[74] Kretschmer et al. selected patients who had vascular surgery in the femoropopliteal region to study the influence of anticoagulants on long-term mortality: they report a significantly better survival in the anticoagulant group compared to placebo after a median follow-up of at least five years.[75] Even taken together, these data still do not convince most clinicians that long-term oral anticoagulation is worthwhile in patients with peripheral arterial obstructive disease (Table 23–8).

Antiplatelet drugs are more readily accepted than anticoagulants, and many practitioners prescribe their patients suffering from peripheral vascular insufficiency aspirin, aspirin-dipyridamole, or (in some countries) ticlopidine. They hope to decrease the incidence of thromboembolic events in other vascular beds, but what is their hope based on?

Large randomized trials with these agents in patients with intermittent claudication are not numerous. The antiserotonin agent ketanserin did not reduce cardiovascular mortality nor the incidence of nonfatal vascular events in the PACK trial, the largest controlled study ever published on pharmacological intervention in claudication patients.[71] The Antiplatelet Trialists Collaboration, on the other hand, calculated in a meta-analysis on 31 randomized trials of antiplatelet therapy involving over 29,000 patients with clinical symptoms of cardiovascular and cerebrovascular disease, that antiplatelet treatment reduced vascular death by 15 per cent and nonfatal myocardial infarction and stroke by 30 per cent ($p < 0.0003$ and $p < 0.0001$, respectively).[81] It appears logical to expect a similar effect in individuals with intermittent claudication, in view of the epidemiological evidence that these patients have coronary and cerebral artery disease as well, and that they have a two- to threefold increase in cardiovascular mortality on long-term follow-up in comparison with an age-matched healthy control group. Further support for a beneficial effect of antiplatelet drugs comes from another, still unpublished, meta-analysis on 28 smaller trials involving patients with peripheral vascular disease, many of whom had undergone surgery. The total number of patients included was 3,864, and 444 vascular events occurred; antiplatelet agents reduced the odds of suffering a vascular event by 25 ± 10 per cent.[76] A recent Swedisch trial (Swedish Ticlopidine Multicentre Study [STIMS]) on 687 patients followed for over five years concluded that the high morbidity and mortality from cardiovascular and cerebrovascular disease in patients with intermittent claudication can be reduced by long-term treatment with ticlopidine.[77]

The local evolution of the atherosclerotic disease in the legs may be influenced by antiplatelet agents as well. There is evidence that aspirin and ticlopidine retard the progression of atherosclerosis and the occurrence of its thrombotic complications in legs of patients with obstructive arterial disease. Schoop et al.[82] randomized 300 patients with a stenosis of the femoral artery in one leg (and an occlusion in the contralateral leg) to receive daily either 1 gram of aspirin, 1 gram of aspirin combined with 225 milligrams of dipyridamole, or placebo. After four years of follow-up the occlusion rate was lower in the two groups treated with the active drugs, but the combination was not superior to the administration of aspirin alone. In addition, antiplatelet therapy did not prevent femoral artery thrombosis in diabetic and hypertensive patients. Hess et al.[6] reported a placebo-controlled, double-blind trial in 199 patients with angiographically studied evolution of peripheral atherosclerosis over a two-year period. Disease progression was most pronounced in the placebo group, less so in the aspirin-treated group (1 gram/day), and least

of all in the aspirin/dipyridamole-treated group (1 gram/225 milligrams, daily). In contrast with the previous study, patients who continued to smoke and those with hypertension benefitted most from active treatment. A similar placebo-controlled randomized trial was conducted with ticlopidine in 114 patients; control angiograms repeated after one year of treatment showed that ticlopidine significantly reduced progression of the disease.[80] Boissel et al.[78] published a meta-analysis on four placebo-controlled trials with ticlopidine in peripheral vascular disease. They found not only a decreased incidence of vascular events with the active substance, but also an improvement of walking distance. Since claudication distance may be influenced by factors other than blood flow, it is uncertain whether this improvement can be taken as proof of a better local evolution of the atherosclerotic disease.

Antithrombotic Therapy in Arterial Surgery

Bypass grafting and thromboendarterectomy are the basic techniques in vascular surgery. For bypass grafting, three materials are widely used: the autologous saphenous vein and two prosthetic grafts, woven or knitted Dacron, and expanded polytetrafluoroethylene (ePTFE or Teflon). The synthetic nature of the prosthetic grafts induces two types of reaction after their implantation. An inflammatory reaction occurs with the adjacent tissues in contact with the outer surface of the graft. This reaction is kept under control by adapting the material used. For instance, the external velours which covers Dacron grafts facilitates the adhesion of adjacent tissues, and the wrapping of Teflon tubes with the same material enhances penetration of fibroblasts and the anchoring of the graft. On the other hand, the circulating blood interacts with the inner surface of the graft. Owing to the absence of a normal endothelium with active biological functions in prosthetic grafts, large proteins rapidly adhere to the artificial surface; in particular, fibrinogen, fibronectin, von Willebrand factor, and thrombospondin. They enhance fibrin and platelet deposition followed by platelet aggregation. Activation of several coagulation factors and complement follows and a thin layer of fibrin spreads over the inner surface. A few cellular elements are trapped within the fibrin film. White cells in turn adhere to exposed receptors on the adsorbed proteins while the red cell concentration, together with other local rheological and hemodynamic factors, largely determines the extent and speed of platelet deposition and aggregation. The organization and transformation of the fibrin layer into a neointima takes a few weeks. In fact, it is rather a pseudointima because no complete endothelialization is observed in humans. The endothelial cells which slide from the native vessel into the prosthesis only penetrate over a short distance beyond the anastomosis. The complete reaction of the inner surface with thickening of the neointima as a final stage may take a few months.

Thromboendarterectomy is followed by a fairly analogous sequence of events. The rough endarterectomized surface is quickly covered with aggregating platelets and later with fibrin, the beginning of pseudointima formation. Smooth muscle cells which originate from the remaining media or from fibroblasts which differentiate, start to proliferate and invade the fibrinous surface. The neoartery takes eight to ten days for complete healing, but it remains a dystrophic vessel: a fibrous tube without endothelium except for the juxta-anastomotic zones. The pseudointima undergoes degenerative phenomena within months to years, with development of new atheromatous plaques and of evolutive complications of atherosclerosis, in particular, ulceration with mural thrombus formation and embolization.

The changes in vein grafts are rather minor in comparison with those in synthetic grafts and on endarterectomized surfaces. They are mainly caused by the changing hemodynamic conditions of the vein when used as an arterial graft: thickening of the intima, hyperplasia of the media, and fibrosis of the adventitia. The caliber of the vein increases progressively. The vein graft is not anchored into the adjacent tissue, and the inflammatory reaction is confined to the anastomic sites. New atherosclerotic lesions develop in a vein graft after several years.

Several problems may arise after implantation of a graft or after a thromboendarterectomy of which early thrombosis, restenosis at the anastomosis, and late occlusion are relevant for the present discussion. Early thrombosis is primarily due to the nonthromboresistant nature of prosthetic materials or endarterectomized surfaces, but additional factors may contribute; for example, technical errors and the unfavorable hemodynamic situation of a poor distal outflow or of an underestimated proximal stenotic lesion. The well-known perioperative thrombotic tendency which is evidenced by platelet hyperreactivity, a decreased level of antithrombin III, a reduced fibrinolytic activity, and elevated fibrinogen and factor VIII levels is enhanced in patients with advanced stages of atherosclerotic disease and augments the risk of early thrombosis.

Intimal hyperplasia is the main cause of stenosis at the anastomotic sutures. It is caused by proliferating smooth muscle cells. Platelet-derived growth factor (PDGF) liberated from platelet deposits on the thrombogenic surface may enhance hyperplasia of the pseudointima, which mainly affects the distal anastomotic site of prosthetic grafts. The progressive reduction of the internal cross section of the graft will result in complete occlusion with thrombus formation as the final event. Progression of the atherosclerotic disease may lead to increasing inflow obstruction and decreasing outflow at the same time and in this way promote occlusion of the graft. New atherosclerotic lesions may develop in the bypass graft as well and result in a late thrombotic occlusion. Embolic complications, on the other hand, are less common; they occur when hemodynamic factors that favor disruption and fragmentation surpass adhesive forces.

In daily practice, the main concern of physicians and surgeons alike is to maintain patency of an arterial reconstruction. For aortoiliac reconstruction, the late results are satisfactory, with fairly high, late patency rates which stress the preponderance of hemodynamic forces over thromboresistance in large-caliber bypasses with a high flow rate. Although Dacron is generally considered to be more thrombogenic than Teflon, it remains the preferred material for aortofemoral grafting, and antithrombotic drugs are rarely prescribed to improve late patency of aortofemoral reconstructions. The situation is more cumbersome for reconstructions that extend below the groin, and the main problems arise when the diameter of the graft drops below 6 millimeters. The number of failures for certain limb salvage bypass grafts in patients with critical ischemia reaches 50 per cent after three months, followed by a slower steady occlusion rate of about 2 per cent per month thereafter.[83] For identical conditions, autologous vein grafts produce better late patency rates than prosthetic grafts, and this explains why the saphenous vein remains the preferred material for distal bypasses.

There are a number of strategies that can conceivably increase long-term patency of vascular grafts.[84] Systematic modification of the chemical composition of prosthetic material is a first direction that is currently being pursued to produce more thromboresistant materials. In addition, resorbable vascular prostheses are being developed that are biodegraded after their implantation with simultaneous invasion of the graft by tissue cells from the host to create a new vessel. The in vitro creation of a vessel by the judicious combination in culture of cellular and noncellular elements is no longer entirely science fiction. A more profane idea is the incorporation of substances such as heparin, prostaglandins, and fibrinolytic agents into biomaterials that degrade at a controlled rate and release those compounds into the circulation for their local action. Finally, endothelial-cell seeding is a method to inoculate endothelial cells harvested from the autologous saphenous vein onto synthetic materials. The aim is a rapid development of a completely endothelialized surface that is more thromboresistant. In humans, endothelial-cell seeding decreases the fixation of indium-labeled platelets onto Dacron and Teflon grafts. Preliminary clinical studies suggest that this technique reduces intimal hyperplasia, but up to now the incidence of early thrombosis is not influenced, and an effect on long-term patency has not been investigated.

What has a clinician to add to this avalanche of advanced technology? Clinicians dispose of a number of substances which intervene in vivo as well as in vitro in the thrombogenic interactions of circulating blood with an artificial surface. For decades, surgeons have satisfactorily used heparin during operations. Prolonged administration of heparin for a few days postoperatively may conceivably prevent early graft thrombosis, but this practice was never considered nor evaluated properly. Dextran-40 infusion for the first postoperative days with the aim of reducing blood viscosity and inhibiting cell adhesion onto the artificial surface appears to diminish the thrombotic risk during the first week after surgery, but the beneficial effect disappears within one month.[85] Some clinicians advocate the use of oral anticoagulants for the first

few months after implantation of a vascular graft, or eventually, their lifelong use if the graft is at high risk of thrombosis. They base their decision on personal clinical experience rather than on controlled clinical trials, although the data obtained by Kretschmer et al.[79] in patients with autologous vein grafts lend some support to their practice. In this study, anticoagulants appeared to favorably influence long-term graft patency and to prolong the life of patients who had undergone femoropopliteal bypass grafting for arterial occlusive disease. However, 12 per cent of treated patients had to discontinue coumarin therapy because of serious bleeding complications.

The popularity of antiplatelet drugs has expanded rapidly since the large trials on their value in cerebral ischemia, after myocardial infarction, and after aortocoronary bypass grafting. Their efficacy in peripheral arterial surgery, however, is less well established. Antiplatelet drugs normalize the shortened platelet survival after aortofemoral Dacron grafting and reduce the deposition of platelets in prosthetic grafts, a measure of thrombogenicity of prosthetic material; they also inhibit thromboxane production after surgery, but it is unclear to what extent they prevent neointimal hyperplasia.

Clinical trials on therapeutic efficacy are not numerous and are usually small. In general, they leave an impression of dissatisfaction and confusion. Bollinger and Brunner[86] reported the results of a prospective study of 120 patients who were followed-up for two years after a successful endarterectomy in the femoropopliteal region. All patients received warfarin for the initial two postoperative weeks. They were then randomized into treatment groups for prophylaxis of reocclusion: aspirin (1 gram/day), aspirin/dipyridamole (1 gram, 225 milligrams/day), or an oral anticoagulant (warfarin). The cumulative patency rate at two years was 84 per cent for the aspirin group, 76 per cent for the aspirin/dipyridamole group, and only 58 per cent for the warfarin-treated patients. Both antiplatelet regimens are significantly superior to warfarin, but the level of hypocoagulability induced by warfarin was probably insufficient. However, endarterectomy in the femoropopliteal region has largely been abandoned by most surgeons in favor of bypass surgery. The Second American College of Chest Physicians Conference on Antithrombotic Therapy evaluated four published trials:[87] the study population is a mixture of patients with vein grafts and prosthetic grafts. Three studies conclude that there is a significant advantage of the antiplatelet treatment, usually aspirin associated with dipyridamol, started before surgery and continued for a variable period, over placebo to maintain patency of the infrainguinal arterial bypass. One trial suggests that the effect is limited to prosthetic grafts and that it is confined to the first postoperative month. The fourth trial followed 100 patients with arterial reconstruction, one third of whom received a prosthetic graft, and found no difference between active drug and placebo, but the treatment was started after surgery only. Despite the weakness of the presented evidence, the American College of Chest Physicians recommends the use of antiplatelet drugs for all infrainguinal arterial prosthesis and for any complex or compromised distal reconstruction, vein graft, or prosthesis. Support for this view is found in the meta-analysis made by the Antiplatelet Trialists Collaboration on 12 randomized trials, including over 2,000 patients with peripheral vascular grafts: antiplatelet drugs reduce the incidence of graft occlusion at the end of the (variable) follow-up period by one third (from 25 to 16 per cent).[76] An optimal protection requires daily administration of 325 milligrams of aspirin to be started before surgery. The association of dipyridamole (225 milligrams/day) is recommended by the American College of Chest Physicians with the argument that this substance augments the antithrombotic effect of aspirin on artificial surfaces in experimental conditions. Surgeons who fear an increased intraoperative blood loss can substitute preoperative aspirin with dipyridamole, although it is unclear whether preoperative dipyridamole alone is efficacious as antithrombotic therapy.

Antithrombotic Therapy in Percutaneous Revascularization Procedures

The balloon catheter used to dilate stenotic arteries overstretches the arterial wall and provokes longitudinal splits and dissections of atherosclerotic plaque and intima which often extend into the media. Platelets rapidly accumulate on sites of intimal disruption to form platelet-rich thrombi. It has been demonstrated in studies with indium-labeled platelets that marked uptake of platelets occurs at the angioplasty site. This platelet accumulation is long standing, and maximal when there is evidence of dissection. Thus the tradition of prescribing antithrombotic agents to patients who undergo percutaneous transluminal angioplasty appears logical even if it was originally based on the fear of rethrombosis rather than on experimental facts. Most centers now advise the use of aspirin or a combination of aspirin/dipyridamole, and many start one or two days before the procedure. During the percutaneous transluminal angioplasty procedure, platelet stimulation and subsequent thrombus formation and activation of the plasma coagulation system is further prevented by intra-arterial or intravenous injection of heparin (3,000 to 5,000 international units).

Data from clinical trials which would support this traditional use of antithrombotic agents during and after percutaneous transluminal angioplasty to decrease the risk of early reocclusion are not available. A German study published in the very early days of percutaneous transluminal angioplasty recommends the use of aspirin on the basis of a similar incidence of rethrombosis with aspirin alone as with the combination aspirin/heparin (4 of 87, and 6 of 90, respectively) whereas the bleeding risk at the puncture site was clearly reduced (6 versus 11). In the same study, four cases of rethrombosis were reported out of an apparently nonrandomized series of 19 patients treated with heparin only.[88] A second German study found much higher early recurrence rates: 30 per cent with aspirin after two weeks versus only 16 per cent with aspirin combined with dipyridamole.[89] Stronger arguments for the periprocedural use of antithrombotic drugs may be found in percutaneous transluminal coronary angioplasty (PTCA), where they decrease the incidence of (a) angiographically detected new thrombi at the angioplasty site, (b) clinically significant thrombi requiring emergency surgery or thrombolysis, and (c) myocardial infarction. The latter effect was obtained with aspirin/dipyridamole started before percutaneous transluminal coronary angioplasty. However, it remains unknown whether data in percutaneous transluminal coronary angioplasty can be extrapolated to peripheral percutaneous transluminal angioplasty.

Properly controlled clinical trials which address the need for long-term pharmacological prevention of restenosis and/or occlusion after peripheral percutaneous transluminal angioplasty are equally rare. Four trials, all taken from the German and Swiss literature, are listed in Table 23–9. Their interpretation is not made easy by the fact that they all compare two regimens of antithrombotic therapy, and only two include a placebo group. The general impression is that the use of antiplatelet agents and/or oral anticoagulants have very little impact on the rate of late recurrence of stenosis and occlusion, but the number of patients studied is too small for a definitive conclusion.

The American College of Chest Physicians Conference on Antithrombotic Therapy[87] issued the following recommendation: (a) use aspirin/dipyridamole before angioplasty, (b) heparin during angioplasty, and (c) again aspirin/dypiridamole for a short period following angioplasty. It is possible that 75 or 100 milligrams/day of aspirin or 325 milligrams on alternate days is as effective as a higher dose of aspirin plus dypyridamole, and produces fewer gastrointestinal side effects.

This whole discussion on the use of antithrombotic therapy in percutaneous transluminal angioplasty might be repeated—mutatis mutandis—for all other forms of percutaneous revascularization if we had data to discuss. In the meantime, most centers apply the same rules as for percutaneous transluminal angioplasty. In addition, the use of antithrombotic agents as discussed here does not take into account the eventual use of aspirin (or ticlopidine) in all patients with peripheral arterial disease with the aim to favorably influence the natural history of the disease (see Antithrombotic Therapy and Natural History of Peripheral Arterial Disease). Whether other compounds may be useful in preventing stenosis after percutaneous transluminal angioplasty is a subject of intensive investigation. A promising attempt is the use of inhibitors of angiotensin-converting enzyme which were found to exert in rats an antiproliferative effect on the smooth muscle cells following vascular injury.[94]

MANAGEMENT OF ACUTE LEG ISCHEMIA

The functional integrity of an extremity depends to a large extent on an adequate blood supply through the main arteries. Sudden arterial occlusion with almost instantaneous and complete interruption of blood flow rapidly jeopardizes the limb's viability and is almost invariably due to arterial thrombosis or arterial embolism. Thrombosis is frequently the end stage of advanced atherosclerosis; the severity of ischemia is inversely related to the degree of preexisting and developed collateral circulation. Thrombosis also occurs with other degenerative or inflammatory diseases, with trauma, and in venous or synthetic grafts. Transection, laceration, and external compression (for example, by bone fragments) lead to occlusive events with trauma, but thrombosis occurs from blunt trauma as well. The daily use of intra-arterial catheters for diagnostic or therapeutic procedures and for monitoring purposes accounts for an increasing number of acute arterial occlusions. Hypovolemia, hyperviscosity, and hypercoagulability as observed in shock, thrombocytosis, polycythemia, and malignant disorders frequently predispose to this complication. More than 80 per cent of arterial emboli arise from the heart: causes

TABLE 23–9. Controlled Secondary Prevention Studies Following Peripheral Percutaneous Transluminal Angioplasty

AUTHORS (YEARS)	FOLLOW-UP	NUMBER	DRUG	RECURRENCE RATE (%)
Staiger et al.[90] (1980)	1 year	39	Placebo	36
		28	Aspirin + dipyridamole	25
		33	Aspirin	21
Heiss et al.[91] (1987)	6 months	67	Placebo	22
		66	Low-aspirin + dipyridamole	27
		66	Aspirin + dipyridamole	21
Mahler et al.[92] (1987)	1 year	51	Coumarins	34
		48	Coumarins + suloctidil	35
Schneider et al.[93] (1988)	1 year	94	Coumarins	31
		103	Ticlopidine	29

include atrial fibrillation associated with valvular disease, prosthetic valves, and mural thrombi in an infarcted or cardiomyopathic dilated left ventricle. Noncardiac causes are arterial aneurysms, ulcerated atherosclerotic lesions, and percutaneous or surgical arterial procedures. Most noncerebral emboli occlude arteries to the lower limbs, while the upper extremity is far less frequently affected. The frequency of embolism is equal in the iliofemoral segment and in the popliteal and tibial area. Rare causes of acute leg ischemia are severe arterial spasm and aortic dissection without distal reentry.

Irrespective of whether an acute arterial occlusion is due to thrombosis or embolism, a number of urgent measures are to be taken. The ischemic leg is placed in a position of about 15 degrees dependency to avoid further impairment to capillary perfusion. Direct heating of the cold leg and mechanical trauma are avoided. Heparin treatment is initiated at a therapeutic dosage to prevent extension of thrombosis or recurrent embolism. Further therapeutic measures will depend on whether the acute occlusion is caused by embolism in a healthy artery or by thromboembolism in an atheromatous artery.

Arterial Embolism in Healthy Arteries

Since the introduction of the Fogarty catheter in 1963, prompt removal of the emboli and of secondary stagnation thrombi with this balloon catheter is the treatment of choice in nearly all patients. The catheter is introduced via the femoral or brachial artery, usually under local anesthesia. The success rate in terms of limb salvage is about 90 per cent, the best results being obtained in patients subjected to early embolectomy (that is, within eight hours). The procedure is simple and the immediate results so convincing that watchful waiting or any other therapeutic approach is irresponsible.

Leg edema may occur after successful revascularization as a result of transsudation of fluid across the capillary membrane, the permeability of which is increased by hypoxia. This complication may induce a compartment syndrome and lead to further damage of the muscle, nerves, and vessels. Fasciotomy may be required.

Thromboembolism in Atheromatous Arteries

Most of the acute arterial thromboses and many of the emboli are superimposed on atheromatous plaques in an already impaired arterial circulation. Nevertheless, in many patients, the Fogarty procedure just described will be tried without delay. However the short- and long-term success rate of thromboembolectomy in these conditions is considerably lower than that for an arterial embolus in a healthy artery. If the Fogarty procedure fails or if it is not advisable, the situation has to be reevaluated and several problems have to be discussed: is expeditious or expectant treatment indicated, is angiography required, and do we have alternatives for surgery?

Many patients have had long-standing stenotic lesions of the occluded vessel with development of sufficient collaterals to retain viability of the extremity. Final occlusion in these patients is frequently not a dramatic event and emergency treatment may not be needed. Elective vascular repair at a later stage offers better perspectives on optimal results in such patients. In addition, a better visualization of run-off vessels is obtained if angiography can be delayed until further collateral circulation has developed, whereas contrast injection in the acute stage correctly localizes the occlusion but frequently fails to show distal vessels. Selective catherization and late exposure of the distal limb may help to obtain adequate images. If expectant treatment is preferred, close monitoring of the condition of the limb is required and continued heparin administration is advised.

Although surgical management remains the treatment of choice for a majority of patients with acute events in atherosclerotic limb arteries, local thrombolysis combined with transluminal angioplasty of the causative stenotic lesion is an alternative in patients in whom a surgical intervention is considered delicate for technical reasons or because of the poor general condition of the patient. However, the success rate of intra-arterial thrombolysis in acute ischemia is not brilliant (see Thrombolytic Therapy), and the main problem is that a few crucial hours may be lost for an endangered limb.

Trauma

In most cases of occlusion caused by trauma, early surgery with appropriate repair of the injured vessel is the preferred treatment. With trauma, the prognosis of the limb is mainly determined by the duration of ischemia. Early thrombectomy is indicated in iatrogenic acute arterial occlusion; thrombolysis is an alternative treatment which can also be applied in children.

Blue Toe Syndrome

A number of patients present with acute and often recurrent pain and ischemia in the toes and fingers, even though the blood supply through the larger arteries appears intact as shown by normal peripheral pulses and systolic pressures. This so-called blue toe (or blue finger) syndrome may be due to obstruction of the microcirculation in patients with essential or secondary thrombocythemia. The platelets of these patients aggregate spontaneously in vitro. Usually, the symptoms respond to symptomatic treatment with aspirin, and skin perfusion improves quickly. The underlying cause of the thrombocytosis needs investigation and proper treatment. Similar but more lasting symptoms of distal ischemia are occasionally caused by peripheral microembolization of atherosclerotic debris or cholesterol emboli originating from ulcerated lesions in proximal arteries. Here, vascular repair without further delay is usually indicated. Anticoagulants do not help to prevent cholesterol emboli and may even produce deleterious effects, possibly by preventing the cementing of cholesterol plaque by fibrin. The important role of fibrin in stabilizing plaques is underlined by the occurence of peripheral cholesterol emboli during thrombolytic treatment (for example, for myocardial infarction).

Prevention of Recurrent Thromboembolism

A normal artery with acute embolic occlusion will remain patent after prompt successful embolectomy. Nevertheless, heparin administration started before or during this procedure is continued and eventually relayed with oral anticoagulants in most patients to prevent new embolic episodes. If the source of embolism can be corrected or eradicated, for example, atrial fibrillation secondary to hyperthyroidism or an aneurysm, anticoagulation will be temporary only. Anticoagulant therapy with heparin or oral anticoagulants reduces the frequency of recurrent emboli by approximately 75 per cent compared with no therapy, but the available evidence comes from retrospective nonrandomized studies.[87]

Prevention of recurrent thromboembolism in diseased arteries is a much more complicated and disputed problem. First, a clear distinction between a thrombotic and an embolic occlusion is frequently difficult to discern in the individual patient, especially in the elderly patient with preexisting atherosclerosis in the limbs. Furthermore, the benefits of antithrombotic therapy have not been definitively and unequivocally established in this clinical condition. Most centers will advise the temporary use of oral anticoagulatnts or antiplatelet agents after thromboembolectomy or thrombolysis in order to prevent early recurrent thromboembolism. Short-term prophylaxis suffices when thrombosis was initiated by a unique incident, such as a puncture or catheter manipulation. Long-term use of these agents is mainly a question of secondary prevention (see Antithrombotic Therapy and Natural History of Peripheral Arterial Disease).

MANAGEMENT OF CHRONIC ISCHEMIA OF THE LEG

Treatment of Intermittent Claudication

PREVENTION

Secondary prevention of progression of atherosclerosis in patients with peripheral arterial occlusive disease of the leg arteries is not restricted to the use of antithrombotic drugs. Reducing the risk factors is probably at least as important. Thus, for decades, patients with intermittent claudication have been exhorted to refrain from cigarette smoking, to follow an appropriate diet, and to have hypertension and diabetes controlled. Abstaining from smoking can even result in an increase of the walking distance (see Atherosclerosis and Thrombosis in Peripheral Arterial Disease: Primary Prevention).

VASCULAR SURGERY OR PERCUTANEOUS TRANSLUMINAL ANGIOPLASTY

Vascular surgery and percutaneous transluminal angioplasty relieve symptoms of ischemia. Therefore, their application should depend first on the severity of the symptoms. Thus, careful evaluation of the handicap for the individual patient is a crucial issue: a walking distance of only 40 meters may be sufficient for an 80-year-old, institutionalized patient, whilst a younger, active person may feel very disabled by a walking distance of 300 meters or even more.

WALKING TRAINING

Daily physical exercise has been shown in several studies to markedly increase the walking distance in patients with intermittent claudication. Larsen and Lassen[95] reported a threefold increase in walking distance after six months of daily leg exercise on a treadmill, as compared with no change in the patients who were randomized to receive placebo tablets but no training program. The sample size, however, was small (only 14 patients), but the data were essentially confirmed in several later studies. Ekroth et al. submitted 148 patients to a six-month training program (three times a week) and obtained a more than doubling of the initial maximal walking distance.[96] In these studies, calf muscle blood flow at rest remained unchanged.

Proposed mechanisms for the effects of training on walking distance include an increase of muscle blood flow during exercise due to development of collateral vessels, redistribution of blood flow within the leg, improved metabolism of muscle cells in trained skeletal muscle, improved rheologic properties of blood, and increased pain tolerance. Up to now, there is little evidence to definitely favor any of these hypotheses.

Whether a planned and supervised training program gives better results than the simple medical advice to regularly walk is unproven, but likely. In the PACK substudy in which all patients were advised to exercise, a significant increase of the pain-free walking distance of 14 per cent at six months and 25 per cent at 12 months was observed in the placebo group.[72] These figures are less than the results reported in studies of imposed, physical training programs (Fig. 23–6). Direct comparative data on the two procedures are not available.

DRUG TREATMENT

Drug treatment of intermittent claudication remains a highly controversial issue. Since vasodilatation as a concept to improve

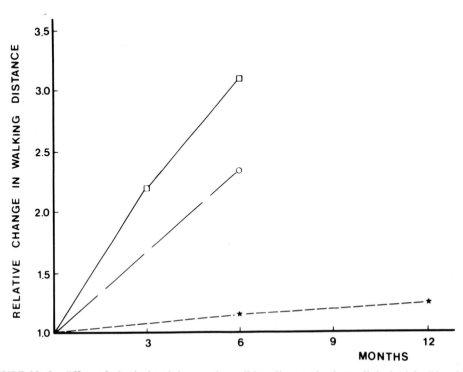

FIGURE 23–6. Effect of physical training on the walking distance in three clinical trials. The change in walking distance with time is expressed as a fraction of the initial walking distance. In two studies (Larsen et al., reference 95, □; and Ekroth et al., reference 96, ○) physical training was imposed and controlled, while in the PACK Claudication Substudy (reference 72, *) walking exercise was only advised to the patients.

symptoms of ischemia almost fell into disgrace, other characteristics of the studied compounds are stressed. For example, pentoxifylline improves red cell deformability, and naftidrofuryl and ketanserin block serotonin-2 receptors.

Cameron et al.[97] analyzed all trials of drug therapy in claudicants which were published during the period 1965 to 1985 and came to a total of 75 trials which had studied 33 different pharmacological agents. They found that (a) treadmill exercise, the most relevant method of evaluating symptoms in this condition, was used in only half of the trials; (b) a significant negative relation between sample size and therapeutic response was observed when analyzing the seven placebo-controlled trials of pentoxifylline, suggesting that the estimated 65 per cent improvement in walking distance was likely to have been biased by nonpublication of negative results; (c) one third of all trials were uncontrolled, most of them (84 per cent) reporting benefit from drug treatment, compared with only 32 per cent of placebo-controlled trials; and (d) one third of trials reported data from less than 20 patients. Thus, the vast majority of published trials on drug treatment of intermittent claudication were unlikely to have made a satisfactory assessment of drug efficacy.

The importance of the sample size is illustrated with the example of ketanserin. This serotonin-2 receptor blocker was reported to increase walking distance in an initial study of 20 patients.[98] However, three subsequent trials using similar design found no effect of the drug in 17,[99] 27,[100] and 179[101] claudicants. Nevertheless, a pooled analysis of these trials still claimed a positive effect of ketanserin.[102] The last word was given by the large-scale PACK claudication substudy on 436 patients who were followed-up for one year, in a double-blind, placebo-controlled design. This trial failed to demonstrate a beneficial effect of ketanserin on walking distance.[72]

This critical assessment should be kept in mind when positive results on claudication distance are reported with new compounds as was recently the case for ticlopidine, an antiplatelet drug, and for L-carnitine, a substance claimed to improve pyruvate utilization and oxidative phosphorylation efficiency in ischemic skeletal muscle. Despite an increasing number of positive randomized, placebo-controlled, and double-blind trials, most authorities would still dispute the efficacy of drug treatment in intermittent claudication.

Treatment of Critical Limb Ischemia

DEFINITION

A strict definition of chronic critical limb ischemia as a condition which endangers the limb is not easy because of its capricious natural history and because of the placebo effect of many therapeutic measures proposed to patients who face an amputation. In the early 1980s, critical ischemia was thought to be present if ischemic pain at rest persisted for at least four weeks and the ankle pressure was below 40 mm Hg, or below 60 mm Hg if skin necrosis already developed.[103,104] This definition did not extend to diabetic patients. A prospective study in Great Britain on 428 ischemic legs in 409 patients reported an overall mortality at one year of 18 per cent, and a 26 per cent amputation rate in survivors.[105] Thus, only 56 per cent of the patients were alive with their two legs one year after their initial presentation with limb ischemia. The study further revealed that patients with pain at rest and ankle pressure below 40 mm Hg had a poorer outcome than those with a pressure above 40 mm Hg; in patients with gangrene this difference was not upheld. A slightly different terminology was therefore proposed to define critical ischemia: (a) rest pain and an ankle pressure lower than 40 mm Hg, or (b) rest pain with ulceration. Diabetics represent a different subset of patients both with regard to clinical presentation and to prognosis after revascularization procedures. Differences may be accounted for by the presence of neuropathy, the increased risk of infection, and the impaired healing response in diabetics. With this background, a European Working Group on Critical Limb Ischemia tried to reach a consensus and adopted the following definition of critical ischemia: persistently recurring rest pain requiring regular analgesia for more than two weeks and/or ulceration or gangrene of the foot and toes, plus ankle pressure below 50 mm Hg and/or toe pressure below 30 mm Hg. For the definition of critical ischemia in diabetics and in patients with calcified arteries, a toe systolic pressure below 30 mm Hg is needed.[106]

ASSESSMENT OF CRITICAL ISCHEMIA

Careful clinical assessment should be complemented by noninvasive measurement of ankle systolic pressure using the Doppler probe. Segmental measurements (at thigh, calf, and ankle levels) may help to define the location of the main obstructive lesions. This method is achievable with very little training. More sophisticated techniques include the measurement of systolic pressure at great-toe level using strain-gauge plethysmography, laser Doppler, and the measurement of transcutaneous oxygen tension using a polarographic probe.

Great-toe systolic pressure is of particular interest in patients (mostly diabetics) with calcified ankle arteries in whom systolic pressures measured at the ankle with the sphygmomanometer are overestimated. Toe pressures lower than 30 mm Hg indicate permanent foot ischemia. Values between 30 and 40 mm Hg are compatible with viability of the limb, but usually do not permit healing of ischemic lesions. If digital ulcers or gangrene are present, transcutaneous oxygen tension may help in assessing the severity of arterial insufficiency, especially in diabetics. Values that are lower than 10 mm Hg on the dorsum of the foot generally indicate critical ischemia of the foot. The response to postural changes or to oxygen breathing has a prognostic value in patients with critical limb ischemia: if the transcutaneous oxygen pressure does not increase above 10 mm Hg, the outlook for the foot appears particularly poor. The method has also been proposed as a useful tool to adequately determine the amputation level.

THERAPEUTIC APPROACH

Ideally, there should be a combined approach to the treatment of patients with critical limb ischemia, involving vascular surgeons, angiologists, diabetes specialists, interventional radiologists, and, in some cases, orthopedic surgeons, in order to define the most appropriate therapeutic approach for the individual patient. Apart from the clinical examination and the noninvasive testing outlined above, an optimal therapeutic decision-making requires an angiographic evaluation of the macrocirculation in most patients. Restoration of the blood supply through the main arteries is the primary therapeutic approach if practicable. The surgical and percutaneous revascularization procedures to achieve this aim are discussed earlier (see Therapeutic Principles to Relieve Arterial Occlusion).

When a first reconstruction fails, reintervention, local thrombolysis, or isolated percutaneous transluminal angioplasty should be considered. However, early thrombotic occlusion of a reopened vessel or a bypass graft may result in premature amputation, eventually at a higher level than was initially anticipated.

Surgical or chemical (with phenol or absolute alcohol) sympathectomy may be proposed in some patients with critical limb ischemia. The procedure usually leads to warming of the foot and some subjective improvement by alleviation of rest pain. Vascular reconstruction is sometimes combined with lumbar sympathectomy in order to improve the run-off in critical ischemia. However, unequivocal evidence that sympathectomy is effective in these two conditions is almost nonexistent. Spinal cord stimulation has been proposed to relieve rest pain and additionally increase skin blood flow,[107] but published data on this method are still too scarce to allow any recommendation.

There is no evidence for the efficacy of primary drug treatment to relieve critical limb ischemia. Anticoagulation, antiplatelet therapy, vasoactive drugs, or fibrinogen-lowering drugs have been proposed, but their efficacy has never been proven in properly designed studies. Prostacyclin, prostacyclin analogues, as well as prostaglandin E_1 act favorably on activated platelets and leucocytes and may improve microcirculation. Although definitive proof for their efficacy in critical ischemia is still lacking, the available evidence may lead to their consideration in patients unsuitable for surgery or percutaneous transluminal angioplasty, except in those requiring immediate amputation. Many years ago, Lassen et al.[108] reported a successful attempt to treat patients with gangrenous foot ulcers by increasing the systemic arterial pressure with sodium chloride and mineralocorticoids. However, increasing the blood pressure in aged, atherosclerotic patients is not devoid of risk, and this therapy was later restricted to ischemic ulcers in young patients with Buerger's disease (thromboangiitis obliterans).[109] In this condition, which was not dealt with in this chapter, intravenous infusion of a prostacyclin analogue, iloprost, was recently shown to favorably influence ulcer healing and amputation rate.[110]

Despite the progress in vascular surgery, percutaneous revascularization procedures, and medical treatment, a number of patients with critical ischemia do not escape from limb amputation. Prognosis of amputees is poor, hospital mortality of below-knee and above-knee amputations being 8 per cent and 18 per cent, respectively.[9] Full mobility is achieved in half of below-knee amputees and only one fourth of above-knee amputees. In diabetics in whom perfusion of the foot has been proven sufficient to allow healing, limited amputations (digital amputation or transmetatarsal amputation) may be tried. Although a distal amputation is always preferable to a proximal amputation, repeated surgical procedures also increase mortality and morbidity, and all means should be used to select the most appropriate amputation level.

REFERENCES

1. Dormandy J, Mahir M, Ascady G, et al. Fate of the patient with chronic leg ischemia. A review article. J Cardiovasc Surg 1989; 30: 50–7.
2. Kannel WB, McGee DL. Update on some epidemiologic features of intermittent claudication: the Framingham study. J Am Geriatr Soc 1985; 33: 13–8.
3. Svendson KH, Kuller LH, Martin MJ, Ockene JK. Effects of passive smoking in the MRFIT. Am J Epidemiol 1987; 126: 783–95.
4. Quick CRG, Cotton LT. The measured effect of stopping smoking on intermittent claudication. Br J Surg 1982; 69(suppl): 24–6.
5. Duffield RGM, Lewis B, Miller NE, Jamieson CW, Brunt JNH, Colchester ACF. Treatment of hyperlipidaemia retards progression of symptomatic femoral atherosclerosis. Lancet 1983; ii: 639–42.
6. Hess H, Mietaschk A, Deichsel G. Drug-induced inhibition of platelet function delays progression of peripheral occlusive arterial disease. A prospective double-blind arteriographically controlled trial. Lancet 1985; i: 415–9.
7. Nevelsteen A, Wouters L, Suy R. Aorto-femoral dacron reconstruction for aorto iliac occlusive disease: a 25-year survey. Eur J Vasc Surg 1991; 5: 179–86.
8. Rutherford RB, Jones DN, Bergentz SE, et al. Factors affecting the patency of infrainguinal bypass. J Vasc Surg 1988; 8: 236–46.
9. European consensus document on critical limb ischaemia. In: Dormandy JA, Stock G, eds. Critical leg ischemia. Its pathophysiology and management. Berlin: Springer-Verlag, 1990:IX–XLVIII.
10. Johnston KW, Rae M, Hogg-Johnston SA, Colapinto RF, et al. 5-year results of a prospective study of percutaneous transluminal angioplasty. Ann Surg 1987; 206: 403–13.
11. Casarella WJ. Percutaneous transluminal angioplasty below the knee: new techniques, excellent results. Radiology 1988; 169: 271–2.
12. Bakal CW, Sprayregen S, Scheinbaum K, Cynamon J, Veith FJ. Percutaneous transluminal angioplasty of the infrapopliteal arteries: results in 53 patients. AJR 1990; 154: 171–4.
13. Mahler F, Katheterinterventionen in der Angiologie. Stuttgart-New York: Georg Thieme Verlag 1990: 1–202.
14. Grüntzig A. Rekanalisation stenosierter Arterien mit dem Dilatationskatheter. München: CEDIP Verlag, 1980.
15. Spence RK, Freiman DB, Gatenby R, et al. Long-term results of transluminal angioplasty of the iliac and femoral arteries. Arch Surg 1981; 116: 1377–86.
16. Freiman DB, Spence R, Gatenby R. Transluminal angioplasty of the iliac and femoral arteries: follow-up results without anticoagulation. Radiology 1981; 141: 347–50.
17. Kumpe DA, Jones DN. Percutaneous transluminal angioplasty. Radiologic viewpoint. Appl Radiol 1982; 11: 29–40.
18. Schneider E, Grüntzig A, Bollinger A. Langzeitergebnisse nach perkutaner transluminaler Angioplastie (PTA) bei 882 konsekutiven Patienten mit iliakalen und femoro-poplitealen Obstruktionen. Vasa 1982; 11: 322–6.
19. Colapinto RF. Long-term results of iliac and femoropopliteal angioplasty. In: Dotter CT, Grüntzig AR, Schoop W, Zeitler E, eds. Percutaneous transluminal angioplasty. Berlin: Springer, 1983: 202–6.
20. Dotter CT, Grüntzig AR, Schoop W, Zeitler E. Percutaneous transluminal angioplasty. Berlin: Springer-Verlag, 1983.
21. Kadir S, White RI, Kaufman SL, et al. Long-term results of aorto-iliac angioplasty. Surgery 1983; 94: 10–4.
22. Gallino A, Mahler F, Probst P, Nachbur B. Percutaneous transluminal angioplasty of the lower limbs: a 5 year follow-up. Circulation 1984; 70: 619–23.
23. van Andel GJ, van Erp WFM, Krepel VM, Breslau PJ. Percutaneous transluminal dilatation of the iliac artery: long-term results. Radiology 1985; 156: 321–3.
24. Kammerlander R. Angioplastie transluminale des artères des membres inférieurs, MD Thesis (under the direction of H. Bounameaux and P.-A. Schneider), Thesis No 9067, University of Geneva, 1989.
25. Krepel VM, van Andel GJ, van Erp WFM, Breslau PJ. Percutaneous transluminal angioplasty of the femoropopliteal artery: initial and long-term results. Radiology 1985; 156: 325–8.
26. Hewes RC, White RI, Murray RR, et al. Long-term results of superficial femoral artery angioplasty. AJR 1986; 146: 1025–9.
27. Schwarten DE, Katzen BT, Simpson JB, Cutliff WB. Simpson catheter for percutaneous transluminal removal of atheroma. AJR 1988; 150: 799–801.
28. Maynar M, Reyes R, Cabrera V, et al. Percutaneous atherectomy as an alternative treatment for postangioplasty obstructive intimal flaps. Radiology 1989; 170: 1029–31.
29. Kensey KR, Nash JE, Abrahams C, Zarins CK. Recanalization of obstructed arteries with a flexible, rotating tip catheter. Radiology 1987; 165: 387–9.
30. Coleman CC, Posalaky IP, Robinson JD, Payne WD, Vlodaver ZA, Amplatz K. Atheroablation with the Kensey catheter: a pathologic study. Radiology 1989; 170: 391–4.
31. Wilms G, Peene P, Baert AL, et al. Laser assisted angioplasty: state of the art and future developments. Front Eur Radiol 1990; 7: 105–20.
32. Siegel RJ, Cumberland DC, Myler RK, Don Michael TA. Percutaneous ultrasonic angioplasty: initial Clinical Experience. Lancet 1989; 2: 772–4.
33. Palmaz JC, Richter GM, Noeldge G, et al. Intraluminal stents in atherosclerotic iliac artery stenosis: preliminary report of a multicenter study. Radiology 1988; 168: 727–31.
34. Quinones-Baldrich WJ, Zierler RF, Hiatt JC. Intraoperative fibrinolytic therapy: An adjunct to catheter thromboembolectomy. J Vasc Surg 1985; 2: 319–26.
35. Becker GJ, Rabe FE, Richmond BD, et al. Low-dose fibrinolytic therapy. Radiology 1983; 148: 663–70.
36. Belkin M, Belkin B, Bucknam C, Straub J, Lowe R. Intra-arterial fibrinolytic therapy. Arch Surg 1986; 121: 769–73.
37. Berni GA, Dandyk DF, Zierler RE, Thiele BL, Strandness E. Streptokinase treatment of acute arterial occlusion. Ann Surg 1983; 198: 185–91.
38. Berridge DC, Earnshaw JJ, Westby JC, Makin GS, Hopkinson BR. Fibrinolytic profiles in local low-dose thrombolysis with streptokinase and recombinant tissue plasminogen activator. Thromb Haemost 1989; 61: 275–8.
39. Earnshaw JJ, Westby JC, Gregson RHS, Makin GS, Hopkinson BR. Local thrombolytic therapy of acute peripheral arterial ischaemia with tissue plasminogen activator: a dose-ranging study. Br J Surg 1988; 75: 1196–200.
40. Fiessinger JN, Vitoux JF, Pernes JM, Roncato M, Aiach M, Gaux JC. Complications of intra-arterial urokinase-lys-

plasminogen infusion therapy in arterial ischemia of lower limbs. AJR 1986; 146: 157–9.

41. Fong H, Downs A, Lye C, Marrow I. Low-dose intra-arterial streptokinase infusion therapy of peripheral arterial occlusions and occluded vein grafts. Can J Surg 1986; 29: 259–62.

42. Giraud C, Joffre F, Puel P, Cerene A. Est-il licite d'utiliser l'association urokinase plasminogène par voie locale dans les ischémies par thrombose poplitée ou sous-poplitée. Haemostasis 1986; 16(suppl 4): 83–6.

43. Graor RA, Olin JW. Regional thrombolysis in peripheral arterial occlusion. In: Julian D, et al., eds. Thrombolysis in cardiovascular disease. Basel-New York: Marcel Dekker, 1989:381–95.

44. Graor RA, Risius B, Denay KM, et al. Local thrombolysis in the treatment of thrombosed arteries, bypass grafts and arteriovenous fistulas. J Vasc Surg 1985; 2: 406–14.

45. Hamelink JK, Elliott BM. Localized intra-arterial streptokinase therapy. Am J Surg 1986; 152: 252–6.

46. Hargrove WC, Barker CF, Berkowitz HD, et al. Treatment of acute peripheral arterial and graft thrombosis with low-dose streptokinase. Surgery 1982; 92: 981–91.

47. Hess H, Mietaschk A, Becker-Linau CH. Actilyse bei peripheren arteriellen Durchblutungstörungen. Hämostaseologie 1988; 8: 219–22.

48. Horvath L, Illes I, Molnar Z. The combined use of transluminal angioplasty and selective clot lysis. Int Angiol 1985; 4: 111–6.

49. Juhan C, Haupert S, Miltgen G. La thrombolyse locale en pathologie artérielle périphérique. Techniques et indications. Sang Thrombose Vaisseaux 1990; 2: 349–53.

50. Karnik R, Slany J. Local thrombolysis in arterial occlusive disease. Int Angiol 1985; 4: 69–71.

51. Hess H, Mietaschk A, Brückl R. Peripheral arterial occlusions: a 6-year experience with local low-dose thrombolytic therapy. Radiology 1987; 163: 753–8.

52. Katzen BT, van Breda A. Low dose streptokinase in the treatment of arterial occlusions. AJR 1981; 136: 1171–8.

53. Koppensteiner R, Minar E, Ahmadi R, Jung M, Ehringer H. Low doses of recombinant human tissue-type plasminogen activator for local thrombolysis in peripheral arteries. Radiology 1988; 168: 877–8.

54. Krupski WC, Feldman RK, Rapp JH. Recombinant human tissue-type plasminogen activator is an effective agent for thrombolysis of peripheral arteries and bypass grafts: preliminary report. J Vasc Surg 1987; 10: 491–500.

55. Lammer J, Pilger E, Neumayer K, Schreyer H. Intra-arterial fibrinolysis: long-term results. Radiology 1986; 161: 159–63.

56. McNamara TO. Role of thrombolysis in peripheral arterial occlusion. Am J Med 1987; 83(suppl 2A): 1–5.

57. Mori KW, Bookstein JJ, Heeney DJ, et al. Selective streptokinase infusion: clinical and laboratory correlates. Radiology 1983; 148: 677–82.

58. Pernes JM, de Almeida Augusto M, Vitoux JF, et al. Local thrombolysis in peripheral arteries band bypass grafts. J Vasc Surg 1987; 6: 372–8.

59. Poredos P, Keber D, Videcnik V. Late results of local thrombolytic treatment of peripheral arterial occlusions. Angiology 1989; 40: 941–7.

60. Rubenfire M, Blevins RD, Cascade PN, Maltzman JB, Goldberg MJ. The systemic fibrinolytic effect of low-dose intra-arterial streptokinase: observations in 12 patients. Radiology 1984; 152: 41–3.

61. Schneider E, Pfyffer M, Von Felten A, Küpperle L, Bollinger A. Lokale Trombolyse mit recombinant tissue plasminogen activator bei akuten und subakuten Beinarterienverschlüssen: Ergebnisse einer Pilotstudie (abstr). Schweiz Med Wochenschr 1988; (188 suppl 23): 11.

62. Sullivan KL, Gardiner GA, Shapiro MJ, Bonn J, Levin DC. Acceleration of thrombolysis with a high-dose transthrombus bolus technique. Radiology 1984; 173: 805–8.

63. Taylor LM, Porter JM, Baur GM, Hallin RW, Peck JL, Eidemiller LR. Intra-arterial streptokinase infusion for acute popliteal and tibial artery occlusion. Am J Surg 1984; 147: 583–8.

64. Traughber PD, Cook PS, Micklos TJ, Miller FJ. Intra-arterial fibrinolytic therapy for popliteal and tibial artery obstruction. AJR 1987; 49: 453–6.

65. Trotty WG, Gilula LA, McClennan BL, Ahmed P, Sherman L. Local dose of intravascular fibrinolytic therapy. Radiology 1982; 143: 59–69.

66. van Breda A, Ratzen BT, Deutsch AS. Urokinase versus streptokinase in local thrombolysis. Radiology 1987; 165: 109–11.

67. Verstraete M, Hess M, Mahler F, et al. Femoro-popliteal artery thrombolysis with intra-arterial infusion of recombinant tissue-type plasminogen activator. Report of a pilot trial. Eur J Vasc Surg 1988; 2: 155–9.

68. Wilms GE, Verhaeghe RH, Pouillon MM, et al. Local thrombolysis in femoropopliteal occlusion: early and late results. Cardiovasc Intervent Radiol 1987; 10: 272–5.

69. Wolfson RM, Kumpe DA, Rutherford RB. Role of intra-arterial streptokinase in treatment of arterial thrombo-embolism. Arch Surg 1984; 119: 697–702.

70. Belkin M, Donaldson MC, Whitlemore AD, et al. Observations on the use of thrombolytic agents for thrombotic occlusion of infrainguinal vein grafts. J Vasc Surg 1990; 11: 289–96.

71. Prevention of Atherosclerotic Complications with Ketanserin Trial Group. Prevention of atherosclerotic complications: controlled trial with ketanserin. Br Med J 1989; 298: 424–30.

72. PACK Claudication Substudy Investigators. Randomized placebo-controlled, double-blind trial of ketanserin in claudicants. Circulation 1989; 80: 1544–8.

73. Hamming JJ, Hensen A, Loeliger EA. The value of long-term coumarin treatment in peripheral sclerosis. Clinical trial (abstr). Thromb Diath Haemorrh 1965; 21: 405.

74. de Smit P, van Urk H. The effect of long-term treatment with oral anticoagulants in patients with peripheral vascular disease. In: Tilsner V, Matthias FR, eds. Arterielle Verschlusskrankheit und Blutgerinnung. Editiones 'Roche', 1987: 211–7.

75. Kretschmer G, Wenzl E, Schemper M, et al. Influence of postoperative anticoagulant treatment on patient survival after femoropopliteal vein bypass surgery. Lancet 1988; 1: 797–9.

76. Antiplatelet Trialists' Collaboration. Final report of the second cycle. 1991 in press.

77. Janzon L, Bergqvist D, Bobergs J, et al. Prevention of myocardial infarction and stroke in patients with intermittent claudication: effects of ticlopidine. Results from STIMS, the Swedish Ticlopidine Multicentre Study. J Int Med 1990; 227: 301–8.

78. Boissel JP, Peyrieux JC, Destors JM. Is it possible to reduce the risk of cardiovascular events in subjects suffering from intermittent claudication of the lower limbs? Thromb Haemost 1989; 62: 681–5.

79. Kretschmer G, Wenzl E, Piza F, et al. The influence of anticoagulant treatment on the probability of function in femoropopliteal vein bypass surgery: analysis of a clinical series (1970 to 1985) and interim evaluation of a controlled clinical trial. Surgery 1987; 102: 453–9.

80. Stiegler H, Hess H, Mietaschk A, Tramppisch HJ, Ingrisch H. Einfluss von Ticlopidin auf die perifere obliterierende Arteriopathie. Dtsch Med Wochenschr 1984; 109: 1240–3.

81. Antiplatelet Trialists' Collaboration. Secondary prevention of vascular disease by prolonged antiplatelet treatment. Br J Med 1988; 296: 320–33.

82. Schoop W, Levy H, Schoop B, Gaentsch A. Experimentelle und klinische Studien zu der sekundären Prävention der peripheren Arteriosklerose. In: Bollinger A, Rhyner K, eds. Thrombozytenfunktionshemmer. Stuttgart: Georg Thieme Verlag, 1983:49–58.

83. Dormandy J. Surgical pharmacotherapy. Leading article. Eur J Vasc Surg 1989; 3: 379–80.

84. Didisheim P. The quest for thromboresistant materials. Semin Thromb Hemost 1989; 15: 240–3.

85. Rutherford RB, Jones DN, Bergentz SE, et al. The efficacy of dextran 40 in preventing early postoperative thrombosis following difficult lower extremity bypass. J Vasc Surg 1984; 1: 765–73.

86. Bollinger A, Brunner U. Antiplatelet drugs improve the pat-

ency rates after femoropopliteal endarterectomy. Vasa 1985; 14: 272–9.

87. Clagett GP, Genton E, Salzman EW. Antithrombotic therapy in peripheral vascular disease. Chest 1989; 95: 128S–39S.

88. Zeitler E, Reichold J, Schoop W, Loew D. Einfluss von acetylsalicylsäure auf das Frühergebnis nach perkutaner Rekanalisation arterieller Obliterationen nach Dotter. Dtsch Med Wochenschr 1973; 98: 1285–8.

89. Hess H, Müller-Fassbender H, Ingrisch H, Mietaschk A. Verhütung von Wiederverschlüssen nach Rekanalisation obliterierter Arterien mit der Katheter-Methode. Dtsch Med Wochenschr 1978; 103: 1994–7.

90. Staiger J, Mathias K, Friederich M, Heiss HW, Konrad S, Spillner G. Perkutane Katheterrekanalisation (Dotter-Technik) bei peripherer arterieller Verschluss-Krankheit. Herz (Kreislauf) 1980; 12: 383–6.

91. Heiss HW, Mathias K, Beck AH, König K, Betzner M, Just H. Rezidivprophylaxe mit Acetylsalicylsäure und Dipyridamol nach perkutaner transluminaler Angioplastie der Beinarterien bei obliterierender Arteriosklerose. Cor Vasa 1987; 1: 25–34.

92. Mahler F, Schneider E, Gallino A, Bollinger A. Combination of suloctidil and anticoagulation in the prevention of reocclusion after femoro-popliteal PTA. Vasa 1987; 16: 381–5.

93. Schneider E, Mahler F, Do DD, Biland L. Zur Rezidivprophylaxe nach perkutaner transluminaler Angioplastie (PTA): Antikoagulation versus Ticlopidin. Vasa 1988; (suppl 20): 355–6.

94. Powell JS, Clozel JP, Müller RK, et al. Inhibitors of angiotensin-converting enzyme prevent myointimal proliferation after vascular injury. Science 1989; 245: 186–8.

95. Larsen OA, Lassen NA. Effect of daily muscular exercise in patients with intermittent claudication. Lancet 1966; ii: 1093–6.

96. Ekroth R, Dahllöf AG, Gundevall B, Holm J, Schersten T. Physical training of patients with intermittent claudication: indications, methods, and results. Surgery 1978; 84: 640–3.

97. Cameron HA, Waller PC, Ramsay LE. Drug treatment of intermittent claudication: a critical analysis of the methods and findings of published clinical trials, 1965–1985. Br J Clin Pharmacol 1988; 26: 569–76.

98. De Cree J, Leempoels J, Geukens H, Verhaegen H. Placebo-controlled double-blind study of ketanserin in treatment of intermittent claudication. Lancet 1984; ii: 775–9.

99. Bounameaux H, Holditch T, Hellemans H, Berent A, Verhaeghe R. Placebo-controlled, double-blind, two-center trial of ketanserin in intermittent claudication. Lancet 1985; ii: 1268–71.

100. Cameron HA, Walker PC, Ramsay LE. Placebo-controlled trial of ketanserin in stable intermittent claudication. Br J Clin Pharmacol 1987; 23: 597–8.

101. Thulesius O, Lundvall J, Kroese A, et al. Ketanserin in intermittent claudication: effect on walking distance, blood pressure and cardiovascular complications. J Cardiovasc Pharmacol 1987; 9: 728–33.

102. Clement DL, Duprez D. Effect of ketanserin in treatment of patients with intermittent claudication: results from 13 placebo-controlled parallel group studies. J Cardiovasc Pharmacol 1987; 10(suppl 3): 589–95.

103. Bell PRF, Challesworth D, DePalma RG, Jamieson C. The definition of critical ischaemia of a limb. Br J Surg 1982; 69: 52.

104. Ad Hoc Committee on Reporting Standards. Suggested standards for reports dealing with lower extremity ischemia. J Vasc Surg 1986; 4: 80–94.

105. Wolfe JHN. The definition of critical ischemia—Is this a concept of value? In: Greenhalgh RM, Jamieson CW, Nicolaides AN, eds. Limb salvage and amputation for vascular disease. Philadelphia: WB Saunders Co., 1988: 3–10.

106. European Working Group on Critical Leg Ischaemia. Second European consensus document on chronic critical leg ischaemia. 1991 Nov(Suppl), in press.

107. Augustinsson LE, Carlsson CA, Holm J, Jivegard L. Epidural electrical stimulation in severe limb ischemia. Pain relief, increased blood flow, and a possible limb-saving effect. Ann Surg 1985; 202: 104–10.

108. Lassen NA, Larsen OA, Sorensen AWS, et al. Conservative treatment of gangrene using mineralocorticoid-induced hypertension. Lancet 1968; 1: 606–9.

109. Krahenbuhl B, Holstein P, Nielsen SL, Tonnesen KH, Lassen NA. Induced hypertension as a therapy in Buerger's disease (thromboangiitis obliterans). Vasa 1975; 4: 407–11.

110. Fiessinger JN, Schafer M. Trial of iloprost versus aspirin treatment for critical limb ischemia of thromboangiitis obliterans. The TAO Study. Lancet 1990; 335: 555–7.

24

PREVENTION OF VENOUS THROMBOSIS AND PULMONARY EMBOLISM

RUSSELL D. HULL, VIJAY V. KAKKAR, and GARY E. RASKOB

Pulmonary embolism remains a leading cause of death in hospital.[1,2] It has been estimated that 100,000 or more hospitalized patients in the United States die each year from massive pulmonary embolism.[3] Many such deaths occur in terminally ill patients, but a significant proportion occur in patients who would otherwise have survived to lead a normal life (for example, patients undergoing elective major orthopedic surgery). In the absence of prophylaxis, the frequency of postoperative fatal pulmonary embolism ranges from 0.1 to 0.8 per cent in patients undergoing elective general surgery,[4-6] from 0.3 to 1.7 per cent in patients having elective hip surgery,[7] and from 4 to 7 per cent in patients undergoing emergency hip surgery.[8,9]

Prevention of fatal pulmonary embolism requires more than an awareness that pulmonary embolism is a leading cause of death after many operations. The clinical diagnosis of both pulmonary embolism and venous thrombosis is insensitive. Consequently, in many cases, a diagnosis of pulmonary embolism is not established until after the patient's death. Although anticoagulant therapy is highly effective, two thirds of patients who die from pulmonary embolism succumb abruptly or within two hours after the acute event,[10] before therapy can be initiated or take effect. Prevention is the key to reducing death and morbidity from pulmonary embolism. It has been estimated that the routine use of effective prophylaxis in patients undergoing elective general surgery could prevent 4,000 to 8,000 postoperative deaths each year in the United States.[11]

Clinical trials have produced major advances in the prevention of venous thromboembolism. Effective prophylaxis is now available for most patient groups. This chapter reviews the current approaches for preventing venous thrombosis and pulmonary embolism. In making specific recommendations, the strength of the evidence from clinical trials is considered. A firm recommendation is made when the following criteria have been met:

1. The clinical trial should be prospective with a concurrent control group.
2. The patients should be randomly allocated to the alternative treatment groups in order to avoid bias in treatment allocation.
3. Comparability of the treatment groups with respect to important prognostic variables should be demonstrated.
4. Properly defined endpoints should be used for the evaluation of effectiveness and safety.
5. Ideally, the study should be double-blind. If a double-blind design is not possible, the endpoints should be interpreted by an independent observer without knowledge of the patients treatment group.
6. A sufficient number of patients should be evaluated to allow valid conclusions.
7. Appropriate statistical methods should be used to analyze the data.

Because of the inaccuracy of clinical diagnosis of both venous thrombosis and pulmonary embolism, it is essential that reliable objective diagnostic methods be used to measure these endpoints. These techniques include I-125-fibrinogen leg scanning, impedance plethysmography, and venography for the diagnosis of venous thrombosis, and ventilation-perfusion lung scanning and pulmonary angiography for pulmonary embolism (or pulmonary embolism confirmed at autopsy).

Much of the data on the incidence of thrombosis and the effectiveness of prophylaxis comes from clinical trials which used I-125-fibrinogen leg scanning as the test for detecting deep vein thrombosis. Leg scanning is highly sensitive to calf vein thrombi and distal thigh thrombi, but is relatively insensitive to thrombi in the iliofemoral venous segment. In most patient groups, including general surgery, urology, neurosurgery, and high-risk medical patients, deep vein thrombosis usually originates in the calf veins, and isolated iliofemoral thrombosis is very uncommon; therefore, most of thrombi in these patients can be detected by leg scanning. In patients undergoing hip surgery, however, isolated iliofemoral vein thrombosis is not uncommon.[115,127] Multiple studies have established that leg scanning is relatively insensitive in hip-surgery patients.[118-120, 127] This remains true when leg scanning is combined with impedance plethysmography; the combined tests fail to detect 23 to 53 per cent of deep vein thrombi in patients undergoing hip surgery.[51, 118-120] Similar findings have been reported recently for B-mode ultrasonography.[121] Therefore, in patients undergoing hip surgery, venography is required in all patients to accurately assess the presence or absence of deep vein thrombosis. The clinical trials in hip-surgery patients in which venography was performed only in patients with positive noninvasive test findings may underestimate the true incidence of deep vein thrombosis.

In this chapter, only those clinical trials that used random allocation with a concurrent control group and appropriate objective endpoints for the assessment of venous thromboembolism are considered. In the context of hip surgery, the clinical trials described are those in which venography was performed in all patients as the diagnostic endpoint for deep vein thrombosis, and the recommendations are based on the findings of these trials.

RISK FACTORS AND CLASSIFICATION OF RISK

Clinical risk factors for venous thromboembolism have been identified[2] and include advanced age (40 years or older), previous venous thromboembolism, recent surgery or trauma, prolonged immobility or paralysis, malignancy, congestive heart failure, obesity, oral contraceptive use, and pregnancy. Certain surgical procedures, such as orthopedic surgery to the lower limbs, or extensive pelvic or abdominal surgery for advanced malignant disease, are associated with a particularly high risk of postoperative venous thromboembolism.

Inherited abnormalities which predispose to venous thromboembolism include deficiencies of antithrombin III, protein C, protein S, or heparin cofactor II, and dysfibrinogenemia. Other conditions which may be associated with venous thromboembolism include abnormalities of the fibrinolytic system, polycythemia vera, and systemic lupus erythematosus.

In general, patients can be classified as low-, moderate-, or high-risk for venous thromboembolism as shown in Table 24–1.

Low-risk patients are: (a) those less than 40 years of age without additional risk factors who have uncomplicated elective abdominal or thoracic surgery or (b) those over the age of 40 without additional risk factors who have minor elective abdominal or thoracic surgery (that is, surgery under general anesthesia for less than 30 minutes).[2] In the absence of prophylaxis, these patients have less than a 10 per cent risk of developing calf vein thrombosis, less than a 1 per cent risk of developing proximal vein thrombosis (popliteal, femoral, or iliac vein thrombosis), and less than a 0.01 per cent risk of fatal pulmonary embolism.

Moderate-risk surgical patients are those over the age of 40 who have elective general abdominal or thoracic surgery performed under general anesthesia that lasts for 30 minutes or longer.[2] The risk of venous thromboembolism in these patients is increased by advancing age, the presence of malignancy, prolonged bed rest, extensive surgical dissection, large bowel surgery, and obesity. In the absence of prophylaxis, patients in the moderate-risk category have a 10 to 40 per cent risk of developing calf vein thrombosis, a 2 to 10 per cent risk of proximal vein thrombosis, and a 0.1 to 0.8 per cent risk of fatal pulmonary embolism.

High-risk surgical patients are those who have a history of recent venous thromboembolism, and those who undergo extensive pelvic or abdominal surgery for advanced

TABLE 24–1. Risk Categories for Postoperative Venous Thromboembolism

| | RISK OF VENOUS THROMBOEMBOLISM (%) | | |
RISK CATEGORY	Calf Vein Thrombosis†	Proximal Vein Thrombosis†	Fatal Pulmonary Embolism
High Risk	40–80	10–30	1–5
General surgery in patients >40 years with recent history of deep vein thrombosis or pulmonary embolism			
Extensive pelvic or abdominal surgery for malignant disease			
Major orthopedic surgery of lower limbs			
Moderate Risk*	10–40	2–10	0.1–0.8
General surgery in patients >40 years lasting 30 minutes or more			
Low Risk	<10	<1	<0.01
Uncomplicated surgery in patients <40 years without additional risk factors			
Minor surgery (that is, <30 minutes) in patients >40 years without additional risk factors			

* The risk is increased by advancing age, malignancy, prolonged immobility, and cardiac failure.
† Venographically confirmed.

malignant disease or major orthopedic surgery to the lower limbs[2] (for example, hip or knee arthroplasty, surgery for fractured hip, tibial osteotomy). In the absence of prophylaxis, these patients have a 40 to 80 per cent risk of developing calf vein thrombosis, a 10 to 30 per cent risk of proximal vein thrombosis, and a 1 to 5 per cent risk of fatal pulmonary embolism.

APPROACHES FOR PREVENTING VENOUS THROMBOEMBOLISM

General Considerations

Two approaches can be taken to prevent fatal pulmonary embolism: (a) *primary prophylaxis* using drugs or physical methods that are effective for preventing deep vein thrombosis and pulmonary embolism, and (b) *secondary prevention* by the early detection and treatment of subclinical venous thrombosis by screening patients postoperatively with objective diagnostic tests that are sensitive for venous thrombosis. Primary prophylaxis is the preferred approach in most patients. Secondary prevention by screening should never replace primary prophylaxis. Screening is reserved for patients in whom effective primary prophylaxis is contraindicated or unavailable. Postoperative screening may also be used to supplement primary prophylaxis in very–high-risk surgical patients, such as those with a history of recent venous thrombosis.

The ideal primary prophylactic approach should be effective, free of clinically important side effects, and well accepted by patients, nurses, and medical staff. It should also be easily administered, inexpensive, and require minimal monitoring.

The primary prophylactic methods that have been evaluated clinically have been directed at one or more of the pathogenic factors for venous thrombosis. These pathogenic factors are the activation of blood coagulation, venous stasis, and venous endothelial damage. The prophylactic methods include anticoagulants that counteract the activation of blood coagulation, mechanical devices that prevent venous stasis by increasing venous flow in the leg veins, and drugs that suppress platelet function and the interaction of platelets with the damaged vessel wall. On theoretic grounds, combined prophylactic approaches that interact against two or more of the pathogenic factors are attractive. For example, the combination of low-dose heparin with intermittent pneumatic leg compression counteracts the activation of blood coagulation and also prevents venous stasis in the leg veins.

Several primary prophylactic approaches have been evaluated by randomized clinical trials and are effective for preventing venous thrombosis and pulmonary embolism. The most extensively evaluated approaches are low-dose subcutaneous heparin,[6,12–33] intermittent pneumatic leg compression,[34–51] oral anticoagulants,[7,8,52–60] and intravenous dextran.[18,23,32,61–68] Other approaches include adjusted-dose subcutaneous heparin,[69] low molecular weight heparin,[70–81] graduated compression stockings,[82–87] and combined modalities such as the combination of the vasoconstrictor dihydroergotamine (DHE) and low doses of heparin,[88–91] graded compression stockings combined with low-dose heparin,[92,93] or intravenous dextran plus intermittent pneumatic compression.[94] Antiplatelet agents,[95–109] such as aspirin, have a very limited role, if any, for preventing venous thromboembolism. Although none of the above approaches meets all of the criteria for an ideal prophylactic approach, most of the criteria are met by low-dose heparin or intermittent pneumatic compression.

Low-Dose Heparin

Low-dose heparin prevents thrombosis by inhibiting the blood coagulation cascade. Heparin markedly accelerates the rate of inhibition by antithrombin III of the coagulation factors XII, XI, IX, X, and thrombin. Because the activation process is amplified by each successive step in the coagulation cascade, much lower doses of heparin are required to inhibit the initiation of blood coagulation than are required for the treatment of established venous thromboembolism.[110]

Low-dose subcutaneous heparin is usually given in a dose of 5,000 units two hours preoperatively, and then postoperatively every 8 hours or every 12 hours. It is one of the approaches of choice for preventing venous thromboembolism in moderate- and high-risk general surgical patients. The effectiveness of low-dose heparin for preventing deep vein thrombosis has been established by multiple randomized clinical trials.[6,12–23,28] In addition, the International Multicentre Trial[6] established the effectiveness of low-dose heparin for preventing fatal pulmonary embolism. In this trial, low-dose heparin prophylaxis resulted in a clinically striking reduction in the frequency of fatal pulmonary embolism (from 0.7 to 0.1 per cent). The results of the International Multicentre Trial are supported by the findings of a recent meta-analysis.[12]

Low-dose heparin is of limited effectiveness in patients undergoing hip[25–27,29] or urologic surgery,[40] and is not the prophylaxis of choice in these two patient groups.

Although low-dose heparin prophylaxis is effective, its acceptance was delayed by the fear that it induces bleeding. This fear is not supported by the data from clinical trials to date. The data indicate that low-dose heparin is not associated with an increased risk of clinically important bleeding in general surgical patients. The eight-hourly regimen may result in an increased frequency of minor wound hematomas,[6] but this is far outweighed by the major clinical benefit of low-dose heparin in preventing fatal pulmonary embolism. Because of the potential for bleeding, however, low-dose heparin should not be used in patients undergoing cerebral or eye surgery.

Low-dose heparin has the advantage that it does not require anticoagulant monitoring and is easily administered.

Adjusted-Dose Heparin

Adjusted-dose subcutaneous heparin is a promising approach for prophylaxis in high-risk patients in whom low-dose heparin is of limited effectiveness or ineffective (for example, hip surgery). Leyvarz and associates reported a randomized trial evaluating adjusted-dose subcutaneous heparin in patients undergoing elective hip replacement.[69] These investigators demonstrated that the shortening of the activated partial thromboplastin time that occurs during the first postoperative week can be restored to normal, and venous thrombosis prevented, by using adjusted doses of subcutaneous heparin. Seventy-nine patients undergoing elective hip arthroplasty were randomly allocated to receive either fixed low-dose (3,500 international units) heparin subcutaneously every eight hours, or to the alternate approach of an initial dose of 3,500 international units, later adjusted to maintain the activated partial thromboplastin time in the upper normal range. Subcutaneous heparin prophylaxis was commenced in both groups two days preoperatively and was continued for at least seven to nine days postoperatively. From the day of surgery to the eighth day postoperatively, patients receiving the adjusted-heparin regimen required progressively more heparin to maintain the activated partial thromboplastin time in the prescribed range. Venography revealed deep vein thrombosis in only 5 of 38 patients (13 per cent) in the adjusted-heparin group compared with 16 of 41 patients (39 per cent) in the fixed low-dose heparin group (p = 0.003). The increased protection provided by adjusted-dose subcutaneous heparin was not associated with an increased frequency of bleeding complications. The number of units of blood transfused, the frequency of postoperative wound hematomas, and the fall in hemoglobin levels were identical in the two groups. These findings suggest that adjusted-dose heparin prophylaxis is an effective and safe method for preventing venous thrombosis in patients undergoing elective total hip replacement. Further randomized clinical trials are required to determine the place of adjusted-dose subcutaneous heparin prophylaxis in other high-risk patient groups.

Low Molecular Weight Heparin

Heparin currently in clinical use is a mixture of glycosaminoglycans, with a mean molecular weight range of 10,000 to 16,000 daltons. In recent years, low molecular weight heparin fractions have been prepared (mean weights of 5,000 to 9,000 daltons). These heparin fractions have the potential advantage of higher bioavailability and a longer half-life of the anticoagulant effect (antiactivated factor X activity) than standard unfractionated heparin. These properties of low molecular weight heparin enable it to be given by once-daily subcutaneous injection. Because low molecular weight heparins differ in their in vivo pharmacologic properties, each low molecular weight heparin fraction must be evaluated independently by clinical trials.

Several low molecular weight heparin fractions have been evaluated by randomized clinical trials in moderate-risk general surgical patients.[70-78] The heparin fractions that have been evaluated include Fragmin, Fraxiparin, Enoxaparin, and Logiparin. The findings indicate that low molecular weight heparin given once daily is as effective or more effective than conventional low-dose heparin given every 8 or every 12 hours.[70-80] Most of the trials documented similar low frequencies of bleeding for low molecular weight heparin and low-dose unfractionated heparin, except for two trials[72,73] using the same heparin fraction which documented an increased risk of clinically minor bleeding complications with the low molecular weight heparin fraction.

The findings of initial randomized trials[79-] [81] indicate that low molecular weight heparin is effective in patients undergoing total hip replacement. Turpie et al. reported a randomized double-blind trial[79] comparing subcutaneous low molecular weight heparin given every 12 hours with a placebo control group. Prophylaxis was begun postoperatively and continued for 14 days. Deep vein thrombosis by venography was present in 4 of 37 patients (11 per cent) given low molecular weight heparin, compared with 20 of 39 patients (51 per cent) given placebo (p = 0.0002). Proximal vein thrombosis was present in 5 per cent of the 37 patients given low molecular weight heparin, compared with 23 per cent of the 39 patients given placebo (p = 0.029). The observed frequency of bleeding complications was 4 per cent in each group.

Planes and colleagues reported a randomized double-blind trial[80] comparing once-daily low molecular weight heparin with low-dose heparin (5,000 units) given every eight hours in patients undergoing elective hip replacement. Prophylaxis was commenced 12 hours preoperatively using low molecular weight heparin, and 2 hours preoperatively with unfractionated heparin. Deep vein thrombosis by venography was present in 27 of 108 patients (25 per cent) given unfractionated heparin, compared with 15 of 120 patients (12.5 per cent) who received low molecular weight heparin (p = 0.03). The incidence of proximal vein thrombosis was also reduced from 18.5 per cent in the unfractionated heparin group (20 of 108 patients) to 7.5 per cent (9 of 120 patients) in the low molecular heparin group (p = 0.014). In the low molecular weight heparin group, two patients had major bleeding and one had minor bleeding, compared with two patients who had minor bleeding in the unfractionated heparin group.

The findings of clinical trials to date indicate that low molecular weight heparin is effective in patients undergoing elective hip replacement, and is associated with a low frequency of bleeding complications. Several issues remain to be resolved, including the need for and timing of preoperative dosing, and the relative effectiveness and safety of low molecular weight heparin compared to other standard approaches such as oral anticoagulant prophylaxis (which is widely used in North America). The relative roles of adjusted-dose subcutaneous heparin, low molecular weight heparin, and oral anticoagulant prophylaxis in patients undergoing hip surgery and in other high-risk patients should be determined by randomized clinical trials over the next few years.

Oral Anticoagulants

Oral anticoagulants prevent thrombosis by inhibiting the synthesis of functionally active vitamin K-dependent coagulation factors II, VII, IX, and X. Multiple studies have established the effectiveness of oral anticoagulants for preventing venous thrombosis confirmed by venography and pulmonary embolism (in all risk categories).[7,8,52-60] In a classic study by Sevitt and Gallagher[52] in patients with fractured hip, oral anticoagulant prophylaxis was associated with a clinically striking and statistically significant reduction in total mortality, owing to a reduction in death from pulmonary embolism (from 10 per cent to 1 per cent). However, the allocation of patients into the treatment groups was not strictly randomized, but was made on the basis of hospital admission date. Two subsequent randomized trials[8,57] have confirmed the findings of Sevitt and Gallagher. Thus, both autopsy and venographic findings indicate that oral anticoagulants are effective for preventing clinically important venous thromboembolism in high-risk patients.

Prophylaxis with oral anticoagulants can be commenced preoperatively, at the time of operation, or in the early postoperative period. Oral anticoagulants commenced at the time of surgery or early postoperatively may not prevent small venous thrombi which form during surgery or soon after surgery, because the anticoagulant effect is not achieved until the third or fourth postoperative day. However, prophylaxis with oral anticoagulants commenced at the time of surgery or in the early postoperative period is effective for inhibiting the extension of these thrombi and has the potential to prevent clinically important venous thromboembolism.

The laboratory test most commonly used to monitor oral anticoagulant therapy is the prothrombin time (PT). The optimal therapeutic range for monitoring with the prothrombin time had been controversial because the clinical trials addressing this issue were performed only recently. This controversy occurred because the different thromboplastin reagents used to measure the prothrombin time vary markedly in sensitivity to

the vitamin K-dependent clotting factors and in response to warfarin.[128] In North America, the thromboplastin reagents are usually obtained from rabbit brain tissue, whereas in the United Kingdom and parts of Europe, the thromboplastin was, until recently, obtained from human brain tissue. The rabbit brain thromboplastins which are available commercially in North America (for example, Simplastin, Dade-C) are generally less sensitive to reductions in the vitamin K-dependent coagulation factors than is standardized human brain thromboplastin. A prothrombin time ratio of 1.5 to 2.0 times control using a rabbit brain thromboplastin such as Simplastin or Dade-C is equivalent to a ratio of 3.0 to 6.0 times control using the standardized human brain thromboplastin widely available in the United Kingdom.[128,129] Conversely, a prothrombin time ratio using standardized human brain thromboplastin of 2.0 to 3.0 times control is equivalent to a ratio of approximately 1.3 to 1.5 times control using a rabbit brain thromboplastin.[128,129]

In order to standardize the prothrombin time for oral anticoagulant monitoring, the World Health Organization (WHO) has developed an international reference thromboplastin from human brain tissue and has recommended that the prothrombin time be expressed as the international normalized ratio (INR). The international normalized ratio is the prothrombin time ratio obtained by testing a given sample using the World Health Organization reference thromboplastin. The international normalized ratio can be calculated for any prothrombin time ratio measured using any thromboplastin reagent if the international sensitivity index (ISI) of the reagent is known. Using the conventional insensitive rabbit brain thromboplastin reagents, a prothrombin time ratio of 1.3 to 1.5 corresponds to an international normalized ratio of 2.0 to 3.0.[128,129] This is the so-called "less intense" therapeutic range.[129]

Oral anticoagulant prophylaxis given in doses that prolong the prothrombin time to 1.5 to 2 times control (using insensitive rabbit brain thromboplastin, corresponding to an international normalized ratio of 3.0 to 4.5), may be associated with a higher frequency of clinically important bleeding complications than the other prophylactic methods in current use. The perceived risk of bleeding complications has limited the acceptance of oral anticoagulant prophylaxis. Recent clinical trials[59,60] in patients undergoing total hip or knee replacement have provided important information about the relationship between the intensity of anticoagulant effect and the effectiveness and safety of oral anticoagulant prophylaxis.

In a randomized clinical trial of 100 patients, Francis et al.[59] compared the efficacy and safety of warfarin sodium with dextran 40 for preventing venous thrombosis in patients undergoing elective total hip or knee replacement. A low dose of warfarin was started 10 to 14 days preoperatively, and the dose of warfarin was adjusted to maintain the prothrombin time (using rabbit brain thromboplastin) between 1.5 and 3 seconds longer than the control at the time of surgery. Immediately after surgery, the dose was increased to prolong the prothrombin time to 1.5 times control. Thus, warfarin was administered in a two-step regimen with the intent to avoid bleeding complications while retaining effectiveness for preventing venous thrombosis. Deep vein thrombosis by venography was present in 11 of 53 patients (21 per cent) who received warfarin, compared with 19 of 37 patients (51 per cent) who received dextran ($p < 0.005$). Proximal vein thrombosis was present in 6 patients (16 per cent) in the dextran group, compared with only 1 patient (2 per cent) in the warfarin group ($p < 0.05$). Postoperative bleeding was similar and infrequent (4 per cent) in both treatment groups.

The above findings are supported by the findings of a more recent randomized trial by Paiement and colleagues.[60] Prophylaxis with warfarin sodium was commenced the night before surgery in a dose of 10 milligrams, followed by 5 milligrams the evening postoperatively, and thereafter the dose was adjusted to maintain the prothrombin time at 1.3 times control using an insensitive rabbit brain thromboplastin (an international normalized ratio of about 2.0). This approach was effective and associated with a low risk of bleeding. Deep vein thrombosis by venography was present in 12 of 72 patients (17 per cent) who received warfarin, compared with 11 of 66 patients (17 per cent) in the control group who received intermittent pneumatic compression. None of the 72 patients given warfarin had major bleeding complications, and only three patients (4 per cent) had minor wound bleeding. Thus, the findings of recent trials[59,60] suggest that by adjusting the warfarin dose to achieve a less intense anticoagulant effect than traditionally used in North America, venous thromboembolism can be prevented with a low risk of bleeding complications.

Oral anticoagulant prophylaxis is relatively inconvenient because it requires careful anticoagulant monitoring with frequent prothrombin times.

Intermittent Pneumatic Leg Compression

Intermittent pneumatic leg compression prevents venous thrombosis by enhancing blood flow in the deep veins of the legs,[111,112] thereby preventing venous stasis. It also increases blood fibrinolytic activity,[113] which may contribute to its antithrombotic properties. Intermittent pneumatic leg compression is effective for preventing venous thrombosis in moderate-risk general surgical patients[34-37] and in patients undergoing neurosurgery,[38,39,42] major knee surgery,[41] and prostatic surgery.[40] In patients undergoing hip surgery, intermittent pneumatic compression of the calf is effective for preventing calf vein thrombosis, but it is relatively ineffective against proximal vein thrombosis.[50] Combined calf and thigh intermittent compression devices have become available in recent years. Sequential compression using calf and thigh cuffs produces greater acceleration of femoral venous blood flow than compression of the calf alone.[112] Recent clinical trials[51,60] indicate that sequential calf and thigh compression is effective for preventing venous thrombosis, including proximal vein thrombosis,[51] in patients undergoing elective total hip replacement.

Intermittent pneumatic leg compression is virtually free of clinically important side effects and offers a valuable alternative in patients who have a high risk of bleeding. It may produce discomfort in the occasional patient, and should not be used in patients with overt evidence of leg ischemia caused by peripheral vascular disease. A variety of well-accepted, comfortable, and effective intermittent pneumatic devices are currently available, which may be applied preoperatively, at the time of operation, or in the early postoperative period. Intermittent pneumatic compression should be continued for the entire period while the patient is confined to bed and until the patient is fully ambulatory.

Graduated Compression Stockings

Graduated compression stockings reduce venous stasis in the limb by applying a graded degree of compression to the ankle and the calf, with greater pressure being applied more distally in the limb. Clinical trials have demonstrated graduated compression stockings to be effective for preventing postoperative venous thrombosis in low-risk general surgical patients,[83] and in selected moderate-risk patients (neurosurgical).[87]

Graduated compression stockings are inexpensive and provide a convenient form of prophylaxis that is free of clinically important side effects. However, the effectiveness of graduated compression stockings for preventing venous thromboembolism in high-risk patients remains uncertain.

Dextran

Dextran is a glucose polymer that was introduced as a volume expander and was subsequently evaluated as an antithrombotic agent. Two sizes of dextran polymer have been used clinically; dextran 70 with a mean molecular weight of 70,000 daltons and dextran 40 with a mean molecular weight of 40,000 daltons. The antithrombotic properties of dextran have been attributed to several actions, including decreased blood viscosity, reduced platelet interaction with the damaged vessel wall, and an increased susceptibility for fibrin clots formed in the presence of dextran to undergo fibrinolysis.[130,131]

Dextran 40, administered intravenously in a volume of 500 milliliters over four to six hours commencing at the time of operation and then daily for two to five days postoperatively, is effective in moderate-risk general surgical patients and in patients undergoing hip surgery.[18,23,32,61–68] Dextran is well tolerated by most patients, but its use may be complicated by volume overload in patients who have impaired cardiac function, particularly in the elderly patient with unrecognized cardiac impairment. Hypersensitivity reactions to dextran occur as an uncommon side effect. In hip surgery patients, dextran may be associated with excessive bleeding when given in doses greater than 500 milliliters during the operation;[94] lower doses were not associated with excessive bleeding.[94]

By comparison with low-dose subcutaneous heparin, the administration of dextran is relatively inconvenient, requiring the maintenance of an intravenous line.

Aspirin

The antithrombotic effect of aspirin has been attributed to its inhibition of platelet function by inhibiting the synthesis of thromboxane A_2 in platelets. It was originally hoped that the antiplatelet action of aspirin would provide effective prophylaxis against postoperative venous thromboembolism. Aspirin prophylaxis, although inexpensive and highly convenient, has limited application, if any, because of its relative ineffectiveness. The randomized clinical trials performed to date have produced conflicting results.[94–108] Aspirin may be effective for preventing venous thrombosis in men undergoing elective hip surgery, but conflicting findings have also been reported in this patient group.

Powers et al. compared aspirin prophylaxis with less intense postoperative warfarin in patients undergoing surgery for fractured hip.[109] The endpoint for effectiveness was venous thrombosis by venography or pulmonary embolism confirmed by a high-probability lung scan or by autopsy. Venous thromboembolism occurred in 13 of 65 patients (20 per cent) given warfarin sodium, compared with 27 of 66 patients (41 per cent) who received aspirin, and with 29 of 63 patients (46 per cent) given placebo ($p = 0.005$). The frequencies of proximal vein thrombosis in the warfarin and aspirin groups were similar (9 per cent and 11 per cent respectively), compared with 30 per cent in the placebo group ($p = 0.001$). The selective effect of aspirin on proximal vein thrombosis observed in this study is consistent with the concept that the pathogenesis of proximal vein thrombosis in hip surgery is contributed to by vessel damage and interaction of platelets with the injured vessel wall. However, the failure of aspirin to affect the overall thrombosis rates limits its value as a prophylactic approach, because 20 per cent of calf vein thrombi extend into the proximal venous segment[114] and may result in clinically important pulmonary embolism.

Based on the reported differential effect of aspirin on platelet thromboxane production and on prostacyclin generation by the vessel wall, it has been suggested that low doses of aspirin may be more effective antithrombotic prophylaxis than medium or high doses. Harris et al. reported a randomized trial[94] comparing the effectiveness of 0.3 gram of aspirin daily with 1.2 grams of aspirin daily for preventing venous thrombosis following elective hip surgery. The overall frequencies of venous thrombosis by venography in the low-dose and high-dose aspirin group were 61 per cent and 60 per cent, respectively. These findings indicate that the lower dose of aspirin has no prophylactic advantage.

Combined Modalities

The use of combined prophylactic approaches (for example, low-dose heparin plus the vasoconstrictor dihydroergotamine, or low-dose heparin plus intermittent pneumatic compression) is based on the concept that venous thromboembolism can be more effectively prevented by counteracting two or more of the pathogenic factors that lead to postoperative venous thrombosis. Currently there are only limited data on the effectiveness of combined prophylactic modalities. The combined approach of low-dose heparin plus dihydroergotamine is more effective in reducing the frequency of venous thrombosis than an equivalent dose of low-dose heparin alone.[88–90] However, this approach is no longer used because of the concern about vasospastic complications from dihydroergotamine. Further clinical trials are required to clarify the role of combined prophylactic approaches.

CHOICE OF PRIMARY PROPHYLAXIS

General Considerations

The choice of primary prophylaxis depends on the patient's risk category and the surgical procedure. The definition of low-, moderate-, and high-risk surgical patients is summarized in Table 24–1. Within the moderate- and high-risk categories, the choice of prophylaxis is influenced by the type of surgical procedure and by the risk of bleeding. The recommended prophylactic approaches for the alternative risk categories and surgical groups are summarized in Table 24–2.

TABLE 24–2. Recommended Prophylactic Approaches for the Alternative Patient Risk Categories and Different Surgical Groups

RISK CATEGORY	Recommended Approach(es)
Low risk	Graduated compression stockings
Moderate risk	
General abdominal or thoracic surgery	Low-dose heparin
	Intermittent compression
	Dextran
Neurosurgery	Intermittent compression
Urologic surgery	Intermittent compression
High Risk	
General abdominal or thoracic surgery	Oral anticoagulants
	Lose-dose heparin (eight-hourly)
	Adjusted-dose heparin
	Any above + intermittent compression
Elective hip surgery	Oral anticoagulants
	Adjusted-dose heparin
	Dextran
	Intermittent compression
	Dextran + intermittent compression
Fractured hip	Oral anticoagulants
	Dextran
Major knee surgery	Intermittent compression

Elective General Abdominal and Thoracic Surgery

In low-risk patients, graduated compression stockings are effective and can be used as the only form of prophylaxis, provided the patient does not develop complications that require continued confinement to bed.

Moderate-risk general surgical patients should be given prophylaxis either with low-dose heparin or with intermittent pneumatic compression. Dextran is effective but is slightly more expensive, and is less convenient because it must be administered by intravenous infusion.

The relative effectiveness of the different prophylactic approaches has not been directly compared in high-risk general surgical patients. Based on the available data, one of the following regimens can be used:

1. Oral anticoagulants begun several days preoperatively, with the prothrombin time (using rabbit brain prothromboplastin) maintained at 1.5 to 3 seconds longer than control at the time of surgery. Postoperatively the dose should be adjusted to maintain the prothrombin time between 1.3 and 1.5 times

control (international normalized ratio 2.0 to 3.0).

2. Low-dose heparin using the eight-hourly regimen.

3. Adjusted-dose heparin, commenced two days preoperatively and adjusted to maintain the activated partial thromboplastin time in the upper normal range.

4. The combination of intermittent pneumatic compression with either heparin or oral anticoagulants as outlined above.

5. Supplementing any of the above four methods of primary prophylaxis with postoperative screening to detect patients who break through prophylaxis.

Hip Surgery

Patients undergoing elective total hip replacement and patients who sustain a fractured hip are at particularly high risk of postoperative venous thromboembolism. Unprotected, 40 to 50 per cent of these patients develop venous thrombosis and 20 to 30 per cent develop proximal vein thrombosis,[51,79,106,109,115-117] between 1 and 5 per cent suffer fatal pulmonary embolism.[7,8,52,59]

At present, the following approaches to primary prophylaxis have been shown to be effective by randomized trials and could be used in patients undergoing elective hip replacement:

1. Oral anticoagulants.

2. Dextran.

3. Adjusted-dose subcutaneous heparin.

4. Intermittent compression using a calf and thigh device.

5. Intravenous dextran plus intermittent pneumatic compression.

Low molecular weight heparin is effective and is clinically available in some European countries, but is not currently available in North America. To date, the results with both low-dose heparin and aspirin prophylaxis have been inconsistent, and neither of these two approaches should be used. Screening with impedance plethysmography or B-mode venous ultrasound plus routine venography at a fixed interval postoperatively will provide early detection of venous thrombosis,[51,118-121] but this approach is expensive and logistically demanding.

In patients undergoing surgery for fractured hip, either warfarin or dextran provides effective protection against venous thromboembolic complications. Patients who sustain a fractured hip are frequently elderly and are at particular risk for volume overload with dextran prophylaxis; in these patients, warfarin is preferred.

Major Knee Surgery

Patients undergoing major knee surgery (for example, total knee replacement, tibial osteotomy) are at high risk for postoperative venous thromboembolism (Table 24–1). In the absence of prophylaxis, 60 to 70 per cent of these patients develop calf vein thrombosis, and 20 to 30 per cent develop proximal vein thrombosis by venography.[41] External pneumatic compression is highly effective in these patients and is the prophylactic measure of choice. An external compression device is available that can be worn under either plaster casts or back slabs and can be applied in the operating room over a bandage and beneath a plaster cast. In most patients external pneumatic compression should be continued for seven to ten days postoperatively, at which time many patients are no longer immobilized, while others have walking plaster casts. In the latter group, prophylaxis should be continued with oral anticoagulants or adjusted-dose subcutaneous heparin until the plaster cast is removed, since these patients remain at risk for developing late venous thromboembolic complications if they are not protected.

Urologic Surgery

Patients having a transurethral resection of the prostate have a 7 to 10 per cent risk of developing I-125-fibrinogen leg scan-detected calf vein thrombosis, while those having retropubic prostatectomy or an equivalent operation have a 25 to 50 per cent chance (moderate risk) of developing fibrinogen leg scan-detected calf vein thrombosis. Low-dose heparin is of limited effectiveness in patients undergoing open prostatectomy. Intermittent pneumatic compression is effective in these patients[40] and is the method of choice.

Neurosurgery

In the absence of prophylaxis, the frequency of venous thromboembolism in patients having neurosurgical procedures varies between 20 and 25 per cent. Anticoagulants are potentially dangerous in this patient group because even minimal intracranial bleeding could have serious consequences. External pneumatic compression is effective in these patients[38,39,42] and is the preferred approach.

COST-EFFECTIVENESS OF PROPHYLAXIS

In many hospitals, the lack of an organized strategy for the prevention of venous thromboembolism has been due, in part, to a reluctance to add new interventions whose cost-effectiveness has not been adequately evaluated. Cost-effectiveness analysis provides a formal method for ranking the alternative prophylactic modalities in terms of both their cost and effectiveness.

The results of cost-effectiveness analysis in general surgical patients[122,123] and in orthopedic patients[124,125] indicate three conclusions. First, the use of "no prophylaxis" is ineffective, resulting in unnecessary loss of life, and is costly owing to the diagnostic and treatment costs incurred by patients who develop venous thromboembolism.[122-125] In both general surgical patients and patients undergoing major orthopedic surgery, the use of effective primary prophylaxis is markedly more cost-effective than the use of no prophylaxis.[122,124] Second, in moderate- to high-risk general surgical patients, primary prophylaxis with low-dose subcutaneous heparin is highly cost-effective for preventing fatal pulmonary embolism. Intermittent pneumatic leg compression is relatively inexpensive, and is the approach of choice in patients at high risk of bleeding. Third, primary prophylaxis with active measures is considerably more cost-effective than secondary prevention by screening,[122,123] because this latter approach necessitates full-dose anticoagulant treatment of large numbers of patients with subclinical venous thrombosis.

In the final analysis, however, the decision to use prophylaxis should be based not on economic grounds but on avoiding the tragic and unnecessary loss of life due to pulmonary embolism.

REFERENCES

1. Dismuke SE, Wagner EH. Pulmonary embolism as a cause of death. The changing mortality in hospitalized patients. JAMA 1986; 255: 2039–42.

2. Consensus Conference. Prevention of venous thrombosis and pulmonary embolism. JAMA 1986; 256: 744–9.

3. Dalen JE, Alpert JS. Natural history of pulmonary embolism. Prog Cardiovasc Dis 1975; 17: 259–270.

4. Skinner DB, Salzman EW. Anticoagulant prophylaxis in surgical patients. Surg Gynecol Obstet 1967; 125: 741–6.

5. Shephard RM, White HA, Shirkey AL. Anticoagulant prophylaxis of thromboembolism in post-surgical patients. Am J Surg 1966; 112: 698–702.

6. International Multicentre Trial. Prevention of fatal postoperative pulmonary embolism by low doses of heparin. Lancet 1975; 2: 45–51.

7. Coventry MB, Nolan DR, Beckenbaugh RD. "Delayed" prophylactic anticoagulation: a study of results and complications in 2,012 total hip arthroplasties. J Bone Joint Surg Am 1973; 55: 1487–92.

8. Eskeland G, Solheim K, Skhorten F. Anticoagulant prophylaxis, thromboembolism and mortality in elderly patients with hip fractures: a controlled clinical trial. Acta Chir Scand 1966; 131: 16–29.

9. Kakkar V, Stamatakis JD, Bentley PG, Lawrence D, DeHass HA, Ward VP. Prophylaxis for post-operative deep-vein thrombosis. JAMA 1979; 241: 39–42.

10. Donaldson GA, Williams C, Scanell J, Shaw RS. A reappraisal of the application of the Trendelenburg operation to massive fatal embolism. N Engl J Med 1963; 268: 171–4.

11. Fratantoni J, Wessler S. Prophylactic therapy of deep-vein thrombosis and pulmonary embolism. DHEW Publ. No. (NIH) 76-866. U.S. Government Printing Office, Washington, D.C., 1975.

12. Collins R, Scrimgeour A, Yusef S, Peto R. Reduction in fatal pulmonary embolism and venous thrombosis by perioperative administration of subcutaneous heparin. N Engl J Med 1988; 318: 1162–73.

13. Gordon-Smith IC, LeQuesne LP, Grundy DJ, Newcombe JF. Controlled trial of two regimens of subcutaneous heparin in prevention of post-operative deep-vein thrombosis. Lancet 1972; 1: 1133–5.

14. Kakkar V, Spindler J, Flute PT, et al. Efficacy of low-doses of heparin in prevention of deep-vein thrombosis after major surgery: a double-blind randomized trial. Lancet 1972; 2: 101–6.

15. Nicolaides AN, Dupont PA, Desai S, et al. Small doses of subcutaneous sodium heparin in preventing deep venous thrombosis after major surgery. Lancet 1972; 2: 890–3.

16. Ballard RM, Bradley-Watson PJ, Johnstone FD, et al. Low doses of subcutaneous heparin in the prevention of deep-vein thrombosis after gynecological surgery. Br J Obstet Gyanaecol. 1973; 80: 469–72.

17. Lahnborg G, Friman L, Bergstrom K, Lagergren J. Effect of low-dose heparin on incidence of post-operative pulmonary embolism detected by photoscanning. Lancet 1974; 1: 329–31.

18. Scottish Study: a multi-unit controlled trial. Heparin versus dextran in the prevention of deep-vein thrombosis. Lancet 1974; 2: 118–20.

19. Albernethy EA, Hartsuck JM. Post-operative pulmonary embolism: prospective study utilizing low-dose heparin. Am J Surg 1974; 128: 739–42.

20. Covey TH, Sherman L, Baue E. Low-dose heparin in post-operative patients. Arch Surg 1975; 110: 1021–6.

21. Rosenberg IL, Evans M, Pollock AV. Prophylaxis of post-operative leg vein thrombosis by low-dose subcutaneous heparin or pre-operative calf muscle stimulation: a controlled clinical trial. Br Med J 1975; 1: 649–51.

22. Gallus AS, Hirsh J, O'Brien SE, McBride JA, Tuttle RJ, Gent M. Prevention of venous thrombosis with small subcutaneous doses of heparin. JAMA 1975; 235: 1980–2.

23. Gruber UF, Duckert F, Fridich R, Torhorts J, Rem J. Prevention of post-operative thromboembolism by dextran 40, low doses of heparin or xantinol nicotinate. Lancet 1977; 1: 207–10.

24. Groote Schuur Hospital Thromboembolus Study Group. Failure of low-dose heparin to prevent significant thromboembolic complications in high-risk surgical patients: interim report of post-operative trial. Br Med J 1979; 1: 1447–50.

25. Morris GH, Henry APJ, Prestion BJ. Prevention of deep-

vein thrombosis by low-dose heparin in patients undergoing total hip replacement. Lancet 1974; 2: 797–800.

26. Hampson WGJ, Harris FC, Lucas HK, et al. Failure of low-dose heparin to prevent deep-vein thrombosis after hip replacement arthroplasty. Lancet 1974; 2: 795–7.

27. Venous Thrombosis Clinical Study Group. Small doses of subcutaneous sodium heparin in the prevention of deep-vein thrombosis after elective hip operations. Br J Surg 1975; 62: 348–50.

28. Gallus AS, Hirsh J, Tuttle RJ, et al. Small subcutaneous doses of heparin in prevention of venous thrombosis. N Engl J Med 1973; 288: 545–51.

29. Manucci PM, Citterio LA, Panajotopoulos N. Low-dose heparin and deep-vein thrombosis after total hip replacement. Thromb Haemost 1976; 36: 157–64.

30. Negus D, Friedgood A, Cox SJ, Peel ALG, Wells B. Ultralow-dose intravenous heparin in prevention of post-operative deep-vein thrombosis. Lancet 1980; 1: 891–4.

31. Moskovitz PA, Ellenberg SS, Feffer HL. Low-dose heparin for prevention of venous thromboembolism in total hip arthroplasty and surgical repair of hip fractures. J Bone Joint Surg Am 1978; 60: 1065–70.

32. Gruber UF, Seldeen T, Brokop T, et al. Incidence of fatal post-operative pulmonary embolism after prophylaxis with dextran-70 and low-dose heparin. Br Med J 1980; 280: 69–72.

33. Clarke-Pearson DL, et al. Venous thromboembolism prophylaxis in gynecologic oncology: a prospective, controlled trial of low-dose heparin. Am J Obstet Gynecol 1983; 145: 606–13.

34. Sabri S, Roberts VC, Cotton LT. Prevention of early post-operative deep-vein thrombosis by intermittent compression of the leg during surgery. Br Med J 1971; 4: 394–6.

35. Hills NH, Pflug JJ, Jeyasingh K, Boardman L, Calman JS. Prevention of deep-vein thrombosis by intermittent pneumatic compression of calf. Br Med J 1972; 1: 131–5.

36. Roberts VC, Cotton LT. Prevention of post-operative deep-vein thrombosis in patients with malignant disease. Br Med J 1974; 1: 358–60.

37. Clarke WB, MacGregor AB, Prescott RJ, Ruckley CV. Pneumatic compression of the calf and post-operative deep-vein thrombosis. Lancet 1974; 2: 5–7.

38. Turpie AGG, Gallus A, Beattie WS, Hirsh J. Prevention of venous thrombosis in patients with intracranial disease by intermittent pneumatic compression of the calf. Neurology 1977; 27: 435–8.

39. Skillman JJ, Collins RR, Coe NP, et al. Prevention of deep-vein thrombosis in neurosurgical patients: a controlled, randomized trial of external pneumatic compression boots. Surgery 1978; 83: 354–8.

40. Coe NP, Collins REC, Klein LA, et al. Prevention of deep-vein thrombosis in urological patients: a controlled, randomized trial of low-dose heparin and external pneumatic compression boots. Surgery 1978; 83: 230–4.

41. Hull RD, Delmore TJ, Hirsh J, et al. Effectiveness of intermittent pulsatile elastic stockings for the prevention of calf and thigh vein thrombosis in patients undergoing elective knee surgery. Thromb Res 1979; 16: 37–45.

42. Turpie AG, Delmore T, Hirsh J, et al. Prevention of venous thrombosis by intermittent sequential calf compression in patients with intracranial disease. Thromb Res 1979; 16: 611–6.

43. Borow M, Goldson H. Post-operative venous thrombosis. Am J Surg 1981; 141: 245–51.

44. Nicolaides AN, Fernandes J, Pollock AV. Intermittent sequential pneumatic compression of the legs in the prevention of venous stasis and postoperative venous thrombosis. Surgery 1980; 87: 69–76.

45. Nicolaides AN, Miles C, Hoare M, Jury P, Helmis E, Venniker R. Intermittent sequential pneumatic compression of the legs and thromboembolism deterrent stockings in the prevention of post-operative deep venous thrombosis. Surgery 1983; 94: 21–5.

46. Butson ARC. Intermittent pneumatic calf compression for prevention of deep venous thrombosis in general abdominal surgery. Am J Surg 1981; 142: 525–7.

47. Hartman JT, et al. Cyclic sequential compression of the lower limb in prevention of deep venous thrombosis. J Bone Joint Surg Am 1982; 64: 1059–62.

48. Caprini JA, et al. Thrombosis prophylaxis using external compression. Surgery 1983; 156: 599–604.

49. Clarke-Pearson DL, et al. Prevention of venous thromboembolism by external pneumatic calf compression in patients with gynecologic malignancy. Obstet Gynecol 1984; 63: 92–8.

50. Gallus A, Raman K, Darby T. Venous thrombosis after hip replacement: the influence of preventative intermittent calf compression and of surgical technique. Br J Surg 1983; 70: 17–9.

51. Hull R, Raskob G, Gent M, et al. Effectiveness of intermittent pneumatic leg compression for preventing deep-vein thrombosis after total hip replacement. JAMA 1990; 263: 2313–17.

52. Sevitt S, Gallagher NG. Prevention of venous thrombosis and pulmonary embolism in injured patients: trial of anticoagulant prophylaxis in middle-aged and elderly patients with fractured neck of femur. Lancet 1959; 2: 981–9.

53. Borgstram S, Greitz T, Vander Linden W, Molin J, Rudics I. Anticoagulant prophylaxis of venous thrombosis in patients with fractured neck of the femur: a controlled clinical trial using venous phlebography. Acta Chir Scand 1965; 129: 500–8.

54. Hamilton HW, Crawford JS, Gardiner JH, Wiley AM. Venous thrombosis in patients with fracture of the upper end of the femur. J Bone Joint Surg Br 1970; 52: 268–9.

55. Pinto DJ. Controlled trial of an anticoagulant (warfarin sodium) in the prevention of venous thrombosis following hip surgery. Br J Surg 1970; 57: 349–52.

56. Hume M, Kuriakose T, Xavier ZL, Turner R. ^{125}I-fibrinogen and the prevention of venous thrombosis. Arch Surg 1973; 107: 803–6.

57. Morris GK, Mitchell JR. Warfarin sodium in the prevention of deep venous thrombosis and pulmonary embolism in patients with fractured neck of femur. Lancet 1976; 2: 869–72.

58. Taberner DA, Poller L, Burslem RW, Jones JB. Oral anticoagulants controlled by the British comparative thromboplastin versus low-dose heparin in prophylaxis of deep vein thrombosis. Br Med J 1978; 1: 272–4.

59. Francis CW, Marder VJ, Evarts M, Yaukoolbodi S. Two-step warfarin therapy: prevention of post-operative venous thrombosis without excessive bleeding. JAMA 1983; 249: 374–8.

60. Paiement G, Wessinger SJ, Waltman WC, Harris WH. Low-dose warfarin versus external pneumatic compression for prophylaxis against venous thromboembolism following total hip replacement. J Arthroplasty 1987; 2: 23–6.

61. Bonnar J, Walsh J. Prevention of thrombosis after pelvic surgery by British dextran 70. Lancet 1972; 1: 614–6.

62. Bonnar J, Walsh JJ, Haddon M. Thromboembolism following radical surgery for carcinoma: prevention by dextran 70 infusion during and immediately after operation. In: Proc 4th Congr Int Soc Thrombosis and Haematostatis, Vienna, 1973:278A.

63. Carter AE, Eban R. The prevention of post-operative deep venous thrombosis with dextran 70. Br J Surg 1973; 60: 681–3.

64. Becker J, Schampi B. The incidence of post-operative venous thrombosis of the legs: a comparative study on the prophylactic effect of dextran 70 and electrical calf muscle stimulation. Acta Chir Scand 1973; 139: 357–67.

65. Kline A, Hughes LE, Campbell H, et al. Dextran 70 in prophylaxis of thromboembolic disease after surgery: a clinically oriented randomized double-blind trial. Br Med J 1975; 2: 109–12.

66. Ahlberg A, Nylander G, Robertson B, Cronberg S, Nilsson IM. Dextran in prophylaxis of thrombosis in fractures of the hip. Acta Chir Scand 1968; 387 (suppl): 83–5.

67. Johnsson SR, Bygdeman S, Eliasson R. Effect of dextran on post-operative thrombosis. Acta Chir Scand 1968; 387 (suppl): 80–2.

68. Evarts CM, Feil EJ. Prevention of thromboembolic disease after elective surgery of the hip. J Bone Joint Surg Am 1971; 53: 1271–8.

69. Leyvraz PF, Richard J, Bachmann F, et al. Adjusted versus

fixed dose subcutaneous heparin in the prevention of deep-vein thrombosis after total hip replacement. N Engl J Med 1983; 309: 954–8.

70. Kakkar VV, Murray WJG. Efficacy and safety of low-molecular-weight heparin (CY216) in preventing postoperative venous thromboembolism: a co-operative study. Br J Surg 1985; 72: 786–91.

71. Koller M, Schoch U, Buchmann P, Largiader F, von Felten A, Frick P. Low molecular weight heparin as thromboprophylaxis in elective visceral surgery. Thromb Haemost 1986; 56: 243–6.

72. Bergqvist D, Burmark U, Frisell J, et al. Low molecular weight heparin once daily compared with conventional low-dose heparin twice daily. A prospective double-blind multicentre trial on prevention of postoperative thrombosis. Br J Surg 1988; 73: 204–8.

73. Bergqvist D, Matzsch T, Brumark U, et al. Low molecular weight heparin given the evening before surgery compared with conventional low-dose heparin in prevention of thrombosis. Br J Surg 1988; 75: 888–91.

74. Caen JP. A randomized double-blind study between a low molecular weight heparin Kabi 2165 and standard heparin in the prevention of deep-vein thrombosis in general surgery. A French multicentre trial. Thromb Haemost 1988; 59: 216–20.

75. Fricker J, Vergres Y, Schach R, et al. Low dose heparin versus low molecular weight heparin (Kabi 2165 Fragmin) in the prophylaxis of thromboembolic complications of abdominal oncologic surgery. Eur J Clin Invest 1988; 18: 561–7.

76. Samama M, Bernard P, Bonnardot JP, et al. Low molecular weight heparin compared with unfractionated heparin in prevention of postoperative thrombosis. Br J Surg 1988; 75: 128–31.

77. The European Fraxiparin Study Group. Comparison of a low molecular weight heparin and unfractionated heparin for the prevention of deep vein thrombosis in patients undergoing abdominal surgery. Br J Surg 1988; 75: 1058–63.

78. Ockelford P, Patterson J, Johns A. A double-blind randomized placebo controlled trial of thromboprophylaxis in major elective general surgery using once daily injections of a low molecular weight heparin fragment (Fragmin). Thromb Haemost 1989; 62: 1046–9.

79. Turpie AG, Levine MN, Hirsh J, et al. A randomized controlled trial of a low-molecular-weight heparin (Enoxaparin) to prevent deep-vein thrombosis in patients undergoing elective hip surgery. N Engl J Med 1986; 315: 925–9.

80. Planes A, Vochelle N, Mazas F, et al. Prevention of postoperative venous thrombosis: a randomized trial comparing unfractionated heparin with low molecular weight heparin in patients undergoing total hip replacement. Thromb Haemost 1988; 60: 407–10.

81. Dechavanne M, Ville D, Berruyer M, et al. Randomized trial of a low-molecular weight heparin (Kabi 2165) versus adjusted-dose subcutaneous standard heparin in the prophylaxis of deep-vein thrombosis after elective hip surgery. Haemostasis 1989; 1: 5–12.

82. Holford CP. Graded compression for preventing deep venous thrombosis. Br Med J 1976; 2: 969–70.

83. Scurr JH, Ibrahim SZ, Faber RG, LeQuesne LP. The efficacy of graduated compression stockings in the prevention of deep-vein thrombosis. Br J Surg 1977; 64: 371–3.

84. Scholz PM, Jones RH, Sabiston DC. Prophylaxis of thromboembolism. Adv Surg 1979; 13: 115–43.

85. Ishak MA, Moreley KD. Deep venous thrombosis after total hip arthroplasty: a prospective controlled study to determine the prophylactic effect of graded pressure stockings. Br J Surg 1981; 68: 429–32.

86. Allan A, Williams JT, Bolton JP, Le Quesne LP. The use of graduated compression stockings in the prevention of postoperative deep vein thrombosis. Br J Surg 1983; 70: 172–4.

87. Turpie AG, Hirsh J, Gent M, Julian D, Johnson J. Prevention of deep-vein thrombosis in potential neurosurgical patients: randomized trial comparing graduated compression stockings alone or graduated compression stockings plus intermittent pneumatic compression with control. Arch Intern Med 1989; 149: 679–81.

88. Kakkar V, Stamatakis JD, Bentley PG, et al. Prophylaxis for post-operative deep vein thrombosis: synergistic effect of heparin and dihydroergotamine. JAMA 1979; 241: 39–42.

89. Multicenter Trial Committee. Dihydroergotamine-heparin prophylaxis of post-operative deep-vein thrombosis. JAMA 1984; 251: 2960–6.

90. Gent M, Roberts RS. A meta-analysis of the studies of dihydroergotamine plus heparin in the prophylaxis of deep vein thrombosis. Chest 1986; 89 (suppl): 396S–400S.

91. Comerota AJ, White JV. The use of dihydroergotamine in the prophylaxis of deep venous thrombosis. Chest 1986; 89 (suppl): 389S–95S.

92. Torngren S. Low dose heparin and compression stockings in the prevention of postoperative deep venous thrombosis. Br J Surg 1980; 67: 482–4.

93. Wille-Jorgensen P, Thorup J, Fischer A, Holst-Christensen J, Flamsholt R. Heparin with and without graded compression stockings in the prevention of thromboembolic complications of major abdominal surgery: a randomized trial. Br J Surg 1985; 72: 579–81.

94. Harris WH, Athanasoulis CA, Waltman AC, Salzman EW. Prophylaxis of deep-vein thrombosis after total hip replacement: dextran and external pneumatic compression compared with 1.2 or 0.3 gram of aspirin daily. J Bone Joint Surg Am 1985; 67: 57–62.

95. O'Brien JR, Tulevski V, Etherington M. Two in-vivo studies comparing high and low aspirin dosage. Lancet 1971; 1: 399–400.

96. Medical Research Council. Report of the steering committee; effect of aspirin on post-operative venous thrombosis. Lancet 1972; 2: 441–4.

97. Renney JT, G, O'Sullivan EF, Burke PF. Prevention of postoperative deep-vein thrombosis with dipyridamole and aspirin. Br Med J 1976; 1: 992–4.

98. Loew D, Brucke P, Simma W, Vinazzer H, Dienstl E, Boehme E. Acetylsalicylic acid, low-dose heparin and a combination of both substances in the prevention of post-operative thromboembolism: a double-blind study. Thromb Res 1977; 1: 81–8.

99. Plante J, Boneu B, Vaysse C, Barret A, Gouzi M, Bierne R. Dipyridamole aspirin versus low doses of heparin in the prophylaxis of deep venous thrombosis in abdominal surgery. Thromb Res 1979; 14: 399–403.

100. Wood EH, Prentice CR, McGrouther DA, Sinclair J, McNicol GP. Trial of aspirin and RA233 in prevention of post-operative deep-vein thrombosis. Thromb Haemost 1973; 30: 18–24.

101. Harris WH, Salzman EW, Athanasoulis C, Waltman AC, Baum S, DeSanctis RW. Comparison of warfarin, low-molecular-weight dextran, aspirin, and subcutaneous heparin prevention of venous thromboembolism following total hip replacement. J Bone Joint Surg Am 1974; 56: 1552–62.

102. Soreff J, Johnsson J, Diener L, Goransson L. Acetylsalicylic acid in a trial to diminish thromboembolic complications after elective hip surgery. Acta Orthop Scand 1975; 46: 246–55.

103. Dechavanne M, Ville D, Viala JJ, et al. Controlled trial of platelet antiaggregating agents and subcutaneous heparin in prevention of post-operative deep-vein thrombosis in high-risk patients. Haemostasis 1975; 4: 94–100.

104. Jennings JJ, Harris WH, Sarmiento A. A clinical evaluation of aspirin prophylaxis of thromboembolic disease after total hip arthroplasty. J Bone Joint Surg Am 1976; 58: 926–8.

105. Morris GK, Mitchell JRA. Preventing venous thromboembolism in elderly patients with hip fractures: studies of low-dose heparin, dipyridamole, aspirin, and flurbiprofen. Br Med J 1977; 1: 535–7.

106. Harris WH, Salzman EW, Athanasoulis CA, Waltman AW, DeSanctis RW. Aspirin prophylaxis of venous thromboembolism after total hip replacement. N Engl J Med 1977; 297: 1246–9.

107. Samatakis JD, Kakkar V, Lawrence D, Bentley PG, Nairn D, Ward V. Failure of aspirin to prevent post-operative deep-vein thrombosis in patients undergoing total hip replacement. Br Med J 1978; 1: 1031.

108. Hume M, Donaldson WR, Suprennant J. Sex, aspirin and venous thrombosis. Orthop Clin North Am 1978; 3: 761–7.

109. Powers PJ, Gent M, Jay R, et al. A randomized trial of less intense postoperative warfarin or aspirin therapy in the prevention of venous thromboembolism after surgery for fractured hip. Arch Intern Med 1989; 149: 771–4.

110. Hull R, Delmore T, Genton E, et al. Warfarin sodium versus low-dose heparin in the long-term treatment of venous thrombosis. N Engl J Med 1979; 301: 855–8.

111. Roberts VC, Sabri S, Beely AH, Cotton LT. The effect of intermittently applied external pressure on the hemodynamics of the lower limb in man. Br J Surg 1972; 59: 223–6.

112. Knight MTN, Dawson R. Effect of intermittent compression of the arms on deep venous thrombosis in the legs. Lancet 1976; 2: 1265–8.

113. Nicolaides AN, Fernandes E, Fernandes J, Pollock AV. Intermittent sequential pneumatic compression of the legs in the prevention of venous stasis and postoperative deep venous thrombosis. Surgery 1980; 87: 69–76.

114. Kakkar VV, Flanc C, Howe CT, et al. Natural history of post-operative deep-vein thrombosis. Lancet 1969; 2: 230–3.

115. Stamatakis JD, Kakkar VV, Sagar S, Lawrence D, Nairn D, Bentley PG. Femoral vein thrombosis and total hip replacement. Br Med J 1977; 2: 223–5.

116. Johnson R, Carmichael JHE, Almond HGA, Loynes RP. Deep venous thrombosis following Charnley arthroplasty. Clin Orthop 1978; 132: 24–30.

117. Nillius AS, Nylander G. Deep-vein thrombosis after total hip replacement: a clinical and phlebographic study. Br J Surg 1979; 66: 324–6.

118. Harris WH, Athanasoulis C, Waltman AC, Salzman EW. Cuff-impedence phlebography and ^{125}I-fibrinogen scanning versus roentgenographic phlebography for diagnosis of thrombophlebitis following hip surgery. J Bone Joint Surg Am 1976; 58: 939–44.

119. Comerota AJ, Katz ML, Grossi RJ, et al. The comparative value of non-invasive testing for diagnosis and surveillance of deep-vein thrombosis. J Vasc Surg 1988; 7: 40–9.

120. Paiement G, Wessinger SJ, Waltman AC, Harris WH. Surveillance of deep-vein thrombosis in asymptomatic total hip replacement patients: impedance phlebography and fibrinogen scanning versus roentgenographic phlebography. Am J Surg 1988; 155: 400–4.

121. Borris L, Christiansen H, Lassen MR, Olsen A, Schott P. Comparison of real-time B-mode ultrasonography and bilateral ascending phlebography for detection of postoperative deep-vein thrombosis following elective hip surgery. Thomb Haemost 1989; 61: 363–5.

122. Salzman EW, Davies GC. Prophylaxis of venous thromboembolism: analysis of cost-effectiveness. Ann Surg 1980; 191: 207.

123. Hull R, Hirsh J, Sackett DL, Stoddart G. Cost-effectiveness of primary and secondary prevention of fatal pulmonary embolism in high-risk surgical patients. Can Med Assoc J 1982; 127: 990–5.

124. Oster G, Tuden RL, Colditz GA. A cost-effectiveness analysis of prophylaxis against deep-vein thrombosis in major orthopedic surgery. JAMA 1987; 257: 203–8.

125. Paiement GD, Bell D, Wessinger SJ, Harris WH. New advances in the prevention, diagnosis and cost-effectiveness of venous thromboembolic disease in patients with total hip replacement. Hip 1987: 94–119.

126. Kakkar VV. Fibrinogen uptake test for detection of deep-vein thrombosis. A review of current practice. Semin Nucl Med 1977; 7: 229–44.

127. Harris WH, Salzmann EW, Athanasoulis CA, et al. Comparison of ^{125}I-fibrinogen count scanning with phebography for detection of venous thrombi after elective hip surgery. N Engl J Med 1975; 292: 665–7.

128. Hirsh J, Poller L, Deykin D, Levine M, Dalen J. Optimal therapeutic range for oral anticoagulants. Chest 1989; 95(suppl): 55–11S.

129. Hull R, Hirsh J, Jay R, et al. Different intensities of oral anticoagulant therapy in the treatment of proximal-vein thrombosis. N Engl J Med 1982; 307: 1676–81.

130. Aberg M, Bergentz SE, Hedneru. The effect of dextran on lysability of ex-vivo thrombi. Ann Surg 1975; 181: 342–45.

131. Tangen O, Wik KO, Almquist IAM. Effects of dextran on the structure and plasmin induced lysis of human fibrin. Thromb Res 1972; 1: 487–92.

25

TREATMENT OF VENOUS THROMBOSIS AND PULMONARY EMBOLISM

SAMUEL Z. GOLDHABER and HERVÉ SORS

Venous thromboembolism is the third most common cardiovascular disease after acute ischemic heart disease and stroke. Pulmonary embolism (PE) accounts for approximately 50,000 deaths per year in the United States. The combination of pulmonary embolism and deep vein thrombosis (DVT) is responsible for about 300,000 United States hospitalizations annually[1] (Fig. 25–1). Data from the National Hospital Discharge Survey indicate that the death rate from pulmonary embolism has not improved since the 1960s[2] (Fig. 25–2).

Heparin accelerates the action of antithrombin III approximately 1,000-fold. This prevents further fibrin deposition (Fig. 25–3) and allows the body's natural fibrinolytic mechanisms to lyse some of the clot that has already formed. Heparin does *not* dissolve thrombus that already exists. One placebo-controlled randomized trial has been carried out in patients with pulmonary thromboembolism.[3] The mortality rate was significantly lower among the patients treated with heparin and the study was discontinued for ethical reasons. No randomized placebo-controlled trial with heparin has been published in deep vein thrombosis.[4]

THE RELATIONSHIP BETWEEN DEEP VEIN THROMBOSIS AND PULMONARY EMBOLISM

Among patients with venographically proven proximal leg deep vein thrombosis, about half endure concomitant pulmonary embolism that is usually clinically silent.[5,6] Approximately 15 to 30 per cent with isolated calf vein thrombosis will have asymptomatic pulmonary embolism,[5,6] a much higher frequency than is generally appreciated. When venous thrombi dislodge, they embolize through the venous system to the pulmonary arterial circulation and may adhere to the bifurcation of the pulmonary artery, forming a "saddle embolus" or, more commonly, occlude a more distal pulmonary vessel. The pathophysiological response to acute pulmonary embolism depends upon the extent to which pulmonary artery blood flow is obstructed, preexisting cardiopulmonary disease, and at least in experimental models, also on the release of vasoactive humoral factors from activated platelets that accumulate at the site of new clot.

ANTICOAGULATION

Pulmonary embolism and symptomatic deep vein thrombosis should be treated with anticoagulation unless the patient is actively bleeding. In particular, one should not withhold anticoagulation from patients with symptomatic deep vein thrombosis that is limited to the calf. Lagerstedt and colleagues[7] studied 51 patients with venographically proven isolated calf vein thrombosis who received a week of intravenous heparin and were then randomized to warfarin or no-warfarin treatment. During the first three months, zero patients in the warfarin group and 29 per cent in the no-warfarin group

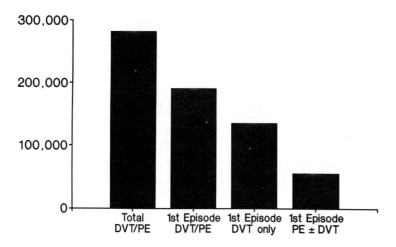

FIGURE 25–1. Estimated number of cases of venous thromboembolism in the United States in 1986, based on a 15-hospital survey in the Worcester, MA area. (Adapted from data in Anderson FA, et al. A population-based perspective of the hospital incidence and case-fatality rates of venous thrombosis and pulmonary embolism: the Worcester DVT Study. Arch Intern Med 1991; in press, with permission.)

suffered recurrent proximal deep vein thrombosis or, in one case, pulmonary embolism. After one year of follow-up, one patient in the warfarin group and 50 per cent in the no-warfarin group experienced recurrent venous thromboembolism.

Initiation of Unfractionated (Standard) Heparin Therapy

The major factors that increase the risk of bleeding during heparin treatment include older age, thrombocytopenia, renal or hepatic failure, concomitant carcinomatosis, and of course, the intensity of anticoagulation.[8] The most frequently overlooked portion of the physical examination is a rectal examination for occult blood. If the history and physical examination are benign, heparin can be started prior to lung scanning or pulmonary angiography. When a stool examination is equivocal (that is, "trace"), we proceed with heparin anticoagulation, but are especially vigilant for potential bleeding complications. However, if a severe bleeding problem is detected, such as active gastrointestinal bleeding, heparin therapy should be withheld. If the diagnosis of pulmonary embolism is confirmed, nonpharmacological treatment with insertion of an inferior vena cava (IVC) filter should be considered.

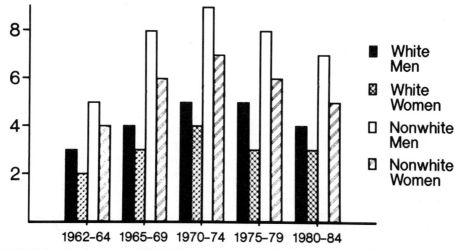

FIGURE 25–2. Death rate peer 100,000 from pulmonary embolism in the United States from 1962 to 1984, based on data from the National Hospital Discharge Survey. (Adapted from data in Lilienfeld DE, et al. Mortality from pulmonary embolism in the United States: 1962 to 1984. Chest 1990;98:1067–72, with permission.)

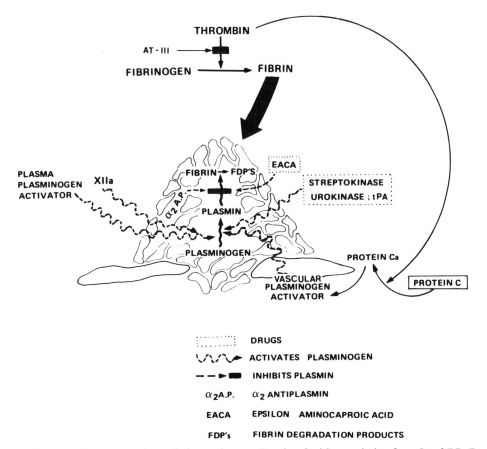

FIGURE 25–3. Lysis versus anticoagulation pathways. (Reprinted with permission from Stead RB: Regulation of hemostasis. In: Goldhaber SZ, ed. Pulmonary embolism and deep venous thrombosis. Philadelphia: WB Saunders Co., 1985;38.)

To manage heparin therapy, we utilize either a modification of the 1989 guidelines published by the American College of Chest Physicians[4] (Table 25–1) or the heparin nomogram developed by McMaster University and the Hamilton Civic Hospitals Research Centre[9] (Table 25–2). A modified approach to these guidelines utilizes an initial heparin bolus of 5,000 to 10,000 units, followed by a continuous infusion of 1,000 to 1,500 units/hour. For heparin, the target activated partial thromboplastin time (APTT) is 1.5 to 2 times the *upper* limit of the control value. The activated partial thromboplastin time should be checked every four to six hours until the target activated partial thromboplastin time range is obtained. When the activated partial thromboplastin time is less than 1.5 times the control, the continuous heparin infusion dose should be increased rapidly, by an increment of at least 25 per cent. Conversely, if an activated partial thromboplastin time level exceeds 3.0 times the control value, a reduc-

tion in the infusion rate of no more than 25 per cent of the dose should be made (see Chapter 8).

Unfortunately, physicians tend to administer inadequate doses of heparin. At Vanderbilt University School of Medicine, 60 per cent of patients with venous thromboembolism did not have a single activated partial thromboplastin time greater than 1.5 times control within the first 24 hours of heparin therapy. Not until day eight of treatment were 90 per cent of the activated partial thromboplastin times within the therapeutic range.[10] When subtherapeutic activated partial thromboplastin times were obtained, physicians responded with modest increases in heparin dosing that were often inadequate to elevate the activated partial thromboplastin time into the therapeutic range. Conversely, when unacceptably high activated partial thromboplastin times were obtained, excessive reduction in heparin dose caused subtherapeutic activated partial thromboplastin

TABLE 25–1. Guidelines for Antithrombotic Therapy with Heparin and Warfarin in Venous Thromboembolism*

Disease suspected	Obtain baseline activated partial thromboplastin time, 1-stage prothrombin time,† and platelet count and give heparin bolus (5–10,000 units) intravenously; order diagnostic test, for example, ventilation-perfusion lung scan, pulmonary angiogram, contrast venogram
Disease confirmed	Give loading dose of heparin (5,000 units) and start constant intravenous infusion at approximately 1,000 units/hour
	Monitor activated partial thromboplastin time at 6 hours and thereafter until the activated partial thromboplastin time is stabilized at 1.5–2 times control value
	Monitor platelet count every 3–4 days while administering heparin
	Start warfarin on day 1 or 2 by instituting the estimated daily maintenance dose (usually 4–10 milligrams)
	After at least 5 days of heparin and 4–5 days of joint therapy, stop intravenous heparin therapy and check 1-stage prothrombin time 4 hours later
	Maintain 1-stage prothrombin time off heparin therapy at 1.3–1.5 times control or pretreatment value
	Full-dose anticoagulation for at least 3 months in patients without continuing risk factors, longer in other patients

* Adapted from Hyers TM, Hull RD, Weg JG. Antithrombotic therapy for venous thromboembolic disease. Chest 1989; 95: 37S–51S, with permission.

† 1.3 times control performed with rabbit brain thromboplastin is roughly equal to 2.0 times control with human brain thromboplastin.

times in more than half of the patients. Thus, it is apparent that the usual practice of administering "blindly" an initial 5,000-unit bolus of heparin followed by an initial infusion of 1,000 units/hour is inadequate anticoagulant therapy for most patients with pulmonary embolism.

Patients with deep vein thrombosis and pulmonary emboli have higher heparin requirements than those who are subsequently proven to have no thrombosis.[11] Among patients with pulmonary embolism, the half-life of heparin is shorter and the clearance of heparin is greater compared with patients who have only deep vein thrombosis.[12]

For pregnant women with venous thromboembolism, we treat initially with continuous intravenous heparin and then use full-dose subcutaneous unfractionated heparin which is continued for the remainder of the pregnancy. With subcutaneous injections, peak standard heparin levels are usually obtained at approximately three hours, and the effect may last as long as 12 hours. To monitor the therapy, the target is a midinterval activated partial thromboplastin time of approximately 1.5 times control. Adjusted full doses of heparin were found to be safe for both the mother and fetus.[13]

In the majority of studies in which continuous and intermittent infusion of heparin have been compared, the frequency of major hemorrhage was lower with continuous intravenous infusion.[4] Also, the patients who received continuous intravenous heparin infusions tended to receive lower total doses of heparin than those allocated to subcutaneous injections. Theoretically, intermittent intravenous heparin administration is disadvantageous because it temporarily causes excessive anticoagulation, as reflected by highly elevated peak activated partial thromboplas-

TABLE 25–2. McMaster Nomogram for Standard Heparin

PARTIAL THROMBOPLASTIN TIME (SECONDS)	BOLUS (UNITS)	HOLD (MINUTES)	RATE CHANGE, (MILLILITERS/HOUR†)	REPEAT PARTIAL THROMBOPLASTIN TIME
<50	5,000	0	+3	6 hours
50–59	0	0	+3	6 hours
60–85	0	0	0	Next AM
86–95	0	0	−2	Next AM
96–120	0	30	−2	6 hours
>120	0	60	−4	6 hours

* From Cruickshank MK, et al. A standard heparin nomogram for the management of heparin therapy. Arch Intern Med 1991; 151: 333–7, with permission.

† 1 milliliter/hour = 40 units/hours when 20,000 units heparin is added to 500 milliliters crystalloid solution; all patients receive an initial 5,000-units bolus and the initial heparin infusion rate is 1,280 units/hour (32 milliliters/hour).

tin times. Therefore, whenever feasible, therapy by continuous intravenous infusion following an initial heparin bolus is to be recommended.

Low Molecular Weight Heparin

Low molecular weight heparins are fractions or fragments prepared from commercial unfractionated heparin. Low molecular weight heparins have an average molecular weight of 4,000 to 8,000 daltons, compared with an average molecular weight of 12,000 to 15,000 daltons for unfractionated heparin (see Chapter 6). Low molecular weight heparin has a longer half-life than unfractionated (standard) heparin and has been less often associated with thrombocytopenia than unfractionated heparin. In a double-blind randomized trial of a low molecular weight heparin (Fragmin) compared with unfractionated heparin, there was a trend in favor of the former for fewer bleeding complications.[14] In a separate study in which another low molecular weight heparin (enoxaparin, Clexane) was compared with unfractionated heparin, among orthopedic patients receiving *prophylaxis* against deep vein thrombosis, the bleeding complication rate was halved although the antithrombotic protection was the same with the two test substances.[15]

Complications of Heparin

Hemorrhage is the major complication of heparin, but nonhemorrhagic side effects should also be kept in mind. A retrospective analysis of anticoagulated patients at Brigham and Women's Hospital found that bleeding correlates with the intensity of therapy[16] (see Chapter 6).

For patients at high risk of bleeding from heparin, the angiographer should be alerted to the possible need to insert an inferior vena cava (IVC) filter on short notice. However, we no longer automatically place an inferior vena cava filter in patients with nonhemorrhagic brain tumors because many of these patients can be anticoagulated safely.[17]

Major bleeding during anticoagulation may unmask a previously·silent lesion, such as bladder or colon cancer. For most cases of moderate bleeding, cessation of heparin therapy will suffice. In the event of life-threatening or intracranial hemorrhage, protamine sulfate can be administered at the time heparin is discontinued. The usual dose of protamine sulfate is approximately 1 milligram per 100 units of heparin, administered slowly (for example, 50 milligrams over 10 to 30 minutes). Protamine sulfate can cause allergic reactions that vary from mild to life threatening.[18]

Coumarin Derivatives

When coumarin treatment is initiated, the level of protein C is lowered and a thrombogenic potential is created. By initiating heparin treatment in adequate doses before protein C suppression and by overlapping heparin and warfarin for four to five days, this theoretically procoagulant effect of warfarin can be counteracted. Therefore, we recommend overlapping heparin and warfarin for four to five days. An Australian study randomized patients to an "early warfarin" or "late warfarin" treatment group. The "early" group started warfarin on average after one day of hospitalization. The "late" group began warfarin after seven days of continuous intravenous heparin. Efficacy and safety were similar in both groups, and early warfarin treatment shortened overall hospital stay by an average of four days.[19] In a more recent randomized trial at McMaster University, patients with deep vein thrombosis were treated either with five days of heparin (with warfarin begun on the first day) or with ten days of heparin (with warfarin begun on the fifth day). The rate of recurrent deep vein thrombosis and bleeding was the same in both groups.[20] Therefore, a practical and safe approach is to treat five to ten days with heparin and to initiate warfarin on the first or second hospital day.

Duration and Intensity of Therapy

In phase I of the Urokinase Pulmonary Embolism Trial (UPET), one fifth of the patients suffered recurrent pulmonary emboli during the first two weeks of therapy.[21] Recurrence appeared to correlate with an inadequate intensity of anticoagulation. The American College of Chest Physicians (ACCP) has recommended sufficient warfarin to prolong the prothrombin time to an international normalized ratio (INR) of 2.0

to 3.0 (Table 25–1). As regards duration of therapy, patients with slowly resolving risk factors (for example, prolonged immobilization) should be treated for at least three months, whereas patients with tumors, antithrombin III or protein C or S deficiency, or recurrent venous thromboembolism should be treated indefinitely (Table 25–1).

Complications

The major toxic effect of warfarin is bleeding that tends to be highly correlated with the intensity of anticoagulation. A study at Brigham and Women's Hospital demonstrated that the risk of bleeding increases as the prothrombin time increases.[22] Of 130 cases of bleeding, 38 per cent were due to remediable lesions, half of which were occult prior to warfarin administration. Therefore, if bleeding occurs when the international normalized ratio is within the recommended range, occult malignancy should be investigated. Minor bleeding with an excessively high international normalized ratio may merely require interruption of warfarin therapy, without administration of vitamin K, or fresh frozen plasma, until the international normalized ratio has returned to the therapeutic range. Extensive investigation of patients with minor bleeding and an international normalized ratio above the therapeutic range is usually not productive.

In Europe, oral vitamin K_1 (phytonadione) (1 to 2 milligrams) is recommended for reversing warfarin in patients without intestinal absorption problems (for example, jaundice). If rapid reversal is needed intravenous vitamin K_1 should be given slowly (1 milligram/minute). Major life-threatening bleeding requires immediate treatment intravenously administered vitamin K_1 and with enough cryoprecipitate or fresh frozen plasma (FFP) (usually 2 units) to achieve immediate hemostasis. To treat less serious bleeding, vitamin K_1 may be administered parenterally.

THROMBOLYTIC THERAPY

Rationale

Among pulmonary embolism patients without prior cardiopulmonary disease, right ventricular afterload increases when pulmonary artery obstruction owing to pulmonary embolism reduces the pulmonary vascular bed by 50 per cent or more. To compensate, right ventricular and pulmonary artery pressures rise. As right ventricular afterload increases acutely, this chamber dilates and becomes hypokinetic, leading to tricuspid regurgitation. As the right ventricle fails, right atrial pressure rises and cardiogenic shock ensues. When cardiac function has been compromised by previous cardiopulmonary illness, relative smaller emboli obstructing only one or two pulmonary segments can already exert a similar hemodynamic effect.

Right ventricular hypertension can displace the interventricular septum toward the left ventricle, resulting in decreased left ventricular diastolic filling and end-diastolic volume.[23] Among 14 patients with acute massive pulmonary embolism, echocardiography revealed that rapid dilation of the right ventricle accounted for the leftward shift of the interventricular septum and reduced left ventricular compliance. During recovery from pulmonary embolism, the interventricular septum returned progressively to a more normal configuration at both end-systole and end-diastole, and the left ventricular diastolic dimension steadily increased. Thus, circulatory failure owing to massive pulmonary embolism was mediated through a profound decrease in left ventricular preload.[24]

Advantages

By relieving the obstruction to pulmonary artery blood flow, thrombolysis can quickly reduce the elevated pulmonary artery pressure and can reverse right ventricular hypertension. Improved right ventricular function leads to better left ventricular function, which helps reverse cardiogenic shock, thereby possibly reducing the mortality rate from massive pulmonary embolism. In addition, by lysing thrombus quickly, these agents can minimize the potentially adverse impact of the neurohumoral response to pulmonary embolism (Table 25–3). Dissolution of the thrombus should normalize pulmonary arterial blood flow and improve pulmonary tissue perfusion which, in turn, should prevent chronic pulmonary hypertension as a late effect of pulmonary emboli and improve the quality of life. However, opinions differ concerning the long-term benefit of thrombolysis in acute pulmonary embolism.[25] Phear showed that serious symptoms related to chronic throm-

TABLE 25–3. Advantages of Thrombolysis

Proven
    Accelerated clot lysis
    Accelerated pulmonary tissue reperfusion
    Improved pulmonary capillary blood volume
Possible
    Reduced mortality
    Reduced recurrent pulmonary embolism
    Accelerated reversal of right heart failure
    Reduced chronic pulmonary hypertension
    Improved quality of life
    Lysis of venous thrombi, origin of pulmonary emboli

boembolism were often found in patients treated with heparin for an acute pulmonary embolism;[26] similarly, others have reported that mild to severe pulmonary hypertension was frequently observed at late follow-up in patients who received conventional anticoagulant therapy for acute or subacute pulmonary embolism.[27,28] However, many patients involved in these studies and who subsequently developed pulmonary hypertension may well have had a chronic thromboembolic disease when first seen, or untreated recurrent pulmonary embolism during the follow-up period. In fact, several retrospective studies have not found evidence for postembolic pulmonary hypertension in any of the survivors of acute pulmonary embolism, despite a follow-up period ranging from one to nine years.[29,30] Moreover, there was no evidence of late death resulting from unresolved pulmonary embolism[29] and nothing to suggest that the form of the initial treatment (that is, conventional anticoagulation, thrombolysis, or pulmonary embolectomy) had any influence on the long-term prognosis.[31] Furthermore, patients initially treated with heparin or streptokinase were indistinguishable with respect to pulmonary hemodynamics and angiography when examined 0.5 to 8.7 years after treatment.[31] Whatever the initial treatment regimen, abnormal perfusion lung scans were frequently observed long after the initial embolism, thereby suggesting that permanent damage or obstruction of small vessels could occur even though the large pulmonary vessels have cleared.[29,30,32] However, the absence of clinical symptoms suggests that such damage has no prognostic significance, at least during the first ten years. In the Urokinase Pulmonary Embolism Trial (UPET) study, the urokinase-treated patients showed greater initial angiographic improvement and more rapid res-

olution of hemodynamic abnormalities during the first few days.[21] Importantly, after one week, the benefit from thrombolytic therapy could not be demonstrated. One year after the treatment, subtle abnormalities of pulmonary function owing to capillary damage were found to be less in the urokinase-treated patients;[33] Nevertheless, the clinical significance of these findings remains unknown and is probably of no consequence.

Recurrent pulmonary embolism can lead to chronic pulmonary hypertension, especially when the diagnosis of pulmonary embolism is initially overlooked. Planned clinical trials will determine whether thrombolytic treatment reduces long-term morbidity from a single acute pulmonary embolism, regardless of size and initial treatment, is minimal.

Immediate clot lysis might salvage patients with massive pulmonary embolism who would otherwise die in cardiogenic shock. It is also possible that by lysing the source of the pulmonary embolism in situ (usually thrombus in the pelvic or deep leg veins), the rate of recurrent pulmonary embolism might be lowered. Thrombolysis in acute pulmonary embolism appears to reverse rapidly the frequently associated right heart failure.[63]

Clinical Experience with Streptokinase and Urokinase

Numerous trials have been conducted with streptokinase and urokinase, the first thrombolytic agents available for clinical use. The main dosage regimens and main characteristics of these trials are summarized in Table 25–4. Although some of these trials were randomized, others were not. Moreover, the dosing regimen of urokinase differed remarkably.[25] Group 1 (high dosage) includes five studies in which urokinase was employed at a maintenance dosage of 4,400 units/kilogram/hour during 12 to 24 hours with or without a loading dose of 4,400 units/kilogram. In all these trials, the total dose of urokinase exceeded 50,000 units/kilogram. Group 2 (moderate dosage) includes six studies in which a maintenance dosage of 1,600 to 2,700 units/kilogram/hour was infused during 12 to 24 hours. The total dose of urokinase in this group ranged from 35,000 to 48,000 units/kilogram. Group 3 (low dosage) comprises these studies in which a single bolus of 15,000 to 20,000 units/kilogram urokinase was used.

TABLE 25–4. Streptokinase and Urokinase Trials in Pulmonary Embolism

TRIAL	NUMBER OF PATIENTS TREATED	LOADING DOSE	MAINTENANCE DOSE/HOUR	TOTAL DOSE*	DURATION (HOURS)
Streptokinase					
Miller[34]	15	600,000	100,000	7,800,000	72
Tibbutt[35]	13	600,000	100,000	7,800,000	72
USPET[36]	54	250,000	100,000	2,650,000	74
Ly[37]	14	250,000	100,000	7,450,000	72
Luomanmaki[38]	10	600,000	100,000	3,800,000	32
Luomanmaki[38]	20	250,000	100,000	3,450,000	32
Ohayon[39]	12	0	200,000	2,000,000	10
Urokinase Group 1					
UPET[21]	82	4,400	4,400	57,200	12
USPET-12[36]	59	4,400	4,400	57,200	12
USPET-24[36]	54	0	4,400	110,000	24
Ohayon[39]	47	0	4,500	54,000	12
UKEP-12[40]	62	4,400	4,400	52,800	12
Goldhaber[41]	23		4,400	110,000	24
Urokinase Group 2					
Brochier[42]	80	0	1,600	38,400	24
Griguer[43]	30	0	1,600	38,400	24
Barberena[44]	11	2,700	2,700	35,100	12
François[45]	32	0	1,600	38,400	24
François[45]	35	0	1,600	38,400	24
Ohayon[39]	18	0	2,000	48,000	24
UKEP-24[40]	67	0	2,000	48,000	24
Urokinase Group 3					
Dickie[46]	9	15,000	0	15,000	
Petitprez[47]	14	15,000	0	15,000	
Stern[48]	161	20,000	0	20,000	

* Expressed in units per Kg for urokinase.

In the high urokinase dosage group, the average effective angiographic improvement attained is 46 per cent. The use of moderate doses of urokinase (group 2) results in an angiographic improvement similar to that obtained with higher doses. Neither the administration of an initial loading dose nor the route of administration (central or peripheral infusion) appear to affect the angiographic and hemodynamic recoveries. In the only randomized study designed to compare a high to a moderate dosage of urokinase, similar rates of thrombolysis were achieved in the two groups.[40] The low-dose bolus regimen of urokinase used in studies of group 3 is appealing because it also produces angiographic improvement similar to the regimens employing larger doses.

Some of the patients in the Urokinase Streptokinase Pulmonary Embolism Trial (USPET) who underwent pulmonary capillary blood volume testing two weeks and one year after enrollment subsequently agreed to be studied with a (research) right heart catheterization and supine bicycle exercise testing, an average of seven years after the pulmonary embolism. Those assigned initially to thrombolysis had high pulmonary capillary blood volumes at one year[33] and preservation of the normal pulmonary vascular response to exercise at seven years.[49] In contrast, patients who had been treated with anticoagulation alone, on average seven years previously, demonstrated a low pulmonary capillary blood volume at one year and a markedly abnormal rise in pulmonary artery pressure and pulmonary vascular resistance when undergoing supine bicycle exercise during right heart catheterization at seven years after randomization. There was a close inverse correlation between low pulmonary capillary blood volume one year after treatment and high pulmonary vascular resistance seven years after therapy. In addition, only one third as many patients with pulmonary embolism randomly allocated to anticoagulation alone and followed-up for an average of seven years were asymptomatic compared with those who had initially been assigned to receive urokinase or streptokinase followed by anticoagulation.

In an uncontrolled observational study of seven patients with massive pulmonary embolism, all of whom were treated with uro-

TABLE 25–5. Contraindications to Thrombolytic Therapy

ABSOLUTE CONTRAINDICATIONS
Active or recent internal bleeding
History of hemorrhagic stroke (ever)
Intracranial or intraspinal disease (for example, neoplasm)
Recent cranial surgery or head trauma

RELATIVE CONTRAINDICATIONS
Major surgery or trauma within 10 days
Biopsy or invasive procedure in a location inaccessible to external compression within 10 days
Nonhemorrhagic stroke within 1 year
Uncontrolled severe hypertension
Severe coagulation defects (for example, platelets <100,000/cubic millimeter)

kinase, follow-up 15 months later demonstrated sustained improvement of pulmonary hemodynamics both at rest and during exercise. On average, pulmonary arterial pressure decreased from 61/23 torr before treatment to 25/8 torr 6 days later, and 24/9 torr 15 months later.[50]

Contraindications

Contraindications to the use of thrombolytic drugs include intracranial or intraspinal disease, recent surgery, or trauma (Table 25–5). It is wise to test the stools for occult blood and not to administer thrombolytic drugs if the examination demonstrates more than a "trace" of blood. Unlike patients with acute myocardial infarction, those with pulmonary embolism appear to have a much wider time "window" for effective use of thrombolysis. Thrombolytic treatment can be considered in patients with any new symptoms or signs within the two weeks prior to presentation.

Clinical Experience with Recombinant Tissue-Type Plasminogen Activator (alteplase)

Thrombolysis for major pulmonary embolism is not routine, even though the Food and Drug Administration approved urokinase (UK), streptokinase (SK) and recombinant tissue-type plasminogen activator (alteplase) for this purpose. The most important reasons for avoiding thrombolysis have been its inconvenience and the fear of major bleeding complications, particularly as pulmonary embolism is often a postoperative complication. However, during the past decade, the successful utilization of tissue-type plasminogen activator in myocardial infarction treatment has reawakened interest in the thrombolytic treatment of pulmonary embolism (Table 25–6).

In 1985, Bounameaux and colleagues[51] published the first case report of alteplase therapy for pulmonary embolism in a 63-year-old man who had undergone a renal transplant five weeks previously. In a subsequent randomized controlled trial of the European Cooperative Study Group, peripheral intravenous and local pulmonary arterial infusion of alteplase were compared among patients with angiographically documented acute, massive pulmonary embolism.[55] Both routes of administration caused similar rates of lysis, bleeding, and induction of a systemic lytic state. Therefore, peripheral administration of alteplase seems to be as effective as locally delivered alteplase.

Two randomized trials[56,57] have compared alteplase plus heparin versus heparin alone, using pretreatment and post-treatment pulmonary angiograms as the primary endpoint. The one published study demonstrated mild improvement in angiographic score among alteplase-treated patients. However, the major bleeding complications that were described underscore the necessity for careful patient selection.

The American Multicenter Venous Thromboembolism Research Group has completed two clinical trials with alteplase. Pulmonary Embolism Trial-1[52–54] was an open-label study of 47 patients with angiographically documented pulmonary embolism which showed that 50 to 90 milligrams of alteplase administered over two to six hours caused clot lysis in 94 per cent of cases. Clot lysis was graded as moderate or marked in 83 per cent and slight in an additional 11 per cent. Among patients with pulmonary artery hypertension, the pulmonary artery pressures decreased during the acute treatment period from 43/17 to 31/13 torr, without any change in systemic arterial pressure. Two thirds of the patients received more than two hours of alteplase. During the third and subsequent hours of alteplase therapy, however, an increased frequency of bleeding, particularly at the femoral vein puncture site used for pulmonary angiography, led to utilization of a more concentrated alteplase dose administered over a shorter period of time

TABLE 25–6. Selected Trials of Alteplase Thrombolysis in Pulmonary Embolism

INVESTIGATORS	FINDINGS
Case Report	
Bounameaux et al.[51] (1985)	30 milligrams/90 minutes resuscitates a patient with massive pulmonary embolism
Case Series	
Goldhaber et al. Pulmonary Embolism Trial 1[52–54] (1986)	47 patients receive alteplase 50–90 milligrams/2–6 hours and 90 per cent have angiographically documented clot lysis within 6 hours
Randomized Trial: Optimal Route to Administer Alteplase	
Verstraete et al. European Cooperative Study Group for Pulmonary Embolism Study I[55] (1988)	34 patients randomized to either local pulmonary arterial or systemic venous infusion of alteplase. Both routes are similarly effective and safe
Randomized Trials: Alteplase versus Heparin	
PIOPED Investigators[56] (1990)	Alteplase 40 milligrams/40 minutes or 80 milligrams/90 minutes improves only slightly the follow-up angiogram at 2 hours (n = 9); one alteplase-treated patient has major gastrointestinal bleeding; heparin-alone-treated patients (n = 4) have no angiographic improvement
PAIMS 2[57] (1991)	Alteplase 100 milligrams/2 hours plus heparin versus heparin alone. Entry requires base-line pulmonary angiography. The principal endpoint is improvement judged on angiogram or obtained at 2 hours after initiation of the assigned therapy
Levine et al.[58] (1990)	58 patients randomized: alteplase (0.6 milligrams/kilogram/2 minutes) versus heparin; on lung scans, 37 per cent mean relative improvement in perfusion (alteplase) versus 19 per cent (heparin) (p = 0.017); no major bleeding
Randomized Trials: Alteplase Versus Urokinase	
Goldhaber et al. Pulmonary Embolism Trial 2[59] (1988)	45 patients randomized to alteplase 100 milligrams/2 hours versus urokinase 2,000 units/pound bolus followed by 2,000 units/pounds/hour for up to 24 hours; at 2 hours, 82 per cent alteplase and 48 per cent urokinase patients had angiographic lysis; 8 of 23 urokinase patients required premature termination of infusion because of groin bleeding (n = 5), hematuria (n = 2), or hematemesis (n = 1); there was **no difference** in plasma fibrinogen levels or in improvement in lung scans between the two treatment groups
Meyer et al.[60] European Cooperative Study Group For Pulmonary Embolism Study II	63 patients randomized to alteplase 100 milligrams/2 hours versus urokinase 2,000 units/pound bolus followed by 2,000 units/pounds/hour for 12 hours; at 2 hours, total pulmonary resistance decreased by 36 per cent in the alteplase group versus 18 per cent in the urokinase group (p = 0.0009); there was no difference between the 2 groups at 12 hours

Reprinted with permission from Goldhaber SZ. Pulmonary embolism thrombolysis. Prog Cardiovasc Dis 1991; 34: 113–34.

in the subsequent trials of the same group of investigators.

Angiographic and hemodynamic improvement was accompanied by normalization in pulmonary perfusion[61,62] and right ventricular function. One day after alteplase, the perfusion defect score for the 19 patients who had follow-up lung scans improved from 0.37 at baseline to 0.16 (a 57 per cent increase in perfusion), utilizing a new semiquantitative scoring system that integrates data from all six views of the perfusion scan.

Come and colleagues performed Doppler echocardiography on seven patients with pulmonary embolism before and after they received alteplase.[63] Within a day of treatment, the right ventricular end-diastolic diameter decreased from an average of 3.9 to 2.0 centimeters. Right ventricular wall motion,

initially graded as mildly, moderately, or severely hypokinetic in one, two, and four patients, respectively, normalized in five and improved to mild hyperkinesis in two. Tricuspid regurgitation was present before lytic therapy in six patients, but was detected after the completion of lytic therapy in only two patients, and had disappeared by restudy five days later in one of these two patients. The early reversal of the hallmarks or right heart failure (right ventricular dysfunction, right ventricular dilatation, and tricuspid regurgitation) suggests that thrombolytic agents might reduce the mortality from acute pulmonary embolism.

Pulmonary Embolism Trial-2 was a randomized trial comparing 100 milligrams of alteplase over two hours versus 2,000 units/pound of urokinase as a bolus followed by

2,000 units/pound/hour for up to 24 hours.[59] The principal endpoints were improvement on the two-hour angiogram and 24-hour lung scan compared with the baseline studies (Fig. 25–4). All 45 patients received the full dose of alteplase, but urokinase infusions were terminated prematurely in 9 of 23 patients, because of allergy in one and uncontrollable bleeding in eight. By two hours, 82 per cent of alteplase-treated patients showed clot lysis compared with 48 per cent of urokinase-treated patients ($p = 0.0008$) (Fig. 25–5). Thrombolysis at angiography was associated with a return of elevated pulmonary arterial pressures toward normal (Fig. 25–6). Thus, in the dosing regimens employed, alteplase was more rapidly effective and safer than urokinase. However, at 24 hours, there was no difference in scintigraphic improvement between alteplase and urokinase patients. Furthermore, at 2 and 24 hours after initiation of thrombolysis, the fibrinogen levels were similar in both treatment groups.

The European Cooperative Study Group undertook a second study of 63 patients with angiographically documented acute, massive pulmonary embolism who were randomized to receive alteplase 100 milligrams over two hours versus urokinase 2,000 units/pound as a bolus followed by 2,000 units/pound/hour for 12 hours.[60] The principal endpoint was reduction in total pulmonary resistance (TPR) after the initial two hours of therapy. At two hours, total pulmonary resistance decreased 36 per cent in the alteplase group compared with 18 per cent in the urokinase group ($p = 0.0009$). After 12 hours, total pulmonary resistance and angiographic improvement was similar in both groups.

Clinical Setting for Thrombolysis

The clinician can now choose from among three Food and Drug Administration-approved thrombolytic regimens for pulmonary embolism (Table 25–7). Urokinase has been used in clinical trials for more than 20 years and is considered the "gold standard" against which newer thrombolytic agents must be compared. The alteplase regimen appears to act most rapidly and is the simplest and most convenient regimen to administer owing to the short two-hour dosing schedule. It is also free of the fever, chills, and flushing that usually characterize a prolonged infusion of streptokinase and, on rare occasions, accompany urokinase. None of the Food and Drug Administration-approved thrombolytic regimens employs concomitant heparin therapy, an important difference from the usual approach to thrombolysis in myocardial infarc-

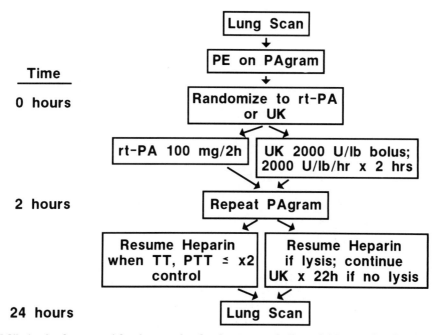

FIGURE 25–4. Study protocol for the completed pulmonary embolism trial-2. (Reprinted with permission from Goldhaber SZ. Tissue plasminogen activator in acute pulmonary embolism. Chest 1989;95:284S.)

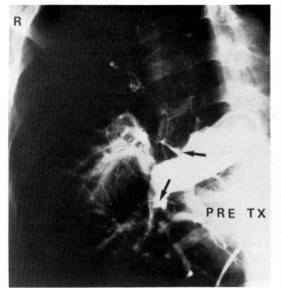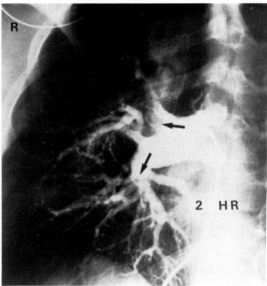

FIGURE 25–5. Pulmonary angiograms (right posterior oblique view) in a 58-year-old man with a five-day history of dyspnea. The left hand panel demonstrates intraluminal thrombus in the right upper and lower lobe arteries (arrows) before treatment. Immediately after two hours of alteplase, the repeat angiogram in the right hand panel demonstrates evidence of clot lysis although some thrombosis persists (arrows). (Reprinted with permission from Goldhaber SZ. Tissue plasminogen activator in acute pulmonary embolism. Chest 1989;95:284S.)

tion. All three regimens employ fixed doses of thrombolytic agents. Therefore, there is no need to obtain laboratory tests during the thrombolytic infusion because no dosage adjustments are made.

Opinions differ on whether it is always necessary to perform pulmonary angiography before initiating thrombolytic therapy; most European centers consider it a rule to obtain a pretreatment diagnostic angiogram, and tolerate only a few exceptions to it.

For patients with high clinical suspicion for pulmonary embolism and high prob-

ability ventilation-perfusion lung scans, there is in the United States increasing acceptance of the concept of proceeding with thrombolytic therapy even when the diagnosis has not been confirmed by angiography. This is particularly the case when the patient is unstable or when angiography is not readily available. However, scans may be misleading and falsely positive in the presence of asthma, chronic pulmonary disease, lung cancer, or prior pulmonary embolism. In these circumstances, further confirmation of the diagnosis with angiography is usually warranted.

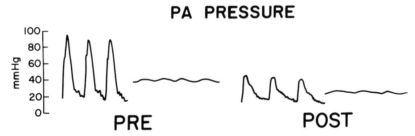

FIGURE 25–6. For the patient whose angiograms are shown in Figure 5, the pulmonary artery pressures were 118/40 (mean pulmonary artery pressure 65) mm Hg before treatment and 53/19 (34) torr after two hours of alteplase. (Reprinted with permission from Goldhaber SZ. Tissue plasminogen activator in acute pulmonary embolism. Chest 1989; 95: 287.)

TABLE 25–7. Food and Drug Administration-Approved Thrombolytic Regimens for Pulmonary Embolism

AGENT	REGIMEN
Streptokinase	250,000 international units as a loading dose over 30 minutes, followed by 100,000 units/hour for 24 hours
Urokinase	2,000 international units/pound as a loading dose over 10 minutes, followed by 2,000 international units/pound/hour for 12–24 hours
Alteplase	100 milligrams as a continuous peripheral intravenous infusion administered over 2 hours

Complications of Thrombolytic Treatment

Trivial superficial oozing at venipuncture or arterial catheter insertion sites may be considered an index of drug efficacy rather than a complication of thrombolytic therapy. Such bleeding can be controlled with manual compression followed by a pressure dressing (Table 25–8). In phase I of the Urokinase Pulmonary Embolism Trial (UPET), severe bleeding, defined as the need for transfusion of more than 2 units of blood or a decrease in hematocrit of more than 10 points, oc-

curred in 27 per cent of the urokinase-treated patients.[21] The large amount of blood drawn for research purposes during the first 24 hours of phase I (about 200 milliliters) contributed to the fall in hematocrit; during phase II,[36] fewer patients (12 per cent) had severe bleeding. In many instances, bleeding occurred at the vascular puncture sites for pulmonary angiography. In the past decade, appropriate patient selection and minimizing the "handling" of patients during the thrombolytic infusion has lessened the bleeding rate. By 1987, the rate of severe bleeding in a multicenter European study of urokinase for pulmonary embolism had decreased to 4 per cent.[40]

Of greatest concern is the risk of intracranial bleeding, which occurs in 2 to 6 of every 1,000 patients treated with thrombolytic therapy. Among patients with a history of migraine, a headache may be precipitated by radiographic contrast agent. The only way to differentiate reliably between an intracranial bleed and a migraine headache is with a head computerized tomographic scan. If intracranial bleeding is suspected, thrombolytic therapy or heparin should be discontinued immediately, and both neurological and neurosurgical consultation should be obtained. An emergent head computerized tomographic scan (without contrast agent) should

TABLE 25–8. Management of Complications From Thrombolytic Therapy*

	MAJOR BLEEDING
Intracranial Bleeding	Discontinue thrombolysis or anticoagulation
	Obtain head computerized tomographic scan
	Consult neurology/neurosurgery
Expanding groin hematoma	Discontinue thrombolysis or anticoagulation
Gross hematuria	Discontinue thrombolysis or anticoagulation
If bleeding continues despite discontinuation of therapy	Order 10 units cryoprecipitate
	Thaw 2 units of fresh frozen plasma
	Reverse heparin with protamine
	Transfuse platelet concentrate if bleeding time is prolonged
	Type and cross-packed red blood cells
	Obtain consultation for endoscopic/surgical control of bleeding
	MINOR BLEEDING
Superficial skin oozing	Apply manual pressure
	Determine if source is vascular puncture site
Gingival oozing	Pack gingiva with gauze
	Dental consult if oozing persists
	ALLERGY
Fever	Acetaminophen 650–1000 milligrams orally
	Hydrocortisone 100 milligrams intravenously
Nausea	Diphenhydramine 25–50 milligrams intravenously
	Lorazepam 1–2 milligrams intravenously
Chills/rigors	Meperidine 50–100 milligrams intravenously

* Reprinted with permission from Goldhaber SZ. Pulmonary embolism thrombolysis. Prog Cardiovasc Dis 1991; 34: 113–34.

be ordered. The head computerized tomographic scan is more sensitive to fresh blood than magnetic resonance imaging scanning. It is to be kept in mind that contrast material can be seen on the noncontrast head computerized tomographic scan for several hours after pulmonary angiography and can simulate intracerebral blood.

Retroperitoneal hemorrhage can also be life threatening because the bleeding is often sustained, brisk, and difficult to diagnose. This complication can occur during the femoral vein catheterization for pulmonary angiography if an artery is inadvertently punctured above the inguinal ligament. Gross hematuria and other internal bleeding can generally be well managed by discontinuing therapy.

If bleeding is brisk or potentially life threatening, 10 units of cryoprecipitate should be given. Each unit contains approximately 200 to 500 milligrams of fibrinogen and 80 units of factor VIII in a volume of 10 to 15 milliliters. A dose of 10 units will increase the fibrinogen level by about 70 milligrams/deciliter and the factor VIII level by about 30 per cent of normal circulating levels. Cryoprecipitate can be thawed rapidly and should be available within ten minutes of a request. In addition, two units of fresh frozen plasma should be ordered. Fresh frozen plasma, which may take 45 minutes to thaw, is a source of factors V and VIII as well as alpha$_2$-antiplasmin, fibrinogen, and other coagulation factors.[18]

Minor allergic reactions owing to streptokinase or, less often, urokinase occur occasionally and are manifested by fever and chills. In an attempt to suppress this reaction, steroids, diphenhydramine, and acetaminophen can be administered prophylactically. If rigors do occur, they can be effectively treated with 50 to 100 milligrams of intravenous meperidine.

Bolus Thrombolysis

The concept of bolus thrombolysis for venous thromboembolism is not new (Table 25–9). In 1974, Dickie et al. described the use of bolus urokinase to treat pulmonary embolism.[46] These investigators employed bolus thrombolysis because most deaths after pulmonary embolism occurred within the first few hours after arrival at the hospital. Ten years later, the outcome of 14 patients with pulmonary embolism treated with 15,000 international units/kilogram of urokinase over ten minutes was described; there was a 34 per cent decrease in pulmonary vascular obstruction within 12 hours after treatment.[47] In addition to anatomic improvement, there was a 20 to 30 per cent decrease in pulmonary artery mean pressure and in total pulmonary resistance within the first three hours after the injection of urokinase. This is an important point, since a prompt decrease in right ventricular strain may be of critical value to unstable patients. The rapid decline in these parameters is probably due to prompt dissolution of thromboemboli in the pulmonary circulation rather than a consequence of a hypothetical vasodilating effect of urokinase on pulmonary vessels. It has been shown that the relationship between total pulmonary resistance and the level of pulmonary vascular obstruction is hyperbolic; a sharp increase in total pulmonary resistance occurs when the pulmonary vascular obstruction exceeds 60 per cent.[61] Therefore, even modest early reperfusion could result in a marked decrease in total pulmonary resistance. This latter

TABLE 25–9. Selected Experimental or Clinical Studies of Bolus Thrombolysis*

MODEL/ INVESTIGATORS	FINDINGS
Dickie et al.[46] (1974)	9 patients receive pulmonary arterial injections of bolus urokinase over 6–10 minutes; repeated daily boluses depended upon clinical response and fibrinogen levels
Petitpretz et al.[47] (1984)	14 patients receive right atrial injections of bolus urokinase 15,000 units/kilogram/10 minutes of urokinase; the greatest hemodynamic improvement occurred during the first 3 hours after the bolus
Levine et al.[58] (1990)	58 patients randomized: alteplase (0.6) milligrams/kilogram/2 minutes) versus heparin; on lung scans, 37 per cent mean relative improvement in perfusion (alteplase) versus 19 per cent (heparin) ($p = 0.017$); no major bleeding

* Reprinted with permission from Goldhaber SZ: Pulmonary embolism thrombolysis. Prog Cardiovasc Dis 1991; 34: 113–34.

finding also emphasizes the lack of sensitivity of the pulmonary angiography to assess the early effects of thrombolytic agents.

Recently, Levine et al. published a clinical study of pulmonary embolism[58] which suggests that weight-adjusted bolus alteplase can achieve comparable efficacy (assessed by pulmonary reperfusion on pretreatment and post-treatment perfusion lung scans) to the efficacy achieved in the alteplase versus urokinase trial[59] and to the pulmonary reperfusion observed in the Urokinase Pulmonary Embolism Trial.[21] Fifty-eight patients with subacute pulmonary embolism were randomized either to alteplase (0.6 milligram/kilogram ideal body weight) as a bolus over two minutes or to placebo. Continuous intravenous heparin therapy was given in the two groups and interrupted only for the duration of the study drug infusion. At 24 hours, the mean relative improvement in the baseline perfusion lung scan defect was 37.0 per cent in alteplase-treated patients compared with 18.8 per cent in the placebo group ($p = 0.017$). There were no major bleeds in either group. For patients who received alteplase, there was a decrease of approximately one-third from the baseline fibrinogen level at 30 minutes.

Thus, a bolus of alteplase Figure 25-7 appears to be a promising treatment strategy for patients with pulmonary emboli. However, its safety and efficacy has not been tested in a randomized controlled trial against a standard Food and Drug Administration-approved regimen for thrombolytic treatment of pulmonary embolism. The use of bolus alteplase (70 mg) in sixty patients with acute myocardial infarction did not induce major bleeding. Nevertheless, bolus thrombolysis warrants intensive investigation with randomized clinical trials.

Contemporary Thrombolysis for Pulmonary Embolism

How often do patients with *subacute* pulmonary embolism have contraindications to thrombolytic treatment? To address this question, a group of 44 institutions across the United States was surveyed for a one-year period. The group was composed of patients with pulmonary embolism confirmed by high-probability lung scan or pulmonary angiography. Of 2,539 patients with pulmonary embolism, 1,314 (53 per cent) would have been acceptable for treatment with thrombolysis,[65] even after excluding patients with the usual contraindications to this therapy (Table 25–10). Thus, thrombolysis appears to have potentially widespread use as a ther-

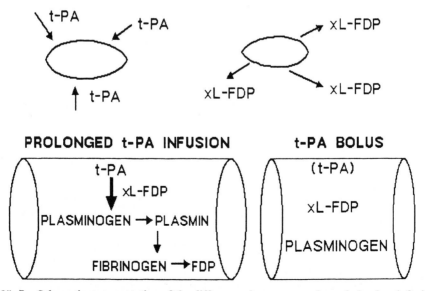

FIGURE 25–7. Schematic representation of the differences between a prolonged alteplase infusion versus a alteplase bolus. xL-FDP = Cross-linked fibrinogen degradation products. (Reprinted with permission from Agnelli G: Rationale for bolus alteplase therapy to improve efficacy and safety. Chest 1990;97:164S.)

TABLE 25–10. Frequency of Exclusion Criteria for Thrombolysis in Patients with Pulmonary Embolism—TIPE Patient Survey*

EXCLUSION CRITERIA	FREQUENCY Number (%)
Risk of blood loss	
Internal or significant bleeding within 6 months	255 (10.1)
Internal surgery or organ biopsy within 10 days	410 (16.2)
Hematocrit of <30 per cent	283 (11.2)
Occult blood in stool	165 (6.5)
Abnormal findings on liver function tests	178 (7.0)
Central nervous system risk	
Cerebrovascular accident or transient ischemic attack	234 (9.2)
Intracranial or intraspinal surgery	148 (5.8)
Intracranial or intraspinal disease	226 (8.9)
Infective endocarditis	9 (0.4)
Severe arterial hypertension	7 (0.3)
Special risks	
Hemorrhagic retinopathy	6 (0.2)
Open heart surgery within 2 weeks	63 (2.5)
Pregnancy	7 (0.3)
Survival	
Expected <1 month	116 (4.6)

* Adapted from Terrin et al. Selection of patients with acute pulmonary embolism for thrombolytic therapy. Thrombolysis in pulmonary embolism (TIPE) patient survey. Chest 1989; 95: 279S–81S, with permission.

apeutic strategy among pulmonary embolism patients. Safety and convenience can be enhanced by delivering shorter, more concentrated infusions.

The principal reason for continued disagreement on indications for thrombolysis in pulmonary embolism is that the advantage of thrombolytic therapy over heparin therapy has not yet been demonstrated definitively with clinically relevant endpoints. It is to be hoped that in the future, a properly designed, international multicenter trial can be undertaken to compare the optimal thrombolytic regimen followed by heparin, with heparin alone. If such a large-scale international study is ever initiated, clinical endpoints might include reduction of mortality, recurrent pulmonary embolism, number of days in the intensive care unit, chronic venous insufficiency, and an improvement in quality of life, including an earlier return to work.

DEEP VEIN THROMBOLYSIS

Thrombolysis for deep vein thrombosis is often precluded by the high frequency of patients who are postoperative or who have gastrointestinal or other major bleeding. It is estimated that only about one in five patients with venographically documented deep vein thrombosis is an acceptable candidate for thrombolysis, even if elderly patients are not excluded from therapy.

The doses of unfractionated and low molecular weight heparin which have been shown to be effective in the treatment of deep vein thrombosis are given in Chapter 5. Thrombolysis for deep vein thrombosis should aid in lysing thrombi in situ, thereby decreasing the frequency of pulmonary embolism. In addition, thrombolysis should minimize damage to venous valves caused by residual thrombus, thereby decreasing the frequency of chronic venous insufficiency. The principal challenge is finding an effective and safe thrombolytic regimen for deep vein thrombosis. Currently, the only Food and Drug Administration-approved thrombolytic treatment of deep vein thrombosis is with streptokinase in a dose of 250,000 units as a 30-minute bolus followed by 100,000 units/hour for 24 to 72 hours. Overviews of randomized trials demonstrate that streptokinase followed by heparin is approximately four times more effective than heparin alone at lysing deep vein thrombosis.[66,67] However, major bleeding complications owing to streptokinase occur about three times more frequently than with heparin alone.

A recently completed American, controlled study in deep vein thrombosis randomizing alteplase and heparin versus heparin alone indicated that the addition of heparin to alteplase does not improve the lysis rate.[68] Surprisingly, heparin did not increase the risk of bleeding from alteplase therapy. This trial employed a low-dose, 24-hour continuous infusion of alteplase.

INFERIOR VENA CAVAL INTERRUPTION

There are three major indications for inferior vena cava filter placement in patients with deep vein thrombosis with or without pulmonary thromboembolism: (a) contraindication to anticoagulation, (b) failure of adequate anticoagulation, and (c) serious bleed-

TABLE 25–11. Percutaneous Insertion of Inferior Vena Cava Filters*

INDICATIONS

Anticoagulation contraindicated in patients with known pulmonary emboli:
Bleeding, or known risk of bleeding (for example, gastrointestinal)
Patients with complications of anticoagulation (for example, central nervous system hemorrhage, heparin-induced thrombocytopenia)
Anticoagulation failure despite adequate therapy (for example, recurrent pulmonary embolism)
Prophylactic for high risk patients:
    Extensive or progressive deep vein thrombophlebitis
    Following surgical pulmonary embolectomy
    Severe pulmonary hypertension; cor pulmonale

CONTRAINDICATIONS†

Severe blood coagulopathy, predisposing to bleeding from the puncture site
Anticipated patient noncompliance with postprocedure rest orders (especially with 24 French filter systems)
Obstructing thrombus along the available route(s) of insertion

* Reprinted with permission from Goldhaber SZ, Grassi CJ. Management of pulmonary embolism. In: Sabiston DC Jr, ed. Textbook of surgery update 8. Philadelphia: WB Saunders Co., 1990: 119.
† Surgical venotomy preferred.

ing during anticoagulation notwithstanding a therapeutic international normalized ratio level.[69–71] In most circumstances, the filter is placed percutaneously, but occasionally, a surgical venotomy is preferred (Table 25–11).

PULMONARY EMBOLECTOMY

Pulmonary embolectomy can be utilized to treat pulmonary emboli in two different clinical settings: (a) when pulmonary embolism is associated with persistent shock,[72–75] and (b) to treat disabling dyspnea in patients with chronic pulmonary hypertension due to occult or recurrent pulmonary emboli.[72,73] Acute pulmonary embolectomy should be reserved for patients in extremis in whom thrombolytic therapy is contraindicated or is failing. Embolectomy should also be considered in patients with massive pulmonary emboli owing to right atrial or right ventricular thrombus in whom an inferior vena caval filter would be useless, particularly when thrombolytic agents fail to lyse these sources of pulmonary embolism.

At the Laënnec Hospital, Paris, 96 consecutive patients with acute massive pulmonary embolism (of 3,000 with confirmed pulmo-

nary embolism) underwent pulmonary embolectomy between 1968 and 1988.[75] Total cardiopulmonary bypass under normothermia and without aortic cross-clamping was utilized in all cases. There were 36 in-hospital deaths (37 per cent), most often due to cardiogenic shock (n = 13), pulmonary hemorrhage (n = 8), and mediastinitis (n = 4), the remaining 11 deaths owing to a variety of causes. Preoperative cardiac arrest and underlying cardiopulmonary disease were two independent predictors of postoperative death. Neither the interval between the first embolic episode and operation nor the initiation of thrombolytic therapy a few hours before operation predicted postoperative death. Long-term follow-up (2 to 144 months; mean 56 months) was available for 55 of the 60 patients discharged from hospital: six had died, and five complained of persistent or severe exertional dyspnea. These results help to assess the perioperative risk in patients undergoing pulmonary embolectomy. They also show that in the few patients who do not benefit from optimal medical therapy, pulmonary embolectomy remains an acceptable procedure in view of the long-term results.

Chronic pulmonary hypertension owing to pulmonary embolism is usually refractory to anticoagulants and thrombolytic agents, but can sometimes be managed with pulmonary thromboendarterectomy.[76] Surgical success leads to a dramatic reduction in symptoms, with associated improvements noted on lung scanning and pulmonary angiography. Pulmonary thromboendarterectomy produces an early marked reduction of pulmonary hypertension which is often sustained.[77]

FUTURE THERAPEUTIC CONSIDERATIONS

Thrombolytic therapy will become more widely utilized in deep vein thrombosis and pulmonary embolism if an optimal dosing regimen of an agent can be found that is both safe and convenient to administer. This will undoubtedly require administering higher concentrations of drug over shorter time periods than has been customary. Other future approaches include development of specific thrombin inhibitors such as hirudin[78] and refinement of low molecular weight heparins.[15]

ACKNOWLEDGMENT: We gratefully acknowledge

the careful review and helpful suggestions of Jack Hirsh, M.D.

REFERENCES

1. Anderson FA Jr, Wheeler HB, Goldberg RJ, et al. A population-based perspective of the hospital incidence and case-fatality rates of venous thrombosis and pulmonary embolism: the Worcester DVT Study. Arch Intern Med 1991; 151: 933–8.
2. Lilienfeld DE, Chan E, Ehland J, et al. Mortality from pulmonary embolism in the United States: 1962 to 1984. Chest 1990; 98: 1067–72.
3. Barritt DW, Jordan SC. Anticoagulant drugs in the treatment of pulmonary embolism. A controlled trial. Lancet 1960; 1: 1309–12.
4. Hyers TM, Hull RD, Weg JG. Antithrombotic therapy for venous thromboembolic disease. Chest 1989; 95: 37S–51S.
5. Doyle DJ, Turpie AGG, Hirsh J, et al. Adjusted subcutaneous heparin or continuous intravenous heparin in patients with acute deep vein thrombosis. Ann Intern Med 1987; 107: 441–5.
6. Huisman MV, Büller HR, ten Cate JW, et al. Unexpected high prevalence of silent pulmonary embolism in patients with deep venous thrombosis. Chest 1989; 95: 498–502.
7. Lagerstedt CI, Olsson C-G, Fagher BO, Öqvist BW, Albrechtsson U. Need for long-term anticoagulant treatment in symptomatic calf-vein thrombosis. Lancet 1985; 2: 515–8.
8. Landefeld CS, Cook EF, Flatley M, et al. Identification and preliminary validation of predictors of major bleeding in hospitalized patients starting anticoagulant therapy. Am J Med 1987; 82: 703–13.
9. Cruickshank MK, Levine MN, Hirsh J, Roberts R, Siguenza M. A standard heparin nomogram for the management of heparin therapy. Arch Intern Med 1991; 151: 333–7.
10. Wheeler AP, Jaquiss RDB, Newman JH. Physician practices in the treatment of pulmonary embolism and deep venous thrombosis. Arch Intern Med 1988; 148: 1321–5.
11. Beaver BL, Young D, Satiani B. Prediction of heparin requirements in acute thromboplastic venous disease. Arch Surg 1985; 120: 436–8.
12. Hirsh J, van Aken WG, Gallus AS, Dollery CT, Cade JF, Yung WL. Heparin kinetics in venous thrombosis and pulmonary embolism. Circulation 1976; 53: 691–5.
13. Ginsberg JS, Kowalchuk G, Hirsh J, Brill-Edwards P, Burrows R. Heparin therapy during pregnancy. Arch Intern Med 1989; 149: 2233–6.
14. Albada J, Nieuwenhuis HK, Sixma JJ. Treatment of acute venous thromboembolism with low molecular weight heparin (Fragmin). Circulation 1989; 80: 935–40.
15. Levine M, Hirsh J, Gent M, et al. Prevention of deep vein thrombosis after elective hip surgery. A randomized trial comparing low molecular weight heparin with standard unfractionated heparin. Ann Intern Med 1991; 114: 545–51.
16. Landefeld CS, Cook EF, Flatley M, Weisberg M, Goldman L. Identification and preliminary validation of predictors of major bleeding in hospitalized patients starting anticoagulant therapy. Am J Med 1987; 82: 703–13.
17. Olin JW, Young JR, Graor RA, Ruschhaupt WF, Beven EG, Bay JW. Treatment of deep vein thrombosis and pulmonary emboli in patients with primary and metastatic brain tumors. Arch Intern Med 1987; 147: 2177–9.
18. Sane DC, Califf RM, Topol EJ, Stump DC, Mark DB, Greenberg CS. Bleeding during thrombolytic therapy for acute myocardial infarction: mechanisms and management. Ann Intern Med 1989; 111: 1010–22.
19. Gallus A, Jackaman J, Tillett J, Mills W, Wycherley A. Safety and efficacy of warfarin started early after submassive venous thrombosis or pulmonary embolism. Lancet 1986; 2: 1293–6.
20. Hull RD, Raskob GE, Rosenbloom D, et al. Heparin for 5 days as compared with 10 days in the initial treatment of proximal venous thrombosis. N Engl J Med 1990; 322: 1260–4.
21. The Urokinase Pulmonary Embolism Trial. A national cooperative study. Circulation 1973; 47 (suppl II): 1–108.
22. Landefeld CS, Rosenblatt MW, Goldman L. Bleeding in outpatients treated with warfarin: relation to the prothrombin time and important remediable lesions. Am J Med 1989; 87: 153–9.
23. Visner MS, Arentzen CE, O'Connor MD, Larson EV, Anderson RW. Alterations in left ventricular three-dimensional dynamic geometry during acute right ventricular hypertension in the conscious dog. Circulation 1983; 67: 353–65.
24. Jardin F, Dubourg O, Gueret P, Delorme G, Bourdarias J-P. Quantitative two-dimensional echocardiography in massive pulmonary embolism: emphasis on ventricular interdependence and leftward septal displacement. J Am Coll Cardiol 1987; 10: 1201–6.
25. Meyer G, Charbonnier B, Stern M, Brochier ML, Sors S. Thrombolysis in pulmonary embolism. In: Julian DG, Kübler W, Norris RM, Swan HJ, Collen D, Verstraete M, eds. Thrombolysis in cardiovascular disease. New York: Marcel Dekker, Inc., 1989: 337–60.
26. Phear D. Pulmonary embolism: a study of late prognosis. Lancet 1960; 2: 832–5.
27. de Soyza NDB, Murphy ML. Persistent post-embolic pulmonary hypertension. Chest 1972; 62: 665–8.
28. Riedel M, Stanek V, Widimsky J, et al. Longterm follow-up of patients with pulmonary thromboembolism. Chest 1982; 81: 151–8.
29. Hall RJC, Sutton GC, Kerr IH. Long-term prognosis of treated acute massive pulmonary embolism. Br Heart J 1977; 39: 1128–34.
30. Sutton GC, Hall RJC, Kerr IH. Clinical course and late prognosis of treated subacute massive, acute minor, and chronic pulmonary thromboembolism. Br Heart J 1977; 39: 1135–42.
31. Lund O, Nielssen TT, Ronne K, et al. Pulmonary embolism: long-term follow up after treatment with full-dose heparin, streptokinase or embolectomy. Acta Med Scand 1987; 221: 61–71.
32. Paraskos JA, Adelstein SJ, Smith RE, et al. Late prognosis of acute pulmonary embolism. N Engl J Med 1973; 289: 55–8.
33. Sharma GVRK, Burleson VA, Sasahara AA. Effect of thrombolytic therapy on pulmonary-capillary blood volume in patients with pulmonary embolism. N Engl J Med 1980; 303: 842–5.
34. Miller GAH, Sutton GC, Kerr IH, et al. Comparison of streptokinase and heparin in treatment of isolated acute massive pulmonary embolism. Br Med J 1971; 2: 681–4.
35. Tibbutt DA, Davies JA, Anderson JA, et al. Comparison by controlled clinical trial of streptokinase and heparin in treatment of life-threatening pulmonary embolism. Br Med J 1974; 1: 343–7.
36. Urokinase-Streptokinase Embolism Trial. Phase 2 results. A cooperative study. JAMA 1974; 229: 1606–13.
37. Ly B, Arnesen H, Eie H, Hol R. A controlled clinical trial of streptokinase and heparin in the treatment of major pulmonary embolism. Acta Med Scand 1978; 203: 465–70.
38. Luomanmaki K, Halttunen PK, Hekali P, et al. Experience with streptokinase treatment of major pulmonary embolism. Ann Clin Res 1983; 15: 21–5.
39. Ohayon J, Colle JP, Tauzin-Fin P, et al. Evolution hémodynamique au cours des fibrinolyses de l'embolie pulmonaire grave. Arch Mal Coeur 1986; 79: 445–53.
40. The UKEP Study: Multicentre clinical trial on two local regimens of urokinase in massive pulmonary embolism. Eur Heart J 1987; 8: 2–10.
41. Goldhaber SZ, Kessler CM, Heit J, et al. Randomised controlled trial of recombinant tissue plasminogen activator versus urokinase in the treatment of acute pulmonary embolism. Lancet 1988; 2: 293–8.
42. Brochier M, Fauchier JP, Griguer P, et al. Le traitement thrombolytique de l'embolie pulmonaire (A propos de 80 cas traités par urokinase). Angéiologie 1976; 28: 299–312.
43. Griguer P, Charbonnier B, Latour F, et al. Plasminogen and moderate doses of urokinase in the treatment of acute pulmonary embolism. Angiology 1979; 30: 1–12.
44. Barberena J. Intraarterial infusion of urokinase in the treatment of acute pulmonary thromboembolism: preliminary observations. AJR 1983; 140: 883–6.
45. François G, Charbonnier B, Raynaud P, et al. Traitement de l'embolie pulmonaire aigue par urokinase comparée à l'as-

sociation plasminogène-urokinase. A propos de 67 cas. Arch Mal Coeur 1986; 79: 435–42.

46. Dickie KJ, de Groot WJ, Cooley RN, et al. Hemodynamic effects of bolus infusion of urokinase in pulmonary thromboembolism. Am Rev Respir Dis 1974; 109: 48–56.

47. Petitpretz P, Simmoneau G, Cerrina J, et al. Effects of a single bolus of urokinase in patients with life-threatening pulmonary emboli: a descriptive trial. Circulation 1984; 70: 861–6.

48. Stern M, Meyer G, Sors H. Urokinase versus tissue plasminogen activator in pulmonary embolism (letter). Lancet 1988; 2: 691–2.

49. Sharma GVRK, Folland ED, McIntyre KM, Sasahara AA. Longterm hemodynamic benefit of thrombolytic therapy in pulmonary embolic disease (abstr). JACC 1990; 15: 65A.

50. Schwarz F, Stehr H, Zimmermann R, et al. Sustained improvement of pulmonary hemodynamics in patients at rest and during exercise after thrombolytic treatment of massive pulmonary embolism. Circulation 1985; 71: 117–23.

51. Bounameaux H, Vermylen J, Collen D. Thrombolytic treatment with recombinant tissue-type plasminogen activator in a patient with massive pulmonary embolism. Ann Intern Med 1985; 103: 64–6.

52. Goldhaber SZ, Vaughan DE, Markis JE, et al. Acute pulmonary embolism treated with tissue plasminogen activator. Lancet 1986; 2: 886–9.

53. Goldhaber SZ, Markis JE, Kessler CM, et al. Perspectives on treatment of acute pulmonary embolism with tissue plasminogen activator. Semin Thromb Hemost 1987; 13: 221–7.

54. Goldhaber SZ, Meyerovitz MF, Markis JE, et al., on behalf of the Participating Investigators. Thrombolytic therapy of acute pulmonary embolism: current status and future potential. JACC 1987; 10: 96B–104B.

55. Verstraete M, Miller GAH, Bounameaux H, et al. Intravenous and intrapulmonary recombinant tissue-type plasminogen activator in the treatment of acute massive pulmonary embolism. Circulation 1988; 77: 353–60.

56. A Collaborative Study by the PIOPED Investigators. Tissue plasminogen activator for the treatment of acute pulmonary embolism. Chest 1990; 97: 528–33.

57. PAIMS 2. Plasminogen Activator Italian Multicenter Study 2. A comparison between rt-PA plus heparin and heparin only in the treatment of pulmonary embolism. 1991 Personal Communication.

58. Levine MN, Hirsh J, Weitz J, et al. A randomized trial of a single bolus dosage regimen of recombinant tissue plasminogen activator in patients with acute pulmonary embolism. Chest 1990; 98: 1473–9.

59. Goldhaber SZ, Kessler CM, Heit J, et al. A randomized controlled trial of recombinant tissue plasminogen activator versus urokinase in the treatment of acute pulmonary embolism. Lancet 1988; 2: 293–8.

60. Meyer G, Sors H, Charbonnier B, et al. The effects of intravenous urokinase versus alteplase on total pulmonary resistance in acute massive pulmonary embolism. A European multicenter double-blind trial. JACC 1991; in press.

61. Safran D, Raynaud P, Dennewald G, Sors H, Even P. Hémodynamique et échanges gazeux dans l'embolie pulmonaire. A propos de 150 cas. In: Goulon M, Rapin M, eds. Réanimation et médecine d'urgence. Paris.

62. Parker JA, Markis JE, Palla A, et al., on behalf of the Participating Investigators. Early improvement in pulmonary perfusion after rt-PA therapy for acute embolism: segmental perfusion scan analysis. Radiology 1988; 166: 441–5.

63. Come PC, Kim D, Parker JA, Goldhaber SZ, Braunwald E, Markis JE, and Participating Investigators. Early reversal of right ventricular dysfunction in patients with acute pulmonary embolism after treatment with intravenous tissue plasminogen activator. JACC 1987; 10: 971–8.

64. Chamone B, Cobbaert C, DeWerf van F, et al. Coronary recanalization rate after intravenous bolus of alteplase in acute myocardial infarction. Am J Cardiol 1991; 68: 161–5.

65. Terrin M, Goldhaber SZ, Thompson B, and the TIPE Investigators. Selection of patients with acute pulmonary embolism for thrombolytic therapy. Thrombolysis in Pulmonary Embolism (TIPE) patient survey. Chest 1989; 95: 279S–81S.

66. Goldhaber SZ, Buring JE, Lipnick RJ, Hennekens CH. Pooled analyses of randomized trials of streptokinase and heparin in phlebographically documented acute deep venous thrombosis. Am J Med 1984; 76: 393–7.

67. Rogers LQ, Lutcher CL. Streptokinase therapy for deep vein thrombosis: a comprehensive review of the English literature. Am J Med 1990; 88: 389–95.

68. Goldhaber SZ, Meyerovitz MF, Green D. Randomized controlled trial of tissue plasminogen activator in proximal deep venous thrombosis. Am J Med 1990; 88: 235–40.

69. Meyer G, Raynaud P, Even P, et al. L'interruption de la veine cave inférieure en pathologie thrombo-embolique. La Presse Méd 1990; 19: 1347–8.

70. Grassi CJ, Goldhaber SZ. Interruption of the vena cava for the prevention of pulmonary embolism: transvenous filter devices. Herz 1989; 14: 182–91.

71. Dorfman GS. Percutaneous inferior vena caval filters. Radiology 1990; 174: 987–92.

72. Clarke DB, Abrams LD. Pulmonary embolectomy: a 25 year experience. J Thorac Cardiovasc Surg 1986; 92: 442–5.

73. Gray HH, Miller GAH, Paneth M. Pulmonary embolectomy: its place in the management of pulmonary embolism. Lancet 1988; 1: 1441–5.

74. Gray HH, Morgan JM, Paneth M, et al. Pulmonary embolectomy for acute massive pulmonary embolism: an analysis of 71 cases. Br Heart J 1988; 60: 196.

75. Meyer G, Tamisier D, Sors H, et al. Pulmonary embolectomy: a 20-year experience at one center. Ann Thorac Surg 1991; 51: 232–6.

76. Daily PO, Dembitsky WP, Iversen S, et al. Risk factors for pulmonary thromboendarterectomy. J Thorac Cardiovasc Surg 1990; 99: 670–8.

77. Moser KM, Auger WR, Fedullo PF. Chronic major-vessel thromboembolic pulmonary hypertension. Circulation 1990; 81: 1735–43.

78. Weitz JI, Hudoba M, Massel D, Maraganore J, Hirsh J. Clot-bound thrombin is protected from inhibition by heparin-antithrombin III but is susceptible to inactivation by antithrombin III-independent inhibitors. J Clin Invest 1990; 86: 385–91.

26

ANTICOAGULANTS DURING PREGNANCY

JEFFREY S. GINSBERG and JACK HIRSH

The use of anticoagulants during pregnancy is problematic because heparin and oral anticoagulant drugs have the potential to produce adverse effects in the mother and fetus. Anticoagulant therapy during pregnancy is indicated for the prevention and treatment of venous thromboembolism and for the prevention and treatment of systemic embolism associated with valvular heart disease or prosthetic heart valves or both. The use of heparin for the treatment of preeclampsia-toxemia[1] and glomerulonephritis,[2] and for the prevention of fetal wastage associated with the lupus anticoagulant,[3] has been reported in small studies, but the efficacy for these conditions is not well established. Most published reports of anticoagulant therapy during pregnancy are small retrospective studies, and therefore, it is difficult to provide definitive recommendations. In this chapter, the fetal and maternal effects of oral anticoagulants and standard heparin will be reviewed and recommendations for their use in patients with venous and cardiovascular disease at risk of thromboembolism.

FETAL EFFECTS OF ANTICOAGULANTS

Heparin is an anionic mucopolysaccharide that does not cross the placenta[4] and is not expected to produce adverse fetal effects, whereas the oral anticoagulants are low molecular weight vitamin K antagonists which cross the placenta and have teratogenic potential.[5] However, a study in which an extensive literature review was performed[6] concluded that approximately one third of pregnancies in which anticoagulant therapy was administered was associated with adverse outcomes regardless of whether heparin or oral anticoagulants were used. The use of coumarin derivatives was associated with warfarin embryopathy, central nervous system abnormalities, fetal hemorrhage, abortions, and stillbirths, so that at most, two thirds of pregnancies resulted in normal infants. On the other hand, heparin therapy during pregnancy was associated with an increase in stillbirths and prematurity and again, only two thirds of pregnancies were normal. Close scrutiny of the literature that was reviewed indicates that a large proportion of the heparin-treated patients had comorbid conditions that are independently associated with adverse fetal outcomes.[7] Thus, 49 of 145 (34 per cent) pregnancies in which heparin was used were associated with severe toxemia, glomerulonephritis, or recurrent abortions. This is attributable to the practice of administering heparin therapy to pregnant women with these conditions. There were 31 (63.3 per cent) adverse fetal outcomes in this subgroup of 49 patients. In contrast, only 4 of the 431 (0.9 per cent) pregnancies associated with oral anticoagulant therapy had comorbid conditions independently associated with adverse fetal outcomes (recurrent abortions). Furthermore, many of the adverse outcomes in the heparin-treated patients were prematurity (gestational age less than 37 weeks) where the infants ultimately suffered no permanent disability or deformity. At worst, these should be considered to be transient adverse outcomes.

In an independent literature review,[8] 186 studies which reported 1,325 pregnancies associated with anticoagulant therapy were identified, including all studies reviewed by Hall et al., and studies identified in a literature search of published articles through 1986. In an attempt to overcome the limitations of the study by Hall et al., four separate analyses were performed. The initial analysis included reported adverse fetal outcomes with all pregnancies included (first analysis). A second analysis was then performed in which all pregnancies that had comorbid conditions independently associated with adverse fetal outcomes were excluded (second analysis). To avoid bias, an obstetrician experienced in high-risk pregnancies compiled a list of comorbid conditions before the data were accumulated and analyzed. Pregnancies associated with these comorbid conditions were excluded from the second analysis regardless of fetal outcomes. A third analysis was then performed by excluding from the second analysis premature births (less than 37 weeks gestation), in which the infant ultimately suffered no permanent deformity or disability. Finally, a fourth subgroup analysis was performed which included only abortions, stillbirths, and neonatal deaths as adverse outcomes in those pregnancies without comorbid conditions. Based on the results of this study it was concluded that the reported high rate of adverse fetal/infant outcomes associated with heparin therapy, but not oral anticoagulant therapy, can be explained by the frequent presence of comorbid conditions and the higher rate of uncomplicated prematurity.

Drawing firm conclusions on the basis of this literature review is difficult because most published studies reviewed were small retrospective reports. A recent retrospective cohort study of 100 consecutive pregnancies associated with standard heparin therapy in 77 women provides reasonable estimates of the fetal and maternal risks of maternal heparin therapy.[9] Heparin was administered in 98 pregnancies for the prevention of venous thromboembolism, and in two pregnancies for the prevention of systemic embolism from prosthetic heart valves. Forty-three of the patients were treated because of acute deep vein thrombosis or pulmonary embolism and received heparin by continuous infusion for 7 to 14 days in doses adjusted to prolong the activated partial thromboplastin time to 55 to 85 seconds. This was followed by full-dose, 12-hourly, subcutaneous injections of heparin, adjusted to prolong a mid-interval (six-hour postinjection) activated partial thromboplastin time to one and a half times control, until term. Fifty-five of the patients received heparin because of previous venous thromboembolism. These patients received heparin 5,000 units 12-hourly by subcutaneous injections until the middle of the third trimester, and then full-dose subcutaneous heparin (see above) until term. Both patients with prosthetic heart valves received full-dose subcutaneous heparin throughout pregnancy. The fetal/infant outcomes are summarized in Table 26–1. The rates of prematurity for Hamilton, Ontario hospitals and of miscarriages, stillbirths, neonatal deaths, and congenital abnormalities for Canada and Ontario, are provided for comparison. The rates of adverse outcomes in the heparin-treated patients are consistent with the rates in the "normal" population, and in absolute terms, are small. However, it is impossible to exclude a small increase in any of the adverse outcomes that could only be detected in a large, randomized, controlled study.

Based on the results of these two studies,[8,9]

TABLE 26–1. Fetal/Infant Outcomes with Full-Dose Subcutaneous Heparin

	CANADA (%)	ONTARIO (%)	HEPARIN-TREATED PATIENTS (%)	95% CONFIDENCE INTERVALS (%)
Prematurity	N/A	6.5–18.5*	11/95† (11.6)	(6.0–20.0)
Miscarriages	16.5	22.4	3/34‡ (8.8)	(1.9–23.7)
Stillbirths	0.4	0.6	3/97§ (3.1)	(0.1–5.9)
Neonatal deaths	0.5	0.5	1/94‖ (1.1)	(0.0–5.9)
Congenital abnormalities	5.3	N/A	1/94‖ (1.1)	(0.0–5.9)

* These are not Ontario rates, but are rates at two of the hospitals in Hamilton.
† Excluding from the original 100 patients, five patients with preterm deaths.
‡ Including only those 34 of the original 100 patients who received heparin during the first 20 weeks.
§ Excluding from the original 100 patients, three patients with miscarriages.
‖ Excluding from the original 100 patients, six patients with antepartum deaths.
N/A = not available.

the fact that no increase in teratogenicity has ever been reported with heparin therapy and the fact that heparin does not cross the placenta, it is unlikely that heparin is fetopathic when administered during pregnancy. On the other hand, coumarin derivatives cross the placenta, and several studies have reported that they have teratogenic potential.

EFFECTS OF COUMARIN DERIVATIVES ON THE FETUS

The reported fetopathic effects of coumarin derivatives include warfarin embryopathy and central nervous system abnormalities. The warfarin embryopathy consists of nasal hypoplasia or stippled epiphyses or both after in utero exposure to oral anticoagulants during the first trimester of pregnancy.[6]

Central nervous system abnormalities that have been reported with oral anticoagulant therapy include: (a) dorsal midline dysplasia characterized by agenesis of the corpus callosum, Dandy-Walker malformations, and midline cerebellar atrophy; (b) ventral midline dysplasia characterized by optic atrophy; and (c) hemorrhage.[6] In the literature review, the warfarin embryopathy occurred in 45 of the 970 pregnancies associated with oral anticoagulant therapy, whereas central nervous system abnormalities were reported in 26 of the 970 pregnancies associated with oral anticoagulant therapy.[8] Unlike warfarin embryopathy, which has only been reported with first trimester warfarin exposure, central nervous system abnormalities can occur following warfarin exposure during any trimester.

Estimating the incidences of warfarin embryopathy and central nervous system abnormalities on the basis of a literature review is likely to be inaccurate because of the problem of case reporting bias. A cohort study of 72 patients[10] is the only prospective study that estimated the incidence of congenital malformations following maternal warfarin therapy for valvular heart disease. The warfarin embryopathy was reported in 10 of 35 infants (28.6 per cent) exposed to warfarin between the 6th and the 12th weeks of gestation, whereas no cases of the warfarin embryopathy occurred in the 19 patients in whom heparin was substituted for warfarin between the 6th and 12th weeks of gestation. There were no central nervous system abnormalities reported. Although this study is relatively small, it suggests that warfarin embryopathy occurs frequently following in utero exposure to coumarin derivatives between 6 and 12 weeks of gestation and can be avoided by withholding coumarin derivatives during this period. Central nervous system abnormalities appear to be an uncommon complication of oral anticoagulant therapy.

Other congenital malformations, including cardiac malformations, hand polydactyly, asplenia, and corneal leukoma, have been rarely reported following oral anticoagulant therapy.[8] It is impossible to be certain if these were chance associations or caused by the oral anticoagulants.

Owing to the fact that oral anticoagulants cross the placenta and enter the fetal circulation, they have the potential to induce an anticoagulant effect in the fetus. This is particularly important at term when the trauma of delivery may cause serious hemorrhage.

MATERNAL EFFECTS OF ANTICOAGULANTS DURING PREGNANCY

The most common maternal complication is hemorrhage. In the cohort study done at McMaster University, Hamilton, Ontario,[9] the incidence of bleeding with long-term heparin therapy was 2 per cent, which is consistent with the rates of bleeding reported with heparin therapy in nonpregnant patients and with warfarin therapy when used for the treatment of venous thrombosis.

Heparin therapy presents a management problem at the time of delivery because of its potential to cause a persistent anticoagulant effect and thus increase the risk of bleeding. In a recent cohort study of pregnant women receiving adjusted-dose subcutaneous heparin therapy at the time of delivery, it was reported that the anticoagulant effect of heparin persisted for up to 28 hours after the last injection of heparin.[11] Thus in women who were being treated with adjusted-dose subcutaneous heparin, the delivery was frequently complicated by a prolonged activated partial thromboplastin time which caused an increased risk of bleeding and cancellation of epidural analgesia. The mechanism for this prolonged anticoagulant effect is not entirely clear. However, one practical way of avoiding an anticoagulant effect during delivery is to discontinue heparin therapy 24 hours prior to elective induction of labor.

This would avoid the problem of having an anticoagulant effect at the time of delivery and reduce the risk of bleeding. If an anticoagulant effect occurs at the time of delivery, judicious use of protamine sulfate to neutralize heparin should be considered.

Heparin-Induced Osteoporosis

Long-term heparin therapy has been reported to cause osteoporosis in both laboratory animals and humans. Up until recently, the true risk of symptomatic osteoporosis to patients treated with heparin therapy was unknown. Two recent studies have provided reasonable estimates of the risk of symptomatic fractures in patients treated with long-term heparin therapy.[12,13] In the first study,[12] a cohort of 61 consecutive premenopausal women previously treated with long-term heparin, and a group of controls matched for age, parity, and duration between the last pregnancy and study entry were evaluated. These patients underwent a questionnaire to determine the incidence of symptomatic fractures and were evaluated with dual-photon absorptiometry of the lumbar spine and single-photon absorptiometry of the wrist. None of the heparin-treated patients had suffered symptomatic fractures (0 of 61, 95 per cent confidence intervals 0.0 to 5.9 per cent), but there was a significantly greater proportion of heparin-treated patients than controls who had reduced bone density. In the second study,[13] 70 patients treated with subcutaneous heparin therapy during pregnancy were evaluated. These patients underwent x-ray of the spine and hip immediately postpartum and again 6 to 12 months postpartum. There were 12 patients with osteopenia and 2 women with multiple fractures of the spine. Reexamination 6 to 12 months postpartum demonstrated that the changes were reversible in most cases. Based on the results of these two studies, it can be concluded that although the risk of symptomatic fractures is low, a subclinical reduction in bone density is a likely consequence of long-term heparin therapy. The implications of these findings are unclear; however, it is possible that such women may be predisposed to fractures in the postmenopausal period.

The mechanism for heparin-induced osteoporosis is not known. It is likely that the risk of osteoporosis is dependent upon the dose of heparin used and the duration of heparin therapy. It is not known whether intervention with agents such as calcium will be successful in preventing the reduction of bone density that occurs with long-term heparin therapy.

Use of Anticoagulants in the Nursing Mother

Heparin is not secreted into breast milk and can be safely administered to nursing mothers.[14] There have been two convincing reports that warfarin does not induce an anticoagulant effect in the breast-fed infant when the drug is administered to a nursing mother.[15,16]

RECOMMENDATIONS

The safety of the fetus is only one of several important considerations when deciding about the best anticoagulant regimen to use in pregnant women. The efficacy of the regimen, the safety of the mother, and the convenience of administration are also important considerations. Although heparin is likely to be safe for the fetus, it is inconvenient because of the need for parenteral administration and can cause maternal bleeding, and when used long term, may cause osteoporosis. On the other hand, although oral anticoagulant therapy is convenient, it can also cause maternal bleeding and is potentially hazardous to the fetus, particularly during the first trimester and at term. For situations in which the efficacy of heparin is established, such as the prevention and treatment of venous thromboembolic disease, heparin should be used. For situations in which the efficacy of heparin is not established, such as the prevention of systemic embolism associated with prosthetic heart valves, deciding upon the best anticoagulant regimen is problematic (see Chapter 11). When such women are seen before conception, they should be advised about the risks of anticoagulant therapy. If pregnancy is still desired, two options can be considered. The first is to use full-dose subcutaneous heparin throughout pregnancy. The second is to use a regimen combining heparin and oral anticoagulants, whereby full-dose subcutaneous heparin is used until the 13th week, followed by warfarin until the middle of the third trimester, and then full-dose heparin until term. This regimen should avoid warfarin embryopathy and anticoagulating the fetus near term. Because no randomized trials comparing these two regimens have been published, a strong recommendation cannot be made.

Patients who develop deep vein thrombosis or pulmonary embolism during pregnancy should be treated with a continuous intravenous infusion of heparin for 5 to 14 days to maintain the activated partial thromboplastin time at 1.5 to 2.5 times control (the equivalent of a heparin level of 0.2 to 0.5 units/milliliter by protamine sulfate titration). This should be followed by subcutaneous heparin administered 12-hourly in a dose that maintains a midinterval activated partial thromboplastin time (6 hours after the morning dose) between 1.5 and 2.5 times control.

Pregnant patients with a history of deep vein thrombosis or pulmonary embolism have a risk of recurrence that is unknown, but has been estimated at 5 to 12 per cent.[17,18] Thus some form of prophylaxis or surveillance seems reasonable. One option is to administer low-dose heparin in subsequent pregnancies during the first two trimesters, and adjusted-dose subcutaneous heparin (see above) during the last trimester. The other option is to withhold anticoagulant prophylaxis and follow-up the patient with serial impedance plethysmography or duplex ultrasonography at weekly intervals.

In women who require long-term anticoagulant therapy and are seen before conception while receiving warfarin therapy, two approaches can be used in converting them to full-dose subcutaneous heparin. Heparin can be initiated immediately or the patient can be left on warfarin, can have weekly pregnancy tests performed, and switched to heparin when pregnancy is achieved. Both approaches have disadvantages. The first may expose the patient to prolonged heparin therapy with an increased risk of osteoporosis if conception is not achieved quickly. The second approach assumes that warfarin therapy is safe during the first six weeks of gestation.

To summarize, when anticoagulants are indicated for the prevention or treatment of venous thromboembolism, heparin is the anticoagulant of choice because it is probably safe and efficacious. When pregnancy is desired in women with prosthetic heart valves, either full-dose subcutaneous heparin throughout pregnancy or a regimen combining heparin and oral anticoagulants can be used.

REFERENCES

1. Howie PWM, Prentice CRM, Forbes CD. Failure of heparin therapy to affect the clinical course of pre-eclampsia. Br J Obstet Gynecol 1978; 82: 711–7.
2. Fairley KF, Adey FD, Ross IC, Kincaid-Smith P. Heparin treatment in severe pre-eclampsia and glomerulonephritis in pregnancy. Perspect Nephrol Hyper 1975; 5: 103–12.
3. Rosove MM, Tabsh K, Howard P, et al. Heparin therapy for prevention of fetal wastage in women with anticardiolipin antibodies and lupus anticoagulant. Blood 1987; 70 (suppl 5): 379.
4. Flessa HC, Kapstrom AB, Glueck MJ, Will JJ. Placental transport of heparin. Am J Obstet Gynecol 1965; 93: 570–3.
5. Becker MH, Genvesser NB, Finegold M, Miranda D, Spackman T. Chondrodysplasia punctata. Is maternal warfarin a factor? Am J Dis Child 1975; 129: 356–9.
6. Hall JAG, Pauli RM, Wilson KM. Maternal and fetal sequelae of anticoagulation during pregnancy. Am J Med 1980; 68: 122–40.
7. Ginsberg JS, Hirsh J. Use of anticoagulants during pregnancy. Chest 1989; 95: 156S–605.
8. Ginsberg JS, Hirsh J, Turner DC, Levine M, Burrow R. Risks to the fetus of anticoagulant therapy during pregnancy. Thromb Haemost 1989; 61: 197–203.
9. Ginsberg JS, Kowalchuk G, Hirsh J, Brill-Edwards P, Burrows R. Heparin therapy during pregnancy: risks to the fetus and mother. Arch Int Med 1989; 149: 2233–6.
10. Iturbe-Alessio I, del Carmen Fonseca M, Mutchinik O, Santos MA, Zajarias A, Salazar E. Risks of anticoagulant therapy in pregnant women with artificial heart valves. N Engl J Med 1986; 315: 1390–3.
11. Anderson DR, Ginsberg JS, Burrows R, Brill-Edwards P. Subcutaneous heparin therapy during pregnancy: a need for concern at the time of delivery. Thromb Haemost 1991; 65: 248–50.
12. Ginsberg JS, Kowalchuk G, Hirsh J, et al. Heparin effect on bone density. Thromb Haemost 1990; 64: 286–9.
13. Dahlman T, Lindvall N, Hellgren M. Osteopenia in pregnancy during long-term heparin treatment: a radiologic survey post partum. Br J Obstet Gynecol 1990; 97: 221–8.
14. O'Reilly R. Anticoagulant, antithrombotic and thrombolytic drugs. In: Gilman AG, et al., eds. The pharmacologic basis of therapeutics. 6th ed. New York: MacMillan, 1980: 1347–66.
15. Orme L'e, Lewis M, DeSwiet M, et al. May mothers given warfarin breast-feed their infants? Br Med J 1977; 1: 1564–5.
16. McKenna R, Cale ER, Vasan U. Is warfarin sodium contraindicated in the lactating mother? J Pediatr 1983; 103 (2): 325–7.
17. Howell R, Fidler J, Letsky E, et al. The risks of antinatal subcutaneous heparin prophylaxis: a controlled trial. Br J Obstet Gynecol 1983; 90: 1124.
18. Badaracco MA, Vassey M. Recurrence of venous thromboembolic disease and use of oral contraceptives. Br Med J 1974; i: 215.

27

DECISION MAKING BASED ON PATHOGENESIS AND RISK

BERNARDO STEIN and VALENTIN FUSTER

Thrombosis and embolism within the circulatory system has been recognized as a major mechanism responsible for cardiovascular morbidity and mortality for more than 50 years. Throughout this period, various antithrombotic drugs have been used for purposes of both prevention and therapy. The vast existing literature is so rapidly supplemented by new data, that confusion may arise among clinicians who confront decisions involving patient management.

Whereas therapeutic recommendations for specific disease entities are provided in several chapters of this book, a rational integration of emerging information requires a conceptual framework based on an understanding of pathogenetic mechanisms and an appreciation of relative risks.[1] In this review we briefly discuss: (a) pathogenesis of thrombosis and embolism in the coronary circulation, cardiac chambers, and valves; (b) stratification of patients into different risk categories; and (c) proposed antithrombotic approach based on concepts of pathogenesis and risk.

PATHOGENESIS OF THROMBOSIS AND EMBOLISM

Coronary Circulation

The endothelial cells that line the entire intimal layer of the cardiovascular system provide it with a surface highly resistant to thrombus formation. Platelets adhere to damaged endothelium or to exposed subendoth-elium in cases of superficial vascular injury. However, when severe injury to the vessel wall occurs, as in cases of atherosclerotic plaque rupture or during angioplasty, components of the medial layer, particularly collagen, become exposed to the circulating blood, which results in marked activation of platelets. This leads to the secretion of additional platelet activators including adenosine diphosphate, thromboxane A_2, and serotonin. Furthermore, vascular damage of this magnitude stimulates the intrinsic and extrinsic coagulation systems, in which the platelet membrane facilitates interactions between clotting factors, leading to the generation of thrombin. Thrombin exerts a positive feedback mechanism on the activation of clotting factors, promotes the formation and polymerization of fibrin, and is a powerful agonist of platelet aggregation. *Platelets and the coagulation system are thus closely interrelated in the genesis of arterial thrombosis.*

Delivery and activation of platelets at the site of injury are dependent on both shear rate and the degree of vessel wall injury. In areas of luminal stenosis, high shear rate promotes contact between blood elements and the vessel wall and favors platelet activation. In cases of superficial vessel injury, platelet deposition and thrombosis can occur, but usually only transiently. In contrast, with deep vessel injury, platelet deposition is considerably enhanced and may lead to fixation of the platelet thrombus to the vascular surface, resulting in persistent vessel occlusion.[2]

In up to two thirds of patients with unstable angina, ischemia results from plaque fissuring, leading to transient vessel occlusion by thrombus. In the other third, ischemia results from vasoconstriction or an increase in myocardial oxygen demand or both. Myocardial infarction is usually associated with more severe plaque disruption and more persistent thrombotic coronary occlusion in the face of inadequate collateral flow (see Chapter 2). In addition, spontaneous or pharmacologic lysis of thrombus occurs in some patients after infarction. The residual thrombus in turn constitutes a powerful thrombogenic surface, which facilitates further activation of platelets and the coagulation cascade. This places patients with acute myocardial infarction at high risk of reocclusion.

Cardiac Chambers

Intracavitary mural thrombi develop frequently in patients with acute myocardial infarction, left ventricular aneurysm, dilated cardiomyopathy, and atrial fibrillation. The pathogenesis of thrombosis may be outlined along the lines established more than a century ago by the pathologist Rudolf Virchow, who defined a triad of precipitating factors: endothelial injury, a zone of circulatory stasis, and a hypercoagulable state.

Soon after acute myocardial infarction, leukocytes infiltrate the endocardium and separate it from the basal lamina.[3] This results in the exposure of subendothelial tissue to intracavitary blood and serves as nidus for thrombus development. In addition, specific endocardial abnormalities have been identified histologically in surgical and postmortem specimens of patients with ventricular aneurysms and in those with idiopathic dilated cardiomyopathy. Endocardial damage may be one of the contributors to thromboembolism commonly seen in these clinical situations.

The presence of blood stasis in hypocontractile or dyskinetic areas promotes the development of left ventricular mural thrombi.[4] Similarly, stasis is important in the development of atrial thrombi, when effective mechanical atrial activity is impaired, as occurs in atrial fibrillation, atrial enlargement, mitral stenosis,[5] and cardiac failure. Stasis is tantamount to conditions of low shear rate, in which *activation of the coagulation system rather than of platelets leads to fibrin formation and con-*

stitutes the predominant pathogenetic mechanism in the development of intracavitary thrombi.

The presence of a hypercoagulable state may explain some situations of thromboembolism, particularly within the venous system. Whether hypercoagulability plays a role in arterial thromboembolism remains to be defined. It is conceivable that rather than a systemic hypercoagulable state being the cause of cardiac or arterial thromboembolism, it is the presence of a thrombus within the cardiac chambers or arterial circulation that provides a thrombogenic surface, thus producing a localized "procoagulant" environment.

The problems of thromboembolism from cardiac chambers prompt analysis of the balance between the effects of regional injury, stasis, and procoagulant factors, which favor thrombus formation; and dynamic forces of the circulation, which are responsible for the migration of thrombotic material into the circulation.[6] For example, whereas stasis favors thrombosis within the sac of a left ventricular aneurysm, its isolation from the circulation protects against embolism.[7] In contrast, in cases of myocardial infarction or dilated cardiomyopathy, the resulting mural thrombus is in contact with the circulating blood, and may be propelled into the left ventricular outflow tract, causing arterial embolism. Thus, factors leading to thrombus formation are not necessarily the same as those that produce systemic embolism, and this apparent paradox must not be neglected in the selection of therapeutic options.

Prosthetic Valves

Once circulation has been restored after implantation of a prosthetic heart valve, platelet deposition begins immediately on the prosthetic device itself, particularly on the endocardium-suture-prosthesis interfaces, and on damaged perivalvular tissue. The exposure of the prosthetic surface to blood components leads to platelet deposition and, more importantly, to activation of the coagulation sequence. When describing the pathogenesis of thromboembolism in prosthetic heart valves, two factors deserve consideration: the nonphysiologic characteristics of the valve, and the abnormalities of the adjacent cardiac chambers, particularly in cases of mitral valve disease. Flow stasis and abnormal hemodynamic characteristics of prosthetic devices *promote mainly thrombin and fibrin generation*; however, platelet activation in areas of high velocity and turbulent flow also occurs.

Bioprosthetic valves are considerably less thrombogenic than their mechanical counterparts, mainly because of the natural properties of the material used in their construction and also because of the characteristics of axial flow profile, leaflet pliability, and axial sinusoidal washout.[8]

In summary, arterial thrombosis involves vascular wall damage and exposure of thrombogenic surfaces, which result in marked activation of both platelets and the coagulation system. In contrast, thrombosis within cardiac chambers occurs predominantly in situations of circulatory stasis and low-shear rate, which favor activation of the coagulation cascade and fibrin formation. Finally, cardiac prosthetic valves lead primarily to activation of the clotting system and, secondarily, of platelets, where mechanical devices are clearly more thrombogenic than bioprosthetic ones.

STRATIFICATION OF THROMBOEMBOLIC RISK

When approaching a patient with (or at risk for) a thromboembolic disorder, the intensity of antithrombotic therapy is not only dictated by the pathogenesis and anatomic location of the process, but is also dependent on the individual's risk of thrombosis or embolism. For the purpose of this analysis, we will discuss three general risk categories. In the high-risk group are patients with a predicted incidence of thromboembolism of more than 6 per 100 patients per year. At medium risk are those with an incidence of thromboembolism that ranges between 2 and 6 per 100 patients per year. Finally, the low-risk group includes those with fewer than 2 episodes per 100 patients per year (Table 27–1).

For thrombosis within the *coronary circulation*, three risk groups are identified: patients at high risk are those with unstable angina, acute myocardial infarction, after thrombolysis for acute myocardial infarction, and during the early phase of myocardial revascularization (coronary angioplasty and aortocoronary bypass surgery). In the medium-

risk category are patients with stable angina pectoris and those in the chronic phase after myocardial infarction, coronary angioplasty, and bypass surgery. The low-risk group consists of individuals in whom antithrombotic therapy for primary prevention is being considered; in these patients, the thrombotic risk is below 1 per cent per year.

With respect to *cardiac chamber* thrombosis and embolism, patients at highest risk are those with atrial fibrillation and cerebral or systemic embolism within the preceding two years. At somewhat lower but still substantial risk, are those with atrial fibrillation and mitral stenosis or uncontrolled hyperthyroidism. At medium risk are patients with atrial fibrillation associated with other forms of organic heart disease including systemic arterial hypertension, coronary cardiomyopathy and valvular disease, (excluding mitral stenosis). In addition, patients in the early phase after anterior infarction and those with dilated cardiomyopathy belong to the medium-risk group. At lowest risk are two groups of patients: those with idiopathic (lone) atrial fibrillation under the age of 60 years, and those with left ventricular aneurysm remote from the acute process of myocardial infarction, in the absence of mobile or protruding mural thrombi (by echocardiography) or diffuse left ventricular dysfunction.

Regarding patients with *valvular prostheses*, those with old mechanical devices (implanted before the mid 1970s) and those with prior embolism are at highest risk. At medium risk are patients with modern mechanical prostheses and those with bioprostheses in the presence of atrial fibrillation. It also includes those who receive a bioprosthetic valve within the first three months after surgery. In the lowest-risk group are patients with bioprostheses along with normal sinus rhythm beyond the first three postoperative months, when the incidence of embolism diminishes considerably.

ANTITHROMBOTIC TREATMENT BASED ON PATHOGENESIS AND RISK

With the foundations established in the foregoing sections of pathogenesis and risk stratification, it is possible to derive a more

TABLE 27–1. Antithrombotic Approach to Cardiovascular Disease Based on Pathogenesis and Risk

LOCATION AND PATHOGENESIS	THROMBOEMBOLIC RISK		
	High (>6% per year)	*Medium (2–6% per year)*	*Low (<2% per year)*
Arterial system	Unstable angina Acute myocardial infarction Myocardial infarction— after thrombolysis Percutaneous transluminal coronary angioplasty— early phase Saphenous vein bypass grafting—early phase	Chronic stable angina Chronic phase after myocardial infarction Percutaneous transluminal coronary angioplasty— chronic phase Saphenous vein bypass grafting—chronic phase	Primary prevention of cardiovascular disease
Platelets + coagulation system	Platelet inhibitor plus anticoagulant*	Platelet inhibitor or anticoagulant (international normalized ratio 2.0–3.0)†	Platelet inhibitor‡
Cardiac chambers	Atrial fibrillation—prior embolism Atrial fibrillation—mitral stenosis	Atrial fibrillation—other forms of organic heart disease Early phase after anterior myocardial infarction Dilated cardiomyopathy	Atrial fibrillation— idiopathic‖ Left ventricular aneurysm (remote from acute myocardial infarction)
Coagulation system > platelets	Anticoagulant (international normalized ratio 3.0– 4.5)§	Anticoagulant (international normalized ratio 2.0–3.0)	Usually no need for therapy
Prosthetic valves	Old mechanical prostheses Mechanical prostheses— prior embolism	Recent mechanical prostheses Bioprostheses—atrial fibrillation	Bioprostheses—sinus rhythm
Coagulation system > platelets	Anticoagulant (international normalized ratio 3.0–4.5) plus platelet inhibitor	Anticoagulant (international normalized ratio 3.0–4.5) in mechanical valves, or 2.0–3.0 in bioprostheses)¶	Usually no need for therapy¶

* Heparin may be used in the acute phase (activated thromboplastin time: 1.5 to 2.0 times control); its value in combination with aspirin is emerging.
† Although both beneficial, platelet inhibitor preferred based on lower cost, toxicity, and ease of administration.
‡ Recommended to men >50 years of age with significant coronary risk factors.
§ Lower anticoagulant dose (international normalized ratio 2.0 to 3.0) may suffice in patients with mitral stenosis.
‖ Patients >60 years of age have higher risk of embolism.
¶ Moderate intensity anticoagulation (international normalized ratio 3.0 to 4.5) recommended to patients with bioprostheses for the first three months after surgery.

rational antithrombotic approach to patients at risk for thromboembolic disorders, as outlined in Table 27–1. The numerical values corresponding to the relative high, medium, and low-risk clinical situations are defined at the top of the columns. These categories should be taken as approximates and even flexible, as distinguishing variables in individual patients preclude classification into rigidly defined groups. An antithrombotic approach is formulated along the lines of anatomic location represented by the horizontal rows in the table. In general, for patients at high risk, aggressive antithrombotic treatment is suggested, whereas for those at low risk, therapy may not even be

necessary. For the medium-risk group, an intermediate approach is recommended.

Coronary Circulation

Activation both of platelets and the coagulation system is fundamental to the pathogenesis of thrombosis within the arterial circulation, particularly the coronary tree. The specific clinical situation may dictate whether a platelet inhibitor, an anticoagulant, or the combination of both is indicated. The patient's risk for thrombosis will determine the intensity of therapy needed.

HIGH RISK

This category includes patients with unstable angina, acute myocardial infarction, and those undergoing coronary revascularization. Patients with unstable angina are at substantial risk of developing myocardial infarction and death. Several randomized trials have clearly demonstrated the efficacy of platelet inhibitory treatment with aspirin[9-12] or with ticlopidine[13] for prevention of myocardial infarction and cardiovascular death. In addition, the results of two other trials[11,14] support the use of heparin during the acute stage. Because a significant proportion of patients with unstable angina progress to myocardial infarction despite treatment with aspirin or heparin, the combination of low-dose (80 milligrams) aspirin plus intravenous heparin has been proposed. Although the advantage of this combination over either agent alone remains unsettled, the results from a recent trial[12] suggest that aggressive antithrombotic treatment with aspirin and intravenous heparin is most beneficial during the first few days after hospitalization. In this trial, a "rebound" increase in coronary events was seen after heparin was stopped. Therefore, there is emerging interest in testing the combination of low-dose warfarin and aspirin in patients with unstable angina. This approach is currently being evaluated in the International Antithrombotic Therapy in Acute Coronary Syndromes (ATACS) trial.[15] Presently, no definite recommendations regarding this combination can be made until the results of the ATACS study become available. Beyond the acute phase, a daily dose of 160 to 325 milligrams of aspirin is recommended.

During the acute phase of myocardial infarction, aspirin has proved unequivocally effective. The results of the Second International Study of Infarct Survival (ISIS-2)[16] showed that aspirin reduces early mortality by one fifth and reinfarction by one half. More significant benefit was seen when aspirin was combined with thrombolytic therapy. Aspirin probably acts by preventing reocclusion and reinfarction after spontaneous or pharmacologically induced thrombolysis. Based on this study,[16] immediate initiation of aspirin therapy is recommended for patients with acute infarction, whether or not a thrombolytic agent is used.

The issue of short-term anticoagulation in acute myocardial infarction for prevention of reinfarction and mortality is still unsettled. Only when the results of randomized trials are pooled[17] does a significant reduction in mortality become apparent. Because of high risk, short term (i.e. six weeks) of a combination of low dose anticoagulation plus aspirin should also be investigated. In combination with aspirin, the role of adjuvant heparin for patients treated with thrombolytic therapy is actively being investigated. Whereas adjuvant intravenous heparin improved early coronary patency rates in several studies,[18-20] the benefit of delayed heparin therapy by the subcutaneous route is still a matter of great controversy, based on the results of recent large, randomized trials.[21-23] Whereas intravenous heparin and oral aspirin are commonly used in patients with acute myocardial infarction treated with alteplase, the therapeutic value of intravenous heparin is currently being tested in a large, multicenter trial.

The risk of vessel occlusion is a major concern in patients undergoing coronary revascularization. Substantial damage to the vessel wall during coronary angioplasty predisposes to acute thrombotic occlusion. Several prospective studies[24-27] have clearly shown that pretreatment with aspirin or ticlopidine significantly reduces the incidence of coronary occlusion and infarction during and after angioplasty. Adequate anticoagulation with intravenous heparin is essential during the procedure, as supported by experimental studies.[28] Given the propensity for thrombotic complications during angioplasty, pretreatment with a platelet inhibitor combined with adequate anticoagulation during the procedure is clearly indicated. Whereas aspirin does not reduce the incidence of restenosis, its long-term use is indicated after angioplasty for prevention of future coronary events in this population at risk.

Coronary bypass surgery can be complicated by early vein graft occlusion, which is mainly thrombotic in nature and in which platelets play a major role. Several large studies[29-32] have documented that aspirin, with or without dipyridamole, and ticlopidine reduce the risk of early graft occlusion when given preoperatively or immediately after surgery. Because preoperative aspirin increases perioperative bleeding, its use before surgery should be avoided whenever possible.

Dipyridamole does not increase intraoperative bleeding, but its antithrombotic value is debatable. More importantly, aspirin should be started immediately after surgery and continued indefinitely. In addition to antiplatelet therapy, intraoperative heparin at large doses is essential for prevention of thrombus formation within the grafts and the extracorporeal system. The use of low-dose aspirin plus warfarin for patients at higher risk for early graft thrombosis is currently being considered. This group includes patients with reduced graft flow or impaired distal coronary run-off associated with diffuse coronary disease or small vessel caliber. Future trials will address the value of this combination.

MEDIUM RISK

Patients with chronic stable angina often receive a platelet inhibitor for prevention of future coronary events. However, evidence supporting antiplatelet therapy for this group of patients has become available only recently. In two preliminary reports,[33,34] long-term aspirin treatment with or without dipyridamole was associated with a lower incidence of myocardial infarction. However, a small increase in stroke was seen in the aspirin group in one of the studies,[34] that requires confirmation by larger trials.

For survivors of myocardial infarction, the search for an effective antithrombotic regimen for secondary prevention has generated enormous controversy. Most trials of platelet inhibitors used after myocardial infarction have disclosed a beneficial trend in terms of reduced mortality and reinfarction. However, when the results of these studies are pooled,[35] it becomes apparent that antiplatelet treatment is associated with a highly significant 25 per cent reduction in cardiovascular events. Aspirin alone appears as effective as it is in combination with dipyridamole, and is more effective than sulfinpyrazone. In addition, its lower cost and ease of administration antiplatelet make aspirin the preferred drug for survivors of myocardial infarction.

The value of chronic anticoagulant therapy for the postinfarction patient has been controversial. However, the results of the Warfarin Reinfarction Study (WARIS),[36] the largest and best conducted trial of anticoagulants after myocardial infarction, clearly show that chronic warfarin treatment reduces the incidence of reinfarction, death, and stroke, with an acceptably low risk of hemorrhage. In addition, results from a randomized trial[37] of patients who were anticoagulated for six years after myocardial infarction showed that continuation of the anticoagulant was associated with a reduction in the incidence of reinfarction and death.

Therefore, for the secondary prevention of postinfarction cardiovascular morbidity and mortality, available evidence supports the use of either aspirin or an oral anticoagulant. Individual variables including age, concomitant diseases, feasibility of close monitoring of the anticoagulant, and geographic distance from the health center are clearly important in determining the most appropriate antithrombotic regimen. In general, aspirin, at a daily dose of 160 to 325 milligrams, offers several advantages in terms of cost, ease of administration, and safety. Warfarin may be indicated for patients intolerant to aspirin, and for those with associated pathology that predisposes to systemic embolism, such as atrial fibrillation or significant left ventricular dysfunction.

LOW RISK

The high prevalence of coronary disease in our society warrants the development and testing of agents for primary prevention. To date, two primary prevention trials[38,39] with aspirin have been published. The American trial[38] showed that aspirin (325 milligrams every other day) reduces the incidence of myocardial infarction by almost 50 per cent in healthy individuals, whereas the smaller, British trial[39] found no benefit from 500 milligrams of aspirin daily. Neither study found a reduction in overall mortality, but aspirin use was associated with a small increase in hemorrhagic stroke. Because of the potential toxicity of chronic inhibition of platelet function, aspirin cannot be universally recommended for primary prevention. Aspirin appears to exert a greater beneficial impact in individuals with a higher likelihood of developing coronary disease, such as those with known risk factors or evidence of atherosclerosis in other vascular territories.[40] Based on a risk-to-benefit analysis, aspirin, for primary prevention, may be recommended to men older than 50 years of age who have significant risk factors for coronary disease. It cannot be overemphasized that risk-factor modification is an essential part of treatment. As regards to aspirin for primary prevention in women, convincing data are not yet available.

The beneficial effects of low-dose warfarin in terms of reduction in coagulation factor VII activity in men considered at high risk for coronary events has been documented.[41] These results have prompted the initiation of a randomized trial comparing low-dose aspirin, low-dose warfarin, and their combination, for primary prevention of cardiovascular disease in this group at risk. The findings of this trial, when available, may have a significant impact on medical practice.

In summary, thrombosis within the coronary system involves both platelet and coagulation factors. For patients at high risk, the combination of a platelet inhibitor and an anticoagulant (in the acute phase) should be considered. For those at medium risk, either a platelet inhibitor or an anticoagulant have proved beneficial, although the former is favored generally, because of lower toxicity and cost. For those at low risk, a platelet inhibitor can be recommended to selected patients.

Cardiac Chambers

Development of thrombi within the left atrium or left ventricle results primarily from blood stasis, which leads to activation of the coagulation system and fibrin formation. Platelet participation in these disorders is generally less important, but may play a role in some clinical situations. Anticoagulants have been the mainstay of antithrombotic therapy for these individuals (Table 27–1).

HIGH RISK

Patients at highest risk are those who have already experienced arterial embolism within the previous two years. These individuals are at substantial risk for recurrent embolism of approximately 10 per cent per year. Therefore, even though prospective randomized studies are lacking and will never be conducted, the increased risk warrants the use of moderate-intensity anticoagulant therapy aimed at an international normalized ratio of prothrombin suppression of 3.0 to 4.5 (equivalent to a prothrombin time of 1.5 to 2.0 times control, using a typical North American thromboplastin reagent).

At somewhat lower but still significant risk for embolism are patients with atrial fibrillation in association with mitral stenosis. Several nonrandomized studies have shown that long-term anticoagulant therapy reduces the incidence of embolism by 25 per cent in this patient population.[42] Whereas most clinicians agree on the need for anticoagulant therapy, the appropriate intensity of treatment is unknown. Because the risk of embolism is substantial, moderate-intensity anticoagulation aimed at an international normalized ratio of 3.0 to 4.5 (prothrombin time of 1.5 to 2.0 using a typical North American thromboplastin) is probably justified. Whether long-term low-dose anticoagulation is equally effective, remains unknown.

In addition, patients with atrial fibrillation and uncontrolled hyperthyroidism are at increased embolic risk and should be anticoagulated until a euthyroid state and reversion to sinus rhythm have been achieved.

MEDIUM RISK

This category includes patients with atrial fibrillation associated with other forms of organic heart disease, also known as nonvalvular atrial fibrillation. This large group of patients has an intermediate but incompletely defined risk for embolism, and accounts for almost one half of cardiogenic strokes. Three recent, large, prospective studies[43–45] have clearly documented the benefits of antithrombotic therapy for patients with atrial fibrillation, in terms of reduction in cerebral and systemic embolism. One trial[43] that included a large proportion of patients of advanced age or with associated left ventricular dysfunction showed that warfarin, but not aspirin, was effective in preventing strokes. In contrast, another study[44] showed that both warfarin or aspirin were effective, but the effect of aspirin was most evident in patients under the age of 75. However, the number of patients older than 75 years was relatively small, which precludes definite conclusions for this subgroup. This question is being investigated by an ongoing clinical trial. Finally, the most recent trial[45] documented that low-intensity anticoagulation for patients with nonvalvular atrial fibrillation is safe and significantly reduces the incidence of stroke and death. Whether warfarin is significantly better than aspirin, and which subgroups of patients stand to gain most from a particular treatment, remains to be determined.

Left ventricular mural thrombi develop in up to one third of patients with acute anterior myocardial infarction. Systemic embolism develops in approximately 10 per cent of patients with a mural thrombus, thus affecting 2 to 5 per cent of patients with anterior infarction. The incidence of embolism is highest in the first weeks after infarction. During this phase, short-term oral anticoagulation has been shown to reduce the embolic rate by 25 to 75 per cent.[46–48] Two recent studies[49,50] showed that medium-dose subcutaneous heparin (12,500 units twice daily) protects patients with anterior myocardial infarction from developing mural thrombosis. Patients with large anterior infarcts, as well as those with myocardial infarction associated with heart failure or atrial fibrillation, should be treated with heparin for several days. Before discharge from the hospital, warfarin therapy should be considered for patients at persistent risk of embolism including those with echocardiographic evidence of mural thrombi or extensive wall-motion abnormalities, those with heart failure, and those with atrial fibrillation. The appropriate duration of anticoagulant therapy for these patients should be determined on an individual basis, depending on whether the aforementioned risk factors for embolism persist.

Patients with dilated cardiomyopathy are also at medium risk for systemic embolism. Based on the results of a retrospective study[51] and of several other observational studies, the use of long-term warfarin therapy may reduce the risk of systemic embolism, and thus should be considered.

In summary, patients at medium risk for embolism from the left atrium or ventricle should receive low-intensity anticoagulant therapy aimed at an international normalized ratio of 2.0 to 3.0 (equivalent to a prothrombin time of 1.3 to 1.5 times control using a typical North American thromboplastin). In addition, recent data suggest that aspirin is also beneficial for some patients with nonvalvular atrial fibrillation,[44] which suggests that platelet thrombi (from the heart, great vessels, or intracerebral arteries) may play a role in the pathogenesis of stroke in some patients.

Low Risk

At the lower end of the risk spectrum are patients younger than 60 years with atrial fibrillation but without associated cardiac pathology (lone or idiopathic fibrillation).[52] In addition, patients with a left ventricular aneurysm remote from acute infarction, who do not have diffuse left ventricular dysfunction or echocardiographic evidence of mobile

or protruding thrombi, are considered at low risk for embolism.[53] For these two groups of patients, chronic anticoagulation is usually unnecessary.

In summary, cardiac chamber thrombosis and embolism are related to blood stasis and predominant activation of the coagulation system. Anticoagulant therapy is recommended for patients at high and medium risk, whereas those at low risk may not require antithrombotic treatment.

Prosthetic Valves

In thromboembolic processes related to heart valve prostheses, activation of the coagulation system predominates over that of platelets. Mechanical valves carry a greater risk of thromboembolism compared to biological devices.

High Risk

In the highest risk category are patients with a mechanical prosthesis who have already suffered an embolic event, because the recurrence rate is high. In addition, patients with old mechanical prostheses, implanted before the mid 1970s, are at high risk. Adequate warfarin therapy, at a dose sufficient to prolong the international normalized ratio to 3.0 to 4.5 (prothrombin time of 1.5 to 2.0 times control using a typical North American thromboplastin) is the most important factor for prevention of thromboembolism. The addition of dipyridamole (300 to 400 milligrams/day) to warfarin may reduce the thromboembolic risk, without increasing the risk of bleeding.[54,55] The combination of aspirin and warfarin was also found effective in two trials,[56,57] but the risk of gastrointestinal bleeding became substantial when aspirin was given at a daily dose of 500 milligrams or more.[55] Therefore, we recommend supplementing warfarin with dipyridamole in high-risk patients with mechanical prostheses.

Medium Risk

This category includes all other patients with mechanical prostheses. They should receive moderate-intensity anticoagulant therapy, aimed at an international normalized ratio of 3.0 to 4.5 (equivalent to a prothrombin time of 1.5 to 2.0 times control using a typical North American thromboplastin). It also includes patients with biologic prostheses, particularly in the mitral position, and especially during the first three months after surgery. Because the thromboembolic risk is highest during the first three postoperative months, some investigators recommend the use of moderate-intensity anticoagulation during this period, aimed at an international normalized ratio of 3.0 to 4.5 (prothrombin time of 1.5 to 2.0 times control using a typical North American thromboplastin). For this group of patients with biological prostheses and in whom atrial fibrillation persists beyond the first three months after surgery, long-term warfarin therapy is recommended, but the dose may be reduced, aiming at an international normalized ratio of 2.0 to 3.0 (prothrombin time of 1.3 to 1.5 times control with a typical North American thromboplastin).

LOW RISK

Patients with a bioprosthetic heart valve who maintain normal sinus rhythm postoperatively and do not have associated left ventricular dysfunction, are at low risk of thromboembolism. This is particularly true for patients with an aortic bioprosthesis. Although anticoagulation is commonly recommended during the first three months after surgery, patients in this low-risk category do not require antithrombotic therapy beyond this period.

In summary, activation, primarily of the coagulation system and secondarily of platelets, occurs in patients with prosthetic cardiac valves. For those at high risk, combination therapy with an anticoagulant at moderate intensity and a platelet inhibitor is recommended. Medium-risk patients can be managed with an anticoagulant alone, and the intensity of therapy will depend on whether the prosthesis is mechanical or biological. Antithrombotic treatment is usually not necessary for patients at low risk beyond the initial postoperative period (Table 27–1).

REFERENCES

1. Stein B, Fuster V, Halperin JL, Chesebro JH. Antithrombotic therapy in cardiac disease: an emerging approach base on pathogenesis and risk. Circulation 1989; 80: 1501–13.
2. Fuster V, Badimon L, Cohen M, Ambrose JA, Badimon JJ, Chesebro JH. Insights into the pathogenesis of acute ischemic syndromes. Circulation 1988; 77: 1213–20.
3. Johnson RC, Crissman RS, Didio LJA. Endocardial alterations in myocardial infarction. Lab Invest 1979; 40: 183–93.
4. Mikell FL, Asinger RW, Elsperger KJ, Anderson WR, Hodges M. Regional stasis of blood in the dysfunctional left ventricle: echocardiographic detection and differentiation from early thrombosis. Circulation 1982; 66: 755–63.
5. Shresta NK, Moreno FL, Narciso FV, Torres L, Calleja HB. Two-dimensional echocardiographic diagnosis of left atrial thrombus in rheumatic heart disease: a clinicopathologic study. Circulation 1983; 67: 341–7.
6. Fuster V, Halperin JL. Left ventricular thrombi and cerebral embolism. N Engl J Med 1989; 320: 392–4.
7. Cabin HS, Roberts WC. Left ventricular aneurysm, intraaneurysmal thrombus and systemic embolus in coronary heart disease. Chest 1980; 77: 586–90.
8. Edmunds LH. Thrombotic and bleeding complications of prosthetic heart valves. Ann Thorac Surg 1987; 44: 430–45.
9. Lewis HD, Davis JW, Archibald DG, et al. Protective effects of aspirin against acute myocardial infarction and death in men with unstable angina: results of a Veterans Administration Cooperative Study. N Engl J Med 1983; 309: 396–403.
10. Cairns JA, Gent M, Singer J, et al. Aspirin, sulfinpyrazone, or both in unstable angina. N Engl J Med 1985; 313: 1369–75.
11. Théroux P, Ouimet H, McCans J, et al. Aspirin, heparin, or both to treat acute unstable angina. N Engl J Med 1988; 319: 1105–11.
12. The RISC Group. Risk of myocardial infarction and death during treatment with low dose aspirin and intravenous heparin in men with unstable coronary artery disease. Lancet 1990; 336: 827–30.
13. Balsano F, Rizzon P, Violi F, et al. Antiplatelet treatment with ticlopidine in unstable angina. A Controlled Multicenter Clinical Trial. Circulation 1990; 82: 17–26.
14. Telford AM, Wilson C. Trial of heparin versus atenolol in prevention of myocardial infarction in intermediate coronary syndrome. Lancet 1981; 1: 1225–8.
15. Cohen M, Adams PC, Hawkins L, Bach M, Fuster V. Usefulness of antithrombotic therapy in resting angina pectoris or non-Q-wave myocardial infarction in preventing death and myocardial infarction (a pilot study from the Antithrombotic Therapy in Acute Coronary Syndromes Study Group). Am J Cardiol 1990; 66: 1287–92.
16. ISIS-2 (Second International Study of Infarct Survival) Collaborative Group. Randomized trial of intravenous streptokinase, oral aspirin, both, or neither among 17,187 cases of suspected acute myocardial infarction: ISIS-2. Lancet 1988; 2: 349–60.
17. Chalmers TC, Matta R, Smith H, Kunzler AM. Evidence favoring the use of anticoagulants in the hospital phase of acute myocardial infarction. N Engl J Med 1977; 297: 1091–6.
18. Hsia J, Hamilton WP, Kleiman N, Roberts R, Chaitman BR, Ross AM. A comparison between heparin and low-dose aspirin as adjunctive therapy with tissue plasminogen activator for acute myocardial infarction. N Engl J Med 1990; 323: 1433–7.
19. Bleich SD, Nichols TC, Schumacher RR, Cooke DH, Tate DA, Teichman SL. Effect of heparin on coronary arterial patency after thrombolysis with tissue plasminogen activator in acute myocardial infarction. Am J Cardiol 1990; 66: 1412–7.
20. European Cooperative Study Group—Phase 6 (ECSG-6). Presented at the XII Session of the European Congress of Cardiology, Stockholm, Sweden, September 1990.
21. Gruppo Italiano per lo Studio della Sopravvivenza nell'Infarto Miocardico. Gissi-II: a factorial randomised trial of alteplase versus streptokinase and heparin among 12,490 patients with acute myocardial infarction. Lancet 1990; 336: 65–70.
22. International Study Group. In-hospital mortality and clinical course of 20,891 patients with suspected acute myocardial infarction randomised between alteplase and streptokinase with or without heparin. Lancet 1990; 336: 71–5.
23. Third International Study of Infarct Survival (ISIS-3). Presented at the Scientific Session of the American College of Cardiology, Atlanta, GA, March 1991.
24. Schwartz L, Bourassa MG, Lesperance J, et al. Aspirin and dipyridamole in the prevention of restenosis after percutaneous transluminal coronary angioplasty. N Engl J Med 1988; 318: 1714–9.
25. White CW, Chaitman B, Lassar TA, et al. Antiplatelet agents

are effective in reducing the immediate complications of PTCA: results from the ticlopidine multicenter trial (abstr). Circulation 1987; 76 (suppl IV): IV–400.

26. Bertrand ME, Allain H, Lablanche JM. Results of a randomized trial of ticlopidine versus placebo for prevention of acute closure and restenosis after coronary angioplasty. The TACT study (abstr). Circulation 1990; 82 (suppl III): III–190.

27. Chesebro JH, Webster MWI, Reeder GS, et al. Coronary angioplasty: antiplatelet therapy reduces acute complications but not restenosis (abstr). Circulation 1989; 80 (suppl II): II–64.

28. Heras M, Chesebro JH, Penny WJ, et al. Importance of adequate heparin dosage in arterial angioplasty in a porcine model. Circulation 1988; 78: 654–60.

29. Chesebro JH, Clements IP, Fuster V, et al. A platelet inhibitor-drug trial in coronary-artery bypass operations: benefit of perioperative dipyridamole and aspirin therapy on early postoperative vein-graft patency. N Engl J Med 1982; 307: 73–8.

30. Limet R, David JL, Magotteaux P, Larock MP, Rigo P. Prevention of aorta-coronary bypass graft occlusion. J Thorac Cardiovasc Surg 1987; 94: 773–83.

31. Goldman S, Copeland J, Moritz T, et al. Improvement in early saphenous vein graft patency after coronary artery bypass surgery with antiplatelet therapy: results of a Veterans Administration Cooperative Study. Circulation 1988; 77: 1324–32.

32. Sanz G, Pajaron A, Alegria E, et al. Prevention of early aortocoronary bypass occlusion by low-dose aspirin and dipyridamole. Circulation 1990; 82: 765–73.

33. Chesebro JH, Webster MWI, Smith HC, et al. Antiplatelet therapy in coronary disease progression: reduced infarction and new lesion formation (abstr). Circulation 1989; 80 (suppl II): II–266.

34. Ridker PM, Manson JE, Gaziano JM, Buring JE, Hennekens CH. Low dose aspirin therapy for chronic stable angina (abstr). Circulation 1990; 82 (suppl III): III–200.

35. Antiplatelet Trialists' Collaboration. Secondary prevention of vascular disease by prolonged antiplatelet treatment. Br Med J 1988; 296: 320–31.

36. Smith P, Arnesen H, Holme I. The effect of warfarin on mortality and reinfarction after myocardial infarction. N Engl J Med 1990; 323: 147–52.

37. Report of the Sixty Plus Reinfarction Study Research Group. A double-blind trial to assess long-term anticoagulant therapy in elderly patients after myocardial infarction. Lancet 1980; 2: 989–94.

38. The Steering Committee of the Physicians' Health Study Research Group. Final report on the aspirin component of the ongoing Physicians' Health Study. N Engl J Med 1989; 321: 129–35.

39. Peto R, Gray R, Collins R, et al. A randomized trial of the effects of prophylactic daily aspirin among male British doctors. Br Med J 1988; 296: 313–6.

40. Fuster V, Cohen M, Halperin JL. Aspirin in the prevention of coronary disease. N Engl J Med 1989; 321: 183–5.

41. Meade TW, Wilhes HC, Stirling Y, Brennan PJ, Kelleher C, Browne W. Randomized controlled trial of low dose warfarin in the primary prevention of ischaemic heart disease in men

at high risk: design and pilot study. Eur Heart J 1988; 9: 836–43.

42. Dunn M, Alexander J, de Silva R, Hildner F. Antithrombotic therapy in atrial fibrillation. Chest 1989; 95(suppl): 118S–27S.

43. Petersen P, Boysen G, Godtfredsen J, Andersen ED, Andersen B. Placebo-controlled, randomised trial of warfarin and aspirin for prevention of thromboembolic complications in chronic atrial fibrillation. The Copenhagen AFASAK Study. Lancet 1989; 1: 175–9.

44. Preliminary report of the Stroke Prevention in Atrial Fibrillation Study. N Engl J Med 1990; 322: 863–8.

45. The Boston Area Anticoagulation Trial for Atrial Fibrillation Investigators. The effect of low-dose warfarin on the risk of stroke in patients with nonrheumatic atrial fibrillation. N Engl J Med 1990; 323: 1505–11.

46. Report of the Working Party on Anticoagulation Therapy in Coronary Thrombosis to the Medical Research Council. Assessment of short-term anticoagulation administration after cardiac infarction. Br Med J 1969; 1: 335–42.

47. Drapkin A, Merskey C. Anticoagulation therapy after acute myocardial infarction. Relation of therapeutic benefit to patient's age, sex and severity of infarction. JAMA 1972; 222: 541–8.

48. Veterans Administration Hospital Investigators. Results of a cooperative clinical trial. JAMA 1973; 225: 724–9.

49. The SCATI (Studio sulla Calciparina nell' Angina e nella Trombosi Ventriculare nell' Infarto) Group. Randomised controlled trial of subcutaneous calcium-heparin in acute myocardial infarction. Lancet 1989; 2: 182–6.

50. Turpie AGG, Robinson JG, Doyle DJ, et al. Comparison of high-dose with low-dose subcutaneous heparin to prevent left ventricular mural thrombosis in patients with acute transmural myocardial infarction. N Engl J Med 1989; 320: 352–7.

51. Fuster V, Gersh BJ, Giuliani ER, Tajik AJ, Brandenburg RO, Frye RL. The natural history of idiopathic dilated cardiomyopathy. Am J Cardiol 1981; 47: 525–31.

52. Kopecky SL, Gersh BJ, McGoon MD, et al. The natural history of lone atrial fibrillation: a population-based study over three decades. N Engl J Med 1987; 317: 669–74.

53. Lapeyre AC, Steele PP, Kazmier FJ, Chesebro JH, Vlietstra RE, Fuster V. Systemic embolism in chronic left ventricular aneurysm: incidence and the role of anticoagulation. J Am Coll Cardiol 1985; 6: 534–8.

54. Sullivan JM, Harken DE, Gorlin R. Pharmacologic control of thromboembolic complications of cardiac-valve replacement. N Engl J Med 1971; 284: 1391–4.

55. Chesebro JH, Fuster V, Elveback LR, et al. Trial of combined warfarin plus dipyridamole or aspirin in prosthetic heart valve replacement: danger of aspirin compared with dipyridamole. Am J Cardiol 1983; 51: 1537–41.

56. Altman R, Boullon F, Rouvier J, et al. Aspirin and prophylaxis of thromboembolic complications in patients with substitute heart valves. J Thorac Cardiovasc Surg 1976; 72: 127–9.

57. Dale J, Myhre E, Storstein O, et al. Prevention of arterial thromboembolism with acetylsalicylic acid: a controlled clinical study in patients with aortic ball valves. Am Heart J 1977; 94: 101–11.

28

DISSEMINATED INTRAVASCULAR COAGULATION

STEVEN M. FRUCHTMAN and JACOB H. RAND

The syndrome of disseminated intravascular coagulation (DIC) has a multitude of etiologies and a variety of clinical presentations. The complexity of the syndrome and its assorted clinical and laboratory presentations makes an all-embracing definition difficult. The central physiological occurrence which marks disseminated intravascular coagulation is the presence of free thrombin in the circulating blood,[1] resulting in fibrin formation in the circulation along with its sequelae.

Diseases of the circulation, as manifested by thrombosis of the coronary and cerebral arteries and pulmonary thromboembolism, are major causes of morbidity and mortality. However, fibrin deposition in the microcirculation is also an important mechanism of disease and needs to be recognized clinically as a cause of ischemia to vital organs, hemorrhage, and potentially, death. Thus, the clinical settings that predispose patients to disseminated intravascular coagulation and its pathophysiology need to be understood so that a rational approach to diagnosis and therapy can be employed.

Schneider, in 1959,[2] described a syndrome in pregnancy associated with acute hemorrhage and a low or absent fibrinogen level and termed this the defibrination syndrome. Initially it was believed that the condition was confined to obstetrical conditions. However, a wide spectrum of clinical settings associated with disseminated intravascular coagulation were subsequently recognized (Table 28–1), and a variety of descriptive terms were commonly employed. The terms consumption coagulopathy,[3] generalized intravascular coagulation,[4] thrombohemorrhagic phenomenon,[5] defibrination syndrome,[6] or consumptive thrombohemorrhagic disorder[7] are expressions used to describe a disease entity that is really not a disease in and of itself, but rather a syndrome associated with a variety of clinical conditions, and which contributes to the morbidity and mortality of the underlying disorder.

EXPERIMENTAL MODELS

Fibrin formation is a normal response to vascular injury. However, the process is usually limited and localized to the site of injury. Disseminated intravascular coagulation may develop when a stimulus to coagulation is either exceptionally powerful, systemic, or constant, especially when the normal inhibitors of blood coagulation are interfered with, as in blockage of the reticuloendothelial system or during inhibition of fibrinolysis.

The Infusion of Thrombin

The intravenous infusion of thrombin into dogs causes a rapid fall in plasma fibrinogen and blood platelet count, as these factors are utilized at a rapid rate.[8] Coagulation factors, particularly factor V and VIII, are also reduced. Circulating activators of fibrinolysis

TABLE 28–1. Etiology and Clinical Settings of Disseminated Intravascular Coagulation

ACUTE DISSEMINATED INTRAVASCULAR COAGULATION

Obstetrics
  Septic and saline-induced abortion
  Abruptio placenta and placenta previa
  Retained dead fetus
  Amniotic fluid embolism
Infections
  Gram-negative sepsis (for example, meningococcemia)
  Gram-positive sepsis (less common)
  Rickettsial (Rocky Mountain spotted fever)
  Protozoal (malaria)
  Viral (congenital rubella)
Shock
  Hypovolemic
  Hypoperfusion
Tissue injury
  Prolonged surgery
  Trauma
  Burns
  Heat stroke
  Anaphylaxis

CHRONIC DISSEMINATED INTRAVASCULAR COAGULATION

Malignant neoplasia
  Solid tumors
  Leukemia (especially promyelocytic leukemia)
Vascular and cardiological disorders
  Giant hemangioma
  Aortic aneurysms
  Valvular heart disease
  Myocardial infarction
  Nonbacterial thrombotic endocarditis
  Cardiopulmonary bypass and left ventricular assist
    devices
Liver disease

decrease initially, and then increase during the recovery period.

During the infusion, generalized uncontrolled bleeding is observed from cut surfaces, and there is evidence for intravascular hemolysis of red blood cells. A characteristic pattern is noted when the animals are sacrificed at various times following the injection of thrombin and the tissues are examined for fibrin. Initially, fibrin cannot be demonstrated by light microscopy, but can be observed on the vascular endothelium of many organs with electron microscopy. As the infusion continues, thrombi occluding the blood vessels become visible with light microscopy. Sacrificing animals and searching for fibrin after the infusion is completed is often futile except in animals pretreated either with thorotrast to block the reticuloendothelial system, or epsilon-aminocaproic acid to inhibit fibrinolysis.[9]

Endotoxin Infusion as a Model for Disseminated Intravascular Coagulation

The generalized Savarelli-Shwartzman phenomena of shock, widespread parenchymatous hemorrhage, and bilateral renal cortical necrosis characteristically follows two spaced intravenous injections of bacterial endotoxin into experimental animals. The first "preparatory" injection causes no clinical effect, while the second "provocative" injection, which may be of a different endotoxin,[10] has to be spaced 6 to 72 hours after the first injection in order to produce the effects. If the second injection is intramuscular, local necrosis is produced at the site of injection. Microscopic examination of the tissues of these animals one hour after the preparatory injection reveals agglutinated masses of platelets and leukocytes in the lung and liver, soon followed by numerous fibrin thrombi in the liver, lungs, and spleen, and new thrombi in the kidney. Virtually every glomerular capillary may be filled with fibrin.

Why two spaced injections are necessary remains an enigma. Under certain circumstances, the response can be seen following a single injection. This can be elicited after reticuloendothelial blockade, inhibition of fibrinolysis, pretreatment with cortisone, and in some animal species, during pregnancy.[11] Continuous infusion of endotoxin for 8 to 14 hours may also produce typical lesions. The clinical effects of the provocative dose may be prevented by prior treatment with heparin, warfarin-type anticoagulants, or by stimulation of fibrinolysis.[12] Leucocytes also appear to play an important role, as prior treatment with chemotherapy to reduce the leucocyte count can prevent the Shwartzman phenomena. The Shwartzman phenomena can be recreated in animals previously rendered leukopenic by using leukocyte transfusions.

The sequence of changes in the blood during the Shwartzman reaction offers better understanding of why certain clinical situations such as infection, pregnancy, or malignancy may predispose these patients to disseminated intravascular coagulation. Early in these settings, fibrinogen, as an "acute-phase protein," can be elevated. Likewise, in the Shwartzman reaction, after the first exposure to endotoxin, there is progressive elevation in fibrinogen levels for 48 hours to levels almost twice as high as baseline levels. Only with the second injection 24 hours later is there an abrupt decrease in fibrinogen. Other factors that are present after the first injection are an increase in circulating leukocytes and a decrease in platelets. The thrombocytopenia becomes more pronounced with the second injection.

The state of the circulation is clearly important in determining the localization of the fibrin deposits. For example, unilateral sympathectomy prevents fibrin deposition in the glomeruli on the denervated side. A similar protective effect has been reported after the administration of alpha-adrenergic blockade.[13] Possibly, vasoconstriction of the afferent arteriole, produced by release of catecholamines from damaged platelets, contributes to congestion and stasis predisposing to fibrin accumulation in the glomeruli. Leukocytes also may contribute to fibrin deposition by synthesizing tissue factor and liberating other vasoactive materials.

DIAGNOSIS OF DISSEMINATED INTRAVASCULAR COAGULATION: THE ROLE OF THE COAGULATION LABORATORY

Normal hemostasis is influenced by (a) the vascular extracellular matrix and alterations in endothelial reactivity, (b) platelets, (c) coagulation proteins, (d) inhibitors of coagulation, and (e) fibrinolysis. Undue bleeding is controlled and the fluidity of blood maintained by the counterbalances of these systems. This brief description is in the context of disseminated intravascular coagulation and its diagnostic laboratory variables.

Blood Vessel

The intact blood vessel is designed to maintain its patency and resist thrombotic occlusion. Among the known mechanisms for this thromboresistance are the prostacyclin synthetic pathway, the endothelium-derived relaxation factor/nitric oxide (EDRF/NO) system, heparan sulfate proteoglycans, the release of tissue plasminogen activator, and the thrombomodulin system.

The injured or disrupted blood vessel promotes thrombus formation. Among the mechanisms for this are the disruption of the intact endothelial layer, which promotes the mechanisms described in the preceding par-

agraph; the stimulation of tissue-factor synthesis; the exposure of tissue factor; the exposure of subendothelial elements to the flowing blood including von Willebrand factor, subendothelial collagens, thrombospondin, and fibronectin; and alterations of the pattern of blood flow in injured vessels.

Platelets

Platelets are cellular elements that serve to plug disrupted areas of the vascular tree and are necessary for the formation of a primary hemostatic plug after injury. The patient with defects in the platelet system, owing either to a deficiency in the quantity of platelets or to abnormal platelet function, usually presents with evidence of skin or mucosal bleeding. Platelets are formed from megakaryocytes, the vast majority of which are present in the bone marrow. Each mature megakaryocyte releases approximately 7,000 platelets into the blood.

Ultrastructural components of the platelets include (a) a glycocalyx coat containing glycoproteins (GPs) necessary for adhesion and aggregation; (b) dense granules containing adenosine diphosphate (ADP), adenosine triphosphate (ATP), serotonin, and calcium; and (c) nondense or alpha granules containing liposomal enzymes, platelet factor 4, thromboglobulin, platelet-derived growth factor, von Willebrand factor, fibrinogen, fibronectin, and platelet factor XIII. The platelet glycocalyx contains a number of glycoproteins which serve as receptors or binding sites for a variety of extracellular matrix materials or adhesive glycoproteins. Glycoprotein Ia serves as a magnesium-dependent collagen receptor. Glycoprotein Ib-IX is a complex ristocetin-dependent receptor for von Willebrand factor. The glycoprotein IIb-IIIa complex is again an integrin complex which recognizes the tripeptide RGD (arginine, glycine, and aspartic acid [Arg-Gly-Asp]) amino acid sequence of fibrinogen, von Willebrand factor, fibronectin, thrombospondin, and vitronectin. The RGD sequence is a critical recognition site for the integrins. Glycoprotein IIb-IIIa also recognizes a non–RGD-containing decapeptide sequence on fibrinogen. Glycoprotein V is the main platelet receptor for thrombospondin.

Coagulation Pathway

The classic coagulation pathway is based on the "waterfall" hypothesis of Davie and

Ratnoff.[14] Coagulation occurs after a series of enzymes or coagulation factors have been activated. This activation can occur through two main routes, designated the extrinsic and intrinsic systems, both converging at the level of factor X into a common pathway. When coagulation is initiated by tissue factor, in the presence of factor VII and calcium, the "extrinsic system" is activated. This system is evaluated by the prothrombin time test. When coagulation is initiated by contact with a negatively charged or damaged surface in the presence of phospholipids, the coagulation factors constituting the "intrinsic system" are activated. This system is evaluated by the activated partial thromboplastin time test. Fibrinogen is converted into fibrin in the common pathway of coagulation. The thrombin time test monitors this conversion of fibrinogen to fibrin. Fibrinogen has a dimeric structure, with each half of the molecule containing three pairs of polypeptide chains: alpha (α), beta (β), and gamma (γ). Thrombin removes two pairs of peptides from the fibrinogen molecule during coagulation; these are called fibrinopeptides A and B and correspond to the N-terminal portions of the α and β chains (Fig. 28–1). Thrombin does not remove the terminal peptides of the gamma chain.

The activity of thrombin is limited by its major inhibitor, antithrombin III. The anticoagulant drug, heparin, complexes with antithrombin III, causing a conformation change which increases its affinity for the active serine center of thrombin and other activated coagulation enzymes and results in marked inhibition of thrombin activity, with decreased formation of fibrin from fibrinogen.

The fibrin clots formed by thrombin's action are highly susceptible to fibrinolysis until

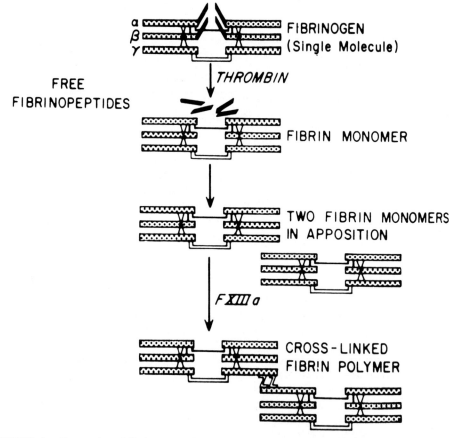

FIGURE 28–1. Conversion of fibrinogen to fibrin. In the presence of thrombin, the fibrinopeptides (*darkened areas*) are split off from fibrinogen. This produces two molecules of fibrinopeptide A, two of fibrinopeptide B, and one of fibrin monomer. Activated factor (F) XIIIa converts the fibrin monomers into cross-linked fibrin polymer.

a further reaction, cross-linking, occurs. In the presence of calcium, factor XIII (which has been activated by thrombin) covalently cross-links adjoining fibrin monomers and converts the fibrin clots into a well-formed, insoluble, and hemostatically effective matrix. Plasmin, the thrombolytic enzyme, may act on fibrinogen or fibrin and produces sequential degradation of these proteins, as will be further discussed.

The thrombin time test is a sensitive indicator of abnormalities of fibrin formation. Prolongation of clotting after the addition of thrombin to plasma is commonly due to (a) the presence of heparin in the patient's blood, (b) the presence of fibrin degradation products interfering with polymerization, (c) hypofibrinogenemia, or (d) dysfibrinogenemia. In cases where heparin is the suspected cause of a prolonged thrombin time but clinical confirmation is absent, the reptilase time is useful. Reptilase, venom from the snake *Bothrops atrox,* cleaves only fibrinopeptide A from the fibrinogen molecule and, unlike thrombin, is not inhibited by heparin. If a prolonged thrombin time is due to the presence of heparin, the reptilase time will be normal. In cases where prolongation is suspected to be due to interference by fibrin degradation products, these products can be measured immunologically for confirmation.

Endogenous Inhibitors of Coagulation

Substances that act as inhibitors of coagulation are also present in plasma. A number of antithrombins have been described, the most important being antithrombin III. Antithrombin III has activity against not only thrombin, but also other serine proteases generated during blood coagulation. Its deficiency in the heterozygous state may result in clinically significant thrombosis, usually appearing after adolescence. The homozygous state may not be compatible with life. As mentioned above, antithrombin III binds to and inactivates thrombin. Heparin works by binding to antithrombin III,[15] which causes a conformational change of the molecule and markedly increases the affinity of antithrombin III for thrombin and other activated coagulation enzymes.

Protein C is another important protein in the regulatory mechanisms of hemostasis.

This system decreases the rate of thrombin formation by inhibiting activated factors V and VIII. The anticoagulant effect of protein C requires the presence of protein S.[16] Protein C also appears to function as a profibrinolytic enzyme, increasing the rate of fibrin degradation by protecting fibrinolysis from plasminogen activator inhibitor-1 (PAI-1). Patients with hereditary deficiencies of protein C who have levels of 60 per cent or less than normal can develop thromboembolic syndromes.[17,18] Individuals born with homozygous protein C-deficiency may develop fatal neonatal purpura fulminans and disseminated intravascular coagulation.[19] Protein C-deficiency may lead to thrombotic complications or skin necrosis when warfarin anticoagulation is initiated.[20]

Heterozygous deficiency of protein S in some families is associated with thromboembolic disease.[21] Activated protein C is inhibited by plasma proteins. The majority of patients with disseminated intravascular coagulation have activation followed by inhibition of protein C. In addition, the majority of disseminated intravascular coagulation-patient plasma contains a higher than normal proportion of protein S in cleaved form, and protein S total antigen levels are found to be low in disseminated intravascular coagulation patients, suggesting that the protein C pathway is activated during disseminated intravascular coagulation.[22]

Fibrinolysis

Fibrinolysis is the mechanism by which fibrin is removed after its role in hemostasis is complete, and results from conversion of plasma proenzyme (plasminogen) into the proteolytic enzyme plasmin. The fibrinolytic system consists of plasminogen and plasmin, together with their activators and inhibitors. Urokinase, isolated from urine, and streptokinase, a bacterial enzyme, along with tissue-type plasminogen are plasminogen activators that have been used in thrombotic disease to produce thrombolysis or recanalize occluded blood vessels. Endogenous plasminogen activators are present in varying concentrations in different body organs. Large amounts are found in the uterine wall and fallopian tubes, although none is present in the placenta.[23] Plasminogen activators are present in other body fluids (for example, milk, tears, saliva, and semen) and may play a role in maintaining the patency of excretory ducts.

Plasmin has a broad spectrum of proteolytic activity. It cleaves arginyl-lysine bonds in a large number of different substrates including hormones, complement and coagulation factors, most prominently fibrinogen and fibrin. Fibrinogen and fibrin absorb plasminogen, and when a fibrin clot forms, plasmin is found in both free and fibrin-absorbed forms; circulating plasminogen is rapidly neutralized by antiplasmin but fibrin-bound plasmin is not. Within the microenvironment of a thrombus, the plasmin incorporated is capable of digesting the fibrin mesh. Freely circulating plasmin will normally be rapidly inactivated by antiplasmins and would, therefore, be unable to degrade its susceptible substrates. Alpha$_2$-antiplasmin and alpha$_2$-macroglobulins are important plasma proteins which neutralize free plasmin. A number of chemical agents have also been shown to inhibit fibrinolysis. These include epsilon-aminocaproic acid (EACA).[24]

Euglobulin Lysis Time. A test used for the evaluation of fibrinolysis is the euglobulin lysis time. Euglobulins are those proteins that precipitate when plasma is diluted in water. The plasminogen activators, plasminogen, plasmin, and fibrinogen are all euglobulins. Antiplasmins and antiplasminogen activators are soluble in water. The euglobulin precipitate is redissolved and thrombin is added to form a fibrin clot. The plasminogen activator activates plasminogen to plasmin. The amount of time required for plasmin to lyse the fibrin clot completely is the euglobulin lysis time. A normal result is a lysis time of longer than two hours. Times shorter than this represent increased fibrinolytic activity.

Degradation of Fibrin and Fibrinogen. The action of plasmin on fibrin or fibrinogen or both, leads (as mentioned earlier) to the formation of a group of soluble protein fragments called fibrin degradation or split products. The immunologic methods usually used for the assay of these fragments do not distinguish among the various degradation products and among those split products derived from fibrin and those derived from fibrinogen. The degradation of fibrin and fibrinogen is a stepwise process, and the molecular size of the resulting fibrin degradation products depends on the duration of the activation of plasmin (Fig. 28–2). Specifically, in the initial step, approximately 20 per cent of the fibrinogen molecule is re-

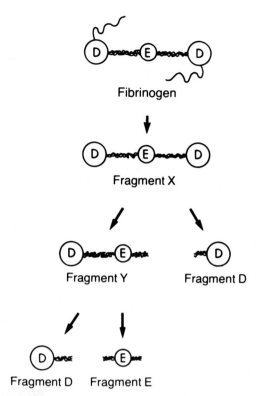

FIGURE 28–2. Degradation of fibrinogen by plasma (see text). (Reprinted with permission from Colman RW, Hirsh J, Marder VJ, Salzman EW. Hemostasis and thrombosis. Basic principles and clinical practice. Philadelphia: JB Lippincott, 1982.)

moved from the C terminal of the alpha chain, yielding fragment X. The proteolysis of fragment X yields fragments D and Y, and with continued proteolysis, smaller fragments D and E are formed. The Thrombo-Wellco test and its analogues use latex particles coated with antibodies to fragments D and E and correlates well with the staphylococcal clumping test, which mainly measures fragments X and Y.[25] The tanned-red cell hemagglutination inhibition test is sensitive to all forms of fibrin degradation products. The D-dimer test is a highly sensitive assay for cross-linked fibrin degradation products and is believed to demonstrate the presence of cross-linked fibrin in the circulation.

Fibrin degradation products are removed from the circulation by the liver, kidney, and the reticuloendothelial system. The half-life of these fragments as a group is approximately nine hours.[26] They impair hemostasis by interfering with platelet function and the polymerization of fibrin, and are typically elevated in disseminated intravascular coagulation.

LABORATORY FINDINGS IN ACUTE, SUBACUTE, AND CHRONIC DISSEMINATED INTRAVASCULAR COAGULATION

Acute Disseminated Intravascular Coagulation

Acute disseminated intravascular coagulation is usually a clinically overwhelming problem characterized by depletion of some coagulation factors and platelets along with concurrent evidence of fibrinolysis. Coagulation factors are depressed because they are consumed or inactivated during the coagulation process or because activated factors are removed by the reticuloendothelial systems. Therefore, there is a marked decrease in fibrinogen. Thrombocytopenia is present and is caused by the consumption of platelets at a rate greater than the bone marrow can compensate for the consumption. Active fibrinolysis occurs, as shown by the increase in concentration of split products of fibrin and fibrinogen; plasma plasminogen concentrations may decrease.[27]

The acute syndrome usually presents with dramatic urgency in the form of unexplained bleeding, shock, or thrombosis occurring in conditions known to be associated with disseminated intravascular coagulation (Table 28–1). For confirmation, important measurements include the plasma fibrinogen, platelet count, prothrombin time, partial thromboplastin time, and fibrin/fibrinogen degradation products. In the typical case, fibrinogen will be substantially reduced. However, since plasma fibrinogen is an acute phase reactant and may be increased in pregnancy, inflammatory disorders, and neoplasia, the amount of fibrinogen has to be compared with that expected for the patient. Therefore, although the fibrinogen may at first be within the usual normal range, the individual patient may be expected to have higher levels. Thus, the clinician should not be misled by a "normal" fibrinogen level. With ongoing consumption, the fibrinogen level may continue to decrease if one does not control the process of disseminated intravascular coagulation.

Subacute and Chronic Disseminated Intravascular Coagulation

In subacute or chronic disseminated intravascular coagulation, the diagnosis may be less obvious and more difficult to make by both clinical and laboratory observations. The number of platelets and levels of coagulation factors in the circulating blood is a dynamic balance between the rate of production and the rate of destruction. In the less severe syndromes, the association of multiple coagulation defects, thrombocytopenia, elevated serum fibrin degradation products, and low fibrinogen may suggest the disorder. However, compensating mechanisms by the bone marrow, liver, and other sites of synthesis of coagulation proteins will have a variable effect so that the absence of one or more of these changes does not exclude the diagnosis. The concentration of some coagulation factors may even be increased if the synthesis processes are fully effective, and traces of thrombin produce a striking activation of factor VIII so that one-stage assays of this factor may give unusually high results.[28] Simple screening tests such as prothrombin, partial thromboplastin, and thrombin times may be normal, prolonged, or even shorter than control times if the coagulation factors are activated. A good example of the possible variability is the platelet count. Thrombocytosis associated with malignancy is well recognized, and a "normal" platelet count may reflect significant peripheral destruction of platelets in a clinical setting that may be associated with thrombocytosis. Therefore, a normal platelet count does not rule out a compensated disseminated intravascular coagulation, and platelet counts may reach supranormal levels when the disseminated intravascular coagulation is controlled.[29]

Studies of platelet and fibrinogen kinetics have helped clarify some of these apparent anomalies. The use of chromium-51-labeled platelets and iodine-125-fibrinogen has assisted in distinguishing between changes in levels caused by altered production, destruction, or distribution. With these techniques, Slichter and Harker[30] showed that malignancy may be associated with increased consumption of both platelets and fibrinogen, the turnover rate being related to the type and extent of the disease. These techniques can also be used to assess the value of various approaches to therapy. However, such techniques are not widely available, and the more conventional coagulation studies remain the basis of evaluation in the majority of patients.

There may be a delay in recognition of chronic disseminated intravascular coagulation because of the complexities already noted. Clinically, obvious bleeding may not be present unless the coagulation factors and platelets are severely depleted, or the patient may present with a focal thrombotic tendency owing to the activation of the clotting system. Thus, in one group of patients with malignancy and various manifestations of thrombosis, isolated venous thrombosis occurred in 113 of 182 patients, and "migratory" venous thrombosis (Trousseau's syndrome), in 96 of these patients.[31] An unusual feature of these chronically ill patients is nonbacterial thrombotic endocarditis, which may be a reflection of chronic disseminated intravascular coagulation.

ROLE OF VASCULAR ENDOTHELIUM IN DISSEMINATED INTRAVASCULAR COAGULATION

As noted above, the intact blood vessel is lined by the endothelial cells, which play an important role in maintaining the integrity of the vascular patency. Endothelial cells play an important role in the regulation of coagulation and fibrinolysis because they are continuously exposed to the coagulation and fibrinolysis factors in the plasma. These activities include maintenance of a continuous lining of the blood vessel which does not encourage platelet adhesion, the generation of prostacyclin and tissue-type plasminogen activator,[32] and the expression of heparin-like glycosaminoglycans and thrombomodulin.[33,34] Endothelial cells synthesize and release activators and inhibitors of platelet aggregation, blood coagulation, and

fibrinolysis. Thus, endothelial cell injury can profoundly influence the balance between these various systems and result in altered hemostasis (Fig. 28–3).

Infectious agents can lead to vascular injury characterized by endothelial cell damage. Septicemia, especially in association with septic shock, is the most frequent disease state associated with disseminated intravascular coagulation, with a lethality of between 40 and 90 per cent.[35] Many of the deleterious consequences of infection can be reproduced in animal models by injecting the infectious agent or endotoxin. Whether endotoxin can cause injury directly to endothelial cells or whether mediators are required for injury to occur is controversial.[36] Endotoxin causes structural and metabolic changes in pulmonary endothelial cells and an increase in permeability of the endothelial layer. Harlan and colleagues[37] have shown that endotoxin or its lipid-A moiety mediates direct, complement-independent endothelial cell cytotoxicity and that this injury is not prevented by inhibitors of protein and prostacylin synthesis. This endothelial injury after incubation with endotoxin in culture is observed with bovine endothelial cells but not with human cells. However, when human endothelial cells in culture are incubated with endotoxin in the presence of granulocytes, these cells adhere to and significantly injure cultured endothelial cells.[38,39] Human endothelial cells also become susceptible to endotoxin-induced cell toxicity when low-density lipoproteins (LDL) are present.[40] After complexing with low-density lipoproteins, endotoxin enters

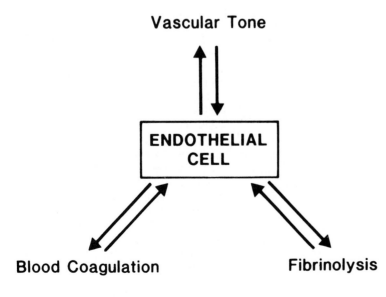

Vascular Tone

ENDOTHELIAL CELL

Blood Coagulation

Fibrinolysis

FIGURE 28–3. Bidirectional action of the endothelial cell with blood, the coagulation, and fibrinolysis systems. (Reprinted with permission from Muller-Berghaus G. Pathophysiologic and biochemical events in disseminated intravascular coagulation: dysregulation of procoagulant and anticoagulant pathways. Semin Thromb Hemost 1989; 15: 58–87.)

endothelial cells and has cytotoxic effects. Gaynor and colleagues[41] showed evidence of endothelial ultrastructural changes and circulating endothelial cells in the blood of rabbits after endotoxin injection. Heparin administration did not prevent development of these lesions, indicating that the endothelial changes may be independent of the abnormalities in the coagulation system, and they interpreted endotoxin-induced disseminated intravascular coagulation as a thrombotic phenomenon which develops at sites of endothelial damage.

In addition to leukocytes, the cytokines produced by lymphocytes influence endothelial cell physiology. The incubation of human umbilical vein endothelial cells with endotoxin increases the binding of T lymphocytes to endothelial cells[42] via activation of the endothelial cells. Soluble products released by lymphocytes are potent regulators of various functions of vascular cells, such as proliferation, migration, production of colony stimulating factor, and expression of class-II histocompatibility (Ia) antigens.[43] Gamma-interferon released from T cells has been shown to regulate the expression of histocompatibility antigens in vascular endothelium.[44] The lymphokine interleukin-1 can substitute for endotoxin in eliciting the local Shwartzman reaction.[45] In addition, the generalized Shwartzman reaction elicited by endotoxin can be prevented by pretreatment with anti-gamma-interferon antibodies.[46] Thus, cytokines produced by lymphocytes influence endothelial cell function and inducers of disseminated intravascular coagulation.

Monocytes and macrophages, via secretion of cachection or tumor necrosis factor (TNF), also play a significant role. The infusion of tumor necrosis factor into animals causes pathophysiological events similar to those observed in animals with septicemia caused by gram-negative organisms: shock and death, microvascular thrombosis, adult respiratory distress syndrome, hemorrhagic diathesis, acute renal tubular necrosis, and adrenal hemorrhage.[47]

CLINICAL SETTINGS

Cardiovascular Disease

The cardiovascular disorder which is most frequently associated with disseminated intravascular coagulation is aortic aneurysm. Fine[48] reported the development of a severe coagulopathy complicating the management of type-1 dissecting aortic aneurysms. Subsequently, many reports of clearly documented disseminated intravascular coagulation associated with the development of vascular aneurysm have appeared. Aneurysms in multiple locations, including aortic arch, ascending thoracic, descending thoracic, thoracoabdominal, total abdominal, and infrarenal abdominal aneurysms, have been reported.

Although the presentation of an abdominal aortic aneurysm may be acute, with sudden onset of abdominal pain, hypotension, and hemodynamic compromise, the presentation of disseminated intravascular coagulation accompanying abdominal aortic aneurysm may also be chronic.[49] Whether clinically manifest or subacute, disseminated intravascular coagulation if present may contribute to the massive hemorrhage associated with this surgery in some patients. Surgery, however, has clearly been documented to be an effective modality of therapy for the disseminated intravascular coagulation associated with an aortic aneurysm. Heparin, given preoperatively, may improve the coagulation profile, and intraoperative coagulation factors and platelets may allow successful surgery.

It is estimated that 4 per cent of patients with aortic aneurysm have clinically overt disseminated intravascular coagulation in the preoperative period, but close to 40 per cent of patients have significant elevation of fibrinogen degradation products.[49] Fibrinogen is an unreliable index of disseminated intravascular coagulation in these patients, and in fact has been noted to be high, low, or normal.[50]

The precise mechanism of initiation of disseminated intravascular coagulation in this setting is not known; however, it is believed that injury to the subendothelial layer of the aortic wall stimulates the deposition of fibrin, and adherence of platelets and activation of the coagulation cascade with secondary fibrinolysis giving rise to the clinical manifestations and laboratory abnormalities. The level of fibrinogen degradation products will slowly decrease in the postoperative period associated with successful surgical therapy and resultant removal of the triggering event for disseminated intravascular coagulation.

MYOCARDIAL INFARCTION

Acute myocardial infarction has been reported as a rare triggering event for the development of chronic, or occasionally even fulminant, disseminated intravascular coagulation. The cause of the development of disseminated intravascular coagulation after acute myocardial infarction is uncertain. The presence of acute, massive myocardial infarction with associated cardiogenic shock may result in hypoxemia, acidosis, and major organ ischemia with resultant tissue injury, thus providing multiple mechanisms for the induction of disseminated intravascular coagulation.

NONBACTERIAL THROMBOTIC ENDOCARDITIS

Nonbacterial thrombotic endocarditis (NBTE), also known as marantic endocarditis and aseptic thrombotic endocardial vegetation, is a common postmortem finding, but there is no general consensus as to its pathogenesis. Nonspecific degenerative changes in the collagenous connective tissue of the cardiac valves and focal erosion of the underlying endocardium could lead to thrombus formation on the valvular surface. Disseminated intravascular coagulation has also been linked to the development of nonbacterial thrombotic endocarditis. The incidence of disseminated intravascular coagulation associated with nonbacterial thrombotic endocarditis has been estimated at 50 per cent.[51] Clinical features of disseminated intravascular coagulation-induced brain injury have included large vessel occlusion with focal neurologic signs of stroke, coma, lethargy, stupor, seizures, and multiple intracerebral hemorrhages. Neurologic manifestations may reflect microvascular thrombosis owing to disseminated intravascular coagulation or embolic occlusion from intracardiac clots. Nonbacterial thrombotic endocarditis is most frequently associated with malignancy, and is also reported with diabetes, tuberculosis, and chronic liver disease.

CAVERNOUS HEMANGIOMAS

The characteristic peripheral vascular disorder capable of triggering disseminated intravascular coagulation is the syndrome of Kasabach and Merrit with cavernous hemangiomas, thrombocytopenia, and hemorrhage. Capillary hemangiomas of various sites have been noted to cause a similar syndrome.

The postulated mechanisms of development of disseminated intravascular coagulation include: (a) localization of platelets within the hemangioma with associated decrease in platelet survival time; (b) concentration of fibrinogen within the hemangiomas, and (c) endothelial cell abnormalities resulting in localized thrombosis and activation of the clotting process that subsequently becomes systemic. In children, the platelet count is usually less than 40,000/cubic millimeter, although it may be normal if the bone marrow can compensate for the peripheral utilization.[52] Severe anemia is a frequent finding, primarily as a result of bleeding into the hemangiomatous lesion, and may require aggressive transfusion and blood component therapy, especially if surgical intervention is contemplated.

HEREDITARY HEMORRHAGIC TELANGIECTASIA

Hereditary hemorrhagic telangiectasia (HHT) may be associated with a hemorrhagic diathesis. This autosomal dominant disorder frequently presents with epistaxis in early childhood. Typical telangiectatic lesions of the skin or mucosa may not appear until the second or third decade of life.

Clinical features may include occult gastrointestinal, genitourinary, pulmonary, or excessive menstrual bleeding, and an approximately 20 per cent incidence of arterial venous fistula of the lungs. Forty to fifty per cent of patients with hereditary hemorrhagic telangiectasia may have laboratory or clinical manifestations of disseminated intravascular coagulation.[53]

Cardiopulmonary Bypass

During the pioneering days of open heart surgery, numerous postoperative complications were reported, including the pump lung syndrome, postperfusion psychosis, renal insufficiency, and fever. In many patients, disseminated intravascular coagulation was proposed as the underlying pathophysiologic derangement. Nonthrombocytopenic purpura associated with splenomegaly, atypical lymphocytosis, and severe purpura fulminans were included among the clinical manifestations of the postcardiopulmonary bypass coagulation defect.

Disseminated intravascular coagulation with manifestations that include severe postoperative hemorrhage may occur in some circumstances after cardiopulmonary bypass. Massive transfusions, cardiac thrombi, severe left ventricular dysfunction, postbypass shock with end-organ ischemia, and perioperative septicemia may all provide the triggering event for a severe coagulopathy in the immediate to subacute postoperative period.

Ventricular Assist Devices and Vascular Prosthesis

More extensive use of the ventricular assist pump as an aid to patients with severe hemodynamic instability or cardiogenic shock has resulted in the demonstration of disseminated intravascular coagulation as a complication of the device. Patients noted to have disseminated intravascular coagulation associated with cardiogenic shock have a poor prognosis. It is frequently difficult to ascertain whether the device itself causes the disseminated intravascular coagulation, or whether other complicating factors such as sepsis, hepatic injury, and pancreatitis are contributing factors in the development of disseminated intravascular coagulation. Intra-aortic balloon pumps may also be associated with the development of thrombocytopenia and low-grade disseminated intravascular coagulation. At times, this can become fulminant, with hemorrhage and aortic or other arterial intramural thrombus formation.[54]

Bleeding after vascular graft replacement is most often attributed to surgical technique. Disseminated intravascular coagulation following vascular graft placement has been reported.[55] The tendency not to suspect an adverse reaction to graft materials is reinforced by the relative inertness of the substances used, either woven or knitted Dacron. However, there are differences in materials used to combine the Dacron together which are the proprietary information of each company. Early recognition of the possibility of disseminated intravascular coagulation following graft placement is important, as survival may depend on rapid replacement of the graft with one from a different manufacturer.[55]

THERAPY

Many of the therapeutic options available in managing patients with disseminated intravascular coagulation are controversial. This is due to the heterogeneity of the underlying disorders causing disseminated intravascular coagulation and the clinical variability of the manifestations of the condition which have not allowed for large randomized trials.

Treatment of the Underlying Cause

This is the cornerstone of management and the most universally accepted principle in the treatment of patients with disseminated intravascular coagulation. In association with infection, specific antimicrobial therapy along with intensive supportive treatment to maintain intravascular volume and organ perfusion are essential. For acutely bleeding patients and those in shock, the maintenance of blood volume is crucial. Evacuation of the uterus in obstetric patients with complications, cytotoxics in malignant disease, and removal of necrotic tissue at surgery are important principles of management. Appropriate and optimal management of underlying cardiologic and vascular disorders, when present, should be the goal of therapy. These are recognized as accepted approaches to therapy. Other aspects of intervention are considered to be more controversial.

Heparin and Other Agents

Because the intravascular generation of thrombin is considered the essential pathogenic factor of consumption coagulopathy, it is a logical therapeutic option to attempt to interfere with thrombin's activity. Heparin should function in this manner to prevent further consumption of the hemostatic proteins and platelets. However, the use of heparin in the management of disseminated intravascular coagulation remains controversial, and widely differing practices exist. Some investigators find that the careful use of heparin is beneficial; others fail to observe improvement in clinical hemostasis or an influence on survival.[56]

Our approach to the use of heparin in disseminated intravascular coagulation is to recognize it as a potentially hazardous drug, but one whose benefit may outweigh its risk in selected patients. If a patient is bleeding or requires a surgical or invasive procedure in the setting of a low fibrinogen level and a low platelet count, it is important to first attempt to improve the level of these factors with transfusion of cryoprecipitate (a source of factor VIII and fibrinogen), fresh frozen plasma (a source of other coagulation proteins), and platelet concentrates. In the setting of active disseminated intravascular coagulation, until the underlying cause can be removed or controlled, it may be very difficult to increase the level of these circulating hemostatic factors with transfusion therapy alone. Therefore, replacement therapy may be given along with a continuous low-dose heparin infusion to interfere with thrombin's action and prolong the half-life of the circulating factors. Sufficient data support low-dose heparin therapy as equivalent to higher-dose therapy in the management of disseminated intravascular coagulation. We recommend heparin at 500 units/hour, and the dosage is adjusted depending upon the clinical disappearance of fibrin degradation products and the increase in the fibrinogen concentration and platelet count seen in monitoring.

There are two situations in which heparin therapy is clearly indicated. The first is the patient with disseminated intravascular coagulation who manifests thrombotic complications of the disorder. The second is the patient with early laboratory evidence for deteriorating disseminated intravascular coagulation who has not yet decompensated to the point of bleeding.

Most obstetric cases of disseminated intravascular coagulation resolve on evacuation of the uterus. Occasionally, the disseminated intravascular coagulation continues and can only be reversed by heparin. Heparin therapy has been reported to be effective in improving clinical hemostasis and the coagulation profile in excessive bleeding associated with giant hemangioma and neoplastic disease, particularly promyelocytic leukemia.

Another possible indication for heparin therapy is evidence of organ ischemia in the setting of disseminated intravascular coagulation. When intravascular volume has been optimized and progressive ischemia to major organs such as the brain or kidney continues, active inhibition of thrombin by heparin to interfere with continued formation of fibrin is probably indicated.

Because heparin's anticoagulant activity depends on the presence of antithrombin III in the blood, heparin may be less effective when antithrombin III is deficient in patients with disseminated intravascular coagulation. Because antithrombin III levels are frequently low in such patients, antithrombin III concentrates have been given along with heparin therapy.[57] These studies suggest that supplementation of antithrombin III in cases of disseminated intravascular coagulation may be a valuable addition to the therapeutic strategies currently employed.

The use of agents such as epsilon-aminocaproic acid (EACA) to block the fibrinolytic component of the syndrome is generally contraindicated. In most discussions of treatment, it is stated that epsilon-aminocaproic acid should be administered only in cases of primary fibrinolysis. This condition is very rare, and it is feared that use of this agent in conditions associated with disseminated intravascular coagulation may precipitate thromboembolic complications and should thus be avoided.

CONCLUSIONS

Disseminated intravascular coagulation is a complex syndrome which is not an independent disease but is incited by a broad spectrum of underlying medical conditions. The first priority, following recognition of the presence of disseminated intravascular coagulation, is the treatment of the primary condition. The paucity of clinical therapeutic trials for disseminated intravascular coagulation do not allow for absolute guidelines. Hematologic support usually involves transfusion therapy. The use of heparin anticoagulant therapy and, possibly, antithrombin III concentrates need to be considered in individual circumstances. There is a crucial need for well-controlled studies for the treatment of this syndrome.

REFERENCES

1. Fruchtman SM, Aledort LM. Disseminated intravascular coagulation. J Am Col Cardiol 1986; 8: 159B–67B.
2. Schneider CL. Fibrin embolism (disseminated intravascular coagulation) with defibrination as one of the end results during placenta abruptio. Surg Gynecol Obstet 1951; 92: 27–34.
3. Lasch HG, Heene DL, Huth K, Sandritter W. Pathophysiology, clinical manifestations and therapy of consumption coagulopathy ("Verbrauchskoagulopathie"). Am J Cardiol 1967; 20: 381–91.
4. Muller-Berghaus G. Pathophysiologic and biochemical events in disseminated intravascular coagulation: dysregulation of procoagulant and anticoagulant pathways. Semin Thromb Hemost 1989; 15: 58–87.
5. Selye H. Thrombohemorrhagic phenomena. Springfield: Thomas, 1966.
6. Merskey C, Johnson AJ, Kleiner GH, Wohl H. The defi-

brination syndrome: clinical features and laboratory diagnosis. Br J Haematol 1967; 13: 528–49.

7. Marder VJ, Martin SE, Brancis CW, Colman RW. Consumptive thrombohemorrhagic disorders. In: Colman RW, Hirsh J, Marder, VJ Salzman EW, eds. Hemostasis and thrombosis. Basic principles and clinical practice. Philadelphia: JB Lippincott Co., 1987: 975–1015.

8. Girolami A, Cliffton EE, Agostino P. Haemorrhagic syndrome in dogs induced by intravenous thrombin. Thromb Diath Haemorrh 1966; 16: 243–56.

9. Margaretten W, Csavossy I, McKay DG. An electron microscopic study of thrombin-induced disseminated intravascular coagulation. Blood 1967; 29: 169–81.

10. Stetson CA Jr. Studies on the mechanism of the Shwartzman phenomenon; certain factors involved in the production of the local haemorrhagic necrosis. J Exp Med 1951; 93: 489–504.

11. McKay DG, Wong T, Galton M. Effect of pregnancy on the disseminated thrombosis caused by bacterial endotoxin. Fed Proc 1969; 19: 246–53.

12. Kliman A, McKay DG. The prevention of the generalized Shwartzman reaction by fibrinolytic activity. Arch Path 1958; 66: 715–9.

13. Muller-Berghaus G, McKay DG. Prevention of the generalized Shwartzman reaction in pregnant rats by α-adrenergic blocking agents. Lab Invest 1967; 17: 276–80.

14. Davie EW, Ratnoff OD. Waterfall sequence for intrinsic blood clotting. Science 1964; 145: 1310–2.

15. Damus PS, Hicks M. Rosenberg RD. Anticoagulant action of heparin. Nature 1973; 246; 355–61.

16. Walker FJ. Regulation of activated protein C by protein S. J Biol Chem 1981; 256: 1128–31.

17. Griffin JH, Evatt B, Simmerman TS, et al. Deficiency of protein C in congenital thrombotic disease. J Clin Invest 1981; 68: 1370–8.

18. Broekmans AW, Veltkamp JJ, Bertina RM. Congenital protein C deficiency and venous thromboembolism—a study of the Dutch families. N Engl J Med 1983; 309: 340–8.

19. Branson HE, Katz J, Marble R, et al. Inherited protein C deficiency and a coumarin-responsive chronic relapsing purpura fulminans syndrome in a neonate. Lancet 1983; 1: 1165–7.

20. Griffin JH. Clinical studies of protein C. Semin Thromb Hemost 1984; 10: 162–5.

21. Schwarz HP, Fischer M, Hopmeir P, Bafard MA, Griffin JH. Plasma protein S deficiency in familial thrombotic disease. Blood 1984; 64: 1297–300.

22. Heeb MJ, Mosler D, Griffin J. Activation and complexation of protein C and cleavage and decrease of protein S in plasma of patients with intravascular coagulation. Blood 1989; 73: 445–61.

23. Albrechsten OK. The fibrinolytic activity of human tissues. Br J Haematol 1957; 3: 284–91.

24. Alkjaersig M, Fletcher AP, Sherry S. E-aminocaproic acid: an inhibitor of plasminogen activator. J Biol Chem 1959; 234: 284–91.

25. Carvalho CA, Ellman LL, Coleman RW. A comparative study of the staphylococcal clumping test and an agglutination test for detection of fibrinogen degradation products. Am J Clin Pathol 1974; 62: 107–14.

26. Fletcher AP, Alkjaersig M, Sherry S. Pathogenesis of the coagulation defect developing during pathologic plasma proteolytic (fibrinolytic) states. I. The significance of fibrinogen proteolysis and circulating fibrinogen breakdown products. J Clin Invest 1962; 41: 896–916.

27. Helegren M, Egberg N, Eklind J. Blood coagulation and fibrinolytic factors and their inhibitors in initially ill patients. Intensive Care Med 1984; 10: 23–8.

28. Penick GD, Roberts HR, Dejanov JF. Covert intravascular clotting. Fed Proc 1965; 24: 835–9.

29. Owen CA Jr, Bowie EJW. Chronic intravascular coagulation syndromes—a summary. Mayo Clin Proc 1974; 499: 673–80.

30. Slichter SJ, Harker LA. Hemostasis in malignancy. Ann NY Acad Sci 1974; 230: 252–61.

31. Sack GH, Levin J, Bell WB. Trousseau's syndrome and other manifestations of chronic disseminated coagulation in patients with neoplasm: clinical, pathophysiologic and therapeutic features. Medicine 1977; 56: 1–37.

32. Loskutoff DJ, Edgington TS. Synthesis of fibrinolytic activator and inhibitor by endothelial cells. Proc Natl Acad Sci USA 1977; 74: 3903–7.

33. Marcum JA, McKenney JB, Rosenberg RD. Acceleration of thrombin-antithrombin complex formation in rat hindquarters via heparin-like molecules bound to the endothelium. J Clin Invest 1984; 74: 341–50.

34. Esmon CT, Owen WG. Identification of an endothelial cell cofactor for thrombin catalyzed activation of protein C. Proc Natl Acad Sci USA 1981; 78: 2249–52.

35. Proctor RA. Clinical aspects of endotoxin shock. In Proctor RA, ed. Handbook of endotoxin. Vol 4. Amsterdam: Elsevier, 1986.

36. Bagby GC Jr, Dinarello CA, Wallace P, Wagner C, Hefeneider S, McCall E. Interleukin 1 stimulates granulocyte macrophage colony-stimulating activity release by vascular endothelial cells. J Clin Invest 1986; 78: 1316–23.

37. Harlan JM, Harker LA, Reidy MA, Gajdusek CM, Schwartz SM, Striker GE. Lipopolysaccharide-mediated bovine endothelial cell injury in vitro. Lab Invest 1983; 48: 269–74.

38. Yamada O, Moldow CF, Sacks T, Craddock PR, Bogaerts MA, Jacob HS. Deleterious effects of endotoxin on cultured endothelial cells: an in vitro model of vascular injury. Inflammation 1981; 5: 115–26.

39. Harlan JM. Leukocyte-endothelial interactions. Blood 1985; 65: 513–25.

40. Morel DW, DiCorleto PE, Chisolm GM. Modulation of endotoxin-induced endothelial cell toxicity by low density lipoprotein. Lab Invest 1986; 55: 419–26.

41. Gaynor E, Bouvier C, Spaet TH. Vascular lesions: possible pathogenetic basis of the generalized Shwartzman reaction. Science 1970; 170: 986–8.

42. Yu C-L, Haskard D, Cavender D, Ziff M. Effects of bacterial lipopolysaccharide on the binding of lymphocytes to endothelial cell monolayers. J Immunol 1986; 136: 569–73.

43. Montovani A, Dejana E. Modulation of endothelial function by interleukin-1: a novel target for pharmacological intervention. Biochem Pharm 1987; 36: 301–5.

44. Pober JS, Gimbrone MA Jr, Cotran RS, et al. Ia expression by vascular endothelium is inducible by activated T cells and by human interferon. J Exp Med 1983; 157: 1339–53.

45. Beck G, Habicht GS, Benach JL, Miller F. Interleukin 1: a common endogenous mediator of inflammation and the local Shwartzman reaction. J Immunol 1986; 135: 3025–31.

46. Billiau A, Heremans H, Van de Kerckhove F, Dillen C. Antiinterferon-γ antibody protects mice against the generalized Shwartzman reaction. Eur J Immunol 1987; 17: 1851–4.

47. Tracey KJ, Beutler B, Lowry SF, et al. Shock and tissue injury induced by recombinant human cachectin. Science 1986; 234: 470–4.

48. Fine NL, et al. Multiple coagulation defects in association with dissecting aneurysm. Arch Intern Med 1967; 119: 522–6.

49. Brieger R, Vreeken J, Stebbe J. Arterial aneurysm as a cause of consumption coagulopathy. N Engl J Med 1971; 285: 152–6.

50. Hardaway RM. What's new: a review of misconceptions concerning fibrinogen. Tex Med 1982; 78: 40–4.

51. Kim HS, Suzuki M, Lie JT, Titus JL. Nonbacterial thrombotic endocarditis (NBTE) and disseminated intravascular coagulation (DIC). Arch Path Lab Med 1977; 101: 65–8.

52. Wacksman SJ, Flessa HC, Glueck HI. Coagulation defects and giant hemangiomas. Am J Dis Child 1966; 111: 71–4.

53. Bick RL, Fekete LF. Hereditary hemorrhagic teleangiectasia and associated defects in hemostasis (abstr). Blood 1978; 52: 179.

54. Al-Mondhiry H, Pierce WS, Richenlacher W. Hemostatic abnormalities associated with prolonged ventricular assist pumping: analysis of 24 patients. Am J Cardiol 1984; 53: 1344–8.

55. Roizen MF, Rodgers GM, Valone FH, et al. Anaphylactoid reactions to vascular graft material presenting with vasodilation and subsequent disseminated intravascular coagulation. Anesthesiology 1989; 71: 331–8.

56. Deykin D. The clinical challenge of disseminated intravascular coagulation. N Engl J Med 1970; 283: 636–44.

57. Sakata Y, Yoshida N, Matsuda I, et al. Treatment of DIC with antithrombin III concentrates. Bibl Haematologica 1983; 49: 307–16.

29

HEMORRHAGIC COMPLICATIONS OF LONG-TERM ANTITHROMBOTIC TREATMENT

MARK N. LEVINE and JACK HIRSH

Vitamin K antagonists are widely used to prevent recurrent thrombosis in patients with established thromboembolism and to prevent thrombosis in individuals with a variety of cardiac disorders. The most common vitamin K antagonist used in North America is warfarin. In other centers, acenocoumarin, dicoumarin, phenprocoumon, and other coumarin derivatives are used. The major complication of anticoagulant therapy is hemorrhage. In this chapter, the incidence of hemorrhage in patients receiving long-term oral anticoagulant therapy (therapy for more than four weeks), and the clinical and laboratory risk factors that predispose to bleeding are discussed. In performing the review of bleeding, conclusions were drawn from results of randomized, controlled trials whenever possible.[1] Hemorrhage was classified as major if it was intracranial or retroperitoneal, if it lead directly to death, or if it resulted in hospitalization or transfusion. All other bleeding episodes were classified as minor.

MECHANISMS OF ORAL ANTICOAGULANT-INDUCED BLEEDING

Vitamin K catalyzes the post-translational carboxylation of glutamic acid residues on several proteins synthesized in the liver. The resulting gamma-carboxyglutamic (Gla) residues bind calcium ions in the presence of membrane phospholipids; an important requirement for the appropriate function of these proteins. The vitamin K-dependent coagulation proteins are factors II, VII, IX, and X (in other chapters, mention is also made of the inhibitors protein C and S). The noncarboxylated forms are inactive because they can no longer form appropriate complexes with calcium and phospholipid, and thus if the carboxylated forms are excessively depleted, thrombin generation is delayed, hemostasis is perturbed, and hemorrhage can result.

There are three major determinants of oral anticoagulant-induced bleeding. These are the intensity of the anticoagulant effect, patient-related comorbid conditions, and the concomitant use of drugs that interfere with hemostasis.

The intensity of the anticoagulant effect is influenced by the dose of warfarin, the patient's vitamin K intake, interindividual variability in anticoagulant response to a given dosage, and other factors that alter the pharmacokinetics and pharmacodynamics of warfarin, of which the most important are concomitant medication and liver disease. The most important patient-related comorbid conditions are an associated lesion (for example, peptic ulcer, carcinoma, and trauma) that predisposes to bleeding and cerebrovascular disease. The most important association of a hemostatic defect is impaired platelet function produced by concomitant aspirin use.

RELATIONSHIP BETWEEN INTENSITY OF ANTICOAGULANT THERAPY AND HEMORRHAGE

A relationship between the intensity of anticoagulant therapy and the risk of bleeding has been reported in patients with deep vein thrombosis, tissue heart valves, and mechanical heart valves (Table 29–1). In patients with venous thrombosis, Hull and colleagues reported a strong relationship between the intensity of warfarin treatment and the risk of bleeding.[2] The patients randomized to receive less intense warfarin (targeted international normalized ratio of 2.0) had significantly less bleeding (4 per cent versus 22 per cent) than those receiving more intense therapy (targeted international normalized ratio of 2.5 to 4.5). In the 13 patients who bled, the international normalized ratio was prolonged to more than three times control value.

In a trial reported by Turpie et al., patients with tissue heart valves were randomized to either standard-intensity warfarin (international normalized ratio of 2.5 to 4.0) or less intense warfarin (international normalized ratio of 2.0 to 2.5).[3] The rate of clinically important bleeding was reduced from 14 per cent in the standard-intensity group to 6 per cent in the low-intensity group without loss of antithrombotic efficacy.

In a recently reported trial, 258 patients with prosthetic heart valves were randomized to either moderate-intensity warfarin (targeted international normalized ratio of 2.65) or high-intensity warfarin (targeted international normalized ratio of 9.0).[4] No difference was detected in the incidence of thromboembolism between the two groups. However, bleeding was more common in the higher-intensity group. Of the 122 patients randomized to the moderate-intensity warfarin, four experienced major bleeding and 22 experienced minor bleeding. In the 125 patients

who received the higher-intensity warfarin, there were nine major bleeds (of which two were fatal intracranial) and 44 minor bleeds. The difference in total and minor bleeding between groups was statistically significant.

RELATIONSHIP BETWEEN RISK OF BLEEDING AND PATIENT RISK FACTORS

Major bleeding is especially likely in patients with ischemic cerebral vascular disease and venous thromboembolism, possibly owing to the higher prevalence of associated risk factors in these conditions.[1] In venous thromboembolism, these comorbid conditions (cancer, recent surgery, and paraplegia) predispose the patient to thrombosis. In cerebral vascular disease, major bleeding is usually intracerebral, possibly because of associated hypertension or the vascular disease per se.

There have been two recent retrospective studies which have examined the risk of bleeding and underlying risk factors. Gurwitz et al. reported a 4.4 per cent rate of major bleeding in 321 patients on long-term oral anticoagulant therapy and found no relationship between age and risk of bleeding.[5] Landefeld et al. reported a 12 per cent rate of major bleeding in 565 patients on long-term oral anticoagulant therapy.[6,7] There were five factors which were known at the start of therapy that predicted independently for bleeding. These were: age 65 years or older, history of stroke, history of gastrointestinal bleeding, atrial fibrillation, and a serious comorbid condition (recent myocardial infarction, renal insufficiency, or severe anemia). In this study, the authors also determined that for each 1.0 increase in the prothrombin time ratio, the odds ratio for major bleeding during the week after the prothrombin time

TABLE 29–1. Relationship Between the Intensity of Anticoagulant Therapy and Hemorrhage

STUDY	INDICATION	TARGETED INTERNATIONAL NORMALIZED RATIO	BLEEDING (%)
Hull[2]	Venous thromboembolism	2.0	4
		2.5–4.5	22
Turpie[3]	Tissue heart valve	2.0–2.5	6
		2.5–4.5	14
Saour[4]	Prosthetic heart valve	2.65	21
		9.0	42

measurement increased by 80 per cent. In addition, there was a suggestion that patients who bled with the prothrombin time in the therapeutic range were subsequently found to have an underlying pathologic lesion as the cause of their bleeding.[6,7]

RISK OF HEMORRHAGE AND CLINICAL DISORDER

Ischemic Cerebral Vascular Disease

There have been six randomized trials conducted which compared oral anticoagulant treatment with either a nontreatment group, a very–low-dose anticoagulant group, or an antiplatelet group[8-15] (Table 29–2). In all cases there was increased bleeding associated with the oral anticoagulant treatment. The risk of bleeding in the anticoagulant group was impressive, and ranged from 11.8 to 39 per cent. The risk of major bleeding (most commonly intracerebral) was also high, being greater than 7 per cent in four out of the six studies.[8,11,12,15] Fatal hemorrhage ranged from 2 to 7 per cent.

Prosthetic Heart Valves

In the published randomized trials of long-term anticoagulant therapy in patients with prosthetic heart valves, oral anticoagulant therapy was compared with a combination of oral anticoagulants and antiplatelet agents[16-20] (Table 29–3). The frequency of bleeding ranged from 1.2 to 10.7 per cent in the patients treated with anticoagulant alone. Major bleeding ranged from 0 to 6.8 per cent. There were no fatal bleeds in one study,[20] but fatal bleeding was as high as 4.1 per cent in another,[18] with most fatal bleeds being intracerebral.

In two of the three studies, there was a significantly greater frequency of bleeding when aspirin was added to warfarin, whereas the addition of dipyridamole did not increase the risk of bleeding.[17,20] Most of the bleeding episodes during combined treatment with anticoagulant and aspirin were gastrointestinal.

Atrial Fibrillation

There have been three randomized trials published recently in patients with atrial fibrillation who received long-term oral anticoagulant therapy[21-23] (Table 29–4). In the study reported by Peterson et al., patients with chronic nonrheumatic atrial fibrillation were randomized to either warfarin (335 patients), aspirin 75 milligrams once daily (336 patients), or placebo (336 patients).[21] The targeted therapeutic range was an international normalized ratio of 2.8 to 4.2. The incidence of thromboembolic complications and vascular mortality was significantly lower in the warfarin group than in the aspirin and placebo groups. Five patients on warfarin had thromboembolic complications compared with 20 patients on aspirin and 21 on placebo. There were 21 warfarin patients (6.3 per cent) who experienced nonfatal bleeding

TABLE 29–2. Ischemic Cerebrovascular Disease

			BLEEDING		
STUDY	TREATMENT	NUMBER OF PATIENTS	Total (%)	Major (%)	Fatal (%)
Baker[11]	Warfarin/Dicumarol	78	31 (39.7)*	10 (12.8)	4 (5.1)
	No therapy	77	5 (6.5)	3 (3.9)	1 (1.3)
Baker,[11] Fisher[13]	Dicumarol	224	88 (39.3)*	18 (8.0)	12 (5.4)
	Placebo	219	10 (4.6)	2 (0.9)	0
Enger[8]	Phenindione	52	10 (19.2)*	4 (7.7)	3 (5.8)
	Placebo	48	0	0	0
Hill[14]	Phenindione (high)	71	15 (21.1)*	5 (7.0)	5 (7.0)
	Phenindione (low)	71	1 (1.4)	1 (1.4)	0
McDowell[9]	Warfarin	95	17 (17.9)*	2 (2.1)	2 (2.1)
	No therapy	105	1 (1.0)	1 (1.0)	1 (1.0)
Olsson[10]	Warfarin	68	8 (11.8)	2 (2.9)	2 (2.9)
	Aspirin plus dipyridamole	67	3 (4.5)	0	0

* $p < 0.01$.

TABLE 29–3. Prosthetic Heart Valves

STUDY	TREATMENT	NUMBER OF PATIENTS	BLEEDING		
			Total (%)	Major (%)	Fatal (%)
Altman[16]	Acenocoumarin plus aspirin (500 milligrams)	57	7 (12.3)	1 (1.7)	1 (1.7)
	Acenocoumarin	65	7 (10.7)	1 (1.5)	1 (1.5)
Chesebro[17]	Warfarin plus aspirin (250 milligrams twice daily)	170	23 (13.5)*	20 (11.8)	3 (1.8)
	Warfarin plus Dipyridamole	180	7 (3.9)	4 (2.2)	0
	Warfarin†	183	9 (4.9)	4 (2.2)	3 (1.6)
Dale[18,19]	Warfarin plus aspirin (500 milligrams twice daily)	75	15 (20.0)*	12 (16.0)	1 (1.3)
	Warfarin	73	6 (8.2)	5 (6.8)	3 (4.1)
Sullivan[20]	Warfarin plus Dipyridamole	79	3 (3.7)	2 (2.5)	2 (2.5)
	Warfarin	84	1 (1.2)	0	0
Turpie[3]	Warfarin	108	15 (13.9)*	5 (4.6)	0
	Warfarin (less intense)	102	6 (5.9)	0	0
Saour[4]	Warfarin (more intense)	125	53 (42.4)*	9 (7.2)*	2 (1.6)
	Warfarin (less intense)	122	26 (21.3)	4 (3.2)	0

* $p < 0.05$.
† Nonrandomized concurrent control.

events, and one warfarin patient had a fatal intracerebral hemorrhage. Two patients on aspirin and none on placebo experienced bleeding.

In the second trial reported by the Stroke Prevention in Atrial Fibrillation Study Group, patients with atrial fibrillation not related to rheumatic or prosthetic valvular heart disease were randomized to either warfarin at a targeted international normalized ratio of 2.0 to 3.5 (201 patients), aspirin 325 milligrams/day (192 patients), or placebo (195 patients).[22] Recruitment to the trial was stopped after 588 patients had been recruited to the study because active therapy with either warfarin or aspirin significantly reduced the risk of thromboembolic events compared to placebo alone. The mean follow-up was 1.13

years. Hemorrhagic events requiring hospital admission, blood transfusion, or surgery occurred at a rate of 1.7 per cent/year in the warfarin group; intracranial hemorrhage occurred at a rate of 0.9 per cent/year, and cerebral hemorrhage at a rate of 0.4 per cent/year. In patients who received placebo, the rate of total bleeding was 1.2 per cent/year with 0.2 per cent/year having intracranial bleeds.

In a recently reported trial from Boston, 420 patients with nonrheumatic atrial fibrillation were randomized to either low-dose warfarin therapy (targeted international normalized ratio of 1.5 to 2.7) (212 patients) or no treatment (208 patients).[23] In this study, bleeding was considered major if it was fatal, intracerebral, or associated with a transfusion

TABLE 29–4. Nonrheumatic Atrial Fibrillation

STUDY	TREATMENT	NUMBER OF PATIENTS	BLEEDING		
			Total (%)	Major (%)	Fatal (%)
Peterson[21]	Warfarin	335	21 (6.3)†	*	1 (0.3)
	Aspirin (75 milligrams)	336	2 (0.6)	*	0
	Placebo	336	0	*	0
SPAF[22]	Warfarin	201	*	1.7%/year	*
	Aspirin (325 milligrams)	192	*	0.9%/year	*
	Placebo	195	*	1.2%/year	*
Boston[23]	Warfarin	212	38 (17.9)	8 (3.8)	1 (4.7)
	No therapy	208	21 (9.6)	8 (3.8)	1 (4.8)

* Not reported in publications.
† $p < 0.05$.

of greater than four units of erythrocytes. There were two major bleeds in the warfarin group (one intracerebral and one gastrointestinal) compared to one in the control group (intrapulmonary hemorrhage); one bleed in each group was fatal. In addition, six warfarin patients experienced bleeding episodes leading to hospitalization or transfusion compared to seven control patients. Thirty-eight warfarin patients had minor bleeds compared to 21 control patients.

Ischemic Heart Disease

There are eight published randomized trials of long-term oral anticoagulant therapy in patients with acute myocardial infarction[24-33] (Table 29-5). In six of these, anticoagulant therapy was compared with placebo or control;[24,25,29-31,33] in the seventh, anticoagulant was compared with aspirin,[27] and in the eighth, anticoagulant was compared with aspirin plus placebo.[28] Anticoagulant therapy was associated with an increased risk of bleeding ranging from 3.8 to 36.5 per cent. The frequency of major bleeding ranged from 0 to 10 per cent, and fatal bleeding ranged from 0 to 2.9 per cent. A number of these randomized trials evaluating long-term oral anticoagulant therapy in patients with myocardial infarction were conducted in the 1970s. The results of these were conflicting, and hence the previous practice of prescribing such patients oral anticoagulant therapy fell out of favor. However, Smith et al. recently reported the results of a randomized trial of oral anticoagulant therapy in patients with acute myocardial infarction which renews interest in the long-term use of oral anticoagulants after myocardial infarction.[24] One thousand two hundred fourteen such patients were randomized to either warfarin (607 patients) or placebo (607 patients). The targeted international normalized ratio was 2.8 to 4.8. There was a clinically impressive and statistically significant reduction in mortality, reinfarction, and cerebrovascular events in patients who received the warfarin. Five patients in the warfarin group (0.8 per cent) had intracranial hemorrhages and three of these were fatal. Eight warfarin patients experienced major extracranial bleeds. There were no major or fatal bleeds in the placebo group. Minor bleeding occurred in 52 of the warfarin patients compared to 25 placebo patients.

Venous Thromboembolism

There have been four randomized trials which have evaluated bleeding during oral anticoagulant therapy in patients with venous

TABLE 29-5. Ischemic Heart Disease

STUDY	TREATMENT	NUMBER OF PATIENTS	BLEEDING		
			Total (%)	Major (%)	Fatal (%)
Sixty-plus[25,26]	Acenocoumarin	439	74 (17.0)‡	18 (4.1)	6 (1.4)
	Placebo	439	6 (1.4)	1 (0.2)	1 (0.2)
EPSIM Group[27]	Oral anticoagulants*	652	104 (16.0)‡	21 (3.2)	8 (1.2)
	Aspirin (500 milligrams three times daily)	651	35 (5.4)	5 (0.8)	4 (0.6)
Breddin[28]	Phenprocoumon	320	12 (3.8)	†	0
	Aspirin (500 milligrams three times daily)	317	9 (2.8)	†	0
	Placebo	309	0	†	0
Meuwissen[29]	Phenprocoumon	68	7 (10.3)‡	0	0
	Placebo	70	0	0	0
Loeliger[30]	Phenprocoumon	128	17 (13.3)‡	1 (0.8)	0
	Placebo	122	7 (5.7)	1 (0.8)	1 (0.8)
Bjerkelund[31,32]	Dicumarol	138	32 (23.2)‡	20 (14.5)	4 (2.9)
	No therapy	139	9 (6.5)	5 (3.6)	1 (0.7)
Harvald[33]	Dicumarol	145	53 (36.5)‡	28 (19.3)	1 (0.7)
	Placebo	170	8 (4.7)	0	0
Smith[24]	Warfarin	607	52 (8.6)	13 (2.1)	3 (4.9)
	Placebo	607	25 (4.1)	0	0

* A number of different oral anticoagulants.
† Not reported.
‡ $p < 0.01$.

TABLE 29–6. Venous Thromboembolism

STUDY	TREATMENT	NUMBER OF PATIENTS	BLEEDING		
			Total (%)	Major (%)	Fatal (%)
Bynum[34]	Warfarin	24	9 (37.5)‡	4 (16.7)	0
	Heparin*	24	1 (4.2)	0	0
Hull[35]	Warfarin	33	7 (21.1)‡	4 (12.1)	0
	Heparin*	35	0	0	0
Hull[36]	Warfarin	53	9 (17.0)‡	3 (5.7)	0
	Heparin†	53	1 (1.9)	0	0
Hull[2]	Warfarin	49	11 (22.4)‡	2 (4.1)	0
	Warfarin (less intense)	47	2 (4.3)	2 (4.3)	0

* Low-dose subcutaneous heparin.
† Adjusted-dose subcutaneous heparin.
‡ $p < 0.01$.

thromboembolism[2,34–36] (Table 29–6). In all of these studies, the dose of warfarin in one group was adjusted to maintain the pro-thrombin time (rabbit brain thromboplastin) at approximately twice control (international normalized ratio of 4.5), while the other group was treated less intensively. In two of the studies, the group on less-intense (non-warfarin) therapy received low-dose unfrac-tionated subcutaneous heparin (5,000 units subcutaneously twice daily);[34,35] in the third trial the comparison group received adjusted-dose subcutaneous standard heparin;[36] and in the fourth trial, the dose of warfarin was adjusted to an international normalized ratio of approximately 2.0.[2] In all four studies, total bleeding (both major and minor) was significantly greater in the more intensely anticoagulated group. Bleeding in patients receiving the more intense warfarin varied from 17 to 37.5 per cent, and major bleeding varied from 4.1 to 16.7 per cent. There were no fatal bleeds.

Summary of Bleeding Risks

Bleeding rates (pooled rates) during long-term anticoagulated therapy are substantial.

For major bleeding, the rates ranged from 2.4 to 8.1 per cent; and for fatal bleeding, 0 to 4.8 per cent (Table 29–7). The highest bleeding rates were seen in patients with cerebrovascular disease and venous throm-boembolism.

TREATMENT OF BLEEDING SECONDARY TO ORAL ANTICOAGULANT THERAPY

The approach to treatment is influenced by whether the prothrombin time is in the targeted therapeutic range at the time of bleeding or by whether it is excessively pro-longed. If hemorrhage occurs when the pro-thrombin time is within the therapeutic range, an underlying cause for bleeding should be sought. Bleeding associated with oral anticoagulants is usually managed by one or more of the following approaches: (a) cessation of anticoagulant therapy, (b) ad-ministration of vitamin K, (c) administration of plasma derivatives containing vitamin K-dependent clotting factors, and (d) volume replacement if indicated. If bleeding is po-

TABLE 29–7. Hemorrhage During Warfarin Therapy

INDICATION	NUMBER OF PATIENTS	MAJOR BLEED (%)	FATAL BLEED (%)
Ischemic cerebrovascular	588	41 (7.0)	28 (4.8)
Prosthetic mechanical heart valves	405	10 (2.4)	7 (1.7)
Atrial fibrillation	748	32 (4.3)	2 (0.3)
Ischemic heart	1890	88 (4.7)	19 (1.0)
Venous thromboembolism	159	13 (8.1)	0 (1.0)

tentially life threatening and the prothrombin time is prolonged, the coagulation defect should be reversed immediately by infusion of fresh frozen plasma or factors II, VII, IX, and X concentrate. The administration of plasma may be problematic in a patient with poor cardiac reserve because of fluid overload. If plasma cannot be given, then the above-mentioned coagulation factor concentrate should be used, except in patients with liver failure. If the prothrombin time is markedly prolonged, but the bleeding is not life threatening, the prothrombin time can be reduced within eight hours by the intravenous or subcutaneous administration of vitamin K. A dose of more than 25 milligrams causes the patient to become refractory to further anticoagulant therapy for days. The dose of five to ten milligrams allows anticoagulant therapy to be continued if indicated. In Europe, vitamin K_1 is mainly used; in the case of bleeding associated with massive overdosage of coumarins or warfarin, 10 milligrams of vitamin K_1 is given intravenously. If the prothrombin time is excessively prolonged without bleeding, then one to two milligrams of vitamin K_1 given orally will suffice, unless the patient has problems with intestinal absorption (for example, obstructive jaundice) in which case vitamin K_1 in low dose, that is, one to two milligrams, can be given subcutaneously or intravenously.

If the prothrombin time is only slightly outside the targeted therapeutic range, and bleeding is not life threatening, the patient can be treated by omitting the next two or three doses of warfarin and by carefully monitoring the patient's progress.

REFERENCES

1. Levine MN, Raskob G, Hirsh J. Hemorrhagic complications of long-term anticoagulant therapy. Chest 1989; 95(suppl 2): 26S–36S.
2. Hull R, Hirsh J, Jay R, et al. Different intensities of oral anticoagulant therapy in the treatment of proximal-vein thrombosis. N Engl J Med 1982; 307: 1676–81.
3. Turpie AGG, Gunstensen J, Hirsh J, Nelson H, Gent M. Randomized comparison of two intensities of oral anticoagulant therapy after tissue heart valve replacement. Lancet 1988; 1: 1242–5.
4. Saour JN, Sieck JO, Mamo LAR, Gallus AS. Trial of different intensities of anticoagulation in patients with prosthetic heart valves. N Engl J Med 1990; 322: 428–32.
5. Gurwitz JH, Goldberg RJ, Holden A, Knapic N, Ansell J. Age-related risks of long term oral anticoagulant therapy. Arch Int Med 1988; 148: 1733–36.
6. Landefeld CS, Rosenblatt MW. Bleeding in outpatients treated with warfarin: relation to the prothrombin time and important remediable lesions. Am J Med 1989; 87: 153–9.
7. Landefeld CS, Goldman L. Major bleeding in outpatients

8. treated with warfarin: incidence and prediction by factors known at the start of outpatient therapy. Am J Med 1989; 87: 144–52.
8. Enger E, Boyesen S. Long term anticoagulant therapy in patients with cerebral infarction. Acta Med Scand 1965; 178(suppl): 7–55.
9. McDowell F, McDevitt E, Wright IS. Anticoagulant therapy: five years experience with the patient with an established cerebrovascular accident. Arch Neurol 1963; 8: 209–14.
10. Olsson JE, Brechter C, Backlund H, et al. Anticoagulant vs. antiplatelet therapy as prophylactic against cerebral infarction in transient ischemic attacks. Stroke 1980; 11: 4–9.
11. Baker RN. An evaluation of anticoagulant therapy in the treatment of cerebrovascular disease: report of the Veterans Administration Cooperative study of atherosclerosis. Neurology 1961; 11: 132–8.
12. Baker RN, Broward JA, Fang HC, et al. Anticoagulant therapy in cerebral infarction: report on cooperative study. Neurology 1962; 12: 823–35.
13. Fisher CM. Anticoagulant therapy in cerebral thrombosis and cerebral embolism. Neurology 1961; 11: 119–31.
14. Hill AB, Marshall J, Shaw DA. A controlled clinical trial of long term anticoagulant therapy in cerebrovascular disease. Q J Med 1960; 29: 597–609.
15. Hill AB, Marshall J, Shaw DA. Cerebrovascular disease: trial of long term anticoagulant therapy. Br Med J 1962; 53: 1003–6.
16. Altman R, Boullon F, Rouvier J, Raca R, de la Fuente L. Aspirin and prophylaxis of thromboembolic complications in patients with substitute heart valves. J Thorac Cardiovasc Surg 1976; 72: 127–9.
17. Chesebro JH, Fuster V, Elveback LR, et al. Trial of combined warfarin plus dipyridamole or aspirin therapy in prosthetic heart valve replacement: danger of aspirin compared with dipyridamole. Am J Cardiol 1983; 51: 1537–41.
18. Dale J, Myhre E, Loew D. Bleeding during acetylsalicylic acid and anticoagulant therapy in patients with reduced platelet reactivity after aortic valve replacement. Am Heart J 1980; 99: 746–51.
19. Dale J, Myhre E, Storstein O, et al. Prevention of arterial thromboembolism with acetylsalicylic acid: a controlled study in patients with aortic ball valves. Am Heart J 1977; 94: 101–11.
20. Sullivan JM, Harken DE, Gorlin R. Pharmacologic control of thromboembolic complications of cardiac-valve replacement. N Engl J Med 1971; 284: 1391–4.
21. Petersen P, Boysan G, Godtfredsen J, Andersan ED, Andersen B. Placebo-controlled randomized trial of warfarin and aspirin for prevention of thromboembolic complications in chronic atrial fibrillation. The Copenhagen AFASAK study. Lancet 1989; 1: 175–9.
22. Special Report. Preliminary report of the Stroke Prevention in Atrial Fibrillation Study. N Engl J Med 1990; 322: 863–8.
23. The Boston Area Anticoagulation Trial for Atrial Fibrillation Investigators. The effect of low dose warfarin on the risk of stroke in patients with non-rheumatic atrial fibrillation. N Engl J Med 1990; 323: 1505–11.
24. Smith P, Arnesen H, Holme I. The effect of warfarin on mortality and reinfarction after myocardial infarction. N Engl J Med 1990; 323: 147–52.
25. Sixty-Plus Reinfarction Study Research Group. A double-blind trial to assess long term anticoagulant therapy in elderly patients after myocardial infarction. Lancet 1980; 2: 989–94.
26. Sixty-Plus Reinfarction Study Research Group. Risks of longterm oral anticoagulant therapy in elderly patients after myocardial infarction. Lancet 1982; 1: 64–8.
27. EPSIM Research Group. A controlled comparison of aspirin and oral anticoagulants in prevention of death after myocardial infarction. N Engl J Med 1982; 307: 701–8.
28. Breddin K, Loew D, Lechner K, et al. Secondary prevention of myocardial infarction: a comparison of acetylsalicylic acid, placebo and phenprocoumon. Haemostasis 1980; 9: 325–44.
29. Meuwissen O, Vervoorn AC, Cohen O, et al. Double blind trial of long term anticoagulant treatment after myocardial infarction. Acta Med Scand 1969; 186: 361–8.
30. Loeliger EA, Hensen A, Kroes F, et al. A double blind trial

of long term anticoagulant treatment after myocardial infarction. Acta Med Scand 1967; 182: 549–66.

31. Bjerkelund CJ. The effect of long term treatment with dicumarol in myocardial infarction. Acta Med Scand 1957; 158(suppl): 1–212.

32. Bjerkelund CJ. Therapeutic level in long term anticoagulant therapy after myocardial infarction: its relation to recurrent infarction and sudden death. Am J Cardiol 1963; 1: 158–63.

33. Harvald B, Hilden T, Lund E. Long term anticoagulant therapy after myocardial infarction. Lancet 1962; 2: 626–30.

34. Bynum LJ, Wilson JE. Low dose heparin therapy in the long term management of venous thromboembolism. Am J Med 1979; 67: 553–6.

35. Hull R, Delmore T, Genton E. Warfarin sodium versus low dose heparin in the long term treatment of venous thromboembolism. N Engl J Med 1979; 301: 855–8.

36. Hull R, Delmore T, Carter C, et al. Adjusted subcutaneous heparin versus warfarin sodium in the long term treatment of venous thrombosis. N Engl J Med 1982; 306: 189–94.

30

COMPUTER-ASSISTED ANTICOAGULATION

HAMSARAJ G. M. SHETTY and PHILIP A. ROUTLEDGE

Because anticoagulant clinics are often delegated to the most inexperienced junior medical staff, anticoagulant control is often poor. This can lead to inadequate efficacy or increased risk of hemorrhage. Computers can be used for several purposes in anticoagulant clinics. First, they can be used to access a database to record patient demographic data, degree of anticoagulation, and dose. Second, they can be used to help to identify situations in which anticoagulant response may be altered. Third, they have been used to help in dose adjustment, both on initiation of therapy and during long-term control.

DATABASE MANAGEMENT

The address and hospital number, age, and sex of the patient may be stored, together with the indication for anticoagulant therapy, the proposed duration of therapy, and the desired target international normalized ratio (INR). Not only does this allow individual patient data to be accessed and displayed in graphical form, but it also allows future audit. The closeness of anticoagulant control can be assessed either in an individual or in groups.

The desired duration of treatment with anticoagulants is particularly important. Many patients remain on warfarin for much longer than originally intended and therefore are exposed to the risks of the treatment without incurring any benefit. Junior and inexperienced staff are often unaware of the variable ranges of international normalized ratio recommended for anticoagulant control in different medical conditions. This information, together with the duration of therapy, can be flagged, and a warning message displayed.

IDENTIFICATION OF RISK SITUATIONS AFFECTING ANTICOAGULANT CONTROL

Several situations are associated with changes in anticoagulant response. For instance, a few days after myocardial infarction or after surgery, anticoagulant requirements fall. Cardiac failure may also be associated with reduced warfarin requirements, as is liver disease and hyperthyroidism.[1] By inputting concomitant medical condition, the prescribing physician may be reminded of these risk situations and warned of their potential significance.

Concomitant drug therapy is also an important determinant of anticoagulant requirements. Warfarin can interact with more drugs than any other agent, and because of its low therapeutic index, such interactions may rapidly lead either to underanticoagulation or, more seriously, to excessive anticoagulation.[2] With the advent of new and even more potent therapeutic agents, new interactions are being recognized on a regular basis. The quinolone group of antibacterials,[3] triazole antifungal agents,[4] and some new hypolipidemic agents[5] have all recently been reported to interact with warfarin in certain circumstances, for example. Computer programs to manage anticoagulant clinics can also identify such drugs by interrogating the user about concomitant drug therapy and can warn the user of the potential for interaction, and the likely direction and magnitude of change in dose requirement.

PREDICTION OF DOSE

In most centers, empirical methods are used to choose warfarin dose. This can cause problems in initiation of anticoagulant therapy, since patients' warfarin requirements may vary up to ten- to 20-fold. When 10 milligrams is given on three successive days, for example, the international normalized ratio is between 2 and 4 in approximately one third of patients.[6] Another third have a higher international normalized ratio, and the remainder an international normalized ratio lower than 2. Excessive anticoagulation owing to large doses of warfarin at this time can increase the risk of bleeding. Avoidance of large loading doses may also reduce the risk of one of the rarer complications of warfarin therapy, skin necrosis.[7]

The first attempt at predicting warfarin requirements was based on thrombotest measurements. It was found that the daily warfarin requirement was correlated with the thrombotest value on the 4th day after a fixed induction dose of 10 milligrams on three successive days.[6] This relationship was sufficiently close to be predictive, and was not affected by whether the patient had concomitant heparin therapy during the first three days.[8] However, with the changeover to international normalized ratio measurement, Fennerty and co-workers modified the induction dose to prevent excessive initial anticoagulation, which might otherwise occur in a third of patients.[9] The international normalized ratio was not affected by heparin infusion, provided the activated partial thromboplastin time was within the recommended range of 1.5 to 2.5 times control.[10] It was therefore possible to adjust the induction dose and yet still predict the maintenance requirements of warfarin with some accuracy. This semiempirical approach can either be used as an algorithm, which can be made available to the prescribing doctor, (for example, on the reverse of the anticoagulant form)[9] (Table 30–1), or can be used as a computer algorithm.

More sophisticated computer-assisted pharmacokinetic/pharmacodynamic models have been developed for induction of warfarin therapy. Some of these models have been evaluated clinically. White et al. evaluated a program which used a pharmacokinetic/pharmacodynamic model and Bayesian forecasting methods to predict warfarin dose for initiation of anticoagulant therapy.[11] Bayesian methods combine population pharmacokinetic parameters with actual observations in individual patients. A prospective randomized study showed that the computer-assisted warfarin dosing was better than those by house-staff physicians who did not routinely manage warfarin therapy. A stable therapeutic dose was achieved 3.7 days earlier using the computer ($p = 0.002$). Only 10 per cent of patients were overanticoagulated using the computer method (versus 41 per cent by the house staff). Predicted maintenance dose resulted in anticoagulation within the therapeutic range in 85 per cent with computer-assisted dosing compared with 42 per cent by house-staff physicians ($p < 0.02$).

Abbrecht et al. evaluated a program based on a maximum drug-induced effect pharmacodynamic model to initiate warfarin therapy. A prospective study comparing ten patients with a control group of ten patients showed that computer-assisted patients required less number of days (4.8 versus 6.8) to first reach prothrombin complex activity values in the 20 to 30 per cent therapeutic range. The delay in achieving therapeutic ranges in computer-assisted patients was attributed to the conservative upper limits set for warfarin dosage in the first few days of therapy. Once the therapeutic range was achieved, however, the computer-assisted patients remained within it for 83 per cent of the time (compared with 60 per cent of the time in controls) and they were much less overanticoagulated.[12]

Computer-assisted methods, both empirical and model based, have been used for predicting warfarin doses during long-term administration. Wilson and James obtained suggested changes in dosing from doctors who prescribed warfarin and used this to construct a relationship between the difference from the target international normalized ratio and the change in dosage.[13] This was incorporated into a computer program which provided recommended doses in terms of previous dose and the current prothrombin time. The program also maintained and updated data file on each patient, recommended the interval before next visit, produced clinic and ambulance lists, and alerted the doctors about the decisions regarding continuation or otherwise of anticoagulant therapy. The

TABLE 30–1. Warfarin Schedule*

WARFARIN DAY	INTERNATIONAL NORMALIZED RATIO PREFERABLE 9–10 AM	WARFARIN DOSE PREFERABLY GIVEN AT 5–6 PM (MILLIGRAMS)
1	<1.4	10.0
2	<1.8	10.0
	1.8	1.0
	>1.8	0.5
3	<2.0	10.0
	2–2.1	5.0
	2.2–2.3	4.5
	2.4–2.5	4.0
	2.6–2.7	3.5
	2.8–2.9	3.0
	3.0–3.1	2.5
	3.2–3.3	2.0
	3.4	1.5
	3.5	1.0
	3.6–4.0	0.5
	>4.0	0

WARFARIN DAY	INTERNATIONAL NORMALIZED RATIO PREFERABLE 9–10 AM	PREDICTED MAINTENANCE DOSE (MILLIGRAMS)
4	<1.4	>8.0
	1.4	8.0
	1.5	7.5
	1.6–1.7	7.0
	1.8	6.5
	1.9	6.0
	2–2.1	5.5
	2.2–2.3	5.0
	2.4–2.6	4.5
	2.7–3.0	4.0
	3.1–3.5	3.5
	3.6–4.0	3.0
	4.1–4.5	Miss out next day's dose then give 2 milligrams
	>4.5	Miss out 2 days doses then give 1 milligram

1. Caution in patients with heart failure, liver disease, or immediately postoperative since their sensitivity to warfarin may vary with time.

2. If international normalized ratio on day 4 is less than 2.0, heparin can be used until the international normalized ratio is within the desired range.

3. If the international normalized ratio on day 3 is 1.4 or greater, the initial doses of warfarin should be reduced and the schedule is not longer relevant.

* For further details see reference 9. (Br Med J 1980;288:1268–70, with permission.)

anticoagulation control achieved by the program was found to be as effective as that done manually.

Wyld et al. used this program (with minor alterations) and showed that it reduced the number of underanticoagulated patients from 14 to 6 per cent in the first 13 months.[14] The number of overanticoagulated patients did not increase in the same period. Ryan and Rose used a program similar to that of Wilson and James, and after six months noted an increase in the mean international normalized ratio from 2.98 to 3.45, and an increase in the proportion of patients in the therapeutic range from 45.3 per cent to 62.9 per cent.[15] They also found that the number of patients below the therapeutic range had dropped to 25.8 per cent from 42.5 per cent, and those who were above it had fallen from 12.3 to 11.3 per cent.

Model-based methods for long-term control of warfarin therapy have been evaluated clinically, but are not widely available. Sawyer and Finn compared a log-linear pharmacodynamic model with a linear pharmacodynamic model and found that in 12 hospitalized patients, a stable dose prediction could be achieved after 6.1 doses with the former and 8 doses with the latter.[16] The mean of the average prediction error for maintenance dose was 0.25 milligram for both models (percentage error ± 12 per cent).

Svec et al. compared the predictive performance of a Bayesian computer program when given from 0 to 5 measured prothrombin ratio.[17] They found that the predictions based on population parameters and one prothrombin ratio feedback were significantly biased, but when four and five prothrombin ratio feedbacks were provided, the predictive performance improved sufficiently to enable them to provide clinically useful dosage guidelines early in the course of warfarin therapy. This study highlighted the need for further delineation of true population-parameter estimates if meaningful dose predictions are to be made.

White and Mungall, in a prospective, randomized trial involving 50 patients, evaluated a computer program based on a pharmacokinetic/pharmacodynamic model plus Bayesian forecasting methods for prediction of steady-state warfarin dose.[18] They found the accuracy of computer-assisted dosage adjustments to be comparable to that of an experienced nurse-specialist.

There have been no studies comparing the accuracy of warfarin dose prediction by empirical with model-based methods, and therefore there is at present no evidence that the latter are more accurate than the former.[19]

OTHER APPROACHES TO ANTICOAGULANT CONTROL

Attempts have been made to encourage patients to measure their own prothrombin time at home using equipment purchased by the patient after appropriate training. This requires considerable input of time and training, however, and the expense of the equipment precludes its use in many patients. Nevertheless, it may have an important role in situations where easy access to anticoagulant laboratory or clinic is not available. Additionally, attempts have been made to train the individuals in adjusting their warfarin therapy, and it has been claimed that this results in control that may be even better than that provided by medical staff. Experience with this approach is limited, however, and again it will be dependent on the ability of the individual to be trained in the control of their own treatment. Finally, many patients

in the United Kingdom have their anticoagulant control performed by their family doctor who takes the blood and sends it to a local laboratory. Whilst this may be convenient for the patient and allows good communication with the patients' personal physician, it does mean that the family doctor may be isolated from sources of information and education on the changing field of anticoagulation. Therefore, the onus is on the physician or surgeon who instituted the therapy to ensure that the general practitioner is adequately informed of the developments in the field (for example, new potential interactions) which may cause concern. Control of anticoagulation by the patient or their family doctor does not preclude the use of methods of dose adjustment, and the empirical models in particular can easily be programmed onto a hand-held calculator for this purpose.

CONCLUSIONS

Anticoagulant control is too crucial to be delegated to inexperienced staff. Computers can help improve the efficiency of anticoagulant clinics by allowing quicker information storage and retrieval and can facilitate audit. They can also be used to identify potential risk situations (for example, interactions) and educate the user concerning situations after anticoagulant response. Empirical or model-based methods may also aid in dose adjustment, and computers are helpful in using the former and essential in using model-based methods. It is likely that computers will take an increasingly important role in clinical use of anticoagulants which have major therapeutic benefits as well as potential risks.

REFERENCES

1. Shetty HGM, Fennerty AG, Routledge PA. Clinical pharmacokinetic considerations in the control of oral anticoagulant therapy. Clin Pharmacokinet 1989; 16: 238–53.
2. Serlin MJ, Breckenridge AM. Drug interaction with warfarin. Drugs 1983; 25: 610–20.
3. Mott FE, Murphy S, Hunt V. Ciprofloxacin and warfarin. Ann Intern Med 1989; 11: 542–3.
4. Yeh J, Soo S, Summerton C, Richardson C. Potentiation of warfarin by itraconazole. Br Med J 1990; 301: 669.
5. Ahmad S. Lovastatin warfarin interaction. Arch Intern Med 1990; 150: 2407.
6. Routledge PA, Davies DM, Bell SM, Cavanagh JS, Rawlins MD. Predicting patients' warfarin requirements. Lancet 1977; ii: 854–1.
7. Cole MS, Minifee PK, Wolma FJ. Coumarin necrosis—a review of literature. Surgery 1988; 103: 271–6.

8. Sharma NK, Routledge PA, Rawlins MD, Davies DM. Predicting the dose of warfarin for therapeutic anticoagulation. Thromb Haemost 1982; 47: 230–1.

9. Fennerty A, Dolben J, Thomas P, et al. Flexible induction dose regimen for warfarin and prediction of maintenance dose. Br Med J 1984; 288: 1268–70.

10. Thomas P, Fennerty A, Backhouse G, Bentley DP, Campbell IA, Routledge PA. Monitoring oral anticoagulants during heparin therapy. Br Med J 1984; 288: 191.

11. White RH, Hong R, Venook AP, et al. Initiation of warfarin therapy: comparison of physician dosing with computer-assisted dosing. J Gen Intern Med 1987; 2: 141–8.

12. Abbrecht PH, O'Leary TJ, Behrendt DM. Evaluation of a computer-assisted method for individualized anticoagulation: retrospective and prospective studies with a pharmacodynamic model. Clin Pharmacol Ther 1982; 32: 129–36.

13. Wilson R, James AH. Computer-assisted management of warfarin treatment. Br Med J 1984; 289: 422–4.

14. Wyld PJ, West D, Wilson TH. Computer dosing in anticoagulant clinics—the way forward? Clin Lab Haematol 1988; 10: 235–6.

15. Ryan PJ, Gilbert M, Rose PE. Computer control of anticoagulant dose for therapeutic management. Br Med J 1989; 299: 1207–9.

16. Sawyer WT, Finn AL. Digital computer-assisted warfarin therapy: comparison of two models. Comput Biomed Res 1979; 12: 221–31.

17. Svec JM, Coleman RW, Mungall DR, Ludden TM. Bayesian pharmacokinetic/pharmacodynamic forecasting of prothrombin response to warfarin therapy preliminary evaluation. Ther Drug Monit 1985; 7: 174–180.

18. White RH, Mungall D. Outpatient management of warfarin therapy: comparison of computer-predicted dosage adjustment to skilled professional care. Ther Drug Monit 1991; 13: 46–50.

19. Holford NHG. Clinical pharmacokinetics and pharmacodynamics of warfarin. Understanding the dose-effect relationship. Clin Pharmacokinet 1986; 11: 483–504.

31

NOVELTIES IN ANTITHROMBOTIC AND THROMBOLYTIC THERAPY:
A Latest Update

MARC VERSTRAETE

BOLUS INTRAVENOUS ADMINISTRATION OF THROMBOLYTIC DRUGS

Bolus Infusion of Streptokinase

Clinical trials with streptokinase conducted in the last decade use a high-dose (1.5 megaunits streptokinase), brief-duration (60 to 90 minutes infusion) drug regimen. Bolus treatment with 0.6 megaunits[1] or 1.5 megaunits streptokinase administered over 10 minutes[2] was apparently associated with a high clinical success rate and a still-acceptable incidence of side reactions. A recent comparative study suggests that 0.75 megaunits streptokinase administered over 30 minutes produces a similar reperfusion rate (indirect evidence) as 1.5 megaunits over 1 hour.[3]

Bolus Administration of Urokinase

Urokinase has been administered intravenously by rapid bolus injection of 500,000, 1.25 million, or 2 million units in two to four minutes in 47 patients (3 groups of 16) with acute myocardial infarction. Repurfusion at 90 minutes was obtained in approximately 50 per cent of the patients without difference between the two highest doses. No adverse effects were noted in this pilot study.[4] With a bolus dose of 2 million units urokinase, the coronary patency was 60 per cent in 30 patients[5] and this dose was well tolerated.[6] With a higher total dose of urokinase (1.5 million-unit bolus, and 1.5 million units over 90 minutes) the coronary patency was 66 per cent in 47 patients at the end of the infusion.

Bolus Administration of Alteplase

Because alteplase is rapidly cleared from the circulation with an initial half-life of only a few minutes, treatment with this thrombolytic drug is usually by infusion. The currently recommended dosage regimen of alteplase for the treatment of acute myocardial infarction is an intravenous infusion of 60, 20, and 20 milligrams hourly over three hours with an initial bolus of 10 per cent of the total dose. With this dosage regimen, the coronary recanalization rate at 90 minutes, which corresponds to the administration of 70 milligrams of alteplase, was 71 per cent in 83 patients.[7]

The biological half-lives of alteplase may be significantly different from their measured plasma half-lives. Indeed, the thrombolytic effect of alteplase was found to be sustained beyond its time of clearance from the circulation in animal thrombosis models[8-11] and in patients with myocardial infarction.[11] Effective thrombolysis after bolus administration or short infusion of alteplase has been reported in animals.[8-10,12,13] As the effect of bolus alteplase on

529

coronary recanalization had not been investigated in patients, we compared in a pilot clinical study the efficacy in terms of angiographic coronary recanalization of alteplase given in a bolus of 50 milligrams (29 patients), 60 milligrams (28 patients), and 70 milligrams (25 patients).[14] Because the highest recanalization rate (72 per cent) was obtained with a 70-milligram bolus of alteplase, the same dose was given in a subsequent trial to a larger number of patients. The recanalization rate was only 48 per cent (95 per cent confidence interval, 37 to 60 per cent) at 90 minutes in 60 patients with, however, a very low reocclusion rate at 14 to 24 hours of 4 per cent.[15] A single 70-milligram bolus injection of alteplase does seem to be less effective than 70 milligrams infused over 90 minutes, which is associated with a recanalization rate of 71 per cent.[7]

ACCELERATED INTRAVENOUS INFUSION OF THROMBOLYTIC DRUGS

Accelerated Infusion of Streptokinase

For years, streptokinase has been infused at an hourly rate of 100,000 international units after a loading dose of 250,000 to 600,000 international units streptokinase administered over 30 to 60 minutes. A high-dose (1.5 million international units), brief-duration intravenous infusion (30 to 60 minutes) was proposed in the early 1980s in patients with acute myocardial infarction with an angiographic reperfusion rate of 62 per cent.[16] This high-dose, brief-duration scheme of streptokinase administration is now the standard regimen in patients with myocardial infarction.

Accelerated Infusion of Alteplase

The dose of alteplase most often used is 100 milligrams administered over three hours (40, 20, and 20 in successive hours). An accelerated administration of the same dose of 100 milligrams over 90 minutes (15-milligram initial bolus, 50 milligrams over 30 minutes and 35 milligrams over 60 minutes) increases the patency rate at 90 minutes from 75 per cent (for the three-hour infusion) to 91 per cent (for the accelerated infusion).[17]

The higher recanalization rate of this accelerated infusion of alteplase has been confirmed with a slightly modified dose regimen (0.75 milligram/kilogram/30 minutes followed by 0.5 milligram/kilogram/60 minutes) which resulted in a patency rate at 90 minutes of 84 per cent in 63 patients, with a reocclusion rate of 5 per cent at predischarge catheterization.[18]

COMBINED INTRAVENOUS ADMINISTRATION OF STREPTOKINASE AND ALTEPLASE

Streptokinase is associated with an activation of the systemic fibrinolytic system, and the circulating plasmin digests fibrinogen and some other coagulation proteins; the reduction of fibrinogen of more than 70 per cent decreases viscosity, which may be important to prevent intermittent and late reocclusion. Furthermore, streptokinase has a longer half-life (approximately 30 minutes) than alteplase (initial half-life, approximately six minutes),[19] because the latter molecule is recognized by the liver primarily through its heavy chain. Combining alteplase with streptokinase provides the potential advantage of rapid coronary thrombolysis with alteplase while substituting a systemic fibrinolytic agent for maintenance infusion. With half the usual dose of alteplase and 1.5 million units streptokinase, a patency rate at 90 minutes of 75 per cent in 40 patients was obtained.[20] Somewhat disappointingly, the angiographically documented reocclusion rate was 8 per cent in this uncontrolled trial. A larger prospective trial in 216 patients with acute myocardial infarction revealed a 90-minute patency rate of 79 per cent with the combined drug regimen (50 milligrams alteplase and 1.5 million units streptokinase) versus 64 per cent with the standard dose of alteplase (100 milligrams over three hours).[21]

COMBINED INTRAVENOUS ADMINISTRATION OF ALTEPLASE AND SARUPLASE

Because the intrinsic fibrin selectivity of alteplase and saruplase is mediated by different molecular mechanisms, their combined effect on clot dissolution might be more than additive. Combination of these drugs in animal models of thrombosis produced significantly greater lysis than could be explained on the basis of their additive effects.[22] In a pilot study in myocardial infarction, a relatively low dose of two-chain alteplase and single-chain urokinase-type plasminogen activator given together induced recanalization of the occluded coronary in almost all patients.[23] This clinical investigation was expanded using 20 milligrams alteplase combined with 10, 15, or 20 milligrams saruplase. In a study in 43 patients with acute myocardial infarction, successful reperfusion (TIMI grades 2 or 3) at 90 minutes was observed in 36 per cent of the total study group.[24] It is obvious that the combination of the two drugs at the doses used is considerably less effective than either drug given alone in their presently recommended doses (100 milligrams alteplase and 80 milligrams saruplase).

COMBINED INTRAVENOUS ADMINISTRATION OF ALTEPLASE AND UROKINASE

Also, various combinations of alteplase with urokinase have been investigated in the United States[18,25,26] and in Europe.[27] Although these combinations did not appear to significantly improve reperfusion velocity or rate when compared with each agent used alone, an encouraging decreased incidence of reocclusion was noted when fibrin-specific alteplase and non–fibrin-specific urokinase are combined.

COMBINED INTRAVENOUS ADMINISTRATION OF SARUPLASE AND UROKINASE

Saruplase (33 to 74 milligrams plus urokinase (250,000 units) were given to patients with acute myocardial infarction.[28–31] No clear improvement in reperfusion was obtained with the combination therapy compared with results in historical controls.[32]

DELETION, DOMAIN SUBSTITUTION, AND HYBRIDS OF ALTEPLASE AND SARUPLASE

Considering that the best therapeutic regimen with thrombolytic agents of the first two generations fail to induce recanalization in approximately 20 percent of treated patients, a third generation of thrombolytic compounds is being designed. The aim is to improve the fibrin affinity or prolong the half-life of novel agents, variants, or hybrids of alteplase or saruplase. A comprehensive review on novel strategies for the improvement of thrombolytic drugs has recently been published.[33]

The fibrin selectivity of alteplase is mediated via its affinity for fibrin which is supported by the finger domain and by the second kringle domain. Several approaches have been made to enhance the fibrin-affinity of alteplase by alteration of the fibrin-binding domain. The rationale for this approach is based on the assumption that mutants of alteplase with enhanced fibrin-affinity would constitute more fibrin-specific thrombolytic agents. Most recombinant variants, designed to mimic the high-affinity lysine-binding site of plasminogen, are unfortunately not endowed with a significant improved thrombolytic potency.[34,35]

Plasmin-resistant mutants of alteplase can be constructed by replacing the arginine of the plasmin sensitive arginine-275–isoleucine-276 peptide bond by glutamic acid or glycine. This compound has in the presence of fibrin a comparable thrombolytic potency as alteplase.[33] This indicates that single-chain alteplase does not have to be converted to a two-chain molecule to gain its full activity.

Mutants of alteplase with altered catalytic efficiency in the presence of fibrin have been made by several groups[33] but did not result in a higher thrombolytic potency in animal models of thrombosis.[35,36]

One of the characteristics of alteplase is its rapid clearance, which results in an initial half-life of approximately six minutes. This is due to two different uptake receptors in the liver: a mannose receptor, mainly in liver endothelial cells, and another unknown receptor in the parenchymal liver cells. Kringle-1 of alteplase contains a high mannose-type oligosaccharide and was on purpose deleted in a novel recombinant construction of the molecule which was restricted to kringle-2 and the protease domain.[37] As this plasminogen activator (BM 06.022) was expressed in *Escherichia coli* cells, it lacks oligosaccharide side-chains. Its half-life in rabbits was 18.9 ± 1.5 minutes compared with 2.1 ± 0.1 minutes for alteplase. The 50 percent effective thrombolytic dose was 163 units/ kilogram for the mutant, and 871 units/

kilogram for alteplase. At equipotent doses, the two plasminogen activators have a similar fibrin specificity.[38] Substitution of a few selected amino acids in the aminoterminal domain of alteplase may yield mutants with significantly slower plasma clearance, possibly with better preservation of specific thrombolytic activity.[33]

Plasminogen activators are inhibited in plasma by specific plasminogen activator inhibitors (PAI), mainly by plasminogen activator inhibitor-1 which rapidly inhibits alteplase. Mutants of alteplase resistant to inhibition by plasminogen activator inhibitor-1 have been reconstructed. In view of the large excess of alteplase over plasminogen activator inhibitor-1 during thrombolytic therapy, resistance of alteplase mutants to plasminogen activator inhibitor-1 may not constitute a major significant progress.

Mutants and plasmin-resistant variants of saruplase have been constructed, but without gaining in thrombolytic potency.[33] A low-molecular-weight derivative of saruplase (molecular weight, 33,000 daltons) with the same thrombolytic activity of the parent molecule, may represent a useful alternative for large-scale production by recombinant DNA technology.[39,40]

Recombinant chimeric proteins containing functional domains of alteplase and of other proteins have been constructed. This approach has mainly been evaluated for chimeras between alteplase and saruplase.[33] For most of these chimeras, information on the in vivo thrombolytic properties is, at present, lacking.

RECOMBINANT STAPHYLOKINASE, A FIBRIN-SPECIFIC THROMBOLYTIC DRUG

In plasma in the absence of fibrin, the plasminogen-staphylokinase complex is rapidly neutralized by alpha$_2$-antiplasmin, thus preventing systemic plasminogen activation. In the presence of fibrin, the lysine-binding sites of the plasminogen-staphylokinase complex are occupied and inhibition by alpha$_2$-antiplasmin is retarded, thus allowing preferential plasminogen activation at the fibrin surface.[41] In animal models of venous thrombosis, recombinant staphylokinase had a comparable thrombolytic potency than streptokinase. The plasma clearance following bolus injection of staphylokinase or streptokinase

in hamsters or rabbits was comparably rapid (1.1 to 1.4 milliliters/minute in hamsters and 14 to 15 milliliters/minute in rabbits) as a result of a short initial half-life (1.8 to 1.9 minutes in hamsters and 1.7 to 2.0 minutes in rabbits).[42]

PLASMINOGEN ACTIVATOR FROM BAT SALIVA

The saliva of the vampire bat (Desmodus rotundus) contains a single-chain plasminogen activator with about 85 percent homology to alteplase, but is missing the kringle-2 domain and plasmin-sensitive cleavage site for conversion to a two-chain form.[43] A smaller molecular form additionally lacks the finger domain.[44] The fibrinolytic activity of the full-length form of the bat plasminogen activator is dramatically 200-fold more selective than alteplase toward fibrin-bound plasminogen.[43,45] As the molecule is lacking the plasmin-sensitive cleavage point, this naturally occurring molecule remains stable in the circulation. The protein is now being produced by recombinant DNA technology in an eukaryotic cell line with a specific activity of about 300,000 units/milligram as compared to alteplase in fibrin plates.[46]

THROMBUS-TARGETED THROMBOLYTIC DRUGS

Thrombi contain both fibrin- and platelet-rich material. Plasminogen activators may be targeted to a thrombus by conjugation with monoclonal antibodies directed against specific epitopes in fibrin or against surface proteins on platelets. Furthermore, bispecific monoclonal antibodies containing one site that recognizes the thrombus and one site that binds the plasminogen activator, may be used to concentrate the therapeutic agent at the surface of the thrombus.

One approach is to target the thrombolytic agent to a fibrin clot by conjugation with monoclonal antibodies which are fibrin-specific and do not cross-react with fibrinogen.[47] Chemical conjugates of two-chain urokinase[47–49] or single-chain urokinase (saruplase)[50] with monoclonal antibodies directed against the NH$_2$-terminal of the Bβ-chain of fibrin, were shown to have a threefold enhanced thrombolytic potency in a plasma milieu in vitro.[49]

A chemical conjugate between recombinant saruplase and a monoclonal antibody (MA-15C5) with a more than 1,000-fold higher affinity for fragment D-dimer of human cross-linked fibrin than for fibrinogen has been prepared.[51,52] This conjugate had a 6.4-fold higher fibrinolytic potency than saruplase in a human plasma milieu in vitro[51] and an eightfold higher thrombolytic efficiency with fourfold slower clearance than unconjugated saruplase in a rabbit jugular vein thrombosis model. The jugular vein clots prepared from human two-chain urokinase obtained after plasmin treatment had a fourfold increase in potency compared to plasmin-derived two-chain urokinase.[53] The single-chain conjugate has a fourfold slower clearance than saruplase as determined from the plasma disappearance after bolus injection, and an eightfold slower clearance as determined from the steady-state plasma levels.[53]

A two-chain derivative of this conjugate was prepared by treatment with thrombin which enhanced in a human plasma milieu in vitro its fibrinolytic potency at least 50-fold with a superior fibrin-specificity to that of thrombin-treated recombinant saruplase.[54] In addition, the latter conjugate is not inhibited by plasma protease inhibitors.

The fibrin-selectivity of the saruplase conjugate was equal or superior to that of saruplase. Experiments in rabbits cannot be extrapolated to humans because the monoclonal antibodies used do not interact with rabbit fibrin and fibrinogen, whereas in humans, interaction of the conjugate with circulating fibrinogen or fibrin(ogen) degradation products may interfere with its thrombolytic potency. It is comforting, however, that human fibrin fragment D-dimer does not influence plasminogen activation by the conjugate in purified systems.[51] Furthermore, similar results were obtained in an autologous.

Chemical conjugates have also been made between single-chain alteplase and a monoclonal antibody specific for the NH_2-terminal part of the Bβ-chain of fibrin (MA-59D8).[49,56] This resulted in a 3.2- to 4.5-fold enhancement of clot lysis in human plasma in vitro and a 2.8- to 9.6-times higher potency than tissue-type plasminogen activator in a rabbit thrombosis model, without causing fibrinogenolysis. Schnee and co-workers have engineered a recombinant version of the alteplase

MA-59D8 conjugate.[57] The MA-59D8 heavy-chain gene was cloned and combined in an expression vector with the sequence coding for a portion of the 2b constant region and for the B-chain of alteplase which contains the catalytic site. This construct was transfected into cloned cells derived from the MA-59D8 hybridoma, which had lost the capacity to express the heavy chain. The chimeric proteins indeed had antifibrin antibody activity and retained plasminogen-activating potential.[57]

Another approach consists of the production of bifunctional antibodies which contain a fibrin-specific monoclonal antibody and an alteplase-specific monoclonal antibody. Such duplex antibodies have been obtained by chemical coupling[58,59] or by recombinant deoxyribonucleic acid technology[60] and were indeed shown to concentrate alteplase at a fibrin matrix.

Monoclonal antibodies that recognize epitopes on the surface of activated platelets, but not of resting platelets, might represent another targeting vector for thrombolytic agents towards platelet-rich thrombi. Bode et al.[61] have chemically coupled two-chain urokinase to a monoclonal antibody that selectively binds to platelet membrane glycoprotein IIb/IIIa with remarkable in vitro enhancement of clot lysis. Also, saruplase was chemically conjugated to a monoclonal antibody (MA-TSPI-1) directed against human thrombospondin, a platelet alpha-granule glycoprotein which is expressed on the surface of stimulated platelets but minimally on the surface of resting platelets.[62]

CONCOMITANT TREATMENT WITH ALTEPLASE AND HIGH-DOSE INTRAVENOUS HEPARIN

There is experimental and clinical evidence that thrombolytic therapy with any thrombolytic agent is associated with activation of the coagulation system and that this activation can largely be blocked by heparin, provided the blood levels are high enough.[63] Clinical trials with alteplase and saruplase have generally been combined with early intravenous heparin.

In a recent trial in patients receiving a three-hour infusion of alteplase, immediate intravenous heparin did not appear to improve the patency rate assessed at 90 minutes after initiation of thrombolytic treatment.[64]

The dosages of heparin used may have been too low, and too few patients were involved in this trial for its effectiveness to be judged. Three other trials revealed a significantly higher patency rate at 18 hours,[65] 60 hours,[66] and 81 hours[67] in patients given alteplase plus immediate intravenous heparin compared to alteplase without heparin. Also, a significantly higher patency rate was obtained when saruplase and intravenous heparin were given concomitantly than when saruplase and placebo were given.[68] The latter four trials are concordant in their conclusion that a higher patency rate after alteplase or saruplase is maintained in the presence than in absence of coadministered intravenous heparin. The important role of intravenous heparin is also evident from the levels of fibrinopeptide A (a sensitive marker of circulating thrombin activity), which are high during treatment with alteplase or streptokinase in the absence of heparin and fall as soon as heparin is added.[69–72] The intravenous heparin infusion can be discontinued 24 hours after alteplase therapy and replaced with an oral antiplatelet regimen without any adverse effects on reinfarction and left ventricular function.[73]

Whether the observed higher patency rate is due to potentiation by heparin of the lytic effect of alteplase or saruplase, or due to inhibition by the anticoagulant of thrombus accretion, could not be differentiated in the experimental animals used so far. This problem has now been circumvented, and it was shown that unfractionated heparin and a low molecular weight heparin (enoxaparin) do not influence the lysis of thrombi by alteplase; the apparent enhancement of thrombolysis in the presence of heparin is due to diminished clot accretion.[74]

In vitro experiments also demonstrate that unfractionated heparin and enoxaparin does not limit the fibrin-selectivity of alteplase by augmenting systemic plasmin generation.

RECOMBINANT HIRUDIN AND SYNTHETIC HIRUDIN-BASED PEPTIDES

Although a powerful anticoagulant, heparin is not the ideal protection against thrombus accretion. When a thrombus forms, thrombin is bound to fibrin and incorporated into the growing thrombus. Both free thrombin in the circulation and fibrin-bound thrombin stimulate new thrombin generation by generating factors V and VIII and by activating platelets. Free and bound thrombin cleave fibrinogen to form fibrin. Free thrombin is readily inhibited by the circulating antithrombin III, particularly when this natural protein is potentiated by heparin, but fibrin-bound thrombin is only to a minor extent inhibited by the antithrombin III-heparin complex. Fibrin-bound thrombin thus continues to activate platelets and fibrinogen in the presence of circulating heparin. In contrast, hirudin, a natural protein produced by leeches, binds to the noncatalytic site in thrombin and also inactivates fibrin-bound thrombin because hirudin does not need to complex with antithrombin III and, being a small molecule, can penetrate the thrombus.[75] Based on in vitro and animal models of thrombosis, hirudin would have a clear advantage over heparin,[74–76] and this hypothesis is presently being tested in patients.

Hirudin, which is now being produced in large quantities by recombinant DNA technology, has another advantage; while heparin used alone at pharmacological concentrations increases platelet adhesion to fibrin and extracellular matrix, hirudin does not. This may be important, particularly after percutaneous transluminal coronary angioplasty.[77]

After intravenous infusion in volunteers, plasma concentrations of hirudin decrease, with a half-life of approximately 0.5 hours in the early phase and about 3.7 hours in the late phase.[75] In order to prolong its action, recombinant hirudin was covalently bound to polyethylene glycol (PEG). This coupling prolongs the in vivo activity of hirudin without loss of activity and selectivity.[78]

The region in the hirudin molecules which inhibits thrombin-catalyzed fibrinogen cleavage is located at the C-terminal end (HIR 54-65). The carboxyterminal dodecapeptide Hir 53-64 comprises a limited domain of hirudin, still showing maximal anticoagulant activity. (for example, hirugen and hirullin P18, a 61-amino-acid hirudin fragment[79]). A 20-mer peptide hybrid (hirulog) has been synthesized, combining the antithrombin activities of D-Phe-Pro-Arg (D-FPR) and the dodecapeptide of hirudin.[80] This hybrid peptide exhibits greater antithrombin efficacy in a baboon model than the present molecules, approaching the potency of D-Phe-Pro-Arg chloromethylketone, but without its toxicity.[81] A synthetic decapeptide (hirudin 55-

65, MDL-28050) was shown to be an effective antithrombotic agent in experimental thrombotic models in mice and rats.[82]

SYNTHETIC THROMBIN INHIBITORS

Argatroban (MCI-9038) is a synthetic thrombin inhibitor that blocks the active site of thrombin and is, like hirudin, independent of antithrombin III for its activity. This molecule is more effective than heparin in reducing platelet deposition at the site of balloon injury produced ex vivo[83] in a canine coronary artery stenosis model[84] and in a rabbit femoral arterial eversion graft model.[85] This molecule accelerates in animal models the reperfusion and lowers the reocclusion rates when compared to standard thrombolytic therapy alone.[86-88]

In human volunteers, steady-state plasma concentrations were achieved after a one-hour intravenous infusion of 1 microgram/kilogram/minute. The elimination half-life was 24 ± 4 minutes. The bleeding time remained unchanged, which opens the possibility of coadministration with aspirin.[88]

Another potent and synthetic selective inhibitor of thrombin is MD-805, which also acts independently of antithrombin III; this compound has been tested in patients with progressing cerebral thrombosis with good tolerability and apparent success.[89]

P-PACK

The "fibrinogen-like" sequence D-phenylalanyl-L-prolyl-L-arginyl chloromethylketone (P-PACK) is a synthetic irreversible thrombin inhibitor; it is in fact an imitation of fibrinopeptide A. This compound markedly reduces or prevents thrombus growth in experimental thrombosis models.[90]

In a baboon arteriovenous model, P-PACK was shown to reduce reocclusion following thrombolysis.[91] The brief local treatment of implanted vascular grafts with high doses of this compound also prevents subsequent thrombus formation without risk or hemorrhage.[92]

Compounds have been synthesized in which the arginine of P-PACK has been replaced by the boronic acid analog of arginine, boroArg; their advantage is the potential oral bioavailability.[93]

PLATELET INHIBITION

As noted above, rethrombosis is partly related to the adequacy of thrombolysis and the residual minimal diameter of the infarct-related artery, but also to the intensity of antiplatelet therapy. The anchored residual thrombus produces not only a persistent stenosis, but also alters the local rheology of blood flow. High shear increases the local concentration of adenosine diphosphate, an inducer of platelet aggregation, and forces more platelets to the periphery of the artery.[94,95] Platelet deposition renders residual mural thrombi more thrombogenic, and in experimental in vivo models, vasoconstriction is directly related to the log of platelet deposition.[96,97] It is remarkable that in experimental studies, antiplatelet agents with no vasodilatatory effects reduce both vasoconstriction and platelet deposition,[96] while vasodilators such as nifedipine or verapamil do not result in decreased platelet deposition.[97]

It has been noted that thrombi trailing distally beyond the area of residual stenosis at early angiography (90 minutes after start of thrombolytic treatment) resolve in about 50 per cent of patients within the following 24 hours, which is most probably related to the continued administration of lytic drugs. However, a further reduction of residual stenosis and improvement in the minimal lumen diameter has been shown at hospital discharge angiography.[98-100] It is remarkable that the median values for minimal luminal diameter, per cent diameter, and area of obstruction of the coronary lesion were not found to be different at hospital discharge in patients randomized to combined treatment consisting of alteplase, intravenous heparin, and aspirin, from those receiving only the last two drugs.[101] Late changes in the size of coronary lesions can be attributed to resorption of hemorrhage, dissolution of residual thrombus due to endogenous thrombolysis, and altered vasomotor tone; it is reasonable to assume that prevention of rethrombus by aspirin and heparin contribute to these effects. Other authors maintain that anticoagulation can contribute to the reduction of residual stenosis of the infarct-related artery at angiography repeated after one month.[102]

Aspirin is the antiplatelet drug most widely used in conjunction with thrombolytic drugs. This drug is also of proven benefit in patients with unstable angina, myocardial infarction, cerebrovascular disease, and after coronary or peripheral artery bypass surgery. This is remarkable because aspirin does not prevent platelet adhesion to exposed subendothelial structures nor does it prevent platelet aggregation induced by thrombin. The proper dose to fully inhibit the synthesis of platelet thromboxane while leaving the endothelial synthesis of prostacyclin largely untouched is still a matter of debate, but 75 milligrams daily seems most probably to be enough.[103]

A thromboxane-synthase inhibitor presents some major advantages when compared to aspirin.[104] Despite its interesting properties, the first clinical trials with thromboxane-synthase inhibitors have been disappointing,[105] to some extent due to the fact that prostaglandin H_2, accumulating during thromboxane-synthase inhibition, can itself interact with the platelet endoperoxide receptor and thereby activate platelets.

The more recently developed thromboxane-receptor antagonists specifically impede the action of both thromboxane and prostaglandin H_2 on their receptor, while leaving the normal pattern of thromboxane and prostaglandin formation unaltered. These drugs give a more reproducible and pronounced inhibition of platelet function and prolong the bleeding time more than thromboxane-synthase inhibitors. Preliminary clinical trials seem to indicate that thromboxane-receptor antagonism may be a more effective antiplatelet therapy than thromboxane-synthase inhibitors[106]; some are very long acting and, moreover, are endowed with an anti-ischemic effect.[107,108]

However, possible drawbacks of this class of compounds are represented by their competitive nature, which could lead to their displacement from receptors by exceedingly high levels of thromboxane A_2 and prostaglandin H_2 generated at localized sites of platelet activation. Furthermore, as compared to thromboxane-synthase inhibitors, thromboxane-receptor blockers do not increase the endogenous production of platelet-inhibitory prostaglandins. Finally, like aspirin and other cyclooxygenase inhibitors and thromboxane-synthase inhibitors, thromboxane-receptor blockers also do not affect platelet activation induced by thromboxane-independent agonists, such as high-dose collagen, thrombin, and to some extent, adenosine diphosphate.[109]

Molecules with the dual activity of inhibiting thromboxane synthase and blocking the receptors for thromboxane and endoperoxides have several advantages, one being that accumulating endoperoxide substrate in the platelets may be donated to the endothelial prostacyclin synthetase at the site of platelet-vascular interaction. Such an agent is ridogrel, which reduces elevated levels of markers of in vivo platelet activation in patients.[110] Ridogrel was also shown to enhance alteplase-induced reperfusion in canine coronary arteries[111–113] and in patients with acute myocardial infarction.[114]

The landmark progress made by molecular cloning of a functional thrombin receptor in human platelets and vascular endothelial cells[115] will open new perspectives in a selective inhibition of thrombin action on platelets, sparing its role in the activation of coagulation components.

COMBINED ANTITHROMBOTIC PREVENTION WITH ASPIRIN AND TICLOPIDINE

Among the numerous compounds decreasing platelet function, aspirin and ticlopidine clearly emerge as the most effective in clinical conditions where the arterial component is pathogenetically relevant. Aspirin acetylates cyclooxygenase in platelets, endothelial and other cells, and renders aspirinated platelets less sensitive to their activation by several agonists such as adenosine diphosphate, adrenaline, and low concentrations of collagen, but not to thrombin or higher concentrations of collagen. Ticlopidine seems to inhibit fibrinogen binding to platelet adenosine diphosphate receptors and would therefore inhibit platelet aggregation induced by most aggregating agents. Clopidogrel, an analogue of ticlopidine, also involves an irreversible inhibition of platelet aggregation affecting specifically adenosine diphosphate-dependent activation of glycoprotein IIb-IIIa. On the basis of these distinct mechanisms of action, a synergism of aspirin and ticlopidine (clopidogrel) is a not unreasonable hypothesis.[116,117] Both drugs increase the bleeding time, an effect which becomes much larger with their combined use. Whether the theoretical antithrombotic benefit would outweigh the risk for hemorrhage can only be resolved in a clinical trial. A suitable test model would be coronary or peripheral artery balloon angioplasty, which is associated with sudden exposure of subendothelial collagen. Either drug used alone offers in this particular condition an inadequate antithrombotic protection which might be offered by their combined use.

MONOCLONAL ANTIBODIES TO PLATELET RECEPTORS

Monoclonal antibodies directed against the platelet glycoprotein receptor IIb-IIIa can prevent aggregation of platelets, irrespective of the pathway of activation.[86,118–120] When compared to heparin, 70 per cent of platelet deposition can be prevented in injured rabbit aortas mounted in a perfusion chamber. This means that 70 per cent of platelet deposition is glycoprotein IIb-IIIa-dependent and 30 per cent is due to platelet subendothelium adhesion. Murine monoclonal antibodies to glycoprotein IIb-IIIa have been shown to shorten the recanalization time even of platelet-rich thrombi[84] and prevent reocclusion in thrombotic models in animals.[121] In patients with stable angina, 7E3 Fab produced marked inhibition of platelet function at single doses of 0.25 milligram/kilogram or more, which can be sustained by continuous infusion.[122] Unfortunately, murine monoclonals against glycoprotein IIb-IIIa can induce murine antimurine antibodies and thrombocytopenia.[86]

Also, a purified peptide-specific monoclonal antibody inhibiting von Willebrand factor binding to glycoprotein IIb-IIIa, without interacting with other adhesive proteins containing the sequence Arg-Gly-Asp, inhibits the deposition of platelets on human atherosclerotic wall.[123]

DISINTEGRINS

Platelet aggregation is dependent on the interaction of the platelet membrane glycoprotein IIb-IIIa complex with macromolecular plasma adhesive glycoproteins, including fibrinogen, von Willebrand factor, fibronectin, and vitronectin. Platelet receptors to these four molecules belong to the superfamily termed "integrins" which are calcium-dependent heterodimers composed of two subunits, one being common to all of them (the beta-subunit). The other two superfamilies of receptors are the immunoglobulin gene superfamily and the selectins.[124]

The relative importance of each protein of the integrin family is less well known; under conditions of high shear stress, binding of von Willebrand factor seems to predominate. Binding studies of integrins to glycoprotein IIb-IIIa have identified a distinct amino acid sequence present in fibrinogen and the other three integrins, which is Arg-Gly-Asp (RGD).

Tigramin, a protein extracted from the snake venom of *Trimeresurus gramineus,* was the first natural compound shown to bind glycoprotein IIb-IIIa complex.[125,126] This group of compounds, termed "disintegrin," inhibit platelet aggregation induced by a large spectrum of agonists including adenosine diphosphate, collagen, thrombin, and sodium arachidonate. Sequence analysis revealed that it is a cysteine-rich, single-chain polypeptide with Arg-Gly-Asp (RGD) sequence near its carboxyterminal end.[127] So far, ten trigamin-like polypeptides (a.o. bitistatin, echistatin, applaggin, kristin) were reported which all have similar properties and highly homologous sequences.[128] These disintegrins are 100 to 2,000 times more potent than cyclic Arg-Gly-Asp peptides.[129] Kristin markedly accelerates reperfusion with alteplase, and complete resolution of experimental coronary thrombi in the dog could be obtained.[130] More recently, cyclic and noncyclic synthetic peptidomimetics have been synthesized which are three orders of magnitude more potent than RGDs, and like the latter, inhibit the binding of all ligands to the glycoproteins IIb-IIIa of stimulated or nonstimulated platelets.[131]

STABLE ANALOGUES OF PROSTACYCLIN

The inherent instability of prostacyclin (PGI$_2$) limits the potential therapeutic usefulness of the compound despite its important biological profile. Consequently, intense efforts have been focused on modifying the prostacyclin molecule to obtain synthetic analogues with greater chemical and metabolic stability and comparable physiological activity.

Iloprost was the first described stable analogue of prostacyclin. This compound protects ischemic myocardium in experimental models of coronary artery reperfusion.[132,133] The combination of iloprost with alteplase did not improve immediate or follow-up coronary artery patency or left ventricular functional recovery compared to alteplase alone.[134] The combination of cicaprost and aspirin exerts significant and synergistic effects in two models of arterial thrombosis,[135] which confirms in vitro findings[136] and has implications for multiple mechanisms for down-regulation of the cyclic adenosine monophosphate pathway.

Beraprost, another stable prostacyclin analogue used in combination with alteplase, does not potentiate thrombolysis in dogs but prevents reocclusion.[137] Another stable analogue is taprostene, which in patients with myocardial infarction results in a higher patency rate than in patients receiving saruplase alone (the two groups were also on intravenous heparin and aspirin). At a dose of over 12.5 nanograms/kilogram/minute, taprostene prevents reocclusion in the first 48 hours in patients with myocardial infarction.[138]

GLYCOSAMINOGLYCAN EXTRACTED FROM SEA CUCUMBER

A depolymerized fragment of the glycosaminoglycan extracted from a sea cucumber (*Stichopus japonicus*) was found to have anticoagulant properties. The compound mainly prevents the activation of prothrombin by inhibition of the generation of prothrombinase complex.[139]

RECOMBINANT ACTIVATED PROTEIN C

Protein C is an endogenous vitamin K-dependent anticoagulant which is activated by the catalytic complex of thrombin and thrombomodulin, a protein released by normal endothelium. Activated protein C acts by inhibiting thrombin formation by means of enzymatic cleavage and destruction of activated coagulation factors V and VIII, thus providing a negative feedback regulation of coagulation. Purified plasma-derived activated protein C has been shown to be a safe and potent antithrombotic agent in venous[140] and arterial[141] models of thrombosis. Recombinant activated protein C is now available;[142] this material was evaluated in a nonhuman primary hemostasis model.[143]

SELECTIVE INHIBITION OF ACTIVATED COAGULATION FACTOR X

A highly selective polypeptide inhibitor of activated coagulation factor X has been iso-

lated from salivary gland extracts of the leech *Haementuria officinalis*. The compound is termed antistasin and is a 199 amino acid protein inducing a reversible, slow-tight binding of activated factor X.[144] A second polypeptide inhibitor was isolated from extracts of the tick *Ornithodoros moubata*.[145,146] The latter is a single-chain acidic polypeptide composed of 60 amino acids, also inhibiting activated factor X in a reversible, slow-tight binding. Both agents are highly selective for factor X, without inhibiting thrombin. Both proteins are now available as a recombinant isoform and are effective in the thrombotic prevention in experimental rabbits.[147] Specific activated factor X inhibition with these agents was shown to enhance alteplase-induced reperfusion and to prevent acute reocclusion in the canine copper coil model of arterial thrombosis.[147]

ENDOTHELIUM RELAXING FACTOR AND NITRIC OXIDE

In the area of endothelium-vascular smooth muscle interaction, the most attention in the past few years has been given to the production and release by endothelial cells of a substance termed endothelium-derived relaxing factor (EDRF). Acetyl choline and other exogenous substances cause the release of endothelium-derived relaxing factor, which is transferred to vascular smooth muscle cells causing vasodilatation. Whether endothelium-derived relaxing factor is identical to nitric oxide (NO), or a closely related nitrosothrol derivative, continues to be challenged.[148,149] Endothelium-derived relaxing factor is negatively charged and is a selective relaxant of vascular smooth muscle cells, whereas nitric oxide is uncharged and will relax a wide variety of nonvascular smooth muscle types. Nitrates generate endothelium-derived relaxing factor and nitric oxide and activate soluble guanylate cyclase and thus elevate cyclic guanosine monophosphate (GMP) levels, causing vasodilatation and inhibition of platelet aggregation.

These two effects are attenuated in atherosclerosis and other situations associated with either loss of endothelium or deficient formation of endothelium-derived relaxing factor.[150] Molsidomine and its metabolite SIN-1, a donor of nitric oxide, are potent vasodilators and inhibit platelet adhesion and aggregation.[151] Furthermore, nitric oxide-generating drugs potentiate the activity of thrombolytic agents in experimental conditions[152] and in volunteers.[153]

ANGIOTENSIN-CONVERTING ENZYME INHIBITORS EARLY AFTER MYOCARDIAL INFARCTION

Several clinical studies have shown that converting enzyme inhibition can improve symptomless left ventricular dysfunction and can possibly prevent congestive heart failure when treatment is started one week after myocardial infarction or later. In a double-blind study, 100 patients with Q wave myocardial infarction, but without clinical heart failure, were randomly allocated to captopril (50 milligrams) or placebo starting 24 to 48 hours after onset of symptoms.[154] Left ventricular volumes measured regularly during three months of treatment revealed a significant difference; furthermore, at three months, a significant intergroup difference also emerged in the change in ejection fraction from baseline.

In the ISIS-4 pilot study, 81 patients with suspected acute myocardial infarction were randomized at a mean of 12.7 hours from pain onset to receive four weeks captopril or isosorbide mononitrate.[155] Both drugs reduced systolic blood pressure, but only captopril resulted in a marked and persistent increase in cardiac output. This appeared to be related to a substantial and sustained reduction in systemic vascular resistance that may help in the myocardial remodeling process. In a similar American pilot study, adjunctive early treatment with captopril to alteplase prevented the increase in end-diastolic volume observed in the first seven days in the placebo group.[156]

REFERENCES

1. Hall GH. Bolus streptokinase after myocardial infarction. Lancet 1987; i: 96–7.
2. Köhler M, Hellstern P, Doenecke P, et al. High-dose systemic streptokinase and acylated streptokinase-plasminogen complex (BRL 26921) in acute myocardial infarction: alterations of the fibrinolytic system and clearance of fibrinolytic activity. Haemostasis 1987; 17: 32–9.
3. Gottlich CM, Cooper B, Schumacher JR, et al. Do different doses of intravenous streptokinase alter the frequency of coronary reperfusion in acute myocardial infarction? Am J Cardiol 1988; 62: 843–6.
4. Cernigliano C, Sansa M, Campi A, Bongo AS, Rossi P. Clinical experience with urokinase in intracoronary thrombolysis. Clin Cardiol 1987; 10: 222–30.
5. Mathey DG, Schofer J, Sheehan FH, Becher H, Tilsner V,

Dodge HT. Intravenous urokinase in acute myocardial infarction. Am J Cardiol 1985; 55: 878–82.
6. O'Rourke M, Gallagher D, Healey J, et al. Paramedic-initiated pre-hospital thrombolyzing using urokinase in acute coronary occlusion (TICO 2) (abstr). J Am Coll Cardiol 1991; 17: 246.
7. Mueller HS, Rao AK, Forman SA. Thrombolysis in myocardial infarction (TIMI): comparative studies of coronary reperfusion and systemic fibrinogenolysis with two forms of recombinant tissue-type plasminogen activator. J Am Coll Cardiol 1987; 10: 479–90.
8. Agnelli G, Buchanan MR, Fernandez F, Van Ryn J, Hirsh J. Sustained thrombolysis with DNA-recombinant tissue type plasminogen activator in rabbits. Blood 1985; 66: 399–401.
9. Badylak SF, Voytik S, Klabunde RE, Henkin J, Leski M. Bolus dose response characteristics of single chain urokinase plasminogen activator and tissue plasminogen activator in a dog model of arterial thrombosis. Thromb Res 1988; 52: 295–312.
10. Clozel JP, Tschopp T, Luedin E, Holvoet P. Time course of thrombolysis induced by intravenous bolus or infusion of tissue plasminogen activator in a rabbit jugular vein thrombosis model. Circulation 1989; 79: 125–33.
11. Eisenberg PR, Sherman L, Jaffe AS. Paradoxic elevation of fibrinopeptide A. Evidence for continued thrombosis despite intensive fibrinolysis. J Am Coll Cardiol 1987; 10: 527–9.
12. Prewitt RM, Shiffman F, Greenberg D, Cook R, Ducas J. Recombinant tissue-type plasminogen activator in canine embolic pulmonary hypertension. Effects of bolus versus short-term administration on dynamics of thrombolysis and on pulmonary vascular pressure-flow characteristics. Circulation 1989; 79: 929–38.
13. Agnelli G. Rationale for bolus t-PA therapy to improve efficacy and safety. Chest 1990; 97 (suppl): 161S–7S.
14. Tranchesi B, Verstraete M, Vanhove P, et al. Intravenous bolus administration of recombinant tissue plasminogen activator to patients with acute myocardial infarction. Coron Artery Dis 1990; 1: 83–8.
15. Tranchesi B, Chamone DF, Cobbaert C, Van de Werf F, Vanhove P, Verstraete M. Coronary recanalization after intravenous bolus of alteplase in acute myocardial infarction. Am J Cardiol 1991 68: 161–5.
16. Neuhaus KL, Köstering H, Tebbe U, et al. High dose intravenous streptokinase infusion in acute myocardial infarction. Z Kardiol 1981; 70: 791–6.
17. Neuhaus KL, Tebbe U, Gottwik M, et al. Intravenous recombinant tissue plasminogen activator rt-PA and urokinase in acute myocardial infarction: results of the German Activator Urokinase Study (GAUS). J Am Coll Cardiol 1988; 12: 581–7.
18. Wall TC, Topol EJ, George BS, et al. The TAMI-7 trial of accelerated plasminogen activator dose regimens for coronary thrombolysis (abstr). Circulation 1990; 82: S538.
19. Verstraete M, Bounameaux H, De Cock F, et al. Pharmacokinetics and systemic fibrinogenolytic effects of recombinant human tissue-type plasminogen activator (rt-PA) in man. J Pharmacol Exp Ther 1985; 235: 506–12.
20. Grines CL, Nissen SE, Booth DC, et al. A new thrombolytic regimen for acute myocardial infarction using combination half dose tissue-type plasminogen activator with full dose streptokinase: a pilot study. J Am Coll Cardiol 1989; 14: 573–80.
21. Grines CL, Nissen SE, Booth DC, et al., and the KAMIT Study Group. A prospective, randomized trial comparing half dose t-PA with streptokinase to full dose t-PA in acute myocardial infarction. Circulation 1991; 82 (in press).
22. Collen D, Stassen JM, Stump DC, Verstraete M. In vivo synergism of thrombolytic agents. Circulation 1986; 74: 838–42.
23. Collen D, Van de Werf F. Coronary arterial thrombolysis with low-dose synergistic combinations of recombinant tissue-type plasminogen activator (rt-PA) and recombinant single-chain urokinase-type plasminogen activator (rscu-PA) for acute myocardial infarction. Am J Cardiol 1987; 60: 431–4.
24. Tranchesi B, Bellotti G, Chamone D, Verstraete M. Effect

of combined administration of saruplase and single-chain alteplase on coronary recanalization in acute myocardial infarction. Am J Cardiol 1989; 64: 229–32.

25. Topol EJ, Califf RM, George BS, et al., and the TAMI Study Group. Coronary arterial thrombolysis with combined infusion of recombinant tissue-type plasminogen activator and urokinase in patients with acute myocardial infarction. Circulation 1988; 77: 1100–7.

26. Califf RM, Topol EJ, Stack RS, et al. An evaluation of combination thrombolytic therapy and timing of cardiac catheterization in acute myocardial infarction: the TAMI 5 randomized trial. Circulation 1991; 83: 1543–56.

27. The Urokinase and Alteplase in Myocardial Infarction Study Group. Combination of urokinase and alteplase in the treatment of myocardial infarction. Coron Artery Dis 1991; 2: 225–35.

28. Karsch KR, Ertl G, Kinkel B, et al. Systemic thrombolysis in acute myocardial infarction with pro-urokinase and urokinase (STAMP): results of a randomized multicenter study (abstr). J Am Coll Cardiol 1990; 15: 3A.

29. Weinheimer CJ, James HL, Kalyan NK, et al. Induction of sustained patency after clot-selective coronary thrombolysis with hybrid-B, a genetically engineered plasminogen activator with a prolonged biological half-life. Circulation 1991; 83: 1429–36.

30. Bode C, Schoenermark S, Schuler G, et al. Efficacy of intravenous urokinase and a combination of pro-urokinase and urokinase in acute myocardial infarction. Am J Cardiol 1988; 61: 971–4.

31. Gulba DCL, Fischer K, Barthles M, et al. Low dose urokinase preactivated natural pro-urokinase for thrombolysis in acute myocardial infarction. Am J Cardiol 1989; 63: 1025–31.

32. Ott P, Fenster P. Combining thrombolytic agents to treat acute myocardial infarction. Am Heart J 1991; 121: 1583–4

33. Lijnen HR, Collen D. Strategies for the improvement of thrombolytic agents. Thromb Haemost 1991; 66: 88–110.

34. Lijnen HR, Nelles L, Van Hoef B, De Cock F, Collen D. Biochemical and functional characterization of human tissue-type plasminogen activator variants obtained by deletion and/or duplication of structural/functional domains. J Biol Chem 1990; 265: 5677–83.

35. Wu Z, Van de Werf F, Stassen T, Matsson C, Pohl G, Collen D. Pharmacokinetics and coronary thrombolytic properties of two human tissue-type plasminogen activator variants lacking the finger-like, growth factor-like, and first kringle domains (amino acids 6-173) in a canine model. J Cardiovasc Pharmacol 1990; 16: 197–203.

36. Collen D, Lijnen HR, Vanlinthout I, Kieckens L, Nelles L, Stassen JM. Thrombolytic and pharmacokinetic properties of human tissue-type plasminogen activator variants, obtained by deletion and/or duplication of structural/functional domains, in a hamster pulmonary embolism model. Thromb Haemost 1991; 65: 174–80.

37. Kohnert U, Rudolph R, Prinz H, et al. Production of a recombinant human tissue plasminogen activator variant (BM 06.022) from Escherichia coli using a novel renaturation technology. Fibrinolysis 1990; 4 (suppl 3): A116.

38. Martin U, Fischer S, Kohnert U, et al. Thrombolysis with an Escherichia coli produced recombinant plasminogen activator (BM 06.022) in the rabbit model of jugular vein thrombosis. Thromb Haemost 1991; 65: 560–4.

39. Stump DC, Lijnen HR, Collen D. Purification and characterization of a novel low molecular weight form of single-chain urokinase-type plasminogen activator. J Biol Chem 1986; 261: 17120–6.

40. Lijnen HR, Nelles L, Holmes W, Collen D. Biochemical and thrombolytic properties of a low molecular weight form (comprising Leu 144 through Leu 411) of recombinant single-chain urokinase-type plasminogen activator. J Biol Chem 1988; 263: 5594–8.

41. Lijnen HR, Van Hoef B, De Cock F, et al. On the mechanism of fibrin-specific plasminogen activation by staphylokinase. J Biol Chem 1991; 266: 1182.

42. Lijnen HR, Stassen JM, Vanlinthout I, et al. Comparative fibrinolytic properties of staphylokinase and streptokinase in animal models of venous thrombosis. Thromb Haemostas, in press.

43. Gardell SJ, Duong LeT, Diehl RE, et al. Isolation, Characterization, and cDNA cloning of a vampire bat salivary plasminogen activator. J Biol Chem 1989; 264: 17947–52.

44. Baldus B, Donner P, Boidal W, Schleuning WD. A novel plasminogen activator from the saliva of the vampire bat Desmodus rotundus. 6th GTH-Kongres, Kiel, 1990.

45. Shebuski RJ, Fujita T, Ramijt DR, et al. Thrombolytic efficacy of I.V. bolus vampire bat salivary plasminogen activator (bPA) in a rabbit model of femoral arterial thrombosis: comparison to tissue-type plasminogen activator (t-PA) (abstr 248). Fibrinolysis 1990; 4(suppl 3): 97.

46. Baldus B, Gehrmann G, Bringmann P, Donner P. Kinetics of Glu-plasminogen activation do not explain the fibrinolytic potency of recombinant desmodus rotundus salivary plasminogen activator α_1 (r DSPA$_{\alpha 1}$) (abstr). Thromb Haemost 1991; 65: 884.

47. Bode C, Matsueda GR, Hui KY, Haber E. Antibody-derived urokinase: a specific fibrinolytic agent. Science 1985; 229: 765–7.

48. Bode C, Runge MS, Newell JB, Matsueda GR, Haber E. Thrombolysis by a fibrin-specific antibody Fab'-urokinase conjugate. J Mol Cell Cardiol 1987; 19: 335–41.

49. Runge MS, Bode C, Matsueda GR, Haber E. Conjugation to an antifibrin monoclonal antibody enhances the fibrinolytic potency of tissue plasminogen activator in vitro. Biochemistry 1988; 27: 1153–7.

50. Bode C, Runge MS, Matsueda GR, Gold HK, Haber E. Can intrinsic tissue-type plasminogen activator be concentrated at the site of a thrombus? (abstr). J Am Coll Cardiol 1987; 9: 81A.

51. Dewerchin M, Lijnen HR, Van Hoef B, De Cock F, Collen D. Biochemical properties of conjugates of urokinase-type plasminogen activator with a monoclonal antibody specific for cross-linked fibrin. Eur J Biochem 1989; 185: 141–9.

52. Declerck PJ, Mombaerts P, Holvoet P, De Mol M, Collen D. Fibrinolytic response and fibrin fragment D-dimer levels in patients with deep vein thrombosis. Thromb Haemost 1987; 58: 1024–9.

53. Collen D, Dewerchin M, Stassen JM, Kieckens L, Lijnen HR. Thrombolytic and pharmacokinetic properties of conjugates or urokinase-type plasminogen activator with a monoclonal antibody specific for cross-linked fibrin. Fibrinolysis 1989; 3: 197–202.

54. Dewerchin M, Lijnen HR, Van Hoef B, De Cock F, Collen D. Characterization of conjugates of thrombin-treated single-chain urokinase-type plasminogen activator with a monoclonal antibody specific for cross-linked fibrin. Fibrinolysis 1990; 4: 19–26.

55. Collen D, Dewerchin M, Rapold HJ, Lijnen HR, Stassen JM. Thrombolytic and pharmacokinetic properties of a conjugate of recombinant single-chain urokinase-type plasminogen activator with a monoclonal antibody specific for cross-linked fibrin in a baboon venous thrombosis model. Circulation 1990; 82: 1744–53.

56. Runge MS, Bode C, Matsueda GR, Haber E. Antibody-enhanced thrombolysis-targeting of tissue plasminogen activator in vitro. Proc Natl Acad Sci USA 1987; 84: 7659–62.

57. Schnee JM, Runge MS, Matsueda GR, et al. Construction and expression of a recombinant antibody-targeted plasminogen activator. Proc Natl Acad Sci USA 1987; 84: 6904–8.

58. Bode C, Runge MS, Newell JB, Matsueda GR, Haber E. Characterization of an antibody-urokinase conjugate. A plasminogen activator targeted to fibrin. J Biol Chem 1987; 262: 10819–23.

59. Charpie JR, Runge MS, Matsueda GR, Collen D, Haber E. Enhancement of fibrinolysis by single chain urokinase (scu-PA) with a bifunctional antibody having both fibrin and scu-PA specificities (abstr). Clin Res 1988; 36: 436A.

60. Haber E, Quertermous T, Matsueda GR, et al. Innovative approaches to plasminogen activator therapy. Science 1989, 243: 51–6.

61. Bode C, Meinhardt G, Runge MS, et al. Conjugation of urokinase to an antiplatelet antibody results in a more potent fibrinolytic agent (abstr 1514). Thromb Haemost 1989; 52: 483.

62. Dewerchin M, Lijnen HR, Stassen JM, et al. Effect of chem-

ical conjugation of recombinant single-chain urokinase-type plasminogen activator with monoclonal antiplatelet antibodies, on platelet aggregation and on plasma clot lysis in vitro and in vivo. Blood 1991; 78: 1005–18.

63. Prins MH, Hirsh J. Heparin as a adjunctive treatment after thrombolytic therapy for acute myocardial infarction. Am J Cardiol 1991; 67: 3A–11A.

64. Topol EJ, George BS, Kereiakes DJ, et al., for the TAMI Study Group. A randomized controlled trial of intravenous tissue plasminogen activator and early intravenous heparin in acute myocardial infarction. Circulation 1989; 79: 281–6.

65. Hsia J, Hamilton WP, Kleiman N, Roberts R, Chaitman BR, Ross AM. A randomized trial of heparin versus aspirin adjunctive to tissue plasminogen activator-induced thrombolysis for acute myocardial infarction. N Engl J Med 1990; 323: 1433–7.

66. Bleich SD, Nichols T, Schumacher R, Cooke D, Tate D, Brinkman D. The role of heparin following coronary thrombolysis with tissue plasminogen activator (t-PA). Am J Cardiol 1990; 66: 1412–7.

67. de Bono DP, Simoons ML, Tijssen J, et al., for the European Cooperative Study Group. Early intravenous heparin enhances coronary patency after alteplase thrombolysis: results of a randomized double blind European Cooperative Study Group. Br Heart J 1991; (in press).

68. Tebbe U. Thrombolysis with recombinant pro-urokinase in acute myocardial infarction: role of heparin. 1991. In press.

69. Eisenberg PR, Sherman L, Rich M, et al. Importance of continued activation of thrombin reflected by fibrinopeptide A to the efficacy of thrombolysis. J Am Coll Cardiol 1986; 7: 1255–62.

70. Rapold HJ, Kuemmerli H, Weiss M, Baur H, Haeberli A. Monitoring of fibrin generation during thrombolytic therapy of acute myocardial infarction with recombinant tissue-type plasminogen activator. Circulation 1989; 79: 980–9.

71. Owen J, Friedman KO, Grossmann BA, Wilkins C, Berke AD, Powers ER. Thrombolytic therapy with tissue-type plasminogen activator or streptokinase induces transient thrombin activity. Blood 1988; 72: 616–20.

72. Rapold HJ, de Bono D, Arnold AER, et al., for the European Cooperative Study Group. Fibrinopeptide A plasma levels and the significance of adequate anticoagulation for coronary patency, recurrent ischemia and left ventricular thrombosis in patients with acute myocardial infarction treated with alteplase. 1991 (submitted for publication).

73. Thompson PL, Aylward PE, Federman J, et al. A randomized comparison of intravenous heparin with oral aspirin and dipyridamole 24 hours after recombinant tissue-type plasminogen activator for acute myocardial infarction. Circulation 1991; 83: 1534–42.

74. Agnelli G. Experimental thrombolysis. In: Myocardial reperfusion and thrombolysis: concepts and controversies. 4th annual symposium of the University of Michigan, March 2, 1991:70–4.

75. Hoet B, Close P, Vermylen J, Verstraete M. Hirudo medicinalis and hirudin. In: Poller L, ed. Recent advances in blood coagulation. Edinburgh: Churchill Livingstone, 1991:223–44.

76. Gray E, Watton J, Cesmeli S, Barrowcliffe TW, Thomas DP. Experimental studies on a recombinant hirudin, CGP 39393. Thromb Haemost 1991; 65: 355–9.

77. Mirshahi M, Soria J, Soria C, Jacob P, Camez A, Steg PG. Hirudin contrary to heparin does not induce platelet adhesion to blood clots and extracellular matrix in vitro (abstr). J Am Coll Cardiol 1991; 16: 51A.

78. Rübsamen K, Hornberger W, Schweden J, Kurfürst M. Pharmacological characteristics of long-acting polyethylene glycol-coupled recombinant hirudin (LU 56471). Geneva 1991.

79. Krstenansky JL, Owen TJ, Yates MT, Mao SJT. Hirudin and hirudin C-terminal domains: structural comparisons and antithrombin properties (abstr). Circulation 1990; 83 (suppl III): 659.

80. Fenton JW II, Witting JI, Bourdon P, Maragamor WCL. Thrombin specific inhibition by a novel hirudin analog (abstr). Circulation 1990; 82 (suppl III): 659.

81. Kelly A, Marzec U, Hanson S, Chao B, Maraganore J, Harker L. Potent antithrombotic effects of a novel hybrid an-

tithrombin peptide in vivo (abstr). Circulation 1990; 82 (suppl III): 603.

82. Broersma RJ, Kutcher LW, Henninger EF, Krstenansky JL, Marshall FN. Antithrombotic activity of a novel C-terminal hirudin analog in experimental animals. Thromb Haemost 1991; 65: 377–81.

83. Kaplan AV, Leung LLK, Leung WH, Grant GW, McDougall IR, Fischell TA. The effects of thrombin inhibition and antiplatelet membrane glycoprotein IIb/IIIa on platelet deposition in an ex vivo angioplasty model (abstr). J Am Coll Cardiol 1991; 17: 51.

84. Yasuda T, Gold HK, Leinbach RC, et al. Lysis of plasminogen activator-resistant platelet-rich coronary artery thrombus with combined bolus injection of recombinant tissue-type plasminogen activator and antiplatelet GPIIb/IIIa antibody (abstr). J Am Coll Cardiol 1990; 82 (suppl III): 277.

85. Jang IK, Gold HK, Leinbach RC, Rivera AG, Fallon JT, Collen D. Persistence of arterial eversion graft patency up to 24 hours following a one hour infusion of argatroban, a selective thrombin inhibitor (abstr). Circulation 1991, 83: 145.

86. Fitzgerald DJ. Platelet inhibition with an antibody to glycoprotein IIb/IIIa. Circulation 1989; 80: 1918–9.

87. Jang IK, Gold HK, Ziskind AA, et al. Differential sensitivity of erythrocyte-rich and platelet-rich arterial thrombi to lysis with t-PA: a possible explanation for resistance to coronary thrombolysis. Circulation 1989; 79: 920–8.

88. Clarke R, FitzGerald GA, Fitzgerald DJ. The human pharmacology of argatroban, a specific thrombin inhibitor (abstr). Circulation 1990; 82 (suppl III): 603.

89. Banner DW, Haavary P. Structural studies of inhibitor binding to the thrombin active site (abstr). Thromb Haemost 1991; 65: 774.

90. Kotze H, Lumsden A, Harker L, Hanson S. In vivo antithrombotic effects of local versus systemic therapy with potent antithrombins (abstr). Circulation 1990; 83 (suppl III): 659.

91. Harker H. Interruption of acute platelet-dependent thrombosis by the synthetic antithrombin D-phenylalanyl-L-propyl-arginyl chloromethylketone. Proc Natl Acad Sci USA 1988; 85: 3184–8.

92. Lumsden A, Kelly A, Dodisdon T, Kotze H, Hanson S, Harker L. Interruption of implanted vascular graft thrombosis by brief local therapy with D-Phe-Pro-Arg Chloromethylketone (D-FPR CH$_2$Cl) (abstr). Circulation 1990; 82 (suppl III): 603.

93. Tapparelli C, Powling M, Gfeller P, Metternich R. Novel boron containing thrombin inhibitor SDZ 217-766: in vitro and in vivo evaluation (abstr). Thromb Haemost 1991; 65: 774.

94. Fuster V, Badimon L, Cohen M, et al. Insights into the pathogenesis of acute ischemic syndrome. Circulation 1988; 77: 1213–20.

95. Chesebro JH, Badimon L, Fuster V. New approaches to treatment of myocardial infarction. Am J Cardiol 1990; 65: 12C–9C.

96. Lam JYT, Chesebro JH, Steele PM, et al. Is vasospasm related to platelet deposition? Relationship in a porcine preparation of arterial artery in vivo. Circulation 1987; 75: 243–8.

97. Lam JYT, Chesebro JH, Fuster V. Platelets, vasoconstriction and nitroglycerin during arterial wall injury: a new antithrombotic role for an old drug. Circulation 1988; 78: 712–6.

98. Chesebro JH, Knatterud G, Roberts R, et al. Thrombolysis in myocardial infarction (TIMI) trial, phase I: a comparison between intravenous tissue plasminogen activator and intravenous streptokinase. Clinical findings through hospital discharge. Circulation 1987; 76: 142–54.

99. Serruys PW, Arnold AER, Brower RW. Effects of continued rt-PA administration on the residual stenosis after initially successful recanalization in acute myocardial infarction: a quantitative coronary angiographic study of a randomized trial. Eur Heart J 1987; 8: 1172–81.

100. Rentrop KP, Feit F, Blanke H, et al. Serial angiographic assessment of coronary artery obstruction and collateral flow in acute myocardial infarction. Circulation 1989; 80: 1166–75.

101. Van Lierde J, De Geest H, Verstraete M, et al. Angiographic assessment of the infarct-related coronary stenosis after spontaneous or therapeutic thrombolysis. J Am Coll Cardiol 1990; 16: 1545–9.

102. Nakagawa S, Hanada Y, Koiwaya Y, et al. Angiographic features in the infarct-related artery after intracoronary urokinase followed by prolonged anticoagulation. Role of ruptured atheromatous plaque and adherent thrombus in acute myocardial infarction in vivo. Circulation 1988; 78: 1335–44.

103. Wallentin L, Nyman I, and the Risk Study Group. Low dose aspirin is an effective treatment of silent myocardial infarction (abstr). Circulation 1990; 82 (suppl III): 200.

104. Gresele P, Deckmyn H, Nenci GG, Vermylen J. Thromboxane synthase inhibitors, thromboxane receptor antagonists and dual blockers in thrombotic disorders. TiPS 1991; 12: 158–63.

105. Fiddler GI, Lumley P. Preliminary clinical studies with thromboxane synthase inhibitors and thromboxane receptor blockers. A review. Circulation 1990; 81: 169–78.

106. Perzborn E, Seuter F. The action of BAY U 3405, a specific thromboxane (Tx) A_2 antagonist, in models of thromboembolism and sudden death (abstr). Thromb Haemost 1991; 65: 1178.

107. Grover GI, Schumacher WA. Effect of the thromboxane A_2 receptor antagonist SQ 30,741 on ultimate myocardial infarct size: reperfusion injury and coronary flow reserve. J Pharmacol Ther 1989; 248: 484–91.

108. Grover GJ, Parham CS, Schumacher WA. The combined antiischemic effects of the thromboxane receptor antagonist SQ 30,741 and tissue-type plasminogen activator. Am Heart J 1991; 121: 426–33.

109. Gresele P, Arnout J, Deckmyn H, Huybrechts E, Pieters G, Vermylen J. Role of proaggregatory and antiaggregatory prostaglandins in hemostasis, studies with thromboxane synthase inhibition and thromboxane receptor antagonism. J Clin Invest 1987; 80: 1435–45.

110. Hoet B, Arnout J, Van Geet C, Deckmyn H, Verhaeghe R, Vermylen J. Ridogrel, a combined synthase inhibitor and receptor blocker, decreases elevated plasma β-thromboglobulin levels in patients with documented peripheral arterial disease. Thromb Haemost 1990; 64: 87–90.

111. Golino P, Ashton JH, McNatt J, et al. Simultaneous administration of thromboxane A_2 and serotonin S_2 receptor antagonists markedly enhances thrombolysis and prevents or delays reocclusion after tissue-type plasminogen activator in a canine model of coronary thrombosis. Circulation 1989; 79: 911–9.

112. Van de Werf F, Wu Z, Stassen TM, De Clerck FL, De Geest H. Dual platelet thromboxane A_2 synthase inhibition/endoperoxide receptor blockade (Ridogrel) and/or aspirin enhance thrombolysis with rt-PA in canine coronary arteries (abstr). J Am Coll Cardiol 1991; 17 (suppl): 227.

113. Van de Water A, Xhonneux R, De Clerck F, Willerson JT. Heparin enhances the synergism between platelet TXA_2 synthase inhibitor/receptor blockade (Ridogrel) and tissue plasminogen activator in lysing canine coronary thrombi (abstr). J Am Coll Cardiol 1991; 17 (suppl): 52.

114. Rapold HJ, Van de Werf F, De Geest H, Sangtawesin W, Vercammen E, Collen D. Pilot study of combined administration of Ridogrel and t-PA in patients with acute myocardial infarction (AMI). J Am Coll Cardiol 1991; 17 (Suppl): 114 (Abstr).

115. Vu TH, Hung DT, Wheaton VI, Coughlin SR. Molecular cloning of a functional thrombin receptor reveals a novel proteolytic mechanism of receptor activation. Cell 1991; 64: 1057–68.

116. De Caterina R, Sicari R, Bernini W, Lazzerini G, Buti Strata G, Granessi D. Benefit/risk profile of combined antiplatelet therapy with ticlopidine and aspirin. Thromb Haemost 1991; 65: 504–10.

117. Lecompte T, Lecribier C, Bouloux C, et al. Potential value of the combination of ticlopidine and aspirin. Effect of the addition of 40 mg daily aspirin to ticlopidine treatment in healthy volunteers (abstr). Thromb Haemost 1991; 65: 1178.

118. Coller BS, Folts JD, Smith SR, Scudder LE, Jordan R. Abolition of in vivo platelet thrombus formation in primates with monoclonal antibodies to the platelet GP IIb/IIIa receptor. Correlation with bleeding time, platelet aggregation and blockade of GP IIb/IIIa receptors. Circulation 1989; 80: 1766–74.

119. Hanson SR, Paretti FI, Ruggeri ZM, et al. Effects of monoclonal antibodies against the platelet glycoprotein IIb/IIIa complex on thrombosis and hemostasis in the baboon. J Clin Invest 1988; 81: 149–58.

120. Yasuda, Gold HK, Fallon JT, et al. Monoclonal antibody against the platelet glycoprotein (GP) IIb/IIIa receptor prevents coronary artery reocclusion after reperfusion with recombinant tissue-type plasminogen activator in dogs. J Clin Invest 1988; 81: 1284–91.

121. Gold HK, Coller B, Yasuda T, et al. Rapid and sustained coronary artery recanalization with combined bolus injection of recombinant tissue-type plasminogen activator and monoclonal antiplatelet GPIIb/IIIa antibody in a canine preparation. Circulation 1988; 77: 670–7.

122. Bhattacharva S, Mackie I, Machin S, et al. Inhibition of platelet function by GPIIb/IIIa (7E3) FAB murine monoclonal antibody: phase-1 clinical studies (abstr). Cardiovasc Drug Ther 1991; 5 (suppl 3): 413.

123. Badimon L, Badimon J, Ruggeri Z, Fuster V. A peptide-specific monoclonal antibody that inhibits von Willebrand factor binding to GPIIb/IIIa inhibits platelet deposition to human atherosclerotic vessel wall (abstr). Circulation 1990; 82 (suppl III): 370.

124. Osborn L. Leukocytes adhesion to endothelium in inflammation. Cell 1990; 62: 3–6.

125. Ouyang C, Huang TF. Platelet aggregation inhibitor from Trimeresurus gramineus snake venom. Biochim Biophys Acta 1983; 757: 332–41.

126. Huang TF, Holt JC, Lukasiewicz H, Niewiarowski S. Trigamin, a low molecular weight peptide inhibiting fibrinogen interaction with platelet receptors expressed in glycoprotein IIb/IIIa complex. J Biol Chem 1987; 262: 16157–63.

127. Huang TF, Holt JC, Kirby EP, Niewiarowski S. Trigamin: primary structure and its inhibition on von Willebrand binding to glycoprotein IIb/IIIa complex on human platelets. Biochemistry 1989; 28: 661–6.

128. Teng CM, Huang TF. Inventory of exogenous inhibitors of platelet aggregation. Thromb Haemost 1991; 65: 624–6.

129. Niewiarowski S, Cook JJ, Stewart GJ, Gould RJ. Structural requirements for expression of antiplatelet activity of disintegrins. Circulation 1990; 82 (suppl III): 370.

130. Yasuda T, Gold HK, Leinbach RC, et al. Enhanced thrombolysis with rt-PA plus kristin, a short acting platelet IIb/IIIa antagonist (abstr). Circulation 1990; 82 (suppl III): 277.

131. Steiner B, Hadvary P, Roux S, Weller T. Selective inhibitors of platelet GPIIb/IIIa (abstr). Thromb Haemost 1991; 65: 948.

132. Chiariello M, Golino P, Cappelli-Bagazzi M, Ambrosio G, Tritto I, Savatore M. Reduction in infarct size by the prostacyclin analogue iloprost (ZK 36374) after experimental coronary artery occlusion reperfusion. Am Heart J 1988; 115: 499–504.

133. Ferrari R, Cargnoni A, Ceconi C, et al. Protective effect of a prostacyclin mimetic on the ischaemic reperfused rabbit myocardium. J Mol Cell Cardiol 1988; 20: 1095–106.

134. Topol EJ, Ellis SG, Califf RM, et al. Combined tissue-type plasminogen activator and prostacyclin therapy for acute myocardial infarction. J Am Coll Cardiol 1989; 14: 877–84.

135. Witt W, Loge O, Müller B, Verhallen PFJ, Baldus B. Combinations of aspirin and oral PGI_2-mimetic cicaprost show synergistic antithrombotic efficacy and reduced gastrointestinal bleeding (abstr). Thromb Haemost 1991; 65: 783.

136. Verhallen PFJ, Kahleyss T, Witt W, Thierach KH. Synergistic inhibition of platelet activation by the prostacyclin-analogue cicaprost and aspirin. Implications for multiple mechanisms for downregulation of the cAMP pathway (abstr). Thromb Haemost 1991; 65: 1283.

137. Saithoh S, Saitho T, Asakura T, Kanke M, Owada K, Maruyama Y. New antiplatelet agent, beraprost (PGI_2 analogue) prevents reocclusion in myocardial infarction model. Circulation 1991; 82 (suppl III): 52.

138. Bär FW, Meyer J, Uebis R, et al. Does taprostene influence patency and reocclusion in myocardial infarction treated with the thrombolytic agent saruplase? (abstr) Circulation 1990; 82 (suppl III): 537.

139. Suzuki N, Kitazato K, Takamatsu J, Saito H. Antithrombotic and anticoagulant activity of depolymerized fragment of the glycosaminoglycan extracted from Stichopus Jaganicus Selenka. Thromb Haemost 1991; 65: 369–73.

140. Emerick SC, Murayama H, Yan SB, et al. Preclinical pharmacology of activated protein C. In Hollenberg JC, Winkenhale J, eds. The Pharmacology and Toxicology of Proteins. New York: Alan R. Liss, Inc. 1987; 351–67.

141. Gruber A, Griffin JH, Harker LA, Hanson R. Inhibition of platelet dependent thrombus formation by human activated protein C in a primate model. Blood 1989; 73: 639–42.

142. Grinnell BW, Berg DT, Walls J, Yan SB. Trans-activated expression of fully gamma-carboxylated recombinant human protein C, an antithrombotic factor. Bio/Technology 1987; 5: 1189–92.

143. Gruber A, Hanson SR, Kelly AB, et al. Inhibition of thrombus formation by activated recombinant protein C in a primate model of arterial thrombosis. Circulation 1990; 82: 578–85.

144. Dunwiddie C, Thornberry NA, Bull HG, et al. Antistasin, a leech-derived inhibitor of factor Xa. J Biol Chem 1989; 264: 16694–9.

145. Waxman L, Smith DE, Acuri KE, Vlassuk GP. Tick anticoagulant peptide is a novel inhibitor of blood coagulation factor Xa. Science 1990; 248: 593–6.

146. Schaffer LW, Davidson JT, Vlasuk G, Siegl PKS. Antithrombotic effect of the factor Xa inhibitor tick anticoagulant peptide (TAP) in a baboon model of acute arterial thrombosis (abstr). Circulation 1990; 82 (suppl III): 660.

147. Vlassuk G, Sitko G, Shebuski R. Specific factor Xa inhibition enhances thrombolytic reperfusion and prevents acute reocclusion in the canine copper coil model of arterial thrombosis (abstr). Circulation 1990; 82: (suppl III): 603.

148. Johns RA. Endothelium-derived relaxing factor: basic review and clinical implications. J Cardioth Vasc Anesth 1991; 5: 69–79.

149. Schini V. Nitric oxide and vascular reactivity. Cor Artery Dis 1991; 2: 293–9.

150. Änggård EE. Endogenous nitrates—implications for treatment and prevention. Eur Heart J 1991; 12 (suppl A): 5–8.

151. Palmer RM, Ferrige AG, Moncada S. Nitric oxide release accounts for the biological activity of endothelium derived relaxing factor. Nature 1987 (1989?); 327: 524–6.

152. Korbut R, Lidbury PS, Vane JR. Prolongation of fibrinolytic activity of tissue plasminogen activator by nitrovasodilators. Lancet 1990; 335: 669.

153. Darius H, Grodzinska L, Hafner G. NO-releasing molsidomine increases fibrinolytic activity in man (abstr). Circulation 1990; 82 (suppl III): 301.

154. Sharpe N, Smith H, Murphy J, Greaves S, Hart H, Gamble G. Early prevention of left ventricular dysfunction after myocardial infarction with angiotensin-converting enzyme inhibitors. Lancet 1991; 337: 872–6.

155. Pipilis A, Flather M, Collins R, Conway M, Sleight P. ISIS-4 pilot study: serial hemodynamic changes with oral captopril and oral isosorbide mononitrate in a randomized double-blind trial in myocardial infarction (abstr). J Am Coll Cardiol 1991; 17: 115.

156. Nabel EG, Topol EJ, Galeana A, et al. A randomized, double-blind, placebo controlled, pilot trial of combined early intravenous captopril and tPA therapy in acute myocardial infarction (abstr). Circulation 1989; 80 (suppl II): II–112.

ACRONYMS IN CARDIOVASCULAR DISORDERS AND THROMBOSIS

AFASAK	Atrial Fibrillation Aspirin Antikoagulation
AFTER	Anistreplase Following Thrombolysis Effect on Reocclusion
AICLA	Accidents Ischémiques Cérébraux Liés à l'Athérosclérose Study
AIMS	APSAC Intervention Mortality Study
AIRE	Acute Infarction Reperfusion Efficacy
AITIA	Aspirin in Transient Ischaemic Attack
AMIS	Aspirin Myocardial Infarction Study
AMPI	Anisoylated Plasminogen Streptokinase Activator Complex in Acute Myocardial Infarction Placebo Controlled Investigation
ANBP	Australian National Blood Pressure Trial
APRICOT	Antithrombotics in the Prevention of Reocclusion In Coronary Thrombolysis
APSIM	APSAC dans l'Infarctus du Myocarde
APSIS	Angina Prognosis Study with Isoptin and Seloken Trial
ARIS	Anturan Reinfarction Italian Study
ARMS	APSAC Reocclusion Multicentre Study
ART	Anturan Reinfarction Trial
ASK	Australian SK Trial in Stroke
ASP Study	Australian Swedish Pindolol Study
ASPECT	Anticoagulants in the Secondary Prevention of Events in Coronary Thrombosis
ASSET	Anglo-Scandinavian Study of Early Thrombolysis
ATACS	Antithrombotic Therapy in Acute Coronary Syndromes
ATEST	Atenolol and Streptokinase Trial
ATIAIS	Anturan Transient Ischemic Attack Italian Study
BAATAF	Boston Area Anticoagulation Trial for Atrial Fibrillation
BARI	Bypass Angioplasty Revascularisation Investigation
BEST	Beta-Blocker Stroke Trial
BH Study	Bogalusa Heart Study
BHAT	Beta-Blocker Heart Attack Trial
BM Study	Belfast Metoprolol Study
BN Study	Belfast Nifedipine Study
BUIC	Balloon-Ultrasound Imaging Catheter
CABRI	Coronary Artery Bypass Revascularisation Investigation
CAFA	Canadian Atrial Fibrillation Anticoagulation Study
CAMIAT	Canadian Amiodarone Myocardial Infarction Arrhythmias Trial
CAPPHY	Captopril Primary Prevention in Hypertension Trial
CAPRIE	Clopidogrel vs Aspirin in Patients at Risk of Ischemic Events

CAPS	Cardiac Arrhythmia Pilot Study
CASCADE	Cardiac Arrest in Seattle Conventional versus Amidarone Drug Evaluation
CASS	Coronary Artery Surgery Study
CAST	Cardiac Arrhythymia Suppression Trial
CATS	Canadian American Ticlopidine Study
CCHD Study	Caephilly Collaborative Heart Disease Study
CDP	Coronary Drug Project
CISS	Canadian Inplantable Defibrillator Study
CITO	Collaboratione Italiana par la Thrombosi in Ortopedia
CLAS	Cholesterol-Lowering Atherosclerosis Study
CLEOPAD	Clopidogrel in Peripheral Arterial Disease
CONSENSUS	Cooperative North Scandinavian Enalapril Survival Study
CRAFT	Catheterization Rescue Angioplasty Following Thrombolysis Study
DART	Diet and Reinfarction Trial
DHCCP	Department of Health and Social Security Hypertension Care Computing Project
DR Study	Diltiazem Reinfarction Study
Dutch IRS	Dutch Invasive Reperfusion Study
DV Trial	Danish Verapamil Trial
EAST	Emory Angioplasty Surgery Trial
EC-COMAC	European Community Concerted Action Programmes
ECAT	European Concerted Action on Thrombosis and Disabilities
ECAT AP Trial	ECAT Angina Pectoris Trial
ECMO	Extra Corporeal Membrane Oxygenation
ECS Study	European Coronary Surgery Study
ECSG	European Cooperative Study Group for rt-PA in Acute Myocardial Infarction
EIS	European Infarction Study
EMERAS	Estudio Multicentrico Estreptoquinasa Republicos Americas Sud
EMIAT	European Myocardial Infarction Amidarone Trial
EMIP	European Myocardial Infarction Project
EMPAR	Enoxaparine Maxipa Prevention of Angioplasty Restenosis
EPSIM	Enquête de Prévention Secondaire de l'Infarctus du Myocarde
ERICA	European Risk and Incidence, a Coordinated Analysis
ESVEM	Electrophysiologic Study Versus Electrocardiographic Monitoring
EWPHE	European Working Party on Hypertension in the Elderly
EXEL	Expanded Clinical Evaluation of Lovostatin
FIPS	Frankfurt Isoptin Progression Study
GABI	German Angioplasty Bypass Investigation
GAMIS	German-Austrian Myocardial Infarction Study
GARS	German-Austrian Reinfarction Study

GAUS	German Activator Urokinase Study
GCP	German Cardiovascular Prevention Study
GEMT	German Eminase Multicenter Trial
GESIC	Grupo Espanol para el Seguimiento del Injerto Aortocoronario
GISSI	Gruppo Italiano per lo Studio della Streptochinasi nell'Infarto Miocardico
GMT	Göteborg Metoprolol Trial
GPP	Göteborg Primary Prevention Trial
GUSTO	Global Utilization of Streptokinase and t-PA for Occluded Coronary Arteries
HAPPHY	Heart Attack Primary Prevention in Hypertension
HART	Heparin Aspirin Perfusion Trial
HDFP	Hypertension Detection and Follow-up Program
HINT	Holland Interuniversity Trial on Nifedipine
HYNON	Cooperative Study on Effectiveness of Non-Drug Treatment in Hypertension
ICIN	Intracoronary Streptokinase Trial of the Interuniversity Cardiology Institute of the Netherlands
IMAGE	International Metoprolol/Nifedipine Angina Pectoris Exercise Trial
IMPACT	International Mexiletine and Placebo Antiarrhythmia Coronary Trial
INTACT	International Nifedipine Trial on Antiatherosclerotic Therapy
IPPPSH	International Prospective Primary Prevention Study in Hypertension
IRS	Invasive Reperfusion Studies
ISAM	Intravenous Streptokinase in Acute Myocardial Infarction Study
ISIS	International Study of Infarct Survival
KAMIT Study Group	Kentucky Acute Myocardial Infarction Trial Study Group
LATE	Late Assessment of Thrombolytic Efficacy
LIMITS	Liquemin in Myocardial Infarction During Thrombolysis with Saruplase
LIT	Lopresor Intervention Trial
LRC-CPPT	Lipid Research Clinics Coronary Primary Prevention Trial
M-HEART	Multi-Hospital Eastern Atlantic Restenosis Trial
MAPHY	Metoprolol Atherosclerosis Prevention in Hypertensives
MARCATOR	Multicenter American Restenosis Cilazapril Angioplasty Trial on Restenosis
MAST-1	Multicenter Acute Stroke Trial = Italy
MDPIT	Multicenter Diltiazem Post-Infarction Trial
MEHP	Metoprolol in Elderly Hypotension Patients
MELODHY	Metoprolol Low Dose in Hypertension
MERCATOR	Multicenter European Restenosis Cilazapril Angioplasty Trial on Restenosis
MIAMI	Metoprolol in Acute Myocardial Thromboangiitis

MILESTONE	Multicenter Iloprost European Study on Endangeitis
MILIS	Multicenter Investigation for Limitation of Infarct Size
MITI Project	Myocardial Infarction, Triage and Intervention Project
MONICA	Monitoring Trends and Determinants in Cardiovascular Disease
MPRG	Multicenter Postinfarction Research Group
MRFIT	Multiple Risk Factor Intervention Trial
NAMIS	Nifedipine Angina Myocardial Infarction Study
NASCET	North American Symptomatic Carotid Endarterectomy Trial
NK Project	North Karelia Project
NM Trial	Norwegian Multicenter Trial
OD1	Italian CNR Multicenter Prospective Study
PACK	Prevention of Atherosclerotic Complications with Ketanserin Trial
PACT	Pro-urokinase in Acute Coronary Thrombosis
PACTE	Prévention des Accidents Thrombo-Emboliques chez les Porteurs de Prothèses Valvulaires Cardiaques
PAIMS	Plasminogen Activator Italian Multicenter Study
PAMI	Primary Angioplasty Myocardial Infarction Trial
PARIS	Persantin-Aspirin Reinfarction Study
PARK	Prevention of Angioplasty Reocclusion with Ketanserin
PARTNER	Peripheral Arterial Disease. Response to Taprostene with New Established Response Criteria
PASS	Practical Applicability of Saruplase Study
PATS	Prehospital Administration of t-PA Pilot Study
PDAY	Pathobiological Determinants in Youth Research Group
PLAC	Pravastatin Limitation of Atherosclerosis in the Coronary Arteries
POSCH	Program On Surgical Control of Hyperlipidaemia
PREMIS	Prehospital Myocardial Infarction Study
PRIMI	Pro-urokinase In Myocardial Infarction
PROCAM	Prospective Cardiovascular Monster Study
PROMISE	Prospective Randomized Mibrinone Survival Evaluation
RAAMI	Rapid Administration of Alteplase in Myocardial Infarction
REPAIR	Reperfusion in Acute Infarction, Rotterdam
RESCUE	Randomized Evaluation of Salvage Angioplasty with Combined Utilization of Endpoints
RISK	Regional Study av Instabil Kranskärssjukdom
RITA	Randomised Intervention Treatment of Angina
ROBUST	Recanalization of Occluded Bypass Graft, Urokinase Study Trial
ROCKET	Regionally Organized Cardiac Key European Trial
SAFE	Safety After Fifty Evaluation
SAMIT	Streptokinase Angioplasty Myocardial Infarction Trial
SCATI	Studio sulla Calciparina nell'Angina e nella Trombosi Ventricolare nell'Infarto

SCRIP	Stanford Coronary Risk Intervention Project
SEPIVAC	Studio Epidemilogica sull'Incidenza delle Vasculopatie Acute Cerebrali
SESAM	Study in Europe of Saruplase and Alteplase in Myocardial Infarction
SHAVE	Steerable Housing for Athero Vascular Excision
SHEP	Systolic Hypertension in the Elderly Program
SIAM	Streptokinase in Acute Myocardial Infarction
SMT	Stockholm Metoprolol Trial
SPAF	Stroke Prevention in Atrial Fibrillation
SPRINT	Secondary Prevention Reinfarction Israeli Nifedipine Trial
SSSS	Scandinavian Simvastatin Survival Study
STAI	Study Ticlopidine in Angor Instable
STAMP	Systemic Thrombolysis in Acute Myocardial Infarction with Pro-urokinase and Urokinase
STEP	Study of Taprostene in Elective PTCA
STIMS	Swedish Ticlopidine Multicentre Study in Patient with Intermittent Claudication
STOP Hypertension	Swedish Trial in Old Patients with Hypertension
SWIFT	Should We Intervene Following Thrombolysis?
TACS	Thrombolysis and Angioplasty in Cardiogenic Shock Study
TACT	Ticlopidine versus Placebo for Prevention of Acute Closure and Restenosis after Coronary Angioplasty Trial
TAMI	Thrombolysis and Angioplasty in Myocardial Infarction
TASS	Ticlopidine Aspirin Stroke Study
TAUSA	Thrombolysis and Angioplasty in Unstable Angina
TEAHAT	Thrombolysis Early in Heart Attack Trial
TEAM	Trial of Eminase in Acute Myocardial Infarction
TENS	Transcutaneous Electrical Nerve Stimulation
TIARA	Timolol en Infarto Agudo, Republica Argentina
TICO	Thrombolysis In Coronary Occlusion
TIMAD	Ticlopidine in Micro Angiopathy of Diabetes
TIMI	Thrombolysis in Myocardial Infarction
TIPE	Thrombolysis in Peripheral Embolism Patient Study
TM Study	The Multifit Study
TOHMS	Trial of Hypertensive Medications Study
TOP	Thrombolysis in Old Patients
TPAT	Tissue Plasminogen Activator Toronto Trial
TPT	Thrombosis Prevention Trial
TRENT	Trial of Early Nifidepine in Acute Myocardial Infarction
UK-TIA Study	United Kingdom Transient Ischemic Attack Study
UNASEM	Unstable Angina Study using Eminase
UPET	Urokinase Pulmonary Embolism Trial
URALMI	Urokinase and Alteplase in Myocardial Infarction Trial
V-HEFT	Veterans Administration Vasodilator Heart Failure Trial
VA-Acme Trial	Veterans Administration Angioplasty Centra Medicine

VA-HEFT	Veterans Administration Heart Failure Trial
WARIS	Warfarin Reinfarction Study
WHA Study	Worcester Heart Attack Study
WWICT	Western Washington Intracoronary Streptokinase Trial
WWIST	Western Washington Intravenous Streptokinase Trial

Index

Note: Page numbers in *italics* refer to illustrations; page numbers followed by t refer to tables.

551

Catheter manipulation, thrombogenic risk of, 435
Cerebral embolism, sources of, *216*
   identification of, by transesophageal echocardiography, 220
  stroke from, with acute myocardial infarction, 227
  with mitral valve prolapse, 194
Cerebral infarction, acute, thrombosis in, 31
  asymptomatic, 219
  ischemic, atherosclerosis and, 71
Cerebral ischemic event, atrial fibrillation and, 21, 225, 232
Cerebrovascular accident. See *Stroke.*
Cerebrovascular disease, as cause of stroke, 410–411
  atherosclerotic, 71, *72*
  classification of, 409–410
  hemorrhage risk with, 516–517, 517t, 520t
  leg arterial atherosclerosis and, 436
  risk factors for, 411–413
  thrombosis in, 29–31
c-fos oncogene, thrombin and, 22
Chest pain, thromboxane A_2 concentration and, 24
Cholesterol, accumulation of, in lipid-filled foam cells, 42
  as restenosis risk factor, 400
  as stroke risk factor, 411
  calcification and, 46
  coronary artery disease and, 368, 377
Chylomicronemia, postprandial, 93
Cigarette smoking, as atherosclerosis risk factor, 72–73, 424
  as peripheral arterial disease risk factor, 32–33
  as restenosis risk factor, 400
  as stroke risk factor, 411
  as thrombogenic risk factor, 27, 80, 377
  fibrinogen levels and, 91, 92–93, 92t
  heart attacks per annum and, 80, 92t
  plaque formation and, 42, 72–73
  platelet function and, 73
Cilazapril, for restenosis, 404
Circadian variation, in thrombogenic risk factors, 27
Claudication, intermittent, frequency of, 31–32
  in peripheral arterial disease, 32
Clofibrate, myocardial infarction reduction with, 91, 92t, 345
Clopidogrel, 536
Clot selectivity, among thrombolytic agents, 311–312
Coagulation. See also *Blood; Hemorrhage; Hemostasis.*
  estrogen and, 91t
  generalized intravascular. See *Disseminated intravascular coagulation.*
  inhibitors of, endogenous, 505
  intravascular disseminated. See *Disseminated intravascular coagulation.*
Coagulation cascade, 82, *83*, 84–85, *123, 133*, 296, 503–505
  activation of, 367
  amplification mechanism of, *125*
  heparin and, 306
  in thrombus formation, 216
  plasminogen activation of, 308
Coagulation disorders, as cerebrovascular disease risk factor, 413
Coagulation factors. See also *Factor* entries; specific factor names.
  activation of, 7–9, 20
  in disseminated intravascular coagulation, 507
  vitamin K-dependent, 6, 7
Cocaine abuse, coronary vasoconstriction from, thrombosis with, 66
Cofactor proteins, 8–9
Collagen, in platelet activation, 7, 17, *18*
  in platelet adhesion, 2, 23
Compression, of leg, for venous thromboembolism prevention, 456, 458t
  with hip surgery, 458
Computer-assisted anticoagulation, 523–526
Computerized tomography, of left ventricular thrombus, 221
Congestive heart failure, as thrombogenic risk factor, 217
Conjunctive agents, 305–309
  development of, 321
Consumption coagulopathy. See *Disseminated intravascular coagulation.*

Coronary angioplasty. See also *Balloon angioplasty.*
  abrupt closure in, 390–391
   incidence of, 393, 394t
   prevention of, 395–397
   restenosis after, *392*
   risk factors for, 393–395
   treatment of, 397–399
  early, for recanalization maintenance, 309–311
  omega-3 fatty acids after, 106t
  percutaneous transluminal, as thromboembolism risk factor, 494t, 495
   complications with, after alteplase therapy, 253
   frequency of, 389
   routine, 389–390
   to prevent occlusion and restenosis, 389–405
  platelet inhibitors during, 104t
Coronary artery, right, rescue angioplasty complications in, 310–311
  status of, in chronic coronary disease, 363–364
Coronary artery bypass. See also *Bypass graft; Cardiopulmonary bypass; Vascular surgery; Vein graft.*
  antithrombotic therapy with, 375–386
  vein graft occlusion after, 495
Coronary artery disease. See also *Heart disease.*
  blood viscosity in, 366
  chronic, antithrombotic therapy in, 367–371
   coronary artery status in, 363–364
   definition of, 363
   progression of, myocardial infarction and, 367
   thrombus formation in, modification and inhibition of, 364–364
   warfarin for, 166t
  heparin for, 152t
  intermittent claudication and, 31
  progressive, hypercoagulability in, 27
Coronary artery lesions, complications of, likelihood of, 394–395, 395t
  in sudden death patients, 239t
  in unstable versus stable angina, 238–239
Coronary artery occlusion, *69*
  and plaques with antifibrin binding, 60
  pathogenesis of, 375–378
Coronary artery plaque, electron micrograph of, *61, 62*
  growth of, temporal sequence of, 69–72
  mural thrombus overlying, *66*, 366
Coronary artery surgery, platelet inhibitors during, 105t, 375–386
Coronary artery thrombosis, 375, *376*
  after deep injury, 364
  cardiac ischemia and, 366–367
  causes of, 81
  cigarette smoking and, 91–93
  circadian variation in, 365–366
  dietary fat intake and, 93
  epidemiology of, 87–91
  genetic contribution to, 93
  hemodynamic factors in, 1–2, 81–82, 365–366
  hypercoagulability and, 82–87
  in acute coronary syndromes, 28–29
Coronary circulation, in thromboembolism formation, 491–497
Coronary death, sudden, mechanisms in, 79
Coronary Drug Project (CDP), 347, 368, 369t
Coronary endothelial injury, combined thromboxane synthase inhibitors and receptor blockers for, 114–115
Coronary stents, for abrupt closure, 398, 405
Coronary syndromes, acute, thrombosis in, 28–29
Coronary thrombolysis. See *Thrombolytic therapy, for myocardial infarction.*
Coumarin. See also *Anticoagulants, oral.*
  drug interactions with, sites of, *143*
  fetal effects of, 487
  for myocardial infarction, in chronic phase, 352
  for venous thromboembolism, 469
  resistance to, congenital, 136
  skin necrosis from, 136
Cyclic adenosine monophosphate, in platelets, drugs that increase, 107–109